SEDATION

A Guide to Patient Management

SEDATION

A Guide to Patient Management

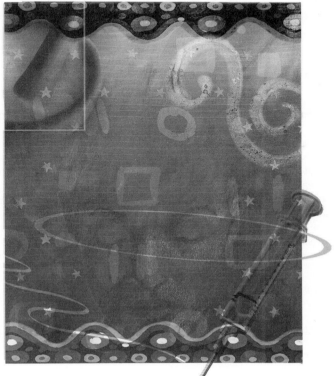

FOURTH EDITION

STANLEY F. MALAMED, DDS

Professor of Anesthesia and Medicine
School of Dentistry
University of Southern California
Los Angeles, California

With 258 *illustrations*
Selected illustrations by Don O'Connor and Oral Health Advantage[sm]
Selected photography by Norman Goldberg

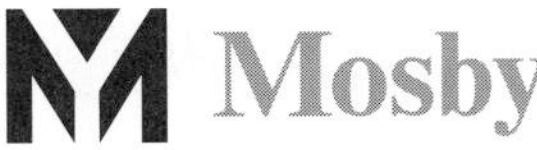

An Affiliate of Elsevier Science

St. Louis London Philadelphia Sydney Toronto

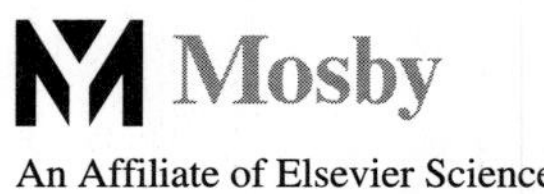

An Affiliate of Elsevier Science

11830 Westline Industrial Drive
St. Louis, Missouri 63146

Sedation: A Guide to Patient Management

ISBN: 0-323-01226-4

NOTICE

Pharmacology is an ever-changing field. Standard safety precautions must be followed, but as new research and clinical experience broaden our knowledge, changes in treatment and drug therapy may become necessary or appropriate. Readers are advised to check the most current product information provided by the manufacturer of each drug to be administered to verify the recommended dose, the method and duration of administration, and contraindications. It is the responsibility of the licensed prescriber, relying on experience and knowledge of the patient, to determine dosages and the best treatment for each individual patient. Neither the publisher nor the author assumes any liability for any injury and/or damage to persons or property arising from this publication.

Previous editions copyrighted 1985, 1989, 1995

International Standard Book Number: 0-323-01226-4

Senior Acquisitions Editor: Penny Rudolph
Senior Developmental Editor: Kimberly Alvis
Publishing Services Manager: Karen Edwards
Designer: Julia Dummitt
Cover Design: Julia Dummitt

KI/MVB
Printed in the United States of America.

Last digit is the print number: 9 8 7 6 5 4 3 2 1

Dedication

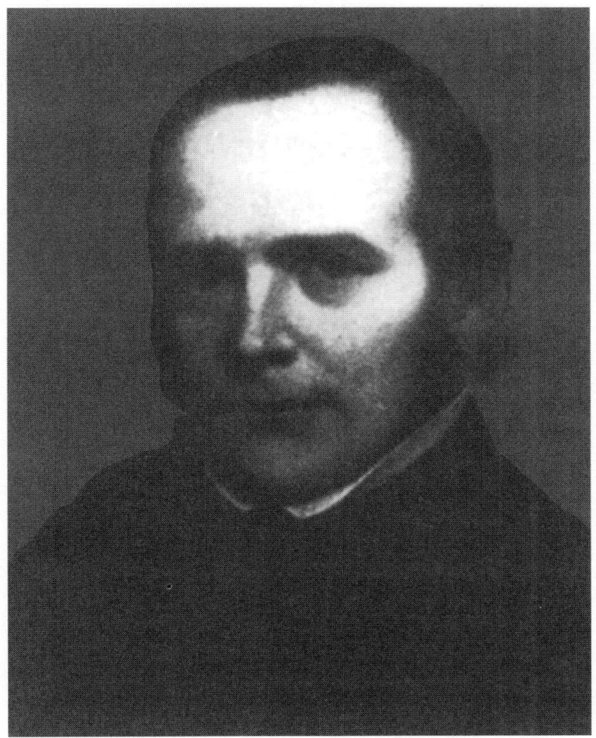

Horace Wells (1815-1848)

To **Francis Foldes, MD**, for having instilled in me an everlasting fascination in the art and science of anesthesiology, and to **Norman Trieger, DMD, MD**, and **Thomas Pallasch, DDS, MS**, for having made possible a career that has provided me with continued challenge, interest, and enjoyment, one that I would change for no other, and to **Horace Wells, DDS**, who 160 years ago discovered anesthesia.

Contributors

Morris S. Clark, DDS
Professor of Oral and Maxillofacial Surgery
Department of Surgical Dentistry
School of Dentistry;
Department of Surgery
School of Medicine
University of Colorado
Denver, Colorado

Christine L. Quinn, DDS, MS
Clinical Professor
Department of Diagnostic and Surgical Sciences
University of California, Los Angeles
School of Dentistry
Los Angeles, California

Kenneth L. Reed, DMD
Clinical Assistant Professor
Department of Oral and Maxillofacial Surgery
Section of Anesthesia and Medicine
School of Dentistry
University of Southern California
Los Angeles, California

Preface

Hartford, Connecticut, December 10, 1844 . . . Almost 160 years ago Samuel Cooley, a clerk in a retail store, ran around a stage in an intoxicated state, little realizing the major role he was playing in forever altering the degree of pain and suffering that patients throughout the world would experience during surgery. Cooley had come to attend a popular science lecture in which advances in science were demonstrated. One demonstration was of the intoxicating effects of "laughing gas," which Cooley volunteered to inhale. Also in attendance that fateful evening was Horace Wells, a local dentist who, on seeing Cooley injure his leg but continue to run about as though nothing had happened, considered there might be a clinical application for this "laughing gas." On the following day, December 11, 1844, nitrous oxide ("laughing gas") was administered to Dr. Horace Wells, rendering him unconscious and able to have a wisdom tooth extracted without any awareness of pain.

The world had forever been changed. But had it?

"In 1845 the New York *Daily Tribune* published a detailed account of an amputation. The operation took place at New York Hospital, a five-acre nest of low brick buildings, located on what is now Lower Broadway. The patient was a young man, cradled tenderly the whole time by his father and at the same time held firmly—and brusquely—in place by the attendants. As the surgeons—there were two—made their cuts, the boy's screams were so full of misery that everyone who could left the room. The first part of the operation complete, the young man watched 'with glazed agony' as the chief surgeon pushed a saw past the sliced muscles, still twitching, and listened as the blade cut through the bone in three heavy passes, back and forth. That was the only noise in the room, for the boy had stopped screaming."[1]

One hundred and sixty years after the discovery of anesthesia so much is taken for granted. Local anesthetics are administered to patients when a surgical procedure might be ever so slightly painful. *Yet in 1844 these drugs did not exist.* When patients require treatment, a variety of techniques are available to help manage their fears—intravenous conscious sedation; intramuscular sedation; oral, rectal, transmucosal, and intranasal sedation; and general anesthesia. *These techniques of drug administration were not available in 1844.*

No longer does a patient about to undergo dental or surgical procedures face that prospect with utter hopelessness and despair. Dentistry has long recognized that many persons are frightened of the dental experience and, to its credit, has taken steps to prepare the dental profession to recognize and manage these patients. In its approach to the management of pain and anxiety, the dental profession has remained in the forefront of all the health-care professions.

Publication of the *Guidelines for the Teaching of Pain and Anxiety Control and the Management of Related Complications* (ADA, 1979) put forth a cohesive document aimed at providing well-constructed standards for teaching the future generations of dental students and dentists safe and effective techniques of managing pain and anxiety. A dentist graduating from a dental school in the United States in the past 25 years has received training (albeit to varying degrees of clinical proficiency) in these important areas. For phobic patients seeking dentists able to manage their dental fears, the search is usually short. More and more dentists promote their ability and desire to "cater to cowards." The public has been the ultimate beneficiary of that chance encounter between Mr. Samuel Cooley and Dr. Horace Wells in December 1844.

This edition of *Sedation: A Guide to Patient Management* is, as were its predecessors, designed for the student of medicine or dentistry on a doctoral, postdoctoral, or continuing dental education level. It is meant to be comprehensive, providing basic concepts needed to fully understand the drugs and techniques and how they work, step-by-step descriptions of the various techniques, and a look at the potential complications and emergencies that might arise. More than anything else, this edition of *Sedation* is designed to be used in conjunction with a course in sedation that provides for the clinical management of patients in a controlled (supervised) environment. Only through this type of program can the techniques described in this book be used safely and effectively in a dental or medical practice.

Changes have occurred in several areas of this edition. In addition to general text and photographic updates of all chapters, Section IV, *Inhalation Sedation,* has been co-authored and rewritten by Dr. Morris Clark. Dr. Clark has lectured extensively on inhalation sedation and is the author of a highly regarded text on the subject: *Handbook of Nitrous Oxide and Oxygen Sedation.*[2] Discussion of the physically compromised patient and anesthetic considerations has been rewritten and expanded into two chapters (Chapters 38 and 39) by Dr. Kenneth Reed.

As stated in previous editions of *Sedation,* the ultimate aim of this book remains the same: to help dental patients, to enable them to receive the quality of care they truly deserve, and to enable them to receive this care in an atmosphere of relaxation, mental ease, and safety.

How times have changed in 160 years!

Stanley F. Malamed

REFERENCES

1. Fenster JM: *Ether day: the strange tale of America's greatest medical discovery and the haunted men who made it,* New York, 2001, HarperCollins.
2. Clark MS, Brunick AL: *Handbook of nitrous oxide and oxygen sedation,* St Louis, 1999, Mosby.

About This Book

This book is divided into eight sections. Section I is introductory, presenting an outline of the "problem" that all members of the dental profession face: the problem of fear and anxiety, which confronts dentists throughout the world on a daily basis.

Section II introduces the concept of sedation and of the spectrum of pain and anxiety control. The dental and medical professions have at their disposal a wide array of techniques that may be used in patient management. The availability of these to the dentist will increase the likelihood of a successful treatment outcome. Also included in Section II are chapters on preoperative physical evaluation of the patient and monitoring of the patient during the various sedative procedures. This section ends with an introduction to two nondrug techniques of sedation: iatrosedation and hypnosis. These techniques are extremely valuable in the management of virtually all patients.

Sections III, IV, and V present an in-depth look at the subject of pharmacosedation. Section III presents discussions of several techniques of sedation, including oral, rectal, and intramuscular (IM). Considerable attention is devoted to the clinical pharmacology of the drugs discussed in an effort to discourage the use of drugs that might be deemed inappropriate for certain procedures and to encourage the use of others that have proved to be safe and effective.

Sections IV and V are each devoted to one technique: Section IV to inhalation sedation and Section V to intravenous (IV) sedation. Because I believe that these are the two most effective and, when used properly, the safest of all sedative procedures, I have presented a complete and up-to-date discussion of these valuable techniques. *It cannot be overemphasized that in the absence of considerable supervised clinical experience the reading of these sections does not constitute preparation adequate to permit anyone to safely use these techniques of drug administration.*

Section VI provides an introduction to general anesthesia, another important method of pain and anxiety control. Training in this area requires a considerably greater length of time: a minimum of 2 years of full-time training.

Section VII addresses the subject of emergencies in the dental office. Preparation for and management of emergencies are reviewed in this section. The most important aspect of training for emergencies—prevention—has been the subject of all of the chapters that precede this section. Although it may appear to some that the subject of emergencies and complications takes up an inappropriately large part of this book, it is my belief that this subject can never be discussed too often or too thoroughly. When the techniques discussed in this book are used properly, the number of emergencies and complications that occur are minimal. Although the absence of complications is our goal, success at achieving this goal does have inherent risks: The doctor may become complacent with a technique that works "all the time" and therefore becomes a little less vigilant. It is at times like this that problems do occur. If the doctor is aware of the possible complications associated with a procedure, then these may be recognized and managed more effectively if and when they do develop.

Finally, Section VIII discusses four groups of "special" patients. Management of the pediatric, geriatric, medically compromised, and disabled patient requires a degree of knowledge and training on the part of the doctor and dental staff beyond that needed for the typical patient. These four groups of patients are not uncommon in the dental office and, unfortunately, present all too many doctors with significant problems during management. It is paramount that the doctor be aware of the subtle changes in treatment protocol that may be required during treatment of these patients. A doctor knowledgeable in the management of these patients will have available a greatly expanded pool of potential patients.

Acknowledgments

Many people have been involved in the development of this fourth edition of *Sedation: A Guide to Patient Management.*

Considering that the first edition of *Sedation* was published in 1985, many of the pictures in this fourth edition required updating. I must thank the photographer, Norman Goldberg, for the excellent quality of the photographs, as well as the two models, Drs. Debbie Kim and Cameron Hulse, for their poise during the often-trying shoot.

Once again I wish to thank Dr. Christine L. Quinn for co-authoring the chapter on the geriatric patient (Chapter 36). She is joined in this edition by two new co-authors: Dr. Morris Clark, who rewrote much of Section IV, Inhalation Sedation (Chapters 11 to 19), and Dr. Kenneth Reed, who rewrote the material on the physically compromised patient (Chapters 38 and 39).

As always, thanks must be proffered to those friendly folks at Mosby, Kimberly Alvis and Penny Rudolph, for doggedly keeping after me to keep those printed pages coming!

Stanley F. Malamed

Note

The treatment modalities and the indications and dosages of all drugs in *Sedation: A Guide to Patient Management* have been recommended in the medical literature. Unless specifically indicated, drug dosages are those recommended for adult patients.

The package insert for each drug should be consulted for use and dosages as approved by the U.S. Food and Drug Administration (FDA). Because standards of usage change, it is advisable to keep abreast of revised recommendations, particularly those concerning new drugs.

Sedation in Dentistry: A Historic Perspective

The words *fear, anxiety,* and *pain* have long been associated with dentistry. Throughout the years the general public has thought, and been taught, that dentistry hurts. The public's image of the dentist has borne this out. Surveys have consistently shown that although dentistry as a profession is highly respected by the public,[1] the image of the dentist as one who enjoys hurting people is still retained by a majority of persons. In a survey of the most common fears of adults, fear of going to the dentist ranked second only to the fear of public speaking (Table 1).[2]

Is this image of the dentist justified? Of course not; indeed, it never truly was. Unfortunately, however, our predecessors in dentistry did not have at their disposal the vast array of equipment and drugs for the management of pain and anxiety that are available today. History has recorded that members of the dental profession have consistently been in the forefront in the research and development of new techniques and medications for the management of pain and anxiety. Horace Wells (a dentist) and William T. G. Morton (dentist and physician), in the 1840s, were the founders of anesthesia and the first to use nitrous oxide (N_2O) (Wells) and ether (Morton) for the management of pain during surgical procedures.[3] Prior to this time, dental care consisted to a great degree of the removal of root tips without any form of anesthetic, except for alcohol, which was frequently used preoperatively (and perhaps still is).[4] Surgery before the introduction of anesthesia consisted almost exclusively of the amputation of limbs that had become infected and gangrenous.[3] As in dentistry, these procedures were of necessity performed without the aid of any form of anesthesia except for landenum, a drink of opium and alcohol.

TABLE 1 Our Most Common Fears

Fear	Percentage
Public speaking	27
Going to dentist	21
Heights	20
Mice	12
Flying	9
Other/no fears	11

From *Dental Health Advisor*, Spring 1987 (survey of 1000 adults).

In the area of intravenous (IV) medications and outpatient general anesthesia, the dental profession again led the way. With the introduction of IV barbiturates in the late 1930s, Victor Goldman and Stanley Drummond-Jackson in England and Adrian Hubbell in the United States pioneered techniques of IV general anesthesia for ambulatory oral surgery patients.[5,6] It was not until the 1970s that the medical profession, realizing the merits of short-stay surgery, began to use these same techniques.[7]

Dentistry has indeed been at the forefront in the fight against pain. Today virtually all dental procedures may be successfully completed in the absence of any patient discomfort through the administration of local anesthetics and/or the use of other techniques (e.g., electronic dental anesthesia). However, the dental consumers, our patients, may not be aware of this, or they may consider that the injection of a local anesthetic is the most traumatic part of the entire dental procedure.[8,9] How then are we to manage these patients?

As dentistry developed, dentists gained the reputation of being "tooth doctors." Dental education was for many years predicated on the fact that the dentist was responsible for the oral cavity of the patient, and dental school curricula illustrated this. Previously, dentists were trained to manage their patients' dental requirements only. The possible interaction between dental treatment and the overall health of the patient was either unknown or ignored.

As medicine became increasingly sophisticated, it became apparent that dental care could and indeed did have a significant affect on the overall health of patients. Dental schools amended their curricula, adding courses in medicine and physical evaluation.[10] The dentist became even more alert to the fact that treatment in the oral cavity could profoundly influence a patient's well-being and conversely that the patient's health could significantly affect the type of dental treatment offered. The use of the patient-completed medical history questionnaire became a standard in the 1950s, followed by the routine recording of vital signs (1970s). The direction in the late 1990s and today is toward more in-depth training in physical evaluation, including heart and lung auscultation.

Unfortunately, until the late 1960s and early 1970s, few dental schools in the United States (the University of Pittsburgh, The Ohio State University, and Loma Linda University being notable exceptions) provided the graduating dentist with a thorough background in the recognition and management of fear and anxiety. Until recently, the dentist could only treat the teeth of a patient who was known to be healthy enough (physically) to withstand the stresses of dental therapy. The "mind" of the patient (the patient's psychological attitude toward dentistry) was almost entirely ignored. The absence, at all levels of education, of training programs in the recognition and management of anxiety implied that anxiety did not exist or that it was of little or no importance. The doctor would treat the patient as well as he or she could given the clinical circumstances, and quite often the quality of the dentistry demonstrated the difficulty in patient management. General anesthesia was always available for those few patients who were absolutely unable to tolerate treatment; however, the most common type of dentistry performed under general anesthesia was exodontia. For conservative dental care, little or no thought was given to the patient's state of mind during treatment.

Under the sponsorship of three organizations—the American Dental Association (ADA), the American Dental Society of Anesthesiology (ADSA), and the American Dental Education Association (ADEA)—five "Workshops on Pain Control" were held (1964, 1965, 1971, 1977, and 1989). From these workshops came the *Guidelines for Teaching the Comprehensive Control of Pain and Anxiety in Dentistry,* which established an outline for three levels of training in various techniques of pain and anxiety control: the predoctoral dental program, the postdoctoral (residency) program, and continuing dental education.[11]

The 1970s saw the establishment by dental schools of viable programs in the area of sedation. Although the level of training still varies considerably from school to school, the dental student today receives, at a minimum, a background in the subject of anxiety and fear of dentistry and the techniques available in their management. Dentists today are aware that many patients are fearful of receiving dental treatment. This awareness is the first step required for the effective treatment of the patient's fears and anxieties. Add to this the almost universal availability of one or more techniques of sedation (usually iatrosedation, oral sedation, and inhalation sedation) and it becomes possible for the dentist to effectively and safely manage virtually all patients seeking care.

In the past few years, however, it has also become quite obvious that some dentists (and physicians) who had not received training in the use of these techniques while in school have begun to use these techniques in their private practices without the benefit of appropriate postgraduate training programs. In all too many cases the result has been death or serious injury to patients.[12,13] Lawmakers in many states have taken action to halt this trend, either by prohibiting dentists from using certain techniques of sedation or anesthesia[14,15] or by requiring a special permit or license if the doctor is to use the techniques.[16] The Dentists Insurance Company (TDIC) in California published a retrospective study of deaths related to drug administration in dental practice.[17] Three major areas of fault were found to be present in almost all instances of negative outcome:

1. Inadequate preoperative evaluation of the patient
2. Inadequate monitoring during the procedure
3. Lack of knowledge of the pharmacology of the drugs being administered

Whenever drugs are administered to a patient, it is essential that the doctor be fully cognizant of these three areas, as well as of any others that are involved in the ultimate safety of a drug technique. Failure to adequately prepare ourselves to administer drugs safely to patients can only result in these techniques being taken forcibly away from us.

One of my goals in preparing this book was to provide the doctor with appropriate background information concerning the various techniques of sedation that are most frequently used in the typical outpatient setting. As was stated in the Preface, this book is not intended to be used as a sole source of knowledge concerning these techniques. Only when used in conjunction with a course of study that involves use of these procedures in the actual management of patients can a doctor become truly capable of safely administering the drugs discussed in this book. Of greater importance perhaps is the level of training required for each of these techniques. At the end of the chapter or section on each technique, recommendations are presented that outline the level of training deemed appropriate for the doctor to be able to use the technique in a safe and effective manner.

As is mentioned throughout this textbook, no single technique of conscious sedation can ever be considered a panacea. Failures are to be expected on occasion with every technique of conscious sedation. Although failures are frustrating for the doctor, they must be considered an unavoidable aspect of any conscious sedation procedure, for as long as some patients retain even the slightest degree of consciousness, they will respond inappropriately to stimulation. It is only with the loss of consciousness (general anesthesia) that a significantly greater success rate can be expected; however, most doctors (both dentists and physicians) do not have the training necessary to use techniques in which unconsciousness is produced purposefully. As the doctor becomes more experienced with the techniques of conscious sedation, failure rates will decrease. Patients will sense a doctor's unease and unfamiliarity with a "new" technique, and this uncertainty is transferred to the patient, thereby decreasing the chance of a successful result. With increased experience, the doctor will become increasingly comfortable with the procedure and so too will the patient, thereby increasing the likelihood of success.

The greater the number of routes of conscious sedation that a doctor has available for patient management, the greater the probability of a successful result. The only way to become successful with these techniques is to receive appropriate supervised training. Acceptable courses are listed semiannually in the *Journal of the American Dental Association*[18] and bimonthly in *Anesthesia Progress.*

REFERENCES

1. Professions with prestige (National Opinion Research Center report on job status), *Washington Post* 115, p WH5, March 31, 1991.
2. *Dental Health Advisor,* Spring, 1987.
3. Bankoff G: *The conquest of pain: the story of anesthesia,* London, 1946, MacDonald.
4. Sykes WS: *Essays on the first hundred years of anaesthesia,* Edinburgh, 1960, E & S Livingstone.
5. Drummond-Jackson SL: Evipal anesthesia in dentistry, *Dental Cosmos* 77:130, 1935.
6. Hubbell AO, Adams RC: Intravenous anesthesia for dental surgery with sodium ethyl (1-methylbutyl) thiobarbituric acid, *J Am Dent Assoc* 27:1186, 1940.
7. White PF: Outpatient anesthesia: an overview. In White PF, ed: *Outpatient anesthesia,* New York, 1990, Churchill Livingstone.
8. Fiset L, Milgrom P, Weinstein P et al: Psychophysiological responses to dental injections, *J Am Dent Assoc* 111:578, 1985.
9. Matsuura H: Analysis of systemic complications and deaths during dental treatment in Japan, *Anesth Prog* 36:219, 1990
10. Curricular guide for physical evaluation, *J Dent Educ* 48:219, 1984.
11. Guidelines for teaching the Comprehensive Control of Pain and Anxiety in Dentistry. Council on Dental Education, American Dental Association, *J Dent Educ* 53:305, 1989.
12. Newcomer K: Dentist waited outside while patient died, *Rocky Mountain News,* August 4, 1992.
13. Child dies in dentist's chair. News2Houston.com, September 8, 2001.
14. Alaska State Board of Dental Examiners, Juneau, AK.
15. Christie B: Scotland to ban general anaesthesia in dental surgeries, *BMJ* 320:598, 2000.
16. Department of State Government Affairs, American Dental Association, 1992.
17. de Julien LF: Causes of severe morbidity/mortality cases, *J Calif Dent Assoc* 11:45, 1983.
18. Council on Dental Education: Continuing education course list for January-June, 2000, Chicago, American Dental Association.

Contents

25 Pharmacology 328

SECTION I

INTRODUCTION

CHAPTER 1

Pain and Anxiety in Dentistry

CHAPTER OUTLINE

August 14, 1984

Dear Dr. Malamed: I am writing to you in hope that you can give me some information on dentists who use conscious sedation in their practice. In reading the *Los Angeles Times* article June 4, 1984 . . . I finally found the right course I could take to get my teeth worked on.

For the last 5 years I have been trying to find a solution to my problem. I have an overwhelming fear of dentists and a very sensitive mouth. When I read the article and found out about various types of anesthesia that are available to dentists, I found light at the end of the tunnel. I do not, however, know how to find these dentists who are trained in the field . . . I would appreciate any help you can give me.

Thank you

The writer of the preceding letter is unusual, not because of her fear of dentistry, but because she was able to write this letter in an effort to seek help for herself.

In the United States it is estimated that somewhere between 6% and 14% of the population (14 million to 34 million people) voluntarily avoid seeking dental care because of their fear of dentistry.[1] These individuals delay treatment until they are in such pain that home remedies are no longer effective. They are categorized as severely anxious patients and represent a dual problem in management, for the doctor will have to treat both the patients' acute dental problem (usually pain and infection) and their psychological emergency. I once gave a speech titled "The Pain of Fear."[2] This title aptly describes the dilemma faced by the acutely fearful dental patient: Fear of pain keeps the patient from seeking needed dental care until the pain, which is exacerbated by this fear, ultimately forces the patient to the dental office. Such patients present the doctor with a significant problem. Attempts to treat these patients without addressing their fear usually lead to great frustration and increased stress for the doctor, as well as an increased level of fear for the patient.[3] Kahn, Cooper, and Mallenger[4] surveyed a group of dentists and reported that 57% of those responding stated that the most stressful factor in their dental practices was the "difficult patient."

Much more typically seen than the person with severe anxiety—the vast majority of those seen in the dental office—is the patient who does not harbor any irrational fears* of dental treatment. However, this patient does experience a degree of heightened anxiety as the scheduled dental appointment nears. This apprehension over the forthcoming dental treatment does not prevent the patient from appearing in the office, for this patient is genuinely concerned about maintaining oral hygiene and does not want to experience the pain of a toothache. This patient is categorized as having low to moderate anxiety and will appear on a regular basis for scheduled care because such a patient knows that avoiding needed dental treatment will only lead to more significant (and painful) problems later. However, while in the dental office, this patient has somewhat sweaty palms and a more rapid heartbeat and admittedly would much rather be somewhere else.

In 1972 the Ad Hoc Committee on Research and Faculty Training in Pain Control in Dentistry[8] reported that "the threat and fear of pain constitutes one of the great obstacles to the acceptance of dental services in the United States, considered by some to be greater than the financial barrier." With the arrival of prepaid dental care and health insurance coverage for many millions of Americans, it has become quite obvious that it is not only the financial aspect of dental care that prevents patients from seeking treatment.

If this is so, then we in the dental profession have been neglecting a very important aspect of the management of our patients. With the great technical advances that have been achieved in dentistry in recent years, almost all areas of dental treatment can be undertaken with greater skill, a greater degree of accuracy, and less trauma, and they can be completed in less time. Yet despite these advances, the problems of fear and anxiety persist.

A large part of the problem can be assumed to be a carryover from the recent past, when many dental patients were severely traumatized both physically and psychologically in the process of receiving routine dental care. Because of the lesser degree of scientific knowledge available at the time, a certain level of discomfort (pain) was to be expected. "Grin and bear it" was a commonly heard cliché.

The traumatized children of that era are the adults of today, and because they carry with them many psychological scars and bitter memories of "going to the dentist," today's dental professional is faced with a multiplicity of management problems when these patients appear for treatment.

Anxious patients present a problem to the dentist not only when they appear for treatment but also when their children require treatment. Anxiety is contagious, and even though the apprehensive adult will usually make every attempt to mask their true feelings about "the dentist" (for it is "childish" to be afraid of the dentist), their feelings usually manage to make themselves evident to their children. Every dentist is familiar with the child who appears at his or her very first dental appointment already "knowing" that the drill is going to hurt. The problem of anxiety and its management in the pediatric patient are discussed more fully in Chapter 35.

This is our problem.

BASIC FEARS

What are the causes of our patients' fear of dentistry? Most persons harbor five universal fears:

1. Fear of pain
2. Fear of the unknown
3. Fear of helplessness and dependency
4. Fear of bodily change and mutilation
5. Fear of death

When the stress of the dental situation is superimposed onto these fears, many patients find themselves unable to successfully cope and they exhibit "dental phobia"—an irrational fear of dentistry and all that it represents.

Each of the aforementioned fears is easily transferred into the dental situation. As will be demonstrated, the *fear of pain* is easily the most significant fear harbored by the typical dental patient. How often does one hear the plaintive question, "Is it going to hurt?" from a patient just before a procedure is to start? In fact, how do most patients select their dentist? Because of the superior quality of dental care or because the doctor has a reputation for being "painless" and caring? Each of us has heard a patient say, "It's nothing personal, Doctor, but I don't like dentists." Milgrom et al. found that patients who were not experiencing dental pain when they appeared for routine treatment fully expected that at some time during their treatment

---

*The terms *fear* and *anxiety* are often used interchangeably, as is the case in this text. However, there is a distinction to be made between them.

Fear tends to be a short-lived phenomenon, disappearing when the external danger or threat passes. It includes a feeling that something terrible is going to happen; physiologic changes, including tachycardia, profuse perspiration, and hyperventilation; and overt behavioral movements such as becoming jittery or shaking. These clinical manifestations comprise what is called the "fight or flight" response.[1,5]

Anxiety, in contrast, is not likely to be dispelled as quickly. The emotional response is usually an internal one and is not readily recognized. Weiss and English[6] define *anxiety* as "a specific unpleasurable state of tension which indicates the presence of some danger to the organism." Anxiety tends to be a learned response, acquired from personal experience or secondarily through the experiences of others. Anxiety arises from anticipation of an event, the outcome of which is unknown.[7]

Milgrom et al.[1] state that a major difference between fear and anxiety is the immediacy of the threat to the person. A response to an immediate threat is fear. Properly used in the dental situation, the term *anxiety* describes reactions that develop in anticipation of or at the thought of dentistry, whereas *fear* refers to the reaction occurring at the dental office.

they would experience pain, and the person most likely to inflict this pain on them was the dentist.[1]

Fear of the unknown is present in varying degrees whenever a person is confronted with a new situation, be it attempting to cross a furnished room for the first time in the dark or facing a new and threatening dental procedure. Fortunately, this fear can be effectively eliminated or at least modulated through an iatrosedative technique (see Chapter 6) called *preparatory communications.* The doctor need merely discuss the planned procedure with the patient, describing in nontechnical and nonthreatening terms the nature of the planned procedure.

The *fear of helplessness and dependency* is, unfortunately, more difficult to eliminate in dentistry. Because of the nature of dental care, the patient is both unable to observe the treatment and is usually placed in a very vulnerable position—the supine position. Most persons experience a sense of unease at this time, especially when they are receiving treatment from a stranger—a doctor or hygienist with whom they are not well acquainted. As the patient becomes more familiar with the doctor or hygienist, this feeling of helplessness should resolve.

In the area of pharmacosedation the fear of helplessness and dependency also appears. Consider that we are asking already apprehensive patients to lie back in the dental chair (a vulnerable position) and to permit virtual strangers to administer drugs that alter their level of consciousness and decrease even further the degree of control they maintain over their body. Examples of ways in which a patient's active participation may be enlisted during certain procedures are presented throughout this book. Such activities increase the patient's sense of being in control, thereby helping allay the feeling of helplessness.

One personality type—the authoritarian—will prove very difficult to manage with the use of pharmacosedation. This individual, the "executive type," is a "take-charge" person who likes to be in complete control of their situation at all times. Where anxiety exists and pharmacosedation is indicated, this patient will prove somewhat more difficult to sedate successfully. The success of pharmacosedation is based, in part, on a patient's desire to simply "let go" and relax. Authoritarian patients often prove unwilling or unable to release control of their mind to the drug(s) being used. The doctor will label this patient as "resistant" or say that the patient "fought the medication."

The *fear of bodily change or mutilation* is common in all aspects of medicine but is especially evident in dentistry. The oral cavity is both a richly innervated and a psychologically important region. All aspects of dental care have potentially great psychological overtones. Though at times these may seem illogical to the doctor, they must be dealt with for treatment to be successful. Changes in the size and shape or configuration of the body may have a profound effect on the patient's overall outlook and attitude toward life. The loss of teeth, for example, in today's society represents the process of growing old, a situation that might prove to be extremely disturbing psychologically to the patient.

The *fear of death* is also ever present. Placed in a vulnerable position in the dental chair, patients next have a multitude of hands and instruments placed into their mouth. Drugs are injected that remove the patient's ability to feel, and then a high-speed handpiece is placed in their mouth, with a bur rotating several hundred thousand times per minute. Many sensations and feelings race through the typical patient's mind at this time: Can I breathe with all this equipment and these hands in my mouth? Will I move my tongue too close to the drill and have it injured? Will the doctor slip and injure me? Add to this the feelings of a patient when the use of conscious sedation is recommended, in light of the many media reports of death and injury related to the use of drugs in dental offices.[9-11]

The fear of death in the dental office has probably been accentuated because of the seeming popularity of this subject in the mass media. Several nationwide television programs (for example, *20/20*) have presented exposés on the dangers of anesthesia and sedation in dentistry.[10,12] Reaction from patients has been as expected: an increased reluctance to permit the doctor to administer any drugs, even local anesthetics and N_2O-O_2 sedation, for their treatment.

DENTAL FEARS

Table 1-1 presents the results of a survey of dental patients who were asked to list, in order of fearfulness, a number of situations that commonly occur in the dental office. As can be seen from this list, virtually every procedure that is performed in the dental office is capable of being viewed as frightening by the patient.[13]

Most of these fear-producing situations are easily understood, for example, extractions and drilling. However, several situations might easily be overlooked by the doctor. Being told that "you have bad teeth" (No. 3), "holding a syringe and needle in front of you" (No. 4), and "dentist laughs as he looks in your mouth" (No. 7) are almost entirely avoidable if the dentist is made aware of them. We all develop habits during our professional careers, most good, but a few of them negative. The manner in which we present ourselves to our patients may be the most important of all the habits we develop. Through the use of proper treatment protocols combined with an appropriate professional attitude and demeanor, these three fear-producing situations may be eliminated or diminished.

TABLE 1-1 Ranking of Dental Situations from the Most Fearful to the Least Fearful

Situation	Total Group	Low-Fear Group	High-Fear Group
Dentist is pulling your tooth	1	1	2
Dentist is drilling your tooth	2	2	1
Dentist tells you you have bad teeth	3	3	3
Dentist holds syringe and needle in front of you	4	4	6
Dentist is giving you a shot	5	5	4
Having a probe placed in a cavity	6	6	5
Dentist laughs as he looks in your mouth	7	7	10
Dentist squirts air into a cavity	8	8	7
Sitting in the dentist's waiting room	9	9	8
Dentist laying out his instruments	10	10	13
Nurse tells you it's your turn	11	12	9
Getting in the dentist's chair	12	11	11
Dentist is putting in the filling	13	13	14
Thinking about going to the dentist	14	15	12
Dentist cleans your teeth with a steel probe	15	14	16
Getting in your car to go the dentist	16	16	15
Dentist looks at your chart	17	17	17
Dentist places cotton in your mouth	18	18	18
Calling dentist to make an appointment	19	19	19
Dental assistant places bib on you	20	20	20
Dentist squirts water in your mouth	21	21	21
Making another appointment with the nurse	22	22	22
Dentist is cleaning your teeth	23	23	23
Dentist asks you to rinse your mouth	24	24	24
Dentist tells you he is through	25	25	25

From Gale E: *J Dent Res* 51:964, 1972.

Our profession has taken great strides toward the elimination of dental pain. With the many excellent local anesthetics available to us today, pain need not be a problem during dental treatment. In fact, with the disposable equipment available today and the use of recommended injection technique, the injection of local anesthetic solution can become virtually 100% painless and atraumatic. Of interest therefore is the finding in Table 1-1 that the statement "dentist holds syringe in front of you" was considered to be more fear provoking than "dentist giving you a shot." The anticipation of the injection produces more fear then the actual injection!

Dental fear does exist. The first step in the management of a patient's fear of dentistry must be the recognition that it is present. All members of the dental and medical office staff must be ever alert to clues that signify the presence of heightened anxiety in a patient. The methods of recognizing the presence of anxiety and fear are discussed in Chapters 4 and 6.

Ignoring the presence of dental fears provokes many negative responses from the patient. One of the most common is the response of the pain reaction threshold to heightened anxiety. Murray[14,15] demonstrated that of the many variables that influence the pain reaction threshold of a patient, anticipation and anxiety appear to be the most important. Apprehensive patients do in fact have a lowered pain reaction threshold. The patient will respond adversely to stimulation (e.g., pressure) that in the more relaxed patient would not be interpreted as painful. When anxiety is reduced or eliminated through psychosedation, the patient's subjective experience of pain declines significantly.[16]

Pain and anxiety are related circularly. According to Schottstraedt,[17] "Pain is a source of anxiety, anxiety is a factor that increases pain, and increased pain incites further anxiety." Ignoring fears and anxieties increases the frustration and stress of the doctor and staff and increases the likelihood of stress-related emergency situations developing in the patient.

Ignoring a patient's fear of dentistry will not make the fears go away. Ignoring a patient's fears of dentistry may, however, make the patient go away. The following is a transcript of an interview with an apprehensive dental patient that illustrates this point:

> I remember when I was in high school, I had a bad experience with a guy who I had to go to like every week for a couple of months and I hated going to this guy because he wasn't very . . . he didn't have very much empathy for . . . at least me . . . I don't know about the rest of his patients. And he kept saying, "Oh, that doesn't hurt . . . Come on, you're just a sissy," which wasn't cool . . . He wasn't just hurting my mouth, but he was hurting my ego . . . and when I was in high school, I just couldn't handle both.
>
> But what he was doing was like he'd give me a prescription of a bunch of sedative pills to take before I went. So I'd take about a double dose, and I'd have to have somebody drive me to the dentist and there I was . . . I don't know if they were like reds (secobarbital) or whatever, but I remember I felt out of it, but I felt uncomfortable. It wasn't a good experience. Going to him really, really, really touched off my fear of going back again because I didn't go back to the dentist for a long time after that.[18]

The remainder of this book is devoted to the various methods involved in the recognition of anxiety and in its management. Today's dental and medical practitioners have at their disposal a plethora of techniques that are quite safe and effective in the management of a patient's fears and anxieties. Many of the techniques discussed involve the administration of drugs to the patient to achieve the desired goal, whereas other techniques may prove effective in the absence of drug administration. It is one of the goals of this book to help the doctor to be able to select the appropriate psychosedative technique for a given patient so that fears of the dental situation may be managed in the least traumatic but still clinically effective manner.

REFERENCES

1. Milgrom P, Weinstein B, Kleinknecht R et al: *Treating fearful dental patients,* Reston, Va, 1985, Reston Publishing.
2. Malamed SF: The pain of fear. Lecture to the California Dental Society of Anesthesiology, October, 1975, San Francisco.
3. Friedman N: Iatrosedation. In McCarthy FM, ed: *Emergencies in dental practice,* ed 3, Philadelphia, 1979, WB Saunders.
4. Kahn RL, Cooper C, Mallenger M: Dentistry: what causes it to be a stressful profession? *Int Rev Appl Psych* 29:307, 1980.
5. Cannon WB: *Bodily changes in pain, hunger, fear and rage,* ed 2, New York, 1929, Appleton-Century-Crofts.
6. Weiss E, English OS: *Psychosomatic medicine,* Philadelphia, 1957, WB Saunders.
7. Pearson RE: Anxiety in the dental office. In Bennett CR, ed: *Conscious-sedation in dental practice,* ed 2, St Louis, 1978, Mosby.
8. National Institute of Health: Report of the Ad Hoc Committee II on research and faculty training in pain control in dentistry, Feb 9-10, 1972.
9. Diamond J, producer: ABC News Show 335, In the dentist's chair, Sept 29, 1983.
10. Newcomer K: Dentist waited outside while patient died, *Rocky Mountain News,* August 4, 1992.
11. Child dies in dentist's chair. News2Houston.com, September 8, 2001.
12. A visit to the dentist. 60 Minutes II, 19 January 1999, CBS Television.
13. Gale E: Fears of the dental situation, *J Dent Res* 51:964, 1972.
14. Murray JB: Psychology of the pain experience. In Weisenberg M, ed: *Pain: clinical and experimental perspectives,* St Louis, 1975, Mosby.
15. Murray JB: The puzzle of pain, *Percep Mot Skills* 28:887, 1969.
16. Jones A, Bentler PM, Petry G: The reaction of uncertainty concerning future pain, *J Abnorm Psychol* 71:87, 1966.
17. Schottstraedt WW: *Psychophysiologic approach in medical practice,* Chicago, 1960, Year Book Medical.
18. Interview, Department of Human Behavior, University of Southern California School of Dentistry, Los Angeles, Calif, 1975.

SECTION II

SPECTRUM OF PAIN AND ANXIETY CONTROL

Sections II through VI present the answer to the problem that was presented in Section I—the problem of fear and anxiety in dentistry. The answer includes all of the techniques that can be termed *conscious sedation,* as well as those termed *general anesthesia;* this terminology is defined in this section.

In Chapter 2 the reader is introduced to the concept of conscious sedation. The term is defined and then discussed in relation to general anesthesia, a state that many persons readily confuse with conscious sedation. The various stages of anesthesia, of which conscious sedation is one, are described.

Chapter 3, The Spectrum of Pain and Anxiety Control, presents the wide range of patient management techniques that are available to the dentist and physician. Advantages and disadvantages of these techniques are discussed and the techniques compared.

Prior to the administration of any drug to a patient, or for that matter prior to treatment of any sort, it is imperative that the doctor fully evaluate the patient to determine his or her ability to withstand the stresses involved in the planned treatment. This evaluation must be even more comprehensive whenever a drug is to be administered to a patient during treatment. In addition, all patients receiving central nervous system (CNS) depressant drugs (conscious sedation or general anesthesia) must be monitored to varying degrees throughout the procedure. Chapters 4 and 5 present extremely important guidelines that should be followed every time drug administration is considered. Failure to properly evaluate a patient before treatment (see Chapter 4) and failure to monitor the patient during treatment (see Chapter 5) have been implicated in many cases of morbidity and mortality.[1] The importance of these two chapters to the safety of the techniques that follow cannot be overstated.

In Chapter 6 the reader is introduced to the first of the two major categories of psychosedation—nondrug techniques. Although several nondrug techniques are available, two, iatrosedation and hypnosis, are used to a greater extent than others. Iatrosedation represents the building block on which the success or failure of all pharmacosedative procedures (techniques involving the administration of drugs) will be based. Whether we are aware of it or not, all doctors use iatrosedation in their office on all of their patients. Hypnosis, on the other hand, is a technique that must be learned in a more formal setting. When used appropriately, its success rate in the management of both pain and fear is quite acceptable.

REFERENCE

1. de Julien LF: Causes of severe morbidity/mortality cases, *J Calif Dent Assoc* 11:45, 1983.

CHAPTER 2

Introduction to Conscious Sedation

CHAPTER OUTLINE

The primary aim of this book is to aid the doctor in the management of pain and anxiety in the dental patient, for it is these two items that, either singly or in combination, produce most of the difficulties associated with patient management.

How may pain and anxiety be managed successfully and safely in the dental office? Pain associated with dental treatment is managed effectively through the administration of local anesthetics at the start of treatment. These chemicals prevent passage of the nerve impulse beyond the site at which they are deposited. Although the tooth or soft tissues have received a noxious stimulus (e.g., drill, curette), the propagated nerve impulse will travel only as far as the site at which the local anesthetic was deposited. The rapid influx of sodium ions into the interior of the nerve (the process responsible for continued propagation of the nerve impulse) is prevented, the impulse is terminated, and the patient experiences no discomfort.

As noted in Chapter 1, however, *fear* of pain is a major deterrent to the delivery of dental care today. Patients who are not in pain fear the visit to the dental office because they believe that at some time during their dental treatment they will be hurt.[1] Fear of pain produces a heightened anxiety in these patients, a factor that may lead to the avoidance of dental care until they are truly in pain.

How can dentistry alter its image of being painful? It is a fact today that virtually all dental care can be completed without discomfort to the patient. With the availability of a wide variety of excellent local anesthetics, it is possible to achieve clinically adequate pain control in almost all situations. The most difficult pain management problems usually occur in endodontically involved teeth and, since the reintroduction of intraosseous anesthesia, only rarely in this situation is effective pain control unattainable.[2,3]

The administration of a local anesthetic is also considered to be a traumatic procedure by most patients and, indeed, by many doctors (see Table 1-1).[4,5] Yet even this aspect of dental care need not be traumatic. Local anesthetic injections may be administered atraumatically anywhere in the oral cavity, including the palate. The technique of the atraumatic injection of local anesthetics is presented in various textbooks of local anesthesia.*

Yet the possibility of pain and the "injection" of local anesthetics are not the only things about

*The reader is referred to the *Handbook of Local Anesthesia*, by S.F. Malamed (St. Louis, ed 4, 1997, Mosby, Inc.), for an in-depth discussion of local anesthesia.

dentistry that induce fear in patients. Doctors with extensive clinical experience have probably heard patients express fear of almost every possible procedure that we are called on to carry out.

How then can we manage these overly fearful patients? The answer is to induce a state of consciousness (or, more precisely, an altered state of consciousness) in which a person is more relaxed and carefree than previously. Over the years many names have been given to this state. Names such as *chemamnesia*,[6] *sedamnesia*,[7] *twilight sleep*,[8] *relative analgesia*,[9] and *co-medication*[10] have been used to describe the state of consciousness that is now called *sedation*.

Many definitions of this important term have been given over the years; however, in 1971, following the Third Pain Control Conference sponsored by the American Dental Association (ADA), American Dental Society of Anesthesiology, and American Association of Dental Schools, the "Guidelines for Teaching the Comprehensive Control of Pain and Anxiety in Dentistry," were published.[11] These guidelines established a standard for the training of dental personnel in this area of patient management. Included in these guidelines were definitions of terms that were adopted to describe the various techniques and levels of consciousness and awareness discussed in the document. The following definitions, extracted from the 1989 revision of this document, are used throughout this book.[12]

general anesthesia The elimination of all sensation, accompanied by the loss of consciousness.

analgesia The diminution or elimination of pain in the conscious patient.

local anesthesia The elimination of sensations, especially pain, in one part of the body by the topical application or regional injection of a drug.

conscious sedation A minimally depressed level of consciousness that retains the patient's ability to independently and continuously maintain an airway and respond appropriately to physical stimulation and verbal command and that is produced by a pharmacological or non-pharmacologic method or combination thereof.

The Academy of Pediatric Dentistry, in its "Guidelines for the Elective Use of Conscious Sedation, Deep Sedation, and General Anesthesia in Pediatric Patients," added another term describing a level of consciousness that lies between sedation and general anesthesia. It is termed *deep sedation*.[13]

deep sedation A controlled, pharmacologically induced state of depressed consciousness from which the patient is not easily aroused and which may be accompanied by a partial loss of protective reflexes, including the ability to maintain a patent airway independently and/or respond purposefully to physical stimulation or verbal command.

One of the most frequent misunderstandings between the doctor and the patient relates to the patient's misinterpretation of the term *sedation*. In the minds of many of our patients, sedation is synonymous with general anesthesia, unconsciousness, and sleep. In addition, I have encountered more than a few health-care professionals, including physicians and dentists, who also misapply or misuse these terms.

Sedation is one of the stages of anesthesia. It is that stage of anesthesia in which the patient is still conscious but is under the influence of a central nervous system (CNS) depressant drug. The definition of *conscious* is extremely important because it provides a baseline description of all the techniques of conscious sedation to be discussed in this book.

conscious Capable of a rational response to command, with protective reflexes intact, including the ability to independently and continuously maintain a patent airway.

The definition of *conscious* was modified in recent years in that the word *rational* was replaced by *appropriate*. This was considered necessary because some patients who receive conscious sedation within the dental or medical office are unable to respond rationally to command. Such persons might include the very young patient or those with physical or mental disabilities. Deaf patients will be unable to respond rationally to the spoken word, but they will be able to respond appropriately, given their disability.

conscious sedation Techniques of pain and anxiety control in which consciousness is retained.

Anesthetic procedures in which consciousness is lost, even for the briefest of times, are considered general anesthesia. General anesthesia is discussed in Chapters 30 and 31.

THE STAGES OF GENERAL ANESTHESIA

In the mid-1840s Francis Plomley described three stages of general anesthesia.[14] In 1847 John Snow added a fourth, overdose.[15] It was not until World War I, however, that Guedel[16] more clearly described the signs and symptoms of the various stages of anesthesia. Guedel's classification of the stages of anesthesia was accepted throughout the world and is considered to be one of the important contributions to the science of anesthesiology. Four stages of anesthesia are described:

I. Stage of analgesia
II. Stage of delirium
III. Stage of surgical anesthesia
IV. Stage of respiratory paralysis

Guedel based his observations on the following parameters:

1. Character of the respirations
2. Eyeball activity
3. Pupillary changes
4. Eyelid reflex (presence or absence)
5. Swallowing or vomiting

Guedel's observations were based primarily on the effects of the gaseous anesthetic ether. As the nature of the practice of anesthesiology evolved over the years, it became obvious that the signs and symptoms described for ether were not always observed with many of the newer agents being developed. In 1943 Gillespie added several new factors to Guedel's criteria[17]:

6. Respiratory response to skin incision
7. Secretion of tears
8. Assessment of pharyngeal and laryngeal reflexes

An overview of the basic pattern of action of general anesthetics (and other CNS depressant drugs) may provide a better understanding of the stages and planes of anesthesia. The basic pattern of action consists of a descending depression of the CNS. CNS depressants (general anesthetics, antianxiety drugs, sedative-hypnotics, opioids, alcohol) first depress the cerebral cortex, producing a loss of sensory function, followed by a loss of motor function. Then the basal ganglia and cerebellum are depressed, followed by the spinal cord and finally the medulla. Medullary depression leads to depression of the respiratory and cardiovascular systems and is the usual cause of death from drug overdose. Guedel's four stages of anesthesia are based on this progressive depression of the CNS: stage I, analgesia or altered consciousness, corresponds to the action of drugs on higher cortical centers (sensory). The various techniques of conscious sedation lie within this stage. Stage II, delirium or excitement, corresponds to the depressant action of drugs on higher motor centers. The patient is unconscious in this stage. Stages I and II comprise the induction stage of general anesthesia. In stage III, surgical anesthesia, spinal reflexes are depressed, producing skeletal muscle relaxation. Stage IV, medullary paralysis, corresponds to depression of respiratory and cardiovascular centers of the medulla, producing first respiratory arrest and then cardiovascular collapse.

The stages of general anesthesia, as defined by Guedel and modified by Gillespie, are now described in greater detail. They are illustrated in Figure 2-1.

Stage I: Analgesia (Conscious Sedation)

The first stage of anesthesia starts with the initial administration of a CNS depressant drug and continues to the loss of consciousness (see Figure 2-1). The patient remains conscious throughout this stage and is capable of responding to command and may therefore provide the administrator with information (concerning, for example, the presence or absence of pain). The portions of the brain of most recent phylogenetic development are depressed earliest, primarily the cerebral cortex. Depression of the cerebral cortex results in diminished intellect, memory, integrative functions, and perception of time and space.

Although this phase is called the stage of *analgesia*, pain may, in fact, be present with the pain reaction threshold unaltered. However, because of the degree of CNS depression, especially depression of the cerebral cortex, the patient's response to noxious stimulation may be diminished.

The techniques of sedation described in this book provide the doctor with a patient who is maintained in stage I of anesthesia. These include the oral, rectal, intramuscular (IM), submucosal, intranasal, inhalation, and intravenous (IV) routes of drug administration. The patient is relaxed and cooperative, with a decreased awareness of his or her surroundings, and may exhibit a diminished response to stimulation.

The patient in stage I is under the influence of the drug but is technically awake. Any person who has ever received nitrous oxide–oxygen (N_2O-O_2) or taken a "sleeping pill" or antianxiety drug such as diazepam or even alcohol has technically been in stage I of anesthesia.

1. Respiration is normal.
2. Eye movements are normal, with voluntary movement possible (e.g., the patient is able to follow the examiner's finger from left to right).
3. Protective reflexes are intact.
4. Amnesia (the lack of recall) may or may not be present. Some techniques (e.g., IV conscious sedation) may provide varying degrees of amnesia, although most will provide little or no amnesia. In some techniques, such as N_2O-O_2 inhalation sedation, amnesia is extremely variable; however, patients will usually exhibit a diminished sense of time. A 2-hour appointment may seem to have been only 15 minutes.

CNS depression that places a patient into the lighter levels of stage I is entirely appropriate for use in outpatient procedures in the dental or medical office. Training is required for the safe and effective use of conscious sedation; however, the degree and length of training are not as extensive or intensive as that required for the administration of general anesthesia. As the depth of CNS depression (sedation) deepens, as may be seen in IM, submucosal, and IV sedation, the patient's ability to respond appropriately, as well as the function of his or her protective reflexes, diminishes. Additional training for the doctor and staff becomes critical, as does an increase in the level of

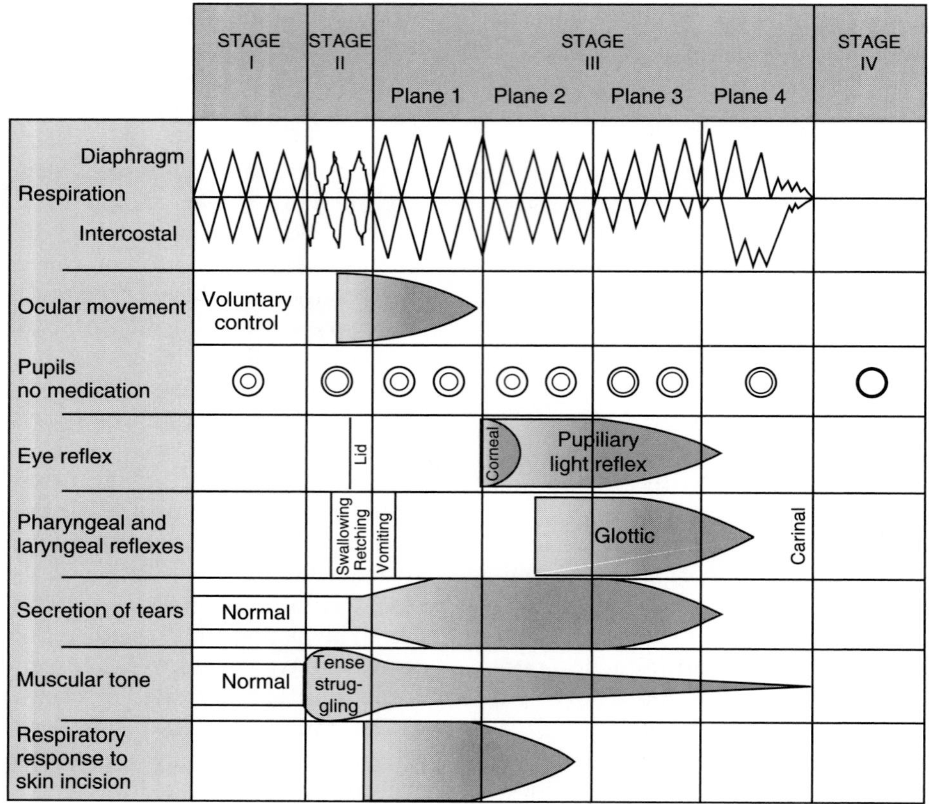

Figure 2-1 Classic signs of unpremedicated diethyl ether anesthesia as described by Guedel and modified by Gillespie. (Redrawn from Allen GD: *Dental anesthesia and analgesia: local and general,* ed 2, Baltimore, 1979, Williams & Wilkins.)

monitoring of the patient. However, the patient in stage I *is* able to maintain a patent airway ("independently and continuously") and to clear the airway should foreign material enter the region of the larynx or pharynx (e.g., cough or swallow).

Once the patient is unable to respond appropriately to command or the protective reflexes are depressed, the patient is technically unconscious; stage I ends and stage II begins.

Unfortunately, there is no objective sign that reliably indicates this transition from stage I to stage II. An oft-used sign of this transition is the eyelid reflex. Gentle stroking of the eyelashes provokes lid closure in the conscious patient. Lack of response to this stimulus is commonly used to denote entry of the patient into stage II of anesthesia. However, some patients in light stage I do not maintain their eyelid reflex.

Stage II: Delirium (Ultralight General Anesthesia)

Stage II of anesthesia is called the stage of *delirium* or *excitement.* When used in outpatient general anesthesia, it is called *ultralight general anesthesia.*

In stage II the degree of CNS depression is greater than that in stage I, and consciousness is lost. Stage II begins with the loss of consciousness and progresses until entry into the stage of surgical anesthesia (stage III).

Early in stage II the respiratory pattern of the patient may be somewhat irregular. As CNS depression deepens, the character of breathing becomes regular once again, marking the end of stage II and entry into stage III. The patient's reflexes may be exaggerated in the earlier part of stage II (the patient overreacts to stimulation). Physical restraints are usually required whenever procedures are carried out in this stage. In response to stimulation, especially noxious stimulation, patients may cry out and move their extremities. Indeed, observers of patients undergoing the extraction of third molars while receiving ultralight general anesthesia with intravenously administered barbiturates often state that they thought the patients were suffering because of their reactions to the stimulation produced during the removal of the teeth. However, quite often the first response of these patients upon regaining consciousness is the question, "When are you going to start?" Amnesia is present in stage II.

Because reflexes are hyperactive in this stage, care must be taken to prevent blood, saliva, or foreign materials from reaching the patient's larynx, where laryngospasm may be provoked (see Chapters 27 and 30). Only procedures of short duration should be contemplated in stage II and then only by persons who have received thorough training in general anesthesia. Trained assistants (doctors or auxiliaries) are responsible for protecting the patient's airway via suctioning and screening off with gauze packing while another trained person is responsible for continued maintenance of a patent airway. Although the patient continues to breathe spontaneously, in the absence of a patent airway, the exchange of O_2 and CO_2 will not occur.

1. Respirations are irregular early in stage II but become more regular as stage II deepens.
2. Eyeballs oscillate involuntarily, a movement termed *lateral nystagmus.*
3. Pupils react to light normally.
4. Skeletal muscle tonus is increased, with muscular rigidity present in some patients early in stage II. Muscle tonus decreases as stage II deepens.
5. The laryngeal and pharyngeal reflexes (swallowing and laryngeal closure) are still quite active early in stage II but become progressively more obtunded as stage II progresses.

Entry into stage II is undesirable when attempting to use conscious sedation techniques. Entry into stage II is an indication that oversedation has occurred. If the doctor has not received adequate training in the recognition and management of the unconscious patient, significant morbidity and even mortality may occur. When stage III (surgical anesthesia) is the goal, it is the practice to induce anesthesia rapidly so as to pass through stage II as quickly as possible, thereby minimizing overreaction to stimulation.

Management of a patient who has inadvertently entered stage II is either to increase the level of CNS depression (administer additional drug) to bring the patient into stage III of anesthesia or to simply maintain the patient in stage II (airway management) and permit a return to stage I as the cerebral blood level of drug is decreased through redistribution.

Stage III: Surgical Anesthesia

Further CNS depression brings the patient to a level at which respiratory regularity once again occurs. This heralds the onset of stage III of anesthesia, a stage that continues until respiration ceases (entry into stage IV). Most surgical procedures are performed at this level of CNS depression.

Entry into stage III is marked by several signs:

1. The respiratory irregularity observed in stage II disappears. Respiration is automatic and involuntary, responding to the level of CO_2 within the blood.
2. Muscular tonus is lost, unlike the increased muscular tonus seen in stage II. The patient's head may now be moved from side to side, and the mouth may be opened with ease.
3. Swallowing and reflex respiratory arrest will not occur if the anesthesiologist suddenly increases the concentration of an inhalational anesthetic. Both of these responses will occur in stage II.

For a more accurate determination of the depth of anesthesia, stage III is divided into four planes. The major differences in physical signs in these planes relates to the character of respiration, the character of eyeball movements, the presence or absence of certain reflexes, and the size of the pupils. The planes of anesthesia were introduced by Gillespie in 1943.[17]

Plane 1 of Stage III. Plane 1 is entered with the return of respiratory regularity. Respirations become full, regular, and automatic and are equally thoracic and abdominal in character.

Eyeballs oscillate slowly during this plane, and the pupils respond to light normally. Pharyngeal reflexes that induce vomiting when an oral airway is inserted are gradually diminished as plane 1 continues. The swallowing, retching, and vomiting reflexes disappear in that order during the induction of general anesthesia and reappear in reverse order on recovery from anesthesia.

Tears are secreted throughout plane 1. The tendency of the patient to breathe deeply and more rapidly with skin incision decreases as plane 1 deepens. Peripheral vasodilation develops in plane 1.

Plane 2 of Stage III. Plane 2 begins when the eyeballs cease to oscillate and become fixed eccentrically. Plane 2 ends when the intercostal muscles weaken and thoracic respiration becomes decreased.

Respiration remains regular, but because the depth of breathing is diminished, tidal volume is decreased.

If patients have not received premedication, pupillary size increases in plane 2 (dilation). However, because of the almost routine administration of preoperative drugs, pupillary signs are inconsistent and are no longer used as reliable indicators of the level of general anesthesia. Opioids produce pupillary constriction, whereas belladonnas, such as atropine, dilate the pupils.

Protective reflexes, such as laryngeal closure (laryngospasm), begin to disappear in plane 2. Secretion of tears diminishes in this plane, and the respiratory response (increased rate and depth) to skin incision disappears.

Plane 3 of Stage III. Plane 3 is entered as thoracic respiration decreases and the abdominal component of respiration increases. This is produced either by the beginning of paralysis of the intercostal muscles or by a weakening of the diaphragm. As plane 3 deepens, intercostal paralysis becomes complete and respiration is produced entirely by the diaphragm. Tidal volume is decreased and inspiration is now of shorter duration than exhalation.

The diaphragm may exhibit excessive or jerking movements during plane 3. During abdominal operations this may interfere with the surgical procedure, leading the surgeon to request a deeper plane of anesthesia. In fact, lightening of the anesthetic level (to plane 2) is all that is required for diaphragmatic movements to become more rhythmical and smooth. Another means of providing the surgeon with a more ideal surgical field is to keep the patient in plane 3 of anesthesia but to assist or control the patient's ventilation.

It is not recommended that plane 3 be used during surgery for extended periods. The upper portions of plane 2 and lower plane 1 are suitable for most procedures once the surgeon has explored the abdomen, exposed the surgical site, and mobilized the organs.

In mid to lower plane 3, pupillary reaction to light is gradually lost. Tear secretion continues to diminish in plane 3.

Plane 4 of Stage III. From the onset of paralysis of the intercostal muscles until respiratory arrest occurs, the patient is in plane 4. Activity of the diaphragm progressively decreases as plane 4 deepens until spontaneous breathing ceases entirely. Pupils dilate and little or no muscle tonus is to be found.

A response known as *tracheal tug* is often encountered in plane 4. Dripps, Eckenhoff, and Vandam[18] state that although there is no single satisfactory explanation for tracheal tug, it may be the result of an attempt by accessory muscles of respiration to augment respiratory exchange.

Stage IV: Medullary Paralysis

Stage IV begins with the onset of respiratory arrest and ends with the cessation of effective circulation (cardiac arrest). Essentially, stage IV is a stage of reversible clinical death. By definition, clinical death occurs with the cessation of effective respiration and circulation. With the application of controlled ventilation and the lightening of the depth of CNS depression, the patient may recover from this overly deep level of anesthesia. Stage IV of anesthesia is rarely sought intentionally. If respiration needs to be terminated temporarily during surgery (as in abdominal surgery in which skeletal muscle relaxation is necessary to enter the abdomen), the patient is maintained in stage III and a muscle relaxant drug such as pancuronium, atracurium, mivacurium, or rocuronium is administered.

Stage IV of anesthesia is seen in the emergency room of the hospital, where drug overdose is treated. Management of the patient in stage IV involves the application of basic and advanced life support, primarily effective ventilation with O_2, until redistribution and biotransformation of the offending drug(s) produce a lower plasma level.

SUMMARY

The reader should be aware of the four classic stages of anesthesia because whenever a technique of conscious sedation involving the administration of a drug is to be used, the patient will enter one or more of these stages. Stage I of anesthesia is called the stage of *analgesia* or the stage of *conscious sedation.* This is the stage in which all of the techniques presented in Sections III, IV, and V may be placed.

The patient in stage I is conscious, but under the influence of the drug(s). The patient is relaxed and cooperative and may be amnesic. Vital signs are minimally altered, protective reflexes are intact, and the patient is able to maintain a patent airway.

In order for a doctor to be able to safely manage a patient in stages II or III of anesthesia, a minimum of 2 full years of training in anesthesiology is necessary. The ability to safely manage the unconscious patient requires a significantly greater period of time to learn well.

Within the practice of dentistry there are indications for the use of stages II and III. Stage II is indicated primarily with outpatient oral surgery procedures, and stage III may be indicated for longer or more traumatic procedures of any type.

The next chapter introduces the many techniques of sedation and general anesthesia available for use by the dental and medical professions for the management of both pain and anxiety. In subsequent parts of this book, each of these techniques are reviewed in considerable depth so as to impart to the reader a degree of knowledge that will, when combined with adequate clinical and didactic training, permit the use of these techniques in a safe and effective manner.

REFERENCES

1. Milgrom P, Weinstein P, Kleinknecht T et al: *Treating fearful dental patients,* Reston, Va, 1985, Reston Publishing.
2. Nusstein J, Reader A, Nist R et al: Anesthetic efficacy of the supplemental intraosseous injection of 2% lidocaine with 1:100,000 epinephrine in irreversible pulpitis, *J Endodont* 24:487, 1998.

3. Parente SA, Anderson RW, Herman WW et al: Anesthetic efficacy of the supplemental intraosseous injection for teeth with irreversible pulpitis, *J Endodont* 24:826, 1998.
4. Gale E: Fears of the dental situation, *J Dent Res* 51:964, 1972.
5. Fiset L, Milgrom P, Weinstein P et al: Psychophysiological responses to dental injections, *JADA* 111:578, 1985.
6. Monheim LJ: *General anesthesia in dental practice,* ed 3, St Louis, 1968, Mosby.
7. Carnow R, Schaffer AB: Application of the concept of augmenter-moderator-reducer to dental patient management. In Spiro SR, ed: *Amnesia-analgesia techniques in dentistry,* Springfield, Ill, 1972, Charles C Thomas.
8. Berns J: Twilight sedation: a substitute for lengthy office intravenous anesthesia, *J Conn State Dent Assoc* 37:4, 1963.
9. Langa H: *Relative analgesia in dental practice: inhalation analgesia with nitrous oxide,* Philadelphia, 1968, WB Saunders.
10. Hamburg HL: *The joy of sedation: a beginner's manual to newer sedative techniques for the dentist and dental student,* Hamburg, NY, 1978, Hamburg.
11. American Dental Association, Council on Dental Education: Guidelines for teaching the comprehensive control of pain and anxiety in dentistry, *J Dent Educ* 36:62, 1972.
12. American Dental Association, Council on Dental Education: Guidelines for teaching the comprehensive control of pain and anxiety in dentistry, *J Dent Educ* 53:305, 1989.
13. Clinical guideline on the elective use of conscious sedation, deep sedation and general anesthesia in pediatric dental patients. *Pediatr Dent* 23:46, 2002.
14. Lee JAA, Atkinson RS: *A synopsis of anesthesia,* ed 5, Baltimore, 1964, Williams & Wilkins.
15. Snow J: *The inhalation of the vapour of ether in surgical operations,* London, 1847, Churchill.
16. Guedel AF: *Inhalation anesthesia: a fundamental guide,* New York, 1937, Macmillan.
17. Gillespie NA: The signs and reflex reactions of the stages of anesthesia, *Anesth Analg* 22:275, 1943.
18. Dripps RD, Eckenhoff JE, Vandam LD: *Introduction to anesthesia,* ed 9, Philadelphia, 1996, WB Saunders.

CHAPTER 3

The Spectrum of Pain and Anxiety Control

CHAPTER OUTLINE

A variety of techniques are available to the dental and medical professional to aid in the management of a patient's fears and anxieties regarding dental care and surgery. To some this statement may be self-evident; however, to others the availability of a variety of techniques may come as something of a surprise. The aim of this chapter is to introduce the concept of the *spectrum of pain and anxiety control*. This spectrum, which is presented graphically in Figure 3-1, demonstrates that there are indeed quite a number of techniques available to manage patients' fears and anxieties. This chapter introduces the various techniques included in this spectrum, and subsequent chapters discuss them in depth.

In Figure 3-1 the vertical bar about three quarters of the way across the spectrum denotes a very significant barrier: the point at which consciousness is lost. All techniques found to the right of the bar fall under the heading of general anesthesia, and all techniques to the left of the bar may be termed *psychosedation, sedation*, or *conscious sedation*.

Techniques of conscious sedation may further be divided into those requiring the administration of drugs to achieve a desirable clinical effect and those that do not. The former are termed *pharmacosedation* techniques, the latter iatrosedation techniques. These terms are further defined at other points in this book.

The bar representing the point at which consciousness is lost is significant in that it identifies a level of training that must be achieved by the doctor before various techniques can even be considered. Without elaborating at this point (educational requirements for specific techniques are discussed in appropriate sections of this book), it may be stated that the absolute minimum of training recommended for the use of general anesthesia is 2 full years. These guidelines for general anesthesia, as well as those for techniques of conscious sedation, have been accepted by the American Dental Association, the American Dental Society of Anesthesiology, and the American Dental Education Association.[1]

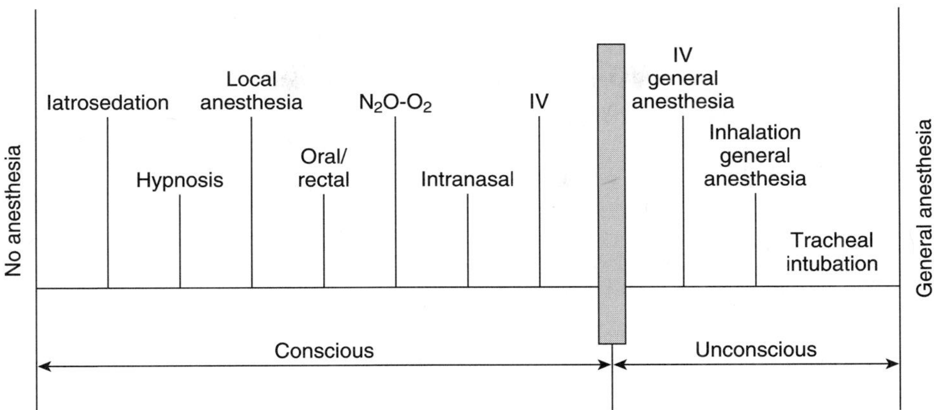

Figure 3-1 Spectrum of pain and anxiety control. Illustration of the range of techniques available in medicine and dentistry for patient management. Vertical bar represents the loss of consciousness.

The duration of time necessary to adequately prepare the doctor to use the various techniques of conscious sedation safely and effectively varies from technique to technique and from doctor to doctor. Many dentists and dental hygienists are fully prepared on graduation from dental school to enter into private practice knowledgeable in the safe and effective use of some of these techniques. Many others, however, will not have this ability, and for them continuing education courses are available.[2] For inhalation sedation with nitrous oxide (N_2O) and oxygen (O_2), a minimum course of 2 to 3 days, including patient management, is recommended; for intravenous (IV) conscious sedation, a much more extensive program, including patient management, is required.[3]

In recent years outpatient surgery in the practice of medicine has greatly increased in popularity. Minor surgical procedures on the limbs, trunk, and face are easily completed with the administration of local anesthetics by general surgeons, dermatologists, and plastic and reconstructive surgeons.[4] Other health professionals, such as podiatrists, are also extensively involved in outpatient surgery.[5] Until recently, however, little consideration was given to the degree of patient anxiety toward this type of surgical procedure. The patient faces these nondental surgical procedures with the same dread as may be seen in dental patients. The techniques and concepts discussed in this book are as appropriate for nondental surgery as they are in dentistry.

Many techniques of pain and anxiety control are available to the health-care professional. Which ones, if any, are used is a very personal choice. Some doctors are comfortable using a technique that others may be quite uncomfortable using. Having several techniques available at his or her disposal enables the doctor to tailor the appropriate conscious sedation technique to a given patient. There is no panacea, nor is any one technique always indicated or always effective. To rely solely on one technique for conscious sedation is to invite occasional failure.

NO ANESTHESIA

The extreme left-hand portion of the spectrum of pain and anxiety control (see Figure 3-1) comprises that small group of patients who require absolutely no conscious sedation or local anesthesia during their dental treatment. Although quite rare, it is probable that a dentist or hygienist will be called upon to treat one or more of these persons at some time. For whatever reason—anatomic, physiologic, psychological, cultural, or religious—these patients either do not feel pain or do not react to it, and they are able to tolerate any form of dental treatment without the need for any sort of drug intervention.

Although such patients may not feel any pain in the course of their treatment, such may not be the case with the dentist or hygienist called on to treat them. The following incident actually took place: The patient, a pleasant 26-year-old woman requiring periodontal surgery (soft tissue), requested that the doctor not use any drugs at all during her treatment because she did not require them. After a futile attempt to dissuade the patient from what was assumed to be a foolhardy course, the doctor agreed to begin the surgical procedure without local anesthesia only if the patient would consent to receive it if at any time during the surgery pain was present. The surgical procedure required approximately 45 minutes to complete, during which time the patient displayed absolutely no evidence of discomfort, to the complete amazement of the (numerous) dental personnel who had gathered around to watch. Vital signs (blood pressure, heart rate, and rhythm) monitored during the procedure demonstrated essentially no deviation from baseline values. Not so with the doctor and assistant. Following the procedure, which proceeded uneventfully, they were bathed in perspiration. The doctor commented that he felt quite uncomfortable throughout the procedure because he knew that the patient *should* be in pain. Indeed, he stopped many times to ask the patient how she was feeling. He also said that he could almost feel the pain for the patient. "I was uncomfortable for the patient," he said. At the next surgical appointment the doctor and assistant were quite pleased when the patient consented to their request to give her local anesthesia for the surgery. When asked why she had changed her mind, the patient stated that she did it for the sake of the doctor and the assistant. She had noticed *their* discomfort at the prior visit and, although she still did not require the pain-controlling drug, felt it prudent to receive it to allow the doctor to be more relaxed during her treatment.

It is important to separate this small group of patients who truly do not require anesthetics from those patients who similarly request that they not receive local anesthesia because they are quite fearful of injections. It is somewhat easier to recognize such a patient prior to starting the planned procedure. However, if the doctor is unable to recognize the patient's anxiety and proceeds to dental treatment, it usually becomes painfully obvious, to both the doctor and the patient, to which group the patient truly belongs.

IATROSEDATION

Iatrosedation, defined as the relief of anxiety through the doctor's behavior, is the building block for all other forms of psychosedation. The term and the technique of *iatrosedation* were created many years ago by Dr. Nathan Friedman, chairman and founder of the Department of Human Behavior, University of Southern California School of Dentistry.[6] Discussed in greater detail in Chapter 6, iatrosedation may briefly be described as a process involving several steps: recognition by the doctor of the patient's anxieties toward dentistry, management of the information gathered by the doctor from the patient, and a commitment by the doctor to aid the patient during dental treatment.

Simply stated, iatrosedation is a technique of communications between the doctor and the patient that creates a bond of trust and confidence. Patients possessing trust and confidence in their doctor (physician, dentist, or other health-care professional) are well on their way to being more relaxed and cooperative, without the need for supplemental pharmacosedation.[7]

Another important benefit of the use of iatrosedation in the practice of medicine and dentistry is the prevention of possible medicolegal complications. Lack of effective communication between the healthcare professional and patient is one of the leading causes of suits brought against medical and dental professionals. In some estimates up to 37% of all malpractice actions are a result of a lack of communication and trust between the doctor and patient.[8]

In some situations iatrosedation alone may remove all of a patient's fears and anxieties concerning the treatment, permitting us to then proceed in a normal manner, without the need for pharmacosedation. More often, however, iatrosedation produces a decrease in the patient's level of anxiety to the point that the use of supplemental pharmacosedation will enable the patient to more readily accept and tolerate the planned treatment.

OTHER NONDRUG PSYCHOSEDATIVE TECHNIQUES

In addition to the technique of iatrosedation, other methods are available to decrease a patient's fear and anxiety about dentistry without the administration of drugs.

Hypnosis has been used for many years for the management of both pain and anxiety. When employed by a trained hypnotherapist, in the proper clinical environment, and on the appropriate patient, hypnosis has proved to be a highly effective means of achieving both a relaxed and a pain-free treatment environment.

Other nondrug techniques for achieving pain and anxiety control are available. Some are not new, having been introduced to the medical and dental professions years ago. Interest in these techniques has waxed and waned over the years. They may prove to be effective in the hands of some medical and dental practitioners. Textbooks that provide in-depth coverage of these potentially valuable procedures are available and recommended.

Nondrug techniques are mentioned here for the sake of completeness. Developments in this field are occurring so rapidly that it is virtually impossible to include all of them in our compendium of available techniques. Nondrug techniques for the management of either pain or anxiety, or both, include acupuncture,[9] acupressure, audioanalgesia,[10] biofeedback,[11] electroanesthesia (transcutaneous electrical nerve stimulation [TENS], electroanesthesia [EA], electronic dental anesthesia [EDA]),[12] and electrosedation.

ROUTES OF DRUG ADMINISTRATION

To this point in discussing the management of treatment-related anxiety, we have not yet employed any technique that requires administration of a drug.

Conscious sedation produced without the administration of drugs is termed *iatrosedation*. The use of drugs to control anxiety is termed *pharmacosedation*. The three methods introduced thus far will permit us to manage but a small percentage of our fearful patients. One advantage possessed by iatrosedative techniques is their ability to increase the effectiveness of any drugs that might be needed for the definitive management of the patient's dental fears. Even though we may have to turn to pharmacosedation, the great majority of patients in whom iatrosedation has been used will require smaller doses of the drug(s) to bring about a comparable degree of conscious sedation.[13]

Drugs may be administered through 14 routes (Table 3-1). The first 13 of these routes are used within the practice of medicine, with the first 10 used in dentistry. The intraperitoneal route is used in veterinary medicine. These routes are as follows:

1. Oral
2. Rectal
3. Topical
4. Sublingual
5. Intranasal (IN)
6. Transdermal
7. Subcutaneous (SC)
8. Intramuscular (IM)
9. Inhalation (pulmonary)
10. Intravenous (IV)
11. Intraarterial (IA)
12. Intrathecal (within the spinal cord)
13. Intramedullary
14. Intraperitoneal

Oral

The oral route is the most common route of drug administration. It possesses advantages over parenteral routes of administration that make it quite useful in various situations involving the management of pain and anxiety. This route, however, has several significant disadvantages that must also be considered.

Advantages include an almost universal acceptance by patients, ease of administration, and relative safety. Patients today are accustomed to taking drugs by mouth, so it is quite rare to encounter an adult objecting to the oral route of administration. The younger child, however, may prove to be an unwilling recipient of orally administered drugs. Unwanted drug effects, such as overdosage, idiosyncrasy, allergy, and drug side effects, may occur whenever a drug is administered by any route, but such reactions are less likely to develop when a drug is administered orally; when they do occur, they are normally less intense than those reactions that develop following parenteral administration. This is not meant to imply that life-threatening situations do not arise following oral drug administration. Indeed, cardiac arrest and anaphylaxis after oral drug administration have been reported.[14,15]

TABLE 3-1 Comparison of Routes of Drug Administration

Route	Cooperation*	First-Pass Effect	Used for Sedation†	Children/ Adults	Titration	Maximum Sedation Level Recommended‡
Topical	2	–	0	na	–	na
Sublingual	2	–	1	–/+	–	1
Intranasal	1	–	2	+/?	–	1
Oral	2	+	1	+/+	–	1
Rectal	1	+	1	+/+	–	1
Transdermal	1	–	1	–/+	–	1
Subcutaneous	1	–	1	+/+	–	1
IM/SM	0	–	2	+/+	–	1
Inhalation	2	–	2	+/+	+	1
Intravenous	2	–	2	+/+	+	2
Intraarterial	2	–	0	na	–	na
Intrathecal (spinal)	2	–	0	na	+	na
Intramedullary	1	–	0	na	+	na
Intraperitoneal	0	–	0	na	–	na

*Key: Cooperation required, 2; cooperation not critical, 1; cooperation not necessary, 0.
†Strongly recommended, 2; somewhat recommended, 1; not recommended, 0.
‡Moderate to deep, 2; light to moderate, 1.
IM, Intramuscular; *na*, not applicable; *SM*, submucosal.

Disadvantages of oral drug administration include a long latent period, unreliable drug absorption, an inability to easily achieve a desired drug effect (titration), and a prolonged duration of action. These are significant disadvantages that serve to limit the clinical use of the oral route in the management of pain and anxiety.

Orally administered drugs must reach the stomach and small intestine, where most absorption into the circulatory system occurs. For most drugs the onset of clinical effectiveness is not noted for approximately 30 minutes, the latent period. Drug absorption continues, and a peak plasma concentration, equivalent to the greatest degree of clinical effectiveness (pain or anxiety relief), is reached. With most orally administered drugs, this maximal clinical effect develops approximately 60 minutes after administration. Because of this slow onset of action and the delay in reaching maximal effect, it is impossible to titrate via the oral route. *Titration is defined as the administration of small incremental doses of a drug until a desired clinical action is observed.* The ability to titrate gives the administrator control over the drug's actions and its ultimate effect. Titration eliminates the need to make an educated "guesstimate" of the appropriate dose of a drug for a patient. The lack of ability to titrate via the oral route of administration is a considerable handicap to the effective use of this technique when central nervous system (CNS) depressant drugs are administered. The clinician must administer a predetermined dose to the patient. This dose will be determined after consideration of a number of factors (discussed fully in Chapter 7). However, once the drug is administered, it becomes virtually impossible to quickly enhance its actions, should the initial dose prove inadequate, or to rapidly reverse its effects, should an undesirable reaction develop.

The duration of action of most orally administered pain- and anxiety-controlling drugs is prolonged, approximately 3 to 4 hours. This duration is unacceptable for most dental procedures (for sedative drugs especially) because the patient will remain under the influence of the drug well into the posttreatment period and therefore be unable to leave the doctor's office unescorted. Patients receiving CNS depressant drugs via the oral route must be advised against operating potentially dangerous machinery or driving a car (see drug package insert for all oral CNS depressants).

Orally administered drugs may be safely and effectively used for the management of pain in the postoperative period and for the management of anxiety in the preoperative period. Because of the significant disadvantages associated with it, the oral route of drug administration is not recommended for routine use in the management of intraoperative pain and anxiety. The oral route of drug administration is more fully discussed in Chapter 7.

Rectal

The rectal route of drug administration is only occasionally employed in dentistry. Its primary use is in pediatric dentistry, where it is more common to encounter patients who are either unwilling or unable to take drugs by mouth.[16,17]

Advantages and disadvantages of the rectal route are similar to those of the oral route of drug administration. Rectal drug administration is discussed more fully in Chapter 8.

The techniques of drug administration that follow are those in which the drug is absorbed directly from its site of administration into the systemic circulation, effectively bypassing the gastrointestinal (GI) tract. Such techniques are given the name *parenteral*, in contradistinction to the oral and rectal routes of administration, in which drugs are absorbed from the GI tract into the enterohepatic circulation before entry into the systemic circulation. These routes are termed *enteral* routes of administration. Common usage of the term *parenteral* usually denotes drug administration by injection with a syringe (e.g., IM, SC, IV). Intranasal and sublingual administration are properly termed parenteral because drug absorption occurs directly into the systemic circulation.

Topical

The absorption of drugs through intact skin is quite poor; however, topically applied local anesthetics can be used to produce anesthesia of tissues where a layer of keratinized skin is absent, such as the mucous membranes of the mouth, nose, throat, trachea, bronchi, esophagus, stomach, urethra, bladder, vagina, and rectum.[18] Topical anesthesia, as used in dentistry, is a highly effective method of relieving some of the fear and pain potentially involved in the administration of injectable local anesthetics.[19] Topical application of drugs other than local anesthetics is not common.

Sublingual

Certain drugs can be administered sublingually; that is, they can be absorbed into the blood through the mucous membranes of the oral cavity. Examples of the clinical use of sublingual drug administration include nitroglycerin for management of anginal pain,[20] aspirin in the prehospital management of suspected myocardial infarction victims,[21] and triazolam for conscious sedation in pediatric patients.[22]

An advantage of sublingual drug administration is that the drug enters directly into the systemic circulation, bypassing the enterohepatic circulation. In this way the drug does not undergo the hepatic first-pass effect in which a percentage of the drug is biotransformed before ever having the opportunity to enter the systemic circulation and to reach its target organ (e.g., brain).[23]

Intranasal

Intranasal (IN) drugs have been used primarily in pediatrics as a means of circumventing the need for injection or oral drug administration in unwilling patients.[24] Absorption of IN drugs occurs directly into the systemic circulation, bypassing the enterohepatic circulation. Clinical trials have demonstrated that the absorption and bioavailability of intranasally administered drugs were close to those of IV administration, with peak plasma levels occurring 10 minutes after administration.[25,26]

Midazolam, a water-soluble benzodiazepine,[24-27] and sufentanil,[27] an opioid analgesic, have received the most attention via the IN route.

Transdermal

The transdermal route is a means of administering a drug, bypassing the GI tract, without the need for injection.[28] The drugs most frequently administered by the transdermal route are scopolamine (primarily for the prevention of motion sickness and postsurgical nausea and vomiting),[29,30] nitroglycerin (for angina pectoris),[31] and nicotine (for smoking cessation).[32] Opioids, such as fentanyl, have also been employed via the transdermal route of administration for postsurgical analgesia.[33]

Transdermal drug administration is considered when a long-term course of drug therapy is necessary. Although rarely necessary in dentistry, there are situations (e.g., after surgery) in which transdermally administered analgesics might prove advantageous. Potential drawbacks to transdermal drug administration include the development of decreased responsiveness to the drug[34] and adverse skin reactions at the site of application.[35]

Subcutaneous

The subcutaneous (SC) route involves the injection of a drug beneath the skin into the subcutaneous tissues. It is useful for the administration of nonvolatile, water- or fat-soluble hypnotic and opioid drugs. Drugs capable of producing irritation, such as diazepam, should not be administered subcutaneously.

The rate of drug absorption into the cardiovascular system varies with the blood supply to the tissue. Subcutaneous tissues have a relatively limited blood supply, so absorption of drugs following subcutaneous administration is usually delayed.

This slow rate of absorption following SC injection limits the effectiveness of this route in dentistry. Other, more rapidly effective and controllable techniques are preferred and available.

Intramuscular

Intramuscular (IM) administration is a parenteral technique that maintains several advantages over enteral techniques, making it potentially useful in the management of pain and anxiety. However, the IM route pales in comparison to other parenteral methods of administration, especially the inhalation and IV routes. Of the four major techniques used in dentistry (oral, IM, inhalation, and IV), IM is the least commonly used.

Submucosal (SM) drug administration is similar to IM administration and is most often employed in pediatric dentistry. Its advantages and disadvantages are similar to those discussed for IM administration, except that the absorption of the drug is somewhat more rapid than that with the IM route.[36] Clinical consequences of this are significant, including a somewhat more rapid onset of drug. Because of this more rapid onset, it is also possible for undesirable drug actions to be noted more rapidly and to be somewhat more intense than those following IM administration. Problems associated with the SM technique are reviewed in Chapter 10.

Advantages of IM administration over enteral routes include a more rapid onset of action (shorter latent period) (approximately 10 minutes) and a more rapid onset of maximal clinical effect (approximately 30 minutes). Another advantage is the usually more reliable absorption of a drug into the cardiovascular system following IM than oral administration. In other words, 50 mg of a drug administered intramuscularly produces a more pronounced clinical effect than the same dose of drug given by mouth or rectally. Patient cooperation is not as essential as it is with most other techniques. This advantage is of particular importance in younger pediatric patients who are unwilling or unable to cooperate during drug administration. The child need be restrained only momentarily while the IM drug is administered.

Disadvantages of IM administration include its 10-minute latent period, a time factor that makes titration impossible. In addition, it is impossible to retrieve or to reverse the effect of the drug should overdose develop, patients may not be willing to accept the injection necessary to administer the drug, the prolonged duration of action (about 2 to 4 hours or more) requires that the patient be accompanied from the doctor's office by a responsible companion, and there is a possibility of injury to the tissues at the site of the injection caused by either the drug or the needle.

Several sites are available for IM injections. Whatever site is selected by the doctor, it is important to become familiar with the anatomy of that area before administering any medication via the IM route.

As with the oral route, the IM route has several significant disadvantages. The IM route is not commonly used in dental practice; however, there are many situations in which this route is valuable. The inability to titrate drugs makes it unwise to attempt to achieve deeper levels of conscious sedation or pain control with this route, unless the drug administrator is well trained in general anesthesia and maintains continual contact with the patient (i.e., does not send the patient home). In adult patients there are limited indications for the administration of pain- and anxiety-controlling drugs via the IM route because the IV route is more effective, reliable, and controllable. One indication is when a longer duration of drug action is desirable, as in postsurgical pain relief or when naloxone is employed following IV drug administration. In patients with disabilities and in recalcitrant children, however, techniques that require any degree of patient cooperation (oral, inhalation, IV) may prove impossible to use effectively, and the IM route may be the only means of conscious sedation available. General anesthesia may prove to be the only alternative treatment available to this patient. IM and SM administration of drugs for pain and anxiety control are discussed further in Chapter 10.

Inhalation (Pulmonary)

A variety of gaseous agents may be administered by inhalation to produce either conscious sedation or general anesthesia. In dental practice, however, the inhalation route is virtually synonymous with the use of N_2O and O_2. Nitrous oxide, the first general anesthetic, has been in clinical use since 1844 in both medicine and dentistry. It is estimated that more than 35% of dentists practicing in the United States use this agent as an aid in patient management.[37] In addition, 13 states (1993 data) have enacted legislation permitting dental hygienists to administer N_2O-O_2.[38]

The advantages and disadvantages discussed here relate to inhalation anesthetics in general and to the use of N_2O-O_2 in particular. The latent period observed in the inhalation route is usually short. Arguably, the inhalation route provides the most rapid onset of clinical action. After rapid passage through the mouth or nose, the trachea, and the lungs, the drug enters into the cardiovascular system. With some inhalation agents, such as N_2O, clinical effects may become noticeable as quickly as 15 to 30 seconds after inhalation. This extremely short latent period is used to advantage to permit titration of the drug to the patient. The ability to titrate is a major reason why N_2O-O_2 inhalation conscious sedation is considered by many to be the most ideal sedative technique currently available. In addition, the administrator of the gases also possesses the ability to reverse the actions of the drug rapidly, should this become necessary. Indeed, the inhalation route is the only one in which drug actions can be quickly adjusted to either increase or to decrease the depth of conscious sedation. With IV conscious sedation, drug action may easily be enhanced; however, it is not possible to lessen the level of conscious sedation unless a specific pharmacologic antagonist is available.

Recovery from inhalation conscious sedation is also quite rapid. In an outpatient medical or dental practice, rapid recovery is important because it permits the doctor to discharge most patients receiving N_2O-O_2 from the office unaccompanied by a responsible adult companion. Most patients may return to their work, drive a motor vehicle, or operate machinery without undue concern for their well-being.

A few disadvantages are associated with the use of the inhalation route. Nitrous oxide is not a very potent anesthetic, and when given with at least 20% O_2 (as it always should be), there will be a certain percentage of patients in whom this technique will fail to produce its desired actions. Patient cooperation is required for the successful use of inhalation conscious sedation, the lack of such cooperation being a significant disadvantage. This will most often be observed in the management of disruptive children and children and adults with disabilities. In the dental setting, patients must be capable of breathing through their noses. As used in the operating room setting, as a component of a general anesthetic, inhalation agents may be administered through both the mouth and nose; this is, of course, not possible in dentistry. Dental patients unable to breath comfortably through their nose will find the use of inhalation conscious sedation quite uncomfortable. Physicians and other health-care professionals employing N_2O-O_2 while treating patients at sites other than the oral cavity (e.g., leg, foot) will be able to use either the nose and/or mouth as a portal of entry for the gaseous agents, an advantage over their dental colleagues.

Two minor disadvantages of the inhalation route include the size and cost of the equipment and the additional training and expense required for the safe administration of N_2O-O_2. It is especially important that all health-care personnel employing inhalation conscious sedation be well trained in all aspects of its clinical application.

N_2O-O_2 inhalation conscious sedation is the technique of choice for most dental procedures and many minor surgical procedures that require intraoperative anxiety control. Pain, however, is not consistently controlled when N_2O-O_2 is employed, and its use as an analgesic, in lieu of local anesthesia, is not recommended primarily because of the high level of effectiveness and safety of local anesthetics and because of the increased incidence of unwanted side effects that may accompany the increased concentration of N_2O that is required to produce profound analgesia. Inhalation conscious sedation is described in depth in Section IV, Chapters 11 through 19.

Intravenous

The IV route of drug administration represents the most effective method of ensuring predictable and adequate conscious sedation in virtually all patients. Effective blood levels of drugs are achieved quite rapidly.

Advantages of IV drug administration include its short latent period of about 20 to 25 seconds (permitting drugs to be titrated) and the ability to rapidly enhance the action of a drug, if necessary. In clinical practice a drug used intravenously for conscious sedation will require approximately 2 to 8 minutes to reach its desired clinical effect. An additional advantage possessed by many intravenously administered drugs used for the management of anxiety is that they provide amnesic periods of varying duration. Dental or surgical procedures that are feared by the patient, such as the injection of local anesthetics, may be carried out during the amnesic period.

Disadvantages of intravenously administered drugs include an inability to reverse the actions of the drugs after they have been injected. Although it is possible to reverse the actions of some drugs (e.g., opioids, anticholinergics, and benzodiazepines) through the use of specific drug antagonists, this is not always the case. The rapid onset of action of intravenously injected drugs, as well as their accentuated clinical actions, lead to more exaggerated problems with overdosage, side effects, and allergic manifestations than are seen with other less effective modes of drug administration. The entire office staff must therefore be well trained in the use of these drugs, as well as in the recognition and management of associated adverse reactions and emergencies.

Patient cooperation is a requirement if venipuncture is to be successful. Many children do not permit venipuncture to be performed; therefore IV conscious sedation is rarely attempted in these disruptive patients. Conversely, a cooperative child, willing to permit a venipuncture, probably does not require as profound a technique as IV conscious sedation for his or her dental care. Intraoral injections of local anesthetics might possibly be carried out with a little more patience on the part of the doctor, and perhaps with another technique of conscious sedation, such as inhalation conscious sedation. However, patients with disabilities (both physical and mental) are usually good candidates for IV conscious sedation. These patients may be incapable of cooperation during dental therapy, but once sedated, they frequently become readily manageable.

IV conscious sedation may not be suitable for all dentists and physicians. Most doctors are uncomfortable with the technique during their early exposure to it; however, they gradually become more comfortable and relaxed as they gain clinical experience. A small percentage, however, remain uneasy with the technique and will be unable to provide dental or surgical care up to their usual standards. It is important to remember that regardless of the route of drug administration used, the quality of dental care delivered should not be compromised.

It is important to remember that regardless of the route of drug administration used, the quality of dental care delivered should not be compromised.

IV conscious sedation is not a panacea. Indeed, no technique of conscious sedation is a panacea. Although the IV route provides the most effective technique of conscious sedation currently available, an occasional patient will be encountered in whom IV drugs prove ineffective. A concern of many involved with the teaching of IV conscious sedation is that intravenously administered drugs will always prove to be effective if a large enough dose is administered. In many cases, however, this course of action will result in the loss of consciousness (general anesthesia, not conscious sedation), and unless the doctor and staff are well versed in managing the unconscious patient, grave complications may develop.

The IV route of administration is most often reserved for the management of the more fearful patient. Drugs and techniques are available that permit the effective management of fear for varying lengths of time. IV drug administration is occasionally used for patients in whom it is difficult to achieve adequate pain control following local anesthetic administration alone. Small doses of opioid analgesics administered intravenously in conjunction with intraoral local anesthesia may produce adequate pain control without increased risk to the patient. IV conscious sedation is discussed in detail in Section V, Chapters 20 through 29.

Thus far we have been able to manage successfully approximately 99% of our dental patients using one or more of the techniques discussed. In the remaining 1%, various factors, such as intense fear or biologic variability, act to produce management failures. General anesthesia is usually required for these patients.

We now approach a very important barrier in the spectrum of pain and anxiety control (see Figure 3-1). When we cross this barrier, we are dealing with the unconscious patient and with general anesthesia. The patient can no longer respond to command, and his or her protective reflexes are no longer operative.

GENERAL ANESTHESIA

The importance of general anesthesia in dentistry is illustrated by the fact that in excess of 5 million persons annually receive general anesthesia on an ambulatory basis in the United States, the overwhelming majority of these in outpatient dental settings (private practice, surgi-centers).[39] About 16% of all general anesthetics administered in the United States annually are administered in conjunction with dental care.[40]

General anesthesia was the first technique of pain and anxiety control introduced into the practice of medicine and dentistry. Though still used extensively in the practice of medicine (although the use of conscious sedation is growing rapidly), its use in dentistry has declined since the introduction of the techniques of conscious sedation. Several advantages to general anesthesia are a rapid onset of action, high effectiveness, and reliability. However, its disadvantages often outweigh its advantages. These include an increased risk to the patient and the requirement of an intensive training program in anesthesiology to prepare the doctor to manage the unconscious patient safely. Most general anesthetics employed in dentistry are used for oral surgery; however, there are many indications for their use in other procedures, such as restorations and hygiene, especially in the disruptive child or in the patient with a disability.[41]

The step from management of the conscious patient (conscious sedation) to management of the unconscious patient (general anesthesia) is a big one, requiring an absolute minimum of 2 full years of training in the principles and techniques of general anesthesia.[42] General anesthesia is further discussed in Section VI, Chapters 30 and 31.

REFERENCES

1. American Dental Association, Council on Dental Education: Guidelines for teaching the comprehensive control of pain and anxiety in dentistry, *J Dent Educ* 36:62, 1972.
2. American Dental Association: *Continuing education directory*, Chicago, 1993, The Association.
3. American Dental Association, Council on Dental Education: *Guidelines for teaching the comprehensive control of pain and anxiety in dentistry, Part III*, Chicago, 1993, The Association.
4. Bernal-Sprekelsen M, Schmelzer A: Local anesthesia of the head and neck, *Anesth Pain Control* 1:81, 1992.
5. Davis JE: Ambulatory surgery . . . how far can we go? *Med Clin North Am* 77:365, 1993.
6. Friedman N: Iatro sedation. In McCarthy FM, ed: *Emergencies in dental practice*, ed 3, Philadelphia, 1979, WB Saunders.
7. Milgrom P: Treatment of the distrustful patient. In Milgrom P, Weinstein B, Kleinknecht R et al, eds: *Treating fearful dental patients*, Reston, Va, 1985, Reston Publishing.
8. Shapiro RS, Simpson DE, Lawrence SL et al: A survey of sued and nonsued physicians and suing patients, *Arch Intern Med* 149:2190, 1989.
9. Santamaria LB: Non-pharmacologic techniques for treatment of post-operative pain, *Minerva Anestesiol* 56:359, 1990.
10. Mayer R: Dental treatment measurements in children using audioanalgesia, *Zahnarztliche Mitteilungen* 81:1370, 1991.
11. Friis-Hasche E, Hutchings B: Psychology of phobias in relation to dental anxiety, *Tandlaegebladet* 94:42, 1990.
12. Status report: transcutaneous electrical nerve stimulation (TENS) units in pain control, Council on Dental Materials, Instruments, and Equipment, *JADA* 116:540, 1988.
13. Malamed SF: A most powerful drug, *J Calif Acad Gen Dent* 4:17, 1979.
14. Safranek DJ, Eisenberg MS, Larsen MP: The epidemiology of cardiac arrest in young adults, *Ann Emerg Med* 21:1102, 1992.
15. Gill CJ, Michaelides PL: Dental drugs and anaphylactic reactions: report of a case, *Oral Surg* 50:30, 1980.
16. Flaitz CM, Nowak AJ, Hicks MJ: Evaluation of anterograde amnesic effect of rectally administered diazepam in the sedated pedodontic patient, *J Dent Child* 53:17, 1986.
17. Mattila MA, Ruoppi MK, Ahlstron-Bengg E et al: Diazepam in rectal solution as premedication in children, with special reference to serum concentrations, *Br J Anaesth* 53:1269, 1981.
18. Norris RL Jr: Local anesthetics, *Emerg Med Clin North Am* 10:707, 1992.
19. Daublaender M, Roth W, Kleeman PP: Clinical investigation of potency and onset of different lidocaine sprays for topical anaesthesia in dentistry, *Anesth Pain Control Dent* 1:25, 1992.
20. Diker E, Ertuerk A, Akguen G: Is sublingual nifedipine administration superior to oral administration in the active treatment of hypertension? *Angiology* 43:477, 1992.
21. American Heart Association Science Advisory and Coordinating Committee: *Aspirin as a therapeutic agent in cardiovascular disease*, Dallas, 1997, American Heart Association
22. Garzone PD, Kroboth PD: Pharmacokinetics of the newer benzodiazepines, *Clin Pharmacokinet* 16:337, 1989.

23. Motwani JG, Lipworth BJ: Clinical pharmacokinetics of drug administered buccally and sublingually, *Clin Pharmacokinet* 21:83, 1991.
24. Saint-Maurice C, Landais A, Delleur MM et al: The use of midazolam in diagnostic and short surgical procedures in children, *Acta Anaesthesiol Scand Suppl* 92:39, 1990.
25. Rey E, Delaunay L, Pons G et al: Pharmacokinetics of midazolam in children: comparative study of intranasal and intravenous administration, *Eur J Clin Pharmacol* 41:355, 1991.
26. Walbergh EJ, Wills RJ, Eckhert J: Plasma concentrations of midazolam in children following intranasal administration, *Anesthesiology* 74:233, 1991.
27. Karl HW, Keifer AT, Rosenberger JL et al: Comparison of the safety and efficacy of intranasal midazolam and sufentanil for preinduction of anesthesia in pediatric patients, *Anesthesiology* 76:209, 1992.
28. Asmussen B: Transdermal therapeutic systems: actual state and future developments, *Methods Find Exp Clin Pharmacol* 13:343, 1991.
29. Scopoderm: transdermal hyoscine for motion sickness, *Drug Ther Bull* 27:91, 1989.
30. Santamaria LB, Fodale V, Mandolfino T et al: Transdermal scopolamine reduces nausea, vomiting and sialorrhea in the postoperative period in teeth and mouth surgery, *Minerva Anesthesiol* 57:686, 1991.
31. Todd PA, Goa KL, Langtry HD: Transdermal nitroglycerin (glyceryl trinitrate): a review of its pharmacology and therapeutic use, *Drugs* 40:880, 1990.
32. McKenna JP, Cox JL: Transdermal nicotine replacement and smoking cessation, *Am Fam Physician* 45:2595, 1992.
33. Calis KA, Kohler DR, Corso DM: Transdermally administered fentanyl for pain management, *Clin Pharm* 11:22, 1992.
34. Parker JO: Nitrate tolerance: a problem during continuous nitrate administration, *Eur J Clin Pharmacol* 38(suppl 1):21, 1990.
35. Hogan DJ, Maibach HI: Adverse dermatologic reactions to transdermal drug delivery systems, *J Am Acad Dermatol* 22(pt 1):811, 1990.
36. Roberts SM, Wilson CF, Seale NS et al: Evolution of morphine as compared to meperidine when administered to moderately anxious pediatric dental patients, *Pediatr Dent* 14:306, 1992.
37. Jastak JT, Donaldson D: Nitrous oxide, *Anesth Prog* 38:172, 1991.
38. Department of Educational Surveys: *Legal provisions for delegating functions to dental assistants and dental hygienists,* Chicago, 1993, American Dental Association.
39. Rosenberg M, Weaver J: General anesthesia, *Anesth Prog* 38:172, 1991.
40. Craig DC, Ponte J: General anaesthesia for dental surgery, *Dent Update* 111:37, 1988.
41. Cichon P, Bader J: Dental care of the handicapped in intubation anesthesia: the outpatient dental care of handicapped patients in intubation anesthesia at a rehabilitation center, *Schweiz Monatsschr Zahnmed* 100:741, 1990.
42. American Dental Association, Council on Dental Education: *Guidelines for teaching the comprehensive control of pain and anxiety in dentistry, Part II,* Chicago, 1992, The Association.

CHAPTER 4

Physical and Psychological Evaluation

CHAPTER OUTLINE

Before a new patient is treated, it is important that the doctor and staff become aware of the patient's medical history. This is true in all situations, regardless of whether or not the patient is to receive drugs for pain or anxiety control. Because dental care can have a profound effect on both the physical and psychological well-being of the patient, it is extremely important for the person treating the patient to know beforehand the most likely problems to be encountered. It has been stated that "when you prepare for an emergency, the emergency ceases to exist."[1] Prior knowledge of a patient's physical status enables the doctor to modify the proposed treatment plan to better meet the patient's limit of tolerance. This is of special importance whenever the administration of a drug for the management of pain or anxiety is planned. The administration of certain drugs used in dentistry is specifically contraindicated in patients with some disease states. Knowledge of these contraindications is critical if potentially serious complications are to be avoided.

GOALS OF PHYSICAL AND PSYCHOLOGICAL EVALUATION

In the following discussion a comprehensive but easy-to-use program of physical evaluation is described.[2] Used as recommended it allows the doctor to assess accurately any potential risk presented by the patient before the start of treatment. The following are the goals that are sought in the use of this system:

1. To determine the patient's ability to tolerate physically the stresses involved in the planned dental treatment
2. To determine the patient's ability to tolerate psychologically the stresses involved in the planned dental treatment

3. To determine whether treatment modifications are indicated to enable the patient to better tolerate the stresses of dental treatment
4. To determine whether the use of psychosedation is indicated
5. To determine which technique of sedation is most appropriate for the patient
6. To determine whether contraindications exist to any of the drugs to be given

The first two goals involve the patient's ability to tolerate the stress involved in the planned dental care. Stress may be of either a physiologic or psychological nature. Patients with underlying medical problems are usually less able to tolerate the usual levels of stress associated with various types of dental care. These patients are more likely to experience an acute exacerbation of their medical problem(s) during periods of increased stress. Such disease processes include angina pectoris, seizure disorders, asthma, and sickle cell disease. Although most of these patients will be able to tolerate the planned dental care in relative safety, it is the obligation of the doctor and staff to determine, first, whether this problem does exist, and second, the severity of the problem.

Excessive stress can also prove detrimental to the nonmedically compromised (e.g., "healthy") patient. Fear, anxiety, and pain produce acute changes in the homeostasis of the body that may prove detrimental. Many "healthy" patients suffer from fear-related emergencies, including hyperventilation and vasodepressor syncope (fainting).

The third goal is to determine whether or not to modify the usual treatment regimen for a patient in order to enable the patient to better tolerate the stress of treatment. In some cases a healthy patient will be psychologically unable to tolerate the planned treatment. Treatment may be modified to minimize the stress faced by this patient. The medically compromised patient will also benefit from treatment modification aimed at minimizing stress. The stress-reduction protocols that are discussed in this chapter are designed to aid the doctor in minimizing treatment-related stress in both the healthy and medically compromised patient.

When it is believed that the patient will require some assistance in coping with his or her dental treatment, the use of psychosedation should be considered. The last three goals involve the determination of the need for use of psychosedation, selection of the most appropriate technique, and selection of the most appropriate drug(s) for patient management.

PHYSICAL EVALUATION

The term *physical evaluation* is used to discuss the steps involved in fulfilling the mentioned goals. Physical evaluation in dentistry consists of the following three components:

1. Medical history questionnaire
2. Physical examination
3. Dialogue history

With the information (database) collected from these three steps, the doctor will be better able to (1) determine the physical and psychological status of the patient (establish a risk factor classification for the patient); (2) seek medical consultation, if indicated; and (3) appropriately modify the planned dental treatment, if indicated. Each of the three steps in the evaluation process are discussed in general terms, with specific emphasis placed on their importance in the evaluation of the patient for whom the use of pharmacosedation is being considered.

Medical History Questionnaire

The use of a written, patient-completed medical history questionnaire is a moral and legal necessity in the practice of both medicine and dentistry. These questionnaires provide the doctor with valuable information about the physical, and in some cases the psychological, condition of the prospective patient.

Many types of medical history questionnaire are available; however, most are simply modifications of two basic types: the "short" form and the "long" form. The *short form* medical history questionnaire provides basic information concerning a patient's medical history and is best suited for use by a doctor with considerable clinical experience in physical evaluation. When using the short-form history, the doctor must have a firm grasp of the appropriate dialogue history required to aid in a determination of the relative risk presented by the patient. The doctor should also be experienced in the use of the techniques of physical evaluation and their interpretation. Unfortunately, most doctors use the short form or a modification of it in their office primarily for convenience to the patient and themselves. The *long form*, on the other hand, provides a more detailed database concerning the physical condition of the prospective patient. It is used most often in teaching situations and represents a more ideal instrument for teaching physical evaluation.

In recent years computer-generated medical history questionnaires have been developed.[3] These questionnaires permit patients to enter their responses to questions electronically on the computer. Whenever a positive response is given, the computer brings up additional questions related to the positive response. In essence the computer asks the questions called for in the dialogue history.

Either form of medical history questionnaire may be used to accurately determine the physical status of the patient. Either form of medical history questionnaire can also prove to be entirely worthless. The ultimate value of a medical history questionnaire rests on the ability of the doctor to interpret its meaning and then to elicit additional information through physical examination and dialogue history. The medical history questionnaire used at the University of Southern California (USC) School of Dentistry (Figure 4-1) has combined the best of both short and long forms.[4]

MEDICAL HISTORY

CIRCLE

1. Are you having pain or discomfort at this time? . . . . . YES NO
2. Do you feel very nervous about having dental treatments? . . . . . YES NO
3. Have you ever had a bad experience in the dental office? . . . . . YES NO
4. Have you been a patient in the hospital during the past two years? . . . . . YES NO
5. Have you been under the care of a medical doctor during the past two years? . . . . . YES NO
6. Have you taken any medicine or drugs during the past two years? . . . . . YES NO
7. Are you allergic to (i.e., itching, rash, swelling of hands, feet or eyes) or made sick by penicillin, aspirin, codeine, or any drugs or medications? . . . . . YES NO
8. Have you ever had any excessive bleeding requiring special treatment? . . . . . YES NO
9. Circle any of the following which you have had or have at present:

Heart Failure	Emphysema	AIDS
Heart Disease or Attack	Cough	Hepatitis A (infectious)
Angina Pectoris	Tuberculosis (TB)	Hepatitis B (serum)
High Blood Pressure	Asthma	Liver Disease
Heart Murmur	Hay Fever	Yellow Jaundice
Rheumatic Fever	Sinus Trouble	Blood Transfusion
Congenital Heart Lesions	Allergies or Hives	Drug Addiction
Scarlet Fever	Diabetes	Hemophilia
Artificial Heart Valve	Thyroid Disease	Venereal Disease (Syphilis, Gonorrhea)
Heart Pacemaker	X-ray or Cobalt Treatment	Cold Sores
Heart Surgery	Chemotherapy (Cancer, Leukemia)	Genital Herpes
Artificial Joints	Arthritis	Epilepsy or Seizures
Anemia	Rheumatism	Fainting or Dizzy Spells
Stroke	Cortisone Medicine	Nervousness
Kidney Trouble	Glaucoma	Psychiatric Treatment
Ulcers	Pain in Jaw Joints	Sickle Cell Disease
		Bruise Easily

10. When you walk up stairs or take a walk, do you ever have to stop because of pain in your chest, or shortness of breath, or because you are very tired? . . . . . YES NO
11. Do your ankles swell during the day? . . . . . YES NO
12. Do you use more than 2 pillows to sleep? . . . . . YES NO
13. Have you lost or gained more than 10 pounds in the past year? . . . . . YES NO
14. Do you ever wake up from sleep short of breath? . . . . . YES NO
15. Are you on a special diet? . . . . . YES NO
16. Has your medical doctor ever said you have a cancer or tumor? . . . . . YES NO
17. Do you have any disease, condition, or problem not listed? . . . . . YES NO
18. WOMEN: Are you pregnant now? . . . . . YES NO
    Are you practicing birth control? . . . . . YES NO
    Do you anticipate becoming pregnant? . . . . . YES NO

To the best of my knowledge, all of the preceding answers are true and correct. If I ever have any change in my health, or if my medicines change, I will inform the doctor of dentistry at the next appointment without fail.

Date *Faculty Signature* *Signature of Patient, Parent or Guardian*

MEDICAL HISTORY / PHYSICAL EVALUATION UPDATE

Date *Addition* *Student / Faculty Signatures*

Figure 4-1 University of Southern California medical history questionnaire. Room is provided on the bottom of the form for the periodic updates of the patient's medical condition.

Although both forms of medical history questionnaire are valuable in the determination of a patient's physical risk during treatment, a decided failing of most available health history questionnaires is the absence of questions relating to the patient's mental attitude toward dentistry. It is recommended therefore that one or more questions be added to the questionnaire relating to this all-important subject. The following questions are included in the USC School of Dentistry adult health history questionnaire:

1. Have you ever had a bad experience in a dental office?
2. Do you feel very nervous about having dental treatment?

It has been my experience that many adult patients are reluctant to express their fears about the proposed treatment to the doctor, hygienist, or assistant for fear of being labeled a "baby." This is especially true of young men, usually younger than 35 years of age. These persons, rather than expressing their fears, will attempt to "take it like a man" or "grin and bear it." Unfortunately, all too often the outcome of such "macho" behavior is an episode of syncope. In situations in which an open admission of their fears before treatment is usually nonexistent, my experience has been that these same patients will volunteer this information in writing if questions are included in the medical history questionnaire. Other means of identifying dental fear and anxiety are discussed later in this chapter.

The USC questionnaire is reviewed here, providing the basic significance of each of the questions as well as their relevance to the possible use of sedation. More detailed discussion of the use of the various techniques of sedation in the presence of specific medical problems is presented in Chapters 37 and 38.

Question 1. Are you having pain or discomfort at this time?

COMMENT: The primary thrust of this question is related to dentistry. The question is asked to determine what it was that actually brought the patient to seek dental care at this time. Should pain or discomfort be present, it may be necessary for the doctor to treat the patient at this first visit; in a more normal (nonemergent) situation, treatment would not begin until subsequent visits.

Question 2. Do you feel very nervous about having dentistry treatment?

Question 3. Have you ever had a bad experience in the dentistry office?

COMMENT: Inclusion of questions relating to a patient's attitude toward dentistry is a significant addition to the medical history questionnaire. Most questionnaires, unfortunately, ignore questioning along this important line. It has been my experience that many adult patients, who would never verbally admit to being fearful, willingly indicate their fears or prior negative experiences on the written questionnaire. In-depth dialogue history must seek to determine the reasons for these positive responses.

Question 4. Have you been a patient in the hospital during the past 2 years?

COMMENT: Knowledge of the reason(s) for hospitalization of the patient greatly helps the doctor to evaluate the patient's ability to safely tolerate the stresses involved in dental treatment.

Question 5. Have you been under the care of a medical doctor during the past 2 years?

COMMENT: As with the previous question, knowledge of any medical problems for which the patient required medical intervention can greatly increase the doctor's ability to evaluate the patient more fully before the start of treatment.

Question 6. Have you taken any medicine or drugs during the past 2 years?

COMMENT: Awareness of any drugs or medications taken by a patient for the control or treatment of a medical disorder is vitally important. It is not uncommon for patients to take medications but be unaware of the medical problem for which it has been prescribed. In addition, many (most) patients do not even know the name of the medication they are taking. For these two reasons, it is essential that the doctor have available one or more means of identifying these medications, which patients may have with them. Several sources are available, including the *Physician's Desk Reference (PDR); Facts and Comparisons; Mosby's Dental Drug Reference*, sixth edition (Gage, 2002)[5]; *Clinical Management of Prescription Drugs* (Long, 1984); and *Mosby's 2002 Nursing Drug Reference* (Skidmore-Roth).[6] The *PDR*, although primarily a compilation of drug package inserts, is a valuable resource, containing a picture section that allows the identification of a drug should the patient not be aware of its name. Online drug reference programs, such as *ePocrates* (www.ePocrates.com) and *Medscape* (www.medscape.com), provide frequently updated information for use on personal data assistants (PDAs).

Knowledge of the drugs and medications being taken by a patient is essential because (1) it permits identification of the medical disorder being treated; (2) there are potential side effects to most drugs, some of which may be of significance in dentistry (e.g., postural hypotension); and (3) drug-drug interactions can develop between a patient's medication and drugs administered during dental treatment. Table 4-1 lists drug-drug interactions involving sedative and anesthetic drugs that are used in dentistry.

Question 7. Are you allergic to (i.e., itching, rash, or swelling of hands, feet, or eyes) or made sick by penicillin, aspirin, codeine, or any drugs or medications?

COMMENT: Question 7 seeks to determine whether the patient has experienced any adverse drug reactions (ADRs). ADRs are not uncommon; the most frequently reported reactions being labeled "allergy." However, true allergic drug reactions are relatively uncommon despite their great frequency in reporting. The doctor must evaluate all ADRs quite thoroughly, especially in those situations in which

TABLE 4-1 Drug-Drug Interactions Involving Sedative/Anesthetic Drugs

Drug	Interacting Agent	Resulting Action
Anesthetics, general	Antidepressants	Hypotension
	Antihypertensives	Hypotension
Barbiturates	Alcohol	Enhanced sedation: ↑ respiratory depression
	Anticoagulants, oral	↓ Anticoagulant effect
	Antidepressants	↓ Antidepressant effect
	β-Adrenergic blockers	↓ β-Blocker effect
	Corticosteroids	↓ Steroid effect
	Digitalis	↓ Digitalis effect
	Doxycycline	↓ Doxycycline effect
	Griseofulvin	↓ Griseofulvin effect
	Phenothiazines	↓ Phenothiazine effect
	Quinidine	↓ Quinidine effect
	Rifampin	↓ Barbiturate effect
	Valproic acid	↓ Phenobarbital effect
Benzodiazepines	Alcohol	Enhanced sedation
	Barbiturates	Enhanced sedation; ↑ respiratory depression
Meperidine	Barbiturates	↑ Central nervous system depression
	Curariform drugs	↑ Respiratory depression
	Monoamine oxidase inhibitors (MAOIs)	Hypertension
Phenothiazines	Alcohol	↑ Sedation
	Guanethidine	↓ Phenothiazine effect
	Levodopa	↓ Levodopa effect
	Lithium	↓ Phenothiazine effect
Sympathomimetic amines (epinephrine)	Antidepressants	↑ Sedation
	Antihypertensives	↓ Phenothiazine effect
	β-Adrenergic blockers	↓ Levodopa effect
	Halogenated anesthetics	↓ Phenothiazine effect
	Digitalis drugs	Hypertension, hypertensive crisis
	Indomethacin	↓ Antihypertensive effect
	MAOIs	Hypertension with epinephrine
		Cardiac dysrhythmias with epinephrine
		↑ Cardiac dysrhythmias
		Severe hypertension
		Hypertensive crisis

Modified from Council on Dental Therapeutics: *JADA* 107:885, 1983.

closely related drugs are to be administered to or prescribed for the patient. Evaluation of alleged allergy and other ADRs is discussed in Chapter 34.

QUESTION 8. **Have you ever had any excessive bleeding requiring special treatment?**

COMMENT: Bleeding disorders, such as hemophilia, can lead to modification in certain forms of dental treatment (e.g., surgery, local anesthetic administration, venipuncture) and must therefore be made known to the doctor before the start of treatment.

QUESTION 9. **Circle any of the following that you have had or have at the present time:**

COMMENT: This question presents a list of the more common illnesses and disorders afflicting the adult population in the United States.

Heart Failure

COMMENT: The severity of heart failure must be determined through the dialogue history. If more serious congestive heart failure (CHF) is present (e.g., dyspnea at rest), the patient will require strict modification of the planned dental treatment, with the possible administration of supplemental oxygen during treatment. Conscious sedation is not contraindicated but should be restricted (if possible) to a "light" level in patients with more severe heart failure (ASA III or IV).

Heart Disease or Attack

COMMENT: Heart attack is the lay term for myocardial infarction. Knowledge of the severity, residual damage, and time elapsed since its occurrence is essential, because treatment modification may be warranted for this patient. Stress reduction is usually indicated.

Angina Pectoris

COMMENT: A history of angina usually indicates the presence of a significant degree of coronary artery atherosclerosis. The risk factor for the typical anginal patient is an ASA III. Stress reduction is strongly recommended in these patients.

High Blood Pressure

COMMENT: Elevated baseline or preoperative blood pressure measurements are occasionally obtained in the dental or surgical environment primarily because of the added stresses associated with dental treatment or surgery. Whenever patients report a history of high blood pressure, the doctor should determine the antihypertensive drug(s) they are taking as well as their side effects and potential drug interactions. Postural (orthostatic) hypotension is a side effect of many antihypertensive drugs. Guidelines for clinical evaluation of risk based on blood pressure determinations are presented later in this chapter (see Table 4-4). The use of stress-reduction techniques is strongly recommended in patients with a history of high blood pressure.

Heart Murmur

COMMENT: Heart murmurs are not uncommon; however, not all murmurs are clinically significant. The doctor should seek to determine whether a murmur is functional (nonpathologic), whether clinical signs and symptoms of either valvular stenosis or regurgitation is present, and whether antibiotic prophylaxis is warranted. The major clinical symptom associated with a significant murmur is undue fatigue. Current regimens for antibiotic prophylaxis are presented in Table 4-2. Sedation may be employed with these patients as deemed necessary.

Rheumatic Fever

COMMENT: A history of rheumatic fever should lead the doctor to an in-depth dialogue history seeking the presence of

TABLE 4-2 American Heart Association Guidelines for Antibiotic Prophylaxis for Bacterial Endocarditis: Prophylactic Regimens for Dental, Oral, Respiratory Tract, or Esophageal Procedures

Situation	Agent	Regimen*
Standard general prophylaxis	Amoxicillin	Adults: 2.0 g Children: 50 mg/kg orally 1 hr before procedure
Unable to take oral medications	Ampicillin	Adults: 2.0 g intramuscularly (IM) or intravenously (IV) Children: 50 mg/kg IM or IV within 30 min before procedure
Allergic to penicillin	Clindamycin	Adults: 600 mg Children: 20 mg/kg orally 1 hr before procedure
	OR Cephalexin† or cefadroxil†	Adults: 2.0 g Children: 50 mg/kg orally 1 hr before procedure
	OR Azithromycin or clarithromycin	Adults: 500 mg Children: 15 mg/kg orally 1 hr before procedure
Allergic to penicillin and unable to take oral medications	Clindamycin	Adults: 600 mg Children: 20 mg/kg IV within 30 min before procedure
	OR Cefazolin†	Adults: 1.0 g Children: 25 mg/kg IM or IV within 30 min before procedure

*Total children's dose should not exceed adult dose.

†Cephalosporins should not be used in individuals with immediate-type hypersensitivity reaction (urticaria, angioedema, or anaphylaxis) to penicillins.

rheumatic heart disease (RHD). If RHD is present, antibiotic prophylaxis is indicated to minimize the risk of subacute bacterial endocarditis (SBE). Additional treatment modification may be desirable to further minimize risk to the patient, depending on the degree of cardiac involvement. The use of the stress-reduction protocols, including sedation, may be necessary in these patients.

Congenital Heart Lesions

Comment: An in-depth dialogue history is called for to determine the nature of the lesion and, of greater significance, the degree of disability (if any) associated with it. Medical consultation may be required, especially if the patient is a child and/or if the defect is uncorrected. Prophylactic antibiotics may be required before treatment. The use of stress-reduction protocols, including sedation, may be necessary in these patients.

Scarlet Fever

Comment: Produced by group A β-hemolytic streptococci, scarlet fever rarely produces cardiovascular sequela such as valvular damage. However, dialogue history should seek to determine the presence of any cardiovascular damage secondary to scarlet fever. The use of the stress-reduction protocols, including sedation, may be necessary in these patients.

Artificial Heart Valve

Comment: With thousands of artificial valves being placed annually in the United States,[7] it is not uncommon to be called upon to provide dental care for these patients. The primary concern of the doctor is to determine which antibiotic regimen for prophylaxis is appropriate for the patient's dental treatment. Medical consultation before the start of therapy is usually recommended in these patients. The use of stress-reduction protocols, including sedation, may be necessary in these patients.

Heart Pacemaker or Implanted Defibrillator

Comment: Pacemakers are implanted beneath the skin of the upper chest or the abdomen, with pacing wires extending into the myocardium. The most frequent indication for the use of a pacemaker is the presence of a clinically significant dysrhythmia. Fixed-rate pacemakers provide the heart with a regular, continuous rate of firing regardless of the inherent rhythm of the heart, whereas the more commonly used demand pacemaker remains inactive while the rhythm of the heart is normal but takes over pacing when the inherent rhythm of the heart becomes abnormal. Although there is little indication for the administration of antibiotics in these patients, medical consultation is recommended before the start of the initial treatment to obtain the recommendations of the patient's physician. The effect of stress on the patient's cardiac rhythm should be ascertained during this consultation, as well as a discussion of the possible use of sedation, if needed, during the patient's dental care.

A growing number of patients have implanted defibrillators, devices that sense the onset of a fatal dysrhythmia (ventricular tachycardia, ventricular fibrillation) and deliver a shock to the myocardium in an attempt to convert the rhythm to one that is more functional.[8] Similar to the pacemaker, the implanted defibrillator is external to the heart and therefore does not require antibiotic prophylaxis. Medical consultation with this patient's primary care physician or cardiologist is recommended before the start of dental care.

Heart Surgery

Comment: This very general term may include any procedure from the placement of a pacemaker to valve replacement to coronary artery bypass surgery to heart transplant. A "yes" response to this question should elicit a vigorous dialogue history. Medical consultation should be considered if there is any uncertainty remaining about the patient's physical condition or about the requirement for sedation during dental care.

Artificial Joint

Comment: The replacement of hips, knees, and elbows with prosthetic devices has become quite common. It is uncertain, however, whether the bacteremia produced during many dental procedures significantly increases the risk of joint infection. For this reason, it is recommended that consultation with the patient's surgeon be obtained prior to the start of any dental procedure. There are no contraindications specifically related to the artificial joint to the use of sedation in these patients.

Anemia

Comment: Determine the nature of the anemia. *Iron deficiency anemia* is relatively common in the adult population, especially among younger women. The concern with anemic patients is the decreased ability of their blood to carry oxygen. This may be of special significance during procedures in which hypoxia is more likely to develop. Although this should never occur during dental care, the use of deeper levels of intramuscular (IM) or intravenous (IV) conscious sedation, without supplemental oxygen administration, is more likely to produce hypoxia, which would be of greater clinical consequence in anemic patients.

Sickle Cell Anemia (see Sickle Cell Disease later in this chapter)

Comment: Sickle cell anemia will be seen in some black patients. A differentiation between sickle cell disease and sickle cell trait must be made. Avoidance of hypoxia is of great importance in these patients.

Methemoglobinemia

Comment: Methemoglobinemia can develop when patients receive large doses of certain drugs, such as the local anesthetic prilocaine.[9,10] Other drugs, including analgesics such as acetanilid and acetaminophen, can produce elevated blood levels of methemoglobin. Patients with congenital methemoglobinemia should not be given any drugs that can further elevate methemoglobin blood levels.

Sedation can be employed in patients with any of these forms of anemia, but the avoidance of hypoxia should be a cardinal concern throughout the procedure.

Stroke

COMMENT: Stroke, or cerebrovascular accident (CVA) or "brain attack," must be evaluated carefully, for patients with a history of CVA (status post-CVA) are also at greater risk when exposed to hypoxic levels of oxygen. When sedation is necessary, only lighter levels, such as those provided by inhalation sedation, are recommended. Transient cerebral ischemia (TCI) (see Fainting or Dizzy Spells) is a prodromal syndrome of CVA and must be evaluated carefully. Medical consultation for both CVA and TIA is suggested.

Kidney Trouble

COMMENT: The nature of the kidney problem should be determined. Treatment modifications, including antibiotic prophylaxis, may be in order for several chronic forms of kidney disease. The use of central nervous system (CNS) depressants and local anesthetics in patients with renal disease is discussed in Chapter 37.

Ulcers

COMMENT: Stomach (peptic) or intestinal (duodenal) ulcers may indicate the presence of acute or chronic anxiety and the patient's possible use of medications such as tranquilizers, H_1 antagonists, and antacids. Knowledge of which drugs are being taken is important before additional drugs are administered during treatment. Sedation may be required for the management of a more fearful patient.

Emphysema

COMMENT: Emphysema is a form of chronic obstructive pulmonary disease (COPD). The emphysematous patient has a decreased respiratory reserve to draw on in the event that the cells of the body require additional oxygen. Oxygen therapy during dental treatment is strongly recommended in patients with more severe emphysema. Only lighter levels of sedation should be used.

Cough

COMMENT: The presence of a chronic cough may be indicative of active tuberculosis or other chronic respiratory disorders, including chronic bronchitis. The administration of CNS depressants, especially those with greater respiratory depressant properties (e.g., barbiturates, opioids) must be evaluated carefully in patients with diminished respiratory reserve.

Tuberculosis

COMMENT: The status of the disease (active or arrested) should be determined before the start of dental treatment. Medical consultation is recommended if doubt persists, with possible modification of dental therapy. Inhalation sedation is not recommended for use in patients with active tuberculosis because of the likelihood of contamination of the rubber goods (mask, tubing, reservoir bag) and the difficulty in sterilizing them. If the doctor treats many patients with tuberculosis, disposable rubber goods for inhalation sedation units are available. Patients can be issued their own set of rubber goods for inhalation sedation.

Asthma

COMMENT: Asthma represents a partial obstruction of the lower airway. The doctor must determine the nature of the asthma (allergic vs. nonallergic), its frequency of occurrence, the causative factors in its onset (e.g., stress), how the patient manages an acute episode, any drugs that the patient may be taking on a regular basis to minimize the risk of an acute episode developing, drugs being used to terminate an acute episode of bronchospasm, and whether hospitalization has been necessary for the patient's asthma.

Sedation is not contraindicated in asthmatic patients. However, certain drugs, such as barbiturates and opioids (especially meperidine), should be avoided, if possible, because their use in asthmatic patients is associated with a greater occurrence of acute bronchospasm. The use of inhalation anesthetics that irritate the respiratory mucosa is contraindicated in these patients. Nitrous oxide–oxygen *is* indicated.

Hayfever

COMMENT: Hayfever indicates the presence of allergy to a foreign protein material (e.g., pollen, cat dander, dust, dirt). Dental treatment with sedation should be avoided, if possible, during periods in which acute exacerbations are more frequent.

Sinus Trouble

COMMENT: Sinus trouble may indicate the presence of allergy (to be pursued via dialogue history) or of an upper respiratory infection (e.g., common cold). Although sedation is not contraindicated, supplemental oxygen administration may be desirable throughout the procedure. Inhalation sedation may be ineffective if the patient has difficulty breathing through his or her nose.

Allergies or Hives

COMMENT: Allergy must be thoroughly evaluated before the start of any dental care and drug administration.

Diabetes

COMMENT: A positive response requires further inquiry to determine the type of diabetes (type 1 [IDDM] or type 2 [NIDDM]), its severity, and the level of control of the diabetes. The patient with diabetes does not usually represent a significant risk during dental therapy or during the administration of drugs for the management of pain or anxiety. The greatest concern relating to the management of this patient relates to the possible effect of dental care on the patient's posttreatment eating habits. Dosages of insulin may require modification (following consultation with the patient's primary care physician) in situations in which the patient cannot maintain a normal food intake.

Thyroid Disease

COMMENT: The presence of clinically evident hyperthyroidism or hypothyroidism should lead the doctor to be more cautious in the administration of certain drug groups (vasopressors [hyperthyroid], CNS depressants [hypothyroid]) to these patients. On most occasions, however, the patient will state that he or she has been hyperthyroid or hypothyroid at one time, but at present, because of either surgical intervention, radiation, or drug therapy, the patient will be functioning at a normal level of thyroid hormone activity (euthyroid). The euthyroid patient does not represent an unusual risk to the administration of anesthetic or sedative drugs.

X-Ray or Cobalt Treatment
Chemotherapy (Cancer, Leukemia)

COMMENT: The presence or prior existence of cancer of the head or neck may require specific modifications in dental therapy. Irradiated tissues may have a decreased resistance to infection and a diminished vascularity with reduced healing capacity. There is no specific contraindication to the administration of any drug for pain or anxiety control. Many patients with cancer may also be receiving long-term therapy with CNS depressants such as antianxiety drugs, hypnotics, or opioids. Consultation with the patient's physician may be in order before treatment is begun.

Arthritis
Rheumatism
Cortisone Medicine

COMMENT: A history of arthritis may be associated with chronic use of salicylates (aspirin) or other nonsteroidal antiinflammatory drugs (NSAIDs), which may alter blood clotting. Arthritic patients may also be receiving long-term corticosteroid therapy, with the possible risk of acute adrenal insufficiency. Such patients may require modification in the dosage of corticosteroids during the period of dental therapy to enable them to respond more appropriately to any additional stress associated with their treatment. An additional consideration relates to the possible difficulty the doctor may have in attempting to place the patient in the recommended position (supine with feet elevated slightly) for sedation. Modification in this position may be necessary to accommodate the patient's physical disability.

Glaucoma

COMMENT: Glaucoma will be of concern for those patients in whom an anticholinergic is to be administered to diminish salivary gland secretions or for their vagolytic actions. Atropine, scopolamine, and glycopyrrolate are contraindicated in these patients.

Pain in the Jaw Joints

COMMENT: Chronic temporomandibular joint (TMJ) pain is seen with increasing frequency today. Evaluation as to the cause(s) should be sought. In the event that the mandibular range of motion is decreased, extreme care must be taken when considering the use of deeper levels of sedation or of general anesthesia to ensure that airway patency can be maintained throughout the procedure.

AIDS
Hepatitis A (Infectious)
Hepatitis B (Serum)
Liver Disease
Yellow Jaundice
Blood Transfusion
Drug Addiction

COMMENT: The preceding diseases are either highly transmissible (human immunodeficiency virus [HIV] and acquired immunodeficiency syndrome [AIDS], hepatitis A and B) or are possible indicators of a state of hepatic dysfunction. When any of these disorders is encountered, the doctor should seek to determine the status of the disease process and of the patient via consultation with the patient's physician.

Most of the drugs that are discussed in this text undergo biotransformation in the liver. The presence of significant liver dysfunction will lead to a decreased rate of drug inactivation and an increased risk of prolonged clinical duration of action, and possibly overdose.

In patients who have undergone blood transfusion or who are admitted (past or present) IV drug abusers, there is a higher-than-normal incidence of liver dysfunction and HIV infection. In addition, IV drug abusers also have a significantly greater risk of valvular damage in the heart and may require antibiotic prophylaxis. The routine use of universal precautions (gloves, masks, glasses) by health care providers minimizes cross-infection during parenteral sedation and general anesthesia.

Hemophilia

COMMENT: Hemophilia and other bleeding disorders must be fully evaluated before the start of any procedure, especially ones in which bleeding may occur. It is prudent to avoid (when possible) the administration of regional nerve blocks in which the risk of positive aspiration of blood is great (inferior alveolar, posterior superior alveolar). In most instances alternative techniques of pain control are available.

The use of parenteral sedation techniques, especially the IV route, is not contraindicated if, in the doctor's opinion, the benefits associated with this procedure outweigh the possible risk of postoperative bleeding.

Venereal Disease (Syphilis, Gonorrhea)
Cold Sores
Genital Herpes

COMMENT: The possibility of the doctor contracting infection is increased when working with these patients. Where oral lesions are present, dental treatment should be postponed, if possible. The use of universal precautions provides the operator with a degree of protection but not absolute protection.

Epilepsy or Seizures

COMMENT: The type(s) of seizure, its frequency, and the drug(s) used to prevent its recurrence should be determined before the start of dental treatment. Stress reduction and other treatment modifications are frequently in order during treatment of these patients because stress is a major precipitating factor of seizures.

The use of sedation is indicated wherever fear or anxiety is noted. Many of the parenteral drugs used for sedation possess anticonvulsant actions. Diazepam, midazolam, or pentobarbital may be administered intravenously to terminate seizures. Their use as sedatives decreases the likelihood of a seizure developing during dental treatment.

Inhalation sedation with N_2O-O_2 may also be used in epileptic patients who exhibit dental fear or anxiety.

Fainting or Dizzy Spells

COMMENT: The presence of chronic postural (orthostatic) hypotension or of symptomatic hypotension or anemia may be detected by this question. Transient ischemic attacks, a form of "prestroke," may also be detected by this question. Further evaluation, including consultation with the patient's physician, is recommended before dental treatment or the use of pharmacosedative techniques.

Nervousness
Psychiatric Treatment

COMMENT: The presence of undue nervousness (in general or specifically related to the planned treatment) and the need for psychiatric care should alert the doctor prior to the start of dental therapy. These patients may be receiving any number of drugs for the management of their disorders, drugs that in some instances interact with other CNS depressants used in dentistry for the control of anxiety (see Table 4-1). Medical consultation is usually desirable in these cases.

Sickle Cell Disease

COMMENT: Sickle cell disease is seen exclusively in the black patient. A sickle cell crisis can be precipitated during periods of unusual stress or when the patient does not receive an adequate supply of oxygen (hypoxia). With a history of sickle cell disease, oxygenation of the patient during dental treatment is strongly recommended and is deemed essential during parenteral sedation techniques.

Bruise Easily

COMMENT: A positive response to this statement may indicate the presence of a bleeding or clotting disorder, which should be evaluated before the start of dental or surgical treatment. Parenteral sedation techniques, as well as regional nerve blocks involving a greater risk of bleeding (e.g., inferior alveolar and posterior superior alveolar nerve blocks), should be avoided until the bleeding or clotting problem is corrected.

QUESTION 10. When you walk up the stairs or take a walk, do you ever have to stop because of pain in your chest, shortness of breath, or because you are very tired?

COMMENT: Although the patient may have indicated in Question 9 that he or she does not have angina or heart failure, clinical signs and symptoms usually associated with these (and other) problems may be present. A positive response to this question should lead the doctor to consider deferring the planned procedure until the patient's physician can be contacted for further evaluation of the patient's status.

QUESTION 11. Do your ankles swell during the day?

COMMENT: CHF immediately comes to mind when one thinks of swelling of ankles (pitting edema or dependent edema); however, several other conditions may produce this sign. These include varicose veins, pregnancy (during the latter stages), and renal dysfunction. In addition, healthy persons who spend much of their time standing on their feet (e.g., letter carriers, police officers) may also exhibit ankle edema.

QUESTION 12. Do you use more than two pillows to sleep?

COMMENT: Persons with more severe CHF exhibit orthopnea, which is an inability to breathe comfortably when lying down. These patients may require additional pillows under their back, in effect propping them up in bed so that they may breathe more comfortably.

The use of more than two pillows (3+ pillow orthopnea) should be considered significant, prompting medical consultation before the start of dental care. Modifications in dental treatment may include altering the position of the dental chair to avoid the supine position. In addition, the use in parenteral sedation of drugs that are known to significantly depress respiration (such as opioid agonists and barbiturates) should be avoided, if possible.

QUESTION 13. Have you lost or gained more than 10 pounds in the past year?

COMMENT: The question refers primarily to any *unexpected* gain or loss of weight (as opposed to dieting). Such weight changes may be observed in patients with heart failure (increased weight with fluid retention) or with metastatic carcinoma (weight loss), among other disorders (hyperthyroidism [loss], hypothyroidism [increase], anorexia nervosa [decrease]). Medical consultation should be considered before any dental care to determine the cause of the change in weight and the significance to the overall physical status of the patient.

***QUESTION 14.* Do you ever wake up from sleep short of breath?**

COMMENT: Paroxysmal nocturnal dyspnea is a clinical manifestation of more severe left-sided heart failure. Medical consultation is recommended. Treatment modifications include positional changes and the possible use of supplemental oxygen.

QUESTION 15. Are you on a special diet?

COMMENT: This question will elicit dietary modifications resulting from certain medical disorders such as diabetes, high blood pressure, elevated cholesterol levels, and heart failure, as well as diets that the patient may be on (either through a physician's consultation or a personal dieting plan) in an attempt to lose or gain weight.

In most situations in which a patient is on a carefully planned and monitored dietary plan, there are no contraindications to the use of any technique of sedation.

QUESTION 16. Has your medical doctor ever said you have a cancer or tumor?

COMMENT: This question refers to comments made previously concerning x-ray or cobalt treatment, as well as chemotherapy.

QUESTION 17. **Do you have any disease, condition, or problem not listed?**

COMMENT: The patient is asked to comment on specific matters not previously discussed. Examples of disorders that might be mentioned at this time that will affect the administration of many common drugs used in dentistry include porphyria, atypical plasma cholinesterase, and malignant hyperthermia (hyperpyrexia).

QUESTION 18. **Women: Are you pregnant now? Are you practicing birth control? Do you anticipate becoming pregnant?**

COMMENT: Pregnancy represents a relative contraindication to extensive elective dental care, particularly during the first trimester. Consultation with the patient's physician is recommended. The use of pharmacosedative techniques should receive careful consideration, weighing the risks versus the benefits to be gained from their use. Of the available techniques, inhalation sedation with N_2O-O_2 is the most highly recommended. Table 4-3 lists many commonly used drugs and their possible fetal effects.

The U.S. Food and Drug Administration (FDA) categorizes drugs based on their potential effects on the fetus. Box 4-1 presents these categories.

After completing the medical history questionnaire (in ink), the patient should sign it. In addition, the doctor should also sign the questionnaire after reviewing it. After any prolonged absence from the dental office (3 months or more), the questionnaire should be updated. The entire history need not be redone, although this would represent the ideal. Only the following questions need be asked:

1. Has there been any change in your general health since your last visit?
2. Are you now under the care of a physician? If so, what is the condition being treated?
3. Are you taking any drug or medicine?

If a positive response is obtained, a detailed dialogue history with the patient should follow. The responses to these questions are recorded on the patient's chart (in the

BOX 4-1 FDA Pregnancy Categories

A Studies have failed to demonstrate a risk to the fetus in any trimester
B Animal reproduction studies fail to demonstrate a risk to the fetus; no human studies available
C Only given after risks to the fetus are considered; animal reproduction studies have shown adverse effects on fetus; no human studies available
D Definite human fetal risks; may be given in spite of risks if needed in life-threatening conditions
X Absolute fetal abnormalities; not to be used anytime during pregnancy because risks outweigh benefits

TABLE 4-3 Known Fetal Effects of Drugs

Drug	Effect
Amobarbital	No adverse effects reported
Anesthetics, local	No adverse effects in dentistry
Atropine	Sympathomimetic effects
Barbiturates	Concentration is greater in fetus than in mother because fetal kidneys are unable to eliminate barbiturate
Bupivacine	Does not cross placenta readily; no adverse effects in dentistry
Chlordiazepoxide	In initial 42 days of pregnancy, congenital abnormalities more frequent
Diazepam	In first trimester, cleft lip and palate increased fourfold
Epinephrine	No adverse effects reported for dental use
Halothane	May be hazardous to pregnant operating room personnel
Hydroxyzine	Hypotonia reported
Lidocaine	No adverse effects reported in dentistry
Meperidine	Decreased neonatal respiration
Mepivacaine	No adverse effects reported in dentistry
Meprobamate	Possible increased congenital abnormalities during first 42 days of pregnancy
Morphine	With chronic use, smaller newborns; withdrawal symptoms noted
N_2O	With few exposures, no adverse effects reported when a 30% oxygen level is maintained and employed as an anesthetic for dental procedures; evidence suggests an increase in spontaneous abortion among wives of heavily exposed (>9 hr/wk) dentists and female chairside assistants; increase in congenital anomalies in offspring of heavily exposed (>9 hr/wk) dental chairside assistants
Pentazocine	Fetal addiction and withdrawl symptoms of hypertonia, tremors, hyperactivity, and inability to feed
Promethazine	Congenital hip dislocation
Prilocaine	No adverse effect reported in dentisty
Scopolamine	No adverse effects reported

Modified from Council on Dental Therapeutics: *JADA* 107:887, 1983.

section for progress notes). Where significant changes are present, the entire questionnaire should be redone.

Physical Examination

The medical history questionnaire is quite important to the overall assessment of a patient's physical and psychological status. However, there are limitations to the questionnaire. For the questionnaire to be valuable, the patient must (1) be aware of the presence of any medical condition and (2) be willing to share this information with the doctor.

Most patients will not knowingly deceive their doctor by omitting important information from the medical history questionnaire, although cases in which such deception has occurred are on record. A patient seeking treatment for an acutely inflamed tooth decides to withhold from the doctor the fact that he had a myocardial infarction 2½ months earlier because he knows that to tell the doctor would mean that he would not receive treatment. Another example is that of an HIV-positive individual withholding this information from the doctor for fear of being refused treatment.

The other factor, a patient's knowledge of his or her physical condition, is a much more likely cause of misinformation on the questionnaire. Most "healthy" persons do not visit their physician regularly for routine checkups. In fact, recent information has suggested that annual physical examination be discontinued in the younger healthy patient because it has not proven to be as valuable an aid in preventive medicine as was once thought.[11] In addition, most patients simply do not visit their physician on a regular basis, doing so instead whenever they become ill. From this premise it therefore stands to reason that the true state of the patient's physical condition may be unknown to the patient. Feeling well, although usually a good indicator of health, is not a guarantor of good health.[12] Many disease entities may be present for a considerable length of time without exhibiting overt signs or symptoms that warn the patient of their presence (e.g., high blood pressure, diabetes mellitus, cancer). When signs and symptoms are present, they are frequently mistaken for other, more benign problems. Although they may answer questions on the medical history questionnaire to the best of their knowledge, patients cannot give a positive response to a question unless they are aware that they do, in fact, have the condition. The first few questions on most histories refer to the length of time since the patient's last physical examination. The value of the remaining answers, dealing with specific disease processes, can be gauged from the patient's responses to these initial questions.

Because of these problems, which are inherent in the use of a patient-completed medical history questionnaire, the doctor must look for additional sources of information about the physical status of the patient. Physical examination of the patient provides much of this information. This consists of the following:

1. Monitoring of vital signs
2. Visual inspection of the patient
3. Function tests, as indicated
4. Auscultation of heart and lungs and laboratory tests, as indicated

Minimal physical evaluation for all potential patients should consist of (1) measurement of vital signs and (2) visual inspection of the patient.

The primary value of the physical examination is that it provides the doctor with important information concerning the physical condition of the patient immediately before the start of treatment, as contrasted with the questionnaire, which provides historical information. The patient should undergo a minimal physical evaluation at the initial visit to the office, before the start of any dental treatment. Readings obtained at this time, called *baseline vital signs*, are recorded on the patient's chart.

Vital Signs. The six vital signs are as follows:

1. Blood pressure
2. Heart rate (pulse) and rhythm
3. Respiratory rate
4. Temperature
5. Height
6. Weight

The techniques of recording vital signs, as well as guidelines for their interpretation, follow.

Blood Pressure

Technique. The following technique is recommended for the accurate manual determination of blood pressure.[13] A stethoscope and sphygmomanometer (blood pressure cuff) are the required equipment. The most accurate and reliable of these devices is the mercury-gravity manometer. The aneroid manometer, probably the most frequently used, is calibrated to be read in millimeters of mercury (mm Hg, or torr) and is also quite accurate, if well maintained. Rough handling of the aneroid manometer may lead to erroneous readings. It is recommended that the aneroid manometer be recalibrated at least annually by checking it against a mercury manometer. Many automatic blood pressure monitoring devices are now available, their cost ranging from under $100 to several thousand dollars. Likewise, their accuracy varies widely.[14] The use of automatic monitors simplifies the monitoring of vital signs, but doctors should be advised to check the accuracy of these devices periodically (comparing values with those of a mercury manometer).

For routine preoperative monitoring of blood pressure, the patient should be seated in the upright position. The arm should be at the level of the heart—relaxed, slightly flexed, and supported on a firm surface (e.g., the arm rest of the dental chair). The patient should be permitted to sit for at least 5 minutes before the blood pressure recording is taken. This will permit the patient to relax somewhat so that the recorded pressure will be closer to the patient's usual baseline reading. During this time, other nonthreatening procedures may be carried out, such as review of the medical history questionnaire.

The blood pressure cuff should be deflated before being placed on the arm. The cuff should be wrapped evenly and firmly around the arm, with the center of the inflatable portion over the brachial artery and the rubber tubing lying along the medial aspect of the arm. The lower margin of the cuff should be placed approximately 1 inch (2 to 3 cm) above the antecubital fossa (the patient should still be able to flex the elbow with the cuff in place). A blood pressure cuff is too tight if two fingers cannot be placed under the lower edge of the cuff. Too tight a cuff will decrease venous return from the arm, leading to erroneous measurements. A cuff is too loose (a much more common problem) if it may be easily pulled off of the arm with gentle tugging. A slight resistance should be present when a cuff is properly applied.

The radial pulse in the wrist should be palpated and then the pressure in the cuff increased rapidly to a point approximately 30 mm Hg above the point at which the pulse disappears. The cuff should then be slowly deflated at a rate of 2 to 3 mm Hg per second until the radial pulse returns. This is termed the *palpatory systolic pressure.* Residual pressure in the cuff should be released to permit venous drainage from the arm.

Determination of blood pressure by the more accurate auscultatory method requires palpation of the brachial artery, located on the medial aspect of the antecubital fossa. The earpieces of the stethoscope should be placed facing forward, firmly in the recorder's ears. The diaphragm of the stethoscope must be placed firmly on the medial aspect of the antecubital fossa, over the brachial artery. To reduce extraneous noise, the stethoscope should not touch the blood pressure cuff or rubber tubing.

The blood pressure cuff should be rapidly inflated to a level 30 mm Hg above the previously determined palpatory systolic pressure. Pressure in the cuff should be gradually released (2 to 3 mm per second) until the first *sound* (a tapping sound) is heard through the stethoscope. This is referred to as the *systolic blood pressure.*

As the cuff deflates further, the sound undergoes changes in quality and intensity. As the cuff pressure approaches the diastolic pressure, the sound becomes dull and muffled and then ceases. The diastolic blood pressure is best indicated as the point of complete cessation of sound. In some instances, however, complete cessation of sound does not occur—the sound gradually fading out. In these instances the point at which the sound became muffled is the diastolic pressure. The cuff should be slowly deflated to a point 10 mm Hg beyond the point of disappearance and then totally deflated.

Should additional recordings be necessary, a wait of at least 15 seconds is required before reinflating the blood pressure cuff. This permits blood trapped in the arm to leave, providing more accurate readings.

Blood pressure is recorded on the patient's chart or sedation/anesthesia record as a fraction: 130/90 R or L (arm on which recorded).

Common Errors in Technique. Some common errors associated with recording blood pressure lead to inaccurate readings (too high or too low) being obtained. Lack of awareness of these may lead to unnecessary referral for medical consultation, added financial burden to the patient, and a loss of faith in the doctor.

1. Applying the blood pressure cuff too loosely produces falsely elevated readings. This probably represents the most common error in recording blood pressure.
2. Use of the wrong cuff size can result in erroneous readings. A "normal adult" blood pressure cuff placed on an obese arm will produce falsely elevated readings. This same cuff applied to the very thin arm of a child or adult will produce falsely low readings. Sphygmomanometers are available in a variety of sizes. The width of the compression cuff should be approximately 20% greater than the diameter of the extremity on which the blood pressure is being recorded (Figure 4-2).
3. An auscultatory gap may be present (Figure 4-3), representing a loss of sound (a period of silence) between systolic and diastolic pressures, with the sound reappearing at a lower level. For example, systolic sounds are noticed at 230 mm Hg; however, the sound then disappears at 198 mm Hg, reappearing at approximately 160 mm Hg. All sound is lost at 90 mm Hg. An auscultatory gap occurred between 160 and 198 mm Hg. In this situation, if the person recording the blood pressure had not palpated (estimated) the systolic blood pressure before auscultation, the cuff might be inflated to some arbitrary pressure, say 165 mm Hg. At this level the recorder would pick up no sound because this lies within the auscultatory gap. Sounds would first be noted at 160 mm Hg, with their disappearance at 90 mm Hg, levels well within therapy limits (see

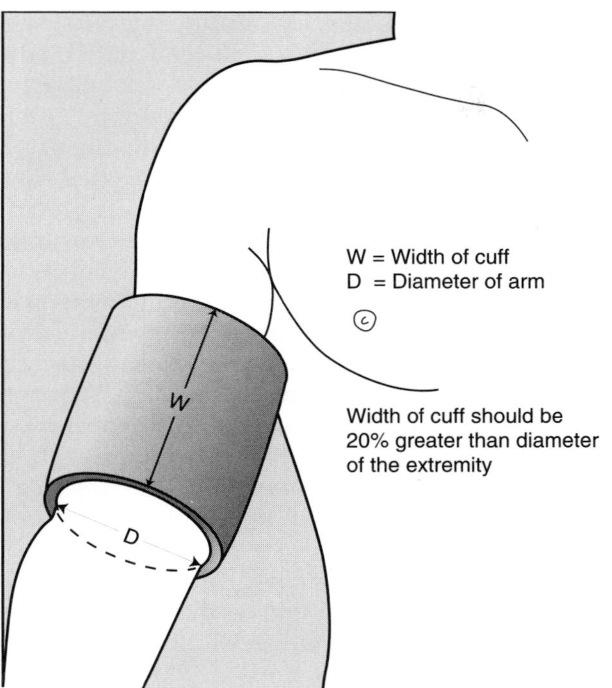

Figure 4-2 Determination of proper size of blood pressure cuff. (Redrawn from Burch GE, DePasquale NP: *Primer of clinical measurement of blood pressure*, St Louis, 1962, Mosby.)

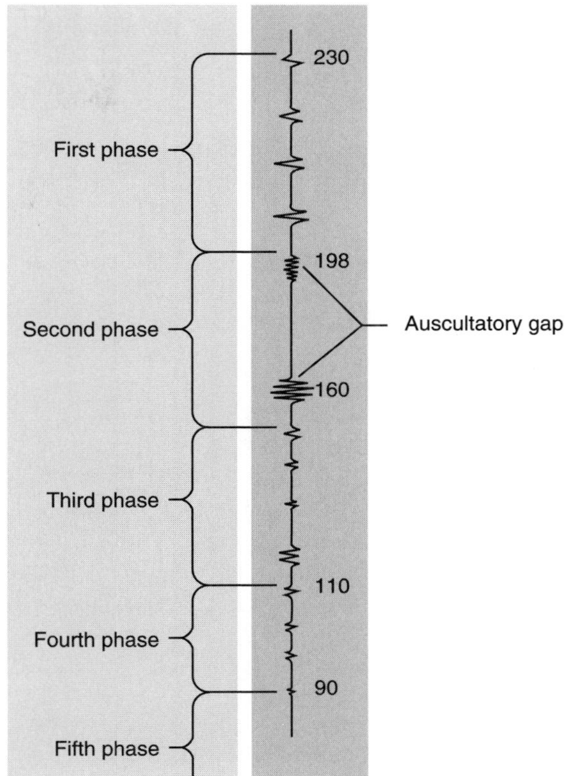

Figure 4-3 Korotkoff sounds illustrating auscultatory gap. Sound is heard at 230 mm Hg, disappears at 198 mm Hg, and reappears at 160 mm Hg. Sound disappears (fifth phase) at 90 mm Hg. (Redrawn from Burch GE, DePasquale NP: *Primer of clinical measurement of blood pressure,* St Louis, 1962, Mosby.)

guidelines for blood pressure, next subsection). In reality, however, this patient has a blood pressure of 230/90 mm Hg, a significantly elevated blood pressure that represents a greater risk to the patient during treatment (in fact, this patient is not considered to be a candidate for elective dental care). Although the auscultatory gap occurs only infrequently, the possibility of error may be eliminated by using the palpatory technique. The pulse *is* present throughout the gap (appearing, in our example, at 230 mm Hg), although the sound is not present. Although there is no pathologic significance to its presence, the auscultatory gap is found most often in patients with high blood pressure.

4. The patient may be anxious. Having one's blood pressure recorded may produce anxiety,[15] causing transient elevations in blood pressure, primarily the systolic pressure. This is even more likely to be noted in a patient who is to receive sedation for management of his or her dental fear. For this reason, it is recommended that baseline measurements of vital signs be obtained at a visit before the actual start of treatment, perhaps the first office visit, when the patient will only be completing various forms. Measurements are more likely to be the norm for the particular patient at this time.
5. Blood pressure is based on the Korotkoff sounds (Figure 4-4) produced by the passage of blood through occluded, partially occluded, or unoccluded arteries. Watching a mercury column or needle on an aneroid manometer for "pulsations" leads to falsely elevated systolic pressures. Pulsations of the dial are noted approximately 10 to 15 mm Hg before the first Korotkoff sounds are heard.
6. Use of the left or right arm will produce differences in recorded blood pressure. A difference of 5 to 10 mm Hg exists normally between arms, the left arm being slightly higher.

Guidelines for Clinical Evaluation. The USC physical evaluation system is based on the American Society of Anesthesiologists (ASA) Physical Status Classification System.[16] It details four risk categories based on a patient's medical history and physical evaluation. The ASA categories for blood pressure recordings in adults are presented in Table 4-4.[17]

For the adult patient with a baseline blood pressure in the ASA I range (<140/<90 mm Hg), it is suggested

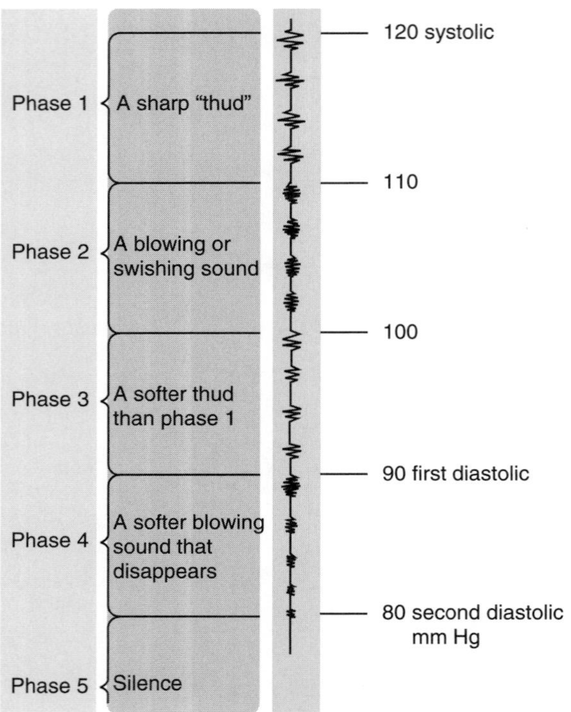

Figure 4-4 Korotkoff sounds. Systolic blood pressure is recorded at the first phase, diastolic blood pressure at the point of disappearance of sound (fifth phase). (Redrawn from Burch GE, DePasquale NP: *Primer of clinical measurement of blood pressure,* St Louis, 1962, Mosby.)

that the blood pressure be recorded every 6 months, unless specific dental procedures demand more frequent monitoring. The parenteral administration of any drug (local anesthesia; IM, IV, or inhalation sedation; or general anesthesia) mandates the more frequent recording of vital signs (see Chapter 5).

Patients with blood pressures in the ASA II, III, or IV categories should be monitored more frequently (e.g., at every appointment), as outlined in the guidelines. Patients with known high blood pressure should also have their blood pressure monitored at each visit to determine whether their blood pressure is adequately controlled. It is impossible to gauge a blood pressure by "looking" at a person or by asking, "how do you feel?" The routine monitoring of blood pressure in all patients according to the treatment guidelines will effectively minimize the occurrence of acute complications of high blood pressure (e.g., hemorrhagic CVA).

When parenteral or inhalation sedation techniques or general anesthesia is to be employed, there is a greater need for obtaining baseline vital signs. One factor that will be used to evaluate a patient's recovery from sedation and ability to be discharged from the office will be a comparison of the posttreatment vital signs with the baseline values.

Still another reason for routine monitoring of blood pressure relates to the management of medical emergencies. After the basic steps of management (P → A → B → C) in each emergency, certain specific steps are necessary for definitive treatment (D). Primary among these is monitoring of vital signs, particularly blood pressure. Blood pressure recorded during an emergency situation provides an important indicator of the status of the cardiovascular system. However, unless a baseline or nonemergency blood pressure measurement had been recorded earlier, the measurement obtained during the emergency is less significant. A recording of 80/50 mm Hg is less ominous in a patient with a preoperative reading of 100/60 mm Hg than if the pretreatment recording were 190/110 mm Hg. The absence of blood pressure is always an indication for cardiopulmonary resuscitation.

The normal range for blood pressure in younger patients is somewhat lower than that in adults. Table 4-5 presents a normal range of blood pressure in infants and children.

Heart Rate and Rhythm

Technique. Heart rate (pulse) and rhythm may be measured at any readily accessible artery (Figure 4-5). Most commonly used for routine measurement are the brachial artery, located on the medial aspect of the antecubital fossa, and the radial artery, located on the radial and ventral aspects of the wrist.

When palpating an artery, one should use the fleshy portions of the first two fingers (index and middle). Gentle pressure must be applied in order to feel the pulsation. Do not press so firmly that the artery is occluded and no pulsation is felt. The thumb ought not to be used to monitor pulse because it contains a fair-size artery.

Guidelines for Clinical Evaluation. Three factors should be evaluated while the pulse is monitored:

1. The heart rate (recorded as beats per minute)
2. The rhythm of the heart (regular or irregular)
3. The quality of the pulse (thready, weak, bounding, full)

The heart rate should be evaluated for a minimum of 30 seconds, ideally for 1 minute. The normal resting heart rate for an adult ranges from 60 to 110 beats per minute. It is often lower in a well-conditioned athlete and elevated in the fearful individual. However, clinically significant disease may also produce slow (bradycardia [<60 per minute]) or rapid (tachycardia [>110 per minute]) heart rates. It is suggested that any heart rate below 60 or above 110 beats per minute (adult) be evaluated (initially via dialogue history). Where no obvious cause is present (e.g., endurance sports, anxiety), medical consultation should be considered.

TABLE 4-4 Guidelines for Blood Pressure (Adult)

Blood Pressure (mm Hg, or torr)	ASA Classification	Dental Therapy Consideration
<140 and <90	I	1. Routine dental management 2. Recheck in 6 months, unless specific treatment dictates more frequent monitoring
140–159 and/or 90–94	II	1. Recheck blood pressure prior to dental treatment for 3 consecutive appointments; if all exceed these guidelines, medical consultation is indicated 2. Routine dental management 3. Stress-reduction protocol as indicated
160–199 and/or 94–114	III	1. Recheck blood pressure in 5 minutes 2. If blood pressure is still elevated, a medical consultation prior to dental therapy is warranted 3. Routine dental therapy 4. Stress-reduction protocol
200+ and/or 115+	IV	1. Recheck blood pressure in 5 minutes 2. Immediate medical consultation if still elevated 3. No dental therapy, routine or emergency,* until elevated blood pressure is corrected 5. Refer to hospital if immediate dental therapy indicated

*When the blood pressure of the patient is slightly above the cut-off for category IV and anxiety is present, the use of inhalation sedation may be employed in an effort to diminish the blood pressure (via the elimination of stress) below the 200/115 level. The patient should be advised that if the N_2O-O_2 succeeds in decreasing the blood pressure below this level, the planned treatment will proceed. However, should the blood pressure remain elevated, the planned procedure will be postponed until the elevated blood pressure has been lowered to a more acceptable range.

TABLE 4-5 Normal Blood Pressure for Various Ages (Figures Have Been Rounded off to Nearest Decimal Place)

Ages	Mean Systolic ±2 SD	Mean Diastolic ±2 SD
Newborn	80 ± 16	46 ± 16
6 mo-1 yr	89 ± 29	60 ± 10*
1 yr	96 ± 30	66 ± 25*
2 yr	99 ± 25	64 ± 25*
3 yr	100 ± 25	67 ± 23*
4 yr	99 ± 20	65 ± 20*
5-6 yr	94 ± 14	55 ± 9
6-7 yr	100 ± 15	56 ± 8
7-8 yr	102 ± 15	56 ± 8
8-9 yr	105 ± 16	57 ± 9
9-10 yr	107 ± 16	57 ± 9
10-11 yr	111 ± 17	58 ± 10
11-12 yr	113 ± 18	59 ± 10
12-13 yr	115 ± 19	59 ± 10
13-14 yr	118 ± 19	60 ± 10

From Nadas AS, Fyler DC: *Pediatric cardiology*, ed 3, Philadelphia, 1972, WB Saunders.
*In this study the point of muffling was taken as the diastolic pressure.

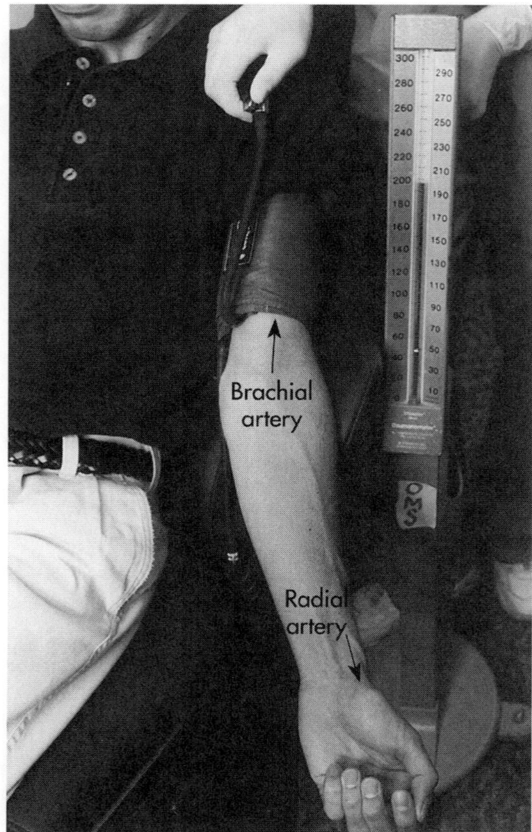

Figure 4-5 Location of brachial artery and radial artery. The brachial artery is located in the medial half of the antecubital fossa; the radial artery is located in the lateral volar aspect of the wrist.

The healthy heart maintains a relatively regular rhythm. Irregularities in rhythm should be confirmed and evaluated via dialogue history and/or medical consultation before the start of treatment. The occasional *premature ventricular contraction (PVC)* is so common that it is not necessarily considered abnormal. PVCs may be produced by smoking, fatigue, stress, various drugs (e.g., epinephrine), and alcohol. Frequent PVCs are usually associated with a damaged or an ischemic myocardium. However, when PVCs are present at a frequency of five or more per minute, especially if they appear at irregular intervals, medical consultation should definitely be sought. Patients with five or more PVCs per minute are considered to be at greater risk for sudden cardiac death (ventricular fibrillation)[18] and are more likely to have implanted automatic defibrillators.[19] Clinically, PVCs detected by palpation appear as a break in a generally regular rhythm in which a longer-than-normal pause (a "skipped beat") is noted, followed by the resumption of a regular rhythm.

A second disturbance of the pulse is termed *pulsus alternans*. It is not truly a dysrhythmia but a regular heart rate that is characterized by a pulse in which strong and weak beats alternate. It is produced by the alternating contractile force of a diseased left ventricle. Pulsus alternans is observed frequently in severe left ventricular failure, severe arterial high blood pressure, and coronary artery disease. Medical consultation is indicated.

Many other dysrhythmias may be noted by palpation of the pulse. The "irregular irregularity" of *atrial fibrillation* is noted in hyperthyroid patients and warrants pretreatment consultation. *Sinus dysrhythmia* is detected frequently in healthy adolescent patients. It is noted as an increase in the heart rate followed by a decrease in rate that correlates with the breathing cycle (the heart rate increases during inspiration, decreases with expiration). Sinus dysrhythmia is not indicative of any cardiac abnormality and therefore does not require pretreatment consultation.

The quality of the pulse is commonly described as full, bounding, thready, or weak. These adjectives relate to the subjective "feel" of the pulse and are used to describe situations such as a "full bounding" pulse (as noted in severe arterial high blood pressure) or a "weak thready" pulse (often noted in hypotensive patients with signs of shock). Table 4-6 presents the range of normal heart rates in children of various ages.

Respiratory Rate

Technique. Determination of respiratory rate must be made surreptitiously. Patients aware that their breathing is being observed will not breathe normally. It is recommended, therefore, that respiration be monitored immediately after the heart rate. The fingers are left on the patient's radial or brachial pulse after the heart rate has been determined; however, the observer counts respirations (by observing the rise and fall of the chest) instead, for a minimum of 30 seconds, ideally for 1 minute.

Guidelines for Clinical Evaluation. Normal respiratory rate for an adult is 14 to 18 breaths per minute. Bradypnea (abnormally slow rate) may be produced by, among other causes, opioid administration, whereas tachypnea (abnormally rapid rate) is seen with fever, fear (hyperventilation), and alkalosis. The most common change in ventilation noted in the dental environment will be hyperventilation, an abnormal increase in the rate and depth of respiration. It is also seen, but much less frequently, in diabetic acidosis. The most common cause of hyperventilation in dental and surgical settings is extreme psychological stress.

Any significant variation in respiratory rate should be evaluated before treatment. The absence of spontaneous ventilation is always an indication for artificial ventilation (P → A → B). Table 4-7 presents the normal range of respiratory rate at different ages.

TABLE 4-6 Average Pulse Rate at Different Ages

Age	Lower Limits of Normal	Average	Upper Limits of Normal
Newborn	70	120	170
1-11 mo	80	120	160
2 yr	80	110	130
4 yr	80	100	120
6 yr	75	100	115
8 yr	70	90	110
10 yr	70	90	110

From Behrman RE, Vaughn VC III: *Nelson textbook of pediatrics*, ed 12, Philadelphia, 1983, WB Saunders.

Blood pressure, heart rate and rhythm, and respiratory rate provide information about the functioning of the cardiorespiratory system. It is recommended that they be recorded as a part of the routine physical evaluation for all potential patients. Recording of the remaining vital signs—temperature, height, and weight—although desirable, may be considered as optional. However, when parenteral drugs are to be administered, especially in lighter weight, younger, or older patients, recording of a patient's weight becomes considerably more important.

Temperature

Technique. Temperature should be monitored orally. The thermometer, sterilized and shaken down, is placed under the tongue of the patient, who has not eaten, smoked, or had anything to drink in the previous 10 minutes. The thermometer remains in the closed mouth for 2 minutes before removal. Disposable thermometers (Figure 4-6) and digital thermometers (Figure 4-7) are equally accurate and easy to use. Forehead thermometers are effective when the patient's behavior will not permit use of an oral thermometer (Figure 4-8).

Guidelines for Clinical Evaluation. The "normal" oral temperature of 37.0° C (98.6° F) is only an average. The true range of normal is considered to be from 36.11° to 37.56° C (97° to 99.6° F). Temperatures vary during the day (from 0.5° to 2.0° F), being lowest in the early morning and highest in the late afternoon.

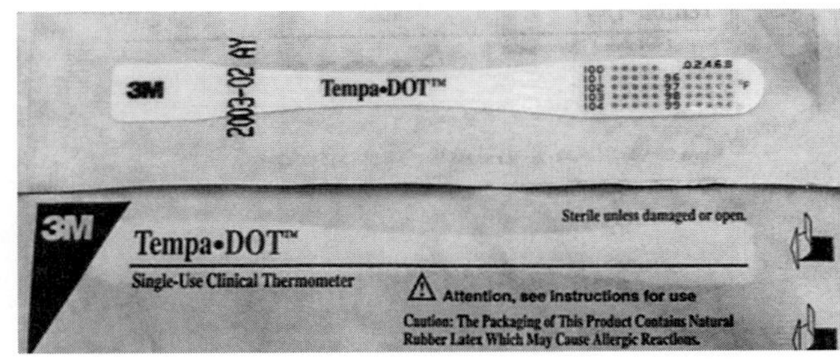

Figure 4-6 Disposable thermometer.

TABLE 4-7 Respiratory Rate by Age

Age	Rate/min
Neonate	40
1 wk	30
1 yr	24
3 yr	22
5 yr	20
8 yr	18
12 yr	16
21 yr	12

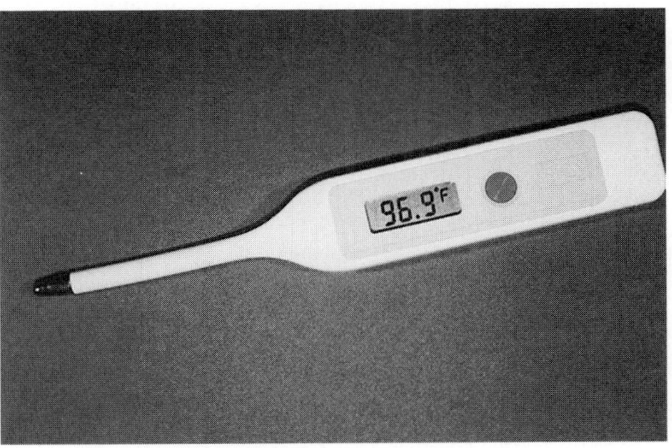

Figure 4-7 Digital thermometer.

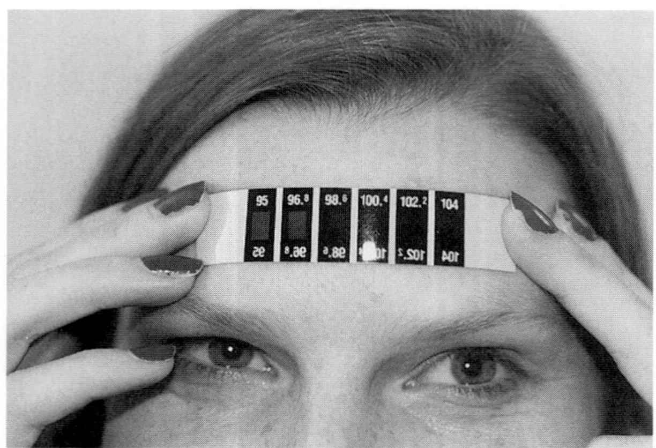

Figure 4-8 Forehead thermometer.

Fever represents an increase in temperature beyond 99.6° F. Temperatures in excess of 101° F (38.33° C) usually indicate the presence of an active disease process. Evaluation of the cause of the fever is necessary before treatment. When dental or periodontal infection is considered to be a probable cause of elevated temperature, immediate treatment (e.g., incision and drainage [I & D], pulpal extirpation, or extraction) and antibiotic and antipyretic therapy are indicated. If the patient's temperature is 40.0° C (104° F) or higher, pretreatment medical consultation is indicated. The planned treatment, especially any treatment involving the administration of CNS depressants, should be postponed, if possible, until the cause of the elevated temperature is determined and treated.

Height and Weight

Technique. Patients should be asked to state their height and weight. The range of normal height and weight is quite variable and is available on charts developed by various insurance companies. New guidelines of range of normal height and weight have been published (Table 4-8).

Guidelines for Clinical Evaluation. Gross obesity or being excessively underweight may indicate the presence of an active disease process. Obesity will be noted in various endocrine disorders such as Cushing's syndrome, whereas extreme loss of weight may be noted in pulmonary tuberculosis, malignancy, and hyperthyroidism. Anorexia nervosa should also be considered in extremely underweight individuals. In all instances where gross obesity or extreme loss of weight is noted, pretreatment medical consultation is recommended.

Excessively tall persons are referred to as *giants,* whereas persons who are decidedly shorter than average are called *dwarfs.* In both instances endocrine gland dysfunction may be present. Medical consultation is usually not necessary for these patients.

Whenever a pharmacosedative technique is to be employed in which titration is not possible (IM, intranasal [IN], or submucosal [SM]), the approximate

TABLE 4-8 Acceptable Weights (in Pounds) for Men and Women*†

	Age	
Height	19-34 Years	35 Years and Older
5′0″	97-128	108-138
5′1″	101-132	111-143
5′2″	104-137	115-148
5′3″	107-141	119-152
5′4″	111-146	122-157
5′5″	114-150	126-162
5′6″	118-156	130-167
5′7″	121-160	134-172
5′8″	125-164	138-178
5′9″	129-169	142-183
5′10″	132-174	146-188
5′11″	136-179	151-194
6′0″	140-184	155-199
6′1″	144-189	159-205
6′2″	148-195	164-210

*Weights based on weighing in without shoes or clothes.
†Source: United States Department of Agriculture and United States Department of Health and Human Resources, 1990.

weight of the patient must be obtained. One method used to determine the appropriate dose of drug for the patient is the patient's lean body weight (see Chapters 9 and 35). It is suggested that the patient be weighed on a scale in the doctor's office rather than relying on the patient to tell you his or her weight.

Visual Inspection of the Patient. Visual observation of the patient provides the doctor with valuable information concerning the patient's medical status and level of apprehension toward the planned treatment. Observation of the patient's posture, body movements, speech, and skin can assist in a diagnosis of possibly significant disorders that may previously have been undetected. Management of many of these patients is discussed in Chapters 37 and 38.

Posture. Patients with CHF and other chronic pulmonary disorders may be forced to sit in a more upright position in the dental chair because of significant orthopnea. The arthritic patient with a rigid neck may need to rotate his or her entire trunk when turning toward the doctor to view an object from the side. Recognition of these factors will better enable the doctor to determine necessary treatment modifications.

Body Movement. Involuntary body movements occurring in conscious patients may connote significant disorders. Tremor is noted in disorders such as fatigue, multiple sclerosis, parkinsonism, hyperthyroidism, and, of great importance to dentistry, hysteria and nervous tension.

Speech. The character of a patient's speech may also be significant. For example, CVA may cause muscle paralysis leading to speech difficulties. Anxiety over impending treatment may also be noted by listening to a patient's speech. Rapid response to questions or a nervous quiver to the voice may indicate the presence of increased anxiety and the possible need for sedation during treatment.

Other disorders may be uncovered by the detection of odors on the patient's breath. A sweet, fruity odor of acetone is present in diabetic acidosis and ketosis. The smell of ammonia is noted in uremia. Probably the most likely odor to be on the breath of a fearful dental patient is that of alcohol. Detection of alcohol on a patient's breath should lead the doctor to consider the possibility of heightened anxiety or of drug abuse. It is recommended that the planned pharmacosedative procedure be canceled in a patient who is "self-medicated."

Skin. The skin is a vast source of information about the patient. It is my belief that the doctor should, as a matter of routine, shake hands on greeting the patient. Much information can be gathered from the feel of a patient's skin. For example, the skin of a very apprehensive person will feel cold and wet, that of a patient with a hyperthyroid condition will be warm and wet, and the skin of a patient with diabetic acidosis will be warm but dry, whereas the hypoglycemic individual is cold and wet to the touch.

Looking at skin is also valuable. The color of the skin is significant. Pallor (loss of normal skin color) may indicate anemia or heightened anxiety. Cyanosis, indicating heart failure, chronic pulmonary disease, or polycythemia, will be most notable in the nail beds and gingiva. Flushed skin may point to apprehension, hyperthyroidism, or elevated body temperature, whereas jaundice may indicate past or present hepatic disease.

Additional factors revealed through a visual examination of the patient include the presence of prominent jugular veins (in a patient seated upright), an indication of possible right-sided heart failure; clubbing of the fingers (cardiopulmonary disease); swelling of the ankles (seen in right heart failure, varicose veins, renal disease, and in the latter stages of pregnancy); and exophthalmos (hyperthyroidism).

For a more complete discussion of the art of observation and its importance in medical diagnosis, the reader is referred to a truly excellent textbook, *Mosby's Guide to Physical Examination.*[20]

Additional Evaluation Procedures. Following completion of these three steps (medical history questionnaire, vital signs, and physical examination), it will occasionally be necessary to follow up with additional evaluation for specific medical disorders. This examination may include auscultation of the heart and lungs, testing for urinary or blood glucose levels, retinal examination, function tests for cardiorespiratory status (e.g., breath-holding test, match test), electrocardiographic examination, and blood chemistries. At present, many of these tests are used in dental offices but do not represent a standard of care in dentistry. However, when general anesthesia or certain sedation techniques are to be used, the level of routine pretreatment evaluation may require some or all of these evaluations.

Dialogue History

After patient information has been collected, the doctor next reviews with the patient any positive responses on the questionnaire, seeking to determine the severity of these disorders and the potential risk they represent during the planned treatment. This process is termed the *dialogue history*, and it is an integral part of patient evaluation. The doctor must put to use all available knowledge of the disease to assess the degree of risk to the patient.

Several examples of dialogue history are presented in the following sections. For a more in-depth description of dialogue history for specific disease states, the reader is referred to *Medical Emergencies in the Dental Office*, fifth edition.[21]

In response to a positive reply to the question "Are you diabetic?" the dialogue history that follows includes the following questions:

1. What type of diabetes do you have (insulin-dependent [type 1] or non–insulin-dependent [type 2])?
2. How do you control your diabetes (oral medications or injectable insulin)?
3. How often do you check your blood or urine for sugar, and what are the measurements (monitoring the degree of control of the disease)?
4. Have you ever required hospitalization for your diabetic condition?

The following is a dialogue history to be initiated with a positive reply to angina pectoris:

1. What precipitates your angina?
2. How frequently do you experience anginal episodes?
3. How long do your anginal episodes last?
4. Describe a typical anginal episode.
5. How does nitroglycerin affect the anginal episode?
6. How many tablets or sprays do you normally need to terminate the episode?
7. Are your anginal episodes stable (similar in nature), or has there been a recent change in their frequency, intensity, radiation pattern of pain, or response to nitroglycerin (seeking unstable or preinfarction angina)?

Dialogue history should be completed for every positive response noted on the medical history. A written note should be included on the questionnaire that summarizes the patient's response to the questions. For example, "heart attack" is circled. Written, by the doctor, next to this on the questionnaire is the statement "June 1999," implying that the patient stated the heart attack occurred in June 1999.

RECOGNITION OF ANXIETY

Thus far the primary thrust of our evaluation of the patient has been the medical history. Few, if any, questions have been directed at the patient's feelings toward the upcoming treatment. The typical medical history questionnaire (long form) has questions that ask "Do you have fainting spells or seizures?" and "Have you had any serious trouble associated with any previous dental treatment?" Most short-form histories contain no questions relating to this important area. Heightened anxiety and fear of dentistry or surgery are stresses that can lead to the exacerbation of medical problems such as angina, seizures, or asthma or to other stress-related problems, such as hyperventilation or vasodepressor syncope. One of the goals of physical evaluation is to determine whether the patient is psychologically able to tolerate the stresses that are associated with the planned dental treatment. Two methods are available to recognize the presence of anxiety. First is the medical history questionnaire, and second is the art of observation.

Earlier in this chapter it was recommended that one or more questions relating to a patient's attitudes toward dentistry be included in the medical history questionnaire. It has been our experience at the USC School of Dentistry that patients who do not verbally admit their fears to their doctor will in fact record such apprehension on the history questionnaire. A positive response to any of these questions should cause the doctor to begin a more in-depth interview with the patient, seeking to determine the reason for their fear of dentistry.

In the absence of such questions or in the absence of a positive response to such questions, careful observation of the patient will enable the doctor and staff members to recognize the presence of unusual degrees of anxiety. Some adult patients do volunteer to the doctor and staff that they are quite apprehensive; however, the vast majority of apprehensive adult patients (both male and female) will do everything within their power to attempt to conceal their anxiety. The usual feeling of patients is that their fear is irrational and probably even a bit childish and that they are the only persons who feel this way. They do not wish to tell the doctor of their fear because they are afraid of being labeled "childish." Because this attitude exists in many adults, all members of the dental and medical office staff should be trained to recognize clinical signs and symptoms of heightened anxiety.

Although there are a number of levels into which anxiety may be subdivided, for the purposes of this discussion, two are discussed: moderate anxiety and severe (neurotic) anxiety.

Patients with severe anxiety usually do not attempt to hide this fact from their doctor. In fact, these persons usually do everything within their power to avoid having to become dental patients. It is estimated that between 14 million and 34 million adults in the United States avoid regular dental care because of their intense fears.[22] These persons constitute the severe anxiety group. When in the dental or medical office, they may be recognized by the following:

1. Increased blood pressure and heart rate
2. Trembling
3. Excessive sweating
4. Dilated pupils

Severely apprehensive and fearful patients most often appear in the dental office suffering from a severe toothache or infection. On questioning, they state that they have had this problem for quite some time, not just a few days, and have exhausted every available means of home remedy (e.g., toothache drops and alcohol), which apparently worked for some time. The reason that they are finally in the dental office is that for the past few nights they have been unable to sleep because of the intense pain that none of their home remedies could alleviate. These patients are driven by their pain to the dental office, where their usual expectation is to have the offending tooth removed. These patients frequently represent a significant management problem. Although they desire to have their problem treated, when the time comes for treatment to begin, their underlying fear of dentistry comes to the forefront, making it almost impossible for them to tolerate the procedure. In addition, and by no means of secondary importance, the doctor is often faced with the unpleasant prospect of either having to extract an acutely inflamed tooth or to extirpate the pulp of an acutely sensitive tooth—two situations in which achieving clinically adequate pain control can be difficult, even in the best of circumstances.

Because of these factors, severely anxious patients will very often be candidates for the use of either IV conscious sedation or general anesthesia. Other techniques, such as oral, IM, or inhalation sedation, used as suggested, will have a diminished likelihood of success, primarily because of their limited effectiveness or the constraints that are properly placed on their use. Younger children with severe anxiety and fear levels are candidates for IM, IN, or IV conscious or deep sedation or for general anesthesia.

It is much more common to see patients with moderate degrees of dental anxiety. Most of these are adult patients who try to hide their fears from the doctor because they believe that, as adults, they should not admit to being afraid of the dentist. Children, on the other hand, being less inhibited and less mature than the typical adult, immediately let the office staff know their feelings toward dentistry. Assuming then that adult patients may attempt to hide their fears, the doctor and staff should remain observant both before and during the planned treatment.

"Front-office" staff (e.g., the receptionist) will be able to overhear patients' conversations in the waiting room, or patients might ask important questions of the receptionist, such as "Is the doctor gentle?" or "Does the doctor use gas?" The receptionist should be trained to inform the doctor or chairside staff immediately whenever a patient makes statements that might indicate an increased degree of concern about their upcoming treatment. This is also true for chairside personnel.

Shaking hands with the patient may lead to a presumption of anxiety when the patient's palms are cold and sweaty, especially when the office is not especially cool. Discussing a patient's prior dental experiences may give an indication of the dental anxiety status. The patient with a history of emergency care only (e.g., extractions or I & D) but who cancels or does not appear for subsequent (more routine) treatment may be a fearful individual. A patient with a history of multiple canceled appointments may also be a fearful patient. This history should be discussed with the patient in an attempt to determine the reasons behind this pattern of treatment (or nontreatment).

The patient, once seated in the chair, should be listened to and watched. Apprehensive patients remain alert and on guard at all times. They sit at the edge of the chair, eyes roaming around the room, taking in everything. They exhibit an unnaturally stiff posture, their arms and legs tense. They may nervously play with a handkerchief or tissue, occasionally being unaware that they are doing so. The "white-knuckle" syndrome may be observed, in which the patient clutches the arm rest of the dental chair tightly enough that their knuckles become ischemic. Diaphoresis (sweating) of the palms and forehead may be noted, explained by the patient as "Gee, it's hot in here!" The moderately apprehensive patient will be overly willing to aid the doctor. Actions are carried out quickly, usually without thinking. Questions to this patient are answered very quickly, usually too quickly.

Once anxiety is recognized, be it through the questionnaire or observation, the patient must be confronted with it. The straightforward approach is surprisingly successful, "Mr. Smith, I see from your medical history that you have had several unpleasant experiences in a dental office. Tell me about them." Or when the anxiety was determined visually, "Mrs. Smith, you appear to be somewhat nervous today. Is something bothering you?" I have been truly astonished at how rapidly patients drop all pretense at being calm once it is known that the doctor is aware of their fears. They usually say, "Doctor, I didn't think you could tell" or "I thought I could handle it." Then, seek to determine the exact source of the patient's fears, such as injections or the drill. Once fears are made known, steps may be taken to minimize the development of adverse situations related to them.

The patient with moderate anxiety will usually prove to be manageable. In most cases psychosedation will be effective in this patient. This may involve the administration of a drug (pharmacosedation) and/or a nondrug form of sedation (iatrosedation). General anesthesia will be needed only rarely for effective management of these patients.

With the information that has now been gathered concerning the patient's past and present medical and dental histories, vital signs, and physical examination, the basic goals of evaluation can now be completed.

DETERMINATION OF MEDICAL RISK

Having completed all of the components of the physical evaluation and a thorough dental examination, the doctor next takes all of this information and answers the following questions:

1. Is the patient capable, physically and psychologically, of tolerating in relative safety the stresses involved in the proposed treatment?
2. Does the patient represent a greater risk (of morbidity or mortality) than normal during this treatment?
3. If the patient does represent an increased risk, what modifications will be necessary in the planned treatment to minimize this risk?
4. Is the risk too great for the patient to be managed safely as an outpatient in the medical or dental office?

In an effort to answer these questions, the USC School of Dentistry developed a physical evaluation system that attempts to assist the doctor in categorizing patients from the standpoint of risk factor orientation.[23,24] Its function is to assign the patient an appropriate risk category so that dental care can be provided to the patient in comfort and with increased safety. The system is based on the ASA Physical Status Classification System, which is described next.

PHYSICAL STATUS CLASSIFICATION SYSTEM

In 1962, the American Society of Anesthesiologists adopted what is now referred to as the *ASA Physical Status Classification System*.[16] It represents a method of estimating medical risk presented by a patient undergoing a surgical procedure. The system was designed primarily for patients about to receive a general anesthetic, but since its introduction the classification system has been used for all surgical patients regardless of anesthetic technique (e.g., general anesthesia, regional anesthesia, sedation). The system has been in continual use since 1962, virtually without change, and has proved to be a valuable method of determining surgical and anesthetic risk prior to the actual procedure.[25] The classification system follows:

ASA I: A patient without systemic disease; a normal, healthy patient

ASA II: A patient with mild systemic disease

ASA III: A patient with severe systemic disease that limits activity but is not incapacitating

ASA IV: A patient with incapacitating systemic disease that is a constant threat to life

ASA V: A moribund patient not expected to survive 24 hours with or without operation

ASA E: Emergency operation of any variety; "E" precedes the number indicating the patient's physical status (e.g., ASA E-III)

When this system was adapted for use in a typical outpatient dental or medical setting, ASA V was eliminated and an attempt made to correlate the remaining four classifications with possible treatment modifications for dental treatment. Figure 4-9 illustrates the USC physical evaluation form on which a summary of the patient's physical and psychological status is presented, along with planned treatment modifications.

In the discussion of the ASA categories to follow, the term *normal*, or *usual*, activity is used, along with the term *distress*. Definitions of these terms follow: *Normal*, or *usual*, activity is defined as the ability to climb one flight of stairs or to walk two level city blocks, and *distress* is defined as undue fatigue, shortness of breath, or chest pain. Figure 4-10 illustrates the ASA classification system based on the ability to climb one flight of stairs. Each of the ASA classifications is reviewed, with specific examples listed.

ASA I

ASA I patients are considered to be "normal and healthy." They are able to carry out normal activity without distress. They are able to walk up a flight of stairs or walk two level city blocks without undue fatigue, shortness of breath, or chest pain.

Review of this patient's medical history, physical evaluation, and any other parameters that have been evaluated indicates no abnormalities (heart, lungs, liver, kidneys, and CNS are within normal limits [WNL]). Physiologically, this patient should be able to tolerate the stresses associated with the planned treatment with no added risk of serious complications. Psychologically, this patient should encounter little or no difficulty in handling the proposed treatment. Healthy patients with little or no anxiety are classified as ASA I. Therapy modifications are usually not warranted in this patient group. The ASA I patient is a candidate for any sedation technique or for outpatient general anesthesia. The ASA I patient represents a green light (go!) for treatment.

ASA II

ASA II patients have "a mild systemic disease"; are healthy, but present with extreme anxiety and fear toward dentistry; or are older (>60 years) or pregnant. ASA II patients are able to complete normal activities but then must rest because of distress. The ASA II

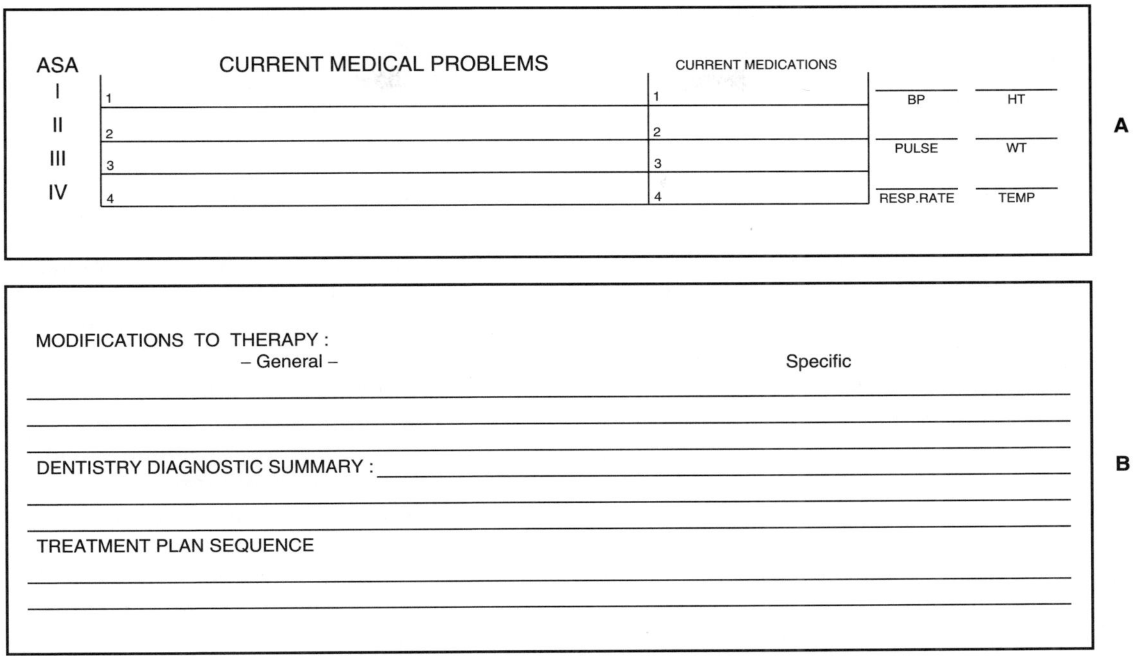

ASA	CURRENT MEDICAL PROBLEMS	CURRENT MEDICATIONS		
I	1	1	BP	HT
II	2	2	PULSE	WT
III	3	3		
IV	4	4	RESP.RATE	TEMP

A

MODIFICATIONS TO THERAPY :
– General – Specific

DENTISTRY DIAGNOSTIC SUMMARY :

TREATMENT PLAN SEQUENCE

B

Figure 4-9 **A,** The physical evaluation section on the health history form provides room for summary of medical problems, vital signs, and ASA classification. **B,** Possible treatment modifications are listed on the patient's chart.

patient can walk up one flight of stairs or walk two level city blocks but must rest at the completion of the task because of distress (chest pain, undue fatigue, or shortness of breath).

ASA II patients are less stress tolerant than ASA I patients. However, they still represent a minimal risk during treatment. Elective treatment is in order, with consideration given for treatment modifications or special considerations, as warranted by the particular condition. Examples of such modifications include using prophylactic antibiotics or sedative techniques, limiting the duration of treatment, and possibly, obtaining medical consultation. There are no general limitations on the use of pharmacosedative procedures for the ASA II patient. Outpatient general anesthesia may be used in ASA II patients. The ASA II patient represents a yellow light (proceed with caution!) for treatment.

Examples of ASA II patients are (1) the healthy, pregnant female; (2) any healthy patient older than 60 years of age; (3) a healthy but extremely phobic patient; (4) the patient with a drug allergy or who is atopic (multiple allergies present); (5) the adult patient with a blood pressure between 140 and 159 mm Hg and/or 90 and 94 mm Hg; (6) the patient with non–insulin-dependent diabetes (NIDDM, or type 2,

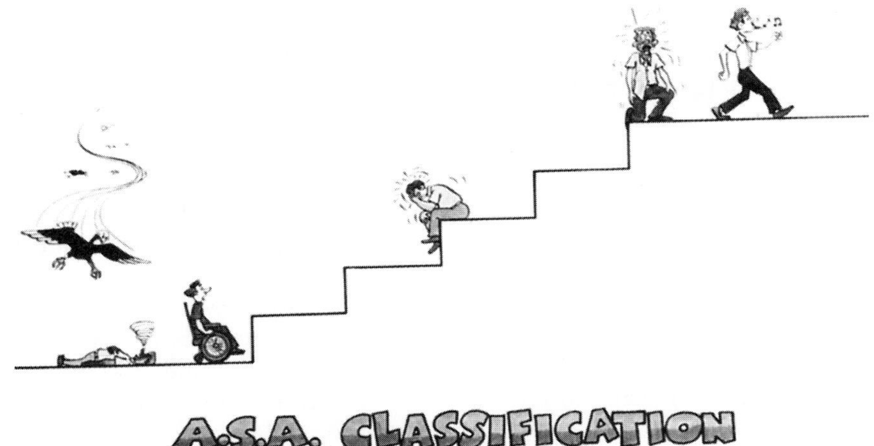

Figure 4-10 ASA classification for congestive heart failure. (Courtesy Dr. Lawrence Day.)

diabetes); (7) the patient with well-controlled epilepsy (no seizures within past year); (8) the patient with well-controlled asthma; and (9) the patient with a history of hyperthyroid or hypothyroid conditions who is under care and presently in a euthyroid condition.

ASA III

ASA III patients have "severe systemic disease that limits activity but is not incapacitating." An ASA III patient is able to walk up a flight of stairs or walk two level city blocks but must stop (at least once) before reaching their goal because of distress.

The ASA III patient does not exhibit signs or symptoms of distress while at rest (e.g., in the waiting room); however, in stressful situations (e.g., dental chair), signs and symptoms develop.

ASA III patients are less able to tolerate stress than those classified as ASA II. Elective dental care is still appropriate; however, the need for stress-reduction techniques and other treatment modifications is increased. Serious consideration must be given to treatment modifications in ASA III patients. Outpatient general anesthesia is not usually recommended for these patients; however, many of the pharmacosedation techniques may be used, although with some potential modification as to the length of procedure and the depth of sedation. ASA III patients represents a yellow light (proceed with caution!) for treatment.

Examples of ASA III patients include (1) the patient with well-controlled insulin-dependent diabetes (IDDM, type 1, diabetes); (2) the patient with symptomatic thyroid disease (hypothyroid or hyperthyroid); (3) the patient who is status post–myocardial infarction more than 6 months with no residual complications; (4) the patient who is status post-CVA more than 6 months with no residual complications; (5) the adult patient with a blood pressure between 160 and 199 mm Hg and/or 95 and 114 mm Hg; (6) the patient with epilepsy, but less well controlled (several seizures or more per year); (7) the asthmatic patient, less well controlled, stress or exercise induced, and/or a history of hospitalization because of status asthmaticus; (8) the patient with angina pectoris (stable angina); (9) the patient with CHF, with orthopnea (more than two pillows) and/or ankle edema; and (10) the patient with COPD (emphysema or chronic bronchitis).

ASA IV

ASA IV patients have "an incapacitating disease that is a constant threat to life." ASA IV patients are unable either to walk up a flight of stairs or walk two level city blocks.

ASA IV patients exhibit signs and symptoms of their medical problem(s) at rest. Seated in the waiting room of the dental or medical office, such patients exhibit undue fatigue, shortness of breath, or chest pain. Patients in this category have a medical problem that is of greater significance than the planned dental treatment. Elective care should be postponed until the patient's medical condition has improved to at least an ASA III. The ASA IV patient represents a significant risk during treatment.

The management of dental emergencies, such as infection and pain, in the ASA IV patient should be treated as conservatively as possible until the patient's physical condition improves. When possible, emergency care should be noninvasive, consisting of the prescription of drugs, such as analgesics for pain and antibiotics for infection. In situations in which it is believed that immediate intervention is required (I & D, extraction, pulpal extirpation), it is recommended that, when possible, the patient receive such care within the confines of an acute care facility (e.g., hospital). Although the risk to the patient is still significant, the chance of survival should an acute medical emergency arise is increased.

The ASA IV patient represents a red light (stop; do not proceed!) for treatment. Examples of ASA IV patients include (1) the patient with unstable angina pectoris (preinfarction angina), (2) the patient who is status post–myocardial infarction less than 6 months, (3) the patient who is status post-CVA less than 6 months, (4) the adult patient who has a blood pressure of 200 mm Hg and/or 115 mm Hg or higher, (5) the patient with uncontrolled dysrhythmias (requires medical consultation), (6) the patient with severe CHF or COPD confining the patient to wheelchair and/or requiring that the patient receive supplemental oxygen therapy, (7) the patient with uncontrolled epilepsy, and (8) the patient with uncontrolled IDDM.

ASA V

An ASA V patient is "A moribund patient not expected to survive 24 hours with or without operation." The ASA V patient is almost always a hospitalized patient with an end-stage disease. The ASA V patient is not a candidate for elective dental care. However, dental treatment is frequently required for the management of any intraoral and dental problems that arise. The nature of the dental care rendered is palliative—the relief of pain and/or infection. The physical condition of the ASA V patient is fragile at best. The use of local anesthetics and other CNS depressants should be undertaken with as much care as possible. ASA V patients should be monitored throughout the procedure.

The ASA V patient represents a red light (stop: do not proceed!) for elective treatment. Examples of ASA V patients include (1) the patient with end-stage cancer, (2) the patient with end-stage heart and/or lung disease, (3) the patient with end-stage renal disease, (4) the patient with end-stage hepatic disease, and (5) the patient with end-stage infectious disease (e.g., AIDS).

The ASA physical evaluation system is quite simple to employ when a patient has an isolated medical problem. However, many patients are seen with histories of several significant diseases. On these occasions the doctor must weigh the significance of each disease and make a judgment as to the appropriate ASA category. The system is not meant to be inflexible but, rather, to function as a relative value system based on the doctor's clinical judgment. When the doctor is unable to determine the clinical significance of one or more disease processes, consultation with the patient's physician or other medical or dental colleagues is recommended. In all cases, however, the ultimate decision of whether to treat or to postpone treatment must be made by the treating doctor. Responsibility and liability rest solely in the hands of the doctor who treats or does not treat the patient.

STRESS-REDUCTION PROTOCOLS

At this point in our pretreatment evaluation of the patient we have reviewed all of the history and physical evaluation data and assigned a physical status classification. Most patients will be assigned an ASA I or ASA II status (85% in most private dental practices), with fewer still being categorized as ASA III (about 14%) and IV.[26]

As has been discussed, every dental or surgical procedure is potentially stress inducing. Such stress may be of a physiologic nature (pain, strenuous exercise) or of a psychological nature (anxiety, fear). In both types, however, one of the responses of the body involves an increased release of catecholamines (epinephrine and norepinephrine) from the adrenal medulla into the cardiovascular system. This results in an increased workload on the cardiovascular system (increased rate and strength of myocardial contraction and an increased myocardial oxygen requirement). Although the ASA I patient may be quite able to tolerate such changes in cardiovascular activity, ASA II, III, and IV patients will be increasingly less able to safely tolerate these changes. The patient with stable angina (ASA III) may respond with an episode of chest discomfort, and various dysrhythmias may develop. Pulmonary edema may develop in patients with CHF. Patients with noncardiovascular disorders may also respond adversely when faced with increased levels of stress. For example, the patient with asthma may develop an acute episode of breathing distress, whereas the epileptic patient may suffer a seizure. Unusual degrees of stress in the ASA I patient may be responsible for several psychogenically induced emergency situations, such as hyperventilation or vasodepressor syncope.

Interviews with fearful dental patients have demonstrated that many begin to worry about their upcoming dental or surgical treatment 1 day or more before the appointment. These persons may be unable to sleep well the night before the appointment, thus arriving for the procedure fatigued and even more stress intolerant. The risk presented by this patient during treatment is increased even more.

The stress-reduction protocols are two series of procedures that, when used either individually or collectively, act to minimize stress during treatment and thereby decrease the risk presented by the patient.[2,27] These protocols are predicated on the belief that the prevention or reduction of stress ought to begin before the start of treatment and continue throughout the treatment period and, if indicated, into the postoperative period.

Stress-Reduction Protocol: Normal, Healthy, but Anxious Patient

1. Recognition of anxiety
2. Premedication with CNS depressant (anxiolytic, hypnotic) the night before the scheduled appointment, as needed
3. Premedication with CNS depressant (anxiolytic, hypnotic) immediately before the scheduled appointment, as needed
4. Appointment scheduled in the morning
5. Minimization of office waiting time
6. Psychosedation during treatment, as needed
7. Adequate pain control during treatment
8. Length of appointment variable
9. Postoperative pain/anxiety control

Stress-Reduction Protocol: Medical Risk Patient (ASA II, III, and IV)

1. Recognition of medical risk
2. Medical consultation before treatment, as needed
3. Appointment scheduled in the morning
4. Preoperative and postoperative vital signs monitored and recorded
5. Psychosedation during treatment, as needed
6. Adequate pain control during treatment
7. Length of appointment variable, but not to exceed patient's limits of tolerance
8. Postoperative pain/anxiety control

Recognition of Medical Risk and Anxiety. Recognition of these factors represents the starting point for the management of stress in the dental or surgical patient. Medical risk assessment will be accurately determined by strict adherence to the measures previously described in this chapter. The recognition of anxiety is often a more difficult task. As has been described, visual observation of the patient, as well as verbal communication, can provide the doctor with clues to the presence of anxiety.

Medical Consultation. Medical consultation should be considered in those situations in which the doctor is uncertain about the degree of risk represented by the patient. Medical consultation is neither required nor recommended for all medically compromised patients. In all cases it must be remembered that a consultation is but a request for additional information concerning a specific patient or disease process. The doctor is seeking information that will aid him or her in determining the degree of risk and which therapy modifications might be beneficial. The ultimate responsibility for the care and safety of the patient rests solely with the person who treats the patient.

Premedication. Many apprehensive patients state that their fear of dentistry or surgery is so great that they are unable to sleep well the night before their scheduled appointment. Fatigued the next day, these patients are less able to tolerate any additional stresses placed on them during their treatment. Should the patient be medically compromised, the risk of an acute exacerbation of the patient's medical problem is significantly increased. In the ASA I patient, such additional stress might provoke a psychogenically induced response. A clinical manifestation of increased fatigue includes a lowered pain reaction threshold, whereby the patient is more likely to respond to any given stimulus as being painful than is a well-rested patient.

Whenever it has been determined that heightened anxiety exists, it should also be determined whether this anxiety interferes with the patient's sleep. Restful sleep the night before a scheduled appointment is desirable. The administration of an oral sedative is one method of achieving this goal. An antianxiety or sedative-hypnotic drug such as diazepam, triazolam, flurazepam, or zolpidem may be prescribed for administration 1 hour before sleep. Appropriate dosages of these and other drugs are discussed in Chapter 7.

As the scheduled appointment approaches, the patient's anxiety level will heighten. In many cases the administration of an antianxiety or sedative-hypnotic drug approximately 1 hour before the scheduled appointment will decrease the patient's anxiety level to a degree such that the thought of dental or surgical treatment is no longer as frightening. Oral drugs should be administered approximately 1 hour before the scheduled start of treatment to permit a therapeutic blood level of the agent to develop. Oral drugs may be taken by the patient while at home or in the dental office. Whenever a CNS depressant drug has been prescribed to be taken by the patient at home, the doctor must advise the patient against driving a car or operating other potentially hazardous machinery. The appropriate use of oral antianxiety or sedative-hypnotic drugs is an excellent means of diminishing preoperative stress. Premedication might also include the need for preoperative antibiotic prophylaxis. Indications and protocols are found in Table 4-2.

Appointment Scheduling. Apprehensive or medically compromised patients are best able to tolerate stress when well rested. For most of these patients the most ideal time to schedule dental treatment is early in the day. This is also the case for apprehensive or medically compromised children.

If treatment is scheduled for the afternoon, the apprehensive patient must contend for many hours with the ominous specter of the dental or surgical appointment, casting a pall over everything the patient does prior to it, allowing him or her more time to think and to worry about it. The patient becomes more anxious, thereby increasing the likelihood of adverse psychogenic reactions. A morning appointment permits this patient to "get it over with" and to then continue with their usual activities unburdened by anxiety.

For the medically compromised patient the situation is somewhat similar. As fatigue sets in, the patient becomes less and less able to tolerate any further increase in stress. An appointment scheduled later in the day following hours at work and perhaps a drive through traffic will present the doctor with a medically compromised patient with little or no ability to handle adequately the additional stress of dental care. An early appointment provides the doctor and the patient with a degree of flexibility in patient management.

Minimization of Waiting Time. Once in the dental or medical office setting, the fearful patient should not be made to remain in the reception area or dental chair for extended periods before treatment begins. It is well known that anticipation of a procedure can induce more fear than the actual procedure.[28] Sitting and waiting allow the patient to smell dental smells, hear dental sounds, and fantasize about the "horrible things" that are going to happen. Cases of serious morbidity and death have occurred in the reception room of dental offices prior to the start of treatment.[29] This factor is of greater significance in the apprehensive patient.

Vital Signs (Preoperative and Postoperative). Before treatment is started on a medically compromised patient, it is recommended that the doctor measure and record the patient's vital signs. (Vital signs may be recorded by a trained auxiliary.) Signs monitored should include blood pressure, heart rate and rhythm, and respiratory rate. Comparison of these preoperative vital signs to the baseline values recorded at a previous visit can serve as an indicator of the patient's physical and emotional status on the day of treatment. Although especially relevant to patients with cardiovascular disease, it is recommended that preoperative vital signs be recorded on all medically compromised (all ASA IV and III and appropriate ASA II) patients. Postoperative vital signs should also be measured and recorded in the dental chart for these same patients.

Psychosedation during Therapy. Should additional stress reduction be deemed appropriate during treatment, any technique of sedation or general anesthesia may be considered. The means of selecting the appropriate technique for a given patient are discussed in subsequent parts of this book. Nondrug techniques include iatrosedation and hypnosis, whereas the more commonly used pharmacosedation procedures include oral, inhalation, IM, IN, and IV sedation. The primary goal of all these techniques is the same: the decrease or elimination of stress in a conscious patient. When used as described in this book, this goal may readily be achieved without additional risk to the patient.

Adequate Pain Control during Therapy. For stress reduction to be successful it is essential that adequate pain control be obtained. The successful management of pain is of greater importance in the medically compromised patient than in the ASA I patient. The potentially adverse actions of endogenously released catecholamines on cardiovascular function in the patient with clinically significant heart or blood vessel disease warrant the inclusion of vasoconstrictors in the local anesthetic solution.[30] Without adequate control of pain, sedation and stress reduction are impossible to achieve.

Duration of Treatment. The duration of treatment is of significance to both medically compromised and fearful patients. In the absence of any medical factors indicating the need for shorter appointments, the length of the appointment should be determined by the doctor after consideration of the patient's desires. In many instances a healthy but apprehensive patient (ASA I) may prefer to have as few dental appointments as possible, regardless of their length. Appointments 3 hours or longer may constitute the preferred management for this otherwise healthy patient (assuming of course, that the doctor, too, is an ASA I or II). However, attempting to satisfy the patient's (or parents' or guardians') desires for longer appointments is inadvisable when the doctor believes that there are appropriate reasons for shorter appointments. Cases of serious morbidity and of death have occurred when the doctor complied with parents' wishes to complete their child's dental treatment in one long appointment.

Unlike the fearful ASA I patient, the medically compromised patient should not be permitted to undergo longer appointments. In a dental chair, 1 hour of treatment is stressful for many persons. Even an ASA I patient may have difficulty tolerating 2- or 3-hour appointments. To permit the higher-risk patient to undergo extended treatments may unnecessarily increase risk. Dental appointments in the medically compromised patient should be shorter and not exceed the limit of the patient's tolerance. Signs that this limit has been reached include evidence of fatigue, restlessness, sweating, and evident discomfort by the patient. The most prudent means of managing the patient at this time is to terminate the procedure as expeditiously as possible and to reschedule the treatment.

Postoperative Control of Pain and Anxiety. Of equal importance to preoperative and intraoperative pain and anxiety control is their management in the posttreatment period. This is especially relevant for the patient who has undergone a potentially traumatic procedure (i.e., endodontics, periodontal or oral surgery, extensive oral reconstruction, or restorative procedures). The doctor must carefully consider any possible complications that could arise during the 24 hours immediately following treatment, discuss these with the patient, and then take steps to assist the patient in managing them. These steps include any or all of the following, when indicated:

1. Availability of the doctor via telephone around the clock
2. Pain control: prescription for analgesic drugs, as needed
3. Antibiotics: prescription for antibiotics, if the possibility of infection exists
4. Antianxiety agents, if in the doctor's opinion the patient may require them
5. Muscle relaxant drugs after prolonged therapy or multiple injections into one area (i.e., inferior alveolar nerve block)

The availability of the doctor by telephone around the clock has become a standard of care in the health professions. With answering services, pagers, cellular phones, and telephone answering machines almost universally available, patients should be able to contact their doctor whenever necessary.

Pain Control. Several studies have demonstrated that unexpected pain is rated as being more uncomfortable than expected pain.[28] Should the possibility of discomfort (pain) following a procedure exist, the patient should be forewarned and an analgesic drug made available. When the possibility of posttreatment pain has not been discussed and it does develop, the patient immediately thinks that something has gone wrong. Such pain is recorded as being more intense and anxiety provoking than pain that is expected (e.g., the patient has been advised of its likelihood) because of the emotional component of unexpected pain, which is not found in pain that is expected.[22] Should posttreatment pain, which has been discussed, fail to materialize, the patient will be all the more relaxed and confident in the doctor's abilities.

Through the use of the steps included in the stress-reduction protocol, patient management has been enlarged to include the preoperative and postoperative periods as well as the intraoperative period. These protocols have made it possible to manage the dental health needs of a broad spectrum of fearful and medically compromised patients with a minimal complication rate. Specific procedures included in the protocols are expanded throughout this book.

REFERENCES

1. Goldberger E: *Treatment of cardiac emergencies*, ed 5, St Louis, 1990, Mosby.
2. McCarthy FM: Stress reduction and therapy modifications, *J Calif Dent Assoc* 9:41, 1981.
3. Berthelsen CL, Stilley KR: Automated personal health inventory for dentistry: a pilot study. *J Am Dent Assoc* 131:59, 2000.
4. McCarthy FM: A new, patient-administered medical history developed for dentistry, *JADA* 111:595, 1985.
5. Gage TW, Pickett FA: *Mosby's dental drug reference*, ed 6, St Louis, 2002, Mosby.
6. Skidmore-Roth L: *Mosby's 2002 nursing drug reference*, St Louis, 2002, Mosby.
7. Little JW: Prosthetic implants: risk of infection from transient dental bacteremias, *Compendium* 12:160, 1991.
8. Fogoros RN: Evidence-based medicine and the implantable defibrillator, *Curr Cardiol Rep* 1:135, 1999.
9. Bardoczky GI, Wathieu M, D-Hollander A: Prilocaine-induced methemoglobinemia evidenced by pulse oximetry, *Acta Anaesthesiol Scand* 34:162, 1990.
10. Wilburn-Goo D, Lloyd LM: When patients become cyanotic: acquired methemoglobinemia, *JADA* 130:826, 1999.
11. Smith DM, Lombardo JA, Robinson JB: The preparticipation evaluation, primary care, *Clin Off Pract* 18:777, 1991.
12. Brady WF, Martinoff JT: Validity of health history data collected from dental patients and patient perception of health status, *JADA* 101:642, 1980.
13. American Heart Association: *Recommendations for human blood pressure determination by sphygmomanometry*, Dallas, 1967, The Association.
14. Zachariah PK, Sheps SG, Smith RL: Clinical use of home and ambulatory blood pressure monitoring, *Mayo Clin Proc* 64:1436, 1989.
15. Manning G, Rushton L, Millar-Craig MW: Clinical implications of white coat hypertension: an ambulatory blood pressure monitoring study, *J Human Hypertens* 13:817, 1999.
16. American Society of Anesthesiologists: New classification of physical status, *Anesthesiology* 24:111, 1963.
17. Malamed SF: Blood pressure evaluation and the prevention of medical emergencies in dental practice, *J Prev Dent* 6:183, 1980.
18. Adgey AAJ, Clements IP, Mulholland HC et al: Acute phase of myocardial infarction: prehospital management of the coronary patient, *Minnesota Med* 59:347, 1976.
19. Damiano RJ Jr: Implantable cardioverter defibrillators: current status and future directions, *J Cardiovasc Surg* 7:36, 1992.
20. Seidel HM, Ball JW, Dains JE et al: *Mosby's guide to physical examination*, ed 5, St Louis, 2002, Mosby.
21. Malamed SF: *Medical emergencies in the dental office*, ed 5, St Louis, 2000, Mosby.
22. Milgrom P, Weinstein B, Kleinknecht R et al: *Treating fearful dental patients*, Reston, VA, 1985, Reston Publishing.
23. McCarthy FM, Malamed SF: *Physical evaluation manual*, Los Angeles, 1975, University of Southern California School of Dentistry.
24. McCarthy FM, Malamed SF: Physical evaluation system to determine medical risk and indicated dental therapy modifications, *JADA* 99:181, 1979.
25. Owens WD, Felts JA, Spitznagel EL Jr: ASA physical status classifications: a study of consistency of ratings, *Anesthesiology* 49:239, 1978.
26. Malamed SF: ASA physical status, unpublished data, 1992.
27. Malamed SF: *The stress reduction protocols: a method of minimizing risk in dental practice*. Paper presented at the fifth annual Continuing Education Seminar in Practical Considerations in IV and IM Dental Sedation, Mt. Sinai Medical Center, Miami, 1979.
28. Corah NL, Gale EN, Illig SJ: Assessment of a dental anxiety scale, *JADA* 97:816, 1981.
29. Matsuura H: Analysis of systemic complications and deaths during dental treatment in Japan, *Anesth Prog* 36:219, 1989.
30. Glover J: Vasoconstrictors in dental anaesthetics contraindication—fact or fallacy, *Aust Dent J* 13:65, 1968.

CHAPTER 5

Monitoring during Conscious Sedation

CHAPTER OUTLINE

The word *monitor* comes from the Latin *monere*, meaning "to remind, admonish." One definition of *monitor* is "to observe and evaluate a function of the body closely and constantly."[1] A second definition is "an apparatus which automatically records such physiological signs as respiration, pulse (heart rate and/or rhythm), and blood pressure in an anesthetized patient or one undergoing surgical or other procedures."[2]

Monitoring of appropriate physiologic functions of a patient, during both sedative procedures and general anesthesia, permits the early detection of adverse side effects that may be produced by drugs or by clinical actions, including, for example, hemorrhage or underventilation.[3] Early detection of these problems allows corrective measures to be instituted at a time when they are more likely to effectively prevent serious complications from developing.

Since the first edition of this book in 1985, there has been a significant increase in emphasis placed on monitoring during conscious sedation and general anesthesia. The first specific, detailed mandatory standards for minimal patient monitoring during anesthesia in medicine were developed by the Risk Management Committee of the Department of Anesthesia, Harvard Medical School, in Boston, Massachusetts, in 1985.[4] Although some of this increased emphasis stemmed from a normal elevation in the standard of care, a major impetus came from studies evaluating critical incidents occurring during anesthesia. It was demonstrated that up to 80% of these critical events were preventable and could be attributed to human error and a lack of vigilance.[5,6] It was believed that the routine application of minimal monitoring devices would enable the detection of subtle physiologic changes, permitting measures to be taken before the situation deteriorated into a catastrophe.[7] In 1986 the American Society of Anesthesiologists (ASA) Committee on Standards of Care[8] developed the *ASA Standards for Basic Intraoperative Monitoring* as a national standard. Prior to the Harvard and ASA standards, formal guidelines for monitoring during conscious sedation in dentistry were limited to but a few states that had previously instituted regulations defining the practice of anesthesia (general anesthesia and conscious sedation) in dentistry, in essence providing guidelines for treatment. There was a considerable increase in implementation of guidelines in the years immediately following their publication. By July 1987, 30 states had enacted regulations governing the use of general anesthesia in dentistry, and 27 were regulating parenteral conscious sedation.[9] By June 1994, these figures had become 48 for general anesthesia and 46 for parenteral sedation.[10] In December 2000, 50 states regulated general anesthesia, 50 parenteral conscious sedation, and 3 oral sedation in children.[11] Specific requirements for monitoring during parenteral conscious sedation or general anesthesia are usually described in these regulations. In addition, specialty organizations within dentistry have produced sedation/anesthesia guidelines for use within their specialty. Guidelines have been forthcoming from the American Association of Oral and Maxillofacial Surgeons,[12] the American Academy of Pediatric Dentistry,[13] and the American Academy of Periodontology.[14] The national governing bodies of dentistry in several countries have also produced guidelines for the use of parenteral sedation and general anesthesia.[15,16]

The Subcommittee on Standards of Care of the American Dental Society of Anesthesiology (ADSA)[17] has created monitoring guidelines that take into account the unique aspects of sedative and anesthetic care delivery in a dental office setting. These guidelines represent an amalgamation of the Harvard and ASA standards and continue to stress the triad of oxygenation, ventilation, and circulation (the **a**irway, **b**reathing, and **c**irculation of basic life support). The ADSA monitoring guidelines are presented in Box 5-1(pp. 58–59).

In a report comparing 43 cases of morbidity and mortality (M & M) from pharmacosedation and general anesthesia in the dental office, the M & M were characterized as occurring in a young, healthy patient in whom multiple pharmacologic agents were used with limited monitoring and resuscitative efforts. Heart rate was *not* monitored in 68%, respiration in 77%, blood pressure in 77%, tissue oxygen saturation in 92%, and heart rhythm in 96%.[18] The authors concluded, and other experts agreed, that lack of adequate monitoring is a key factor in the majority of morbid and mortal events.[18,19] If, as Jastak[19] has stated, "subtle *trends* in vital signs are not detected because appropriate monitoring is not used, the morbid event eventually recognized by the practitioner is often the last in a series of physiologic distress signals, and, of course, results in the clinician's response being too little and too late." The implementation of monitoring guidelines has been associated with improved anesthesia care and a downward adjustment of anesthesia malpractice insurance premiums.[20,21]

An apparatus that measures a physiologic function may correctly be termed a *monitor* only if it delivers an audible or visual warning when the function being measured falls outside of predetermined parameters (e.g., systolic blood pressure <90 mm Hg or >200 mm Hg). In the absence of a warning system the device is more truly a measuring *instrument* than a *monitor.* The effectiveness of the monitor usually rests with the person administering the conscious sedation or general anesthesia.

Because the terms *monitoring* and *measurement* are so frequently used interchangeably, the term *monitoring* is used throughout this chapter. Many techniques and devices are available to assist in monitoring the sedated or anesthetized patient. In general, these devices are designed to measure the functioning of the following:

Central nervous system (CNS)
Respiratory system
Cardiovascular system
Temperature

Devices are termed *invasive* and *noninvasive.* When possible, monitors should be noninvasive. Indeed, for routine monitoring, noninvasive monitoring is essential. Invasive devices hurt, their placement is time-consuming, they are costly, and their use has unacceptable risks in many instances.[3] Invasive monitors include arterial lines for measurement of blood gases and lines for central venous pressure. Although they provide highly accurate measurements of important physiologic parameters, there is an increased risk associated with their use in that complications are more likely to develop because of the very nature of the techniques. In addition, invasive monitors are often quite time-consuming to prepare for use. In the outpatient dental or surgical environment, where only conscious sedation techniques are employed, the use of invasive monitors is rarely justified. However, in cases in which inpatient general anesthesia is to be used, particularly when the patient is classified as ASA IV, III, or II (see Chapter 4), the use of additional, highly accurate monitoring procedures is warranted. Noninvasive monitors are easier to use and are not associated with increased risk. Some may suffer from a diminished level of accuracy (compared with invasive monitoring of the same physiologic parameter). However, devices such as the pulse oximeter and capnograph (end-tidal carbon dioxide [CO_2] monitors) have been shown, by and large, to be quite accurate. For outpatient conscious sedation techniques used in dentistry and medicine, noninvasive devices prove to be quite acceptable for monitoring of patients during and after treatment. The requirements of the ideal monitoring device are as follows[22]:

1. Safe
2. Reliable
3. Noninvasive
4. Easily interpreted display
5. Easy to calibrate
6. Stable
7. Portable

8. Easily integrated with other monitoring equipment
9. No technical aid required
10. Inexpensive

In the pages that follow, monitoring devices ranging in price from but a few dollars to several thousand dollars are described. Our goal in monitoring the sedated or anesthetized patient is to increase patient safety during the procedure. As will be evident as we proceed, it is not necessary to use sophisticated and expensive equipment to achieve this goal.

ROUTINE PREOPERATIVE MONITORING

Before treatment of any dental or medical patient, vital signs should be recorded as a part of the routine pretreatment patient evaluation (see Chapter 4). Vital signs recorded at this pretreatment visit include blood pressure, heart rate and rhythm, and respiratory rate. Additional vital signs to be monitored as indicated include temperature, height, and weight.

These values should be recorded on the patient's chart (Figure 5-1) and serve as baseline values, against which values obtained during treatment may be compared. Baseline vital signs should be recorded at a nonthreatening time when they are likely to be more nearly "normal" for that patient. A patient's initial visit to a dental office, a time when no invasive dental procedure is planned, is likely to provide reliable baseline values.

Pulse (Heart Rate and Rhythm)

Monitoring of the pulse (heart rate and rhythm) is reviewed in Chapter 4. Monitoring of the pulse is recommended for all patients as a part of their routine preoperative evaluation. Values below 60 or greater than 110 beats per minute (in the adult) should be evaluated before treatment is started.

Preoperative recording of the heart rate and rhythm should be made whenever any drug (including local anesthetic) is to be administered. Monitoring of the heart rate and rhythm at *regular intervals* is desirable during parenteral conscious sedation techniques, such as intramuscular (IM), intranasal (IN), and intravenous (IV) sedation. Monitoring of these vital signs every 15 minutes (q15min) or every 5 minutes (q5min) is suggested. Specific time frames are discussed later in this chapter, but a basic rule of thumb is that the greater the CNS depression is and the less able a patient is to respond appropriately to verbal command, the more frequently vital signs must be evaluated.

In techniques of deep sedation in which a more profound level of CNS depression is sought (IM), *continuous monitoring* of the pulse is considered mandatory. Continuous monitoring of the pulse is also mandatory for all forms of general anesthesia.

The heart rate and rhythm may be measured manually or by electronic methods. When the heart rate is recorded manually, the fleshly portions of one or two fingers are gently placed over a superficial artery for at least 30 seconds (preoperative recording). When monitoring takes place during conscious sedation or general anesthesia, a period of 10 to 15 seconds is usually employed, although 30 seconds is suggested. Arteries that are accessible for monitoring of the pulse are listed in Table 5-1. The radial and brachial arteries are most often used in routine situations. The superficial temporal artery is frequently used during general anesthesia. The facial or labial arteries are accessible when working in or around the oral cavity. Palpation of the carotid artery is usually reserved for emergency situations.

It is suggested that the doctor palpate a large artery on the patient at the start of a procedure so that he or she will know its precise location at a later time when, perhaps, conditions have deteriorated and the pulse may be weak or absent. The feel of a strong, regular pulse beneath one's fingers during a deep sedation or general anesthesia case is greatly reassuring to the doctor!

A rough but consistent estimate of systolic blood pressure may be obtained via palpation of three of the aforementioned arteries. Where the radial artery pulse is palpable, the systolic blood pressure is at least 80 mm Hg. A brachial artery pulse will be palpable at a systolic pressure of 70 mm Hg, and a carotid artery pulse is present at a systolic reading of 60 mm Hg. Therefore, if both the carotid and brachial pulses are

ASA	CURRENT MEDICAL PROBLEMS	CURRENT MEDICATIONS		
I	1	1	BP	HT
II	2	2	PULSE	WT
III	3	3	RESP.RATE	TEMP
IV	4	4		

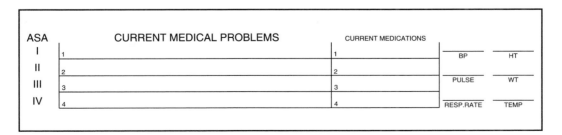

Figure 5-1 Baseline vital signs are recorded on the right side of the patient's chart.

BOX 5-1 American Dental Society of Anesthesiology Guidelines for Intraoperative Monitoring of Patients Undergoing Conscious Sedation, Deep Sedation, or General Anesthesia

The terminology recognized by the American Dental Association (ASDA) for various methods of delivery of nonregional anesthetics and sedatives and the anticipated clinical effect has been previously approved by the House of Delegates in 1985. These include, but are not limited to, the following: enteral, parenteral, conscious sedation, deep sedation, and general anesthesia. The standards endorsed by the ADSA in these guidelines apply to all nonregional dental anesthesia care. They are designed to encourage a high level of quality care in the dental office setting. It should be recognized that emergency situations may require that these standards may be modified on the basis of the judgment of the clinician(s) responsible for the delivery of anesthesia care services. Changing technology; individual states' rules, regulations, or laws; and regulations developed by the parent organization, the American Dental Association, may also supersede the standards listed herein. It should also be recognized that there may be certain situations whereby the standards may be clinically impractical* (e.g., combative patient, emergency surgery) and that adherence to the standards is no guarantee of successful outcome.

When the intention of the practitioner responsible for delivery of anesthesia care is to maintain a state of conscious sedation in a patient, it is that practitioner's responsibility to assess continually that level of sedation. If a change is observed, the type of intraoperative monitoring and the number of personnel present must be consistent with the level of anesthesia.

Standard I: Qualified Personnel

Qualified personnel shall be present in the operating room during the anesthesia period.

Objectives

1. During conscious sedation, a minimum of two qualified persons (e.g., doctor and assistant trained to monitor appropriate physiologic parameters) should be present.
2. Because deep sedation and general anesthesia are often indistinguishable entities with regard to the levels of consciousness or unconsciousness, a minimum of three qualified persons must be present during deep sedation and general anesthesia. There should be one person whose sole responsibility is monitoring and recording vital signs continually. This person may be classified as an anesthesia assistant, anesthesia technician, nurse, physician, or dentist.
3. In the event of special circumstances (e.g., an emergency in another location, radiation exposure to personnel), a modification in the number of personnel present may be made according to the best judgment of the clinician responsible for the patient under anesthesia. However, at no time should the monitoring of the patient be interrupted.

Standard II: Oxygenation

During the anesthesia period, the oxygenation of the patient shall be continually evaluated and ensured.

Objective

Adequate oxygen concentration must be delivered through inspired gases to be delivered to the body tissues.

Methods

Inspired gas. Fail-safe mechanisms (e.g., automatic nitrous oxide turnoff) must be used on delivery systems before the entry of the gas mixture to the patient's respiratory system. If an anesthesia machine that is capable of delivering more than 80% nitrous oxide (i.e., <20% oxygen) is used, then low-oxygen alarms and oxygen analyzers should be used.

Blood oxygenation. The color of mucosa, skin, or blood should be evaluated on a continual basis. In certain circumstances (e.g., deep sedation, general anesthesia), mechanical monitors should be used to supplement clinical signs. Pulse oximetry is strongly encouraged during deep sedation and general anesthesia, especially in pediatric patients.

Standard III: Ventilation

During the anesthesia period, the ventilation of the patient shall be continually evaluated. When inhalation agents other than nitrous oxide are used, continuous observation of the patient is required.

Objective

The exchange of oxygen and carbon dioxide from the lungs must be adequately maintained.

Methods

1. During conscious sedation, clinical signs, including chest excursion, auscultation of breath sounds, and movement of the reservoir bag on the gas machine (except when a nasal cannula is being used), should be continually monitored. Auscultation of breath

*In certain circumstances the clinician in charge of the delivery of monitored anesthesia care may waive the requirements. Documentation in the patient's chart or anesthesia record is recommended.

BOX 5-1 American Dental Society of Anesthesiology Guidelines for Intraoperative Monitoring of Patients Undergoing Conscious Sedation, Deep Sedation, or General Anesthesia—cont'd

sounds can be performed by a precordial or suprasternal stethoscope.

2. During deep sedation and general anesthesia, clinical signs, including chest excursion, auscultation of breath sounds, and movement of the reservoir bag on the gas machine, must be continuously monitored.
3. During endotracheal anesthesia, breath sounds and chest excursion must be verified after intubation and monitored continually. The use of a capnograph to measure carbon dioxide levels is encouraged.*

Standard IV: Circulation

During the anesthesia period, the circulation and its related organ (e.g., heart) should be evaluated.

Objectives

Adequate perfusion of blood must be maintained to permit the exchange of oxygen from the blood to the tissues and carbon dioxide from the tissues to the blood.

Methods

1. When conscious sedation is being used, a blood pressure reading should be made before its use and after its use before discharge.
2. A blood pressure device must be used to continually monitor systolic and diastolic pressure during deep sedation and general anesthesia. The pulse rate should be measured by either peripheral palpation or by mechanical devices. Both the pulse and blood pressure should be properly recorded at regular intervals during deep sedation and general anesthesia.
3. The electrocardiogram should be used to continuously display cardiac rhythm during deep sedation* and must be used during general anesthesia throughout the anesthesia period.

Standard V: Body Temperature

During the anesthesia period, the patient's body temperature may need to be evaluated.

Objective

Body temperature should be maintained at or as near to normal as possible. Certain types of anesthetic agents are more commonly associated with excessive body temperature changes. Low body temperatures, although generally less likely to develop during dental or office-type anesthesia, may cause a delay in drug metabolism and patient recovery. High body temperatures may cause a hypermetabolic state and increase oxygen consumption.

Methods

1. An enteral or transcutaneous device should be readily available to monitor body temperature during or after general anesthesia.
2. During general anesthesia, when anesthetic agents that are frequently implicated in malignant hyperthermia (e.g., depolarizing muscle relaxants and volatile gaseous agents) are used, monitoring body temperature continually is encouraged.

Terminology

Anesthesia period: Period of time beginning with placement of a needle, mask, or solution into or onto the body until patient has regained sufficient reflexes to be transferred to the recovery area

Conscious sedation: A minimally depressed level of consciousness that retains the patient's ability to maintain the airway independently and continuously and to respond appropriately to physical stimulation and verbal command; produced by pharmacologic and nonpharmacologic methods, alone or in combination

Continual: Repeated regularly and frequently in steady succession

Continuous: Prolonged without any interruption at any time

Deep sedation: A controlled state of depressed consciousness, accompanied by partial loss of protective reflexes, including inability to respond purposefully to verbal command; produced by pharmacologic or nonpharmacologic methods, alone or in combination

Enteral: A route of drug administration in which the drug is placed directly into the gastrointestinal tract, from which absorption occurs across the entire membrane; includes oral and rectal administration

General anesthesia: A controlled state of unconsciousness accompanied by partial or complete loss of protective reflexes, including inability to maintain an airway independently and to respond purposefully to physical stimulation or verbal command; produced by a pharmacologic or nonpharmacologic method, alone or in combination

May or could: Indicates freedom or liberty to follow a suggested alternative

Parenteral: A route of administration of a drug in which the agent passes by the gastrointestinal tract; includes injections, inhalation, and topical routes

Qualified personnel: Persons with training and credentials to perform specific tasks

Regional anesthesia: Elimination of sensations, especially pain, in one part of the body by topical application or local injection of a drug

Shall or must: Indicates imperative need and/or duty: an indispensable item; mandatory

Should: Indicates the recommended manner to obtain the standard; highly desirable

TABLE 5-1 Arteries Employed for Pulse Determination

Artery	Location
Radial	Ventrolateral wrist
Brachial	Medial antecubital fossa
Carotid	Groove between trachea and sternocleidomastoid muscle in neck
Labial	Upper lip
Facial	Cheek
Superficial temporal	Anterior to tragus of ear

present but the radial pulse is absent, it can be stated that (barring anatomic anomalies) the systolic blood pressure is greater than 70 mm Hg (brachial) but less than 80 mm Hg (appearance of radial). This technique is used almost exclusively in emergency situations in which a blood pressure monitoring apparatus is not immediately available or in which it is impossible to hear the sounds produced.

Pulse monitors provide a continuous measurement of the heart rate. These devices usually involve a simple electromechanical or optical transducer that is placed on a patient's fingertip or earlobe. A photoelectric beam is interrupted by the flow of blood through the finger following each contraction of the heart. This interruption produces a visual and/or audio signal.

In addition to their primary function(s), many monitoring devices such as the pulse oximeter, automatic vital signs monitor, and the electrocardiograph (ECG) also measure the heart rate. Either a digital display or a graph on the oscilloscope is provided. Recommendations for heart rate monitoring are found in Tables 5-2 and 5-3.

Blood Pressure

The technique of recording blood pressure is presented in Chapter 4. Monitoring blood pressure is

TABLE 5-2 Recommended Monitoring for Adult Patients

	Technique															*General anesthesia*					
Monitor	Local Anesthesia			Oral			IM/IN			Inhalation			IV			Outpatient			Inpatient		
	Pr	*In*	*Po*	*Pr*	*In*	*Po*	*Pr*	*In*	*Po*	*Pr*	*In*	*Po*	*Pr*	*In*	*Po*	*Pr*	*In*	*Po*	*Pr*	*In*	*Po*
Heart rate	**	0	*	**	0	*	**	**	**	**	**	**	**	**	**	**	**	**	**	**	**
								q5min			q5min			Cont.			Cont.			Cont.	
Blood pressure	**	*	*	**	*	*	**	**	**	**	*	**	**	**	**	**	**	**	**	**	**
								q5min			q5min			q5min			q5min			q5min	
ECG	0	0	0	0	0	0	*	*	0	0	0	0	*	*	*	**	**	**	**	**	**
Respiration	**	0	0	**	0	0	**	**	**	**	*	**	**	**	**	**	**	**	**	**	**
	V			V			V	PT	V	V	V	V	V	PT	V	V	PT	V	V	PT/E	V
Oximetry	0	0	0	0	*	0	*	**	**	0	0	0	*	**	**	**	**	**	**	**	**
Temperature	*	0	0	*	0	0	*	0	0	*	0	0	*	0	0	**	*	*	**	**	*

0, Not essential; *, optional; **, recommended; *Pr*, preoperative; *In*, intraoperative; *Po*, postoperative; *Cont.*, continuous; *V*, visual; *PT*, pretracheal stethoscope; *E*, esophageal stethoscope

HEART RATE: Heart rate may be monitored by palpation in both the preoperative and postoperative periods; however, it is suggested that when the heart rate is monitored intraoperatively, an electrical monitor providing a continuous reading be used. Devices such as the pulse meter, pulse oximeter, capnograph, and ECG provide continuous heart rate monitoring.

BLOOD PRESSURE (BP): When the recommendation for monitoring BP is **, I suggest the BP cuff be kept on the patient's arm throughout the entire procedure.

ELECTROCARDIOGRAPH (ECG): The ECG provides continuous monitoring of the electrical activity of the heart and the heart rate.

RESPIRATION: Visual monitoring implies a casual observation of the movements of the patient's chest for 30 to 60 seconds. PT, pretracheal stethoscope, provides instantaneous evaluation of breath sounds as well as respiratory rate. E, the esophageal stethoscope, is inserted into the esophagus during general anesthesia, providing excellent sound quality for both heart and lung sounds.

OXIMETRY: Oximetry provides continuous monitoring of arterial oxygen saturation.

TEMPERATURE: Preoperative temperature monitoring may be done manually, but if intraoperative monitoring of body temperature is required, it is more readily achieved continuously via a rectal or esophageal probe.

TABLE 5-3 Recommended Monitoring for Pediatric Patients

	Technique															*General anesthesia*					
Monitor	Local Anesthesia			Oral			IM/IN			Inhalation			IV			Outpatient			Inpatient		
	Pr	*In*	*Po*	*Pr*	*In*	*Po*	*Pr*	*In*	*Po*	*Pr*	*In*	*Po*	*Pr*	*In*	*Po*	*Pr*	*In*	*Po*	*Pr*	*In*	*Po*
Heart rate	**	0	*	**	**	**	**	**	**	**	**	**	**	**	**	**	**	**	**	**	**
					Cont.			Cont.			Cont.			Cont.			Cont.			Cont.	
Blood pressure	**	*	*	**	**	**	**	**	**	**	**	**	**	**	**	**	**	**	**	**	**
					q5min			q5min			q5min			q5min			q5min			q5min	
ECG	0	0	0	0	0	0	*	*	0	0	0	0	*	*	*	**	**	**	**	**	**
Respiration	**	0	0	**	**	**	**	**	**	**	**	**	**	**	**	**	**	**	**	**	**
	V			V	PT		V	PT	V	V	V/PT	V	V	PT	V	V	PT	V	V	PT/E	V
Oximetry	0	0	0	**	**	**	*	**	**	0	0	0	*	**	**	**	**	**	**	**	**
Temperature	*	0	0	*	0	0	*	*	*	*	0	0	*	*	*	**	**	**	**	**	**

Refer to footnotes to Table 5-2.

the second method, along with the heart rate and rhythm, of determining the status of a patient's cardiovascular system. Blood pressure levels should be determined on a routine basis for all potential patients as a part of their pretreatment physical evaluation. For adult patients a blood pressure of 200 mm Hg systolic or 115 mm Hg diastolic or higher represents an ASA IV risk, requiring medical consultation and management *before* the start of elective dental or surgical care. Blood pressure values for younger patients will vary, being somewhat lower than usual adult values. Table 4-5 presents representative blood pressures for children.

Patients with an ASA I blood pressure determination at their first office visit have their blood pressure rechecked every 6 months when their medical history is updated or on those occasions when the planned treatment necessitates the administration of drugs such as sedatives and/or local anesthetics. Blood pressure should be monitored and recorded before, and in some cases after, drug administration.

Whenever conscious sedation techniques are used, particularly those in which more profound levels of CNS depression are obtainable, such as the parenteral techniques (IM, SM, IV), blood pressure must be monitored more frequently. Specifically, it is recommended that blood pressure be recorded immediately after the administration of any drug and then at least every 15 minutes for the duration of the procedure. The deeper the level of sedation and the less able the patient is to respond appropriately to verbal command, the greater the requirement is for blood pressure monitoring. During deep sedation and general anesthesia, blood pressure is monitored and recorded every 5 minutes.

Several methods exist to monitor blood pressure. The preferred method involves auscultation through the use of a stethoscope and sphygmomanometer (blood pressure cuff). The blood pressure cuff is applied to the patient's upper arm and left in place throughout the procedure. It should be placed on the arm closest to the person assigned to monitor the blood pressure (assistant or doctor). However, where an IV infusion is in place, the blood pressure cuff should, whenever possible, be placed on the opposite arm to prevent a temporary occlusion of the IV line whenever the cuff is inflated. The same is true where a pulse oximeter is being used. Inflation of the blood pressure cuff will temporarily occlude blood flow through the finger, and the pulse oximeter alarm will be activated.

In some situations, particularly with markedly obese individuals, it may be extremely difficult, if not impossible, to determine blood pressure accurately by auscultation. If this is the case, a palpatory blood pressure may be used. After locating the radial artery in the wrist, the examiner should rapidly inflate the blood pressure cuff until the pulse disappears, continuing to inflate for an additional 20 to 30 mm Hg. While keeping his or her fingers over the radial artery, the examiner slowly decreases the pressure in the cuff until a pulse is felt. A relatively accurate systolic blood pressure may be obtained in this manner; however, no diastolic pressure is obtainable. When this technique is used, a note should be entered in the anesthesia record, such as BP: 130 mm Hg (palpation).

Blood pressure may also be monitored by automatic devices. Some devices simply require the inflation of the blood pressure cuff, after which the cuff's deflation is automatic. Pressure is released slowly, and auditory (beeping) and visual (flashing light) monitors announce the systolic and diastolic pressure (and in many cases the heart rate too). Digital readouts are available on most of these devices, and many also provide a printed record. Until recently, the accuracy of many of these devices was suspect. For these devices to provide accurate readings, the sensor (equivalent to a stethoscope head) had to be placed precisely over the brachial artery and the patient had to sit still. Any extraneous movement produced erroneous measurements. The most accurate automatic blood pressure monitoring equipment costs several thousand dollars (United States). In recent years second-generation devices have appeared that are significantly more reliable than the earlier models. In addition, the cost of these instruments has become more reasonable. Most of the newer blood pressure monitors can be programmed to record blood pressure at regular intervals (e.g., every 30 seconds, every 2 minutes, every 4 minutes). Some devices combine several functions. The device shown in Figure 5-2 integrates blood pressure, heart rate, ECG, oxygen saturation, and temperature into one unit.

Yet another means of monitoring blood pressure is through the direct cannulation of an artery. The level of accuracy obtained with this method is unsurpassed by any noninvasive technique previously discussed. The need for this degree of accuracy in blood pressure monitoring during outpatient conscious sedation and general anesthetic procedures is not great considering the limitations we impart on the type of patients treated as outpatients. Indirect techniques of blood pressure monitoring prove quite adequate for ASA I, II, and III patients. Direct monitoring of arterial blood pressure is indicated both in general anesthetic procedures involving a greater degree of risk (e.g., neurosurgery, cardiac surgery) and when the degree of risk presented by the patient (ASA IV or V) is significant. Recommendations for monitoring blood pressure during various techniques of sedation and general anesthesia are found in Tables 5-2 and 5-3.

Electrocardiography

The ECG (Figure 5-3) monitors both the heart rate and rhythm and provides warning of the development of changes in the electrical activity of the myocardium. Although 12 leads may be used, standard lead I (right arm → left arm) or lead II (right arm → left leg) are most commonly used during anesthesia because they permit excellent detection of dysrhythmias.

Use of the ECG as a tool for monitoring during dental, surgical, and anesthetic procedures has increased dramatically since the 1970s. With the availability of clip-on wrist leads (Figure 5-4), the ease with which the ECG may be employed has greatly increased its value in many procedures. A number of textbooks on basic electrocardiography are available and enable the reader to become proficient at interpreting ECG tracings.[23] Normal sinus rhythm is illustrated in Figure 5-5.

Although not recommended for use in all procedures, the ECG does increase one's ability to detect possibly significant changes in the functioning of the myocardium at a time when corrective treatment may usually restore a normal rhythm.

The appearance of dysrhythmias is more likely during general anesthesia than during conscious sedation. Two common causes of dysrhythmias are (1) hypoxia, leading to myocardial ischemia, and (2) endogenous catecholamine release, secondary to inadequate pain

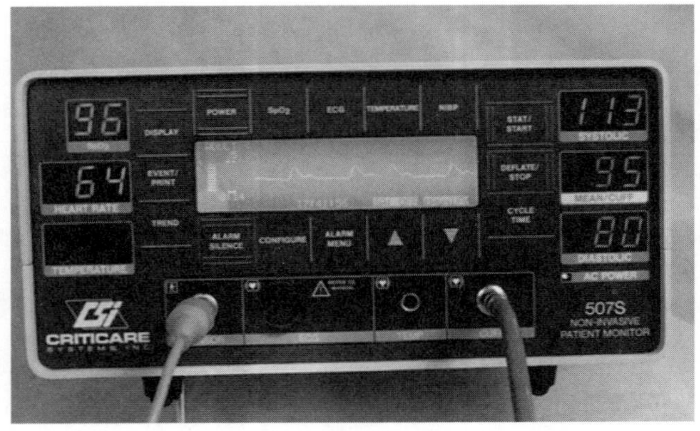

Figure 5-2 Criticare 507 monitor.

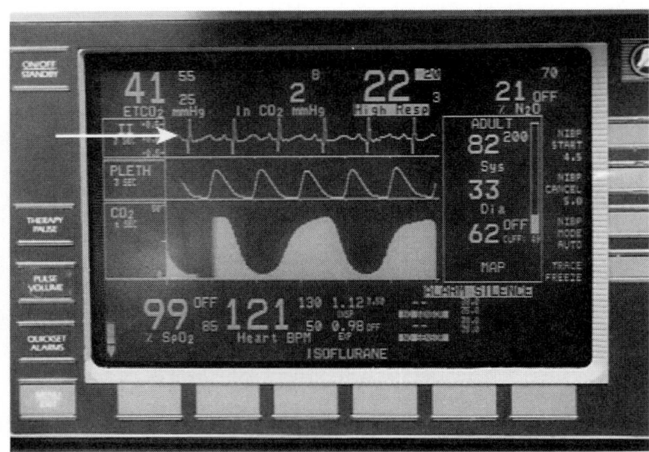

Figure 5-3 Vital signs monitor, includes ECG (*arrow*).

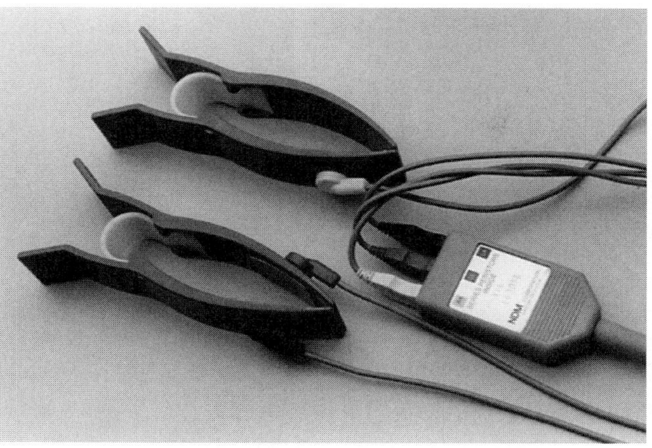

Figure 5-4 Clip-on wrist leads for ECG.

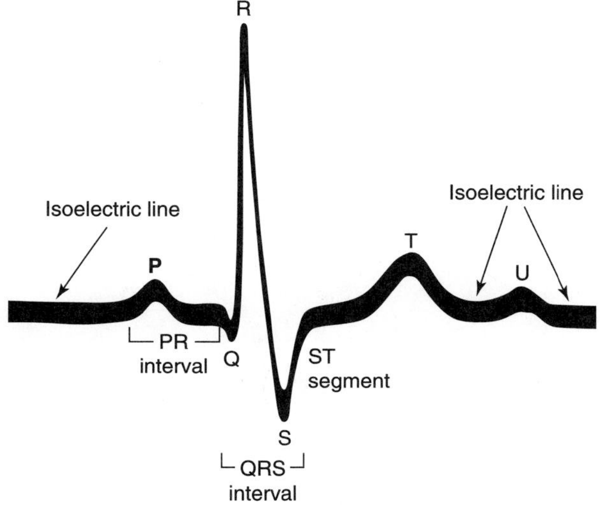

Figure 5-5 Normal electrocardiographic components of the cardiac cycle. (From Phillips RE, Feeney MK: *The cardiac rhythms*, Philadelphia, 1973, WB Saunders.)

control or too light a level of CNS depression. Management of dysrhythmias secondary to these causes, which are usually readily correctable, is done through (1) ensuring airway management and ventilation, (2) providing adequate pain control (e.g., local anesthesia), or (3) increasing the level of anesthesia (greater CNS depression). Recommendations for the use of the ECG during sedation and anesthesia are found in Tables 5-2 and 5-3.

Respiration

Of at least equal, if not greater, importance than monitoring cardiovascular function during sedative and general anesthetic procedures is monitoring respiratory status. Because the drugs used to provide conscious sedation or general anesthesia are CNS and respiratory depressants to a greater degree than they are cardiovascular depressants, respiratory changes are usually observed well before cardiovascular changes. Alterations in cardiac rhythm (dysrhythmias) observed on the ECG in the ASA I or II patient are likely to be produced by myocardial ischemia, which is most often secondary to respiratory depression or inadequate ventilation produced by the drugs that have been administered.

Over the years I have become adamant in my advocacy of respiratory monitoring as an imperative during parenteral conscious and deep sedation and general anesthetic techniques. Morbidities and mortalities have occurred because of respiratory depression (or arrest) that went unrecognized for too long.[24,25] Casual monitoring of respiratory adequacy by observation of the rise and fall of the patient's chest or by observation of the color of oral mucous membranes is unreliable and cannot be recommended as the sole method of monitoring in those techniques in which more profound levels of sedation or the loss of consciousness are possible.[17]

Respiratory adequacy may be crudely monitored by (1) determining the respiratory rate, (2) observing the rise and fall of the chest wall, (3) observing the color of the mucous membranes (oral membranes and fingernail beds), and (4) observing the inflation and deflation of the reservoir bag—if inhalation sedation or oxygen is being administered (and if the patient is breathing through his or her nose, not breathing through the mouth).

It must always be remembered that ***movement of the chest wall*** is not an absolute guarantee of air exchange between the lungs and the external environment. Chest wall movement indicates that a mechanical effort is being made to exchange air and that respiratory arrest has not occurred. The airway may be obstructed (e.g., tongue, foreign body) with no air exchange in the presence of spontaneous respiratory efforts. In addition, respiratory efforts normally indicate that cardiac arrest has not yet occurred because the primary cause of cardiac arrest during conscious sedation and general anesthesia is the occurrence of acute dysrhythmias resulting from ischemia of the myocardium secondary to either respiratory arrest or airway obstruction.

> Respiratory arrest usually occurs before cardiac arrest.

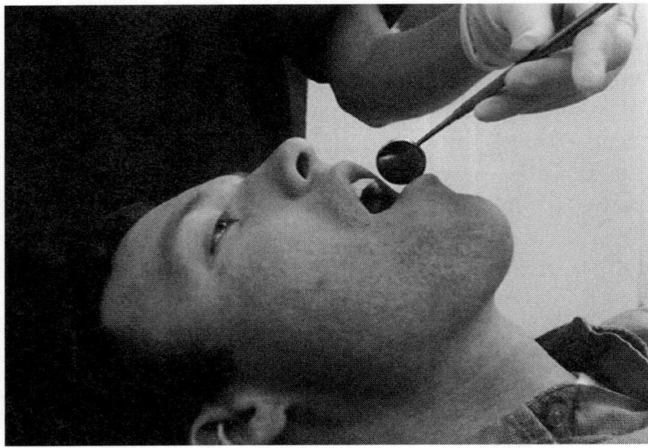

Figure 5-6 Fogging of mirror indicates exchange of air.

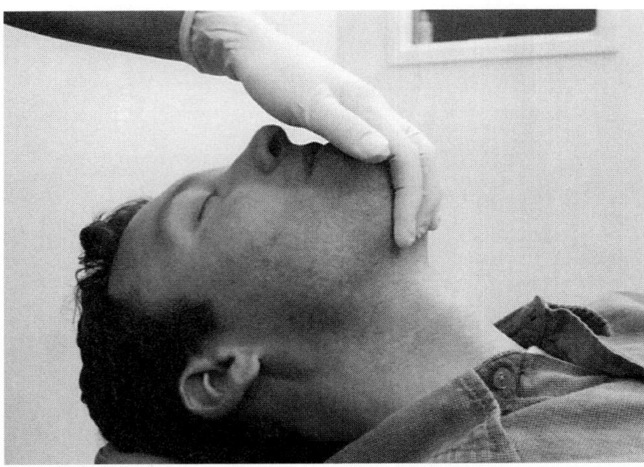

Figure 5-7 Hand held in front of patient's mouth and nose to feel exchange of air.

Observing the ***color of mucous membranes*** as a respiratory monitor is unreliable because cyanosis is not observed until sometime after the patient has become hypoxic. In addition, placement of a rubber dam is indicated during many dental procedures, especially in patients receiving parenteral conscious or deep sedation or general anesthesia. The rubber dam covers the lips and intraoral soft tissues, obviating this as a means of monitoring.

Visualization of the reservoir bag on an inhalation sedation unit or anesthesia machine is a valid method of determining air exchange if an airtight seal of the mask is maintained. The reservoir bag partially deflates during inhalation and reinflates with exhalation. However, if leakage occurs around the sides of the nasal hood or if the patient begins to mouth breathe, the reservoir bag will cease to inflate and deflate during breathing.

While operating in the patient's oral cavity, the doctor, hygienist, or assistant is able to determine if air is being exchanged by the patient. A mirror held in the patient's mouth or in front of his or her nose will fog over if air is being exchanged (Figure 5-6). More effective is holding a hand in front of the patient's mouth and nose so that air is felt on the palm of the hand if exchange of air is occurring (Figure 5-7).

Several excellent and inexpensive devices are available for use in monitoring respiratory function. Two such devices are the precordial/pretracheal stethoscope and the esophageal stethoscope. In addition, these devices provide a means of monitoring heart sounds and rate.

The *precordial/pretracheal stethoscope* is extremely valuable as a monitoring device during both general anesthesia and sedation. A weighted stethoscope head is secured with tape (Figure 5-8) to either the precordial (Figure 5-9) or pretracheal (Figure 5-10) region on the patient's chest. Used as a pretracheal stethoscope, the weighted head is placed in the midline of the neck over the trachea, just superior to the sternal notch. It lies above the lower end of the trachea, at or just slightly above its bifurcation into the right and left mainstem bronchi. Tubing connects this stethoscope to a binaural or monaural (Figure 5-11) earpiece. The custom monaural earpiece is preferred because of its comfort and because it permits the user to carry on normal conversation while continually listening for the sounds associated with the exchange of air. Custom earpieces can usually be obtained from companies that manufacture hearing aids.*

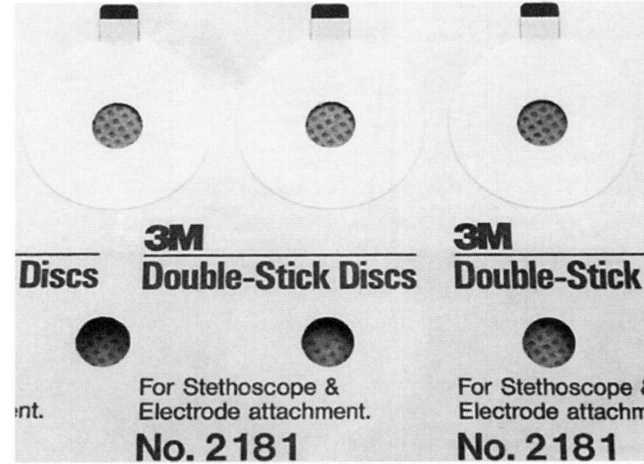

Figure 5-8 Double-sided tape for pretracheal stethoscope.

*Miracle Ear:–1-800-896-6400 (United States), www.miracle-ear.com.

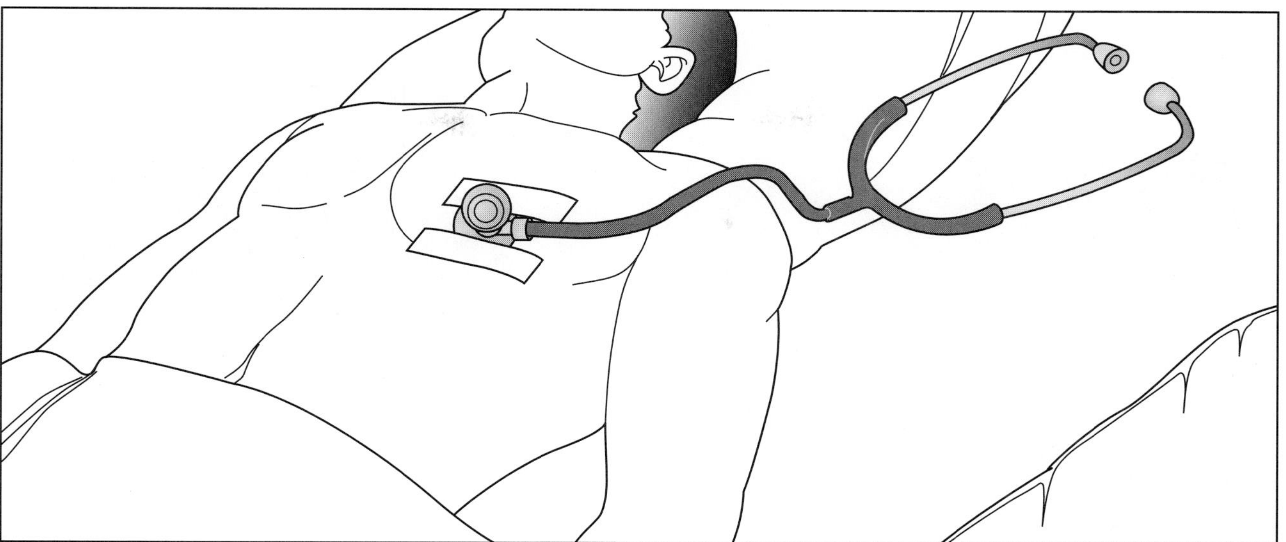

Figure 5-9 Precordial stethoscope provides an excellent monitor of both heart and respiratory sounds. (Redrawn from Dripps RD, Eckenhoff JE, Vandam LD: *Introduction to anesthesia*, ed 3, Philadelphia, 1967, WB Saunders.)

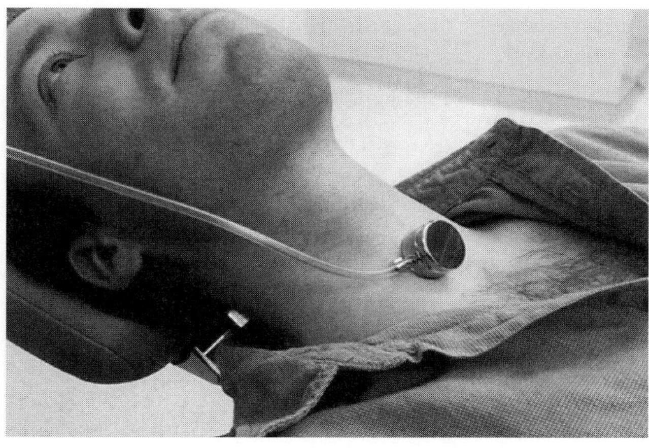

Figure 5-10 Pretracheal stethoscope on patient's neck.

Heart sounds are more easily heard when a weighted stethoscope head is placed in the precordial region, but in some cases heart sounds may overwhelm the more subtle sounds of respiration. Placement in the pretracheal region allows easier recognition of respiratory sounds, but the intensity of heart sounds is diminished. My preference is to place the stethoscope head in the pretracheal region, because my primary goal in the use of this device is to monitor respiration. The weighted stethoscope head is available in adult and pediatric sizes (Figure 5-12). When placed in the pretracheal region with double-sided adhesive discs, the pediatric head is adequate for both children and adults. The heavier adult stethoscope head is often uncomfortable for both children and adults.

The *esophageal stethoscope* is placed into the patient's esophagus through his or her nose or mouth. Heart, as well as breath, sounds will be heard quite well because of the proximity of the stethoscope to the lungs and heart (see Figure 31-13). For obvious reasons, the esophageal stethoscope cannot be used during sedative procedures because the conscious patient is unable to tolerate placement of this tube. The esophageal stethoscope is an extremely valuable monitoring device during general anesthesia. In dental procedures in which a general anesthetic is used, the well-lubricated esophageal stethoscope is inserted through the patient's nose so that it will not interfere with the operative procedure. As with the precordial/pretracheal stethoscope, the esophageal stethoscope may be attached to a monaural custom earpiece or a binaural stethoscope.

When breathing is being monitored, two elements should be considered: (1) the rate of breathing and (2) the sounds of breathing. The ***rate*** in breaths per minute is obtained by counting breaths for 15 or 30 seconds and multiplying by 4 or 2. The most frequent disturbances in respiratory rate are an overly rapid rate (tachypnea) and an unusually slow rate (bradypnea). Tachypnea may indicate the presence of anxiety (e.g., hyperventilation), a pathologic condition (e.g., diabetic acidosis and ketosis), or elevated CO_2 levels, whereas bradypnea is noted after the administration of larger doses of the opioid agonist analgesics (see Chapter 25).

The recognition of abnormal breath sounds is of vital importance. Normal, unobstructed airflow is relatively quiet, a smooth "***whooshing***" sound being

A

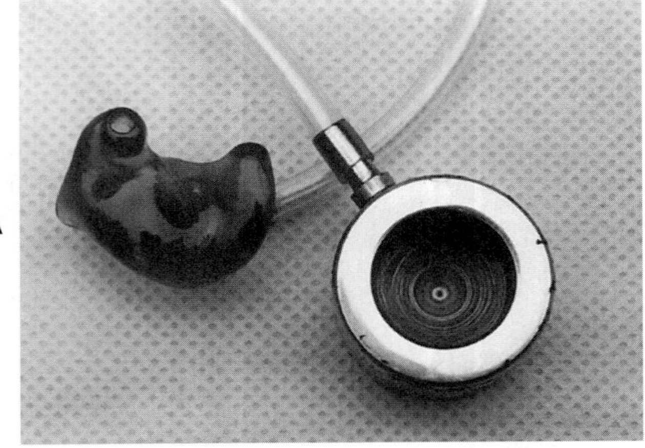

B

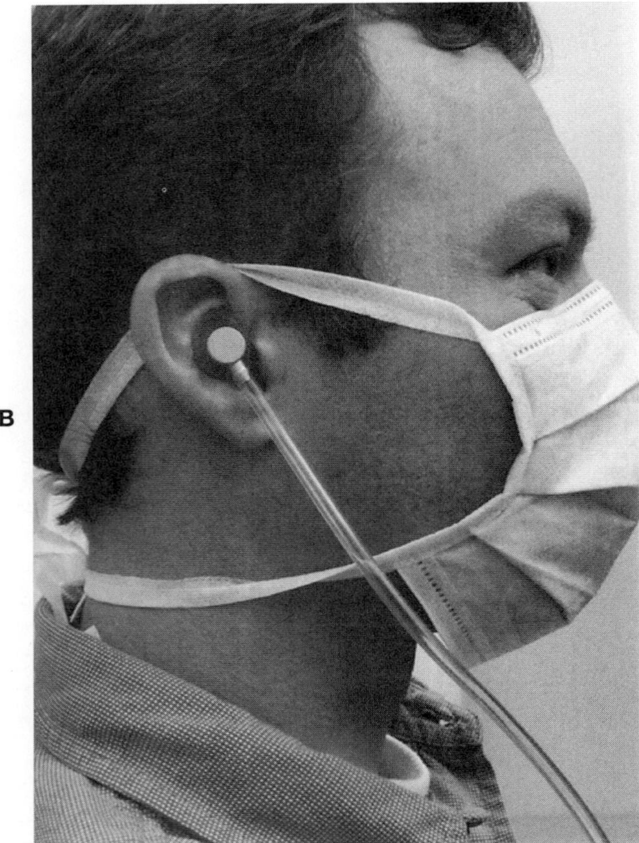

Figure 5-11 **A,** Custom-molded earpiece and pretracheal stethoscope. **B,** Molded earpiece for pretracheal stethoscope.

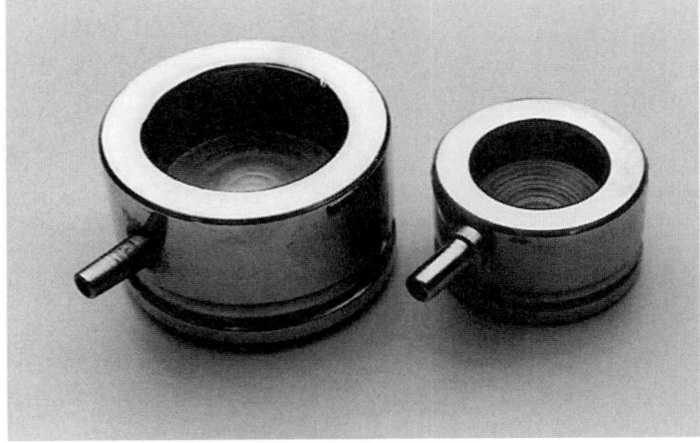

Figure 5-12 Adult *(left)* and pediatric *(right)* weighted stethoscope heads.

heard in the earpiece. The presence of a quiet whooshing sound is indicative of a patent airway and should serve as a comforting influence on the doctor. Silence in the earpiece, on the other hand, is ominous and must trigger an immediate response. Respiratory obstruction (in the presence of exaggerated ventilatory movements) or respiratory arrest (no chest movements) may have developed and must be corrected immediately. Or it may merely be that the stethoscope has become disconnected from the patient! The use of the pretracheal, precordial, or esophageal stethoscope decreases the time required for recognition of this potentially serious problem, allowing corrective measures to start more quickly.

Wheezing indicates partial obstruction in the lower airways (i.e., bronchioles) and is termed *bronchospasm* (see Chapter 34). Management is required, but bronchospasm is not the immediate, acutely life-threatening situation that a total airway obstruction represents. ***Snoring*** or the sound of fluid (a ***gurgling*** sound) indicates the presence of partial obstruction of the upper airway. Snoring most often results when the base of the tongue falls against the posterior wall of the pharynx, whereas the bubbling, gurgling, or crackling sound of fluid indicates the presence of a liquid (i.e., blood, saliva, water, or vomitus) in the airway. Management of snoring requires elevation of the mandible (head-tilt/chin-lift), which lifts the base of the tongue off of the pharyngeal wall.

When foreign matter is present in the airway of a sedated or unconscious patient, three problems may develop: (1) aspiration of foreign matter into the trachea or bronchi, with possible development of infection; (2) obstruction of the airway; and (3) laryngospasm. When the presence of fluid (or other foreign matter) is suspected, immediate management requires suctioning of the posterior pharynx. With removal of this material, normal breath sounds should return. Table 5-4 describes breath sounds and their management. Recommendations for monitoring of respiration during sedative and general anesthetic procedures are found in Tables 5-2 and 5-3.

TABLE 5-4 Causes of Partial Airway Obstruction

Sound Heard	Probable Cause	Management
Snoring	Hypopharyngeal obstruction by the tongue	Repeat head-tilt/chin-lift
Gurgling	Foreign matter (blood, water, vomitus) in airway	Suction airway
Wheezing	Bronchospasm	Bronchodilator (via inhalation, only if conscious; IM, IV if unconscious)
Crowing (high-pitched)	Laryngospasm (partial)	Suction airway; + pressure O_2

Pulse Oximetry

Monitoring breath sounds and the rate of respiration, although important to patient care during sedation and anesthesia, does not provide an absolutely accurate assessment of the adequacy of ventilatory efforts. Clinically unsuspected hypoxemia occurs considerably more frequently than was thought prior to introduction of oximetry.[25-27] In one study, 53% of 296 adults who received anesthesia demonstrated hypoxia (arterial O_2 saturation [Spo_2] 86% to 90%) during routine surgical procedures.[25] Severe hypoxemia (Spo_2 <81%) was detected in 20% of the patients, yet 70% of these episodes were not detected visually by the anesthetist. McKay and Noble[26] found that 6% of a series of 5000 patients who received anesthetic involved critical incidents, 29 of which involved Spo_2 readings under 75%. Cote et al.,[27] in a single-blind study of 402 pediatric anesthetics, examined the effect of withholding the oximeter and/or capnograph data from the anesthesia team. They identified 59 major desaturation events (Spo_2 <85% for >30 seconds) in 43 patients and 130 minor desaturations (Spo_2 <95% for >60 seconds). Of the 43 major events, 41% were first diagnosed by the oximeter, 13 by the anesthesiologist, and 5 by the capnograph. The authors conclude that "the pulse oximeter is far superior to either the capnograph or clinical judgment in providing the earliest warning of desaturation events."[27] It is thus apparent that monitoring of the blood gases (oxygen [O_2] and CO_2) provides more accurate analysis of the effectiveness of ventilation during anesthesia and sedation.

Until recently, determination of arterial O_2 and CO_2 levels necessitated invasive techniques that were potentially uncomfortable for the patient and that required technical skill, the availability of expensive equipment, and the expenditure of considerable time. Such techniques were, and are, used during major surgical procedures or on high-risk patients, but their use during outpatient procedures was essentially unknown.

In outpatient procedures involving parenteral sedation, a knowledge of the oxygen saturation of arterial blood is adequate for clinical purposes, especially in situations in which alveolar ventilation is apt to be constant, as in ASA I, ASA II, and most ASA III patients. A simple noninvasive assessment of arterial oxygenation is clearly advantageous in these situations. The pulse oximeter provides this level of monitoring (Figure 5-13; see also Figure 5-2).

A function of the pulse oximeter—indeed its primary function during sedation and general anesthesia—is the detection and quantification of hypoxemia. Pulse oximeters measure the oxygen saturation of arterial blood. *Oxygen saturation* refers to the amount of oxygen carried by hemoglobin. Expressed as a percentage, oxygen saturation is the amount of oxygen carried compared with the total oxygen-carrying capacity of hemoglobin. Breathing ambient air at sea level, normal Spo_2 is 95%; at an altitude of 5000 feet (e.g., Denver, Colorado), 92%; and at 10,000 feet (e.g., Mexico City, Mexico), approximately 88%.

The pulse oximeter is designed to operate on the assumption that hemoglobin exists in two principal forms in the blood: (1) oxygenated (with O_2 molecules

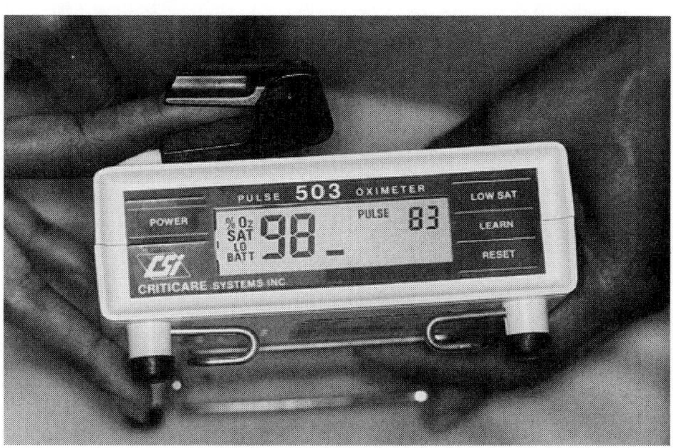

Figure 5-13 Pulse oximeter.

loosely bound) = HbO_2 and (2) reduced (with no O_2 molecules bound) = Hb. Spo_2 is defined as the ratio of oxygenated hemoglobin (HbO_2) to total hemoglobin (HbO_2 + Hb):

$$Spo_2 = \frac{HbO_2}{HbO_2 + Hb}$$

The pulse oximeter measures the absorption of selected wavelengths of light (660 nm and 910 nm or 940 nm) as they pass through living tissue, such as the fingertip, toe, or earlobe (Figure 5-14). HbO_2 and Hb absorb these wavelengths of light to differing degrees. The relative percentages of these two hemoglobins are calculated within the oximeter, and the Spo_2 is displayed on the screen.[28]

The pulse oximeter allows the setting of parameters for all monitored functions (Spo_2, heart rate) above and below which both an audible and visual alarm is triggered (e.g., <90% Spo_2, <50 or >120 beats per minute heart rate). The accuracy of pulse oximeters varies from unit to unit,[29,30] but in general, the statement by manufacturers of oximeters that the devices are accurate within ±3% at Spo_2 values greater than 70% has been confirmed.[31-34] Various other factors, such as the presence of ambient light reaching the sensor,[35] skin pigmentation,[36] the presence of nail polish or acrylic nails,[37] vasoconstriction of the skin due to cold,[38] and motion artifact,[39] may induce error into the observed reading. In 63 dental visits, 87% to 90% of the 235 desaturation episodes recorded were due to patient movement.[39] In addition, although the response of the oximeter to changes in arterial oxygen saturation is ever more rapid than direct visualization of mucous membranes, there is a time lag between change in respiratory function (e.g., the onset of acute airway obstruction) and its detection by the oximeter. This time lag varies with the placement of the probe (finger, toe), from oximeter to oximeter,[40] and with the temperature of the extremity on which the probe is located.[41] It is estimated that the time lag averages between 20 and 60 seconds on a typical pulse oximeter, using the finger as the site of monitoring.[42]

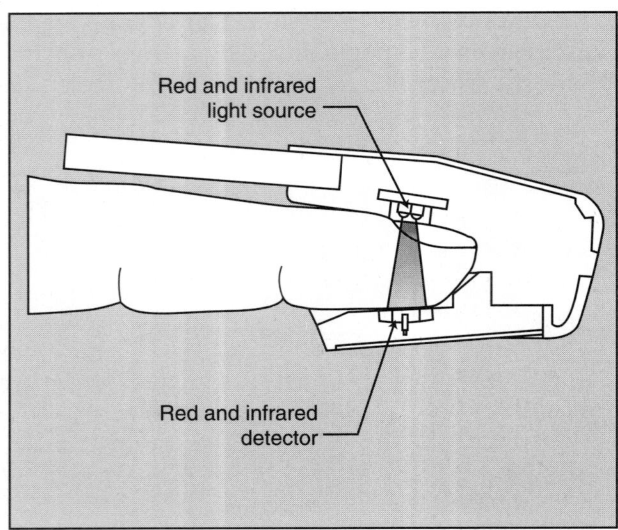

Figure 5-14 Pulse oximeter measures wavelengths of light passing through finger.

Use of pulse oximetry has become the standard of care during general anesthesia, whether for inpatients or outpatients.[4,8,17] Pulse oximetry is also standard of care during ultralight general anesthesia[11] and deep sedation.[12] Although pulse oximetry is highly recommended for conscious sedation, its use is not, at present, the standard of care.[17] In my own practice, I consider the pulse oximeter to be an essential part of the armamentarium for all parenteral sedation cases. Where state regulation governs the administration of oral sedative drugs to pediatric patients, use of pulse oximetry is mandated.[43] Used in conjunction with the pretracheal stethoscope, pulse oximetry permits respiratory function of the sedated or anesthetized patient to be accurately and continuously evaluated, adding a level of increased safety to the procedure.

Does pulse oximetry increase patient safety during anesthesia? Severinghaus[28] concluded that "pulse oximetry *probably* did contribute to the increasing safety of anesthesia. In one sense, however, this change may have come through the device's educational role in promoting vigilance and awareness of inadequacies in technique."

Carbon Dioxide Monitoring

Noninvasive CO_2 monitors have been developed and have become increasing popular.[44] Using the principle of infrared absorption, these devices monitor the levels of inspired and end-tidal CO_2, providing visual displays as a percentage (%) or millimeters of mercury (mm Hg). Response of the CO_2 monitor is virtually instantaneous, assessing every breath taken by the patient (Figure 5-15).[45] Arterial oxygen saturation and respiratory rate are also provided. Audible and visual alarms alert the operator if end-tidal CO_2 values are less than or greater than the selected parameters (<23 mm Hg, or 3%; >51 mm Hg, or 6.5%) or if apnea occurs. When nitrous oxide (N_2O) is administered concurrently, the percentage of N_2O is also displayed. Although still not in common use in outpatient conscious sedation, end-tidal CO_2 monitoring has become increasingly recommended in outpatient general anesthesia[46] because it provides yet another noninvasive means of increasing the safety of our patients. With the

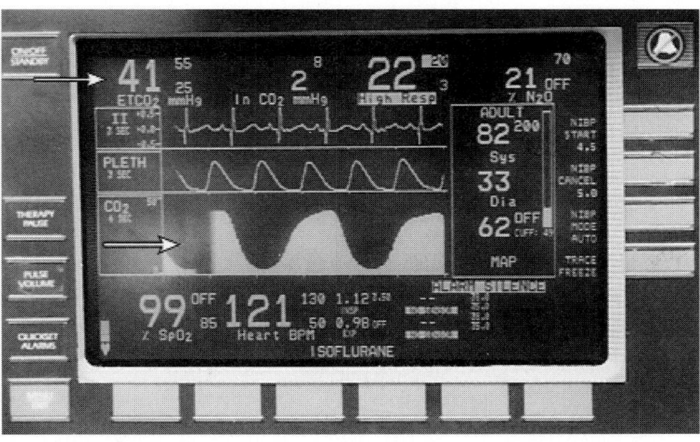

Figure 5-15 Vital signs monitor, includes CO_2 *(arrows)*.

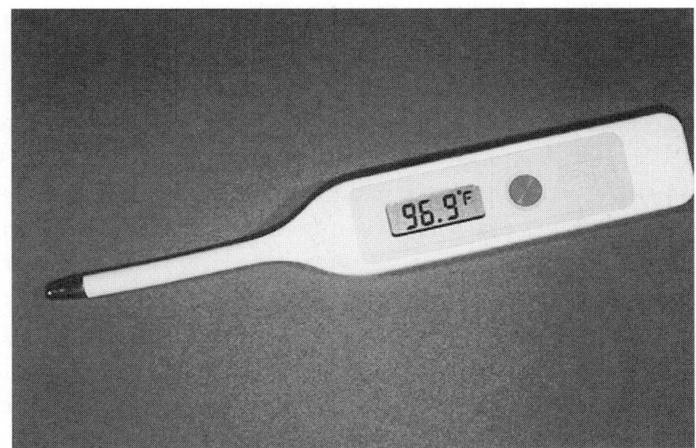

Figure 5-16 Digital thermometer.

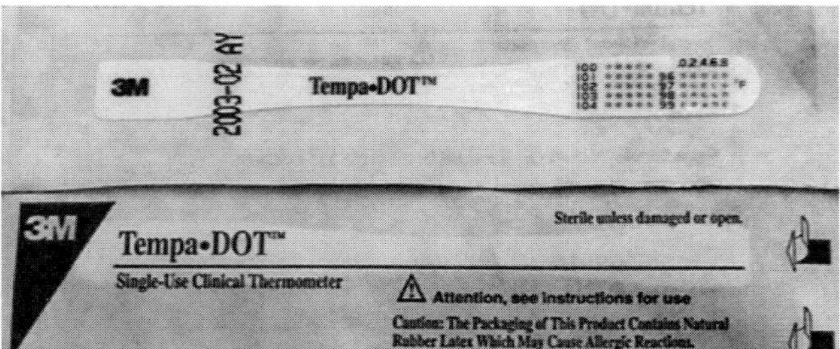

Figure 5-17 Disposable thermometer.

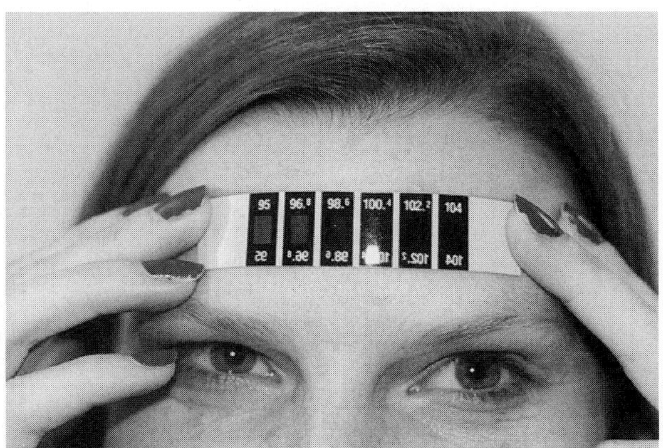

Figure 5-18 Forehead thermometer.

development of future generations of CO_2 monitors, their use during conscious sedation, deep sedation, and general anesthesia in outpatients is likely to increase.

Temperature

Monitoring of the patient's body temperature during parenteral sedation is not usually as critical as are the cardiovascular and respiratory parameters already discussed. However, it is important to determine whether a patient has elevated temperature before the start of the planned treatment. Fever increases the workload of the cardiovascular and respiratory systems. Heart rate increases with an increase in body temperature, as does respiratory rate. The patient's ability to tolerate stress decreases.

Temperature is most often monitored orally or rectally. In the dental office the most practical method of routinely monitoring temperature is the oral route. Nondisposable thermometers may be used, as may disposable units. When a nondisposable thermometer is employed, it is placed in the sublingual area for 3 to 5 minutes before reading the temperature. The patient should not have had any hot or cold liquids or foods in his or her mouth immediately before temperature monitoring. Digital, nondisposable thermometers are also available, providing a rapid assessment of body temperature (Figure 5-16). Disposable thermometers using a system of chemicals that melt and recrystallize at specific temperatures have made the monitoring of temperature extremely simple and sanitary. When the unit is placed sublingually, the dots change color, within approximately 30 seconds, according to the patient's temperature (Figure 5-17). When patient compliance is lacking and it is desirable to record the temperature preoperatively, a forehead thermometer may be used, being held firmly against the dry forehead for about 15 seconds. Color changes in the strips occur, indicating the patient's temperature. Because forehead temperatures are lower than oral temperatures, the forehead thermometer has been adjusted to accommodate this difference (of about 4.5° F, or 2.5° C) (Figure 5-18).

Invasive monitors of body temperature during general anesthesia are available. Probes monitoring rectal or esophageal temperature are most often employed.

The esophageal temperature probe is frequently included as a part of the esophageal stethoscope.

The importance of monitoring temperature intraoperatively during general anesthesia is based on the need to prevent severe hypothermia, which develops as body heat is dissipated during abdominal and thoracic surgery, and to monitor the possible development of malignant hyperthermia (hyperpyrexia), a serious complication during general anesthesia. Monitoring of the body temperature is a standard of care in pediatric general anesthesia.[4,8] Tables 5-2 and 5-3 present my recommendations for monitoring of body temperature during sedation and general anesthesia.

Other Monitoring Devices and Techniques

Other monitoring devices and techniques are available. However, the necessity of using them during the typical outpatient procedure on an ASA I, II, or III patient in the dental or medical office environment is questionable.

These additional procedures include monitoring of *central venous pressure* (CVP) as a measure of right-side heart filling pressures as a guide to intravascular volume. A high CVP indicates circulatory overload (as in CHF), whereas a low CVP indicates reduced blood volume. Monitoring CVP necessitates the passage of a catheter from either the subclavian or the internal jugular vein approximately 10 to 15 cm to the junction of the superior and inferior venae cava and the right atrium. CVP monitoring is not recommended for use in the ASA I, II, or III patients undergoing "elective" treatment under general anesthesia.

The level of CNS depression may be monitored through the use of the (noninvasive) *electroencephalogram* (EEG). Predictable changes are noted in the EEG with different anesthetic agents.[47] The need for EEG monitoring during sedative and most outpatient general anesthetic procedures is minimal, and it is not recommended.

Before reviewing the various techniques of sedation and general anesthesia with recommendations for monitoring for each, it must be emphasized that the most important system to monitor is the CNS, the one which is targeted for depression in our techniques. Therefore the most important technique of patient monitoring during any conscious sedation technique remains direct communication between the patient and the doctor. The ability of the sedated patient to respond *appropriately* to command is an integral part of the definition of consciousness presented in Chapter 2. Lack of such an appropriate response is a call for immediate action to determine (and correct) the cause of the lack of response. Direct communication with the patient is a means of determining the level of functioning of the CNS. Because virtually all drugs used in conscious sedation and/or general anesthesia act primarily by depressing the CNS (this is, in fact, their raison d'être), it is appropriate that the importance of monitoring the CNS be recognized. Monitoring of the respiratory and cardiovascular systems, although important, is considered secondary to CNS monitoring during conscious sedation (e.g., oral benzodiazepine or N_2O-O_2 inhalation sedation). As the level of CNS depression increases in moderate to deep sedation, the patient's ability to respond appropriately is increasingly diminished, warranting an intensification of monitoring of "other systems"—respiratory and cardiovascular. Generalizing to a slight degree, most drugs used during conscious sedation and general anesthesia (CNS depressants) depress breathing to a greater degree—at sedative doses—than they depress the cardiovascular system; thus my emphasis on more intensive monitoring of respiratory function than of the cardiovascular system during sedation. With the loss of consciousness, however, effective communication with the patient is lost and the doctor must rely solely on respiratory and cardiovascular monitoring to assess the patient's clinical status.

Monitoring the pediatric patient proves to be somewhat more difficult if the patient presents a significant management problem. When oral, IN, or IM sedation is to be employed, the patient may be combative, crying, or screaming, making it virtually impossible for the recommended baseline vital signs to be obtained. Although determining these parameters may be difficult or impossible, there actually is little necessity to monitor the vital signs of the patient during the immediate preoperative period when he or she is extremely active, because the patient's baseline vital signs have (hopefully) been recorded at the preoperative visit to the office. Monitoring of the patient, pediatric as well as adult, becomes increasingly more important when the patient, under the influence of the administered CNS depressant drugs, becomes quiescent and cooperative. Once this state is achieved (when dental care can commence), the doctor must become ever more vigilant in monitoring the parameters recommended (CNS, respiratory, cardiovascular). As with the sedated adult patient, monitoring of respiration becomes ever more critical as the level of sedation deepens. Some pediatric sedation techniques include the administration of opioid agonists, often in combination with other CNS depressants. Respiratory depression is a significant concern in these patients. The probability that the unmanageable pediatric patient has been placed into a physical restraint, such as the Pedi-Wrap or papoose board, increases the likelihood of respiratory depression while decreasing the team's ability to monitor respiration. A rubber dam used to isolate the oral cavity may also be in place, restricting mouth breathing as well as hindering visualization of oral mucous membranes. The use of a pretracheal stethoscope and pulse oximeter is therefore considered essential whenever parenteral pediatric sedation or more profound oral sedation is employed.

RECORDKEEPING

A written record must be prepared for each patient during the administration of sedative or anesthetic drugs. Such records serve several purposes:

1. As a trend plot of vital values
2. As an aid to the clinician's memory
3. As documentation of a patient's response to the administration of drugs and the operative procedure
4. Nonclinically, as a legal document

Records maintained for sedative and general anesthetic procedures are essentially identical; however, a basic difference in these records is the frequency and level of monitoring. Figures 5-19 and 5-20 illustrate records available for use in sedation and general anesthesia.

Sedation Record

In the sedation form (see Figure 5-19) patient identification is presented on the top of the record. The upper left portion of the record is a summary of the preoperative evaluation (medical history and baseline vital signs) (Figure 5-21). Intraoperative monitoring and drug administration data are found at the

Patient's Name: S.S. #: Age: DATE ___/___/___

Medical Hx: CVS
Respiratory System
CNS
Liver
Kidneys
Other

Current Medications:

Allergy:

Base Line Vital Signs:
Date of V.S.:
B.P.: P.R.:
R.: T.:
Ht.: Wt.:
Age:

ASA: I, II, III, IV

Reason for Sedation:

Evaluator:

Name of Driver:

IV started at ______ a.m./p.m.
Venipuncture Site______
Type of Needle ______
IV d/c'd at ______ a.m./p.m.
IV solution & Volume______ML

DRUGS ADMINISTERED
– SUMMARY –

DRUGS DISCARDED
– SUMMARY –

PREOPERATIVE time	INTRAOPERATIVE time	time	time	time	time	POST-OP time	DISCHARGE time
Blood Pressure							
Heart Rate							
Respirations							
O_2 LPM							
N_2O LPM							
(mg)							
(mg)							
(mg)							
(mg)							
(mg)							
(mg)							
(mg)							

List all drugs and route of administration (IV, IM)

DENTISTRY TREATMENT

Start ____ Finish ____
Name of person discharged to: ______
Post-Op Medications (if any) ______

Additional Monitoring: *(check as appropriate)*
precordial stethoscope ______ pulse oximeter ______
ECG ______ automatic blood pressure ______

COMMENTS

Student Doctor: ______ AMED Faculty: ______ ☐ Informed Consent
IV Student: ______ Assistants: ______ ☐ Post-Operative Instructions

SAM/USC/SOD
02/85

Figure 5-19 Sedation record.

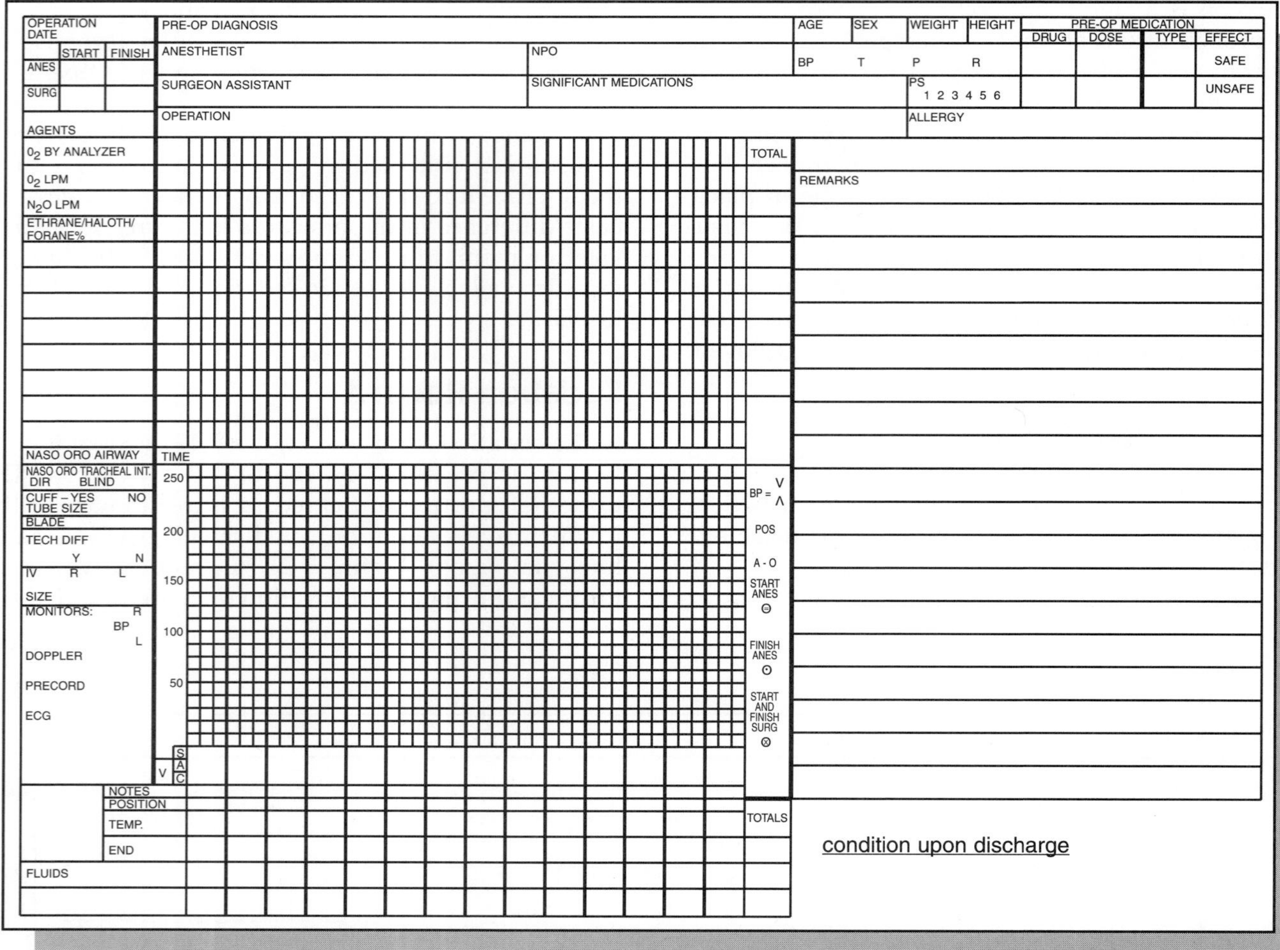

OPERATION DATE | PRE-OP DIAGNOSIS | AGE | SEX | WEIGHT | HEIGHT | PRE-OP MEDICATION: DRUG | DOSE | TYPE | EFFECT
START | FINISH | ANESTHETIST | NPO | BP | T | P | R | SAFE
ANES
SURG | SURGEON ASSISTANT | SIGNIFICANT MEDICATIONS | PS 1 2 3 4 5 6 | UNSAFE
AGENTS | OPERATION | ALLERGY
O_2 BY ANALYZER | TOTAL
O_2 LPM | REMARKS
N_2O LPM
ETHRANE/HALOTH/FORANE%
NASO ORO AIRWAY | TIME
NASO ORO TRACHEAL INT. DIR BLIND | 250 | BP = V Λ
CUFF – YES NO TUBE SIZE
BLADE
TECH DIFF Y N | 200 | POS
IV R L | 150 | A - O
SIZE | START ANES ⊖
MONITORS: BP R L | 100
DOPPLER | FINISH ANES ⊙
PRECORD | 50 | START AND FINISH SURG ⊗
ECG
V | S A C
NOTES
POSITION
TEMP. | TOTALS
END | condition upon discharge
FLUIDS

Figure 5-20 Anesthesia record, which may be used for sedation or general anesthesia.

bottom portion of the chart (Figure 5-22). Time is noted on the top column, and directly below are spaces for recording vital signs and dosages of drugs administered. The names of *all* drugs administered, including local anesthetics, are listed, with the milligram dose or flow rate (liters per minute) of gases placed in the appropriate column. At the conclusion of the procedure the right side of the chart is completed (Figure 5-23), summarizing the drugs administered and discarded, site of needle puncture (if appropriate), fluids administered, dental treatment rendered, and additional comments.

We recommend as a minimum that ***vital signs*** be recorded on the chart:

1. Preoperatively
2. Intraoperatively: after the administration of any drug and every 5 to 15 minutes during treatment
3. Immediately postoperatively
4. Before discharge

Immediately below the operative record, the monitors used during the procedure are identified (see Figure 5-22). Monitoring recommendations are presented in the chapters on specific conscious sedation and general anesthesia techniques. Recommendations for monitoring from the American Dental Society of Anesthesiology are found in Box 5-1.

A summary of the procedure (needles used, IV/IM site, type of IV infusion, and volume administered) and drugs administered is located on the upper right side, immediately below which is a list of total drug doses administered and the amount (milligrams) of drug discarded (see Figure 5-23). The lower right side lists the dental treatment completed, start and finish times, name of the person to whom the patient is discharged (if appropriate), and comments of interest concerning the procedure. The purpose of the comment section is to provide helpful hints that may improve the quality of subsequent sedation procedures on the same patient. For

Patient's Name: JANE DOE S.S. #: 000-00-0000 Age: 15 DATE 7 / 5 / 02

Medical Hx: CVS 0
Respiratory System ASTHMA
CNS 0
Liver 0
Kidneys 0
Other 0

Current Medications: VENTOLIN

Allergy: NKDA

Base Line Vital Signs:
Date of V.S.: 6-30-02
B.P.: 110/66 P.R.: 90
R.: 16 T.: 98.4
Ht.: 5'2 Wt.: 104
Age: 15

ASA: I, (II), III, IV

Reason for Sedation: FEAR & ANXIETY

Evaluator: MALAMED

Name of Driver: MRS. DOE

IV started at ______ a.m./p.m.
Venipuncture Site ______
Type of Needle ______
IV d/c'd at ______ a.m./p.m.
IV solution & Volume ______ ML

DRUGS ADMINISTERED – SUMMARY –

DRUGS DISCARDED – SUMMARY –

PREOPERATIVE time	INTRAOPERATIVE time	time	time	time	time	POST-OP time	DISCHARGE time
Blood Pressure							
Heart Rate							
Respirations							
O_2 LPM							
N_2O LPM							
List all drugs and route of administration (IV, IM) (mg)							
(mg)							
(mg)							
(mg)							
(mg)							
(mg)							
(mg)							

DENTISTRY TREATMENT
Start ____ Finish ____
Name of person discharged to: ______
Post-Op Medications (if any) ______

Additional Monitoring: (check as appropriate) precordial stethoscope ______ ECG ______ pulse oximeter ______ automatic blood pressure ______

COMMENTS

Student Doctor: ______ AMED Faculty: ______ ☐ Informed Consent
IV Student: ______ Assistants: ______ ☐ Post-Operative Instructions

Figure 5-21 Preoperative records for sedation.

example, it might be noted that the only readily apparent site for venipuncture was the right antecubital fossa or that midazolam was somewhat ineffective in producing sedation but changing to diazepam markedly improved the procedure. The doctor then signs the form, which is placed into the patient's dental or medical chart.

General Anesthesia Record

Because the patient receiving general anesthesia is unconscious and unable to respond to verbal or physical stimulation, intensified monitoring is mandatory. As described in the preceding section, the frequency and intensity of monitoring are increased as CNS depression increases. Several vital functions (e.g., heart rate and rhythm, respiration, SaO_2, temperature [and increasingly, end-tidal CO_2]) are monitored continuously, whereas others, including blood pressure, are monitored at intervals of approximately 5 minutes. A typical record used in general anesthesia is presented in Figure 5-20. Each of the small, thin vertical lines is an interval of 5 minutes; the thicker, darker lines represent 15 minutes. Drug administration is listed chronologically, as is the performance of specific procedures, such as the start of anesthesia, the start of surgery (i.e., incision made), specific intraoperative procedures, the termination of surgery, and the termination of anesthesia.

Examples of completed sedation and general anesthesia records are presented in Figures 5-24 and 5-25. The anesthesia record also provides an area for monitoring of the patient during the postoperative period in the anesthesia recovery room.

Recordkeeping is an important aid to the doctor in reconstructing events that occurred during a sedative or general anesthetic procedure. Review of records can provide the doctor with information regarding a patient's prior response to certain drugs or procedures, possibly alerting the doctor to modify treatment or drug therapy at subsequent appointments. In addition, well-kept written documentation

Patient's Name: S.S. #: Age: DATE ___/___/___

Medical Hx: CVS
Respiratory System
CNS
Liver
Kidneys
Other

Current Medications:

Allergy:

IV started at ______ a.m./p.m.
Venipuncture Site______
Type of Needle ______
IV d/c'd at ______ a.m./p.m.
IV solution & Volume______ML

Base Line Vital Signs:
Date of V.S.:
B.P.: P.R.:
R.: T.:
Ht.: Wt.:
Age:

ASA: I, II, III, IV

Reason for Sedation:

Evaluator:

Name of Driver:

DRUGS ADMINISTERED
– SUMMARY –

DRUGS DISCARDED
– SUMMARY –

PREOPERATIVE time 0930	INTRAOPERATIVE 0935 time	0950 time	1005 time	1020 time	time	POST-OP 1025 time	DISCHARGE 1100 time
Blood Pressure 110/64	116/68	110/60	106/58	104/58		108/60	106/58
Heart Rate 88	96	82	84	84		88	84
Respirations / O_2 sat 98	99	98	98	99		98	98
O_2 LPM	4 ———			6			
N_2O LPM	2 ———			1 Ø			
MIDAZOLAM (mg) IV	3						
MEPERIDINE (mg) IV	25						
LIDOCAINE (mg) IM		72					
(mg)							
(mg)							
(mg)							
(mg)							

List all drugs and route of administration (IV, IM)

DENTISTRY TREATMENT

Start ___ Finish ___
Name of person discharged to: ______
Post-Op Medications (if any) ______

Additional Monitoring: (check as appropriate) precordial stethoscope _X_ ECG ___ pulse oximeter _X_ automatic blood pressure _X_

COMMENTS

Student Doctor: ______ AMED Faculty: ______ ☐ Informed Consent
IV Student: ______ Assistants: ______ ☐ Post-Operative Instructions

Figure 5-22 Intraoperative records for sedation.

Patient's Name: S.S. #: Age: DATE ___/___/___

Medical Hx: CVS
Respiratory System
CNS
Liver
Kidneys
Other

Current Medications:

Allergy:

IV started at 0935 (a.m.)/p.m.
Venipuncture Site (R) ANTECUBITAL F.
Type of Needle 21 g CATHETER
IV d/c'd at 1025 (a.m.)/p.m
IV solution & Volume D5(E 130) ML

Base Line Vital Signs:
Date of V.S.:
B.P.: P.R.:
R.: T.:
Ht.: Wt.:
Age:

ASA: I, II, III, IV

Reason for Sedation:

Evaluator:

Name of Driver:

DRUGS ADMINISTERED
– SUMMARY –
MIDAZOLAM 3mg IV
MEPERIDINE 25mg IV
LIDOCAINE 72mg IM (oral)

PREOPERATIVE time	INTRAOPERATIVE time	time	time	time	time	POST-OP time	DISCHARGE time
Blood Pressure							
Heart Rate							
Respirations							
O_2 LPM							
N_2O LPM							
(mg)							
(mg)							
(mg)							
(mg)							
(mg)							
(mg)							
(mg)							

List all drugs and route of administration (IV, IM)

DRUGS DISCARDED
– SUMMARY –
MIDAZOLAM 2mg
MEPERIDINE 25mg

DENTISTRY TREATMENT
Restorative

Start 0955 Finish 1020
Name of person discharged to: MRS DOE
Post-Op Medications (if any) n/a

Additional Monitoring: (check as appropriate) precordial stethoscope ___ ECG ___ pulse oximeter ___ automatic blood pressure ___

COMMENTS
Good veins –
Responds well to midazolam + meperidine

Student Doctor: JONES AMED Faculty: MALAMED ☒ Informed Consent
IV Student: SMITH Assistants: LOPEZ ☒ Post-Operative Instructions

SAM/USC/SOD 02/85

Figure 5-23 Postoperative summary.

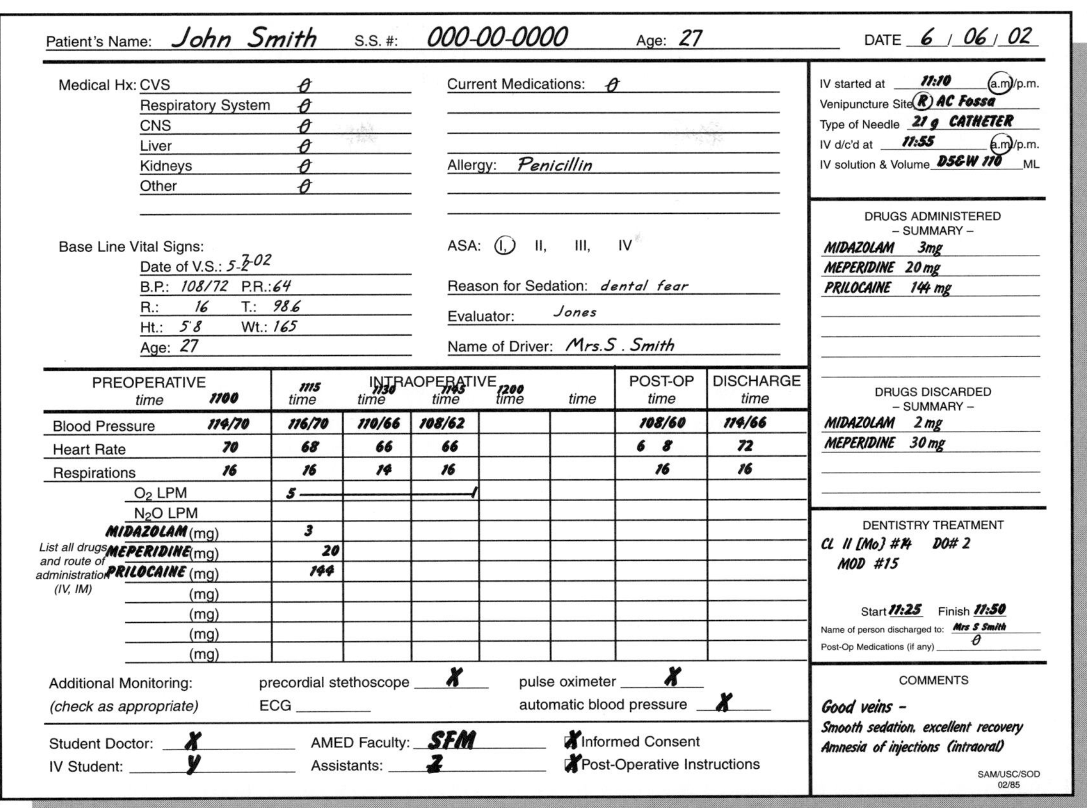

Patient's Name: John Smith S.S. #: 000-00-0000 Age: 27 DATE 6 / 06 / 02

Medical Hx: CVS θ
Respiratory System θ
CNS θ
Liver θ
Kidneys θ
Other θ

Current Medications: θ

Allergy: Penicillin

IV started at 11:10 (a.m.)/p.m.
Venipuncture Site (R) AC Fossa
Type of Needle 21 g CATHETER
IV d/c'd at 11:55 (a.m.)/p.m.
IV solution & Volume D5&W 110 ML

Base Line Vital Signs:
Date of V.S.: 5-7-02
B.P.: 108/72 P.R.: 64
R.: 16 T.: 98.6
Ht.: 5'8 Wt.: 165
Age: 27

ASA: (I), II, III, IV
Reason for Sedation: dental fear
Evaluator: Jones
Name of Driver: Mrs. S. Smith

DRUGS ADMINISTERED – SUMMARY –
MIDAZOLAM 3mg
MEPERIDINE 20 mg
PRILOCAINE 144 mg

	PREOPERATIVE time 1100	INTRAOPERATIVE time 1115	time 1130	time 1145	time 1200	time	POST-OP time	DISCHARGE time
Blood Pressure	114/70	116/70	110/66	108/62			108/60	114/66
Heart Rate	70	68	66	66			68	72
Respirations	16	16	14	16			16	16
O_2 LPM		5 ———	———	———				
N_2O LPM								
MIDAZOLAM (mg)		3						
MEPERIDINE (mg)		20						
PRILOCAINE (mg)		144						
(mg)								
(mg)								
(mg)								
(mg)								

List all drugs and route of administration (IV, IM)

DRUGS DISCARDED – SUMMARY –
MIDAZOLAM 2 mg
MEPERIDINE 30 mg

DENTISTRY TREATMENT
CL II [Mo] #14 DO# 2
MOD #15
Start 11:25 Finish 11:50
Name of person discharged to: Mrs S Smith
Post-Op Medications (if any) θ

Additional Monitoring: (check as appropriate)
precordial stethoscope X pulse oximeter X
ECG ____ automatic blood pressure X

Student Doctor: X AMED Faculty: SFM X Informed Consent
IV Student: Y Assistants: Z X Post-Operative Instructions

COMMENTS
Good veins -
Smooth sedation, excellent recovery
Amnesia of injections (intraoral)

SAM/USC/SOD 02/85

Figure 5-24 Completed sedation record.

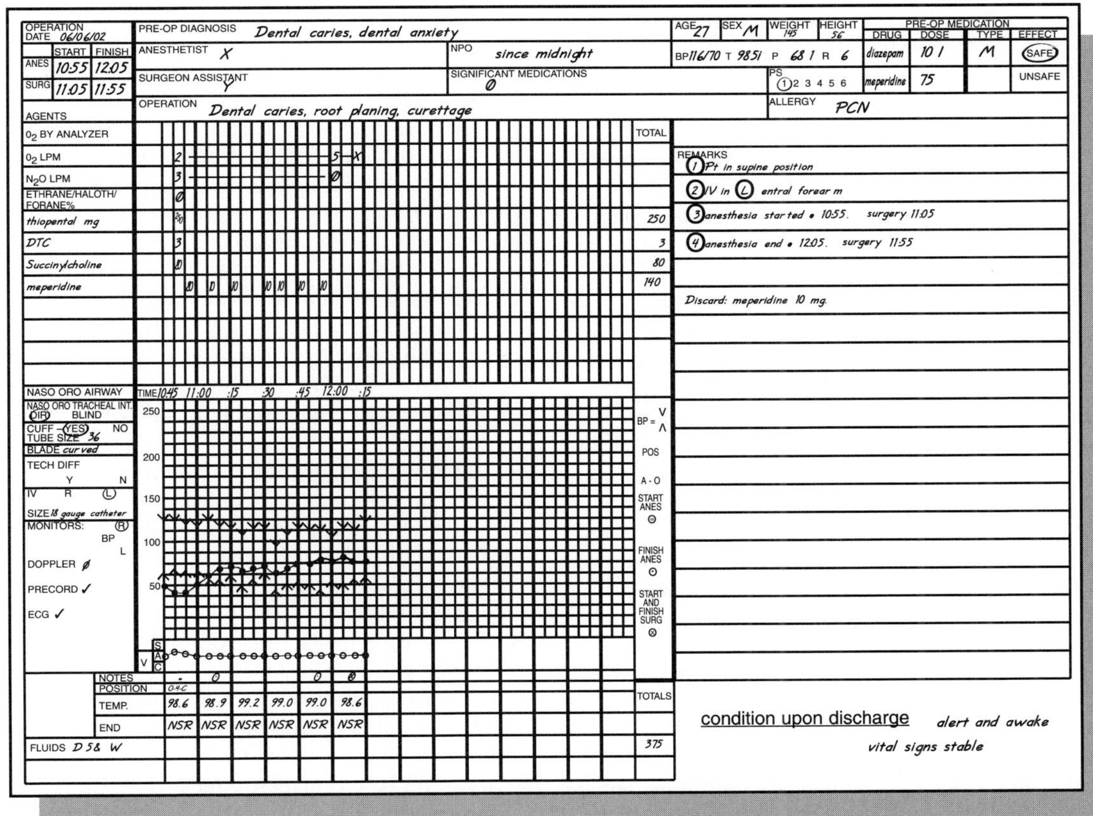

OPERATION DATE 06/06/02
PRE-OP DIAGNOSIS Dental caries, dental anxiety
AGE 27 SEX M WEIGHT 145 HEIGHT 56

	START	FINISH
ANES	10:55	12:05
SURG	11:05	11:55

ANESTHETIST X
NPO since midnight
BP 116/70 T 98.51 P 68 / R 6
SURGEON ASSISTANT Y
SIGNIFICANT MEDICATIONS θ
PS (1) 2 3 4 5 6
OPERATION Dental caries, root planing, curettage
ALLERGY PCN

PRE-OP MEDICATION

DRUG	DOSE	TYPE	EFFECT
diazepam	10 /	M	(SAFE)
meperidine	75		UNSAFE

AGENTS		TOTAL
O_2 BY ANALYZER		
O_2 LPM	2 ——— 5 — X	
N_2O LPM	3 ——— θ	
ETHRANE/HALOTH/FORANE%	θ	
thiopental mg	250	250
DTC	3	3
Succinylcholine	80	80
meperidine	20 10 10 10 10 10 10 10 10 10	140

REMARKS
(1) Pt in supine position
(2) IV in (L) entral forearm
(3) anesthesia started • 10:55. surgery 11:05
(4) anesthesia end • 12:05. surgery 11:55
Discard: meperidine 10 mg.

TIME 10:45 11:00 :15 :30 :45 12:00 :15

NASO ORO AIRWAY
NASO ORO TRACHEAL INT. (OIF) BLIND
CUFF (YES) NO
TUBE SIZE 36
BLADE curved
TECH DIFF Y N
IV R (L)
SIZE 18 gauge catheter
MONITORS: (R) BP L
DOPPLER θ
PRECORD ✓
ECG ✓

BP = V Λ
POS
A - O
START ANES ⊙
FINISH ANES ⊙
START AND FINISH SURG ⊗

NOTES	•	θ			θ	θ
POSITION	0→C					
TEMP.	98.6	98.9	99.2	99.0	99.0	98.6
END	NSR	NSR	NSR	NSR	NSR	NSR

FLUIDS D 5 & W TOTALS 375

condition upon discharge alert and awake vital signs stable

Figure 5-25 Completed anesthesia record.

will greatly assist in a doctor's defense, should a claim be made against the doctor or facility.

Because of the potential value of the written sedation or anesthesia record, it is important that these records not be altered after the fact. In addition, it is essential that these records be kept in ink, not pencil. Should an error or omission be noted after the fact, and it becomes necessary to add, change, or delete something from the written record, a single line should be drawn through the error (without obscuring it, which would only increase suspicion), and the correction entered and initialed. If this occurs at a later date, include both the time and date of the correction. The record should remain with the patient's medical or dental chart as a part of the permanent record.

REFERENCES

1. *Mosby's medical, nursing, & allied health dictionary*, ed 6, St Louis, 2002, Mosby.
2. *Dorland's illustrated medical dictionary,* ed 29, Philadelphia, 2000, WB Saunders.
3. Gravenstein JS, Paulus DA: *Monitoring practice in clinical anesthesia,* Philadelphia, 1982, Lippincott.
4. Eichhorn JH, Cooper JB, Cullen DJ et al: Standards for patient monitoring during anesthesia: Harvard Medical School, *JAMA* 256:1017, 1985.
5. Cooper JB, Newbower RS, Long CD: Preventable anesthesia mishaps: a study of human factors, *Anesthesiology* 49:399, 1978.
6. Keenan R, Bozan CP: Cardiac arrest due to anesthesia, *JAMA* 253:2373, 1985.
7. Emergency Care Research Institute: Death during general anesthesia, *J Health Care Technol* 1:155, 1985.
8. Standards for basic intra-operative monitoring, *ASA Newslett* 50:13, 1986.
9. American Dental Association: Department of State Government Affairs, Chicago, 1987, The Association.
10. American Dental Association: Department of State Government Affairs, Chicago, 1992, The Association.
11. American Dental Association: Department of State Government Affairs, Chicago, 2000, The Association.
12. American Association of Oral and Maxillofacial Surgeons, Committee on Anesthesia: *Office anesthesia evaluation manual,* ed 4, Rosemont, Ill, 1991, The Association.
13. Guidelines for the elective use of conscious sedation, deep sedation, and general anesthesia in pediatric patients, *Pediatr Dent* 7:334, 1985.
14. American Academy of Periodontology, Subcommittee on Anxiety and Pain Control of the Pharmacotherapeutics Committee: *Guidelines for the use of conscious sedation in periodontics,* Chicago, 1990, The Academy.
15. General anaesthesia, sedation and resuscitation in dentistry. Report of an Expert Working Party, prepared for the Dental Advisory Council. London, March 1990.
16. Thompson I: Emergency treatment in Australia, *J Anesth Pain Contr Dent* 1:167, 1992.
17. Rosenberg MB, Campbell RL: Guidelines for intraoperative monitoring of dental patients undergoing conscious sedation, deep sedation, and general anesthesia, *Oral Surg* 71:2, 1991.
18. Krippaehne JA, Montgomery MT: Morbidity and mortality from pharmacosedation and general anesthesia in the dental office, *J Oral Maxillofac Surg* 50:691, 1992.
19. Jastak JT: Discussion: morbidity and mortality from pharmacosedation and general anesthesia in the dental office, *J Oral Maxillofac Surg* 50:698, 1992.
20. Eichhorn JH, Cooper JB, Cullen DJ et al: Anesthesia practice standards at Harvard: a review, *J Clin Anesth* 1:55, 1988.
21. Holzer JF: Liability insurance issues in anesthesiology, *Int Anesthesiol Clin* 27:205, 1989.
22. Lawler PG: Monitoring during general anesthesia. In Gray TC, Nunn JF, Utting JE, eds: *General anesthesia,* London, 1971, Butterworth.
23. Dubin DB: *Rapid interpretation of EKG's,* ed 4, Tampa, Fla, 1989, Cover Publishing.
24. Tiret L, Nivoche Y, Hatton F et al: Complications related to anaesthesia in infants and children: a prospective survey of 40,240 anaesthetics, *Br J Anaesth* 61:263, 1988.
25. Moller JT, Johannessen NW, Berg H et al: Hypoxaemia during anaesthesia: an observer study, *Br J Anaesth* 66:437, 1991.
26. McKay WPS, Noble WH: Critical incidents detected by pulse oximetry during anesthesia, *Can J Anaesth* 35:265, 1988.
27. Cote CJ, Rolf N, Liu LM et al: A single-blind study of combined pulse oximetry and capnography in children, *Anesthesiology* 74:980, 1991.
28. Severinghaus JW, Kelleher JF: Recent developments in pulse oximetry, *Anesthesiology* 76:101, 1992.
29. Severinghaus JW: History and recent developments in pulse oximetry, *Scand J Clin Lab Invest Suppl* 214:105, 1993.
30. Kelleher JF: Pulse oximetry, *J Clin Monit* 5:37, 1989.
31. Ralston AC, Webb RK, Runciman WB: Potential errors in pulse oximetry: I. Pulse oximeter evaluation, *Anaesthesia* 46:202, 1992.
32. Webb RK, Ralston RC, Runciman WB: Potential errors in pulse oximetry: II. Effects of changes in saturation and signal quality, *Anaesthesia* 46:207, 1991.
33. Severinghaus JW, Naifeh KH, Koh SO: Errors during profound hypoxia in 14 pulse oximeters, *J Clin Monit* 5:72, 1989.
34. Taylor MB, Whitwam JG: The accuracy of pulse oximeters: a comparative clinical evaluation of five pulse oximeters, *Anaesthesia* 43:229, 1988.
35. Costarino AT, Davis DA, Keon TP: Falsely normal saturation reading with the pulse oximeter, *Anesthesiology* 67:830, 1987.
36. Ries AL, Prewitt LM, Johnson JJ: Skin color and ear oximetry, *Chest* 96:287, 1989.
37. Cote CJ, Goldstein EA, Fuchsman WH et al: The effect of nail polish on pulse oximetry, *Anesth Analg* 67:683, 1988.
38. Langston JA, Lassey D, Hanning CD: Comparison of four pulse oximeters: effects of venous occlusion and cold-induced peripheral vasoconstriction, *Br J Anaesth* 65:245, 1990.

39. Wilson S: Conscious sedation and pulse oximetry: false alarms? *Pediatr Dent* 12:228, 1990.
40. Mendelson Y: Pulse oximetry: theory and applications for noninvasive monitoring, *Clin Chem* 38:1601, 1992.
41. Severinghaus JW, Spellman MJ Jr: Pulse oximeter failure thresholds in hypotension and ischemia, *Anesthesiology* 73:532, 1990.
42. Severinghaus JW, Kelleher JF: Recent developments in pulse oximetry, *Anesthesiology* 76:1018, 1992.
43. Board of Dental Examiners: *Pediatric oral conscious sedation regulations,* Sacramento, CA, January 2001, The Board.
44. Gudipati CV, Weil MH, Bisera J et al: Expired carbon dioxide: a noninvasive monitor of cardiopulmonary resuscitation, *Circulation* 77:234, 1988.
45. Benumof JL: Interpretation of capnography. *AANA Journal* 66:169, 1998.
46. Vascello LA, Bowe EA: A case for capnographic monitoring as a standard of care. *J Oral Maxillofac Surg* 57:1342, 1999.
47. Rampil IJ: A primer for EEG signal processing in anesthesia, *Anesthesiology* 89:980, 1998.

CHAPTER 6

Nondrug Techniques: Iatrosedation and Hypnosis

CHAPTER OUTLINE

In Chapter 3 the concept of sedation was described, using the terms *psychosedation, iatrosedation,* and *pharmacosedation.* Definitions of these terms are presented at this time to provide groundwork for the remaining sections of this book.

The overall concept of *sedation* was originally defined as "the calming of a nervous, apprehensive individual, through the use of systemic drugs, without inducing the loss of consciousness."[1] Although this definition is essentially accurate, it requires further clarification. This is so because clinical techniques exist that act to diminish a patient's fears and anxieties toward dentistry and surgery without the use of drugs. In addition, the term *sedation,* implying relaxation of the mind, is too broad of a term because it is possible to specifically "relax" or "sedate" the function of other organs, for example, the heart (through the use of beta-blocking drugs, for example). Therefore the more specific term *psychosedation* is suggested when discussing the management of fear and anxiety. The term *psychosedative* describes a drug capable of producing relaxation of the patient's mind (e.g., central nervous system [CNS] depression). The two major categories of psychosedative techniques are *iatrosedative* techniques and *pharmacosedative* techniques.

Iatrosedation is defined in both a general and a more specific manner. The general definition of *iatrosedation* is those techniques of psychosedation not involving the administration of drugs. This chapter presents an introduction to these extremely valuable patient management techniques. The following are included in these techniques:

- Acupressure
- Acupuncture
- Audioanalgesia
- Biofeedback
- Electronic dental anesthesia (EDA)
- Electrosedation
- Hypnosis

Iatrosedation and hypnosis are discussed in this chapter because they are both important components of the doctor's armamentarium against pain and anxiety. The reader interested in the other techniques just listed is referred to specific references cited for each: acupressure,[2] acupuncture,[3] audioanalgesia,[4] biofeedback,[5] EDA,[6] and electrosedation.[7]

IATROSEDATION

Iatrosedation was defined in general terms as any technique of anxiety reduction in which no drug was given. At this point a more specific definition of this same term is presented:

iatrosedation The relief of anxiety through the doctor's behavior.

This definition of the term *iatrosedation* was formulated by Dr. Nathan Friedman, for many years the chairman of the Section of Human Behavior at the University of Southern California School of Dentistry. The word is derived from the Greek prefix *iatro,* meaning "pertaining to the doctor," and the word *sedation,* meaning "the relief of anxiety."[8]

The basic concept on which the technique of iatrosedation is based is rather simple: The behavior of the doctor and staff has a profound influence on the behavior of the patient. Other names have been applied to this concept, including "suggestion," "chairside/bedside manner," and "the laying on of hands." The underlying premise of all these techniques is similar: One can use himself or herself to aid in relaxing the patient.

How important is iatrosedation in the overall concept of psychosedation? I have received extensive training in the administration of drugs for pharmacosedation and general anesthesia, yet I have received no formal training in any aspect of psychology or human behavior. It would appear, therefore, that I should have a strong bias toward the use of techniques requiring drug administration. When I first started my training in anesthesiology in 1969 this was true. However, in the ensuing years I have become acutely aware that iatrosedation is an integral part of the success (or possible failure) of every procedure that we in medicine and dentistry attempt. The success or failure of every pharmacosedative procedure also hinges on the use of iatrosedation.

Two classic studies illustrate the importance of human behavior in the control of pain and anxiety. In the first, Egbert et al.[9] demonstrated the value of the preoperative visit by the anesthesiologist to patients about to undergo surgery the next day. Patients were placed in one of three groups.

Group 1 received a preoperative visit from the anesthesiologist but no preoperative drug for sedation before surgery. The purpose of the preoperative visit was to discuss the upcoming events with the patients and to answer any questions they might pose so as to allay their fears. The group 2 received a sedative—pentobarbital—1 hour preoperatively but no preoperative visit from the anesthesiologist. Group 3 received both the visit from the anesthesiologist and the preoperative pentobarbital.

Results of the study demonstrated that patients in the first group were alert on arrival in the operating room but were quite calm. They did not appear apprehensive. Patients in the second group were drowsy (the effect of the pentobarbital) but did not appear to be calm. In fact, they appeared quite concerned with the activities occurring around them. The third group, receiving both the visit and medication, were both drowsy and calm.

A second study by Egbert[10] once again demonstrated the value of iatrosedative techniques in patients undergoing surgery. Patients scheduled for abdominal surgery were placed in one of two groups.

Patients in group 1 were not told about postoperative discomfort (pain) following abdominal surgery. Patients were told that analgesics would be available if they were required. Patients in group 2 ("special care patients") were told that postoperative discomfort following abdominal surgery was quite usual and normal. The type of discomfort was described, as was its probable location. These patients were also told that analgesics would be available should they be required.

During the postoperative recovery period, patients in group 1 required twice the number of doses of analgesics for their discomfort as the patients who had been prepared for the discomfort. It appears that when pain is expected and is considered normal, the patient is better able to tolerate it. Put another way, it might be stated that pain that is expected by a patient simply does not hurt as much as unexpected pain. A significant anxiety component is noted with unexpected pain, a reaction that is not present with pain that is expected (is normal). It is this anxiety (the fear that the presence of pain means that something is wrong) that makes the patient experience even more and greater discomfort. A second interesting finding in this study was that patients in the "special care" group recovered from their surgical procedure more rapidly and were discharged from the hospital an average of 2.7 days earlier than the patients in group 1. This may be because of the diminished requirement for analgesic drugs in the second group, leading to a reduction in drug-related side effects and complications that might impede recovery and discharge from the hospital.

These two studies by Egbert demonstrate the power of communication. I have been witness to many such demonstrations during the use of sedative drugs in dental practice. Unfortunately, not all communication works to the benefit of the doctor. This next case illustrates this point.

❖ Case Study 1: The Power of Communication ❖

A patient received inhalation sedation with nitrous oxide (N_2O) and oxygen (O_2) for root planing and curettage. The doctor performing the procedure was working with a dental assistant. The patient was receiving approximately 35% N_2O, was quite well sedated, and had a degree of soft tissue analgesia. Treatment was proceeding well despite the patient's earlier anxiety and sensitivity of the tissues. Approximately 20 minutes into the procedure the doctor, who had been conversing casually with the dental assistant throughout the procedure, made the comment, "Gee, I haven't done one of these (root planing) in about 15 years." Almost immediately, the patient grabbed the nasal hood, pulled it off his nose, sat up, and told the doctor he wanted to go home. The patient did not want to be treated by anyone in whom he did not have confidence (even a doctor who was quite capable of doing the procedure well). An offhand remark, meant for the ears of the dental assistant, had destroyed the patient's confidence in the doctor. Another example of the power (albeit negative) of communication.

❖ Case Study 2: Lack of Communication ❖

Yet another example of the power of communication, or the lack of communication, is that of a young man, age 26, who admits to being quite uncomfortable with dental treatment. He stated that his previous doctor would walk into the treatment room, tell him to open his mouth, and immediately start treatment, without ever saying hello. The patient was very aware of this and became uncomfortable with his overall care. This doctor suggested that perhaps the patient would be more comfortable if he took a sedative before his next appointment. The patient told us that his treatment was even more uncomfortable than it had been previously because, under the influence of the medication, he was even more aware of the doctor's lack of concern for him as a person. Following this treatment the patient sought another doctor.

Communication is a powerful ally to the health professional. As these last cases illustrate, even when pharmacosedation is used, communication must never be ignored. Effective communication makes the drugs administered even more effective.

In the motion picture *The Doctor*,[11] a successful surgeon falls ill and enters into the contemporary health care system as a patient experiencing, as never before, the trials and tribulations that befall patients every day in the hospitals and medical centers of America. Through his negative experiences the physician learns the value of communication and the importance of empathy in dealing with patients. This award-winning and highly successful film was based on a true story. Incoming residents in family practice medicine at the Long Beach (California) Veterans Administration Hospital begin their hospital career as patients being admitted to the hospital, undergoing the routines all patients face (hospital gowns, blood tests, impersonal attitudes by hospital staff).[12] Much of the commercial success of *The Doctor* was thought to be the fact that audiences (all potential patients) felt that the message of the film struck home. The medical profession, to its credit, has recognized that the great emphasis placed in medical education upon the "scientific process" leads to the isolation of the physician from the patient and has begun to take steps to right the perceived wrongs. In a recent paper, Spiro[13] states that "medical students lose some of their empathy as they learn science and detachment, and hospital residents lose the remainder in the weariness of overwork and in the isolation of the intensive care units that modern hospitals have become." Medical schools have begun to modify their curricula, including in them new programs on communication and human behavior, designed to prevent the impersonalization of the physician.[14]

Similar programs have been in place for years in many dental schools throughout the United States and other countries. Yet in the highly competitive world that is dentistry today, it is often the patient who gets lost in the shuffle. I abhor the increasing use of the term *client* when discussing our *patients*. The importance of effective communication among the doctor and staff and patient can never be overemphasized. Interestingly, in the venue of continuing dental education, among the most popular programs offered are those in practice management—how to have a successful dental practice.[15] The theme of communication is paramount in all these programs.

Preparatory Communication

In the studies by Egbert,[9,10] examples were presented of preparatory communication. Preparatory communication is aimed at minimizing or eliminating a patient's fear of the unknown, one of our most prominent fears. Within the realm of dentistry, patients possess many fears that are based on hearsay. Patients faced with the prospect of endodontic therapy become hysterical because of their conception of "root canal work." The thought of the "nerve" being removed from a tooth is an unpleasant one to most persons. However, if the doctor spends but a few moments prior to the start of the endodontic treatment describing what is to be done or if educational pamphlets are available to the patient, such fears will be allayed. What is endodontic therapy? It may be described as the removal of tissue from the tooth, followed by shaping and filling of the tooth (or canal) with an inert material. When root canal therapy is described in this manner, it appears much less traumatic to the patient.

A few moments spent with a patient describing the planned procedure, before the start of a new mode of treatment, serves to allay most of the patient's anxieties. Terms used to describe the treatment should be nonthreatening if preparatory communication is to be effective in decreasing fear. Explaining an endodontic procedure by stating that "we will give you a shot of anesthetic and then remove the nerve from the tooth" only succeeds in increasing a patient's fears. The art of semantics therefore plays an important role in communication between the doctor and patient. Friedman discusses the use of euphemistic language, which is the substitution of mild or inoffensive words for those that may offend or suggest something unpleasant.[8] The word *euphemism* is derived from the Greek *eu* (well) and *phanai* (to speak).

Euphemistic Language

The dental vocabulary is replete with threatening words, examples of which are presented here:

Hurt, pain
Needle, shot, injection
Cut
Cauterize
Extract
Drill
Scalpel
Operatory
Nerve

Most health professionals, especially dentists, are acutely aware of the need to avoid using threatening words. However, occasions do arise when their use seems inescapable. For example, during the administration of a nasopalatine nerve block (perhaps the most difficult intraoral injection to administer atraumatically on a consistent basis), the patient might feel some pain (a negative word). Should the doctor tell the patient before the injection, "You will probably feel some *pain* during this injection" or "This *shot* will probably hurt a little"? The answer is no, at least not in the manner described. When it is expected that there will be pain, a nonthreatening term, such as *discomfort,* can be substituted. The statement "I will be doing this slowly; if there should be some discomfort please raise your hand and I will stop immediately" relays the same information but does not traumatize the patient psychologically, as does the preceding statement.

Examples of other terms that may be substituted for more traumatic ones are *discomfort* or *feel,* in place of *hurt* or *pain,* as in, "I don't expect you to feel this" instead of "This won't hurt." The only word heard by the patient is "hurt." *Novocain* or *local anesthetic,* in place of *needle, shot,* or *injection,* as in "We're going to give you a local anesthetic now," is preferable to "We're going to give you a shot (or injection) now." Canadian dentists have used the word *freeze* in this situation ("I am going to freeze you now") with great success. In essence the message delivered to the patient who is about to receive an injection of a local anesthetic is nonthreatening.

In pediatric dentistry, euphemistic language has always been an important means of describing to the younger, less mature patient the instruments and procedures that are to be used. The injection (administration) of a local anesthetic is described as "spraying sleepy water on a tooth," a saliva ejector is called a "vacuum cleaner," and preparation of a tooth with a drill is described as "tickling the tooth." Although the words used for adults may be different, the concept is the same. Describe the procedure in a way that lessens, not heightens, a patient's anxiety. *Remove* may be substituted for *extract* or *extirpate.* That is, "Tissue will be removed from the tooth" instead of "We will have to extirpate the nerve." *Handpiece* is used in place of *drill,* and *treatment room* may be substituted for *operatory.*

Euphemistic Language in Sedation. Throughout this book examples of euphemistic language are offered as they relate to the use of pharmacosedation. In describing the feelings a patient will experience during a sedative procedure or the equipment that is used to deliver the drugs to the patient, less threatening words or phrases are substituted for potentially traumatic ones. An excellent example deals with the administration of diazepam, a drug commonly used to obtain light levels of conscious sedation via the intravenous (IV) route. Because diazepam is not water soluble, propylene glycol is used as a solvent. Propylene glycol can produce irritation of vein walls as the drug is injected. Some patients may experience this irritation only slightly or even not at all, whereas others may considered it quite uncomfortable. It is suggested that the person administering IV diazepam caution (e.g., advise) the patient before its administration that there is a possibility of discomfort. Should the doctor fail to tell the patient and a painful sensation does occur, the patient may become quite apprehensive, fearing that something is wrong. This possibility can be eliminated by forewarning the patient. The manner in which this potential "feeling" is described is important. Stating that the patient will experience a painful sensation or that there will be a burning sensation as the drug is injected is likely to put the patient on the alert, increasing an already heightened anxiety level. The patient might ask, "Why, if this drug is going to hurt when it is being injected, is the doctor using it at all?" I have found it best to tell the patient receiving IV diazepam that "You may experience a slight warmth in your arm as the drug is administered. This is entirely normal and will pass within a few seconds." In this manner the patient is prepared but not frightened.

Inhalation sedation with N_2O-O_2 is commonly called *gas, laughing gas, sweet air,* or *medicated air* by doctors who believe that the chemical names may be too threatening to their patients.[16] Yet another euphemistic term relating to sedation comes to mind: With the recent media avalanche of headlines concerning the illicit use of drugs, such as cocaine and narcotics, the very word *drug* has acquired a negative connotation. Use of the word *medication* relays the desired message in a more professional and less intimidating manner.

Iatrosedation: Staff and Office

The entire dental staff must be alert to the appropriate use of language, for much of a patient's contact in the office will be with persons other than the doctor. In addition, the demeanor of the receptionist, chairside personnel, and all others will add to or detract from the environment in the office. Sedation does not just magically happen when a patient sits down in the dental chair. As was demonstrated in the stress-reduction protocols (see Chapter 4), the recognition and management of anxiety must start before the actual treatment. A receptionist is just as important in the management of anxiety as are chairside personnel. The receptionist is trained to answer the telephone "with a smile," to help reassure the apprehensive patient, and to relay such information to the doctor and other chairside personnel. The apprehensive patient is on the alert for clues on entering the dental office. A positive attitude on the part of the staff, as well as a relaxed environment within the office, will help allay the patient's fears. A busy, high-pressure office where staff members are constantly running about in a frenzy is not conducive to relaxation. The use of striking colors and loud rock music will also detract from a sedative environment (although patients' musical tastes do vary considerably). Conversely, a low-pressure, relaxed office staff, combined with a toned-down color scheme (earth colors) and a more moderate type of music, provides a warm, cheerful environment that adds to the sedative effect of any drugs that may subsequently be administered.[17]

Once the patient arrives in the dental office, his or her presence should be acknowledged within a minute or two. Even when the doctor may be somewhat delayed in scheduling, the patient should be informed of this and not kept waiting for no apparent reason. The patient should be escorted to the (dental) treatment room (the term *operatory* or *surgery* is threatening to many patients) and seated in the dental chair. At this point the dental assistant can aid the patient's level of comfort by simply adjusting the chair and headrest as may be desired by the patient or by offering the patient a facial tissue. An attitude of concern or empathy should be relayed by the assistant to the patient to help establish lines of communication. On entering the treatment room the doctor should always greet the patient, shake hands (personal touches like this are greatly appreciated by the patient, as well as being an aid in recognition of anxiety [cold, sweaty palms]), and spend a moment or two talking before starting treatment. I have been astounded by the number of fearful patients who have stated that the major reason they left a doctor was because "the doctor didn't care about me as a person." A few words spoken to the patient before and during treatment help establish a better working relationship between the treatment team and the patient.

I was present when a dental student was interviewing an apprehensive patient whom he was seeing for the first time. The student had reviewed the patient's medical history questionnaire and was seeking to determine the causes of the patient's fears of dentistry. The audio portion of the tape of this interview demonstrated that the student was quite adept at obtaining the necessary information and at transmitting his desire to work with the patient to help him diminish his dental fears. However, when seen on video, the entire interview was considered a failure. The student doctor, asking all of the appropriate questions and expressing his concern for the patient, was standing with his back toward the patient and reading from a prepared list of questions. At no point during this 20-minute interview did the patient ever see the doctor's face for more than a few seconds at a time!

Clinical Demeanor

Why does a patient select one dentist over another? Most patients select a dentist after discussion with friends and relatives. Commonly expressed reasons for selection include the comments that this doctor "is good" or "is painless." It appears, therefore, that one of the primary considerations used in the selection process is a doctor's clinical demeanor.[18] This does not always mean that the technical quality of the dentistry is superior; it does, however, mean that the doctor "cares about the patients" and makes an effort to be gentle and to provide painless treatment.

Friedman[8] has stated that "the more threatening an instrument, the more significant your manner of wielding it" becomes to the patient. A gentle touch is appreciated over a rough appearance. Expressions of concern, verbal or nonverbal, during treatment aid in allaying a patient's fears. A simple statement such as "If for any reason you would like me to stop, simply raise your hand and I will stop immediately" tells the patient of the doctor's concern. A new patient may test this system several times to be certain the doctor was truthful but, once convinced, will relax and permit treatment to continue.

The Goal of Iatrosedation

The ultimate goal of iatrosedation is to minimize the patient's requirement for pharmacosedation. Another goal is to open lines of communication so that the patient will not be inhibited from expressing true feelings or desires to the doctor or staff members. When patients are able to express their fears to the doctor before treatment begins, it becomes that much more simple to manage them during the treatment.

Iatrosedation is an effective technique; however, it may not be adequate by itself to remove the fears of dentistry harbored by all patients. The use of supplemental pharmacosedation may be necessary in the initial phases of patient management. Iatrosedation effectively minimizes the depth of pharmacosedation required to reach a desired clinical level of relaxation, and/or it maximizes the effectiveness of the pharmacosedative technique used.

By communicating with our patients, we can begin the process of fear reduction during our initial contact. Through the establishment of rapport with the patient we are able to determine the level of pharmacosedation (if any) required to manage the patient's dental fears and make more effective use of any drugs we might employ. The following case study serves to point up the objectives of iatrosedation.[19]

❖ Case Study 3: Objectives of Iatrosedation ❖

The patient, a 24-year-old college student, had purposely avoided dental treatment in the past until forced by pain to seek help. His anxieties were related to the sound of the dental handpiece and originated in childhood, when the patient was treated by a dentist who did not use local anesthesia. The patient associated the sound of the handpiece with the pain of "drilling." The patient arrived at the University of Southern California School of Dentistry Emergency Clinic with acute pulpitis of the mandibular right first molar.

The patient admitted to an extreme fear of dentistry and stated that despite his pain, he could not tolerate dental treatment. At the first treatment visit IV diazepam, 19 mg, was administered (via titration) to sedate the patient, and after mandibular anesthesia was obtained, the pulp was extirpated without incident. The patient later stated that he had "enjoyed" the dental appointment and wished to become a regular clinic patient.

At subsequent appointments the patient did require the use of pharmacosedative techniques. However, at the end of eight dental visits, spanning a period of 3 months, the patient no longer required the use of pharmacosedation for his dental care. This is the goal to be sought. Through the combined use of iatrosedation and pharmacosedation, in many cases it is possible to achieve this goal by reeducating the fearful patient. This goal may easily be accomplished in those practices in which patients remain for many years, such as in general dental practice, pediatric dentistry, and periodontics. Because of the shorter treatment periods required in oral surgery and endodontics, this same goal is somewhat more elusive, although it is still achievable.

As stated in Chapter 2, the goal in initially using pharmacosedation as an aid in patient management is to eventually eliminate its need. The technique of iatrosedation will, of course, be used with each and every patient who appears in the office seeking treatment at each and every appointment.

HYPNOSIS

Hypnosis has been defined as a "special trancelike state in which the subject's attention is focused intensely on the hypnotist, while attention to other stimuli is markedly diminished."[20] Barber and Mayer[21] define hypnosis as "an altered state of consciousness characterized by narrowed, heightened attention, and the capacity for producing alterations in memory and perception."

Franz Anton Mesmer (1734-1815), a graduate of the University of Vienna School of Medicine, did much work on the subject of animal magnetism. His work became the subject of controversy throughout Europe, and his Magnetic Institute in Paris attracted many influential and rich persons. Banned from Paris, Mesmer moved his institute, along with its ardent followers, to Switzerland. Animal magnetism, or mesmerism, as it came to be known, was an early form of hypnotism, and as such was instrumental in the development of a new awareness of the possibilities of making people insensitive to pain. James Esdaile in India performed 73 painless surgical operations using mesmerism; however, the medical communities of the day remained unconvinced of its value, and mesmerism remained a controversial topic within the medical community and among the public for many years to come.[22]

In 1837 the first reported case of a tooth extraction using mesmerism was published.[23] It was not until 1843 that the term *hypnotism* was introduced by James Braid.

At the end of the nineteenth century and the beginning of the twentieth century, the foundations of hypnosis were elucidated by Jean-Martin Charcot (1825-1893) and others. Sigmund Freud initiated the use of hypnosis as a therapeutic tool in psychoanalysis, a role that it still maintains today.[22]

Hypnosis in Dentistry

As with iatrosedation, hypnosis serves as a means of providing relaxation without the need for drug administration. In addition, hypnosis serves as a means of providing clinically acceptable pain control in some patients, making it a potentially valuable technique in dentistry.

Barber[24] lists the following possible uses of hypnosis in dentistry:

- Patient relaxation
- Anxiety reduction
- Orthodontics (aid in overcoming fear of orthodontics)
- Maintenance of comfort during prolonged treatments
- Modification of noxious dental habits (e.g., thumb sucking)
- Reduction of the need for anesthesia or analgesia
- Postoperative analgesia
- Substitution for premedication in general anesthesia
- Control of reflexes and autonomic processes (i.e., gagging, nausea, salivary flow, bleeding)
- Management of difficult patients

Hypnosis is an effective technique as an aid in helping patients overcome their fears of various procedures. Hypnotic suggestion has proven valuable in eliminating the fear of injections (both intraoral and IV/intramuscular), and the claustrophobic feeling some patients experience when the N_2O-O_2 inhalation sedation nasal hood is placed over their nose.[25] When venipuncture is difficult to achieve because of a patient's fear of needles, hypnosis may prove effective in eliminating or minimizing the fear.[26]

In many cases hypnosis can be used in place of other, more conventional techniques of pain and anxiety control.[27] When hypnosis is successful, even local anesthetics for pain control may not be required. Postoperative complications and discomfort may be minimized through the effective use of posthypnotic suggestion, thereby decreasing a patient's requirement for analgesics and other drugs with their attendant side effects.[21]

The Success of Hypnosis

Although folklore acknowledges that only 25% of the population is "susceptible" to hypnosis, reports on the success of hypnosis in clinical practice are more positive. Beecher[28] reported that hypnosis is an effective substitute for anesthesia in all but approximately 20% of the surgical population tested. Barber and Mayer,[21] using a technique of hypnotic induction called *rapid induction analgesia,* reported that test subjects were able to "dramatically alter their awareness of experimental dental pain, irrespective of hypnotic susceptibility. . . . Ninety-nine percent of unscreened dental patients were able to undergo normally painful dental procedures using only hypnosis, as induced by rapid induction analgesia."

Education in Hypnosis

Although some dental schools include training in hypnosis as a part of their curricula, most practicing dentists have not received training in the effective use of this potentially valuable technique. Two professional groups offer clinical workshops in hypnosis throughout the United States. The reader is referred to them for additional information and training in hypnosis.*

SUMMARY

In conclusion, I must restate the vital importance of iatrosedation in the everyday practice of medicine and dentistry. Iatrosedation must be employed by each of us whenever we are in contact with other human beings, be they our patients, staff, or simply other persons we come into contact with. Our behavior and our appearance provide these persons with a sense of "like" or "dislike" toward us. For a practice of dentistry or medicine to be successful, an attitude of caring must become an integral part of office philosophy. In the absence of this caring attitude, patients feel isolated and alienated, increasing their own anxiety levels and producing additional management difficulties for the staff. The successful use of iatrosedation will enhance the effectiveness of the pharmacosedative techniques that will be discussed in the chapters to follow.

---

*American Society of Clinical Hypnosis, 130 East Elm Court, Suite 201 Roselle, IL 60172-2000; phone: 630-980-4740; fax: 630-351-8490; e-mail: info@asch.net; web site: www.asch.net.

Society for Clinical and Experimental Hypnosis, SCEH Central Office, Washington State University, PO Box 642114, Pullman, WA 99164-2114; fax: 509-335-2097; e-mail: sceh@pullman.com; web site: http://sunsite.utk.edu/IJCEH/scehframe.htm.

REFERENCES

1. Council on Dental Education: *Guidelines for teaching the comprehensive control of pain and anxiety in dentistry,* Chicago, 1993, American Dental Association.
2. Smith LS: Evaluation and management of the muscle contraction headache, *Nurs Pract* 13:20, 1988.
3. Wong T: Use of electrostimulation of acupuncture points in general dental practice, *Anesth Prog* 36:243, 1989.
4. Mayer R: Stress, anxiety and audio-analgesia in dental treatment measured with the aid of biosignals, *Deutsche Zahnarztliche Zeitschrift* 44:692, 1989.
5. Elmore AM: Biofeedback therapy in the treatment of dental anxiety and dental phobia, *Dent Clin North Am* 32:735, 1988.
6. teDuits E, Geopferd S, Donly K et al: The effectiveness of electronic dental anesthesia in children, *Pediatr Dent* 15:191, 1993.
7. Treschinskii AI, Aznaurian SK, Trotsevich VA: Changes in autonomic homeostasis during anesthesia induction in patients operated on for congenital cleft palate, *Stomatologiia* 70:59, 1991.
8. Friedman N: Iatrosedation. In McCarthy FM, ed: *Emergencies in dental practice,* ed 3, Philadelphia, 1979, WB Saunders.
9. Egbert L, Battit G, Turndoff H et al: Value of the preoperative visit by an anesthetist, *JAMA* 195:553, 1963.
10. Egbert LD: Reduction of post-operative pain by encouragement and instruction of patients: a study of doctor-patient rapport, *N Engl J Med* 270:825, 1964.
11. Ziskin L, producer: *The Doctor,* Hollywood, 1991, Touchstone Films (film).
12. LBVA hospital program, Long Beach, Calif.
13. Spiro H: What is empathy and can it be taught? *Ann Intern Med* 116:843, 1992.
14. Matthews DA, Feinstein AR: A review of systems for the personal aspects of patient care, *Am J Med Sci* 295:159, 1988.
15. *Continuing education directory,* Chicago, 1993, American Dental Association.
16. Shedlin M, Wallechinsky D: *Laughing gas, nitrous oxide,* Berkeley, Calif, 1973, And/Or Press.
17. Schmierer A: Use of relaxation sound tracks in the dental office, *Zahnarztliche Praxis* 42:286, 1991.
18. Friedman H: The doctor-patient relationship in an intravenous-sedation practice, *Anesth Prog* 23:48, 1976.
19. Malamed SF: A most powerful drug, *J Calif Acad Gen Dent* 4:17, 1979.
20. Seltzer S: *Pain control in dentistry, diagnosis and management,* Philadelphia, 1978, Lippincott.
21. Barber J, Mayer D: Evaluation of the efficacy and neural mechanism of a hypnotic analgesia procedure in experimental and clinical dental pain, *Pain* 4:41, 1977.
22. Lyons AS, Petrucelli RJ: *Medicine: an illustrated history,* New York, 1978, Harry N Abrams.
23. Ring ME: *Dentistry: an illustrated history,* New York and St Louis, 1985, Harry N Abrams and Mosby.
24. Barber J: Acupuncture and hypnosis in dentistry. In Allen GD, ed: *Dental anesthesia and analgesia (local and general),* ed 2, Baltimore, 1979, Williams & Wilkins.
25. DiBona MC: Nitrous oxide and hypnosis: a combined technique, *Anesth Prog* 26:17, 1979.
26. Morse DR, Cohen BB: Desensitization using meditation-hypnosis to control "needle" phobia in two dental patients, *Anesth Prog* 30:83, 1983.
27. Hilgard ER: Pain: its reduction and production under hypnosis, *Proc Am Philosoph Soc* 115:470, 1971.
28. Beecher HK: *Measurement of subjective responses,* New York, 1959, Oxford University Press.

SECTION III

ORAL, RECTAL, AND INTRAMUSCULAR SEDATION

In this, and in subsequent sections, the techniques of pharmacosedation are described in detail. Major sections are devoted to inhalation and intravenous (IV) sedation, two of the most useful pharmacosedative techniques. In this section three routes of drug administration are discussed in depth, oral, rectal, and intramuscular (IM), each of which can prove to be quite effective within the practice of dentistry for the management of pain, fear, and anxiety. Three other potentially valuable routes of drug administration, sublingual, transdermal, and intranasal (IN), are reviewed in Chapter 9.

The oral, rectal, and IM techniques are frequently referred to as *premedication,* whereas the term *sedation* is commonly applied to inhalation and IV techniques. *Premedication* is defined as "any sedative, tranquilizer, hypnotic, or anticholinergic drug administered before anesthesia."[1] A deciding factor as to whether a technique will be considered premedication or sedation is the latent period of the technique. The latent period is the period of time that elapses between the administration of a drug and its onset of clinical activity.

In both inhalation and IV drug administration, the latent period is quite short, well under 60 seconds. However, in oral, rectal, IM, and IN drug administration, the latent period may range from 10 minutes to more than 30 minutes.

Each of these routes of drug administration may be used to provide sedation and is referred to that way throughout this text because they all accomplish the stated goal of sedation: "relaxation of an apprehensive person without inducing the loss of consciousness." It is in their clinical application that the distinction between premedication and sedation has developed. The term *sedation* is used to describe techniques in which clinical actions develop more rapidly, and the term *premedication* is used to describe those techniques with a more gradual onset of action. The term *sedation* is used throughout this text in our discussion of all techniques of patient relaxation.

REFERENCE

1. *Mosby's medical, nursing, & allied health dictionary,* ed 6, St Louis, 2002, Mosby.

CHAPTER 7

Oral Sedation

CHAPTER OUTLINE

The oral route is the oldest route of drug administration and still the most commonly used. It is also the safest, most convenient, and most economical method of drug administration. The oral route may be used quite effectively in dentistry for the reduction of stress before or during dental treatment and as a means of managing preoperative and postoperative pain. Although other routes of administration may be more reliable and more effective in producing a desired clinical effect, the oral route still maintains a valued place in dentistry's armamentarium against pain and anxiety.

ADVANTAGES

The oral route possesses several advantages over other routes of drug administration:

1. Almost universal acceptability
2. Ease of administration
3. Low cost
4. Decreased incidence of adverse reactions
5. Decreased severity of adverse reactions
6. No needles, syringes, or equipment
7. No specialized training

Most adults do not object to taking drugs by mouth. For better or for worse, we have become a "pill-popping" society, a fact that makes the prescription of an anxiety-reducing drug before dental treatment all the more palatable to the patient. An important exception to this is the young, immature child, who may prove unwilling to accept any drugs by mouth.

Oral drugs are exceptionally easy for the doctor to administer. In most cases the drug prescribed for premedication will be taken by the patient at home. In an increasing number of situations, the doctor may elect to administer an oral drug to the patient personally on his or her arrival in the dental office, to better ensure proper dosage and time of administration. In either case the administration of drugs via the oral route requires only that the doctor have knowledge of the pharmacologic action of the drug being administered, its side effects, potential drug-drug interactions, and any contraindications to its administration. No special equipment, personnel, or advanced training is required for the safe use of the oral route (in the adult patient).

The cost of most oral drugs is usually quite low, especially for the small number of doses employed in dentistry. Although there is significant variation in the cost of drugs, the oral form of a drug is usually significantly less expensive than its parenteral counterpart.

Complications are always possible when drugs are administered, regardless of the route of administration. Drug idiosyncrasy, allergy, and overdose, as well as other adverse actions, can and do occur. Drug-related side effects are less likely to develop after enteral drug administration (i.e., oral, rectal) than after parenteral drug administration. In addition, adverse reactions following oral administration are often much less intense than those noted following parenteral administration of the same drug. This is not to imply that serious complications do not occur following oral drug administration. Berger, Green, and Melnick[1] reported cardiac arrest following oral diazepam intoxication, and Gill and Michaelides[2] described an anaphylactic response to oral penicillin. Other serious adverse reactions to orally prescribed drugs have been reported.[3]

The convenience of the oral route is a primary reason for its popularity. This technique can be employed with minimal risk if the doctor prescribing the drug(s) is knowledgeable of (1) the pharmacologic actions of the drug; (2) its indications, contraindications, precautions, side effects, and dosage; and (3) the medical history of the patient, especially as it relates to prior drug use, specific contraindications to the use of particular drugs, and prior reactions to the drug to be administered. No special equipment (e.g., needles, syringes), no additional personnel, and no advanced educational training are required when oral drugs are used in adult patients.

The aforementioned advantages make the use of orally administered drugs quite compelling. However, there are, as with all routes of drug administration, some distinct disadvantages that effectively limit the clinical use of this route of drug administration.

DISADVANTAGES

Disadvantages associated with the oral route include the following:

1. Reliance on patient compliance
2. Prolonged latent period
3. Erratic and incomplete absorption of drugs from the gastrointestinal (GI) tract
4. Inability to titrate
5. Inability to readily lighten or deepen the level of sedation
6. Prolonged duration of action

When prescribing drugs for oral administration, the doctor must rely on the patient to take the drug as prescribed (the proper dose at the proper time). Although most patients will medicate themselves properly, some do not. This potential problem, termed *noncompliance,* is significant in medicine, especially in relation to long-term drug administration (e.g., antihypertensive drugs). The Council on Patient Information and Education estimates that 35% to 50% of all prescriptions dispensed by doctors are taken incorrectly by patients and that 1 in 5 patients never even bothers to have the prescription filled. One in seven stops taking the drug too soon. Noncompliance rates among patients older than 65 years are more than 55%.[4] Although noncompliance is not as critical a problem in the dental situation, the administration of too small or too large a dose, too soon or too late, may significantly alter the drug's effectiveness during the treatment period. A common form of noncompliance is the taking of a dose larger than that prescribed, the patient's rationale being that "if one (tablet or capsule) is good, then two or more will be better." This type of thinking leads to oversedation, overdose, and other unwanted and unpleasant complications. Fortunately (in this situation, at least), the erratic and incomplete absorption of orally administered drugs minimizes the development of serious problems from drug overadministration.

On many occasions I have observed this phenomenon in pediatric dental practice: A parent or guardian administers a tablespoon of drug instead of a teaspoon, or a larger dose than desired, because the child did not take all of the first dose. Significant overdose, with attendant respiratory depression, can develop in this manner if the administered drug is a central nervous system (CNS) depressant. The consequences of these actions are formidable, with potential morbidity or mortality being the result. This has led to the enactment of legislation in a number of states (Ohio, Florida, and California, as of December 2000) that restricts the use of oral conscious sedation in patients younger than 13 years of age to doctors who have received appropriate education and training in this patient population.[5]

The doctor prescribing oral drugs for the management of anxiety must never forget that these drugs are CNS depressants and that excessive CNS depression (e.g., oversedation or general anesthesia) is always possible. To minimize concern over patient noncompliance, the doctor should (1) tell the patient, or the parent or guardian, exactly how much of the drug to take and at what time to take it; (2) write these instructions down and give them to the patient; (3) make sure the prescription is clearly marked with these same instructions; (4) prescribe only the dose the patient is to take (this is warranted even though prescriptions for larger numbers of tablets or capsules are less expensive per item than are single doses); and (5) record the instructions given to the patient, as well as the drug and its dose, in the patient's chart. When the patient a child or is known to be unreliable, the patient can be asked to appear in the dental office 1 hour before the scheduled treatment, and the drug is given to the patient by the doctor.

Another disadvantage of the oral route is its relatively long latent period (the period following administration before a clinical effect is observed). Most orally administered drugs have a latent period of approximately 30 minutes. At this time (30 minutes), the blood (plasma) level of the drug is at the minimal (therapeutic) level required for clinical activity to be observed. Absorption of oral drugs occurs primarily from the small intestine with less absorption from the stomach (alcohol and aspirin are significant exceptions). Drug absorption into the cardiovascular system continues, and the blood level of the drug increases until a maximal level is reached. With most oral drugs, peak blood levels occur approximately 60 minutes following ingestion or 30 minutes following the onset of clinical activity. Peak blood level is equated clinically with maximal drug action (i.e., most intense analgesia or sedation).

In addition to a long latent period, most oral drugs are absorbed erratically and incompletely from the GI tract, which makes consistent clinical results difficult to achieve. A number of factors act to influence absorption of drugs from the GI tract as follows:

1. Lipid solubility
2. pH of the gastric tissues
3. Mucosal surface area
4. Gastric emptying time
5. Dosage form of the drug
6. Drug inactivation
7. Presence of food in the stomach
8. Bioavailability of the drug
9. Hepatic "first-pass" effect

Absorption

Both the lipid solubility of the drug and the pH of the gastric tissues affect drug absorption from the GI tract. Lipid-soluble drugs are absorbed more rapidly than non–lipid-soluble drugs. Gastric fluid has a pH of approximately 1.4. Drugs that are organic acids, such as aspirin, freely diffuse across the gastric mucosa into the circulatory system. Drugs that are bases, codeine, for example, are poorly absorbed from the highly acid environment of the stomach. As gastric fluid leaves the stomach to enter the small intestine, its pH changes dramatically as a result of the addition of biliary, intestinal, and pancreatic secretions. In the intestinal environment, with its pH of approximately 4.0 to 6.0, the absorption of aspirin is slowed, whereas absorption of the more basic codeine is accelerated.

Primary absorption of most drugs occurs from the small intestine rather than the stomach. This is true even for drugs such as aspirin because although the lower gastric pH favors its absorption, more than 90% of the absorption of aspirin occurs in the small intestine. The architecture of the small intestine is the primary reason for this. The process of absorption is facilitated by the small intestine's considerable surface area, consisting of microvilli, villi, and the folds of Kerckring. The stomach, by contrast, is a relatively smooth organ, poorly adapted for absorption.

Because the small intestine is the primary site for drug absorption, it is important to get the drug through the mouth, esophagus, and stomach and into the small intestine as rapidly as possible. The removal of foods and other substances from the stomach occurs by contraction of the antrum of the stomach. The time required for a substance to be expelled from the stomach is the *gastric emptying time.* Liquids, when taken alone, require approximately 90 minutes to be removed, and a mixed meal of food and liquids requires about 4 hours to reach the duodenum. Liquids are discharged from the stomach into the duodenum at a rate of 10 ml per minute. The presence of fat in the stomach significantly retards gastric emptying time. It is therefore recommended, as a general rule, that oral drugs be taken with a glass of water (approximately 8 oz) in the absence of food. In this manner the drug's delivery to the duodenum is maximized, permitting more reliable absorption. Anxiety is another factor that delays gastric emptying. It is estimated that gastric emptying time can be delayed by as much as two times in the fearful patient,[6] thereby delaying the onset of action of antianxiety drugs. Thus a negative cycle is established. Oral antianxiety drugs are administered 1 hour before treatment to lessen the patient's fear of impending dental or surgical care, yet the very fear that we are seeking to manage inhibits the absorption of the drug into the cardiovascular system. This helps explain why, in the presence of extreme fear, orally administered drugs may prove ineffective despite having been administered as directed by the doctor.

Drugs administered in aqueous solution are more rapidly absorbed than those given as an oily solution or in tablet or capsule form. The tablet or capsule must first dissolve in the gastric fluid before absorption can occur. Once it has dissolved, the size of the resulting particles of drug is important. The smaller the particle is, the greater is the rate of drug absorption.[7] There is, in fact, significant variation in the clinical effectiveness of different forms (i.e., liquid, capsule, tablet) of the same drug (see the next section, Bioavailability).

Some drugs, such as morphine, cannot be administered orally because a significant level of drug inactivation occurs before they reach the cardiovascular system. Although the acidity of the stomach is the major cause of this, intestinal contents can also affect the actions of oral drugs. The hepatic first-pass effect is also involved. Drugs absorbed from the GI tract (stomach, intestine, colon) are first delivered to the liver via the hepatic portal system before entering into the systemic circulation. The liver is rich in enzymes that biotransform certain drugs into pharmacologically inactive byproducts. A prime example of this is the antidysrhythmic drug lidocaine. Lidocaine is so completely transformed via hepatic first-pass effect that the drug is essentially useless when administered orally.[8] However, modifying the chemical structure of lidocaine produced the chemical analog tocainide, which is clinically effective as an oral antidysrhythmic.[9] In the area of drugs used for anxiety reduction, there is a subtle (but not clinically significant) hepatic first-pass effect noted with the opioid analgesics.

The presence of food in the stomach decreases absorption of drugs into the cardiovascular system by increasing gastric emptying time, and if the drug is bound to food, it will not be available for absorption.[10] As mentioned previously, it is recommended that oral drugs be ingested with a full glass of water and in the absence of food (unless a drug specifically requires that it be administered along with food as a means of minimizing gastric upset).

Bioavailability

Two tablets from different manufacturers of the same dosage of the same drug are said to be *chemically* equivalent. If the ensuing blood levels of the drugs are equivalent, they are said to be *biologically* equivalent. They are *therapeutically* equivalent if they are equally effective therapeutically. Drugs that are chemically equivalent are not necessarily biologically or therapeutically equivalent. These differences are termed *bioavailability.* Differences in bioavailability of drugs are most often seen with oral preparations. The difference in absorption of chemically equivalent drugs is related to differences in the size of particles or shape of crystals and to the rates of disintegration and dissolution of the drugs.

The slow onset of clinical activity of oral drugs prevents their titration. Ability to titrate a drug permits individualization of drug dosages for all patients. Undersedation or oversedation should not occur where titration is possible. The ability to titrate a drug to clinical effect is one of the greatest safety factors in drug administration. Unfortunately, the 30-minute latent period and 60-minute delay for the drug to reach peak blood level (for most oral drugs) preclude titration. Care must be exacted to avoid underadministration or overadministration of orally administered CNS depressant drugs.

Another disadvantage of orally administered drugs is the inability to either lighten or deepen the level of sedation rapidly. Should the effect of the drug prove inadequate, a second dose may be given; however, the same time factors (30 and 60 minutes) will be required to achieve full benefit of the drug, making this option unattractive. If, on the other hand, the effect of the initial dose proves too intense, there is no effective means of reversing it. This *lack of control* over the actions of the drug seriously impairs the usefulness of this technique in a typical outpatient dental environment.

The duration of clinical action of most oral drugs is approximately 3 to 4 hours. For the typical 1-hour dental appointment, this duration of action is entirely too long. Unfortunately, however, there is no means of reversing the clinical action of the orally administered drug. The patient will remain under the influence of the drug well into the postoperative period and be unable to leave the dental office unescorted. Patients receiving oral CNS depressants for stress reduction must always be cautioned against driving or operating potentially hazardous machinery. If patients receive oral sedative drugs at home before their dental appointment, they must be similarly cautioned.

RATIONALE FOR USE

When the advantages and disadvantages of the oral route are compared, it becomes obvious that a number of significant disadvantages are associated with the use of this technique. These combine to produce a route of drug administration in which the administrator has little control over the ultimate clinical action of the drug.

This lack of control over drug action is a potential problem every time a drug is administered orally. This is particularly so when the drug is a CNS depressant, as are those used in stress reduction. The potential for oversedation, respiratory depression, and loss of consciousness must always be considered when administration of an oral drug for anxiety relief is contemplated.

Despite the negative factors associated with oral sedation, there is considerable need in dentistry for orally administered drugs for stress reduction. The primary use of the oral route is in the management of anxiety before the dental procedure. However, because of the lack of control over the ultimate drug action, it is strongly suggested that only lighter levels of sedation be sought via the oral route. Light levels of sedation may prove adequate to reduce anxieties that develop before the dental appointment but may prove inadequate in diminishing the fears occurring once the patient enters the dental office and commences treatment. It is possible to produce deeper levels of sedation with the oral route. However, the clinician must always keep in mind the lack of control over drug action and the wide range of individual responses to a given drug dose. The possibility of overdose, respiratory depression, impaired consciousness, or unconsciousness is increased as the degree of CNS depression increases. Persons untrained in the management of the unconscious airway ought not attempt to achieve deeper levels of sedation by the oral route. In addition, the doctor prescribing or administering oral drugs must possess a thorough knowledge of the drug's actions, contraindications, side effects, and precautions. The doctor must also be capable of prompt recognition and management of any adverse reaction that might develop (e.g., unconsciousness). If deeper levels of sedation are required, a more controllable technique of sedation (i.e., inhalation or IV) should be considered.

What then represents the rational use of the oral route in a typical dental practice? From the standpoint of safety it is important that the clinician never seek to achieve a level of sedation beyond which he or she is comfortable (has been trained to use) and is capable of recognizing and managing any undesirable side effects that might develop. For these reasons, the rational use of oral sedation includes only lighter levels of sedation. Deeper levels of sedation should be restricted to more controllable techniques or, when indicated via the oral route, should be employed only by a doctor with prior experience or training in the technique of deep oral sedation and who is fully prepared to manage any adverse reactions that might develop.

The most common use of oral sedation is for the relief of anxiety in the hours immediately preceding a dental appointment. An antianxiety or sedative-hypnotic drug is used to reduce anxiety so that the patient will appear in the dental office for the scheduled appointment. More controllable techniques may be used at this time for intraoperative sedation. When using oral drugs for this purpose, the clinician must remember to caution the patient against driving or operating hazardous machinery. If the patient has taken the drug at home, he or she should be advised against driving a car and should be accompanied to the office (driven) by a responsible adult. For medicolegal purposes this should also be noted in the patient's chart.

A second use for oral sedation is one that is often overlooked by a busy clinician. As noted earlier (see Chapter 4), not only do patients with fears of dentistry or surgery become apprehensive immediately before their appointment, often their anxieties start to build the *day before* the scheduled appointment. These persons might be unable to sleep the night before the appointment as they anticipate their upcoming "ordeal" and will be fatigued when they appear in the dental office the next day, a factor leading to a lowering of the pain reaction threshold. An antianxiety or hypnotic drug taken 1 hour before sleep (1 hr hs) the night before the appointment helps ensure a restful night's sleep and a more fit patient during treatment.

Other uses of the oral route in dentistry include the administration of drugs to inhibit salivary secretions (antisialagogues), drugs to prevent or to manage nausea (antiemetics), and antibiotics.

DRUGS

A large number of drugs may be administered orally in the management of anxiety. The overwhelming majority of these are classified as either antianxiety or sedative-hypnotic drugs. Other drug groups that may be used for this purpose are histamine blockers and opioids.

Before we discuss these drugs, a word is in order regarding the appropriate dosages to be used. The clinician must use as much information as is available to make an informed decision regarding the appropriate dose to administer, particularly when using the oral route. Information available to the clinician includes the patient's medical history, age, weight, and previous drug reactions. In addition, the clinician must determine the degree of anxiety present and the level of sedation sought. After consideration of these factors, a drug dose is determined.

A source of information regarding recommended dosages of drugs is the drug package insert or publications such as *Facts and Comparisons*,[11] *Mosby's Drug Consult*,[12] or *Mosby's Dental Drug Reference*, sixth edition.[13] Online sources of drug information are readily available for downloading onto a desktop computer or handheld device.* An advantage of online drug data resources is that they are updated on a regular basis.

A common problem associated with the use of recommended doses is that they often lead to inadequate anxiety reduction in the dental or surgical setting. There is a reasonable explanation for this: The package insert recommends a certain dose of a drug to induce sedation or sleep in a nonstress situation, such as the home environment. The dose of a drug that would effectively relax an apprehensive individual at home will probably prove ineffective when the stresses of

*ePocrates is available at www.ePocrates.com, Medscape is available at www.medscape.com, and *Mosby's Drug Consult* is available at www.mosbysdrugconsult.com.

the dental office environment are added. For this reason, the doses recommended for oral sedation in this chapter and in many textbooks of pediatric dentistry may be somewhat higher than those in the package inserts.[12,13]

Many antianxiety and sedative-hypnotic drugs for oral administration are produced in three dosage forms. When a dosage is chosen for stress reduction in dental practice, these three dosage forms correlate with the normal distribution ("bell-shaped") curve (Figure 7-1). The middle dosage form is the "average" dose, producing clinically effective results (in nonstress situations) in approximately 70% of persons receiving it. The largest dosage form is for persons in whom the average dose proves to be ineffective or who have a greater degree of anxiety. The smallest dosage form is for persons in whom the average dose provides too intense a clinical effect, for persons with less anxiety, for elderly patients, or for debilitated patients. It must be remembered that the added stresses associated with dental or surgical treatment will increase the percentage of patients requiring larger than "usual" doses for management of their treatment-related fears.

Although titration (individualization of drug dosages) is not possible with orally administered drugs—a significant impediment to their safe use—it is possible in situations in which oral drugs are to be used over multiple appointments to *titrate by appointment.* This concept was introduced to me by Dr. Ronald Johnson, then chairman of the Department of Pediatric Dentistry at the University of Southern California.[14] Quite simply, titration by appointment means that the doctor will assess the efficacy of sedation achieved at the first appointment with a given drug dosage and, if necessary, will increase or decrease the dosage of drug(s) administered at subsequent appointments. Therefore, over a period of two to three visits, the appropriate dosage for that patient can be achieved (titrated). Titration by appointment is discussed more fully in the chapter on pediatric sedation (see Chapter 35).

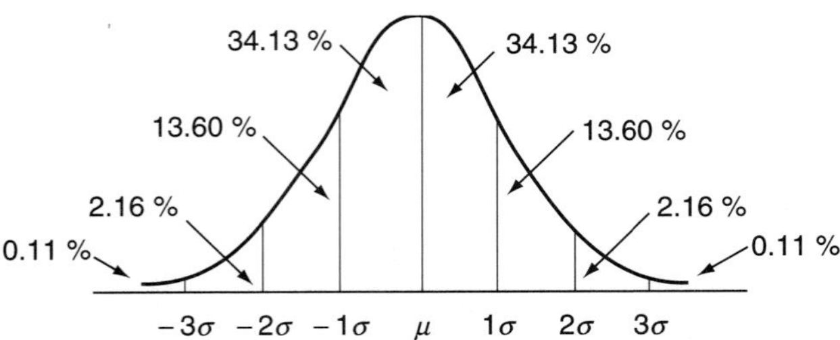

Figure 7-1 Normal distribution curve ("bell-shaped" curve). Persons will respond to drug dosages in dissimilar ways. Approximately 2.5% of persons will be extremely resistant to a "usual dose," and 2.5% will be quite sensitive to the same dose. (From Bennett CR: Anesth Prog 30:106, 1983.)

In the remainder of this chapter, drugs that are administered orally for sedation are reviewed. Drugs are discussed by their therapeutic category as follows:

1. Sedative-hypnotics
   a. Barbiturates
   b. Benzodiazepines
   c. Nonbenzodiazepines
2. Antianxiety drugs
3. Histamine blockers
4. Opioid analgesics

SEDATIVE-HYPNOTICS

Sedative-hypnotics are drugs that produce either sedation or hypnosis, depending on the dosage of the drug administered and the patient's response to it. Lower dosages of these drugs produce a calming effect (sedation), usually associated with a degree of drowsiness and motor incoordination (ataxia), whereas higher dosages produce hypnosis (a state resembling physiologic sleep).

Sedative-hypnotics are commonly divided into two groups: barbiturates and nonbarbiturate sedative-hypnotics. Alcohol, probably the most frequently used sedative-hypnotic, is discussed first.

Ethyl Alcohol

Alcohol has long been used by apprehensive patients as a means of medicating themselves before dental care. Each and every one of us in dentistry has had occasion to manage a patient who was quite well premedicated with alcohol (*not* prescribed by the doctor!). The very fact that patients believe that they require some form of sedation to "handle" their dental treatment should alert the dental office staff to the probable presence of anxiety (or of a drug abuse problem). The doctor should seek to determine the underlying dental fears harbored by such patients and take the steps necessary to correct or alleviate them.

As common a drug as alcohol may be, its use as a sedative in dentistry has never been popular. In 1923, Niels Bjorn Jorgensen, considered by many to be the "father of sedation in dentistry," first used medicinal alcohol in the management of the fearful adult patient. Jorgensen administered 4 oz of medicinal alcohol, with excellent results. Jorgensen later prescribed aromatic elixir USP in a flavored base, which became known as *Jorgensen's elixir.*[15]

McCarthy and Hayden[16] reviewed the history of alcohol, presenting a protocol for its use as a sedative in dentistry. McCarthy[17] has stated that many doctors have employed alcohol in their offices, virtually all with resounding success.

With the introduction of many newer pharmacologic drugs capable of more specific CNS depression than alcohol, its use as a pretreatment sedative has decreased. The reader interested in the administration of alcohol for sedation is referred to the McCarthy and Hayden paper for a detailed discussion of the technique.[16]

Barbiturates

The barbiturates represented the first truly effective drugs for the management of anxiety that were widely prescribed. Barbiturates are generalized CNS depressants, depressing the cerebral cortex, the limbic system, and the reticular activating system (RAS) at therapeutic blood levels. These actions produce a reduction in the anxiety level, decreased mental acuity, and drowsiness. At higher dosages, depression of the medulla occurs, leading to respiratory depression and possible cardiovascular depression. Barbiturates are capable of producing any level of CNS depression, ranging from light conscious sedation through hypnosis, general anesthesia, coma, and death.[18,19]

Pharmacology

Central Nervous System. Barbiturates produce a reversible depression of all excitable tissues, the CNS being remarkably sensitive. As previously mentioned, barbiturates produce a dose-related depression of the CNS, ranging from mild sedation to death. The reticular formation, a complex network of neurons, nuclei, and neural pathways extending through the brainstem from the medulla to the thalamus, is especially sensitive to barbiturate-induced depression. The reticular formation is sometimes called the *ascending reticular activating system* (ARAS) and is important in the maintenance of sleep and wakefulness. It appears that the major action of the barbiturates is on the ARAS.

Barbiturates commonly exert a clinical effect that exceeds the expected clinical duration of the drug. For example, an oral dose of secobarbital may produce a sedative action for only 3 to 4 hours, but there may be a subtle hangover effect consisting of mood alteration (irritability), drowsiness, and impaired judgment and this may persist for many hours.

Barbiturates lack the ability to obtund the sense of pain; in other words, they do not possess analgesic properties. Patients receiving noxious stimuli after having received barbiturates for sedation often hyperreact to the stimulus. Patients in pain who receive barbiturates may become aroused, agitated, and even dysphoric. Fortunately, this property of hyperalgesia is not shared by the nonbarbiturate sedative hypnotics. This increased response to pain in patients receiving barbiturates should concern dentists and physicians who are considering their use for sedation. Effective pain control must be provided whenever barbiturates are used. If this is not possible, other sedative drugs should be used in their place.

Barbiturates are capable of preventing or terminating convulsive episodes, such as those occurring in grand mal epilepsy or local anesthetic overdose.[20] To be effective, however, the barbiturate must be administered intravenously. A notable exception is phenobarbital, a drug that has been administered orally for many years in the preventive management of grand mal epilepsy.

Respiratory System. Barbiturates are respiratory depressants. At sedative doses there is little noticeable effect on respiration; however, at hypnotic levels or higher, a progressive depression of respiration is noted. These actions of the barbiturates are reviewed in the section on IV sedation.

Cardiovascular System. At oral doses normally used for sedation or hypnosis, barbiturates do not exhibit significant cardiovascular effects. Barbiturate-induced depression of the cardiovascular system is not usually seen until a significant degree of CNS and respiratory depression has developed.

Liver. In the therapeutic dosage range, barbiturates do not impair normal hepatic function; however, in patients who are hypersensitive to the barbiturates, severe liver damage can develop from therapeutic dosages.

Prolonged use of barbiturates produces a nonspecific increase in the activity of the hepatic microsomal enzyme system. The resultant rise in levels of these enzymes causes an increase in the rate at which many drugs (e.g., barbiturates) are metabolized. The induction of hepatic microsomal enzymes can give rise to drug-drug interactions. For example, barbiturates shorten the prothrombin time of patients receiving anticoagulants,[21] and the potency of digitoxin may be decreased by acceleration of its conversion to digoxin.[22] One of the more dangerous side effects of barbiturates on the liver is their ability to increase the synthesis of porphyrins. In patients who have acute intermittent porphyria, barbiturates may precipitate an episode of acute abdominal pain, nerve demyelination, paralysis, and death. Barbiturates are absolutely contraindicated in patients with acute intermittent porphyria.[23]

Termination of Clinical Activity. The processes responsible for termination of the clinical activity of barbiturates are redistribution of the drug, biotransformation, and renal excretion. All three produce a decrease in the plasma level of the drug and result in its removal from its primary site of action in the CNS.

Redistribution is responsible in large part for the short duration of clinical action noted with the intravenously administered barbiturates thiopental, methohexital, and thiamylal. The drug undergoes redistribution from the brain to other tissue compartments, where it is stored and slowly rereleased into the cardiovascular system, ultimately undergoing metabolic transformation when it reaches the liver. The slow release of the barbiturate from its storage site (liver or fat) may be responsible for the hangover effect seen with many barbiturates.

Barbiturates that do not undergo metabolic transformation in the liver are excreted from the body unchanged in the urine. The long-acting barbiturate barbital has approximately 65% to 90% of its total dose removed from the body in this manner, whereas about 50% of a hypnotic dose of phenobarbital or aprobarbital is handled in this manner.

Most barbiturates are eliminated from the body through biotransformation into inactive metabolites. The liver is the primary site for this process. Thiobarbiturates may undergo a small portion of their metabolism in the kidney and brain. The presence of hepatic microsomal enzymes affects the rate of metabolic degradation of barbiturates. Although these enzymes may be present at normal levels in patients with some hepatic diseases, cirrhotic patients may demonstrate an increased sensitivity to the barbiturates. Barbiturates must be administered with caution to patients with hepatic damage. Initial dosages should be decreased. The plasma half-lives (the time required for blood levels of the drug to fall by half) of the barbiturates vary significantly (Table 7-1).

Tolerance. Tolerance develops to the barbiturates, especially when they are administered on a long-term basis, a situation of minimal significance in dentistry. Persons addicted to barbiturates are often resistant (they hyporespond to the dose administered) to the hypnotic effects of the barbiturates and other depressants; however, tolerance to the hypnotic effects does not increase the lethal dose of the drugs. A hypnotic dose of a barbiturate taken daily for 2 weeks or longer will, at the end of this period, be ineffective in producing or maintaining sleep. Larger doses of the drug will be required to produce the same clinical effect observed with a smaller dose 2 weeks earlier. Of all the sedative-hypnotics (both barbiturate and nonbarbiturate) discussed in this chapter, only the benzodiazepines flurazepam and triazolam do not produce this tolerance.[24]

Dependence. Barbiturates produce both psychological and physical dependence (addiction). Methods of minimizing this problem include prescribing no more than the recommended dose of the drug and terminating the use of the drug at the earliest possible time. Within the realm of dentistry this is not very difficult to achieve.

TABLE 7-1 Classification of Barbiturates

Generic	Proprietary	Half-Life
Ultrashort-acting		
Hexobarbital	Sombulex	5 hours
Methohexital sodium*	Brevital, Brietal	3.5 to 6 hours
Thiamylal sodium*	Surital	—
Thiopental sodium*	Pentothal	3 to 8 hours
Short-acting		
Pentobarbital sodium*	Nembutal	21 to 42 hours
Secobarbital sodium*	Seconal	20 to 28 hours
Intermediate-acting		
Amobarbital	Amytal	14 to 42 hours
Butabarbital	Butisol	—
Long-acting		
Phenobarbital	—	24 to 96 hours

*Intravenous agents.

Oral Barbiturates in Dentistry. The barbiturates are classified as sedative-hypnotics, which at different dosage levels produce different levels of CNS depression manifested as relaxation (sedation) or drowsiness (hypnosis). Barbiturates are normally categorized by their duration of clinical action following an average oral dose (when possible). The *long-acting* (16 to 24 hours of clinical CNS depression) and the *intermediate-acting* (6 to 8 hours) *barbiturates* produce clinical levels of sedation far too long for the usual dental or surgical appointment. The long-acting barbiturates, such as phenobarbital, are commonly used as anticonvulsants or when long-term sedation is necessary; the intermediate-acting barbiturates are used as "sleeping pills" in specific types of insomnia (such as when a person has no difficulty in falling asleep but encounters difficulty in remaining asleep).

Short-acting barbiturates (3 to 4 hours' duration of action), most notably pentobarbital and secobarbital, are better suited for dental situations. They are also used for insomnia when the patient has difficulty in falling asleep but once asleep has no difficulty remaining asleep. Most of the *ultrashort-acting barbiturates* are used intravenously for the rapid induction of general anesthesia. The most frequently employed ultrashort-acting barbiturates are thiopental (Pentothal), thiamylal (Surital), and methohexital (Brevital, Brietal).

The barbiturates possess numerous disadvantages. In the years since the introduction of more effective and pharmacologically specific antianxiety drugs, barbiturate use has declined.[25] This laudable trend should continue as evidence accumulates regarding the adverse properties of barbiturates, including dose-related respiratory depression, the potential for habituation and addiction, the development of tolerance, and drug-drug interactions. In addition, the barbiturates are the drugs most often implicated in suicide attempts.[26]

Another important consideration in the use of barbiturates in dentistry is their lack of ability to obtund pain without inducing a concurrent decrease in the level of consciousness. In sedative doses the barbiturates actually increase a patient's response to noxious stimuli. Barbiturates ought not be administered to patients who are in pain or in whom pain is expected to occur (e.g., postoperatively).[27]

Of the dozen or so barbiturates in use clinically, only three (the short- and ultrashort-acting drugs) are of any value in dentistry, and even then only in isolated instances. The IV barbiturates, the intermediate-acting, and the long-acting barbiturates are of little value in contemporary dentistry for preoperative anxiety reduction. The two drugs of potential value when administered orally in dentistry and surgery are pentobarbital and secobarbital.

Contraindications. Barbiturates are contraindicated in cases of hypersensitivity (allergy), uncontrolled pain, known addiction to sedative-hypnotics, latent or manifest porphyria or familial history of intermittent porphyria, and presence of respiratory disease when dyspnea or obstruction is present. Barbiturates should be avoided in patients with severe hepatic dysfunction.

Pregnancy and Lactation. Barbiturates readily cross the placenta and, if administered during pregnancy, may have a depressant effect on the fetus. In addition, barbiturates are found in the milk of nursing mothers; therefore their use should be avoided during lactation.

Drug-Drug Interactions. Barbiturates may decrease the potency of the coumarin anticoagulants. Patients receiving both groups of drugs should undergo more frequent prothrombin determinations. The systemic actions of exogenous hydrocortisone and endogenous cortisol may also be diminished.

Care must be exercised when administering barbiturates to patients receiving other CNS depressant drugs because of the possibility of additive respiratory depression. These drugs include analgesics, other sedatives or hypnotics, alcohol, and antianxiety drugs.

Pentobarbital. Pentobarbital sodium is classified as a short-acting barbiturate. Its onset of action after oral administration is approximately 15 to 30 minutes, with a 3- to 6-hour duration of action. The half-life of pentobarbital is 21 to 42 hours. The therapeutic index (the ratio of the median lethal dose to median effective dose) of pentobarbital is relatively high, which is unusual for barbiturates. For this reason, as well as for its shorter duration of action, pentobarbital is preferred over most other barbiturates for sedation before dental or surgical care. Pentobarbital is available in dosage forms of 50- and 100-mg capsules. The average dose recommended for adult preoperative sedation is 100 mg, 1 hour before the scheduled appointment. Pentobarbital is packaged in white and yellow capsules. The name *yellow jackets* is frequently applied to this drug in the illicit drug market.

Pentobarbital	
Pregnancy category	D (see Box 4-1)
Lactation	?
Metabolism	Liver
Excretion	Urine
DEA schedule	II

Availability. Pentobarbital sodium (generic): 50- and 100-mg capsules. Nembutal sodium (Abbott): 50- and 100-mg capsules. Pentobarbital is a controlled substance in Schedule II.

Secobarbital. Secobarbital is a short-acting barbiturate with a half-life of 20 to 28 hours. Its onset of action develops within 15 to 30 minutes, with a duration of action of 3 to 6 hours. The therapeutic index of secobarbital is lower than that of pentobarbital, increasing the likelihood of unwanted side effects. The recommended dose for preoperative sedation is 100 to 200 mg taken 1 hour before the scheduled treatment. Secobarbital comes in distinctive red capsules, from which is derived its street name of *reds.*

Availability. Secobarbital sodium (generic): 50- and 100-mg capsules. Seconal sodium (Lilly): 30-, 50-, and 100-mg capsules. Seconal elixir (Lilly): 440 mg secobarbital per 100 ml. Secobarbital is a controlled substance in Schedule II.

Secobarbital	
Pregnancy category	D
Lactation	S
Metabolism	Liver
Excretion	Urine
DEA schedule	II

Summary. The short-acting barbiturates secobarbital and pentobarbital are appropriate for preoperative anxiety control and, on rare occasions, for more profound intraoperative sedation when more controllable techniques are not available or may be contraindicated. The latter use of these drugs cannot be recommended unless the doctor is capable of recognizing and managing any adverse reactions that might develop after administration of these drugs. Oversedation, noted as decreased cooperativeness and/or respiratory depression, is the most frequently observed clinical sign. Barbiturates should be used for sedation only when other, more effective antianxiety drugs (e.g., benzodiazepines) have proved to be ineffective or are unavailable.

Effective sedation with the barbiturates results in drowsiness. The patient *must* be accompanied by an adult and must be warned against operating a motor vehicle or dangerous machinery for the balance of the day.

Benzodiazepine Sedative-Hypnotics

Many other drugs share with barbiturates the ability to produce a state of hypnosis. These *nonbarbiturate sedative-hypnotics* have many of the same disadvantages as barbiturates. The only two ways in which these drugs differ from barbiturates are that (1) they are less potent than barbiturates and (2) they are not cross-allergenic with barbiturates. Drugs included in this category are listed here by their major classification:

1. Benzodiazepines
   a. Flurazepam
   b. Temazepam
   c. Triazolam
   d. Lorazepam
   e. Midazolam
2. Nonbenzodiazepine sedative-hypnotics
   a. Zolpidem
   b. Zaleplon
3. Chloral derivatives
   a. Chloral hydrate

Benzodiazepines. The benzodiazepines include some drugs categorized as sedative-hypnotics and others categorized as anxiolytics. All benzodiazepines have hypnotic effects to a degree; however, the incidence of side effects and the duration of action of some benzodiazepines preclude their use in this area. The pharmacology of this important therapeutic drug group is reviewed in depth in the section on oral antianxiety drugs.

One of the primary benefits gained from using benzodiazepines instead of barbiturates as sedative-hypnotics is the decreased occurrence of the hangover effect that so often accompanies the barbiturates. Additional benefits include a minimal effect on the hepatic microsomal enzyme system and the fact that pharmacologically the benzodiazepines present less of a risk to the patient than do the barbiturates. Six benzodiazepines have received significant attention as sedative-hypnotics: flurazepam, temazepam, triazolam, lorazepam, midazolam, and nitrazepam.

Flurazepam. Flurazepam, like most other benzodiazepines, has been demonstrated to produce its clinical action on the hypothalamus and the amygdala. Because of the lack of hepatic microsomal enzyme induction, the dose of flurazepam required to induce sleep does not increase with prolonged administration. Following oral administration, flurazepam is rapidly absorbed and distributed; peak plasma levels develop within 30 to 60 minutes. Because flurazepam is biotransformed in the liver, the drug should be used with caution in patients with hepatic dysfunction. The half-life of flurazepam is 47 to 100 hours.

The incidence of side effects occurring with flurazepam administration is approximately 7%. The most frequently reported side effects include dizziness, drowsiness, lightheadedness, staggering, and ataxia. The hangover effect so often seen with barbiturates is infrequent with flurazepam.

The clinical effectiveness of a 15- to 30-mg dose of flurazepam has been demonstrated in controlled trials to be equivalent to that of 100 mg of secobarbital, 100 mg of pentobarbital, 50 mg of amobarbital, 500 mg of glutethimide, and 500 and 1000 mg of chloral hydrate.[28]

Contraindications. The use of flurazepam is contraindicated in patients with hypersensitivity (allergy) to benzodiazepines and in pregnant women.

Warnings. Patients should be cautioned against operating motor vehicles or hazardous machinery and combining other CNS depressant drugs, such as alcohol, with flurazepam.

Drug Interactions. Additive CNS depressant actions may develop when flurazepam is administered to patients taking other CNS depressants, such as alcohol, barbiturates, or opioids.

Dosage. The usual dose of flurazepam is 30 mg taken 1 hour before bedtime. In elderly or debilitated patients, a 15-mg dose is recommended.

Availability. Dalmane (Roche): 15- and 30-mg capsules. Flurazepam is a controlled substance in Schedule IV.

Flurazepam	
Pregnancy category	X
Lactation	NS
Metabolism	Liver
Excretion	Urine
DEA schedule	IV

Temazepam. Temazepam is absorbed slowly after oral administration. Onset occurs within 20 to 30 minutes; however, peak plasma levels require 2 to 3 hours (whereas flurazepam reaches peak levels at 30 minutes to 1 hour). The mean plasma half-life is 10 hours, and there are no significant active metabolites. The primary clinical use of temazepam is for patients having difficulty remaining asleep once they fall asleep. Because of its slow onset of action, temazepam is not effective in patients having difficulty falling asleep.

Contraindications, warnings, and drug interactions are similar to those for flurazepam (discussed previously).

Dosage. The usual dose is 30 mg 1 hour before bedtime. The 15-mg dosage form should be used initially in elderly and debilitated patients.

Availability. Restoril (Sandoz): 15- and 30-mg capsules. Temazepam is a controlled substance in Schedule IV.

Temazepam	
Pregnancy category	X
Lactation	NS
Metabolism	Liver
Excretion	Urine
DEA schedule	IV

Triazolam. Triazolam is another benzodiazepine derivative. It was approved for marketing as a hypnotic in 1982 and has become the most prescribed psychoactive drug in the United States.[29] Triazolam is valuable in dentistry because of its short half-life of 1.5 to 5.5 hours and the fact that it has no active metabolites.[30] Peak plasma levels develop at 1.3 hours (following oral administration). Very little residual drowsiness (hangover) is noted with triazolam.

Triazolam has been used in dentistry as an effective oral drug in the management of pretreatment anxiety.[31,32] Several recent trials have evaluated its effectiveness in pediatric populations.[33,34] The use of oral triazolam in pediatric anxiety control is discussed more fully in Chapter 35.

Contraindications. Triazolam is contraindicated in pregnant patients.

Warnings. Overdosage of triazolam may develop at four times the recommended therapeutic dosage. Patients receiving triazolam must be cautioned against operating machinery or driving a motor vehicle and against the simultaneous ingestion of alcohol and other CNS depressant drugs.

Anterograde amnesia, of varying intensity, and paradoxical reactions have been reported following therapeutic doses of triazolam.[35] Cases of "traveler's amnesia" have been reported by persons taking triazolam to induce sleep while traveling, such as during an airplane flight.[36] In some of these cases, insufficient time was allowed for the sleep period before awakening and before beginning activity. Triazolam (Halcion) has received some extremely negative press.[37,38] Great Britain, following reports of several serious complications, including suicide, banned the prescription of triazolam.[39] Following discussion of the safety and potential hazards posed by triazolam, the U.S. Food and Drug Administration (FDA) decided against issuing any prohibitions on the prescription of this drug in the United States.[40]

Drug Interactions. Additive CNS depressant actions may develop when triazolam is administered to patients receiving other CNS depressants such as alcohol, barbiturates, or opioids.

Adverse Reactions. The most common adverse side effects noted after triazolam administration are drowsiness (14.0%), headache (9.7%), dizziness (7.8%), and nervousness (5.2%).[41]

Dosage. A hypnotic dose of 0.25 mg 1 hour before bedtime or 1 hour before dental treatment is adequate for most patients, and a dose of 0.125 mg may be sufficient for selected patients. A dose of 0.5 mg should be reserved for patients who do not respond adequately to a smaller dose because the risk of several adverse reactions increases with the size of the dose administered.

In elderly or debilitated patients, the recommended dose is 0.125 to 0.25 mg. The initial dose in this group should be 0.125 mg.

Availability. Halcion (Upjohn): 0.125- and 0.25-mg tablets. Triazolam is a controlled substance in Schedule IV.

Triazolam	
Pregnancy category	X
Lactation	?
Metabolism	Liver
Excretion	Urine
DEA schedule	IV

Lorazepam. Lorazepam is absorbed slowly after oral administration; peak plasma levels develop in 2 hours, and the mean half-life is 12 hours. The drug was marketed in 1977 under the trade name of Ativan. Lorazepam is also available for parenteral administration. Orally, the drug is effective as an antianxiety and hypnotic drug. It is one of the few benzodiazepines not possessing active metabolites. Hepatic dysfunction (hepatitis, cirrhosis) does not alter the manner in which lorazepam is handled by the liver.

Contraindications. Lorazepam is contraindicated in patients with known sensitivity to benzodiazepines and with narrow-angle glaucoma.

Warnings. Lorazepam is not recommended for patients with a primary depressive disorder or psychosis. Patients receiving lorazepam must be cautioned against operating machinery or driving a motor vehicle and against the simultaneous ingestion of alcohol and other CNS depressant drugs.

Drug Interactions. Additive CNS depressant effects develop with the concurrent administration of other CNS depressant drugs, such as opioids, barbiturates, and alcohol.

Adverse Reactions. The most frequently observed side effects of lorazepam are sedation (15.9%), dizziness (6.9%), weakness (4.2%), and ataxia (3.4%).[42]

Because of the greater possibility of unwanted sedation with lorazepam than with other benzodiazepines, its use in the immediate preoperative period should be discouraged unless the doctor desires this effect and if arrangements have been made for the patient to be escorted from the office by an adult companion. The use of lorazepam the evening before treatment to ensure a restful night's sleep appears more reasonable.

Dosage. The usual adult dosage of lorazepam is from 2 to 6 mg in two or three divided doses. The largest dose should be taken 1 hour before bedtime. For anxiety the initial dose is from 2 to 3 mg per day in two to three doses. Elderly or debilitated patients should receive an initial dose of 1 to 2 mg per day in divided dosages. The safety and efficacy of lorazepam in patients younger than 12 years has not been established (as is true for most drugs). For preoperative anxiety control or as an aid to sleep before dental or surgical treatment, a single dose of 2 to 4 mg may be given 1 hour before sleep or the appointment.

Availability. Ativan (Wyeth): 0.5-, 1-, and 2-mg tablets. Ativan is a controlled substance in Schedule IV.

Lorazepam	
Pregnancy category	D
Lactation	NS
Metabolism	Liver
Excretion	Urine
DEA schedule	IV

Midazolam. Midazolam is available in an oral dosage form for use as a sedative-hypnotic. It is prepared as a syrup in a concentration of 2 mg/ml.

The absorption and onset of clinical action of midazolam are more rapid than those of benzodiazepines, with which it has been compared.[43,44] Peak action after oral administration occurs within 30 minutes.[45] Monti et al.[46] concluded that a 15-mg oral dose of midazolam was appropriate for patients demonstrating difficulty in falling asleep and that a 30-mg dose was appropriate in patients having difficulties in staying asleep. The actions of midazolam are less apparent after 8 hours than those of other benzodiazepines.[43] Hildebrand et al.[47] concluded that absorption of midazolam is better with oral than intramuscular administration. The clinical pharmacology of midazolam is discussed in more detail in Chapters 10 and 25. Midazolam has been employed orally as premedication before surgical procedures in medicine[48] as well as in dentistry for adults[49,50] and dentistry for children.[51-54]

The usual adult oral dosage of midazolam when used to help induce sleep is 15 mg taken 1 hour before bedtime. Wahlmann, Dietrich, and Fischer[49] administered a dose of 7.5 mg preoperatively for anxiety control in adults before oral surgery with little success, whereas Luyk and Whitley,[50] using the same dose, demonstrated significant anxiolysis, amnesia, and patient preference. Using a 10-mg dose of the parenteral form of midazolam orally, Turner and Paech[48] found the drug to be equal to a 20-mg dose of oral temazepam in anxiolysis and sedation preceding day-case gynecologic surgery. In pediatrics, oral doses of midazolam have proven effective in dosages ranging from 0.2 mg/kg[53] to 0.4 mg/kg[56,57] to 0.5 mg/kg[51,54,55] to 0.75 mg/kg.[56]

Contraindications. Contraindications are similar to those of other benzodiazepines and include narrow-angle glaucoma, severe respiratory disease (COPD), congestive heart failure (CHF), and impaired renal or hepatic function.

Dosage. For procedural sedation in pediatrics in patients older than 6 months of age, the recommended dosage of midazolam syrup is 0.25 to 0.5 mg/kg. Maximum should not exceed 20 mg/dose.

Availability. As Versed as a 2.0 mg/ml syrup. In other countries, midazolam is available as 7.5-mg tablets.

Midazolam	
Pregnancy category	D
Lactation	?
Metabolism	Liver
Excretion	Feces and urine
DEA schedule	IV

COMMENT: The benzodiazepines are the preferred drugs for the management of preoperative anxiety in the dental setting. This is also the case in situations in which nighttime sedation is desirable. The primary advantage of the benzodiazepines over other sedative-hypnotics, especially the barbiturates, is their relative safety. The benzodiazepines have proved to be relatively innocuous when taken alone in intentional or accidental overdosage.[58] In addition, the benzodiazepines do not produce clinically significant hepatic microsomal enzyme induction, nor do they interact as significantly with other drugs, such as the coumarin anticoagulants, as do the barbiturates.

The benzodiazepines most preferred for their hypnotic effects, either for sleep the evening before treatment or for preoperative sedation, are flurazepam (30 or 15 mg) and triazolam (0.125 and 0.25 mg). With the introduction of an oral preparation, midazolam has become an attractive drug for preoperative sedation in children.

Nonbenzodiazepine Anxiolytics/Hypnotics

Zolpidem (Ambien). Zolpidem tartrate is a nonbenzodiazepine sedative-hypnotic of the imidazopyridine class used for the short-term management of insomnia. It was approved for use in the United States in 1993.

Actions. Although zolpidem is unrelated structurally to benzodiazepines, it interacts with a gamma aminobutyric acid (GABA)–benzodiazepine receptor complex and shares some of the pharmacologic properties of benzodiazepines. It is a strong sedative with only mild anxiolytic, myorelaxant, and anticonvulsant properties. It has been shown to be effective in inducing and maintaining sleep in adults.[59]

Following oral administration, zolpidem is rapidly absorbed from the GI tract, having an onset of action of 45 minutes and a peak effect seen in 1.6 hours. It is metabolized in the liver, with an elimination half-life of 2.6 hours. Zolpidem is converted into inactive metabolites eliminated primarily through renal clearance. Zolpidem is one of a few CNS depressants that is recommended for administration during pregnancy (pregnancy category B; see Box 4-1).

Precautions. Respiratory depression is not usually seen in healthy patients receiving hypnotic doses of zolpidem. If it is used in patients with compromised respiratory function, the likelihood of depressed respiratory drive is increased.[11,60]

Contraindications. Contraindications include a history of hypersensitivity to zolpidem. Zolpidem should be used cautiously in patients with acute intermittent porphyria or impaired renal or hepatic function, in addiction-prone patients, and during pregnancy and lactation.

Adverse Effects. Adverse effects most commonly observed (>3%) include dizziness, drugged feelings, headache, allergy, back pain, headache, drowsiness, lethargy, nausea, dyspepsia, diarrhea, myalgia, arthralgia, and dry mouth.[11,60]

Availability. Zolpidem tartrate (Ambien, Searle): 5- and 10-mg tablets.

Dosage: Adult. 10 mg PO hs.

Dosage: Pediatric. The safety and efficacy of zolpidem have not been established in children.

Dosage: Geriatric. Elderly and debilitated patients may be especially sensitive to the effects of zolpidem. An initial dosage of 5 mg orally is recommended in these patients.

Zolpidem	
Pregnancy category	B
Lactation	S
Metabolism	Liver
Excretion	Feces and urine
DEA schedule	IV

Zaleplon (Sonata, Wyeth-Ayerst Laboratories). Zaleplon is another nonbenzodiazepine sedative-hypnotic of the imidazopyridine class used for the short-term management of insomnia.[61,62]

Actions. Pharmacologically and pharmacokinetically, zaleplon is similar to zolpidem. Both are hypnotic agents with short half-lives, and both have been demonstrated to interact with GABA receptors. Zaleplon appears to be absorbed and eliminated more rapidly than zolpidem.

Precautions. No precautions are known, according to the manufacturer.

Contraindications. Use with caution in patients who demonstrate hypersensitivity to this class of drugs, in patients with impaired hepatic function, in elderly patients, in pregnant patients, in those with pulmonary disease, and in those with a history of drug abuse.

Adverse Effects. Dependency and abuse are potential problems associated with prolonged administration. More common adverse reactions include drowsiness, amnesia, paresthesias, abnormal vision, dizziness, headache, hangover effect, rebound insomnia, and confusion.

Dosage: Adult. 5 to 10 mg orally 1 hour before sleep.

Dosage: Pediatric. The safety and efficacy of zaleplon have not been established in children.

Availability. Zaleplon (Sonata): 5- and 10-mg capsules.

Zaleplon	
Pregnancy category	C
Lactation	NS
Metabolism	Liver
Excretion	Other
DEA schedule	IV

Chloral Derivatives

Chloral Hydrate. Several drugs classified as chloral derivatives may be used for hypnosis or sedation. Within the practice of dentistry, one of these drugs, chloral hydrate, is a popular drug for the management of anxiety, particularly in pediatric dentistry. Chloral betaine and triclofos sodium are other less commonly used members of this group.

Chloral hydrate, first synthesized in 1832, was the first member of the hypnotic group of drugs. With the introduction of the barbiturates, interest in chloral hydrate waned; however, there has been a renewal of interest in it since the 1950s. Chloral hydrate is available for oral administration as a syrup.

Chloral hydrate is quite irritating to skin and mucous membranes. It also produces GI irritation in a high percentage of patients.[63] Gastric upset may be minimized by diluting the drug or by following the drug immediately with a full glass (8 oz) of water or milk. In pediatric dentistry particularly, the syrup is especially useful. Unfortunately, the elixir has an unpleasant taste, which may be masked by mixing the drug with a suitable liquid such as ginger ale or fruit juice.

Chloral hydrate does not possess any analgesic properties; therefore the drug should not be administered to patients who are in pain because their response may be quite exaggerated. The effects of a therapeutic dose of chloral hydrate on blood pressure and respiration are negligible, similar to those occurring in normal sleep.[64] Chloral hydrate is rapidly absorbed through the GI tract into the cardiovascular system and undergoes metabolic degradation in the liver and kidneys into its active form, trichloroethanol. Other chloral derivatives, chloral betaine and triclofos sodium, undergo metabolic degradation into chloral hydrate and then into trichloroethanol. Trichloroethanol is thought to be the active metabolite responsible for the CNS depressant effects of these three drugs. The chloral derivatives may be administered safely to patients with hepatic and renal dysfunction. The half-life of chloral hydrate is 7 to 9.5 hours.

Among the untoward effects produced by the irritating properties of chloral hydrate are an unpleasant taste, gastric upset, nausea, vomiting, and flatulence. Other CNS effects considered uncomfortable are lightheadedness, ataxia, and nightmares.[65] Hangover is a much less common occurrence than with barbiturates. Chloral hydrate, although not metabolized by the hepatic microsomal enzyme system, does accelerate the metabolism of drugs such as the coumarin anticoagulants. The toxic oral dose reported for chloral hydrate is 10 g, although death has been reported with as little as 4000 mg (4 g). More important in clinical situations is the dose of chloral hydrate based on patient body weight. The usual oral dose is 50 mg/kg (or about 25 mg/lb) of body weight, with a suggested range of 40 to 60 mg/kg.[63,64,66,67] In a survey of pediatric residency programs it was determined that chloral hydrate in doses between 25 and 100 mg/kg is the most common drug used for sedation.[68]

Reports of overdose following chloral hydrate administration in pediatric dentistry are rare but have included cases of life-threatening hypotension and respiratory arrest following estimated doses of 86 and 118 mg/kg.[64,69] The GI upset produced by chloral hydrate proves to be advantageous when accidental overdosage occurs. With doses larger than 60 mg/kg, vomiting is frequently noted, thus diminishing the absorption of chloral hydrate from the GI tract and limiting the degree of overdose observed.[63]

Following oral administration the onset of action of chloral hydrate is rapid; drowsiness or a rousable sleep usually developing within 30 to 45 minutes. Duration of action is 2 to 5 hours.

Chloral hydrate is useful as a sedative before dental care and to assist the patient in achieving a restful night's sleep before a scheduled treatment. It is an especially useful drug in debilitated, elderly, and younger patients. Chloral hydrate appears to be less effective when given in smaller doses or when used for dental care in older patients with disabilities.[70-72]

Contraindications. Allergy to chloral hydrate or other chloral derivatives, severe hepatic or renal dysfunction, severe heart disease, and gastritis are contraindications. Chloral hydrate should not be prescribed to nursing women because the drug does appear in breast milk.

Warnings. Prolonged use of chloral hydrate may be habit forming. This is unlikely to occur in dental situations because of the manner in which the drug is prescribed.

Drug Interactions. As with the barbiturates, chloral hydrate must be used with caution in patients who are concurrently receiving the coumarin anticoagulants. Prothrombin times should be monitored on a more frequent basis. Doses of chloral hydrate should be decreased in patients receiving other CNS depressant drugs, such as alcohol, opioids, and barbiturates, because additive CNS depression will develop.

Precautions. Chloral hydrate should be used with caution in patients with severe cardiovascular disease, because large doses (significantly greater than therapeutic) may further depress the myocardium. In therapeutic dosages there is no contraindication to the administration of this drug in patients with cardiovascular disease.

Adverse Reactions. The most frequently reported adverse effect of chloral hydrate is gastric irritability. The only other adverse reaction, reported on occasion, is the occurrence of a skin rash.

Dosage. The dosages presented here are for the adult patient. The use of chloral hydrate in pediatric dentistry is presented in Chapter 35.

The hypnotic dose of chloral hydrate is 500 to 1000 mg taken 15 to 30 minutes before bedtime. The usual dose for sedation in a nondental setting is 250 mg; however, when chloral hydrate is administered for surgery or dental procedures, doses of 500 to 1500 mg may be required.

When the capsule form of chloral hydrate is prescribed, the drug should be taken with a full (8-oz) glass of water. If administered as an elixir or syrup, chloral hydrate should be mixed in one half glass of water, ginger ale, or fruit juice.

Availability. Chloral hydrate (generic): 250- and 500-mg capsules; 500 mg/5 ml (tsp) syrup; 500 mg/5 ml (tsp) elixir.

Chloral Hydrate	
Pregnancy category	C
Lactation	S
Metabolism	Liver
Excretion	Urine, primarily
DEA schedule	IV

ANTIANXIETY DRUGS

Antianxiety drugs are used to manage mild to moderate daytime anxiety and tension. Drugs in this group share a similar CNS depressant action: At therapeutic dosages they produce a mild degree of anxiolysis without impairing the patient's mental alertness or psychomotor performance. Groups of drugs that are commonly categorized as antianxiety drugs are as follows:

1. Benzodiazepines
   a. Chlordiazepoxide
   b. Diazepam
   c. Oxazepam
   d. Clorazepate
   e. Prazepam
   f. Halazepam
   g. Alprazolam

For the management of mild to moderate levels of anxiety, the benzodiazepine antianxiety drugs are much preferred to the barbiturates because the latter group much more commonly produces the undesirable side effect of loss of alertness. Intentional and unintentional overdosage occurs much more readily with barbiturates, and undesirable actions are noted at dosages just slightly above the usual therapeutic levels. Benzodiazepine antianxiety drugs have a wider therapeutic dosage range and thus are less likely to produce unwanted side effects.

Although termed *antianxiety drugs,* a more appropriate name for these drugs might be *sedative-antianxiety drugs,* for all drugs in this group possess sedative properties as well as antianxiety actions.

The antianxiety drugs have, in the past, been known by other names, such as *minor tranquilizers, anxiolytics, ataractics, anxiolytic sedatives,* and *psychosedatives.* The general category "antianxiety drugs" has become accepted for this group of drugs.

Benzodiazepines

The benzodiazepines are the most effective drugs currently available for the management of anxiety. They also possess skeletal muscle relaxant properties and are anticonvulsants. More than 2000 benzodiazepines have been synthesized since 1933. Chlordiazepoxide was the first benzodiazepine introduced (1960). In

2001, in the United States, 12 benzodiazepines were available, 7 of which were categorized as antianxiety drugs. These included alprazolam, chlordiazepoxide, clorazepate, diazepam, halazepam, and oxazepam. Estazolam, flurazepam, lorazepam, midazolam, quazepam, temazepam, and triazolam were classified as sedative-hypnotics, and clonazepam was approved for use only as an anticonvulsant.

The benzodiazepines are one of the most popular classes of drugs available today. Diazepam has remained one of the most prescribed drugs in the United States since 1977. Approximately 30% of all psychotropic drug prescriptions are for benzodiazepines (100 million prescriptions annually). Furthermore, it is estimated that between 5% and 15% of adults in the United States take some form of antianxiety drug. More than one third of hospital inpatients receive a benzodiazepine during their hospitalization. In recent years the overuse and possible misuse of benzodiazepines have come under scrutiny. However, in the dental or surgical situation, rational drug-prescribing habits minimize potential misuse of this very important class of antianxiety drugs.

Pharmacology

Mode of Action. The benzodiazepines have depressant effects on subcortical levels of the CNS. The specific anxiolytic effect of benzodiazepines is a result of their actions on the limbic system and the thalamus, those areas of the brain involved with emotions and behavior. Benzodiazepines have been called *limbic system sedatives* because they impair neuronal discharge in the amygdala and amygdala-hippocampus nerve transmission. Benzodiazepines depress the limbic system at doses smaller than those depressing the RAS and the cerebral cortex. The barbiturates and other sedative-hypnotics, on the other hand, do not exhibit this selective depression, producing instead a generalized depression of the CNS.

Specific receptors for benzodiazepines have been isolated within the spinal cord and the brain. The location of these receptors parallels that of GABA, the major inhibitory neurotransmitter in the brain, and of glycine, the major inhibitory neurotransmitter in the spinal cord.[63] Benzodiazepines act by intensifying the physiologic inhibitory effects of GABA by interfering with GABA reuptake.[73-75]

One of the most significant features of the benzodiazepines as a group is the very wide margin of safety between therapeutic and toxic doses. Ataxia and sedation develop only at doses beyond those required for antianxiety effects.

Central Nervous System. The principal behavioral effects of the benzodiazepines are the following:

1. Reduction of hostile and aggressive behavior (frequently termed *taming*)
2. Attenuation of the behavioral consequences of frustration, fear, and punishment (termed *disinhibition,* this is the most consistently observed behavioral action of the benzodiazepine antianxiety drugs)

It is interesting that when aggression and hostility are held in check by fear and anxiety, the ingestion of a benzodiazepine or other anxiolytic drug may produce a "paradoxic" increase in aggression. Other CNS depressants, such as the barbiturates, produce these same effects, but only at doses that produce drowsiness and motor incoordination. The benzodiazepines commonly achieve this action without these side effects.[76]

Other CNS actions of the benzodiazepines include skeletal muscle relaxant properties and anticonvulsant effects.[77,78] The site of action of the muscle relaxant properties of benzodiazepines is yet to be determined; however, it is thought that the effect is central rather than peripheral. Skeletal muscle relaxation appears to be caused by a combination of central depression of the brainstem reticular formation and depression of polysynaptic spinal reflexes.[77,79] Anticonvulsant actions of benzodiazepines are produced by a depression of epileptiform discharge in the cerebral cortex and an enhancement of electrical activity of Purkinje cells. For effective anticonvulsant activity, the benzodiazepines must be administered intravenously (although intramuscularly administered midazolam has terminated seizures).[80] Diazepam and clonazepam are currently approved for anticonvulsant therapy.

Respiratory System. All sedative-hypnotics and antianxiety drugs (including benzodiazepines) are potential respiratory depressants. At usual therapeutic oral dosages in healthy patients, the benzodiazepines, administered alone, do not produce clinically significant respiratory depression and do not potentiate the depressant effects of opiates. Cases of significant respiratory depression and respiratory arrest following oral benzodiazepine ingestion have been reported.[81,82]

Cardiovascular System. Following oral administration to a healthy patient (American Society of Anesthesiologists [ASA] I), benzodiazepines produce virtually no changes in cardiovascular function. Indeed, the benzodiazepines are frequently used in the management of anxiety and depression associated with cardiac disease. They are preferred to the barbiturates and other sedative-hypnotics in this situation, primarily because they do not produce unwanted degrees of CNS depression or restlessness and because they do not produce cardiovascular depression at therapeutic levels.[83]

Liver. The benzodiazepines undergo biotransformation in the liver (see following section); however, they do not stimulate the induction of hepatic microsomal enzymes. Potentially hazardous drug interactions, such as those observed between the barbiturates and coumarin anticoagulants, are not observed with benzodiazepines. In addition, patients with hepatic dysfunction may receive the benzodiazepines without increased risk of side effect, regardless of the cause of the hepatic dysfunction.

Absorption, Metabolism, Excretion. Following oral administration, all benzodiazepines are absorbed relatively rapidly and reliably from the GI tract. The rate at which maximum plasma levels develop exhibits significant variation among the different benzodiazepines and among individuals. Approximate time for peak plasma levels following oral administration of several benzodiazepines is shown in Table 7-2.

Benzodiazepines undergo biotransformation in the liver. There is considerable variation in the half-lives of these drugs: Diazepam's elimination half-life is 20 to 70 hours, whereas triazolam's is 1.5 to 5.5 hours. In addition, many of the benzodiazepines have biotransformation products that are pharmacologically as active as the parent drug (Table 7-3).

Chlordiazepoxide has a plasma half-life of between 24 and 48 hours and has as intermediate metabolites two pharmacologically active chemicals, desmethylchlordiazepoxide and demoxepam. The half-life of diazepam ranges between 20 and 70 hours (frequently quoted as "1 hour per year of age"). Pharmacologically active metabolites of diazepam include desmethyldiazepam (half-life of 96 hours), temazepam, and oxazepam. Flurazepam, with a plasma half-life of 2.3 hours, has an active metabolite with a half-life of 47 to 100 hours. Medazepam has three active metabolites: diazepam, desmethyldiazepam, and desmethylmedazepam; prazepam (half-life 63 to 70 hours) has among its metabolites desmethyldiazepam and oxazepam. Desmethyldiazepam is a metabolite of clorazepate.

TABLE 7-2 Onset of Peak Plasma Levels Following Oral Administration of Benzodiazepines

Drug	Peak Plasma Level (hr)
Flurazepam	0.5-1
Midazolam	0.5
Triazolam	1.3
Medazepam	1-2
Alprozolam	1-2
Oxazepam	1-4
Nitrazepam	2
Diazepam	2
Lorazepam	2
Halazepam	2
Temazepam	2-3
Chlordiazepoxide	4
Prazepam	4-6

TABLE 7-3 Properties of Benzodiazepines

	Peak Plasma Level (hr)	Half-Life (hr)	Active Metabolites
Alprazolam	1-2	12-15	No
Chlordiazepoxide	4	24-48	Yes
Clorazepate	1	48	Yes
Clonazepam	1-2	18-50	Yes
Diazepam	2	20-70	Yes
Flunitrazepam	—	13.5-36	Yes
Flurazepam	0.5-1	2.3	Yes
Halazepam	2	14	Yes
Lorazepam	2	12	No
Medazepam	1-2	—	—
Midazolam	0.5	1.2-12.3	No
Nitrazepam	2	18-28	No
Oxazepam	1-4	5.7-10.9	No
Prazepam	4-6	63-70	Yes
Temazepam	2-3	10	No
Triazolam	1.3	1.5-5.5	No

Nitrazepam, oxazepam, lorazepam, midazolam, triazolam, temazepam, and alprazolam are biotransformed into pharmacologically inactive metabolites. The combination of rapid absorption from the GI tract (1 to 4 hours), short elimination half-life (5.7 to 9 hours), and inactive metabolites make oxazepam an attractive drug for the management of anxiety within the dental or surgical environment. Lorazepam, on the other hand, with a slow rate of absorption (2 hours) and a half-life of 12 hours (range 9 to 24 hours), is less appealing. Triazolam, with a rapid onset of action and short half-life (1.5 to 5.5 hours), is ideally suited as a hypnotic in dentistry.[31,32,34]

All benzodiazepines are excreted in the feces and urine. The percentage of urinary excretion varies from 80% for flurazepam and oxazepam to 22% for prazepam.

Dependence. Psychological and physiologic dependence may develop to benzodiazepines.[84] The incidence of physiologic dependence is considerably less than that of psychological dependence. It is unlikely to develop unless the patient takes doses much greater than therapeutic over long periods of time. Within the dental setting, there is little likelihood of this occurring.

Oral Benzodiazepines in Dentistry. The benzodiazepines represent the most nearly ideal drugs for the management of anxiety. In the dental and surgical setting the benzodiazepines remain the drugs of choice via the oral route for the management of mild to moderate pretreatment anxiety and apprehension in the adult patient. Many benzodiazepines are currently available, and many more will surely become available in the future. Because there are significant differences in the onset of action and the duration of action among these drugs, the choice of a specific drug should be made only after consideration of the needs of both the patient and the doctor.

Although there are indications for the use of other drugs in specific instances, the drugs most ideally suited for pretreatment anxiety control via oral administration in the dental and surgical setting are oxazepam and diazepam. For patients requiring sedation (hypnosis) to sleep restfully the evening before their treatment, flurazepam and triazolam are preferred.

Contraindications. Allergy, psychoses, and acute narrow-angle glaucoma are contraindications. Benzodiazepines may be administered to patients with open-angle glaucoma who are receiving appropriate therapy.

Warnings. Patients must be advised against driving a motor vehicle or operating hazardous machinery. Other CNS depressants, such as alcohol, opioids, and barbiturates, should be avoided while benzodiazepines are being administered. There is some evidence that the use of benzodiazepines (particularly chlordiazepoxide and diazepam) during the first trimester of pregnancy increases the risk of congenital malformations (e.g., cleft palate).[85] Benzodiazepines cross the placental barrier and are excreted in breast milk.

Benzodiazepines in Children. Use of oral diazepam tablets in children younger than 6 months of age is not recommended. Oral diazepam has been used successfully in pediatric dentistry. Recommended pediatric doses range from 0.15 to 0.3 mg/kg.[86,87] Midazolam, a sedative-hypnotic, is recommended in an oral dose of 0.2 to 0.5 mg/kg. Oral forms of chlordiazepoxide and oxazepam are not recommended for children younger than 6 years. Clorazepate is not recommended in patients younger than 18 years. This is a common statement in the drug package insert of many drugs and is a reflection of an inadequate volume of research data on these age groups. A more in-depth discussion of the use of oral benzodiazepines can be found in Chapter 35.

Drug Interactions. Patients should be advised against the concurrent use of benzodiazepines and other CNS depressants. This includes alcohol; other psychotropic drugs such as phenothiazines, opioids, barbiturates, and monoamine oxidase (MAO) inhibitors; and other antidepressants.

Precautions. Drug dosages should be decreased in elderly or debilitated patients. Initial dosages should be small, with subsequent increases if warranted, as judged by the patient's response (titration by appointment). In this way, the adverse effects of drowsiness and ataxia may be minimized.

Adverse Reactions. The most frequently reported adverse reactions following oral benzodiazepine administration for anxiolysis include transient drowsiness (especially in the elderly or debilitated), fatigue, and ataxia.

Paradoxic reactions, although rare, may occur and consist of excitement, hallucinations, insomnia, and rage.[76] Discontinuance of drug administration leads to termination of these effects.

Chlordiazepoxide. Chlordiazepoxide was synthesized by Leo Sternbach in 1955. When tested in 1957, it was demonstrated to possess hypnotic and sedative properties, as well as skeletal muscle relaxant and anticonvulsant actions. The chemical is inactivated when exposed to ultraviolet light; thus it is marketed as a capsule. Chlordiazepoxide may also be used parenterally; however, because of its lack of stability, it must be prepared immediately before injection. Other benzodiazepines, such as diazepam, midazolam, and lorazepam, are more stable and are preferred to chlordiazepoxide when parenteral administration is required.

On February 24, 1960, the FDA approved the marketing of the first benzodiazepine, chlordiazepoxide, under the brand name Librium.

When administered orally, chlordiazepoxide is absorbed well from the GI tract; however, peak plasma levels of the drug do not develop for up to 4 hours. Although adequate anxiety reduction may develop within 1 to 2 hours, the slow onset of anxiolysis makes chlordiazepoxide less attractive than other, newer benzodiazepines in the management of mild to moderate anxiety in the pretreatment period in surgery and dentistry.

Hypotension and syncope have been observed after large oral doses of chlordiazepoxide, and there have been reports of usual oral doses exacerbating ventilatory failure in patients with chronic bronchitis.[88] Long-term use of larger than usual doses may produce physical or psychological dependence, or both.

Dosage. The adult dosage of chlordiazepoxide for relief of mild to moderate anxiety is 5 or 10 mg three to four times daily. For relief of severe anxiety and tension, the dosage is 20 or 25 mg three to four times daily. The dosage for elderly patients or patients with debilitating disease is 5 mg two to four times daily. The recommended dosage for preoperative apprehension and anxiety is 5 to 10 mg three to four times daily on the day before treatment or surgery.

Chlordiazepoxide is not recommended for use in children younger than 6 years. For older children, treatment should be initiated with the smallest possible dose and increased as required: 5 mg two to four times daily to start, increased to 10 mg two to three times daily, if needed.

Availability. Chlordiazepoxide (generic), Librium (Roche), SK-Lygen (Smith Kline and French): 5-, 10-, and 25-mg capsules. Chlordiazepoxide is a controlled substance in Schedule IV.

Chlordiazepoxide	
Pregnancy category	D
Lactation	NS
Metabolism	Liver
Excretion	Urine
DEA schedule	IV

Diazepam. Diazepam was synthesized in 1959; it was found to be equitoxic to chlordiazepoxide but to have greater antianxiety, skeletal muscle–relaxing, and anticonvulsant properties. Marketed in December 1963 as Valium, diazepam quickly became one of the most prescribed drugs in the United States. By 1966 diazepam was one of the 50 most prescribed drugs, and by the 1970s it was the leader among prescription drugs, a position it retained until recently.

Following oral administration, diazepam is rapidly absorbed from the GI tract, achieving peak plasma levels within 2 hours. The drug may be administered 1 hour before treatment because 90% of the maximal clinical effect develops within this time. Because of its prolonged plasma half-life (20 to 70 hours) and the presence of active metabolites, cumulation of effect may develop with prolonged oral administration of diazepam. However, in the typical dental or surgical situation in which not more than one or two doses are prescribed, this effect does not occur. Diazepam is highly effective in the preoperative management of apprehension and mild to moderate anxiety. Its rapid onset of action makes it an appropriate drug for use in dental or surgical situations.

Patients receiving diazepam at home must be cautioned against operating a motor vehicle. They must be driven to the medical or dental facility by a responsible adult companion, who can later drive them back home. Failure to warn a patient about this potential hazard may lead to legal action should a problem develop before or after treatment. That such problems do occur is seen in a study by Murray, in which 68 automobile drivers taking oral diazepam were monitored for a 3-month period. During this time, 16 of them were involved in accidents, an incidence 10 times greater than that expected.[89] Impaired motor function produced by the benzodiazepine was presumed to be the basis for the increase.

Dosage. The adult dosage for tension and anxiety states is 2 to 10 mg two to four times daily. For elderly patients or those with debilitating disease (ASA III or IV), recommended dosages are 2 to 2.5 mg once or twice daily to start; the dosage can then be increased if needed. The suggested dose for premedication is 5 to 10 mg 1 hour before bedtime or treatment.

Diazepam is not recommended for children younger than 6 months of age. For older children the recommendation is 1 to 2.5 mg three to four times daily, with the dose being increased if needed. Recommended pediatric doses range from 0.15 to 0.3 mg/kg.[86,87]

Availability. Valium (Roche): 2-, 5-, and 10-mg tablets, and as Valrelease in 15-mg capsules. Diazepam is also available generically. Diazepam is a controlled substance in Schedule IV.

Diazepam	
Pregnancy category	D
Lactation	NS
Metabolism	Liver
Excretion	Urine
DEA schedule	IV

Oxazepam. Oxazepam, synthesized in 1961, was marketed in 1965 under the proprietary name Serax. It possesses a short elimination half-life (5.7 to 10.9 hours) and no active metabolites. Oxazepam is therefore quite attractive in situations in which short-term anxiety control is required, such as during surgery or dentistry. The incidence of drowsiness is low, usually developing in persons receiving doses of 60 mg or more daily. Other side effects are similar to those for other members of this drug group.

Oxazepam is rapidly and reliably absorbed after oral administration, with peak plasma levels developing within 1 to 4 hours. This, in combination with the lack of active metabolites and a short half-life, makes oxazepam a preferred benzodiazepine for use as an antianxiety drug in dentistry.

Dosage. The adult dosage for mild to moderate anxiety and tension is 10 to 15 mg three to four times daily. For elderly patients the initial dosage is 10 mg three times daily, increased if needed to 15 mg three to four times daily.

An absolute dosage has not been established for children younger than 12 years. Oxazepam should not be taken by patients who are younger than 6 years.

Availability. Serax (Wyeth): 10-, 15-, and 30-mg capsules; 15-mg tablets. Oxazepam is a controlled substance in Schedule IV.

Oxazepam	
Pregnancy category	D
Lactation	NS
Metabolism	Liver
Excretion	Urine
DEA schedule	IV

Clorazepate. Clorazepate (also spelled chlorazepate) is available in the form of two salts: monopotassium and dipotassium salts. The dipotassium salt was marketed in 1972 as Tranxene, and clorazepate monopotassium was marketed in 1972 as Azene (no longer marketed). The monopotassium salt reaches peak plasma levels following oral administration in approximately 1 hour, and the dipotassium salt requires 1 to 2 hours. The plasma half-life of both forms is approximately 48 hours.

Clorazepate itself cannot be absorbed from the GI tract. The chemical is hydrolyzed in the stomach to its active form, desmethyldiazepam, which is then absorbed, producing the clinical actions of the drug. The rate and extent of absorption of clorazepate from the GI tract depend on gastric pH. Antacid therapy significantly decreases the absorption of clorazepate. Clorazepate is useful in dental and surgical situations; however, oxazepam, because it possesses a shorter half-life, is preferred.

Dosage. The usual adult dosage of dipotassium salt is 15 to 60 mg daily, divided into two to four doses, or in one dose (15 mg) 1 hour before bedtime. The dose for preoperative anxiety control is 15 mg of the dipotassium salt 1 hour before treatment.

For elderly or debilitated patients, the initial dose of dipotassium salt is 7.5 to 15 mg. Adequate information is not available to establish a dosage in patients younger than 18 years.

Availability. Clorazepate dipotassium, Tranxene (Abbott): 3.75-, 7.5-, and 15-mg tablets. Tranxene-SD (Abbott): 11.25- and 22.5-mg tablets. Clorazepate is a controlled substance in Schedule IV.

Clorazepate	
Pregnancy category	C
Lactation	NS
Metabolism	Liver
Excretion	Feces and urine
DEA schedule	IV

Alprazolam. Alprazolam is another benzodiazepine derivative being marketed as an antianxiety drug. It reaches peak plasma levels within 1 to 2 hours (orally) and has a half-life of 12 to 15 hours, with no active metabolites.

Dosage. The adult dosage for anxiety reduction is 0.25 to 0.5 mg three times a day. The dosage for elderly or debilitated patients is 0.25 mg two or three times daily. Modification in dosage may be appropriate as based on patient response.

Availability. Xanax (Upjohn): 0.25-, 0.5-, 1.0-, and 2.0-mg tablets. Alprazolam is a controlled substance in Schedule IV.

Alprazolam	
Pregnancy category	D
Lactation	NS
Metabolism	Liver
Excretion	Urine
DEA schedule	IV

Several other oral benzodiazepines have been mentioned, but because they are unavailable at this time in the United States or their primary indication is not anxiolysis, they are not reviewed in this section. These drugs include the following:

- Nitrazepam (Mogadon), discussed under sedative-hypnotics
- Flurazepam (Dalmane, Roche), discussed under sedative-hypnotics
- Midazolam (Hynovel, Dormicum, Versed), discussed under sedative-hypnotics
- Medazepam (Nobrium), an antianxiety drug not available in the United States
- Flunitrazepam (Rohypnol), a hypnotic not available in the United States
- Clonazepam (Klonopin, Roche), an anticonvulsant drug
- Lorazepam (Ativan, Wyeth), discussed under sedative-hypnotics
- Triazolam (Halcion, Upjohn), discussed under sedative-hypnotics
- Temazepam (Restoril, Sandoz), discussed under sedative-hypnotics

For the management of milder degrees of anxiety arising in the dental and surgical environment, there is probably no more effective group of drugs than the benzodiazepines. Pharmacologically, they offer significantly greater safety than the sedative-hypnotics, especially the barbiturates. Although respiratory and cardiovascular depression are possible following oral administration of benzodiazepines, these are unlikely to develop. The most frequently observed side effect is a degree of sedation.

As safe and as frequently administered as the benzodiazepines may be, it must be remembered that the patient must always be cautioned against driving a car when these drugs have been administered. Motor coordination may be subtly depressed, a condition that could have serious consequences for both the patient and the doctor.

Although any of the benzodiazepines may be employed therapeutically in dentistry, it is my opinion that for the management of mild to moderate preoperative anxiety on the day of the dental or surgical treatment, diazepam (in a dose of 5 to 10 mg) or oxazepam (in a dose of 15 to 30 mg) is the most practical. When used to aid in the induction of sleep (hypnosis) in a fearful patient the night before the appointment, flurazepam (in a dose of 30 mg) or triazolam (in a dose of 0.25 to 0.5 mg) is suggested. Table 7-4 summarizes the availability of the benzodiazepines.

HISTAMINE (H_1) BLOCKERS (ANTIHISTAMINES)

Sedation and hypnosis are known side effects of some drugs used primarily for other purposes. Such effects occur with many of the histamine blockers, drugs used primarily in the management of allergies, motion sickness, and parkinsonism. Several histamine blockers demonstrate this property and in fact are marketed primarily as sedative-hypnotics. These drugs include methapyrilene, pyrilamine, diphenhydramine, promethazine, and hydroxyzine.

Methapyrilene and pyrilamine are available as nonprescription sedative-hypnotics, usually in combination with scopolamine. Diphenhydramine in 25-mg capsules has been approved by the FDA as a nonprescription preparation.

The two histamine blockers most frequently used for their sedative-antianxiety properties are promethazine and hydroxyzine. In dentistry these drugs have proved to be quite useful, primarily in pediatric dentistry.

Promethazine

Promethazine is a phenothiazine derivative commonly used as an antiemetic for management of nausea and vomiting, for preoperative sedation, for sedation and the relief of apprehension and anxiety, to produce a light sleep from which the patient is easily aroused, and in the management of various forms of allergic reaction.

Promethazine was marketed in 1951 under the brand name Phenergan. Its first reported use in dentistry was in 1959, when it was used in conjunction with meperidine and chlorpromazine in the lytic cocktail (DPT: Demerol, Phenergan, Thorazine). Its primary function in this cocktail was to serve as an antiemetic to control nausea and vomiting commonly produced by opioids.

In dentistry, promethazine is frequently used in pediatric sedation. In a 1973 survey of drug use in pediatric dentistry, promethazine was the fourth most frequently employed solo premedicant and the most commonly used combination drug (with meperidine).[90] More recent surveys find the use of promethazine to remain high, ranking third as a solo premedicant and remaining first (with meperidine) as a combination drug.[91]

TABLE 7-4 Availability of Benzodiazepines (Oral)

Generic	Proprietary	Class	Availability (mg)	Dose* (mg)
Alprazolam	Xanax	AA	0.25, 0.5, 1	0.25-0.5
Chlorazepate with monopotassium	Azene	AA	3.25, 6.5, 13	13
Chlorazepate with dipotassium	Tranxene	AA	3.75, 7.5, 15	15
Chlordiazepoxide	Librium, SK-Lygen, Libritabs	AA	5, 10, 25	10
Clonazepam	Klonopin	AC	0.5, 1, 2	n/a
Diazepam	Valium	AA	2, 5, 10	10
Flunitrazepam	Rohypnol	SH	2	0.25-2
Flurazepam	Dalmane	SH	15, 30	30
Halazepam	Paxipam	AA	20, 40	20-40
Lorazepam	Ativan	SH, AA	0.5, 1, 2	2-4
Medazepam	Nobrium	AA	5, 10	5-10
Midazolam	Dormicum	SH	15	15-30
Nitrazepam	Mogadon	SH	5	2.5-10
Oxazepam	Serax	AA	10, 15, 30	15-30
Prazepam	Centrax	AA	5, 10	10-20
Temazepam	Restoril	SH	15, 30	30
Triazolam	Halcion	SH	0.25, 0.5	0.25-0.5

AA, Antianxiety; *AC*, anticonvulsant; *n/a*, not applicable; *SH*, sedative-hypnotic.
*For nighttime sedation or preoperative anxiety control.

Promethazine is a member of a group of drugs termed *phenothiazines*, a group of drugs classified as *antipsychotics* (formerly termed *major tranquilizers*). The primary use of these drugs (Table 7-5) is to decrease agitation, hostility, combativeness, and hyperactivity. They are also useful in the management of nausea and vomiting, and some members have potent antihistaminic actions. Promethazine differs structurally from the antipsychotic phenothiazines by the presence of a branched side chain and no ring substitution. It is believed that this structural difference is responsible for the lack of antipsychotic action. Promethazine is an H_1 receptor-blocking drug, providing antihistaminic, antiemetic, and sedative effects.

All phenothiazines produce some degree of sedation (CNS depression). The action of these drugs is quite different from that of the barbiturates and other sedative-hypnotics. Two major differences are that (1) phenothiazines, in large doses, do not produce unconsciousness or depress respiration or the cardiovascular system, and (2) the phenothiazines are not addictive.[92,93]

On the negative side, all phenothiazines are capable of producing extrapyramidal reactions. They usually develop early in phenothiazine therapy and most

TABLE 7-5 Phenothiazines

Generic	Proprietary	Sedative Action
Chlorpromazine	Thorazine	High
Promethazine	Phenergan	High
Thioridazine	Mellaril	High
Prochlorperazine	Compazine	Moderate
Promazine	Sparine	Moderate
Trifluoperazine	Stelazine	Moderate
Perphenazine	Trilafon	Low to moderate

often prove quite benign; however, they may require treatment. The incidence of extrapyramidal reactions is greatest with perphenazine, prochlorperazine, and trifluoperazine and lowest with promethazine and thioridazine.[94]

Four types of extrapyramidal reaction may be observed. *Akathisia* (motor restlessness) refers to the compelling need of the patient to be in constant motion. The patient feels the need to get up and walk or continuously move about. *Acute dystonias* include perioral spasms (protrusion of the tongue), mandibular tics, facial grimacing, hyperextension of the neck and trunk, and clonic convulsions. These reactions may be accompanied by hyperhidrosis, pallor, fever, and increased anxiety. *Parkinsonism,* which consists of tremors, rigidity, shuffling gait, postural abnormalities, masklike facies, and hypersalivation, may also occur. *Tardive dyskinesia* represents a late-appearing neurologic syndrome associated with antipsychotic drug use. It is more common in older patients and is characterized by choreiform movements of the face, trunk, and extremities.

Management of extrapyramidal reactions involves the discontinuance of the offending drug and the possible administration of an antiparkinsonism drug such as diphenhydramine (Benadryl, 50 mg IM or IV in adults) or trihexyphenidyl (Artane, 5 to 15 mg daily, orally).[95]

Many phenothiazines act on the cardiovascular system to produce postural (orthostatic) hypotension and a reflex tachycardia. This is most common with chlorpromazine. The phenothiazines undergo metabolic degradation in the liver and are excreted in the urine and feces.

Contraindications. Known allergy to phenothiazines is a contraindication to the use of promethazine and other phenothiazines.

Warnings. Patients receiving other CNS depressants should be aware of the additive effects of the phenothiazines. These drugs should either be eliminated or their dosages reduced.

Precautions. Patients must be advised against operating a motor vehicle or potentially hazardous machinery. Phenothiazines must be used with caution in patients with a history of convulsive disorders because they may lower the seizure threshold.

Children with acute disease, such as chicken pox, measles, and gastroenteritis, appear much more susceptible to extrapyramidal reactions, especially dystonias, than do adults.

Adverse Reactions. The most frequently reported adverse reactions to phenothiazines include dryness of the mouth, blurring of vision, and less commonly, dizziness. Oversedation is the most frequently observed side effect of promethazine. In general, the phenothiazines have a high therapeutic index and are remarkably safe drugs. Extrapyramidal reactions are the most significant side effects of these drugs.

Dosage. The adult dose for sedation is 25 to 50 mg 1 hour before treatment; for preoperative sedation, 50 mg 1 hour before bedtime. In children the dose for sedation is 12.5 to 25 mg 1 hour before treatment.

For preoperative sedation in pediatric dentistry, the traditional dose recommendation for promethazine is 2.2 mg/kg when used alone and 1.1 mg/kg when used in combination with other CNS depressants.[96]

Availability. Promethazine (generic): 12.5-, 25-, and 50-mg tablets. Phenergan (Wyeth): 12.5-, 25-, and 50-mg tablets; 6.25 mg/5 ml (1.5% alcohol) syrup; 25 mg/5 ml (1.5% alcohol) syrup fortis.

Promethazine	
Pregnancy category	C
Lactation	NS
Metabolism	Liver
Excretion	Feces and urine
DEA schedule	Not controlled

Hydroxyzine

Hydroxyzine is derived from a group of drugs called *diphenylethanes.* Although classified as a histamine (H_1) blocker, hydroxyzine also possesses sedative, antiemetic, antispasmodic, and anticholinergic properties. Two forms of the drug are available: hydroxyzine hydrochloride (Atarax) and hydroxyzine pamoate (Vistaril). Hydroxyzine is the most popular oral sedative in the practice of pediatric dentistry, with 50% of the responding pedodontists using one or both drugs.[90,91]

The sedative actions of hydroxyzine are not produced by cortical depression. It is thought to suppress some hypothalamic nuclei and to extend its actions peripherally into the sympathetic portion of the autonomic nervous system.

Following oral administration, hydroxyzine is rapidly absorbed from the GI tract, with clinical actions observed within 15 to 30 minutes. Maximal clinical actions develop in 2 hours, with an approximate duration of action of 3 to 4 hours.

The oral liquid form of hydroxyzine hydrochloride (Atarax) is more pleasant tasting to most patients than the liquid form of hydroxyzine pamoate (Vistaril). This fact is of particular importance in pediatric dentistry.

When these drugs are administered in combination with opioids or barbiturates, their dosage should be decreased by 50% because the depressant actions of opioids and barbiturates are potentiated by hydroxyzine.

Indications for the use of hydroxyzine include providing total management of long-term anxiety and tension, managing anxiety and tension in which the causative stress is temporary (e.g., dental or other surgical procedures), providing preoperative sedation, allaying of apprehension and anxiety in the cardiac-risk patient, and managing nausea and vomiting. Hydroxyzine is metabolized in the liver and excreted in the urine.

In dental practice the use of hydroxyzine as a sole drug is limited to the management of children with mild to moderate fear. It is often used in combination with either meperidine or chloral hydrate for management of more fearful pediatric patients.

The incidence of side effects is quite low, with transient drowsiness being observed most commonly. Fatal overdosage with hydroxyzine is extremely uncommon, and withdrawal reactions after long-term therapy have never been reported.

Contraindications. Contraindications include previous hypersensitivity to hydroxyzine.

Drug Interactions. Hydroxyzine will potentiate the CNS depressant actions of drugs such as barbiturates, opioids, alcohol, sedative-hypnotics, and antianxiety drugs. Dosages of these drugs should be decreased by 50% when they are administered concurrently with hydroxyzine.

Precautions. Patients receiving hydroxyzine must be warned against operating a motor vehicle or hazardous machinery. Children receiving hydroxyzine should be kept under observation by their parent or guardian for the remainder of the day.

Dosage. The adult dosage ranges from 25 mg three times a day to 100 mg four times a day. The dosage for children younger than 6 years is 2 mg/kg daily orally in divided doses every 6 to 8 hours. The dosage for children 6 to 12 years is 12.5 to 25 mg orally every 6 to 8 hours. The dose for preoperative drug in adults is 50 to 100 mg 1 hour preoperatively.

In pediatric dentistry the oral dose of hydroxyzine is 1.1 to 2.2 mg/kg when it is used as a sole drug for anxiety control. When it is administered in conjunction with other CNS depressants, such as meperidine or chloral hydrate, the dose of hydroxyzine should be reduced by 50%.[96]

Availability. Hydroxyzine hydrochloride, Atarax (Roerig): 10-, 25-, 50-, and 100-mg tablets; 10 mg/5 ml (0.5% alcohol) syrup. Hydroxyzine pamoate, Vistaril (Pfizer): 25-, 50-, and 100-mg capsules; 25 mg/5 ml oral suspension.

Hydroxyzine	
Pregnancy category	C
Lactation	NS
Metabolism	Liver
Excretion	Urine
DEA schedule	Not controlled

OPIOIDS (NARCOTICS)

Opioids are classified as strong analgesics. Their primary indication for use is the relief of moderate to severe pain. Beneficially, opioids alter a patient's psychological response to pain and suppress anxiety and apprehension. Many opioids are used parenterally as preanesthetic drugs because of their sedative, antianxiety, and analgesic properties. On the other hand, many anesthesiologists prefer to administer sedative-hypnotics or antianxiety drugs preoperatively unless pain is present. In the absence of pain, opioids administered alone frequently produce dysphoria instead of sedation. To achieve antianxiety and sedative effects, opioids ought not be administered via the oral route. Absorption following oral administration is not as consistent as it is with parenteral administration, and the incidence of unwanted side effects (postural hypotension, nausea, and vomiting) is considerably greater. The resulting sedative effect varies significantly from patient to patient. Respiratory and cardiovascular depression may be noted and, if present, can result in airway obstruction, hypoventilation, and hypotension. Oral opioid administration should be reserved for the management of *pain* when milder analgesics have proved ineffectual.

SUMMARY

The oral route of drug administration may be used successfully for the relief of mild to moderate degrees of apprehension and anxiety. Because of inherent difficulties attendant in achieving precise levels of sedation, it is recommended that only light levels of sedation be sought by the oral route.

A large number of drugs are presently available for the relief of anxiety via oral administration. This chapter describes only commonly used drugs in dentistry and surgery and those that appear most applicable in the outpatient environment. In general, these drugs belong to a small number of drug groups: the antianxiety drugs, the sedative-hypnotics, and the histamine blockers.

Although all drugs may be employed by the knowledgeable, well-trained doctor, the more prudent will restrict their prescribing habits to a limited number of drugs with which they are familiar. From the practical point of view, the benzodiazepines have virtually supplanted the barbiturates as the drugs of choice for preoperative management of anxiety in dentistry and surgery. Although many benzodiazepines are available, oxazepam and diazepam are the most frequently employed and are highly recommended for management of milder levels of anxiety in dentistry. Flurazepam and triazolam, classified as sedative-hypnotics, are useful for mild to moderate anxiety and are administered the evening before treatment and occasionally on the day of treatment.

Two newer drugs, zolpidem and zaleplon, appear efficacious in the management of pretreatment anxiety. At present, their use in dentistry is minimal. Only time will tell where they stand in the dental armamentarium against fear and anxiety. Other drug groups should be considered for use where the benzodiazepines are contraindicated or have proved ineffective and when other more controllable techniques of pharmacosedation are unavailable.

Ease of drug prescription is a minor factor in selection of a suitable drug for premedication but one that must be considered. Among the drugs discussed in this chapter, the benzodiazepines and chloral hydrate are placed in Schedule IV on the Controlled Substances Schedule; Schedule II drugs include amobarbital, pentobarbital, and secobarbital.

REFERENCES

1. Berger R, Green G, Melnick A: Cardiac arrest caused by oral diazepam intoxication, *Clin Pediatr* 14:842, 1975.
2. Gill CJ, Michaelides PL: Dental drugs and anaphylactic reactions: report of a case, *Oral Surg* 50:30, 1980.
3. Johnson AG, Seideman P, Day RO: Adverse drug interactions with nonsteroidal anti-inflammatory drugs (NSAIDs): recognition, management and avoidance, *Drug Safety* 8:99, 1993.
4. Brody JE: Personal health: ignoring the doctor's orders has become a costly and deadly epidemic, *New York Times* cxli:B-6, Sept 16, 1992.
5. California State Board of Dental Examiners: Use of oral conscious sedation for pediatric patients, Sections 1647.10-1647.17, Sacramento, 2000.
6. Magni G, Cadamuro M, Borgherini G et al: Psychological stress and gastric emptying time in normal subjects, *Psychol Rep* 68:739, 1991.
7. Sugito K, Ogata H, Goto H et al: Gastric emptying rate of drug preparations. III. Effects of size of enteric microcapsules with mean diameters ranging from 0.1 to 1.1 mm in man, *Chem Pharm Bull* 40:3343, 1992.
8. Wedlund PJ, Wilkinson GR: Hepatic tissue binding and the oral first-pass effect, *J Pharm Sci* 73:422, 1984.
9. Lucas WJ, Maccioli GA, Mueller RA: Advances in oral anti-arrhythmic therapy: implications for the anaesthetist, *Can J Anaesth* 37:94, 1990.
10. Zimmermann T, Leitold M: The influence of food intake on gastrointestinal pH and gastric emptying time: experience with two radiotelemetring methods (Heidelberg pH capsule system and Flexilog 1010), *Int J Clin Pharmacol Ther Toxicol* 30:477, 1992.
11. *Drug Facts and Comparisons (Pocket Edition)—2000,* ed 4, Philadelphia, 2000, Lippincott Williams & Wilkins.
12. Wright GZ: Pharmacotherapeutic approaches to behavior management. In Wright GZ, ed: *Behavior management in dentistry for children,* Philadelphia, 1975, WB Saunders.
13. Anderson JA, Vamm WF Jr, Dilley DC: Pain and anxiety control, part II: pain reaction control—conscious sedation. In Pinkham JR, ed: *Pediatric dentistry: infancy through adolescence,* ed 3, Philadelphia, 1999, WB Saunders.
14. Johnson R: Personal communications, 1992.
15. Jorgensen NB, Hayden J Jr: *Premedication, local and general anesthesia in dentistry,* Philadelphia, 1967, Lea & Febiger.
16. McCarthy FM, Hayden J Jr: Ethyl alcohol by the oral route as a sedative in dentistry, *JADA* 96:282, 1978.
17. McCarthy M: Personal communication, 1978.
18. Harvey SC: Hypnotics and sedatives: the barbiturates. In Goodman IS, Gilman A, eds: *Pharmacological basis of therapeutics,* ed 5, New York, 1990, Macmillan.
19. Felpel LP: Sedative-hypnotics and central nervous system stimulants. In Yagiela JA, Neidle EA, Dowd FJ, eds: *Pharmacology and therapeutics for dentistry,* ed 4, St Louis, 1998, Mosby.
20. Bleck TP: Convulsive disorders: status epilepticus, *Clin Neuropharm* 14:191, 1991.
21. Rehse K, Kapp WD: Structure activity relationships in oral anticoagulants: barbituric acids and quinolones, *Arch Pharm* 315:502, 1982.
22. Leslie SW: Sedative-hypnotic drugs: interaction with calcium channels, *Alcohol Drug Res* 6:371, 1985-1986.
23. Pimstone NR: Hematologic and hepatic manifestations of the cutaneous porphyrias, *Clin Dermatol* 3:83, 1985.
24. DeTullio P, Kirking DM, Zacardelli DK et al: Evaluation of long-term triazolam use in ambulatory Veterans Administration Medical Center population, *Drug Intell Clin Pharm* 23:290, 1989.
25. Warneke LB: Benzodiazepines: abuse and new use, *Can J Psychiatry* 36:194, 1991.
26. Melander A, Henricson K, Stenberg P et al: Anxiolytic-hypnotic drugs: relationships between prescribing, abuse and suicide, *Eur J Clin Pharmacol* 41:525, 1991.
27. Nembutal sodium, drug information sheet, Chicago, 1993,Abbott Laboratory.
28. Loeffler PM: Oral benzodiazepines and conscious sedation: a review, *J Oral Maxillofac Surg* 50:989, 1992.

29. Greenblatt DJ: Pharmacology of benzodiazepine hypnotics, *J Clin Psychiatry* 53(suppl):7, 1992.
30. Garzone PD, Kroboth PD: Pharmacokinetics of the newer benzodiazepines, *Clin Pharmacokinet* 16:337, 1989.
31. Young ER, Mason D: Triazolam: an oral sedative for the dental practitioner, *Can Dent Assoc J* 54:511, 1988.
32. Lieblich SE, Horswell B: Attenuation of anxiety in ambulatory oral surgery patients with oral triazolam, *J Oral Maxillofac Surg* 49:792, 1991.
33. Meyer ML, Mourino AP, Farrington FH: Comparison of triazolam to a chloral hydrate/hydroxyzine combination in the sedation of pediatric dental patients, *Pediatr Dent* 12:283, 1990.
34. Quarnstrom FC, Milgrom P, Moore PA: Experience with triazolam in preschool children, *J Anesth Pain Control Dent* 1:157, 1992.
35. Greenfield DP: What about Halcion? *N J Med* 88:889, 1991 (editorial).
36. Bixler EO, Kales A, Manfredi RL et al: Next-day memory impairment with triazolam, *Lancet* 337:827, 1991.
37. Medawar C, Rassaby E: Triazolam overdose, alcohol, and manslaughter, *Lancet* 338:1515, 1991.
38. Schneider PJ, Perry PJ: Triazolam: an "abused drug" by the lay press? *Drug Intell Clin Pharm* 24:389, 1990.
39. Myrhed M: Background and current status. Halcion (triazolam) banned in England—Sweden investigates, *Lakartidningen* 88:4035, 1991.
40. Wysowski DK, Barash D: Adverse behavioral reactions attributed to triazolam in the Food and Drug Administration's Spontaneous Reporting System, *Arch Intern Med* 151:2, 1991.
41. Halcion, drug package insert, Kalamazoo, 1990, The Upjohn Company.
42. Ativan, drug package insert, Radnor, Pa, 1992, Wyeth-Ayerst Laboratories.
43. Castleden CM, Allen JG, Altman J et al: A comparison of oral midazolam, nitrazepam, and placebo in young and elderly subjects, *Eur J Clin Pharmacol* 32:253, 1987.
44. Jochemsen R, van Rijn PA, Hazelzet TG et al: Comparative pharmacokinetics of midazolam and loprazolam in healthy subjects after oral administration, *Biopharm Drug Dispos* 7:53, 1986.
45. Langlois S, Kneeft, JH, Chouinard G et al: Midazolam: kinetics and effects on memory, sensorium, and haemodynamics, *Br J Clin Pharmacol* 23:273, 1987.
46. Monti JM, Alterwain P, Debellis J et al: Short-term sleep laboratory evaluation of midazolam in chronic insomniacs: preliminary results, *Arzneimittelforschung* 37:54, 1987.
47. Hildebrand PJ, Elwood RJ, McClean E et al: Intramuscular and oral midazolam: some factors influencing uptake, *Anaesthesia* 38:1220, 1983.
48. Turner GA, Paech M: A comparison of oral midazolam solution with temazepam as a day case premedicant, *Anaesth Intens Care* 19:365, 1991.
49. Wahlmann UW, Dietrich U, Fischer W: The question of oral sedation using midazolam in outpatient dental surgery, *Deut Zahnarzt Z* 47:66, 1992.
50. Luyk NH, Whitley BD: Efficacy of oral midazolam prior to intravenous sedation for the removal of third molars, *Int J Oral Maxillofac Surg* 20:264, 1991.
51. Parnis SJ, Foate JA, vander Walt JH et al: Oral midazolam is an effective premedicant for children having day-care anaesthesia, *Anaesth Intens Care* 20:9, 1992.
52. Payne KA, Coetzee AR, Mattheyse FJ: Midazolam and amnesia in pediatric premedication, *Acta Anaesthesiol Belg* 42:101, 1991.
53. Hennes HM, Wagner V, Bonadio WA et al: The effect of oral midazolam on anxiety of preschool children during laceration repair, *Ann Emerg Med* 19:1006, 1990.
54. Feld LH, Negus JB, White PF: Oral midazolam preanesthetic drug in pediatric outpatients, *Anesthesiology* 73:831, 1990.
55. Weldon BC, Watcha MF, White PF: Oral midazolam in children: effect of time and adjunctive therapy. *Anesth Analg* 75:51, 1992.
56. Tolksdorf W, Eick C: Rectal, oral and nasal premedication using midazolam in children aged 1-6 years: a comparative clinical study, *Anaesthetist* 40:661, 1991.
57. Molter G, Altmayer P, Castor G, Buech U: Oral premedication with midazolam in children, *Anaesthesiol Reanim* 16:75, 1991.
58. Miller NS, Gold MS: Benzodiazepines: a major problem; introduction, *J Subst Abuse Treat* 8:3, 1991.
59. Salva P, Costa J: Clinical pharmacokinetics and pharmacodynamics of zolpidem: therapeutic implications, *Clin Pharmacokinet* 29:142, 1995.
60. Karch A: *Lippincott's nursing drug guide, 2000 edition,* Philadelphia, 2000, Lippincott Williams & Wilkins.
61. Zaleplon. *Am J Health-System Pharm* 57:430, 2000.
62. Drover D, Lemmens H, Naidu S et al: Pharmacokinetics, pharmacodynamics, and relative pharmacokinetic/pharmacodynamic profiles of zaleplon and zolpidem, *Clin Ther* 22:1443, 2000.
63. Moore P, Haupt M: Sedative drugs in pediatric dentistry. In Dionne RA, Phero JC, eds: *Management of pain and anxiety in dental practice,* New York, 1992, Elsevier.
64. Nordenberg A, Dalisle G, Izukawa T: Cardiac arrhythmias in a child due to chloral hydrate ingestion, *Pediatrics* 47:134, 1971.
65. Greenberg SB, Faerber EN, Aspinall CL et al: High-dose chloral hydrate sedation for children undergoing MR imaging: safety and efficacy in relation to age, *AJR Am J Roentgenol* 161:639, 1993.
66. Judish GF, Andreasen S, Bell EB: Chloral hydrate sedation as a substitute for examination under anesthesia in pediatric ophthalmology, *Am J Ophthalmol* 89:560, 1982.
67. Thompson JR, Schneider S, Ashwal S et al: The choice of sedation for computed tomography in children: a prospective evaluation, *Neuroradiology* 143:475, 1982.
68. Cook BA, Bass JW, Nomizu S et al: Sedation of children for technical procedures: current standard of practice, *Clin Pediatr* 31:137, 1992.
69. Troutman KC: Misuse of chloral hydrate in sedating a pediatric patient, ADSA Mortality and Morbidity Conference, ADSA Annual Meeting, Boston, 1984.
70. Moore PA: Therapeutic assessment of chloral hydrate premedication for pediatric dentistry, *Anesth Prog* 31:191, 1984.
71. Smith RC: Chloral hydrate sedation for handicapped children: a double-blind study, *Anesth Prog* 24:159, 1977.
72. Barr ES: Oral premedication in children, *Anesth Analg* 41:201, 1962.

73. Richter JJ: Current theories about the mechanisms of benzodiazepines and neuroleptic drugs, *Anesthesiology* 54:66, 1981.
74. Study RE, Barker JC: Cellular mechanisms of benzodiazepine action, *JAMA* 247:2147, 1982.
75. Tallman JF, Paul SM, Skolnick P et al: Receptors for the age of anxiety: pharmacology of the benzodiazepines, *Science* 207:274, 1980.
76. Greenblatt DJ, Miller LG, Shader RI: Benzodiazepine discontinuation syndromes, *J Psychiatr Res* 24(suppl):73, 1990.
77. Oreland L: The benzodiazepines: a pharmacological overview, *Acta Anaesthesiol Scand* 88(suppl):13, 1988.
78. Lacey DJ: Status epilepticus in children and adults, *J Clin Psychiatry* 49(suppl):33, 1988.
79. Simiand J, Keane PE, Biziere K et al: Comparative study in mice of tetrazepam and other centrally active skeletal muscle relaxants, *Arch Int Pharmacodyn Ther* 297:272, 1989.
80. Mayhue FE: IM midazolam for status epilepticus in the emergency department, *Ann Emerg Med* 17:643, 1988.
81. Classen DC, Pestotnik SL, Evans RS et al: Intensive surveillance of midazolam use in hospitalized patients and the occurrence of cardiorespiratory arrest, *Pharmacotherapy* 12:213, 1992.
82. Daneshmend TK, Bell GD, Logan RF: Sedation for upper gastrointestinal endoscopy: results of a nationwide survey, *Gut* 32:12, 1991.
83. Greenblatt DJ, Shader RI: *Benzodiazepines in clinical practice*, New York, 1974, Raven Press.
84. Edwards JG, Cantopher T, Olivieri S: Benzodiazepine dependence and the problems of withdrawal, *Postgrad Med* 66(suppl):27, 1990.
85. Laegreid L, Olegard R, Conradi N et al: Congenital malformations and maternal consumption of benzodiazepines, *Dev Med Child Neurol* 32:432, 1990.
86. Badalaty MM, Houpt MI, Koenigsberg SR et al: A comparison of chloral hydrate and diazepam sedation in young children, *Pediatr Dent* 12:33, 1990.
87. Palma-Aguirre JA, Rodriguez-Palomares C: Indications and contraindications for analgesics and antibiotics in pediatric dentistry, *Practica Odontol* 10:11, 1989.
88. Jacobsen D, Frederichsen PS, Knutsen KM et al: Clinical course in acute self-poisonings: a prospective study of 1125 consecutive hospitalized patients, *Hum Toxicol* 3:107, 1984.
89. Murray JB: Effects of Valium and Librium on human psychomotor and cognitive functions, *Genet Psychol Monogr* 109:167, 1984.
90. Wright GZ, McAulay DJ: Current premedicating trends in pedodontics, *J Dent Child* 40:185, 1973.
91. Wright GZ, Chiasson RC: The use of sedation drugs by Canadian pediatric dentists, *Pediatr Dent* 9:308, 1987.
92. Jones KF: Preoperative drugs in operative dentistry for children, *J Dent Child* 36:93, 1969.
93. Pautola A, Elomaa M: The use of promethazine and diazepam in dental treatment of apprehensive children, *Suom Hammaslaak Toim* 67:226, 1971.
94. Skorin L Jr, Onofrey BE, DeWitt JD: Phenothiazine-induced oculogyric crisis, *J Am Optometr Assoc* 58:316, 1987.
95. Lopez-Rois F et al: Drug-induced extrapyramidal syndrome: apropos of 22 cases, *Anales Esp Pediatr* 26:91, 1987.
96. ADA Publishing: *ADA guide to dental therapeutics*, ed 2, Chicago, 2000, American Dental Association.

CHAPTER 8

Rectal Sedation

CHAPTER OUTLINE

Interest in the rectal route of drug administration has increased in anesthesiology and, to a lesser extent, in dentistry in recent years.[1] Historically, the rectal route of drug administration was used for the administration of smoke ("fumigation") for resuscitation[2] and the administration of anesthetics. An ether boiler for rectal application was developed in 1847 by Pirogoff.[3] With the advent of more reliable routes of drug administration (e.g., intravenous [IV] and inhalation), use of the rectal route decreased.

Certain situations remain in which rectal drug administration may be valuable. These include the administration of a drug to a patient who is unwilling or unable to take drugs orally. In most instances this is a child or an adult with a disability requiring conscious sedation either to permit treatment to proceed[4-6] or as a preliminary to the induction of general anesthesia.[7-9] Another situation in which rectal drugs are warranted is the administration of antiemetics to patients with nausea and vomiting. Although parenteral administration is preferred (if the patient is present in the office where the drug may be injected), rectal administration can be used if the patient objects to injection or if the patient is at home. Another indication for rectal administration of drugs is analgesics for postoperative control of pain.[10]

ADVANTAGES

Advantages of the rectal route include a relatively rapid onset of clinical activity; a decreased incidence and intensity of drug-related side effects; the lack of a needle, syringe, or other equipment; the avoidance of an injection; ease of administration (many children who vehemently object to the oral route will not object to this route); and its low cost.

In the past it was thought that rectally administered drugs were absorbed directly into the systemic circulation via the vena cava, bypassing the enterohepatic circulation and thereby eliminating the hepatic first-pass effect, which so influences the clinical activity of most drugs administered enterally.[11] The superior rectal vein empties into the inferior mesenteric vein and thence into the portal system. The middle and inferior rectal veins empty into the internal iliac vein and the inferior vena cava.[12,13] However, it has been demonstrated that hepatic clearance is *the* main factor affecting bioavailability of rectally administered drugs.[1] This may be because blood flow occurs through anastomoses that interconnect the superior, middle, and inferior rectal venous systems, thereby producing a hepatic first-pass effect with rectally administered drugs. Other potential factors, such as adsorption by feces, intraluminal degradation by microorganisms, metabolism within the mucosal cell, and lymphatic drainage, do not significantly affect the fate of rectally administered drugs.

Comparing the oral, nasal, and rectal administration of the water-soluble benzodiazepine midazolam, Tolksdorf[7] found that children aged 1 to 6 years accepted the oral drug better than rectal or nasal but that the rectally administered midazolam had the most rapid onset of action and fewest side effects in the postoperative period. In several studies, peak levels of clinical action were noted rapidly after rectal administration. Roelofse et al.[4] noted good anxiolysis, sedation, and cooperation 30 minutes after rectal administration of midazolam, whereas Kraus et al.[14] noted peak plasma levels of midazolam at 7.5 minutes.

DISADVANTAGES

Disadvantages of the rectal route include inconvenience to the administrator and the patient, variable absorption of some drugs from the large intestine, possible irritation of the intestines by some drugs, inability to reverse the action of the drug easily, prolonged recovery with some drugs, and an inability to titrate precise individual dosages.

The primary use of rectal drug administration in both medicine and dentistry is management of uncooperative patients, whether children or adults. The drug may be administered to the patient by a parent at home 1 hour before the appointment; however, it is strongly suggested that rectally administered central nervous system (CNS) depressants be administered in the medical or dental office by the doctor or a staff person. Signs and symptoms of sedation develop rapidly with many rectal drugs, clinical sedation being evident at 15 to 30 minutes.[4,14] Because the possibility of oversedation exists, it would be beneficial for the patient to be in an environment where oversedation could be easily managed. An automobile en route to the doctor's office is not a desirable location.

Because of the lack of control over the clinical actions of the drug, rectal administration ought not to be used in an effort to achieve deeper levels of conscious sedation unless the doctor is well versed in general anesthesia and in airway management in the unconscious patient. The recommended use of rectal sedation is for the induction of light to moderate sedation when other, more controllable methods of anxiety control (IV, inhalation) may be used if needed during treatment. Rectally administered drugs may provide a level of patient management adequate for many procedures, such as root planing and curettage[5] and restoration or extraction of primary teeth,[6] but it may prove inadequate for procedures such as radiographs, which require a patient to remain immobile during exposure.[15]

The administration of rectal drugs is often considered difficult for the administrator and uncomfortable for the patient. Of 80 children receiving rectal premedication, deWaal, Huisman, and Veerman[16] reported that 66 (82.5%) accepted rectal instillation well, 12 (15%) moderately well, and 2 (2.5%) poorly.

The patient receiving rectal drugs for sedation should receive supplemental oxygen and be monitored via pulse oximetry and pretracheal stethoscope. Personnel and equipment for resuscitation must always be available.

DRUGS

Many drugs are administered rectally. Ideally, a rectally administered drug will be available as a suppository, although in several cases (e.g., with midazolam), drug formulations designed for parenteral administration have been successfully employed. Historically, the two major drug groups that have been employed rectally are the barbiturates and opioids.

1. Barbiturates
   a. Phenobarbital
   b. Secobarbital
   c. Pentobarbital
   d. Thiopental
   e. Methohexital
2. Opioids
   a. Hydromorphone
   b. Oxymorphone
3. Promethazine
4. Chloral hydrate
5. Benzodiazepines
   a. Diazepam
   b. Midazolam
6. Ketamine

Phenobarbital

Phenobarbital is classified as a long-acting barbiturate. It is a relatively safe drug for sedation of infants and younger children. It is also indicated for use in patients with prolonged vomiting or who experience convulsive states, as well as in general when oral sedatives cannot be administered. The prolonged duration of action of phenobarbital restricts its use in surgery and in dentistry.

Dosage. The usual dosage for children is 1 to 6 mg/kg body weight daily in three divided doses.

Availability. Phenobarbital sodium (generic): 8-, 16-, 32-, 65-, 100-, and 130-mg suppositories. Hypnette (Fleming): 8- and 16-mg suppositories. Phenobarbital is classified as a Schedule II drug.

Secobarbital

Secobarbital sodium is a short-acting barbiturate sedative-hypnotic. It is recommended for preoperative sedation or for helping a patient obtain a restful night's sleep before a dental appointment. It may be used in both children and adults.

Dosage. For adults the usual dose is 120 to 200 mg 1 hour before bedtime or before the scheduled dental appointment. The usual pediatric dose is 15 to 60 mg for infants up to 6 months of age, 60 mg for children 6 months to 3 years old, and 60 to 120 mg for older children.

Availability. Secobarbital sodium (generic): 8-, 50-, 65-, 100-, 130-, and 195-mg suppositories. Seconal sodium (Lilly): 30-, 60-, 120-, and 200-mg suppositories. Secobarbital is classified as a Schedule II drug.

Pentobarbital

Pentobarbital sodium is another short-acting barbiturate sedative-hypnotic that is available in suppository form. Its applications are similar to those of secobarbital sodium. Because of its relatively short duration of action (3 to 4 hours), pentobarbital is an excellent choice for sedation via the rectal route.

Dosage. Refer to Table 8-1 for dosage information.

Availability. Pentobarbital sodium (generic): 16-, 32-, 65-, 130-, and 195-mg suppositories. Nembutal sodium (Abbott): 30-, 60-, 120-, and 200-mg suppositories. Pentobarbital is classified as a Schedule II drug.

TABLE 8-1 Pentobarbital Dosage

Age (Weight)	Usual Dose
Adults (average to above average weight)	120-200 mg
Children	
2 months to 1 year (10-20 lb)	30 mg
1-4 years (20-40 lb)	30-60 mg
5-12 years (40-80 lb)	60 mg
12-14 years (80-110 lb)	60-120 mg

Data from Pentobarbital package insert, Chicago, 1992, Abbott Laboratories.

Thiopental

Thiopental sodium is an ultrashort-acting CNS depressant commonly used for the induction of general anesthesia via the IV route. It is also available as a rectal suspension for use in achieving deep sedation. Its primary use is in the uncooperative patient in whom other techniques of sedation are unavailable and the duration of the planned procedure is short (not more than 15 minutes). The effective dose of thiopental for deep sedation is 44 mg/kg, which is approximately 10 times the IV dose for general anesthesia.[11] Giovannitti and Trapp[11] recommend that once sedation has been achieved rectally, an IV infusion be established and maintained throughout treatment. If the planned treatment cannot be completed in 15 minutes, other sedative drugs should be administered intravenously before the patient becomes uncooperative.

Because of the pharmacology of the barbiturates in general and the uncertainty of drug response following rectal administration, thiopental is not recommended for use by anyone who has not had thorough training in general anesthesia and in maintenance of the unconscious airway. Larsson et al.[17] reported elevated PCO_2 levels after rectal induction of anesthesia with either thiopentone (thiopental, 30 mg/kg) or methohexitone (methohexital, 20 or 30 mg/kg). The authors concluded that the use of rectal induction of anesthesia with barbiturates carries an increased risk of hypoventilation in infants younger than 2 years of age.

Dosage. The recommended dose for preoperative sedation is 1 g/75 lb body weight (1 g/34 kg).[18] This is equivalent to 13.5 or 29.4 mg/kg. The total dose should not exceed 1000 to 1500 mg in children weighing 75 lb or more and 3000 to 4000 mg in adults weighing more than 200 lb. A cleansing enema is rarely required before administration of pentobarbital. The volume administered rarely induces defecation. The effective dose for deep sedation is 44 mg/kg.[11]

Availability. Pentothal (Abbott) rectal suspension: 400 mg/g of suspension. Thiopental is classified as a Schedule IV drug.

Methohexital

Methohexital (Brevital, Brietal), like thiopental, is an ultrashort-acting barbiturate. IV methohexital produces ultralight general anesthesia of a somewhat shorter duration than thiopental. Methohexital has also been used via rectal instillation for premedication before the induction of general anesthesia in children.[1,19-22] As mentioned in the discussion of rectal thiopental, the use of rectal barbiturates for sedation or induction of anesthesia carries an increased risk of respiratory depression (hypoventilation).[17]

Dosage. A dose of 20 mg/kg of methohexital is the usually recommended rectal dose for premedication as a sole agent. A dose of 10 mg/kg of methohexital following intramuscular (IM) atropine and meperidine produces equal results.[22]

Availability. Methohexital is classified as a Schedule IV drug.

Hydromorphone

Hydromorphone is an opioid analgesic whose primary indication is the relief of pain. One of the advantages of hydromorphone is a low incidence of nausea and vomiting. Sleep occurring following its administration is a result of the relief of pain, not hypnosis.

Hydromorphone administered rectally provides long-lasting pain relief. The onset of action of the drug occurs within 30 minutes, and it has a duration of action of 4 to 5 hours.

Dosage. The usual dose is 3 mg 1 hour before bedtime.[23]

Availability. Dilaudid (Knoll): 3-mg suppositories. Hydromorphone is classified as a Schedule II drug.

Oxymorphone

Oxymorphone is a rapid-acting opioid analgesic used primarily for the management of pain. It also produces sedation and is therefore indicated for use in preoperative sedation. Following oral or rectal administration, the onset of action occurs within 30 minutes; the duration of action is approximately 6 hours.

Dosage. The usual adult dosage is 5 mg every 4 to 6 hours.[24] The safe use of oxymorphone in children younger than 12 years has not been established.

Availability. Numorphan (DuPont): 5-mg suppositories. Oxymorphone is classified as a Schedule II drug.

Promethazine

The pharmacology of promethazine, a phenothiazine derivative, has been discussed in the section on oral sedation (see Chapter 7). Promethazine may also be administered rectally for preoperative sedation and in the management of nausea and vomiting.

Dosage. The usual adult dose is 25 to 50 mg 1 hour before bedtime. For preoperative sedation of adults, the dose is 50 mg 1 hour before treatment. For sedation of children the usual dose is 12.5 to 25 mg 1 hour before treatment.

Availability. Phenergan (Wyeth): 12.5-, 25-, and 50-mg suppositories.

Chloral Hydrate

Chloral hydrate, a nonbarbiturate sedative-hypnotic, has been reviewed in Chapter 7. Chloral hydrate is also used rectally for preoperative sedation.

Dosage. For adults for preoperative sedation or to aid in falling asleep the night before dental treatment, the usual dose is 650 to 1300 mg 1 hour before treatment or bedtime. The dosage for children is discussed in Chapter 34

Availability. Rectules (Fellows): 650- and 1300-mg suppositories. Chloral hydrate is classified as a Schedule IV drug.

Diazepam

Diazepam has been used rectally for two specific purposes in medicine: management of epilepsy[25] and management of anxiety in a variety of clinical settings, including in terminal cancer patients[26] and in adults for sedation during oral surgery.[27] The pediatric use of rectal diazepam has been well received.[28] Mattila et al.[29] stated that the rectal solution of diazepam is a faster and more effective and reliable alternative to either tablets or suppositories and to the uncertain IM injection of diazepam. Diazepam is not available at this time in the United States in a rectal formulation. However, it is available in this form in many countries, where its administration rectally has been well accepted.

Flaitz, Nowak, and Hicks[30] reported on the effective use of rectally administered diazepam for pediatric sedation in dentistry. Using the IV formulation of diazepam, a dose of 0.6 mg/kg was administered rectally. Effective levels of both sedation and anterograde amnesia were found in most patients. A potential complication of the rectal administration of diazepam is intestinal irritation, the incidence of which is thought to be quite low.[31]

Midazolam

Midazolam, a water-soluble benzodiazepine, has received considerable attention as a rectally administered drug for premedication or sedation.* Various doses of rectal midazolam have been used, ranging from 0.2 to 5.0 mg/kg. It appears that a rectal dose of approximately 0.35 mg/kg[4,14,36] to 0.5 mg/kg[7,16] provides a rapid onset of action, a high level of successful sedation, with minimal intraoperative or postoperative complications. Roelofse et al.[4] observed that 23% of the 60 patients receiving rectal midazolam exhibited disinhibition reactions, particularly those receiving a dose of 0.45 mg/kg. Reactions observed included agitation/excitement, restlessness/irritation, disorientation/confusion, and emotional/crying responses.

Midazolam is not available in a rectal formulation. The parenteral formulation of midazolam has been used, with 2 ml of midazolam diluted with 8 ml of distilled water.[16] This volume is then instilled behind the anal sphincter with a suitable plastic applicator. Midazolam has not been observed to produce irritation of the rectal mucosa.

Studies in which vital signs and other physiologic parameters were monitored after the rectal administration of midazolam show no clinically significant changes in arterial blood pressure, heart rate, oxyhemoglobin saturation, or end-tidal carbon dioxide concentrations.[9,32]

Availability. Midazolam is not available as a rectal formulation, nor is it recommended for rectal administration in the United States. Several European countries (e.g., France and Switzerland) have approved the pediatric use of midazolam via rectal administration.[40] Midazolam is classified as a Schedule IV drug.

Ketamine

Ketamine, a cyclohexane derivative, is classified as a dissociative anesthetic. First reported in 1969, ketamine produces a surgical-depth anesthesia by interrupting afferent impulses reaching the cerebral cortex.[41] During dissociative anesthesia, patients appear to be awake—their eyes may be open, their mouths moving—yet they are incapable of purposefully reacting to environmental stimulation with appropriate motor responses.[42] The pharmacology of ketamine is discussed in greater detail in Chapter 31. Although used primarily via the IM and IV routes, ketamine has also been administered rectally for premedication or sedation.[1,35,39] Holm-Knudsen, Sjogren, and Laub[35] used 10 mg/kg ketamine and 0.2 mg/kg midazolam for induction of general anesthesia in healthy 2- to 10-year-olds and reported that no cases of rectal irritation or unpleasant dreams occurred and that postoperative analgesia was good. vander Bijl, Roelofse, and Stander[39] also administered rectal ketamine (5 mg/kg) and midazolam (0.3 mg/kg) to patients 2 to 9 years old. They reported that 30 minutes after administration of the two drugs, good anxiolysis, sedation, and cooperation were obtained in most patients. The group that received midazolam alone appeared to be more efficacious and had fewer adverse effects than the group that received ketamine alone (but no statistical difference was noted).[39]

A commonly reported side effect of ketamine, via any route of administration, is vivid dreams or hallucinations.[43] Such adverse events are rarely noted in pediatric patients, who generally tolerate ketamine anesthesia quite well. Ketamine should not be used by doctors who have not been trained in general anesthesia and in the management of the airway of the unconscious patient.

Lytic Cocktail

The lytic cocktail is a combination of meperidine (Demerol), promethazine (Phenergan), and chlorpromazine (Thorazine), also known as *DPT.* Used intramuscularly, DPT was frequently used in hospitals (especially in the emergency room) during painful procedures. The efficacy of this mixture is poor, especially when compared with alternative approaches, and it has been associated with a high frequency of adverse effects.[44,45] It has been used rectally in pediatric patients. A dose of 0.07 ml/kg was administered to patients ranging in age from 1 to 12 years.[46] One milliliter of lytic cocktail contains 28 mg meperidine, 7 mg promethazine, and 7 mg chlorpromazine. Satisfactory sedation was achieved before operation in most patients, but following the operation, rectally premedicated patients were less sedated than a control group that received IM DPT.

That the lytic cocktail has fallen into disfavor is noted in the U.S. Department of Health and Human Services' *Clinical Practice Guideline on Acute Pain Management.*[47] Their conclusion is that the lytic cocktail "is not recommended for general use and should be used only in exceptional circumstances."

COMPLICATIONS OF RECTAL ADMINISTRATION

Several complications are associated with rectal administration of drugs. Primary among these is the

*References 4, 6, 7, 9, 14-16, 32-39.

initiation of a bowel movement by instillation of a large volume of fluid into the rectum.[11] The incidence of this complication is not documented, but it is estimated to occur in 5% to 10% of patients receiving rectal drugs.[11]

Irritation of rectal mucosa, even to the extent of ulceration, is possible with certain drugs and with prolonged rectal administration.[48] Long-term rectal administration of acetylsalicylic acid has produced rectal ulceration. However, even single-dose rectal instillation has produced rectal irritation.

The potential for oversedation or the loss of consciousness (general anesthesia), both with attendant risk of airway obstruction produced by the relaxed tongue, must be considered whenever rectally administered drugs are intended to provide deep sedation. This risk is increased when barbiturates, opioid agonists, or ketamine is used. The occurrence of oversedation, inadvertent general anesthesia, or airway obstruction is decreased when rectal benzodiazepines are employed.

SUMMARY

The use of rectally administered drugs has increased in popularity in many countries, especially since the introduction of midazolam. Clinical trials have demonstrated that drugs administered rectally are usually well accepted, are well tolerated, and provide a relatively rapid onset of action with a minimum of adverse effects or complications. Rectally administered drugs provide an alternative to the oral and parenteral routes, which might prove difficult to employ or be contraindicated in certain populations such as pediatric patients and patients with disabilities.

Rectal sedation should be considered only by doctors who are knowledgeable in the pharmacology of the drug(s) to be administered and in the potential side effects and complications of the technique and drug(s) and who are adept in the management of the unconscious patient and airway. In addition, I strongly recommend that supplemental oxygen be administered to all patients receiving deep sedation via rectal drugs, that an IV infusion be maintained throughout the procedure, and that monitoring of the patient be continuous, including pulse oximetry and a pretracheal stethoscope.

Where rectal sedation is to be employed, I suggest the drug be administered in the office to ensure proper dosing and monitoring after administration. Whenever possible, the use of benzodiazepines, midazolam or diazepam, should be considered. Opioids, barbiturates, ketamine, and especially the lytic cocktail ought not be given rectally unless specific indications for their administration exist and adequately trained personnel are available to manage the patient during and after the sedation.

REFERENCES

1. Jantzen JP, Diehl P: Rectal administration of drugs: fundamentals and applications in anesthesia, *Anaesthesist* 40:251, 1991.
2. American Heart Association: National Academy of Sciences and National Research Council standards for cardiopulmonary resuscitation (CPR) and emergency cardiac care (ECC), *JAMA* 227(suppl):833, 1974.
3. Sykes WS: *Essays on the first hundred years of anaesthesia*, Edinburgh, 1960, ES Livingstone.
4. Roelofse JA, vander Bilj P, Stegmann DH et al: Preanesthetic medication with rectal midazolam in children undergoing dental extractions, *J Oral Maxillofac Surg* 48:791, 1990.
5. Diner MH, Fortin RC, Marcoux P: Behavioral influences of rectal diazepam in solution on dental patients with mentally and physically handicapping conditions, *Spec Care Dent* 8:19, 1988.
6. Kraemer N, Krafft T, Kinzelmann KH: Treatment of deciduous teeth under rectal midazolam sedation, *Deut Zahnarzt Z* 46:609, 1991.
7. Tolksdorf W, Eicj C: Rectal, oral and nasal premedication using midazolam in children aged 1-6 years: a comparative clinical study, *Anaesthesist* 40:661, 1991.
8. Kasaba T, Nonoue T, Yanagidani T et al: Effects of rectal premedication and the mother's presence on induction of pediatric anesthesia, *Masui Jpn J Anesthes* 40:552, 1991.
9. Spear RM, Yaster M, Berkowitz ID et al. Preinduction of anesthesia in children with rectally administered midazolam, *Anesthesiology* 74:670, 1991.
10. Maunuksela EL, Ryhaenen P, Janhunen L: Efficacy of rectal ibuprofen in controlling postoperative pain in children, *Can J Anaesth* 39:226, 1992.
11. Giovannitti JA, Trapp LD: Adult sedation: oral, rectal, IM, IV. In Dionne RA, Phero JC, eds. *Management of pain and anxiety in dental practice*, New York, 1991, Elsevier.
12. De Boer A, De Leede L, Breimer D: Drug absorption by sublingual and rectal routes, *Br J Anaesth* 56:69, 1984.
13. De Boer A, Moolenaar F, Leede L et al: Rectal drug administration: clinical pharmacokinetic considerations, *Clin Pharmacokinet* 7:285, 1982.
14. Kraus GB, Gruber RG, Knoll R et al. Pharmacokinetic studies following intravenous and rectal administration of midazolam in children, *Anaesthesist* 38:658, 1989.
15. Coventry DM, Martin CS, Burke AM: Sedation for paediatric computerized tomography: double-blind assessment of rectal midazolam, *Eur J Anaesthesiol* 8:29, 1991.
16. deWaal FC, Huisman J, Veerman AJ: Rectal premedication with midazolam in children: a comparative clinical study, *Tijdschr Kindergeneesk* 56:82, 1988.
17. Larsson LE, Nilsson K, Andreasson S et al: Effects of rectal thiopentone and methohexitone on carbon dioxide tension in infant anesthesia with spontaneous ventila-

tion, *Acta Anaesthesiol Scand* 31:227, 1987.
18. Pentothal rectal syringe package insert, Chicago, 1992, Abbott Laboratories.
19. Bjorkman S, Gabrielsson J, Quaynor H et al: Pharmacokinetics of IV and rectal methohexitone in children, *Br J Anaesth* 59:1541, 1987.
20. Quaynor H, Corbey M, Bjorkman S: Rectal induction of anaesthesia in children with methohexitone, *Br J Anaesth* 57:573, 1984.
21. Liu L, Gaudreault P, Friedman P et al: Methohexital plasma concentrations in children following rectal administration, *Anesthesiology* 62:567, 1985.
22. Karhunen U: Sleep effect of rectal methohexital (10 mg/kg) in children premedicated for anaesthesia, *Dev Pharmacol Ther* 11:92, 1988.
23. Dilaudid drug package insert, Whippany, NJ, 1989, Knoll Pharmaceuticals.
24. Numorphan drug package insert, Garden City, NY, 1985, DuPont Multi-Source.
25. Dhillon S, Ngwane E, Richens A: Rectal absorption of diazepam in epileptic children, *Arch Dis Child* 57:264, 1982.
26. Ehsanullah RS, Galloway DB, Gusterson FR et al: A double-blind crossover study of diazepam rectal suppositories, 5 mg and 10 mg, for sedation with advanced malignant disease, *Pharmatherapeutica* 3:215, 1982.
27. Lundgren S: Serum concentration and drug effect after intravenous and rectal administration of diazepam, *Anesth Prog* 34:128, 1987.
28. Knudsen F: Plasma-diazepam in infants after rectal administration in solution and by suppository, *Acta Paediatr Scand* 66:563, 1977.
29. Mattila MA, Ruoppi MK, Ahlstrom-Bengg E et al: Diazepam in rectal solution as premedication in children, with special reference to serum concentrations, *Br J Anaesth* 53:1269, 1981.
30. Flaitz CM, Nowak AJ, Hicks MJ: Evaluation of anterograde amnesic effect of rectally administered diazepam in the sedated pedodontic patient, *J Dent Child* 53:17, 1986.
31. Lundgren S, Rosenquist J: Comparison of sedation, amnesia, and patient comfort produced by intravenous and rectal diazepam, *J Oral Maxillofac Surg* 42:646, 1984.
32. Roelofse JA, de V Joubert JJ: Arterial oxygen saturation in children receiving rectal midazolam as premedication for oral surgical procedures, *Anesth Prog* 37:286, 1990.
33. Piotrowski R, Petrow N: Anesthesia induction in children: propofol in comparison with thiopental following premedication with midazolam, *Anaesthesist* 39:398, 1990.
34. Molter G, Castor G, Altmayer P: Psychosomatic, sedative and hemodynamic reactions following preoperative administration of midazolam in children, *Klin Padiatr* 202:328, 1990.
35. Holm-Knudsen R, Sjogren P, Laub M: Midazolam and ketamine for rectal premedication and induction of anesthesia in children, *Anaesthesist* 39:255, 1990.
36. Roelofse JA, Stegmann DH, Hartshorne J et al: Paradoxical reactions to rectal midazolam as premedication in children, *Int J Oral Maxillofac Surg* 19:2, 1990.
37. Tolksdorf W, Bremerich D, Nordmeyer U: Midazolam for premedication of infants. A comparison of the effect between oral and rectal administration, *Anasthesiol Intensivmed Notfallmed* 24:355, 1989.
38. Saint-Maurice C, Esteve C, Holzer J et al: Better acceptance of measures for induction of anesthesia after rectal premedication with midazolam in children: comparison of results of an open and placebo-controlled study, *Anaesthesist* 36:629, 1987.
39. vander Bijl P, Roelofse JA, Stander IA: Rectal ketamine and midazolam for premedication in pediatric dentistry, *J Oral Maxillofac Surg* 49:1050, 1991.
40. Moore PA: Pediatric medication with rectal midazolam in children undergoing dental extractions. Discussion, *J Oral Maxillofac Surg* 48:797, 1990.
41. Corssen G, Groves EH, Gomez S et al: Ketamine: its place in anesthesia for neurosurgical diagnostic procedures, *Anesth Analg* 48:181, 1969.
42. Jeffers GE, Dembo JB: Deep sedation. In Dionne RA, Phero JC, eds: *Management of pain and anxiety in dental practice*, New York, 1991, Elsevier.
43. Becsey L, Malamed S, Radnay P et al: Reduction of the psychotomimetic and circulatory side effects of ketamine by droperidol, *Anesthesiology* 37:536, 1972.
44. Benusis KP, Kapaun D, Furnam LJ: Respiratory depression in a child following meperidine, promethazine, and chlorpromazine premedication: report of a case, *J Dent Child* 46:50, 1979.
45. Nahata N, Clotz M, Krogg E: Adverse effects of meperidine, promethazine, and chlorpromazine for sedation in pediatric patients, *Clin Pediatr* 24:558, 1985.
46. Laub M, Sjogren P, Holm-Knudsen R et al: Lytic cocktail in children: rectal versus intramuscular administration, *Anaesthesia* 45:110, 1990.
47. US Department of Health and Human Services: *Clinical practice guideline: acute pain management: operative or medical procedures and trauma*, Publication No. 92-2, Rockville, Md, 1992, US Department of Health and Human Services, Public Health Service, Agency for Health Care Policy and Research.
48. van Hoogdalem E, de Boer AG, Breimer DD: Pharmacokinetics of rectal drug administration, part I. General considerations and clinical applications of centrally acting drugs, *Clin Pharmacokinet* 21:11, 1991.

CHAPTER 9

Sublingual, Transdermal, and Intranasal Sedation

CHAPTER OUTLINE

In recent years efforts have been directed at seeking alternative routes of drug administration for use where traditional routes are unavailable or where patient cooperation is lacking. Such situations include younger children or infants (the "precooperative patient"), where cooperation does not exist; older patients requiring long-term drug therapy, where noncompliance with administration recommendations is a significant problem; and victims of burns, trauma, or life-threatening emergencies, where other routes of administration are not present, yet rapid onset of drug action is necessary.

Three routes of drug administration, sublingual (SL), transdermal, and intranasal (IN), are discussed. These techniques are becoming increasingly popular in many areas of medicine.

Transdermal drug administration is most often used for sustained-action drug administration, for example, scopolamine as an anti–motion sickness therapy, whereas *SL* and *IN* drug administration provide a considerably more rapid onset of clinical action.

SUBLINGUAL SEDATION

SL drug administration has a long history. Indeed, SL administration of nitroglycerin tablets has been the recommended route for management of anginal pain for decades. SL placement of nitroglycerin tablets usually provides relief from anginal discomfort within 2 minutes.

An advantage of SL drug administration is that the drug enters directly into the systemic circulation, almost entirely bypassing the enterohepatic circulation. This avoids the hepatic first-pass effect, in which a percentage of the drug is biotransformed before ever having the opportunity to enter the general circulation and to reach its target organ (e.g., brain).[1-3] Harris and Robinson[4] have stated that SL drug delivery provides rapid absorption and good bioavailability for some drugs, although this site is not well suited to sustained-delivery systems. Patient cooperation is important to the success of the SL route of administration, which minimizes its use in many pediatric and other uncooperative patients.[5]

Among the drugs that have been used sublingually are nitroglycerin in the management of angina pectoris, acute pulmonary edema, and acute myocardial infarction[6]; heparin in the prophylaxis of atherosclerotic disease[7]; nifedipine, a calcium channel blocker, for the management of acute hypertensive urgencies and emergencies[8-14]; opioids, such as meperidine and buprenorphine, for relief of pain in cancer[15,16] or following abdominal or gynecologic surgery[5,17]; and sedatives for premedication and conscious sedation.[18-20]

Nitroglycerin

Nitroglycerin is administered sublingually in the management of anginal discomfort. Rapid SL absorption provides venodilation within 2 minutes. The rapidity of onset and degree of vasodilation observed make nitroglycerin the drug of choice for the management of angina pectoris. Side effects of SL nitroglycerin are few and usually not severe. However, in certain individuals SL nitroglycerin has provoked severe side effects. Brandes, Santiago, and Limacher[21] report on 35 cases of nitroglycerin-induced hypotension, bradycardia, apnea, and unconsciousness and conclude that this is a drug-induced effect of nitroglycerin that is independent of the route of administration and is unpredictable. They recommend close monitoring whenever nitroglycerin is administered.

Therapeutic advantage may be taken of the hypotensive side effect of nitroglycerin in the management of acute hypertensive episodes. Acute hypertensive episodes are classified as either "urgencies" or "emergencies," the level of blood pressure elevation determining the classification. Hypertensive emergencies involve significantly greater blood pressure elevations and require more aggressive and immediate treatment than do hypertensive urgencies.[8] Although nitroglycerin has been used effectively sublingually, the calcium channel blocker nifedipine has received considerably more attention in management of both hypertensive urgencies and emergencies. SL nifedipine is rapidly absorbed, leading to improved myocardial perfusion, increased coronary blood flow, and decreased coronary vascular resistance.[9] A capsule of nifedipine is punctured several times (in the dental office an explorer or small round bur will be sufficient for this purpose), placed under the tongue, and sucked on by the patient. Nifedipine SL has been used in the management of clonidine overdose, which produces severe hypertension and altered mental status. SL nifedipine (20 mg) produces a rapid decline in blood pressure and improved mental status.[10] As with nitroglycerin, SL nifedipine used for management of acute hypertensive episodes may produce symptomatic hypotension in some patients.[13] Vital signs should be monitored closely whenever SL nifedipine is used. Recent evidence has demonstrated that SL nifedipine may cause serious dose-dependent adverse effects.[14]

Opioids

Four studies have reported on the efficacy of SL administration of opioids. Kortilla and Hovorka[17] compared SL buprenorphine with intramuscular (IM) oxycodone as a preanesthetic medication. Preoperatively the SL opioid produced less drowsiness and sedation and alleviated patients' apprehension significantly less than oxycodone. However, in the recovery room, moderate to severe pain was more common with oxycodone than with SL buprenorphine. SL buprenorphine was as effective as IM oxycodone for pain relief. However, two patients receiving SL opioids developed severe respiratory depression postoperatively. The authors concluded that SL opioids can provide good postoperative pain relief for gynecologic procedures performed under anesthesia but that patients must be monitored because of the potential for respiratory depression. In a similar study, Carl et al.[5] compared SL and IM buprenorphine and IM meperidine for pain control following major abdominal surgery. Patients receiving SL buprenorphine were significantly more conscious in the immediate postoperative period than either IM group, yet all three groups demonstrated equal pain relief. Sedation and nausea were the most common complications in all three groups. Three cases of IM meperidine and one of IM buprenorphine required intermittent positive-pressure ventilation (IPPV) for respiratory depression. They concluded that SL opioids are useful for postoperative pain and exhibited administrative advantages when patients were able to cooperate. Two studies have looked at the use of opioids for the long-term relief of cancer pain, concluding that SL morphine has enabled patients whose cancer pain is refractory to traditional methods of drug delivery to obtain satisfactory control of their symptoms.[15,16]

Oral Transmucosal Fentanyl Citrate (Fentanyl "Lollipop")

Fentanyl has also been formulated as a lozenge or lollipop (Fentanyl Oralet, Abbott Laboratories). Originally designed for use in long-term pain management in cancer patients,[22,23] oral transmucosal fentanyl citrate (OTFC) has recently demonstrated advantages in the management of moderate to severe postoperative pain[24] and as a preoperative sedative in children.[25,26] The use of oral transmucosal fentanyl citrate has been studied as an alternative to oral and parenteral medication in younger or older patients who are unwilling or unable to tolerate orally administered drugs.[27-34] Although several dosages have been evaluated, most studies indicated that a dose of

15 to 20 μg/kg provides the optimal sedation and anxiolysis preoperatively.[27,28] Acceptance of the lollipop was reported as universal in most studies, a significant advantage over most other forms of drug administration.[27-31] The objective onset of sedation was noted to develop from 10 minutes[29] to 30 minutes[27] following administration of the lollipop. After beginning OTFC, 60% of patients became drowsy or sedated in 12 to 30 minutes.[31] When volunteers were asked to rapidly suck the lollipop (as opposed to permitting it to passively dissolve), a more rapid onset of a pleasant feeling (the first subjective sensation) was observed. However, the onset of subjective sedation or analgesia was no more rapid than with passive dissolution.[28]

The use of fentanyl lollipops is not without the potential for side effects. Significant decreases in respiratory rate and arterial oxygen saturation (Spo_2) have been reported.[2,27,29,33] Management of these episodes of opioid-induced respiratory depression was simple: reminding the patient to breathe.[27] Other side effects noted with some frequency included pruritis[27,30,33] in 80%[27] to 90%[30] of patients preoperatively and 33% to 70% postoperatively[27]; postoperative nausea (30% to 58%[27]); and vomiting (50% to 83%),[27,30,32-33] which was not significantly reduced by the prophylactic administration of the antiemetic droperidol.[32]

The conclusion reached by most authors is that OTFC is a reliable means of inducing rapid, noninvasive preoperative sedation for pediatric outpatients undergoing short operations[32,34] or in the emergency room.[31] They further observe that OTFC use is associated with potentially significant reductions in respiratory rate and Spo_2 and a high incidence of postoperative nausea and vomiting and pruritus.[32] In the absence of controlled clinical trials in dental outpatients, it seems prudent, at this time, to withhold recommendation of this method of opioid administration for preoperative sedation in dentistry.

Sedatives

Several studies have reported on the use of the SL route for preoperative sedation. Two have compared the SL administration of a benzodiazepine with oral administration. Gram-Hansen and Schultz,[18] administering 2.5 mg lorazepam either orally or sublingually before gynecologic surgery, found a maximal plasma concentration at 40 minutes orally and 60 minutes after SL administration. Garzone and Kroboth,[19] looking at alprazolam and triazolam, found peak concentrations that occurred earlier and were higher following SL versus oral administration. SL lormetazepam (2.5 mg) followed in 35 minutes by intravenous (IV) diazepam (10 mg) was compared with SL placebo followed in 35 minutes by IV diazepam (10 mg) in patients undergoing surgical removal of impacted third molars.[20] A rapid onset of sedation was noted after SL lormetazepam administration, whereas the course and duration of postoperative sedation, measured using standard psychometric tests, were similar following both treatments. Surgeons' ratings indicated that SL lormetazepam was comparable to IV diazepam, but patients' ratings indicated greater satisfaction with and preference for IV diazepam. Significant anterograde amnesia was found following both treatments. The authors indicate that SL lormetazepam may have a role in anesthesia as a premedicant and for conscious sedation.

Conclusions

The SL route of drug administration possesses possible uses in dentistry in two distinct areas. First, for the management of preoperative fears and anxiety, the use of certain drugs, such as benzodiazepines, appears to provide a level of conscious sedation comparable to that achieved with orally administered drugs. The onset of action also appears comparable to that of oral drugs. The second possible use for SL administration in dentistry is in management of postoperative pain. SL opioid administration appears to provide adequate pain relief with less sedation than IM opioids. The potential for opioid-induced respiratory depression is still present; therefore the usual postoperative monitoring practices must be continued when SL opioids are used. Patient cooperation is essential for SL delivery of drugs to be effective. Therefore the use of SL administration in younger children or any uncooperative patient is not recommended.

TRANSDERMAL SEDATION

The administration of drugs through the skin (transdermally) has existed for a long time. In the past the most commonly applied systems were topically applied creams and ointments for dermatologic disorders. The occurrence of systemic side effects with some of these formulations is indicative of absorption through the skin. In a broad sense the term *transdermal delivery system* includes all topically administered drug formulations intended to deliver the active ingredient into the general circulation.[35] Serious consideration for the transdermal delivery of drugs for systemic therapy began with a number of revolutionary ideas in the early 1970s.[36] It is only since the 1980s, however, that modern transdermal therapeutic systems (TTS) have been successfully marketed.[37] Drugs such as nitroglycerin (angina),[38] scopolamine (anti–motion sickness),[39,40] clonidine (high blood pressure),[41] estradiol (postmenopause),[42] and nicotine (smoking cessation)[43] are the current prominent representatives that have met expectations regarding therapeutic benefits based on TTS applications. The use of opioids via TTS for pain management has also met with considerable clinical success.[44,45]

A major advantage of TTS is the avoidance of the hepatic first-pass effect. Other advantages include simplified dosage regimens, enhanced compliance, reduced side effects, and improved disease therapy.[46]

The intact skin provides an efficient barrier against percutaneous absorption of drugs.[47] This barrier function can be ascribed to the structure of the stratum corneum, which consists of alternating lipoidal and hydrophilic regions, making intact skin relatively impermeable. This impermeability of skin is associated with its dual functions as a protective barrier against invasion by microorganisms and the prevention of the loss of physiologically essential substances such as water. Elucidation of factors that contribute to this impermeability has made the use of skin as a route for controlled systemic drug delivery possible.[35] For drugs for systemic therapy to be delivered through the skin, skin permeability must be enhanced by either modifying the drug molecules or applying skin permeation enhancers to reduce the barrier property of the skin.[48] Traditionally, enhancement of skin permeability is achieved by either improvement of drug lipophilicity and the partition of drugs into the skin or through direct actions of skin permeation enhancers on the chemical structure and/or composition of lipids and proteins in the stratum corneum.

A number of transdermal delivery systems are currently employed that allow for effective absorption of drugs (of low molecular mass) across the skin.[49] The most widely used system is the membrane-permeation-controlled system. A second system is the microsealed system, a partition-controlled delivery system that contains a drug reservoir with a saturated suspension of the drug in a water-miscible solvent homogeneously dispersed in a silicone elastomer matrix. A third system is the matrix-diffusion-controlled system, and a fourth system is the gradient-charged system. Nitroglycerin TTS is based on a multilayered laminated polymeric structure. A layer of vinyl chloride copolymer or terpolymer containing the drug is sandwiched between two or more layers of polymeric films. Nitroglycerin is released from the device at a controlled rate by a process of diffusion through the reservoir and one of the outer layers, which can function as a rate-controlling membrane.[50] Advanced transdermal systems are being developed, including iontophoretic and sonophoretic systems, thermosetting gels, prodrugs, and liposomes.[35] Penetration enhancers such as Azone may allow the delivery of larger molecules such as proteins and polypeptides.

Systemic and localized side effects may be noted with the use of transdermal drug delivery systems. These have included skin inflammation and allergy[37,48,51] and drug tolerance.[38,52] Side effects produced by the drug are similar to those noted with other routes of drug delivery.

The onset of clinical activity of TTS-administered drugs is slow, hence the primary use of this technique for sustained-release drug therapy. After application of a transdermal fentanyl patch, fentanyl is absorbed into the skin beneath the patch, where a depot forms in the upper skin layers. Plasma fentanyl concentrations are barely detectable for about 2 hours after patch placement. From 8 to 12 hours after patch placement, however, plasma fentanyl concentrations approximate those achieved with equivalent IV doses.[45]

Opioids

Interest in the use of transdermal drug delivery systems in dentistry centers on postoperative pain control. Opioids, particularly fentanyl, have received attention in the management of both chronic (cancer) and acute (postoperative) pain.

Mosser[44] describes the unique pharmacokinetics of the transdermal system, including a prolonged time to peak analgesic effect, a long elimination half-life, and the skin depot concept, and recommends fentanyl over parenterally administered opioids in the treatment of cancer pain. Calis, Kohler, and Corso[45] also recommend fentanyl TTS for management of chronic cancer-related pain. The use of TTS for acute postoperative pain is not as well accepted. Although Clotz and Nahata[53] state that the transdermal fentanyl patch seems to provide the same degree of analgesia as a continuous IV infusion, Calis, Kohler, and Corso[45] state that the overall efficacy and safety of the transdermal fentanyl system for the treatment of postoperative pain has not been adequately evaluated.

Antiemetics

A second area in which TTS drug delivery systems have potential utility in dentistry is the delivery of antiemetic drugs. Swallowed blood is a potent emetic following oral surgical procedures. In addition, the administration of opioid analgesics during the surgical procedure or postoperatively is associated with an increased likelihood of nausea and vomiting.

Scopolamine was one of the first drugs employed transdermally in the management of motion sickness.[54] When it is administered transdermally, its duration of effect is 72 hours compared with a 3- to 6-hour duration when administered orally or parenterally. Transdermal administration is associated with a lower incidence of side effects than orally or parenterally administered scopolamine. The most commonly observed side effects following transdermal administration have been dry mouth, drowsiness, and impairment of ocular accommodation, including blurred vision and mydriasis. Systemic side effects, such as adverse central nervous system (CNS) effects, difficulty in urinating, rashes, and erythema, have been reported only occasionally. The efficacy of transdermal scopolamine in preventing nausea and vomiting in postsurgical patients was evaluated by Schuh, Tolksdorf, and Hucke.[55] Scopolamine has a well-documented postoperative antiemetic effect. One study has demonstrated a 50% reduction of emetic symptoms compared with placebo.[56] In this study of cholecystectomy patients (a procedure with a high incidence of postoperative emesis), the antinausea and antiemetic effect of scopolamine TTS was insufficient and significantly less than that seen with IV droperidol (7.5 mg).[55] In the droperidol group, 45% of patients did not have nausea, and vomiting occurred in only 25%, whereas in the scopolamine TTS group, only 15% did not become nauseous and 50% vomited. Further study is warranted to determine the efficacy of transdermal scopolamine as an antiemetic following oral surgical procedures.

Conclusions

Transdermal drug delivery systems provide an easy, reliable mechanism of administering drugs when rapid onset is not important. Transdermal drug delivery bypasses the enterohepatic circulation, thereby providing a more reliable clinical action. With many drugs, the efficacy of transdermal delivery is equivalent to that of a continuous IV infusion, yet in a noninvasive system.

It appears that the transdermal use of opioids might prove advantageous in dental situations in which long-term pain control is required but patient compliance is suspect. Drug-related side effects following transdermal delivery, although less common, are the same as those noted when other administration techniques are used. Oversedation and respiratory depression must be considered whenever opioids are employed. Use of transdermal opioids should be reserved for clinical situations in which patient monitoring can be ensured throughout the drug's delivery. The use of transdermal scopolamine as an antiemetic following dental surgery requires additional research before its use can be recommended.

INTRANASAL SEDATION

A relatively recent addition to the drug administration armamentarium, IN drugs have been used primarily in pediatric patients as a way to circumvent the need for injection or oral drug administration in unwilling patients.[57,58] Absorption of IN drugs occurs directly into the systemic circulation, avoiding the enterohepatic circulation.[59,60] Clinical trials have demonstrated that rates of absorption and bioavailability of IN drugs are close to those with IM administration, with peak plasma levels of the agent occurring approximately 10 minutes after administration.[60-67] Midazolam, a water-soluble benzodiazepine,[57,58,60-68] and sufentanil,[68,69] an opioid analgesic, have received the most attention regarding administration via the IN route.

Midazolam

Midazolam has been demonstrated to provide a consistent level of CNS activity following IN administration.[58,61-68] A dose of 0.2 mg/kg appears to be the most effective in pediatric patients for premedication before general anesthesia,[64-65,68,70] with somewhat larger doses recommended for sedation adequate to permit treatment.[71]

The mean IN absorption rates (t_{max}) of flurazepam, midazolam, and triazolam were 1.7, 2, and 2.6 times faster, respectively, than those achieved with oral dosing.[72] When children accept oral administration at all, they appear to accept it better than drugs administered intranasally.[70] IN drugs are administered by either the parent or the doctor using a 1- or 3-ml syringe without a needle and with the child seated on the parent's lap. Some children are temporarily distressed at the instillation of the fluid (drug) into the nose, but all rapidly settled down again in the presence of their parents.[57] An undiluted solution of the drug should be used to avoid large volumes of liquid being instilled into the nose and possibly entering the pharynx and producing coughing or sneezing, with attendant expulsion of the drug and decreased absorption. Rose, Simon, and Haberer[67] found IN midazolam to be slightly more effective than oral diazepam as preanesthetic medication in children, producing anxiolysis and sedation with rapid onset. Buenz and Gossler[64] suggest that with the advent of a more concentrated solution of midazolam (>5 mg/ml), IN application is also conceivable as a premedication in adults.

The IM and IN routes of midazolam administration have been compared. There were no significant differences in the onset of sedation (12.42 ± 4.07 minutes for IM; 15.26 ± 7.99 minutes for IN), the degree of sedation, and in the response to venipuncture.[65] Theissen et al.[73] compared IM and IN midazolam for sedation in adults before endoscopy of the upper gastrointestinal tract. Sedation was equivalent in both groups, with three patients (n = 10) in the IM group experiencing retrograde amnesia (0 in the IN group). No significant differences in the degrees of anterograde amnesia were noted in either group. IN administration of midazolam was concluded to be a simple, nontraumatic, well-tolerated alternative to the IM route of sedation for bronchoscopy in adults.

Several studies have compared IN midazolam to IV midazolam. The half-life of midazolam is similar (2.2 hours IN vs. 2.4 hours IV) following IM and IV administration in children ages 1 to 5 years.[63] At 10 minutes following IN administration, the mean plasma concentration of midazolam was 57% of that in the IV group.[66]

An additional finding noted by one observer was the association of IN instillation of midazolam with a sense of euphoria that occurred almost immediately. This effect was not observed when midazolam was administered by other routes.[70]

Two studies used IN midazolam for procedures akin to dental care. In one, IN midazolam was employed in adults for sedation during upper gastrointestinal endoscopy, and it compared well to IM midazolam.[73] Only two patients (n = 20) receiving IM or IN midazolam had a bad opinion of their experience, as compared with four of the nine receiving placebo. IN midazolam was used for sedation before ophthalmologic examination in children ranging in age from 3.5 months to 10 years.[71] An IN midazolam dose of 0.35 to 0.5 mg/kg provided a rapid onset of sedation that was adequate in all cases to permit ocular examination. In all of the IN midazolam studies reported, oxygen saturation was monitored throughout the procedure, including recovery. No instances of significant desaturation were reported.

IN midazolam in a dose of approximately 0.2 mg/kg appears to be an acceptable alternative to both oral and IM administration of midazolam for premedication before additional IV sedation or general anesthesia. A larger dose, 0.35 to 0.5 mg/kg, may be necessary if the IN drug is the sole route of sedative administration. It may be of significant value as an alternative in cases in which IM sedation is necessary, such as venipuncture in the uncooperative child or adult. When more profound and more controllable levels of sedation are desired, the IV route is recommended. IN midazolam provides the level of sedation adequate to permit separation of the child from the parent and to enable the patient to tolerate venipuncture with minimal distress.

My own clinical experience using IN midazolam (a dose of 0.2 mg/kg) in a pediatric population has shown that use of an aerosol spray (similar to a nasal decongestant spray) is better tolerated by patients than a syringe. Use of a syringe often results in the fluid leaking into the patient's throat, precipitating crying and coughing. The clinical efficacy of IN midazolam appears to be similar to that of IM midazolam in both speed of onset and ability to separate the patient from his or her parent. However, as with other nontitratable techniques, there were occasions when IN midazolam demonstrated little or no clinical effect.

Sufentanil

Sufentanil via IN administration was one of the first drugs to receive attention for preoperative sedation.[68,69] Both IV and IN sufentanil (IV and IN dose of 15 μg) had rapid onset of action and limited duration.[74] At 10 minutes, all patients (n = 8) in the IV group were sedated, compared with only two in the IN group. However, no significant differences in sedation were observed in either group at 20 to 60 minutes. These findings are in agreement with measured plasma levels of sufentanil, which are significantly lower following IN than IV administration at 5 and 10 minutes, being 36% and 56% of those after IV dosing, respectively. From 30 minutes on, plasma concentrations were virtually identical following both IN and IV sedation. An important finding was a clinically significant decrease in arterial oxygen pressure ($Pa{O_2}$) at 5 minutes after IV administration of sufentanil that was not observed following IN administration.[74] In a pediatric trial (including children ages 6 months to 7 years) for premedication, doses of 0.15, 0.30, and 0.45 μg/kg of sufentanil were administered intranasally before induction of general anesthesia.[75] Patients receiving sufentanil were more likely to separate willingly from their parents and to be judged as calm at or before 10 minutes compared with placebo-treated patients. However, patients receiving 0.45 μg/kg had a higher incidence of vomiting in the recovery room and during the first postoperative day. Relative to IN midazolam, IN sufentanil was accepted more readily by children but produced a significantly greater incidence of decreased $Pa{O_2}$.[57]

IN sufentanil produces a euphoric effect in addition to anxiolysis and sedation.[75] Its onset of action is similar to that of midazolam. However, the potential decrease in $Pa{O_2}$ and the increased potential for nausea and vomiting following IN sufentanil administration call for intensified monitoring (oximetry and visual observation) during both the perioperative and postoperative periods. The use of IN midazolam does not appear to be associated with either of these two clinical actions.

Conclusions

The IN route of drug administration appears to be of potential value in dentistry. A rapid onset of action enables IN drugs to be used when speed is of the essence, such as for premedication of the uncooperative child. Although some degree of cooperation is necessary, IN drugs are more readily administered than oral drugs when no patient cooperation is available. Use of an aerosol spray for drug administration is preferred to a syringe. As a noninvasive technique, IN administration has few of the potential side effects and complications that are associated with IM drug administration (see Chapters 3 and 10).

Two drugs, sufentanil and midazolam, have received the most study to date and have been demonstrated to be quite effective intranasally. The IN use of sufentanil is associated with the potential development of significant opioid-related side effects such as nausea, vomiting, and respiratory depression. The benzodiazepine midazolam provides clinical actions that are similar to sufentanil's but is not associated with its side effects. Intensive monitoring should be used whenever IN drugs are administered.

REFERENCES

1. Aliberti G, D'Erasmo E, Oddo CM et al: Effect of the acute sublingual administration of ketanserin in hypertensive patients, *Cardiovasc Drugs Ther* 5:697, 1991.
2. DeBoer A, DeLeede L, Breimer D: Drug absorption by sublingual and rectal routes, *Br J Anaesth* 56:69, 1984.
3. Motwani JG, Lipworth BJ: Clinical pharmacokinetics of drug administered buccally and sublingually, *Clin Pharmacokinet* 21:83, 1991.
4. Harris D, Robinson JR: Drug delivery via the mucous membranes of the oral cavity, *J Pharm Sci* 81:1, 1992.
5. Carl P, Crawford ME, Masden NB et al: Pain relief after major abdominal surgery: a double-blind controlled comparison of sublingual buprenorphine, intramuscular buprenorphine, and intramuscular meperidine, *Anesth Analg* 66:142, 1987.
6. Schneider W, Bussmann WD, Hartmann A et al: Nitrate therapy in heart failure, *Cardiology* 79(suppl 2):5, 1991.
7. Kanabrocki EL, Bremner WF, Sothern RB et al: A quest for the relief of atherosclerosis: potential role of intrapulmonary heparin—a hypothesis, *Q J Med* 83:259, 1992.
8. Gonzalez-Ramallo VJ, Muino-Miguez A: Hypertensive crises and emergencies: the concept and initial management, *Ann Med Intern* 7:422, 1990.
9. Cohn PF: Effects of calcium channel blockers on the coronary circulation, *Am J Hypertens* 3(pt 2):299, 1990.
10. Dire DJ, Kuhns DW: The use of sublingual nifedipine in a patient with clonidine overdose, *J Emerg Med* 6:125, 1988.
11. Garcia JY Jr, Vidt DG: Current management of hypertensive emergencies, *Drugs* 34:263, 1978.
12. Bauer JH, Reams GP: The role of calcium entry blockers in hypertensive emergencies, *Circulation* 75(pt 2):V174, 1987.
13. Wachter RM: Symptomatic hypotension induced by nifedipine in the acute treatment of severe hypertension, *Arch Intern Med* 147:556, 1987.
14. Ishibashi Y, Shimada T, Yoshitomi H et al: Sublingual nifedipine in elderly patients: even a low dose induces myocardial ischaemia, *Clin Exp Pharmacol Physiol* 26:404, 1999.
15. Ripamonti C, Bruera E: Rectal, buccal, and sublingual narcotics for the management of cancer pain, *J Palliative Care* 7:30, 1991.
16. Shepard KV, Bakst AW: Alternate delivery methods for morphine sulfate in cancer pain, *Cleve Clin J Med* 57:48, 1990.
17. Korttilla K, Hovorka J: Buprenorphine as premedication and as analgesic during and after light isoflurane-N_2O-O_2 anaesthesia: a comparison with oxycodone plus fentanyl, *Acta Anaesthesiol Scand* 31:673, 1987.
18. Gram-Hansen P, Schultz A: Plasma concentrations following oral and sublingual administration of lorazepam, *Int J Clin Pharmacol Ther Toxicol* 26:323, 1988.
19. Garzone PD, Kroboth PD: Pharmacokinetics of the newer benzodiazepines, *Clin Pharmacokinet* 16:337, 1989.
20. O'Boyle CA, Barry H, Fox E et al. Controlled comparison of a new sublingual lormetazepam formulation and IV diazepam in outpatient minor oral surgery, *Br J Anaesth* 60:419, 1988.
21. Brandes W, Santiago T, Limacher M: Nitroglycerin-induced hypotension, bradycardia, and asystole: report of a case and review of the literature, *Clin Cardiol* 13:741, 1990.
22. Portenoy RK, Payne R, Coluzzi P et al: Oral transmucosal fentanyl citrate (OTFC) for the treatment of breakthrough pain in cancer patients: a controlled dose titration study, *Pain* 79:303, 1999.
23. Rhiner M, Kedziera P: Managing breakthrough cancer pain: a new approach, *Home Healthcare Nurse* 17(suppl): quiz 13, 1999.
24. Lichtor JL, Sevarino FB, Joshi GP et al: The relative potency of oral transmucosal fentanyl citrate compared with intravenous morphine in the treatment of moderate to severe postoperative pain, *Anesth Analg* 89:732, 1999.
25. Ginsberg B, Dear RB, Margolis JO et al: Oral transmucosal fentanyl citrate as an anaesthetic premedication when dosed to an opioid effect vs total opioid consumption, *Paediatr Anaesth* 8:413, 1998.
26. Dsida RM, Wheeler M, Birmingham PK et al: Premedication of pediatric tonsillectomy patients with oral transmucosal fentanyl citrate, *Anesth Analg* 86:66, 1998.
27. Streisand JB, Stanley TH, Hague B et al: Oral transmucosal fentanyl citrate premedication in children, *Anesth Analg* 69:28, 1989.
28. Stanley TH, Hague B, Mock DL et al: Oral transmucosal fentanyl citrate (lollipop) premedication in human volunteers, *Anesth Analg* 69:21, 1989.
29. Stanley TH, Leiman BC, Rawal N et al: The effects of oral transmucosal fentanyl citrate premedication on preoperative behavioral responses and gastric volumes and acidity in children, *Anesth Analg* 69:328, 1989.
30. Nelson PS, Streisand JB, Mulder SM et al: Comparison of oral transmucosal fentanyl citrate and an oral solution of meperidine, diazepam, and atropine for premedication in children, *Anesthesiology* 70:616, 1989.
31. Lind GH, Marcus MA, Mears SL et al: Oral transmucosal fentanyl citrate for analgesia and sedation in the emergency department, *Ann Emerg Med* 20:1117, 1991.
32. Friesen RH, Lockhart CH: Oral transmucosal fentanyl citrate for preanesthetic medication of pediatric day surgery patients with and without droperidol as a prophylactic anti-emetic, *Anesthesiology* 76:46, 1992.

33. Feld LH, Champeau MW, van Steennis CA et al: Preanesthetic medication in children: a comparison of oral transmucosal fentanyl citrate versus placebo, *Anesthesiology* 71:374, 1989.
34. Ashburn MA, Streisand JB, Tarver SD et al: Oral transmucosal fentanyl citrate for premedication in paediatric outpatients, *Can J Anaesth* 37:857, 1990.
35. Ranade VV: Drug delivery systems. 6. Transdermal drug delivery, *J Clin Pharmacol* 31:401, 1991.
36. Merkle HP: Transdermal delivery systems, *Methods Find Exp Clin Pharmacol* 11:135, 1989.
37. Asmussen B: Transdermal therapeutic systems: actual state and future developments, *Methods Find Exp Clin Pharmacol* 13:343, 1991.
38. Todd PA, Goa KL, Langtry HD: Transdermal nitroglycerin (glyceryl trinitrate): a review of its pharmacology and therapeutic use, *Drugs* 40:880, 1990.
39. Scopoderm: transdermal hyoscine for motion sickness, *Drug Ther Bull* 27:91, 1989.
40. Parrott AC: Transdermal scopolamine: a review of its effects upon motion sickness, psychological performance, and physiological functioning, *Aviat Space Environ Med* 60:1, 1989.
41. Lowenthat DT, Matzek KM, MacGregor TR: Clinical pharmacokinetics of clonidine, *Clin Pharmacokinet* 14:287, 1988.
42. Balfour JA, Heel RC: Transdermal estradiol: a review of its pharmacodynamic and pharmacokinetic properties, and therapeutic efficacy in the treatment of menopausal complaints, *Drugs* 40:561, 1990.
43. McKenna JP, Cox JL: Transdermal nicotine replacement and smoking cessation, *Am Fam Physician* 45:2595, 1992.
44. Mosser KH: Transdermal fentanyl in cancer pain, *Am Fam Physician* 45:2289, 1992.
45. Calis KA, Kohler DR, Corso DM: Transdermally administered fentanyl for pain management, *Clin Pharm* 11:22, 1992.
46. Geraets D, Burke T: Sustained-release dosage forms, *Iowa Med* 80:141, 1990.
47. Wiechers JW: The barrier function of the skin in relation to percutaneous absorption of drugs, *Pharm Weekbl* (sci ed) 11:185, 1989.
48. Xu P, Chien YW: Enhanced skin permeability for transdermal drug delivery: physiopathological and physiochemical considerations, *Crit Rev Ther Drug Carrier Syst* 8:211, 1991.
49. Karzel K, Liedtke RK: Mechanisms of transcutaneous absorption: pharmacologic and biochemical aspects, *Arzneimittelforschung* 39:1487, 1989.
50. Shah KR, Ng S, Zeoli L et al: Hercon technology for transdermal delivery of drugs, *J Biomater Appl* 1:239, 1986.
51. Hogan DJ, Maibach HI: Adverse dermatologic reactions to transdermal drug delivery systems, *J Am Acad Dermatol* 22:811, 1990.
52. Anderson KA: A practical guide to nitrate use, *Postgrad Med* 89:67, 1991.
53. Clotz MA, Nahata MC: Clinical uses of fentanyl, sufentanil, and alfentanil, *Clin Pharm* 10:581, 1991.
54. Clissold SP, Heel RC: Transdermal hyoscine (scopolamine): a preliminary review of its pharmacodynamic properties and therapeutic efficacy, *Drugs* 29:189, 1985.
55. Schuh R, Tolksdorf W, Hucke H: Transdermal scopolamine or droperidol in the prevention of postoperative nausea and vomiting in cholecystectomy patients, *Anasthesiol Intensivmed Notfallmed* 22:261, 1987.
56. Palazzo MG, Strunin L: Anaesthesia and emesis. I: Etiology, *Can Anaesthet Soc J* 31:1788, 1984.
57. Wilton NCT, Leigh J, Rosen DR et al: Preanesthetic sedation of preschool children using intranasal midazolam, *Anesthesiology* 69:972, 1988.
58. Saint-Maurice C, Landais A, Delleur MM et al: The use of midazolam in diagnostic and short surgical procedures in children, *Acta Anaesthes Scand (Suppl)* 92:39, 1990.
59. Sarkar MA: Drug metabolism in the nasal mucosa, *Pharmaceut Res* 9:1, 1992.
60. Fukuta O, Braham RL, Yanase H, Kurosu K: Intranasal administration of midazolam: pharmacokinetic and pharmacodynamic properties and sedative potential, *ASDC J Dent Child* 64:89, 1997.
61. Rey E, Delaunay L, Pons G et al: Pharmacokinetics of midazolam in children: comparative study of intranasal and intravenous administration, *Eur J Clin Pharmacol* 41:355, 1991.
62. Walbergh EJ, Wills RJ, Eckhert J: Plasma concentrations of midazolam in children following intranasal administration, *Anesthesiology* 74:233, 1991.
63. Rey E, Delaunay L, Pons G et al: Pharmacokinetics of midazolam in children: comparative study of intranasal and intravenous administration, *Eur J Clin Pharmacol* 41:355, 1991.
64. Buenz R, Gossler M: Intranasal premedication of young children using midazolam (Dormicum): clinical experience, *Anaesthesiol Intensivmed Notfallmed Schmerzther* 26:76, 1991.
65. de Santos P, Chabas E, Valero R et al: Comparison of intramuscular and intranasal premedication with midazolam in children, *Rev Esp Anesthesiol Reanimac* 38:12, 1991.
66. Walbergh EJ, Wills RJ, Eckhert J: Plasma concentrations of midazolam in children following intranasal administration, *Anesthesiology* 74:233, 1991.
67. Rose E, Simon D, Haberer JP: Premedication with intranasal midazolam in pediatric anesthesia, *Ann Fr Anesth Reanim* 9:326, 1990.
68. Karl HW, Keifer AT, Rosenberger JL et al: Comparison of the safety and efficacy of intranasal midazolam and sufentanil for preinduction of anesthesia in pediatric patients, *Anesthesiology* 76:209, 1992.
69. Vercauteren M, Boech E, Hanegreefs H et al: Intranasal sufentanil for pre-operative sedation, *Anaesthesia* 43:270, 1988.
70. Tolksdorf W, Eick C: Rectal, oral and nasal premedication using midazolam in children aged 1-6 years: a comparative clinical study, *Anaesthetist* 40:661, 1991.
71. Gobeaux D, Sardnal F, Cohn H et al: Intranasal midazolam in pediatric ophthalmology, *Cah Anesthesiol* 39:34, 1991.
72. Lui CY, Amidon GL, Goldberg A: Intranasal absorption of flurazepam, midazolam, and triazolam in dogs, *J Pharm Sci* 80:1125, 1991.

73. Theissen O, Boileau S, Wahl D et al: Sedation with intranasal midazolam for endoscopy of the upper digestive tract, *Ann Fr Anesth Reanim* 10:450, 1991.
74. Helmers JH, Noorduin H, van Peer A et al: Comparison of intravenous and intranasal sufentanil absorption and sedation, *Can J Anaesth* 36:494, 1989.
75. Henderson JM, Brodsky DA, Fisher DM et al: Pre-induction of anesthesia in pediatric patients with nasally administered sufentanil, *Anesthesiology* 68:671, 1988.

CHAPTER 10

Intramuscular Sedation

CHAPTER OUTLINE

The intramuscular (IM) route of drug administration is a parenteral technique in which the drug enters the cardiovascular system without first passing through the gastrointestinal (GI) tract. Parenteral techniques possess an advantage over enteral techniques (oral, rectal) in that the drug does not first have to pass through the enterohepatic circulation before entering the systemic circulation. This eliminates several disadvantages of the oral route, including a possible hepatic first-pass effect, presence of food in the stomach, and delayed gastric emptying. The advantages and disadvantages of the IM route were discussed in Chapter 3 and are summarized in Box 10-1.

Probably the most significant negative aspect of using the IM route is an inability to titrate the drug to a desired clinical effect. The doctor is unable to consistently predict the proper dose to administer in any given patient, leading to the use of an "educated guesstimate" based on a number of factors to be discussed shortly. Although the dose is often appropriate, situations occur in which the calculated dose proves ineffective, leading to an inability to treat the patient. More significant, however, are those occasions when the calculated dose has proved too great for the patient, leading to possibly dire consequences for both the patient and the doctor.[1-4]

The IM route of drug administration is indicated for use in almost any patient; however, several factors must be considered in determining the depth of sedation that can (and should) safely be sought via this route. As mentioned, inability to titrate is a prime negative consideration, as is the inability to rapidly reverse the actions of the drug.

Suggested uses of the IM route in the dental office include the following:

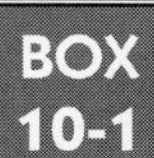

BOX 10-1 Advantages/Disadvantages of Intramuscular Drug Administration

Advantages	*Disadvantages*
Rapid onset of action (15 minutes)	Inability to titrate (15-minute onset)
Maximal clinical effect (30 minutes)	Inability to reverse drug action
More reliable absorption (than oral, rectal)	Prolonged duration of drug effect
Patient cooperation not as essential	Injection needed
	Possible injury from injection

1. The adult patient when other, more controllable, parenteral routes (intravenous [IV], inhalation) are unavailable
2. The precooperative pediatric patient in whom other routes have proved ineffective
3. The disruptive handicapped adult or child patient in whom other routes have proved ineffective
4. The disruptive pediatric patient or adult or child with a disability for use as premedication before the use of IV sedation or general anesthesia
5. The administration of emergency drugs to any patient in whom the IV route is unavailable

The last factor, the administration of emergency drugs, is the reason I believe that all dental personnel should be trained to administer drugs intramuscularly. Although IV drug administration is more rapidly effective, in an emergency situation the IM route may be the only practical route immediately available.

The level of central nervous system (CNS) depression sought via the IM route will vary considerably, from lighter levels of anxiolysis (in a frightened but otherwise healthy adult) to deeper levels of sedation (in the unmanageable child or adult or patient with a disability in whom the only alternative to IM sedation is general anesthesia). It must be stated here (as it is over and over again throughout this text) that the doctor administering drugs to a patient must know his or her limitations in drug usage. Important factors in deciding the depth of sedation to which a patient may safely be brought include (1) the physical status of the patient, (2) the training of the doctor and staff, and (3) the availability of trained personnel and equipment for the prompt and effective management of any emergency situation that might conceivably arise as a result of the use of a drug or coincident with its use. Deep sedation must not be employed by a doctor who is not well versed in the art and science of anesthesiology and in the management of the unconscious airway.

All 50 states in the United States require a doctor employing parenteral (IM/IV) conscious sedation to obtain a special permit from the state board of dental examiners. State requirements for parenteral conscious sedation permits vary, but all take into account the degree of education in the technique, preparedness for emergencies, and demonstrated clinical proficiency.[5]

In the healthy adult there are few indications for IM conscious sedation. Most adults, although not "liking it," will tolerate an IM injection of a drug. If the patient can psychologically tolerate this traumatic event (the "sticking of a needle into the skin"), then the IV route of administration is preferred. The IV route is more controllable than is the IM route. If a needle is to be inserted into a patient's body for the purpose of administering a CNS depressant drug, it is much preferred, for reasons of safety and effectiveness, to administer such drugs intravenously. IV administration offers immensely more control over the drug's actions, and in many cases unwanted reactions to the drug can be quickly reversed (e.g., with the administration of naloxone or flumazenil). In the absence of superficial veins, elective venipuncture and IV conscious sedation are contraindicated; the inability to breathe through the nose or adverse clinical experience in the past with inhalation sedation contraindicates nitrous oxide–oxygen (N_2O-O_2). In these situations IM conscious sedation in an adult patient should receive serious consideration.

In the child the IM route is more frequently indicated. Both IV and inhalation conscious sedation require a degree of patient cooperation for success to be achieved. The overtly disruptive child will neither permit a venipuncture nor allow a nasal hood to be placed and secured over his or her nose, thereby dooming these two valuable techniques to failure. In such a situation the IM route may be the only sedative route with a likelihood of success. Failure of the IM technique most likely means that the patient will have to receive dental care under general anesthesia.

Some patients with physical or mental disabilities, both pediatric and adult, are unable to tolerate dental care in the usual manner and are therefore candidates for sedative techniques. Although many of these patients are manageable with oral, inhalation, or IV conscious sedation, disruptive patients with disabilities may require IM drug administration as a means of calming them before the use of other, more controllable sedative techniques.

Another use of the IM route in dentistry is the administration of nonsedative drugs. These drugs may also be administered orally or rectally; however, because of the increased reliability of absorption and greater efficacy noted with the IM route, this technique should be considered when these drugs are used. Drugs commonly administered via this route are the anticholinergics (atropine, scopolamine, glycopyrrolate) and the antiemetics (trimethobenzamide, chlorpromazine). These drugs are discussed later in this chapter. The suggested uses of IM drug administration in dentistry are presented in Box 10-2.

SUBMUCOSAL SEDATION

A variation on IM drug administration called *submucosal (SM) administration* has been use in pediatric dentistry.[6] In the SM technique a CNS depressant drug is injected into the mucous membrane in either the maxillary or mandibular buccal fold. An advantage of SM administration over IM administration is a slightly more rapid onset of clinical action.[7,8] However, this same rapid onset of action may also be associated with a more rapid appearance of undesirable drug actions, such as respiratory depression. As originally developed, the SM route was used for the administration of opioid agonists such as alphaprodine.[9] The technique has fallen into disfavor because of a significant number of serious adverse reactions that were noted in conjunction with the SM administration of alphaprodine.[1-3,6] The SM route is discussed in greater detail in Chapter 35.

SITES OF INTRAMUSCULAR DRUG ADMINISTRATION

Four sites are available for IM drug administration.[10-12] Proper site selection varies from patient to patient and is an important factor in the safety of this technique. The sites most commonly chosen for the administration of IM drugs are the following:

1. Gluteal area
2. Ventrogluteal area
3. Vastus lateralis
4. Deltoid area

Each potential site for IM drug administration has specific advantages and disadvantages that must be considered before final site selection is made.

Gluteal Area

The upper outer quadrant of the gluteal region is the most commonly used site for IM drug administration in adults.[13] The gluteus maximus is the muscle most commonly injected.

The gluteal region extends superiorly to the anterior superior iliac spine (Figure 10-1). With this as a landmark, the region is divided into quadrants. The upper outer quadrant is the most anatomically safe because it is at a distance from the sciatic nerve and the superior gluteal artery.[14] The lower inner aspect of the upper outer quadrant is the preferred site within this quadrant.

The gluteal region in the adult can accept 4 to 8 ml of solution.[11,14] In addition, the skin of this region is relatively thin and is more easily penetrated by the needle.

The upper inner quadrant is unacceptable as an IM injection site because it contains the roots of the sacral plexus. The lower inner quadrant contains the sciatic nerve. Ceravolo et al.[13] report a nerve injury rate of up to 8% following IM injection into the gluteal region.

For injection into the upper outer quadrant, the patient should be lying face down on a bed or examining table with the toes in and arms hanging off the table.[15] This permits maximal relaxation. Although this site is also used with the patient standing, it is not as highly recommended because the muscles do not

BOX 10-2 Recommended Use of the Intramuscular Route

For Sedation in the Following Types of Patients

1. The adult patient, when inhalation and IV routes are unavailable
2. The disruptive pediatric or adult patient in whom other routes have proved ineffective
3. The disruptive child or adult with disabilities in whom other routes have proved ineffective

Uses of the Intramuscular Route

1. Premedication before IV sedation or general anesthesia in the precooperative pediatric patient or adult or pediatric patient with disabilities
2. Administration of antiemetics or anticholinergics
3. Administration of emergency drugs when intravenous administration is not available

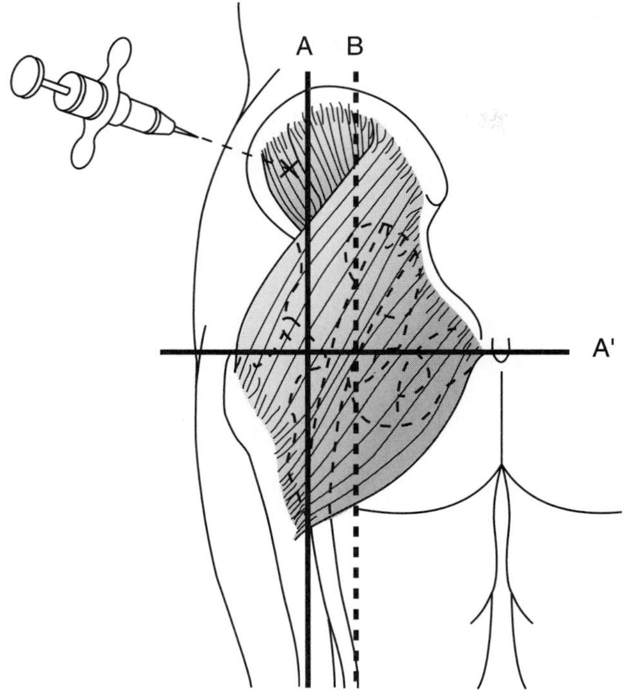

Figure 10-1 Gluteal region, divided into quadrants. The upper outer quadrant is the recommended site for intramuscular injection. Lines *A* and *A'* represent boundaries in classic intramuscular technique. Line *B* demonstrates the ease with which a landmark may be displaced, increasing the risk of sciatic nerve injury.

relax as well in this position. Muscle tissue that is contracted does not accommodate the injected fluid, forcing it upward into the subcutaneous tissues, where absorption is less reliable and slower and where certain chemicals are more likely to produce tissue irritation and damage. In addition, the administration of IM drugs into contracted muscle is thought to be more uncomfortable than IM injection into relaxed muscle.[12]

Of the four available IM injection sites, the gluteal region is the least well perfused, having 20% lower perfusion than the deltoid.[16] Because perfusion is the rate-limiting step in the absorption of IM drugs, the rate of onset of action of drugs administered in the gluteal region is somewhat slower than that when alternative sites are used.[11,14]

The gluteal region requires a degree of patient disrobing for the injection to be properly administered. This may, in some instances, limit the utility of the gluteal region in the adult patient within the dental office; however, with assistance from the parent/guardian, this site may readily be employed in the pediatric patient with little or no loss of modesty.

Ventrogluteal Region

The ventrogluteal region lies in close proximity to the gluteal region. Its primary use is for IM injection in patients who are bedridden and unable to lie face down.[14]

The site is located among three bony landmarks that are usually quite readily palpated. These are the anterior superior iliac spine, the iliac crest, and the greater trochanter of the femur. Anatomically, this region lies at some distance from the sciatic nerve and other anatomically important structures.[15]

For this site to be properly used, the anterior superior iliac spine is located with the tip of the index finger (Figure 10-2). The left hand is pressed onto the hip with the palm of the hand over the greater trochanter and the fingers pointed toward the patient's head. The index and middle fingers are spread as far as possible, forming a V, with the tip of the ventrally placed finger pressed down on the soft tissue over the anterior superior iliac spine, preventing movement of the skin. The needle puncture is made between these fingers and aimed just below the iliac crest.

The ventrogluteal region in an adult is capable of managing 4 to 8 ml of solution. This site is rarely used in the typical dental office situation. Where bedridden patients are treated, this IM site warrants consideration.

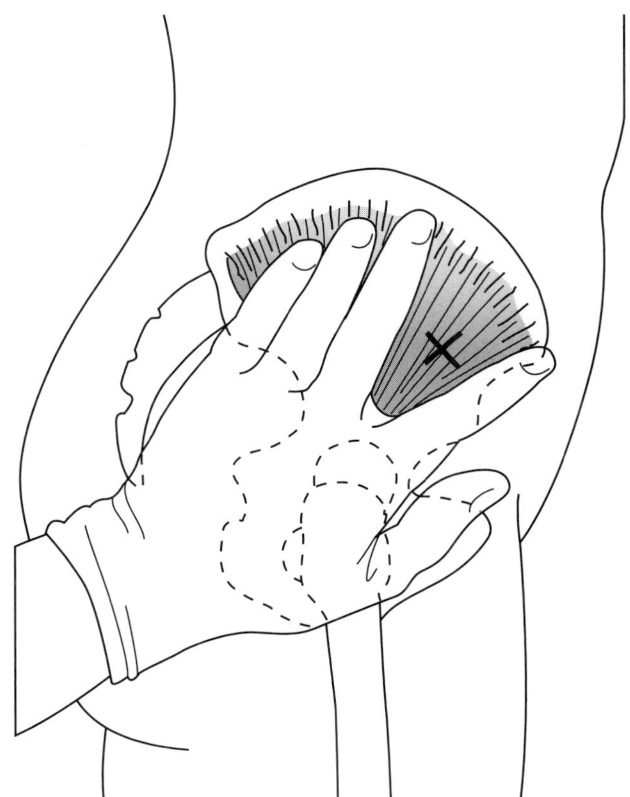

Figure 10-2 Ventrogluteal region. Index finger locates anterior iliac spine, index and middle fingers spread apart forming a V. Needle puncture occurs between fingers (X) and is aimed toward the iliac crest.

Vastus Lateralis

The anterior aspect of the thigh is probably the safest region in which to deposit IM drugs. Although not of consequence in the typical dental situation, the vastus lateralis can accommodate volumes of solution up to 15 ml, whereas the gluteal and ventrogluteal can accommodate approximately 4 to 8 ml each before muscle distortion and dissection occur, leading to increased pain during and after injection.

The site for injection in the vastus lateralis muscle is a narrow rectangular band running along the anterior lateral aspect of the thigh (Figure 10-3). The region begins approximately one handbreadth above the knee and runs to the same distance below the greater trochanter of the femur.[15]

Anatomically, the vastus lateralis site contains no structures of importance (Figure 10-4). Overly deep penetration of the needle may strike the femur, resulting in discomfort and possible needle breakage. All significant anatomic structures are located on the medial and posterior aspects of the thigh (the femoral artery and vein and the sciatic nerve).

This site is strongly recommended for use in small children.[11] Injection in the gluteal muscles is contraindicated in children who have not yet begun to walk because of the lack of maturity and development of their gluteal musculature. The gluteal region ought not to be chosen until at least 1 full year after the child has begun to walk.[17]

Some degree of disrobing is required when the vastus lateralis site is used. The site is more readily accessible in the woman wearing a skirt or dress, but it is of absolute importance that a female assistant be present with the doctor in the treatment room throughout the time that the injection is given. In any patient wearing pants or slacks, a greater degree of disrobing is required, a fact that might discourage use of this site. In the pediatric patient the vastus lateralis may readily be employed with assistance from the patient's parent or guardian.

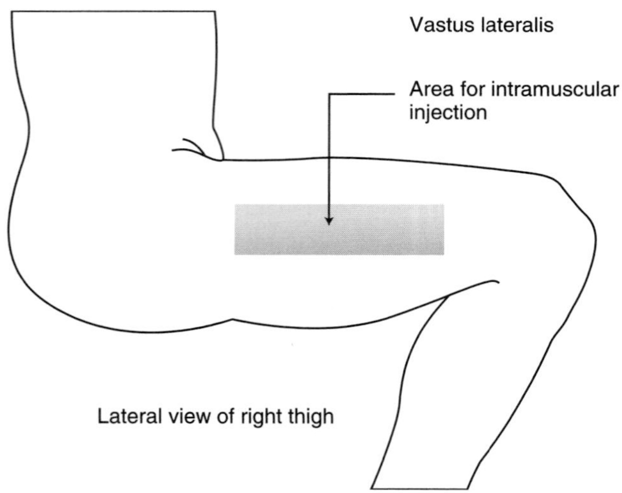

Figure 10-3 Location of the vastus lateralis site on anterior lateral aspect of thigh, the preferred site for intramuscular drug administration in infants and children.

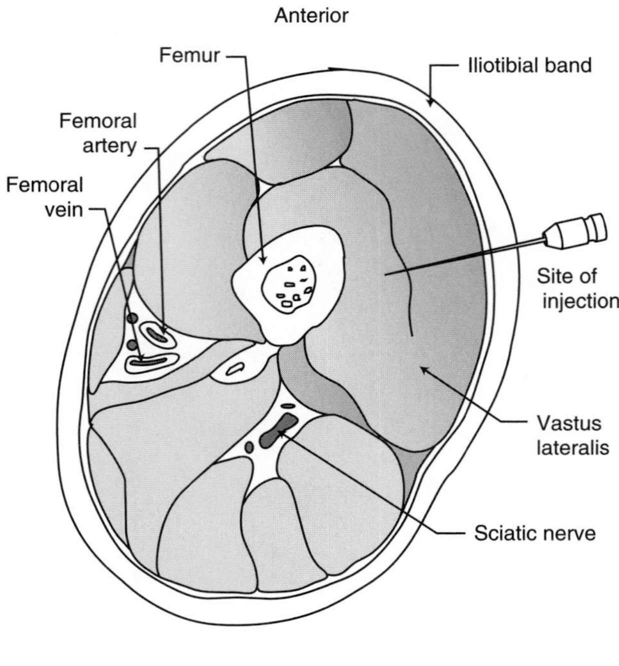

Figure 10-4 Cross section through vastus lateralis injection site illustrating location of anatomically significant structures.

In adult or larger pediatric patients who are unmanageable (e.g., combative) and when IM drug administration is considered mandatory, IM injection into the vastus lateralis muscle through the patient's clothing is appropriate. Although sterile technique cannot be maintained in this situation, it is unlikely that complications will be noted. This consideration is of especial importance when a life-threatening situation develops (e.g., anaphylaxis) and immediate drug therapy is warranted (e.g., epinephrine).

The vastus lateralis muscle is capable of receiving 8 to 15 ml of injected drug (in adults) without distortion or dissection of muscle fibers. This represents the largest available reservoir for IM drugs in the adult body.

Deltoid

The deltoid muscle is easily accessible in the upper third of the arm. The injection is given between the upper and lower portions of the deltoid muscle (Figure 10-5), thereby avoiding the radial nerve.

The boundaries of the deltoid region form a rectangle. The superior border is formed by the lower edge

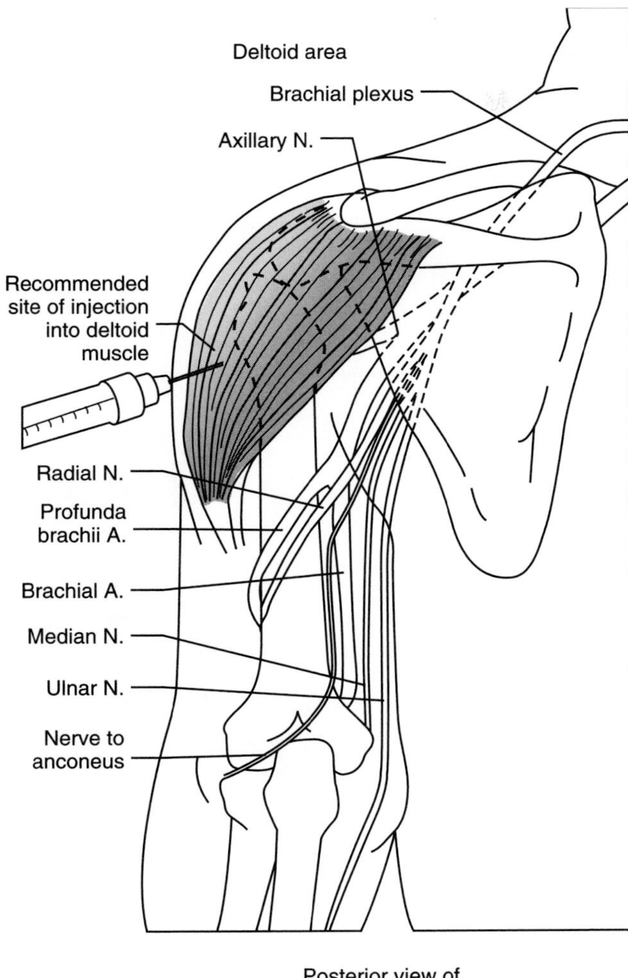

Figure 10-5 Middeltoid injection site in upper third of arm.

of the acromion (the outward extension of the spine of the scapula). The inferior boundary lies opposite the axilla or armpit. The side boundaries are two lines drawn parallel to the arm, about one third to two thirds of the way around the lateral aspect of the upper arm.

Advantages of the deltoid region include easy access in most patients. It is important that the patient not be permitted to simply roll up the shirt sleeve to expose the injection site, for if the sleeve is tight, it may not permit visualization of the entire site, in which case the injection might be administered inferior to the desired area and in too close proximity to the radial nerve. The patient should be required to remove the shirt or blouse to expose the entire injection site. A female assistant must be with the doctor (male or female) if the patient is female. Another positive factor in the deltoid region is more rapid absorption of the injected drug into the cardiovascular system than is seen with any of the other IM injection sites. Perfusion is 20% greater in the deltoid region than in the gluteal region.[14] The deltoid region is not recommended for use in the infant or child who has not yet begun to walk.[11]

The degree of disrobing required to visualize the injection site is not usually of significance in the deltoid region, making this the most easily used IM injection site in dentistry. This site may be used with the patient lying down, sitting, or standing.

Probably the only negative feature of this site, other than the anatomy, is its lack of size; it is able to accommodate only up to 4 ml of solution (adult). However, this is not of significance in dentistry because it is rare to ever administer more than 3 ml intramuscularly. Giovannitti and Trapp[18] suggest the deltoid muscle as the preferred site for IM sedation in the dental environment.

Site Selection

Selection of the site for IM injection in dentistry is predicated on several factors, including the size (age) of the patient, degree of patient cooperation, and volume of solution to be injected. In the younger (smaller) pediatric patient, the preferred site for IM injection is the vastus lateralis, whereas in older children the vastus lateralis and the deltoid regions are recommended. In the adult the preferred sites for IM injection are the deltoid region, vastus lateralis, and both gluteal injection sites. Table 10-1 compares the four IM injection sites.

ARMAMENTARIUM

Very few items are required for IM drug administration. Included in this list are the following:

1. Sterile, disposable syringe (1 to 2 ml) with needle (18, 20, or 21 gauge) of appropriate length
2. Alcohol sponges
3. Sterile gauze
4. Band-Aid type of bandage
5. Desired drug

There is a very real concern for self-inflicted puncture injuries among health-care professionals with possible infection with either human immunodeficiency virus (HIV) or hepatitis.[19-22] Syringes and other devices (e.g., the "sharps" container) have been developed to permit IM drug administration with a minimum risk of needlestick injury.[23-25] These "safe syringes" prevent accidental needlestick following drug administration through a self-locking sheath that covers the exposed (and contaminated) needle.

TECHNIQUE

The appropriate injection site for the IM injection must be selected. After disrobing the patient, if necessary, the doctor must carefully palpate the site on every

TABLE 10-1 Comparison of Intramuscular Injection Sites

IM Injection Site	Perfusion*	Maximum Volume for Adult (ml)	Infant	Child	Adult
Vastus lateralis	2	8-15	+	+	+
Gluteal/ventrogluteal	3	4-8	–	–	+/–
Deltoid	1	4	–	–	+

*1, Most vascular; 3, least vascular

patient to determine the precise anatomic landmarks. Visual examination alone should never be relied on to determine landmarks. From the point of view of propriety (and medicolegally), it is important that the doctor have another staff member present in the treatment room during the injection, especially if the patient is of the opposite sex from the doctor. The following are step-by-step instructions for the administration of an IM injection[11,15,26]:

1. Cleanse the skin thoroughly using a suitable antiseptic (e.g., isopropyl alcohol). Apply friction while cleansing the area with a circular motion from the injection site outward. The antiseptic should be permitted to dry before injection. Injection into a moistened area may introduce antiseptic into the tissues, which will lead to discomfort and possibly to tissue irritation.
2. Grasp the tissue to be injected with one hand, keeping the tissue taut. Holding the syringe in a dartlike grasp, introduce the needle to its appropriate depth (deep within muscle tissue) with one quick motion. Although the depth of insertion will vary from patient to patient, the needle should not be inserted, for safety reasons, more than approximately three fourths of its length into tissue (Figure 10-6).
3. With the needle at its proper depth, aspirate, pulling the plunger of the syringe back slightly to determine whether the needle tip lies within the lumen of a blood vessel. Rotate the syringe a quarter turn and reaspirate to ensure that the needle tip was not lying against the wall of a vessel. If blood appears in the syringe at any time, withdraw the syringe from the tissue and prepare a different injection site. In the uncooperative pediatric or adult patient, it may prove difficult or impossible to perform this step as described. Aspiration should be performed whenever possible before IM injection.
4. Following negative aspiration, inject the drug slowly. In most IM injections the solution flows quite easily into the tissues. Rapid injection produces increased patient discomfort and should be avoided. Release the pressure that has been maintained on the tissues during needle insertion. Maintaining the pressure during injection of the drug may force solution to backtrack along the path of needle insertion into the subcutaneous tissues, where tissue irritation may occur, or out of the tissue through the injection site. Release of pressure prevents this from occurring.
5. Holding a dry sterile gauze in the other hand (non–syringe-holding hand), slowly withdraw

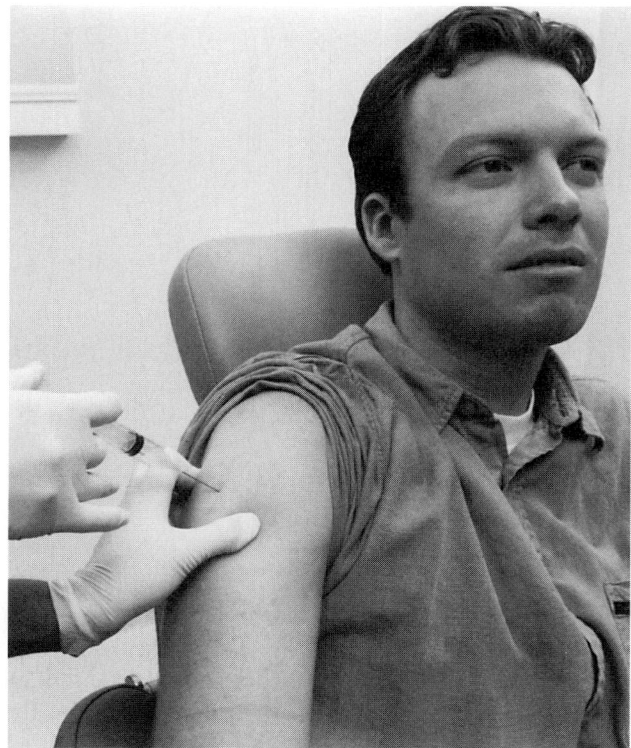

Figure 10-6 Area to be injected is grasped with one hand, holding tissue taut, while the syringe, held in a dartlike grasp, is inserted to the proper depth.

the needle from the tissue. Place the dry gauze over the puncture point for approximately 2 minutes to prevent bleeding. A bandage can be placed over the site at this time. Care must be taken with the now-contaminated needle to prevent accidental percutaneous puncture of the treating staff. The used needle/syringe should be disposed of in a sharps container.

6. Massage or rub the injection site to increase the blood flow through the area and speed up drug absorption.
7. Record in the patient's chart the date, time of injection, site of injection, drug used, and dose.
8. Observe the patient during the post–IM injection period for the onset of sedation and/or undesirable actions (e.g., syncope, overdose, allergy).

COMPLICATIONS

Although rare, complications can arise after IM drug administration. In most cases the complication appears to be directly related to the site of needle entry and drug deposition.[27,28]

The needle itself is capable of producing injury to structures through which it passes. Nerve damage, consisting of paralysis (usually of the sciatic nerve in gluteal injection), hyperesthesia, or paresthesia, has been reported after IM injection. In addition, inadvertent IV and intraarterial (IA) drug administration have occurred, as well as air embolism, periostitis, and hematoma. Many of these complications have potentially serious consequences and, of course, steps should be taken to prevent their occurrence. Knowledge of anatomy and proper injection technique will minimize these complications.

The drugs that are administered intramuscularly are, in some cases, capable of producing injury to the tissues into which they are deposited. Injuries such as *abscess, cyst* and *scar formation,* and *necrosis* and *sloughing of skin* at the injection site may occur. Although these are potential complications with all drugs, there are a few drugs that, because of their pH or viscosity, are more apt to produce these problems. These drugs include diazepam and hydroxyzine. Improper injection technique, specifically when the drug has not been injected deep into the muscle or when the tissue is kept taut following the injection of the drug with leakage of the drug into the subcutaneous tissues as the needle is withdrawn, is a common cause of this problem.

Nerve injury of any type is managed conservatively. In many cases the injury may not be noted by the patient for several days following the IM injection or, in the case of a younger patient or a patient with a disability, possibly for several months, thus emphasizing the importance of precise recordkeeping. The site of injection should always be recorded when an IM drug is given. When injury is detected, the patient should return to the office so that the nature and extent of the injury may be noted on the chart. Unless the injury is severe, the management of choice for most nerve injury is "tincture of time." Most minor traumatic nerve injuries resolve with time. In most instances normal function returns within 6 months. The patient should be advised of this time factor at the onset. A few cases of nerve injury do not resolve completely within 6 months and require additional time (an unknown duration) or may never return completely to normal function. Periodic examination of the patient during this time span (e.g., once every month) is recommended to keep the doctor informed of any progress and to keep the patient aware of the doctor's concern.

Discomfort secondary to the injury should be manageable with milder analgesics, such as aspirin, acetaminophen, or another nonsteroidal antiinflammatory drug (NSAID). If more potent analgesics are required, consultation with a physician is recommended because this might indicate a greater degree of injury.

If the injury appears more severe at the onset, the patient should be referred to a physician, preferably a neurologist, for examination. Medical management usually is consistent with that described. Referral to a physician should also be given serious consideration if the patient appears to be dissatisfied with the progress of his or her recovery or with the management of the injury by the "dental doctor." Before referral of the patient to the physician, a telephone call from the dentist, explaining the circumstances surrounding the case, is appropriate.

Although legal action following nerve injury does occur, the percentage of such cases is extremely small. A patient who is satisfied with the treatment is less likely to initiate a legal action than the patient who believes that the care rendered is below the usual standard.

Inadvertent IV or *IA* drug administration ought never occur. Proper IM technique recommends aspiration before injection of the drug. The presence of blood in the syringe indicates a positive aspiration. The doctor should remove the syringe from the injection site, apply pressure to the site to prevent hematoma, and reinject the patient at a different location.

Because the drugs administered for sedation are CNS depressants, clinical signs and symptoms attending this complication (accidental IV or IA administration) are related to the degree of CNS depression that develops. This may range from a slightly oversedated patient—one who is conscious but sedated to a degree beyond which the doctor feels comfortable—to the patient who may be unconscious but breathing (requiring airway management), to the unconscious patient whose breathing is quite depressed or who may be apneic. This latter patient requires airway management with controlled ventilation. The pharmacology and the cerebral blood level of the drug(s) injected determine the severity of the reaction that develops. Some antianxiety drugs, such as benzodiazepines (e.g., midazolam) and hydroxyzine, although capable of producing significant CNS depression, are less likely to than are barbiturates and opioids.

Management of an oversedated patient consists primarily of airway maintenance (*A*, airway) and, when necessary, assisted or controlled ventilation (*B*, breathing). In addition, some drugs, such as the opioids and benzodiazepines, have pharmacologic antagonists that may be administered in these circumstances. Their use, and a more detailed discussion of the management of the oversedated patient, is found in Chapters 27 and 34.

Air embolism has been reported after IM drug administration. With proper technique in loading a drug into a syringe, there ought not be any air remaining in its barrel. In addition, avoidance of inadvertent intravascular injection (see previous discussion) will prevent this occurrence.

Periostitis is an inflammation of the periosteum. If acute, it may be associated with severe pain and suppuration and is usually secondary to infection. The condition usually becomes chronic in nature and is characterized by tenderness and swelling of the tissues overlying the bone. It may also be produced by the inadvertent striking of the needle against the periosteum during insertion. Proper technique involves grasping the tissue being injected between the fingers, pulling it away from the bone, and inserting the needle to the proper depth (varying from patient to patient and from site to site). This technique minimizes the development of periostitis.

If the patient complains of soreness, tenderness, and swelling at the site of an IM injection 2 days or more following injection, the complaint should be evaluated by bringing the patient to the office, examining the area, and if need be, seeking a medical consultation. Management of milder degrees of periostitis involve "tincture of time" and the maintenance of good relations with the patient. If signs of suppuration and swelling appear, antibiotics are indicated (usually penicillin). Medical consultation should be sought in this situation.

Hematoma is, by definition, a tumor consisting of effused blood. It develops following puncture of a blood vessel, either an artery or a vein. Clinically, a small but gradually enlarging swelling, bluish in color, will be observed at the site of needle insertion, either during injection or, more commonly, after withdrawal of the syringe from the tissues. Management consists of pressure applied directly to the site of bleeding for a minimum of 2 to 5 minutes. If the site subsequently becomes sore, heat can be applied to it (but not less than 4 hours after the bleeding ceases) and mild analgesics administered. The effused blood is gradually resorbed into the cardiovascular system, a process requiring 7 to 10 days. Heat should not be applied to the site of a hematoma within the first few hours because heat produces vasodilation, which may restart the bleeding.

An *abscess* may occur after IM injection if either the needle or the solution injected was contaminated. Management consists of antibiotics (penicillin) and immediate medical consultation. Prevention consists of sterile technique in handling both drugs and equipment.

Cyst formation, scarring, and *necrosis* and *sloughing* of tissues may also occur. Although several factors may be responsible for these, many are produced by the tissues' reaction to the injected drug. Drugs that are irritating to the tissues are more commonly involved in these complications. Superficial injection of drugs is another cause of this problem. Management should consist of referral to a physician, preferably a dermatologist. Complications of IM injections are listed in Box 10-3.

DETERMINATION OF DOSAGE

The factors that influence the way in which a drug acts in a given patient are discussed in Chapters 3 and 7. With IM administration of CNS depressants, the influence of these various factors becomes quite important. How then can the informed clinician safely determine the appropriate IM dose of the drug or

BOX 10-3 Complications of Intramuscular Injections

- Nerve injury
  - Paralysis
  - Paresthesia
  - Hyperesthesia
- Intravascular injection
  - Intravenous
  - Intraarterial
- Air embolism
- Periostitis
- Hematoma
- Abscess
- Cyst and scar formation
- Necrosis and sloughing of skin

drugs that are to be administered to a patient for intraoperative sedation?

Most IM drugs have their dosages determined, in large part, by the body weight of the patient. Although this is far from an absolute guarantee of proper dosage, in most cases a therapeutically effective result will occur. Other factors that must be considered in determining dosage include the degree of anxiety, the level of sedation desired, the patient's age and health status, prior response of the patient to CNS depressant drugs, and the education and experience of the drug's administrator.

For the adult patient, dosages for the drugs discussed are based primarily on body weight, expressed in milligrams per pound (mg/lb) or milligrams per kilogram (mg/kg). From this calculated dose the doctor will decrease or increase the actual dosage administered as determined from the other factors mentioned. For example, a patient weighing 150 pounds is to receive a drug, the recommended dose of which is 0.5 mg/lb. The calculated dose of this drug for the patient is therefore 75 mg. If the patient were a healthy individual (American Society of Anesthesiologists [ASA] I), this dose would be appropriate; however, if this patient is older, has a history of cardiovascular or other serious systemic disease, or has a history of overreaction to average drug dosages, a smaller dose (e.g., 50 mg) might be administered. The level to which the drug dosage is decreased is left to the clinical judgment of the doctor administering it. Conversely, an ASA I patient demonstrating high levels of anxiety, with a history of hyporesponding to CNS depressant drugs, might be administered a dose somewhat greater than that determined strictly by body weight.

In the pediatric patient the same factors must be considered in determining drug dosage. The patient's age is often considered in determining the dosage of a drug. For example, for a given drug the dose for a 3-year-old patient may be 12.5 mg, whereas the dose for a 4-year-old is 25 mg. Dosages based solely on the patient's age are apt to lead to inaccuracies because patients of the same age will vary considerably in physical stature and body weight. The patient's age should not be the primary factor by which the dose of a drug is determined.

Several rules have been in use for years in the determination of pediatric drug dosages. *Clark's rule* takes the weight of the child in pounds and divides it by 150 (the weight of the average adult in pounds). The resultant fraction is multiplied by the adult dosage of the drug.

Clark's rule:

$$\text{Pediatric dose} = \frac{\text{Weight of child (lb)}}{150} \times \text{Adult dose}$$

Young's rule divides the age of the child in years by the age of the child plus 12 and then multiplies this number by the adult dose.

Young's rule:

$$\text{Pediatric dose} = \frac{\text{Age of child (yr)}}{\text{Age} + 12} \times \text{Adult dose}$$

A factor that has proved even more accurate in determining effective pediatric dosages is the body surface area of the patient. Table 10-2 permits a determination of the approximate surface area of the patient. The pediatric dosage is determined as a percentage of the usual adult dosage, based on the average adult surface area of 1.73 m^2.

Most of the drugs discussed in this chapter have their dosages presented on a milligram per pound or kilogram of body weight basis. Although not the most accurate method available, this remains the most frequently employed method of determining IM drug dosage. The reader may employ the surface area method of determining pediatric dosages for any drug listed in this book by simply referring to Table 10-2.

Dosages based on body weight (e.g., 1 mg/kg or 0.5 mg/lb) are determined by the middle of the "bell-shaped" curve (see Figure 7-1). Approximately 70% of patients respond appropriately to this dose, with 15% being undersedated. Unfortunately, another 15% respond in an exaggerated manner—oversedation.

The degree of education and experience of the drug administrator has a significant bearing on the level of CNS depression to which the patient may safely be taken, which will obviously influence the dosage of drug administered. Doctors who have completed residency training in anesthesiology will be better able to administer larger doses of drugs to patients in a safe manner than doctors who have merely completed a short postgraduate program. All dental personnel involved in patient management should be adept in monitoring vital signs and in recognizing and managing life-threatening emergencies, including the ability to perform basic life support.

Determination of Intramuscular Dose

Body weight
Degree of anxiety
Level of sedation desired
Age
Health status
Prior response to CNS depressant drugs
Education and experience of drug administrator
Surface area (pediatric patient)

DRUGS

A myriad of drugs are available for the management of anxiety via IM administration. The level of sedation

TABLE 10-2 Determination of Children's Doses from Adult Doses on the Basis of Surface Area

Weight (kg)	Weight (lb)	Approximate Surface Area (m^2)	Approximate Percentage of Adult Dose*
2	4.4	0.15	9
4	8.8	0.25	14
6	13.2	0.33	19
8	17.6	0.40	23
10	22.0	0.46	27
15	33.0	0.63	36
20	44.0	0.83	48
25	55.0	0.95	55
30	66.0	1.08	62
35	77.0	1.20	69
40	88.0	1.30	75
45	99.0	1.40	81
50	110.0	1.51	87
55	121.0	1.58	91

From Modell W: *Modell's drugs in current use and new drugs*, ed 34, New York, 1988, Springer.
*Based on average adult surface area of 1.73 m^2.

may vary from lighter levels (conscious sedation) to levels approaching unconsciousness (deep sedation). Although certain drugs are more apt to produce more profound sedation than others, any of the following drugs listed can produce overly deep sedation. When IM drug dosage is being determined, it must always be remembered that the administrator cannot control the drug's action, that titration is not possible, via this route. Care and prudence must be exercised whenever IM drugs are administered to any patient, but especially to pediatric, geriatric, or medically compromised patients. Box 10-4 lists drugs that are commonly given via IM administration in dentistry. As will be noted with specific drugs, different levels of training are recommended for their safe use. In some situations the doctor should have received training in general anesthesia and be capable of managing the unconscious airway before ever considering the use of the drug in question.

Antianxiety Drugs and Sedative-Hypnotics

In this group of drugs—antianxiety and sedative-hypnotics—I have included the benzodiazepines, barbiturates, and histamine blockers, drugs commonly used for light to moderate levels of conscious sedation when given as solo agents. However, it is not uncommon to combine one of the drugs in this category with an opioid analgesic to provide deeper levels of sedation. When this is done, it is necessary for the doctor and all staff members to have been thoroughly trained in general anesthesia and patient monitoring.

Chlordiazepoxide. Chlordiazepoxide (Librium) is one of a number of benzodiazepines available for parenteral administration. Patients receiving chlordiazepoxide parenterally should be cautioned against the operation of a car or other potentially hazardous machinery for the remainder of the day.

Because the parenteral preparation of chlordiazepoxide is not very stable, it is prepared for use immediately before its administration. Two milliliters of an IM diluent (provided with the drug) is injected into the ampule of chlordiazepoxide powder (100 mg). The solution is agitated slowly and gently until the powder is completely dissolved. This provides a solution of chlordiazepoxide at 50 mg/ml.

Chlordiazepoxide should be administered deep into muscle to minimize discomfort and to optimize absorption. It is recommended that the drug be deposited slowly into the upper outer quadrant of the gluteus muscle.[29] Any unused drug should be discarded. Following parenteral administration deep into muscle, the onset of action will be approximately 15 minutes. Maximal clinical effect arises 30 minutes following injection, with a gradual decrease in clinical action over the next 3 to 5 hours.[30]

Because of the necessity to prepare chlordiazepoxide immediately before injection, it is rarely employed in

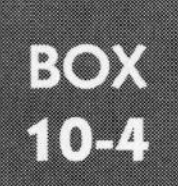

BOX 10-4 Frequently Used Drugs Via Intramuscular Administration for Sedation

Antianxiety Drugs and Sedative-Hypnotics
Chlordiazepoxide
Diazepam
Lorazepam
Midazolam

Histamine Blockers (Antihistamines)
Promethazine
Hydroxyzine

Barbiturates
Secobarbital
Pentobarbital

Opioid Analgesics
Morphine
Meperidine
Fentanyl

Opioid Agonist/Antagonists
Pentazocine
Butorphanol
Nalbuphine

Dissociative Anesthetic
Ketamine hydrochloride

Anticholinergics
Atropine
Scopolamine
Glycopyrrolate

dentistry for IM sedation. Other benzodiazepines are more readily available for parenteral administration.

Dosage. The usual adult dose for preoperative sedation is 50 to 100 mg 1 hour before treatment. The usual dose for elderly or debilitated patients is 25 to 50 mg 1 hour before treatment. Chlordiazepoxide injectable is not recommended in patients younger than 12 years.

Availability. Librium (Roche): 5-ml dry-filled ampule containing 100 mg chlordiazepoxide hydrochloride in dry crystalline form; 2-ml ampule of Special Intramuscular Diluent containing 1.5% benzyl alcohol, 4% polysorbate 80, 20% propylene glycol, 1.6% maleic acid, and sodium hydroxide (to adjust pH to 3.0). When prepared for injection, the concentration of the chlordiazepoxide is 50 mg/ml. Chlordiazepoxide is classified as a Schedule IV drug.

Diazepam. Before the introduction of midazolam, diazepam (Valium) was commonly administered via the IM route in preoperative anxiety control in the hospital setting. It may also be given in dentistry via this route, but because of the availability of the IV route and the advantages of IM midazolam, diazepam is infrequently used IM in dentistry.

Another reason for the infrequent use of diazepam IM was the results of early studies on the absorption of diazepam from IM injection sites. Diazepam injectable is an extremely lipophilic drug, and early studies on absorption of IM diazepam were conflicting.[31-34] Peak plasma levels were noted 60 minutes after oral dosing, whereas IM dosing required 90 minutes.[34] Absorption of diazepam from IM injection sites may be slow or incomplete or both because of its lipophilic nature. However, a more recent report indicates that IM diazepam absorption appears to be more rapid when the drug is injected into the deltoid rather than the gluteal or vastus lateralis muscle groups.[35] The most likely explanation is the higher blood flow per gram of tissue in the deltoid muscle group.[33] In the gluteal area the depth of injection may be a factor in the completeness of absorption of diazepam. Given equal doses of diazepam via the oral and IM routes, the oral dose will be absorbed more completely than the IM dose, and in many cases the rate of onset will be shorter via the oral route than with the IM route.[34] However, diazepam deposited deeply into muscle (preferably the deltoid) can produce satisfactory sedation in most patients.

Contraindications. Parenteral diazepam should be avoided in patients with known hypersensitivities to it or other benzodiazepines, in patients with acute narrow-angle glaucoma, and in patients with narrow-angle glaucoma unless they are receiving appropriate therapy.

Warnings. When used in combination with other CNS depressants, particularly opioid analgesics, the dosage of the opioid should be decreased by approximately one third to minimize the occurrence of oversedation or of other more serious complications.

Diazepam should not be given during the first trimester of pregnancy because an increased risk of congenital malformations has been observed. Diazepam crosses the placental barrier, potentially producing depression of the fetus. Its use in pregnancy is not recommended.

Injectable diazepam dosages should be decreased when patients are receiving other CNS depressants, such as barbiturates, phenothiazines, opioids, and alcohol. Elderly and debilitated patients usually require decreased dosages of diazepam to achieve a desired clinical effect.

Dosage. The usual adult dose for preoperative sedation is 10 mg 30 minutes to 1 hour before treatment. The preferred injection site for diazepam is the deltoid muscle. Regardless of the IM injection site, diazepam should be deposited deep into muscle to prevent discomfort and provide more reliable absorption. The dose for elderly or debilitated patients is 2 to 5 mg 30 minutes to 1 hour before treatment. The dose of parenteral diazepam for children should not exceed 0.25 mg/kg of body weight, administered deep into the gluteal or deltoid regions. For example, a child weighing 20 kg (44 lb) will receive a dose of 5 mg IM diazepam. Since the introduction of midazolam, the IM use of diazepam has markedly diminished.

Availability. Valium (Roche): 5 mg/ml in 2-ml ampules and 10-ml vials; 5 mg/ml in 2-ml preloaded syringes. Injectable diazepam also contains 40% propylene glycol, 10% ethyl alcohol, 5% sodium benzoate, benzoic acid, and 1.5% benzyl alcohol. Diazepam is classified as a Schedule IV drug.

Diazepam	
Pregnancy category	D
Lactation	NS
Metabolism	Liver
Excretion	Urine
DEA schedule	IV

Lorazepam. Lorazepam (Ativan) is another benzodiazepine available for use parenterally. Its action following parenteral administration is primarily that of sedation rather than anxiolysis. A potential benefit of IM lorazepam is that it frequently provides a degree of amnesia. This lack of recall is maximal within 2 hours of IM injection.

Because the agent is virtually insoluble in water, its onset of action may prove to be prolonged in some patients, although, as with diazepam, the onset of action will be about 15 minutes in most patients. Peak plasma levels of lorazepam are seen in 60 to 90 minutes.[36] The duration of action of lorazepam following IM administration is approximately 6 to 8 hours. The major side effect is excessive sleepiness and a prolonged amnesic period.

Odugbesan and Magbagbeola[37] recommend that the IV route be preferred to IM for administration of lorazepam, providing a somewhat more rapid onset of activity. Patients receiving lorazepam IM must not be permitted to leave the dental office unescorted and must be advised of the possibly enhanced CNS depressant actions of other agents such as opioids, alcohol, and barbiturates. Because of the prolonged duration of action of lorazepam, it is seldom used in the outpatient practice of dentistry.

Warnings. Lorazepam should not be administered to pregnant patients because it may increase the risk of congenital malformation. Patients must be advised against driving a car or operating hazardous machinery for a period of 24 to 48 hours, a period of time that may severely limit the usefulness of this agent in an ambulatory dental patient.

Precautions. Additive CNS depression is observed when lorazepam is administered concurrently with barbiturates, alcohol, opioids, phenothiazines, antidepressants, scopolamine, and monoamine oxidase inhibitors (MAOIs). When scopolamine is used concurrently with lorazepam, the incidence of hallucinations and irrational behavior is increased. The use of IM lorazepam has resulted in discomfort at the injection site, including a sensation of burning, or observed redness. The overall incidence of burning and pain is about 17% immediately after the injection and 1.4% 24 hours later. Of patients receiving IM lorazepam, 2% had redness immediately after the injection and 0.5% noted redness after 24 hours.[36]

Dosage. The usual adult dose of lorazepam for preoperative sedation is 0.05 mg/kg (0.025 mg/lb) to a maximum of 4 mg. The drug should be administered undiluted deep into the muscle mass. If dilution is desired (it is not recommended for IM injection), sterile water for injection, sodium chloride injection, and 5% dextrose injection are compatible solutions. The use of lorazepam in patients younger than 18 years is not recommended because of insufficient data.

Availability. Ativan (Wyeth): 2 and 4 mg/ml in 10-ml vials. The drug should be stored in a refrigerator. Lorazepam is classified as a Schedule IV drug.

Lorazepam	
Pregnancy category	D
Lactation	NS
Metabolism	Liver
Excretion	Urine
DEA schedule	IV

Midazolam. Midazolam (Versed, Dormicum, Hypnovel) is a water-soluble benzodiazepine approved for use in the United States in 1986. It is well absorbed following IM administration and is frequently administered as an alternative to opioid agonists as a means of managing pretreatment anxiety. In my clinic, IM midazolam has been used with great success as a sole agent or in conjunction with IV midazolam in the management of patients with disabilities (adult and pediatric) as well as in the management of behavioral problems in pediatric dentistry.[38,39] These techniques are described in detail in Chapters 35 and 38. Midazolam provides a degree of retrograde amnesia in many patients following IM administration.[40]

Warnings. Midazolam, like other CNS depressants, may produce respiratory depression. This is especially likely to occur in patients who are receiving other CNS depressants (opioids, barbiturates) concurrently and in patients with preexisting cardiopulmonary disease. Special care must be taken whenever midazolam is administered to these patients.

Dosage. For use in the extremely fearful pediatric or handicapped patient, I have employed an IM dose of 0.15 mg/kg.[38,39] Dosages should be decreased in the presence of cardiorespiratory disease or other indicators of increased responsiveness to benzodiazepines. Continuous monitoring of the patient is essential once the drug is administered.

Availability. Versed (Roche Labs): 1 and 5 mg/ml in 2- and 5-ml ampules. Midazolam is classified as a Schedule IV drug.

Midazolam	
Pregnancy category	D
Lactation	?
Metabolism	Liver
Excretion	Feces and urine
DEA schedule	IV

The benzodiazepines chlordiazepoxide and lorazepam are seldom used in dentistry via the IM route. The primary dental indication for the use of lorazepam IM might be a patient about to undergo a long dental appointment (lasting longer than 3 hours) or one in whom a degree of amnesia is desired. Diazepam has received considerable use as an IM agent for preoperative sedation, although primarily in hospital situations rather than in dentistry. When injected deep into muscle, especially the deltoid, it appears to be an effective preoperative sedative. Midazolam, a water-soluble benzodiazepine, has proved to be a very effective IM sedative agent, especially in the pediatric and handicapped population.

Histamine Blockers (Antihistamines)

Two drugs classified as histamine blockers are commonly administered via the IM route for sedation before dental treatment. Although used primarily in pediatric dentistry, they may also be used effectively in the adult patient.

The pharmacology of these drugs, promethazine and hydroxyzine, is reviewed in Chapter 7, because these drugs are also effective anxiolytics when administered orally. In this chapter the clinical pharmacology of these drugs following IM administration is presented.

Promethazine. Promethazine hydrochloride, a phenothiazine derivative, is frequently employed via the IM or IV route for the management of anxiety. Other indications for use of promethazine include the management of allergic reactions and motion sickness, as an antiemetic, and as a preoperative sedative.[41]

Subcutaneous injection is contraindicated because promethazine produces localized tissue irritation that could lead to necrosis and sloughing. Deep IM injection is preferred to subcutaneous administration. The risk of this complication is considerably diminished with IM administration because of the superior vascularity of muscle. Onset of action following IM administration is rapid (10 to 15 minutes). Duration of action, however, is quite long: The patient usually feeling the effects of the drug for up to 24 hours. If the patient is a child, a parent must be cautioned to watch the child during this time, not permitting bicycle riding or participation in any hazardous activities. The adult patient must also be cautioned and advised not to drive a car or operate hazardous machinery for 24 hours.

Because the degree of sedation produced by IM promethazine as a sole IM agent will be mild, it is common to administer an opioid along with promethazine when more profound sedation is desired. Occasionally, promethazine is administered in combination with a barbiturate and an atropine-like agent. This latter combination is commonly used as premedication for the hospitalized patient about to undergo surgery and general anesthesia. It is extremely important to remember that when promethazine is combined with an opioid, the dose of the opioid must be decreased by 25% to 50%; if it is combined with a barbiturate, the barbiturate dose must be reduced by 50%. Promethazine may produce additive effects with other CNS depressants, or the effect may be one of potentiation. In either case the administration of "average" doses of both CNS depressants is likely to result in excessive degrees of CNS and possible respiratory depression.

In addition to its H_1-receptor–blocking actions, sedative, and antiemetic effects, promethazine also has anticholinergic properties. Promethazine is therefore not recommended for patients with narrow-angle glaucoma, prostatic hypertrophy, stenosing peptic ulcer, pyloroduodenal obstruction, or bladder neck obstruction. Because these medical problems are rarely mentioned on the typical medical history questionnaire, the doctor considering the use of promethazine must question the patient specifically about these problems.

When used as a sole drug in pediatric dentistry, promethazine is effective in the management of children with lesser degrees of anxiety. It is not, however, effective in the management of children with extreme apprehension or of the disruptive, unmanageable child. In these situations promethazine will be combined with other CNS depressants, most commonly opioids, such as meperidine. A discussion of the use of these drugs in combinations is presented in Chapter 35.

Dosage. The usual dose of promethazine for adults for preoperative sedation is 25 to 50 mg 1 hour before treatment. The dose as an antiemetic is 12.5 to 25 mg every 4 hours. The dose for children for preoperative sedation is 0.5 mg/lb or 1.0 mg/kg, not to exceed 50 mg.

Availability. Phenergan (Wyeth-Ayerst): 25 and 50 mg/ml.

Promethazine	
Pregnancy category	C
Lactation	NS
Metabolism	Liver
Excretion	Feces and urine
DEA schedule	Not controlled

Hydroxyzine. Hydroxyzine hydrochloride is available for parenteral administration. The drug is not recommended for IV, IA, or subcutaneous administration because of adverse reactions that have occurred after its administration via these routes.[42]

Advantages of hydroxyzine in dentistry include its antiemetic and sedative actions and the fact that it potentiates the CNS depressant actions of opioids and barbiturates, permitting their dosages to be decreased by as much as 50%.

As with promethazine, hydroxyzine as a sole agent will prove effective in management of lesser degrees of anxiety; however, unless combined with opioids, barbiturates, or inhalation sedation (N_2O-O_2), hydroxyzine will be ineffective in more severe anxiety. Patients must be cautioned not to drive a car or to operate hazardous machinery for up to 24 hours following administration of IM hydroxyzine hydrochloride.

Because of possible tissue irritation following hydroxyzine injection, the preferred IM injection site in adults is the upper outer quadrant of the buttock or the vastus lateralis; in children the vastus lateralis is preferred.[43] The deltoid region should not be used until it is well developed (adults and teenagers), and the lower and middle third of the upper arm should never be used because of the risk of radial nerve injury.

Dosage. The usual adult dose of hydroxyzine for preoperative sedation is 25 to 100 mg 1 hour before treatment. The dose for use as an antiemetic is 25 to 50 mg. The dose for children for preoperative sedation is 0.5 mg/lb (1.0 mg/kg) 1 hour before treatment. The antiemetic dose for children is 0.5 mg/lb (1.0 mg/kg).

Availability. Vistaril (Pfizer): 25 and 50 mg/ml in 1-ml ampules and 10-ml multiple-dose vials.

Hydroxyzine	
Pregnancy category	C
Lactation	NS
Metabolism	Liver
Excretion	Urine
DEA schedule	Not controlled

Promethazine and hydroxyzine are effective drugs for IM conscious sedation. Used primarily in pediatric dentistry and then usually in conjunction with opioids, promethazine and hydroxyzine can be employed with success in the adult patient. Although the dosage range is quite wide, the doctor will select the appropriate dose of the drug after consideration of the factors discussed previously in this section. When used as sole drugs, their greatest efficacy is in the patient exhibiting milder levels of anxiety or one in whom only a light level of conscious sedation is desired.

Barbiturates

Two barbiturates, secobarbital and pentobarbital, are administered via the IM route for preoperative sedation. The depth of sedation achieved with either of these drugs usually is more profound than that seen previously with the benzodiazepines or histamine blockers. Caution is advised when barbiturates are used IM because of the lack of control maintained over the drug's effect and the respiratory depressant properties of the barbiturates.[44] Use of barbiturates is recommended only by doctors with the knowledge and ability to adequately monitor, recognize, and manage any adverse actions involved with use of these drugs. The pharmacology of these drugs is discussed in Chapter 7.

Secobarbital. Secobarbital is a short-acting barbiturate that produces clinical activity within 10 to 15 minutes after IM administration. Its duration of sedative action is approximately 3 to 4 hours.

A potential drawback to the use of secobarbital is that the drug begins to hydrolyze on exposure to moisture in the air or in aqueous solution. For this reason, the drug should be administered within 30 minutes of being withdrawn from its container. For IM administration the most practical concentration of secobarbital is 50 mg/ml.

Dosage. The usual dose for adults or children for preoperative sedation is 1.0 mg/lb of body weight. For lighter levels of sedation or anxiety control, the dose may be decreased to 0.5 to 0.75 mg/lb.

Availability. Secobarbital sodium: 50 mg/ml in 1-, 2-, 10-, 20-, and 30-ml vials. Seconal sodium (Lilly): 250-mg ampule dry powder (dilute with 5 ml of sterile water for injection); 50 mg/ml in 20-ml vial or 2-ml disposable syringe. Secobarbital is classified as a Schedule II drug.

Secobarbital	
Pregnancy category	D
Lactation	NS
Metabolism	Liver
Excretion	Urine
DEA schedule	IV

Pentobarbital. Pentobarbital, like secobarbital, is a short-acting barbiturate used to produce sedation. This drug is discussed in much greater depth in the section on IV sedation as a component of the Jorgensen technique. It may also be administered intramuscularly; however, solutions of pentobarbital are quite alkaline and have the ability to injure tissues into which they are deposited. IM pentobarbital must be administered deep into a large muscle mass, such as the upper outer quadrant of the gluteal region. The onset of action develops within 10 to 15 minutes, the duration of action is 3 to 4 hours.[45]

The parenteral solution is composed of pentobarbital sodium, propylene glycol 40%, alcohol 10%, and water for injection at a pH of 9.5. Use of pentobarbital is contraindicated in patients with allergy to any barbiturate or those with porphyria.

Although pentobarbital is frequently used alone, when it is administered in conjunction with other CNS depressants (e.g., opioids), the dose of the opioid must be decreased to prevent possible oversedation or respiratory depression. Use of pentobarbital with opioids should be limited to the doctor who has received training in patient monitoring and in recognition and management of the unconscious patient.

Dosage. Dosage should be calculated on the basis of age, weight, and the patient's condition. The usual adult dose is 150 to 200 mg; the child's dose frequently ranges from 25 to 80 mg. In all cases the drug is administered approximately 15 to 30 minutes before the scheduled appointment.[45]

Availability. Pentobarbital sodium (generic): 50 mg/ml in 1-, 2-, 5-, 20-, 30-, and 50-ml vials; 120 mg/ml in 10-ml vials; 130 mg/ml in 10-ml vials; 325 mg/ml in 10-ml vials. Nembutal sodium (Abbott): 50 mg/ml in 2-, 5-, 20-, and 50-ml vials. Pentobarbital is classified as a Schedule II drug.

Pentobarbital	
Pregnancy category	D
Lactation	?
Metabolism	Liver
Excretion	Urine
DEA schedule	II

The short-acting barbiturates secobarbital and pentobarbital are occasionally administered via the IM route for preoperative sedation. Although they are effective, the doctor must be aware of the potential for respiratory depression and excessive sedation that is inherent in the use of barbiturates. When these drugs are combined with other CNS depressants, the possibility of undesirable actions increases. The entire chairside staff must be fully prepared to recognize and manage any possible complications.

Opioid Agonists

The opioid agonists (OAs), although classified as strong analgesics, are commonly used for the management of anxiety in both medicine and dentistry. Although opioids may be employed as solo agents in this regard, this is uncommon; more often they are administered conjointly with nonopioid CNS depressants such as benzodiazepines, barbiturates, or histamine blockers to provide a greater depth of sedation than the latter drugs can produce by themselves.

The administration of opioids by any route of administration, but particularly parenterally, must be approached with caution. As discussed under the pharmacology of these potent drugs, a significant number of potentially serious side effects and drug-drug interactions may be observed following opioid administration. Although the incidence of most side effects is dose related, many serious problems have been encountered following dosages well within the "normal" range. Because OAs are quite potent, the doctor is cautioned to be absolutely certain, beyond any degree of doubt, that his or her entire staff is fully prepared, both mentally and technically, to recognize and manage any opioid-induced complications. Without this preparation opioid analgesics should not be used.

There is a need for opioids in dentistry. OAs are valuable in the management of postoperative discomfort following surgical procedures. In this regard the most practical route of administration often is the oral route, although most OAs possess a significant hepatic first-pass effect and are more effective following parenteral administration. However, it may be more prudent to forgo parenteral administration of OAs in the ambulatory outpatient setting. If a drug-related problem develops following patient discharge, assistance might not be immediately available. Parenteral administration of OAs for postoperative discomfort in the hospitalized, nonambulatory patient is much more practical and is indeed the most common method of administration.

Another use of OAs in dentistry is in the management of more intense degrees of anxiety and fear. All OAs, as CNS depressants, possess the ability to produce a state of sedation, and advantage may be taken of this to aid in patient management. The use of opioid agonist analgesics as solo drugs for the management of anxiety is not always the most effective approach. Larger doses of the OAs must be administered to achieve a desired level of sedation when they are administered alone than when OAs are administered concurrently with other nonopioid CNS depressants. Adverse effects of the OAs are potentially more serious than those of nonopioids (although even nonopioids may produce morbidity and mortality) and are dose related. It simply makes sense (1) to avoid the use of OAs unless there is a definite reason for their use and (2) to use the smallest clinically effective dose of the OA.

An ever-growing number of OAs has been introduced into clinical practice. However, a small group of these drugs probably represents 99% of all OAs used in medicine and dentistry. These include meperidine and fentanyl (and its congeners alfentanil and sufentanil). To these must be added the opioid agonist/antagonists exemplified by pentazocine, butorphanol, and nalbuphine.

Pharmacology. Morphine, although not commonly used in dentistry because of its prolonged duration of action, is recognized as the prototypical opioid agonist. Its pharmacology is reviewed in some depth as being representative of the entire group. Other OAs used in dentistry are discussed later, and the differences in their actions from those of morphine are pointed out.

Mechanism of Action. A significant body of research exists concerning the mechanisms of action of OAs. Four major stereospecific receptors for OAs and opioid antagonists have been located within the CNS, the spinal cord, the trigeminal nucleus, the brainstem solitary nuclei and area postrema of the medulla, the medial thalamus, the limbic system (amygdala), and the periaqueductal gray matter of the mesencephalon (brainstem).[46] The periaqueductal gray matter has been identified as a site important to opioid-induced analgesia, as well as to the perception of pain. In addition to the discovery of these receptors, endogenous opioid-like substances called *enkephalins* and *endorphins* have been isolated.[47] Both possess potent opioid-like properties and have received extensive examination as to their role in the management of pain.

Mu receptors are thought to be responsible for supraspinal analgesia, respiratory depression, euphoria, and physical dependence; *kappa* receptors are associated with alterations in affective behavior; *sigma* receptors are involved in the dysphoria, hallucinations, and vasomotor stimulation associated with some opioids; and *delta* receptors appear to modulate the actions of the mu receptors.[48-50] Table 10-3 summarizes the actions of these four opioid receptors. OAs are drugs that bind with the mu, kappa, and delta fibers. Opioid agonist/antagonists (OAAns) possess either agonist or antagonist actions at the various receptors, and opioid antagonists (OAns) possess antagonist actions at the receptors.

It is likely that OAs and the endogenous opioids (endorphins and enkephalins) act to alter pain perception and pain reaction by inhibiting neuronal activity at their receptor sites through a decrease in sodium conductance through ion channels in nerve membranes. That opioid receptors are found in certain areas of the CNS in greater abundance than in others

TABLE 10-3 Classification of Opioid Receptors

Receptor	Effect	Agonist	Antagonist
mu_1	Supraspinal analgesia	β-Endorphin Morphine	Naloxone Pentazocine
mu_2	Depression of ventilation	Morphine Meperidine	Naloxone
	Indifference or euphoria	Sufentanil Alfentanil	
	Miosis Bradycardia Hypothermia Physical dependence	Fentanyl	
delta	Modulates mu	Leuenkephalin	Metenkephalin
kappa	Miosis Sedation Analgesia	Dynorphin Pentazocine Butorphanol	
sigma	Dysphoria Tachycardia Tachypnea Mydiasis	Ketamine? Pentazocine	Naloxone

lends credence to this theory. OAs modify both components of the pain experience: the perception of pain and the reaction of the patient to pain. The presence of opioid receptors within the substantia gelatinosa of the spinal cord, the trigeminal nucleus, and the periaqueductal gray matter provides a reasonable explanation of the effect of OAs on pain perception, and the identification of opioid receptors located within the amygdala of the limbic system and the medial thalamus aids in explaining their effects on the reaction to pain. Patients receiving OAs may still perceive pain, but their reaction to it is usually diminished. The side effect of nausea and vomiting is explained by the presence of opioid receptors within the area postrema of the medulla, and their presence within the solitary nuclei explains the antitussive, hypotensive, and GI effects of OAs. The two primary areas influenced by morphine are the CNS and the GI tract, the only areas in which opioid receptors have been found.

Central Nervous System Effects. Morphine produces analgesia, drowsiness, mood changes, and mental clouding. Of significance is the fact that morphine produces analgesia without inducing the loss of consciousness. Following a therapeutic dose of morphine (10 to 15 mg) to patients in pain or feeling anxiety or fear, any or all of these may disappear. Pain may be diminished in intensity or eradicated completely, accompanied frequently by drowsiness. The extremities become quite heavy, the body becomes warm, itching develops on the face (most frequently the nose or upper lip), and the mouth becomes dry. Some patients may become euphoric.

Interestingly, when the same dose of morphine is administered to a pain-free patient, the reaction may not be as pleasant. Many patients report dysphoria rather than euphoria, consisting of increased anxiety or fear and frequently of nausea or vomiting.

With increased doses (15 to 20 mg), the subjective effects of morphine are increased. Drowsiness is increased, euphoria (when present) is accentuated, and patients in severe pain not relieved by smaller doses report relief. The side effects of nausea, vomiting, and respiratory depression are also accentuated.

Morphine and other OAs appear to be much more effective in the relief of dull, aching, continuous pain than that of a sharp, intermittent nature. Patients often report that they still feel the pain but that it no longer bothers them. It appears that the OAs primarily affect those systems responsible for the affective responses to noxious stimuli. Therefore, when patients no longer respond to pain in the usual manner, their ability to tolerate the noxious stimulus may be dramatically increased, although their ability to perceive the pain is relatively unaltered.

Pupillary Responses. Morphine and many other OAs produce a dose-related constriction (miosis) of the pupil. Although the pupil still responds to changes in light, miosis produced by morphine is evident even in total darkness. Marked miosis and pinpoint pupils are considered pathognomonic of OA overdose. Atropine (and related agents) administered concurrently with OAs counteracts morphine-induced miosis.

Respiratory Responses. Morphine and other OAs produce a dose-related respiratory depression. Respiratory depression is observed even at therapeutic doses of morphine and is the most significant undesirable effect of the opioid agonists. Opioid-induced respiratory depression is a major factor in many instances of morbidity and mortality occurring following IM or IV sedation.[18]

Morphine depresses the responsiveness of the medullary respiratory centers to carbon dioxide (CO_2), as well as depressing the pontine and medullary centers that regulate respiratory rhythm and rate. Clinically, it is observed that the rate, minute volume, and tidal exchange are all depressed by opioid agonists. Normal respiratory rates of 16 to 20 breaths per minute may decrease to as few as 3 to 4 breaths per minute following overdose. Maximal respiratory depression following morphine administration develops 7 minutes after IV administration, 30 minutes after IM administration, and 90 minutes after subcutaneous administration. Respiratory depression may be present for up to 4 to 5 hours after morphine administration.

All OAs are capable of producing respiratory depression. When equianalgesic doses are administered, the degree of respiratory depression is not significantly different from that produced by morphine.[51]

Nausea and Emetic Actions. Nausea and vomiting produced by morphine and other OAs result from direct stimulation of the chemoreceptor zone for emesis, located in the area postrema of the medulla. This emetic effect is counteracted by opioid antagonists.

It is significant that the incidence of nausea and vomiting is considerably greater in ambulatory patients than in recumbent patients. Nausea occurs in approximately 40% and vomiting in 15% of ambulatory patients receiving 15 mg morphine subcutaneously. It is probable that the emetic effect is produced in part by a peripheral effect on the vestibular apparatus of the ear and by orthostatic hypotension.[52]

Because most dental patients are ambulatory, the potential for nausea and vomiting following OA administration in dentistry is increased. Reversal of the OA with an antagonist before discharge of the patient might be considered as a means of minimizing this occurrence, but it must be remembered that the continued presence of the OA in the blood in the immediate postoperative period will aid in the management of any pain that might develop. In addition, it has been found that reversal of OAs not only reverses their adverse actions (respiratory depression, nausea, vomiting) but also reverses their analgesic actions. Routine reversal of OAs by opioid antagonists before patient discharge is not recommended. Use of opioid antagonists should be reserved for those few situations in which their administration is essential to a patient's safety. Probably the most effective means of minimizing the occurrence of nausea and vomiting following opioid administration is to minimize the dose administered to the patient because this complication is dose related.

Cardiovascular Effects. Morphine in therapeutic doses has virtually no effect on blood pressure and heart rate or rhythm when patients are in the supine position.[51] Actions on the cardiovascular system do not develop until doses well into the overdose range are administered, and even then, the cardiovascular system is not affected to a great degree. The most significant factor in hypotension developing following OA overdose is hypoxia. In the presence of opioid overdose with adequate oxygenation, the blood pressure usually is maintained within normal limits.

Postural (orthostatic) hypotension does increase in incidence and severity with increasing doses of morphine and other OAs, a factor to be considered in the usual dental office environment. This is thought to be a result of peripheral vasodilation occurring as a result of histamine release associated with OA administration. Whenever the patient is shifted from a recumbent to a more upright position, the ability of the cardiovascular system to respond to the effect of gravity will be depressed by the OA. Slower changes in patient positioning are essential to prevent or minimize postural hypotension. Minimizing OA doses further diminishes the incidence of this dose-related situation. Postural hypotension is most likely to be noted with morphine and meperidine (which provoke the greatest release of histamine).

Another result of OA histamine release is the possible development of pruritus at the site of administration. This effect is responsible for the flushed feeling and itching that develop in some patients following IV administration. This is discussed in detail in the section on IV sedation.

OAs have little or no effect on the myocardium, producing either an increase in heart rate or no change. The cerebral circulation, likewise, is little affected by therapeutic doses of morphine. However, in the presence of respiratory depression and elevated CO_2 levels, cerebral blood vessels dilate, and intracranial pressure increases.

Gastrointestinal Tract Effects. Morphine produces constipation by decreasing motility of the stomach, duodenum, and colon, as well as diminishing both pancreatic and biliary secretions. Because morphine increases biliary tract pressure, its use in patients with biliary colic may produce an increase in pain rather than relief.

Smooth Muscle Effects. Morphine and other OAs increase smooth muscle tonus throughout the body, such as in the ureter, urinary bladder, uterus, and bronchioles. Although therapeutic doses of OAs do not produce significant bronchospasm, their administration to patients with asthma may aggravate this condition, possibly precipitating bronchospasm. OAs ought to be avoided in patients with a history of asthma (a relative contraindication).

Tolerance, Physical Dependence, and Abuse Potential. The development of tolerance and physical dependence following repeated use is a characteristic of all opioid agonists. This represents one of the limiting factors in the use of these drugs. Within dentistry the potential for producing addiction in a patient through use of OAs for sedation is quite unlikely to develop; however, the presence of OAs within the office does increase the potential for unauthorized use of the drugs by persons unassociated with the dental office (after-hours robbery) or, unfortunately, by dental personnel themselves. Although it is not as significant a problem in dentistry as within the medical community, opioid abuse by health-care professionals does occur and must be scrupulously guarded against.

Because opioid agonists are Schedule II drugs, they must be stored in a locked cabinet or storage area. Precise records as to the use of these drugs are mandatory so that anyone can determine the fate of a package of OAs. These records are reviewed in the section on IV sedation.

Absorption, Distribution, Biotransformation, and Excretion. OAs are rapidly absorbed following subcutaneous, submucosal (SM), or IM injection (Table 10-4). Because of a significant hepatic first-pass effect, parenteral doses of OAs are considerably more effective than equal doses administered orally (only 30% of an oral dose of morphine reaches the systemic circulation).

Morphine leaves the blood rapidly and is distributed to the kidney, liver, lungs, and spleen. The major portion of the drug is found in skeletal muscle. Accumulation of the drug in tissues is rare, and within 24 hours the tissue concentration of morphine is quite low.

The OAs undergo biotransformation within the liver and are excreted in the urine. Only a small fraction of the administered dose is found unmetabolized in the urine.

Contraindications. The only absolute contraindication to the use of morphine is the presence of allergy.

Warnings. OAs should not be administered to patients with head injury or increased intracranial pressure because of the respiratory depressant actions of these drugs and their ability to increase intracranial pressure. Within the typical dental environment, this is an unlikely occurrence.

Morphine and other OAs should be used cautiously, if at all, in patients with asthma, chronic obstructive pulmonary disease (COPD), or any degree of respiratory depression, hypoxia, or hypercarbia. Even usual therapeutic doses of OAs in these patients may significantly decrease respiratory drive while simultaneously increasing airway resistance to the point of producing apnea.

TABLE 10-4 Comparison of Opioid Agonists and Opioid Agonist/Antagonists Via Intramuscular or Submucosal Injection

	Onset (min)	Peak Action (min)	Duration (hr)	Adult Dose	Pediatric Dose (mg/kg)
Opioid Agonists					
Morphine	20	30-90	Up to 7	5 to 15 mg	0.1-0.2
Meperidine	10-15	30-60	2-4	50 to 100 mg	1-2
Fentanyl	5-15	30	1-2	0.05 to 0.1 mg	—
Opioid Agonist/ Antagonists					
Pentazocine	15-20	—	3-5	30 mg	—
Butorphanol	10	30-60	3-4	2 to 4 mg	—
Nalbuphine	15	—	3-6	10 mg/70 kg	—

Patients receiving OAs must be cautioned against operating motor vehicles or other hazardous machinery. Orthostatic hypotension, nausea, and vomiting are more likely to develop in ambulatory patients receiving OAs.

OAs cross the placenta and may produce fetal respiratory depression. The use of OAs in the pregnant patient should be considered only following consultation with the patient's physician and only if other techniques and drugs are unavailable. The benefit versus the risk of drug administration should always be considered.

Drug Interactions. OAs must be used with caution in patients who are receiving other CNS depressants, such as other OAs, phenothiazines, benzodiazepines, sedative-hypnotics, tricyclic antidepressants, and alcohol. Exaggerated clinical effects, including respiratory depression, hypotension, profound sedation, and unconsciousness, may and have developed.

The use of meperidine in patients receiving MAOIs is contraindicated because patients have experienced unpredictable, severe, occasionally fatal reactions. Because the therapeutic actions of the MAOIs may continue for 14 days after their discontinuance, meperidine should not be used until at least 2 weeks following the last dose of the MAOI. A list of these drugs is presented in Table 7-3. The reactions are of two types. Some responses involve unconsciousness, severe respiratory depression, cyanosis, and hypotension, resembling acute opioid overdose. Other responses are characterized by hyperexcitability, convulsions, tachycardia, hyperpyrexia, and hypertension. The use of opioid antagonists in the management of these reactions has not always proved effective.

Precautions. Doses of OAs must be decreased in patients who are elderly or debilitated or are known to be sensitive to CNS depressants. Among these are patients with cardiovascular, pulmonary, or hepatic disease. Doses should also be decreased in patients with hypothyroid conditions, alcoholism, convulsive disorders, asthma, Addison's disease, and prostatic hypertrophy or urethral stricture.

OAs may aggravate preexisting convulsions in patients with seizure disorders. Convulsions may develop in patients without a history of seizures if the OA is administered in a dose considerably above that recommended because of the development of tolerance.

Adverse Reactions. The most significant adverse reaction associated with the administration of OAs is respiratory depression. Respiratory depression is dose dependent; however, some degree of depression is usually present even with therapeutic doses of most OAs. All aspects of respiration are depressed, but probably the most observable change is respiratory rate, which will be reduced significantly from the normal adult range of 16 to 20 breaths per minute to as little as 3 to 4 breaths per minute. Respiratory rates below 8 breaths per minute following administration of OAs should be evaluated carefully, and if necessary, treatment instituted to correct the situation. In addition to respiratory depression, respiratory arrest, cardiovascular depression, and cardiac arrest have been noted following OA administration.

Among the more common side effects of the OAs are lightheadedness, dizziness, nausea, vomiting, and diaphoresis (sweating). These appear to be more common in ambulatory patients. Because most of these effects are dose related, the use of smaller doses, as recommended in this book, should minimize the development of these undesirable effects. If side effects develop despite use of smaller doses, the ambulatory patient should be advised to lie down and avoid unnecessary positional changes, a maneuver that often alleviates the symptoms.

Other adverse reactions associated with OAs include euphoria, dysphoria, headache, insomnia, agitation, tremor, uncoordinated muscular movements, transient hallucinations, disorientation, visual disturbances, dry mouth, constipation, biliary tract spasm, flushing of the face, tachycardia, bradycardia, palpitation, faintness, syncope, urinary retention, reduced libido, pruritus, urticaria, skin rashes, and edema. In other words, the OAs are capable of producing just about any and every side effect that most other drugs (or even nondrugs) may produce.

Overdose. Overdose produced by opioids is manifested by respiratory depression, primarily a decrease in the rate and tidal volume of breathing. In more profound overdose the patient may lose consciousness, with pupils becoming constricted (miosis), muscles flaccid, and skin cold and clammy. Bradycardia or hypotension or both may be present. Respiratory arrest may develop.

The primary goal in the management of overdose from any OA is airway maintenance (*A,* airway) and the delivery of oxygen to the lungs, cardiovascular system, and brain (*B,* breathing). Ventilation may need to be assisted or indeed controlled by the person managing the patient. Once a patent airway is established and oxygenation assured, the administration of an opioid antagonist may be considered (*D,* definitive care). Naloxone is the drug of choice, administered by the IV route, if possible, or IM, if necessary. Other drugs and measures that may be considered are oxygen, IV fluids, and vasopressors. More specific details of management of drug-related overdose are discussed in Chapter 27.

Morphine. The pharmacology of morphine has been discussed at great length in the preceding section. Morphine is used as the sulfate (frequently abbreviated as MS). Following IM or subcutaneous administration, the onset of action develops within 20 minutes, with a peak effect noted between 30 and 90 minutes. Unfortunately for most dental situations, the average duration of clinical effect of morphine sulfate is approximately 7 hours. Approximately 90% of the dose administered is excreted within 24 hours, primarily in the urine.

Morphine is employed primarily as an analgesic, but it is also used commonly as a preoperative sedative before surgery and general anesthesia. Morphine is absorbed more reliably following parenteral administration than oral administration primarily because of a significant hepatic first-pass effect.

Dosage. The usual adult dose of morphine for preoperative sedation is 5 to 15 mg 30 minutes preoperatively. The usual dose for children for preoperative sedation is 0.1 to 0.2 mg/kg (0.05 to 0.1 mg/lb).

Availability. Morphine sulfate: 8, 10, and 15 mg/ml in 1-ml ampules; 15 mg/ml in 20-ml vials. Morphine is classified as a Schedule II drug.

Morphine	
Pregnancy category	C
Lactation	?
Metabolism	Liver
Excretion	Urine
DEA schedule	II

Meperidine. Meperidine was first synthesized in 1939 and was studied as an atropine-like agent.[51] Its analgesic properties quickly became recognized, and its atropine-like properties are today listed under side effects of the drug.

Following IM or subcutaneous administration, the onset of action of meperidine is more rapid than that of morphine (10 to 15 minutes), and its duration of action is somewhat shorter (2 to 4 hours). Maximal effectiveness develops between 30 and 60 minutes. Meperidine is probably the most commonly used opioid agonist in dentistry, its clinical onset and duration of action being quite amenable to the typical dental appointment. With doses of 80 to 100 mg, meperidine is equianalgesic with 10 mg morphine sulfate. Meperidine is approximately half as effective orally as parenterally.

Peak respiratory depression following IM administration of meperidine develops in 1 hour with a return toward normal at 2 hours, although measurable respiratory depression may be noted for up to 4 hours. Opioid antagonists readily reverse opioid-produced respiratory depression. As with morphine sulfate, meperidine produces virtually no untoward effect on the cardiovascular system at therapeutic doses. Ambulatory patients are more likely to experience postural hypotension. Although IV meperidine may produce a tachycardia, IM meperidine seldom does. Meperidine produces less smooth muscle spasm, less constipation, and less depression of the cough reflex than equianalgesic doses of morphine sulfate.

Dosage. The usual adult dose for preoperative sedation is 50 to 100 mg intramuscularly 30 to 90 minutes before treatment. The usual dose for children for preoperative sedation is 0.5 to 1.0 mg/lb (1 to 2 mg/kg) intramuscularly 30 to 90 minutes before treatment.

Availability. Meperidine: 25 mg/ml in 1-ml ampules; 50 mg/ml in 1-ml ampules and 30-ml vials; 75 mg/ml in 1- and 1.5-ml ampules; 100 mg/ml in 1-, 2-, 20-, and 30-ml ampules and vials. Demerol (Sanofi Winthrop): 25, 50, 75, and 100 mg/ml ampules and vials. Meperidine is classified as a Schedule II drug.

Meperidine	
Pregnancy category	C
Lactation	?
Metabolism	Liver, mostly
Excretion	Urine
DEA schedule	II

COMMENT: For IM administration of meperidine and other OAs, it is reasonable to employ one of the more concentrated dosage forms of the drug (e.g., 50 mg/ml) to minimize the volume of solution injected. On the other hand, when administered intravenously, more dilute concentrations of these same drugs are recommended to minimize the risk of mistakenly administering too large a dose.

Meperidine with Promethazine. Meperidine (Demerol) is combined with the phenothiazine/histamine blocker promethazine (Phenergan) to produce a drug combination that is commonly employed in pediatric dentistry. The pharmacology of the individual drugs has been discussed. This drug combination came into being because several clinical studies demonstrated that promethazine potentiated the analgesic and sedative properties of the opioid agonist meperidine. The dose of meperidine necessary to produce clinically effective sedation or analgesia could be reduced by almost 50% when promethazine was added.[53]

The combination is clinically useful in pediatric dentistry, not because of its analgesic actions but because the mixture produces more sedation than is seen with either drug alone. It is available in both oral and injectable forms, but its primary effectiveness has been in IM administration. Following IM administration, the combination produces a clinical effect within 15 to 30 minutes, with a duration of action of 3 to 4 hours.

Dosage. The usual adult dose for preoperative sedation is 25 to 50 mg of each component (1 to 2 ml) 15 to 30 minutes before treatment. Although the *Physician's Desk Reference* indicates a recommended dose for children of 0.5 mg/lb of body weight,[54] many pediatric dentistry textbooks indicate a smaller dose: 0.02 mg/kg (0.01 mg/lb) intramuscularly 15 to 30 minutes preoperatively.[55,56]

Availability. Mepergan (Wyeth): 25 mg meperidine and 25 mg promethazine per milliliter. Mepergan is classified as a Schedule II drug.

Mepergan	
Pregnancy category	N/A
Lactation	NS
Metabolism	Liver
Excretion	Urine
DEA schedule	II

Alphaprodine. Alphaprodine is a synthetic opioid analgesic introduced in 1949 as Nisentil. Its initial primary indications were in obstetrics as an analgesic during labor and delivery, urologic procedures, and surgical procedures. Dentistry became interested in alphaprodine because of its advantages over meperidine: its rapid onset and shorter duration of action. Alphaprodine became quite well accepted in pediatric dentistry, where it was one of the most used drugs in the management of the disruptive child.

Unfortunately, alphaprodine in dentistry was associated with an incidence of morbidity and mortality quite out of proportion to its use. Although most of these cases were the result of the administration of inappropriate doses of the drug, as well as an absence of adequate patient monitoring, the manufacturer of alphaprodine, Roche Laboratories, voluntarily withdrew Nisentil from the American market in September 1980.[57] Following a series of retrospective studies,[6,8,58] alphaprodine was reintroduced. Following its reintroduction, a number of additional serious incidents were reported,[4,59] and alphaprodine was again voluntarily withdrawn from the market in 1986. Alphaprodine is no longer available for clinical use in the United States or Canada, although it is available in other parts of the world.

Most serious complications resulting from the administration of alphaprodine were attributed to several factors as follows:

1. Inappropriate dosage of alphaprodine
2. Combinations of CNS depressants administered
3. Inadequate monitoring of patient
4. Lack of preparedness in emergency management

Fentanyl. Fentanyl is a rapid-onset, short-duration OA with qualitative clinical actions similar to those of morphine and meperidine. Fentanyl is significantly more potent, however, with a dose of 0.1 mg being equianalgesic to 10 mg morphine and 75 mg meperidine. In other words, 1 mg of fentanyl is equianalgesic with 100 mg morphine or 750 mg meperidine.[60]

As do other OAs, fentanyl produces a dose-related respiratory depression. However, respiratory depression produced by fentanyl may be of longer duration than its analgesic action. Fentanyl appears to produce less nausea and vomiting than do most other OAs. Other OA actions are also observed: miosis, bradycardia, bronchoconstriction, and euphoria. A potentially serious reaction to fentanyl administration is muscular rigidity ("chest wall rigidity"), which is quite rare, developing primarily after IV administration and involving most muscles, but particularly the muscles of the chest wall and muscles of respiration.[61] Chest wall rigidity is discussed in depth in the section on IV sedation.

Fentanyl is used primarily via the IV route, either alone or as the opioid component of Innovar (consisting of fentanyl and droperidol), for the induction and maintenance of neuroleptanesthesia (see Section VI). In addition, fentanyl is used to provide sedation preoperatively or postoperatively as an analgesic.

The onset of action of fentanyl following IM administration is 5 to 15 minutes; maximal effect develops within 30 minutes, and the duration of action is approximately 1 to 2 hours. These figures demonstrate that fentanyl is an OA whose clinical actions are quite well suited to the typical, short (1-hour) dental or surgical appointment. Fentanyl, in the proper hands, is a useful drug for the management of pain and anxiety, via either the IV or IM route.

Dosage. The usual adult dose for preoperative sedation is 0.05 to 0.1 mg intramuscularly 30 to 60 minutes preoperatively. The dosage must be decreased in elderly and debilitated patients, as well as in patients who have received other CNS depressants. Fentanyl is recommended for IV administration, but there is no recommended dose for children via the IM route.[62]

Availability. Sublimaze (Janssen): 0.05 mg/ml in 2- and 5-ml ampules. Fentanyl is classified as a Schedule II drug.

Fentanyl	
Pregnancy category	C
Lactation	NS
Metabolism	Liver
Excretion	Urine
DEA schedule	II

Alfentanil, sufentanil, and remifentanil are congeners of fentanyl that are gaining popularity in short procedures. They are similar to fentanyl in most properties. The primary use of alfentanil, sufentanil, and remifentanil is via the IV route. They are discussed in greater detail in Chapter 25.

The opioid agonist analgesics just presented are those most frequently given intramuscularly in both medicine and dentistry in the management of anxiety in the preoperative period. From the practical point of view, the most useful OAs for most dental procedures would be those possessing the shortest duration of action: alphaprodine and fentanyl, sufentanil, and alfentanil. With the loss of alphaprodine from our IM armamentarium, other short-acting OAs must be evaluated for efficacy and safety. The IM administration of fentanyl and its congeners has not received much attention with dentistry. Their primary use is via IV administration, where their short duration makes them appropriate for many short procedures. Meperidine, with its longer history of use and its longer duration of action, is the most commonly used opioid agonist in dentistry and medicine, being administered either IM or IV. In pediatric dentistry meperidine was used less often than alphaprodine, primarily because of its longer duration of action, but it is much more commonly employed today. Morphine, although an excellent agent, is rarely used IM in outpatient dentistry and surgery because of its long duration of action.

Opioid Agonist/Antagonists

Three opioid agonist/antagonists (OAAs) are available for IM and IV use. These drugs differ from the OAs in that they possess not only opioid-like properties (agonist) but also opioid antagonist properties. The systemic effects described earlier for morphine, as the prototypical opioid, represent agonistic actions. Antagonistic actions include (1) prevention of agonist effects if administered before or simultaneously with the OA, (2) reversal of agonist effects if administered after the OA, and (3) precipitation of acute withdrawal syndrome almost immediately in the opioid-dependent individual. One compound, naloxone, is considered a pure antagonist and is an important drug in the management of opioid overdose. Its actions and use are described in Chapter 25. Pentazocine, butorphanol, and nalbuphine are drugs with mixed agonist and antagonist activities and are discussed next.

Pentazocine. Pentazocine is a product of research aimed at developing an effective analgesic with little or no abuse potential. It possesses agonistic properties as well as very weak antagonistic actions (1/50th as potent as nalorphine as an antagonist). Its actions mimic those of morphine, including a sense of euphoria. Since its introduction in the 1960s, many instances of psychological and physical dependence to pentazocine have been documented. Because of its antagonistic properties, the administration of pentazocine to opioid-dependent persons may precipitate acute withdrawal syndrome, an action not produced by opioid agonists.[63]

The action of pentazocine on the cardiovascular system differs somewhat from that of morphine. With large doses, blood pressure and heart rate are seen to rise. Other actions of pentazocine, such as those on uterine smooth muscle and the GI tract, mimic those of morphine.

Pentazocine is approximately one third as potent as morphine following IM administration, 10 mg of morphine sulfate being equianalgesic to 30 mg pentazocine. Pentazocine is metabolized in the liver and has a half-life of approximately 12 hours. Following IM administration, the onset of action develops within 15 to 20 minutes. Duration of action is approximately 3 to 5 hours.[64]

Side effects, including respiratory depression, *warnings,* and *contraindications* to the use of pentazocine are similar to those for morphine and the other opioids. Pentazocine-induced respiratory depression may be antagonized by naloxone.

Dosage. The usual adult dose for preoperative sedation is 30 mg intramuscularly or subcutaneously 15 to 30 minutes before treatment. IM administration is preferred to subcutaneous administration because of possible tissue irritation and damage associated with subcutaneous administration. The administration of pentazocine in children younger than 12 years is not recommended.[65]

Availability. Talwin (Sanofi Winthrop): 30 mg/ml in 1-, 1.5-, 2-, and 10-ml ampules. Pentazocine is classified as a Schedule IV drug.

Pentazocine	
Pregnancy category	C
Lactation	?
Metabolism	Liver
Excretion	Urine
DEA schedule	IV

Butorphanol. Butorphanol is a potent analgesic with an onset of action within 10 minutes following IM administration; it reaches a peak level of clinical activity at 30 to 60 minutes and has a duration of analgesia of 3 to 4 hours. An opioid agonist/antagonist, its antagonistic actions are approximately 30 times those of pentazocine and about 1/40th those of naloxone. In analgesic properties, butorphanol is 3.5 to 7 times more potent than morphine (2 mg = 10 mg).[66]

Side effects of butorphanol are similar to those of other OAs, including the possibility of respiratory depression. Although 2 mg of butorphanol does produce respiratory depression equivalent to that produced by 10 mg of morphine, increasing doses of butorphanol to 4 mg and greater does not appreciably increase the degree of respiratory depression. This one factor should make butorphanol (and nalbuphine) an important drug in dentistry's armamentarium against anxiety and pain. Although the magnitude of respiratory depression observed with butorphanol appears not to be dose related (above the 2-mg dose), the duration of respiratory depression is dose related. Naloxone rapidly reverses respiratory depression produced by butorphanol.[67]

Cardiovascular effects of butorphanol are similar to those of pentazocine, including increased blood pressure and heart rate. In addition, butorphanol increases cardiac workload by increasing pulmonary artery pressure, left ventricular end-diastolic pressure, and pulmonary vascular resistance. For these reasons, the use of butorphanol is contraindicated in patients with recent myocardial infarction, coronary insufficiency, or ventricular dysfunction.[65]

Butorphanol has received attention in both medicine and dentistry as a drug for preoperative sedation. It may be administered either intravenously or intramuscularly.

Dosage. The usual adult dose for preoperative sedation is 2 mg intramuscularly 15 to 30 minutes before treatment. Doses larger than 4 mg are not recommended because of a lack of sufficient information.[65]

Availability. Stadol (Mead Johnson): 1 and 2 mg/ml in 1- and 2-ml vials. Butorphanol is classified as a Schedule IV drug.

Butorphanol	
Pregnancy category	C
Lactation	S
Metabolism	Liver, extensively
Excretion	Urine
DEA schedule	IV

Nalbuphine. Nalbuphine is another analgesic possessing opioid agonist/antagonist properties. Nalbuphine is equipotent with morphine on a milligram basis. Following IM administration, onset of action is noted within 15 minutes, with a duration of action of from 3 to 6 hours. The plasma half-life of nalbuphine is 5 hours. The opioid antagonistic activity of nalbuphine is one fourth that of nalorphine and 10 times that of pentazocine.[68]

As with butorphanol, the *actions, side effects, contraindications,* and *warnings* are similar to those of opioid agonists. The one major difference in pharmacology between butorphanol and nalbuphine is the absence of any increased cardiovascular workload with nalbuphine. Its use is not contraindicated in cardiovascular-risk patients.[69]

At the usual IM therapeutic dose of 10 mg (for a 70-kg patient), nalbuphine produces respiratory depression equivalent to 10 mg morphine sulfate. Increasing the dosage of nalbuphine does not appreciably increase the degree of respiratory depression. Naloxone readily reverses respiratory depression produced by nalbuphine.

Dosage. The usual adult dose of nalbuphine for preoperative sedation is 10 mg/70 kg 15 to 30 minutes before the procedure. The dose should be adjusted, based on the patient's physical and emotional status, the depth of sedation desired, the patient's age, and the presence of other CNS depressants. Because of a lack of clinical experience, the administration of nalbuphine to patients younger than 18 years is not recommended.[69]

Availability. Nubain (DuPont): 10 mg/ml in 1-, 2-, and 10-ml ampules. Nalbuphine is not classified as a schedule drug.

Nalbuphine	
Pregnancy category	?
Lactation	?
Metabolism	Liver
Excretion	Feces and urine
DEA schedule	Not controlled

Opioid agonist/antagonists offer the significant advantage over the OAs (morphine, meperidine, fentanyl) of a ceiling effect in dose-related respiratory depression. Although this action will not be of great significance in the doses usually employed for conscious sedation in dentistry (up to 2 mg butorphanol or 10 mg nalbuphine), accidental overadministration of these drugs is less likely to result in serious respiratory depression or respiratory arrest. As with the opioid agonists, the doctor using OAA drugs must be prepared to both recognize and manage any unwanted side effects produced by these agents. Their presumed safety is not an excuse to forgo routine patient monitoring during the procedure. To do so is an invitation to disaster.

Nonsteroidal Antiinflammatory Drugs

Ketorolac. Ketorolac is an NSAID possessing appropriate solubility and minimal tissue irritation, making it suitable for IM injection. Ketorolac, as a potent NSAID, relieves pain through inhibition of arachidonic acid synthesis at the cyclooxygenase level and possesses no central opioid effects.[70] Ketorolac has analgesic potencies comparable to those of morphine, with the following IM equivalence: 30 to 90 mg ketorolac = 6 to 12 mg morphine.[71] Ketorolac is indicated for the short-term (up to 5 days) management of moderately severe acute pain that requires analgesia at the opioid level. It is not indicated for minor or chronic painful conditions. Increasing the dose beyond the label recommendations will not provide better efficacy but will result in increasing risk of developing serious adverse events. It is useful by itself or in combination with opioids, decreasing the required dose of opioid by approximately 45%.[70,72] It is especially useful when opioids are contraindicated, especially to prevent respiratory depression and sedation. When ketorolac proves to be ineffective in pain management, opioids should be considered.[73]

Dosage. Following IM administration, onset occurs within 10 minutes and peak blood levels are reached in 45 to 50 minutes, with a duration of approximately 6 hours.[72,74] Ketorolac is administered as a 30- to 60-mg IM loading dose followed by 15 or 30 mg IM every 6 hours, with a maximum first-day dose of 150 mg and 120 mg on subsequent days up to a recommended maximum of 5 days. The lower dosage range is recommended for elderly patients, patients weighing less than 50 kg, and patients with impaired renal function.[72]

Availability. Toradol (Syntex): 15 mg/ml Tubex cartridge-needle unit, 1-ml syringe; 30 mg/ml 1- and 2-ml syringe.

Ketorolac	
Pregnancy category	C
Lactation	S
Metabolism	Liver, mostly
Excretion	Urine, primarily
DEA schedule	Not controlled

Dissociative Anesthetic

Ketamine. Ketamine, a phencyclidine derivative, is administered parenterally to produce a state called *dissociative anesthesia*.[75] Following administration, the patient becomes mentally dissociated from the environment. Phencyclidine is used in veterinary medicine and was a popular drug of abuse known as *angel dust*. Ketamine may be used to produce a state of general anesthesia (its primary use) or, in subanesthetic doses, to induce a state resembling sedation. Within 5 to 8 minutes following IM administration, the patient loses consciousness. Recovery of consciousness occurs within 10 to 20 minutes, but it is several hours before the patient has recovered fully. The state of unconsciousness produced by ketamine differs significantly from that produced by more traditional general anesthetics. Dissociative anesthesia is described in Chapters 25 and 31.

Pharmacology. Ketamine exerts its dissociative effects by interrupting the cerebral association pathways and by depression of the thalamocortical tracts. The reticular activating system, the limbic system, and the medulla are but little affected.

The cardiovascular system is stimulated following ketamine administration (most general anesthetics depress the cardiovascular system). Increases occur in the mean arterial pressure, heart rate, and cardiac output, brought about by direct stimulation by ketamine. The median elevation in blood pressure following IM ketamine is about 20% to 25% above preanesthetic levels. Airway patency is easily maintained following ketamine administration because muscle tonus is actually increased, in direct contrast to decreased muscle tonus seen with other general anesthetics. Protective reflexes are also maintained, but there is some degree of diminution of their effectiveness. Administration of overly large doses of ketamine may produce apnea.[76] The administrator of ketamine must remain ever vigilant during patient treatment with this drug. Ketamine undergoes biotransformation in the liver into alcohols, which are excreted in the urine.

The use of ketamine is contraindicated in patients with high blood pressure, severe psychiatric disorders, increased intracranial pressure, epilepsy, arteriosclerotic heart disease, or cerebrovascular accident.[77]

Probably the major adverse action observed following ketamine administration is the development of unpleasant dreaming, confused states, and frightening or upsetting hallucinations during recovery. These are more likely to occur in adults than in children. When they do occur in children, they are usually less intense than those in adults.[78]

Ketamine should never be used, in either anesthetic or subanesthetic doses, by a doctor untrained in anesthesiology. The differences between a ketamine-induced state of general anesthesia and the more traditional stage III anesthesia may tempt unqualified people to believe that they are able to safely employ this drug in their practice. Rest assured that this is not the case! I have had more than 1000 case experiences with ketamine and can attest to the fact that this drug can, although it is only on very rare occasion, produce some very severe and frightening situations. Doctors not fully prepared for these reactions will be unable to respond to them effectively, much to their patient's detriment. The reader is referred to Chapters 25 and 31 for a more complete discussion of ketamine, its dosages and availability, and the concept of dissociative anesthesia.

Ketamine	
Pregnancy category	D
Lactation	NS
Metabolism	Liver
Excretion	Kidney
DEA schedule	III

Anticholinergic Drugs

The anticholinergic drugs atropine, scopolamine, and glycopyrrolate are also called *cholinergic blocking agents, belladonna alkaloids,* and *antimuscarinic drugs.* Commonly employed in general anesthesia, anticholinergics are also frequently used in dentistry. Their primary use in dentistry is for the reduction of salivary flow. In addition, their vagolytic actions are effective in the prevention or management of bradycardia. These drugs may be administered subcutaneously, intramuscularly, or intravenously. Anticholinergics act as competitive antagonists of the postganglionic receptor located at the neuroeffector junction of the parasympathetic nervous system.[79]

Pharmacology

Eye. The anticholinergics block parasympathetic receptors in the sphincter of the iris and the ciliary muscle, producing dilation of the pupil (mydriasis) and an inability of the eye to accommodate (cycloplegia). There is little effect on intraocular pressure, except in patients with narrow-angle glaucoma, in whom significant increases in intraocular pressure may result. Narrow-angle glaucoma represents a contraindication to use of these agents.

Respiratory System. Administration of anticholinergics removes the parasympathetic nervous system's control over bronchial smooth muscle, leaving it under sole control of the sympathetic nervous system, which produces bronchodilation. Secretion of all glands within the oral cavity, pharynx, and respiratory tract is inhibited. Anticholinergics are frequently used before the induction of general anesthesia to minimize the risk of laryngospasm. This desirable action is a result of the decrease in secretions within the respiratory tract.

Salivary Glands. All parasympathetically mediated salivary secretions are completely inhibited by these agents. It is not uncommon for the patient receiving an anticholinergic to complain to the doctor that his mouth is overly dry, making it difficult to swallow or to speak.

Gastrointestinal Tract. The anticholinergic agents inhibit GI motility.

Cardiovascular System. The actions of the vagus nerve on the heart are diminished when anticholinergics are administered. This is termed the *vagolytic effect* and is of importance during the induction and maintenance of general anesthesia. There is an increase in heart rate following administration of usual therapeutic doses (0.4 to 0.6 mg) of atropine and scopolamine. Glycopyrrolate does not produce this effect to the same degree.

Urinary Tract. Anticholinergic drugs inhibit contractions of the bladder and ureter and produce dilation of the pelvis of the kidney, all of which act to produce urinary retention. In the presence of prostatic hypertrophy, this retention is more likely to develop.

Body Temperature. The anticholinergics inhibit sweating through their action on the cholinergic fibers of the sympathetic nervous system that innervate sweat glands. Body temperature rises following their administration. Elevation in temperature is the most serious and potentially life-threatening result of overdosage of these agents.

Motion Sickness. Anticholinergics have been used for centuries in the management of motion sickness. They appear to act on the vestibular end organs, the cerebral cortex, or both. Scopolamine is more effective as an anti–motion sickness agent than is atropine. Scopolamine is available for this use in the form of a transdermal patch (see Chapter 9).

Absorption, Metabolism, and Excretion. Anticholinergics are rapidly absorbed following IM administration. The liver is primarily responsible for their biotransformation, and the kidney is the main route of excretion. The half-life of atropine is 4 hours.

Contraindications. Anticholinergics are contraindicated in patients with glaucoma (acute narrow angle), adhesions between the iris and the lens of the eye, and asthma. Their use in patients with prostatic hypertrophy is contraindicated because of the risk of urinary retention.

Drug Interactions. Anticholinergics should be used with caution in patients receiving other drugs possessing anticholinergic actions. These include tricyclic antidepressants, antipsychotics, histamine blockers, and antiparkinsonism drugs.

Adverse Reactions. Although there is great potential for individual variation in response to these drugs, Table 10-5 shows the usual pattern of adverse response to atropine.

Atropine. Atropine sulfate is commonly used in general anesthesia, both preoperatively and during the surgical procedure. Its primary functions during this time are (1) the inhibition of secretions within the respiratory tract, thereby minimizing the risk of laryngospasm but not preventing it, and (2) the vagolytic action of the drug on the heart, minimizing the occurrence of vagally induced bradycardia. Atropine is more effective than scopolamine as a vagolytic agent but does not possess the CNS depressant or amnesic actions of scopolamine; however, these actions of scopolamine are not observed following IM administration but only after IV administration.

The recommended adult parenteral dose of atropine (0.4 to 0.6 mg) does not produce an increase in intraocular pressure and is not contraindicated in patients with glaucoma. If such an increase in pressure does develop, it may be counteracted with topically applied pilocarpine. Following IM administration, atropine produces clinical actions within 10 to 15 minutes, with a duration of action of 90 minutes.

Dosage. The usual adult dose is 0.4 to 0.6 mg intramuscularly 10 to 20 minutes before treatment. For children the following dosage schedule for parenteral atropine is recommended in the drug product insert[83]:

7-16 lb	0.1 mg
17-24 lb	0.15 mg
24-40 lb	0.2 mg
40-65 lb	0.3 mg
65-90 lb	0.4 mg
Over 90 lb	0.4-0.6 mg

Availability. Atropine sulfate: 0.3, 0.4, 0.5, 0.6, 1.0, and 1.3 mg/ml. Atropine is not classified as a schedule drug.

Atropine	
Pregnancy category	C
Lactation	S
Metabolism	Other
Excretion	Urine
DEA schedule	Not controlled

TABLE 10-5 Adverse Response to Atropine

Dose	Response
0.5 mg	Slight drying of mouth, bradycardia, inhibition of sweating
1.0 mg	Greater dryness of nose and mouth, increased thirst, slowing then acceleration of the heart, slight mydriasis
2.0 mg	Very dry mouth, tachycardia with palpitation, mydriasis, slight blurring of near vision, flushed dry skin
5.0 mg	Increase in above symptoms, disturbance of speech, difficulty in swallowing, headache, hot dry skin, restlessness
10.0 mg and above	Above symptoms to extreme degree, ataxia, excitement, disorientation, hallucinations, delirium, coma*

*"Red as a beet, dry as a bone, and mad as a hatter" describes the patient during an anticholinergic overdose.

Scopolamine. Scopolamine hydrobromide possesses the same pharmacologic properties as atropine, but in some cases to differing degrees. The vagolytic action of scopolamine is less than that of atropine, as is its effect in producing mydriasis. In addition, whereas atropine produces a stimulation of the CNS, scopolamine depresses the cerebral cortex. Scopolamine possesses a more intense drying effect than atropine.

In dentistry, scopolamine is primarily used for its ability to produce sedation and amnesia (as a component of the Jorgensen technique of IV conscious sedation). Following IM administration, the onset of action is 10 to 15 minutes, with a duration of action of approximately 90 minutes.

A possible side effect of scopolamine is the occurrence of excitement, restlessness, disorientation, and delirium during the postoperative recovery period.[81] This does not occur with atropine or glycopyrrolate. Emergence delirium, as it is known, is more likely to be observed in the very young or older adult patient, and it may be treated effectively with physostigmine (1 to 3 mg IV or IM). Emergence delirium is more common following IV than IM scopolamine administration; it is discussed more fully in Chapter 27.

Dosage. The usual adult dose is 0.32 to 0.65 mg 10 to 15 minutes before the procedure. The dose for children 6 months to 3 years old is 0.1 to 0.15 mg; for children 3 to 6 years old, 0.15 to 0.2 mg; for children 6 to 12 years old, 0.2 to 0.3 mg.[82]

Availability. Scopolamine hydrobromide: 0.3, 0.4, and 0.6 mg/ml. Scopolamine is not classified as a schedule drug.

Scopolamine	
Pregnancy category	C
Lactation	S
Metabolism	Liver
Excretion	Urine
DEA schedule	Not controlled

Glycopyrrolate. Glycopyrrolate (introduced in 1961) is similar in many ways to atropine and scopolamine. Following IM administration, glycopyrrolate acts within 10 to 15 minutes, exerts a maximal effect in 30 to 45 minutes, and has a duration of action of approximately 7 hours, considerably longer than that of the other anticholinergics.

Because glycopyrrolate is a quaternary ammonium compound, it does not pass through lipid membranes such as the blood-brain barrier, as do atropine and scopolamine (tertiary amines, which pass easily through lipid membranes). Glycopyrrolate does not produce sedation or emergence delirium.

The drying effect of a 0.2-mg dose of glycopyrrolate is equal to that of 0.4-mg atropine. Glycopyrrolate offers the same vagolytic action as atropine and scopolamine; however, and importantly, glycopyrrolate does not produce tachycardia or dysrhythmias as frequently as the other anticholinergics. This action may be significant in the cardiac-risk patient receiving these drugs (a beneficial effect) or in situations in which the doctor wishes to increase a too-slow heart rate (glycopyrrolate would not be indicated). Glycopyrrolate offers an attractive alternative to atropine and scopolamine when long-duration drying action is desired during dental procedures.

Dosage. The usual adult dose is 0.1 to 0.2 mg intramuscularly 30 to 60 minutes before treatment. The dose for children is between 0.004 and 0.01 mg/kg 30 to 60 minutes before treatment.[83]

Availability. Glycopyrrolate hydrobromide (Robinul, Robins): 0.2 mg/ml. Glycopyrrolate is not classified as a schedule drug.

Glycopyrrolate	
Pregnancy category	B
Lactation	NS
Metabolism	Unknown
Excretion	Feces, primarily
DEA schedule	Not controlled

The anticholinergics are most often used in conjunction with parenterally administered CNS depressants. The primary goal in their use is a reduction in salivary secretions, leading to the production of a dry operating field; a secondary goal during IM sedation is the vagolytic actions of the drug. CNS depression produced by scopolamine via the IM route is usually insignificant compared with the other drugs being used. Although all three drugs are effective and safe when used in therapeutic dosages, scopolamine should not be used if the sole aim in using an anticholinergic is the production of a dry field or its vagolytic actions. Atropine or glycopyrrolate are more appropriate in this regard. Scopolamine is indicated for use when a degree of CNS depression or amnesia is desired, although IV administration produces a much more reliable effect than does IM administration. In addition, scopolamine has the disturbing ability to produce emergence delirium; the other anticholinergics do not. Table 10-6 compares the actions of the anticholinergics.

TABLE 10-6 Comparison of Anticholinergic Actions

	Atropine	Scopolamine	Glycopyrrolate
Effect on secretions	Effective	Effective	Effective
Vagolytic action	Effective	Less than atropine	Effective
Tachycardia, dysrhythmias	Yes	Yes	Less likely
Effect on eye	Mydriasis	Less than atropine	Mydriasis
Effect on central nervous system	Stimulates	Depresses cortex	Stimulates

BOX 10-5 Drugs Used in Intramuscular Sedation

Group A	*Group B*	*Group C*
Diazepam*	Morphine†	Atropine
Lorazepam†	Meperidine	Scopolamine
Midazolam	Alphaprodine§	Glycopyrrolate†
Promethazine	Fentanyl	
Hydroxyzine*	Alfentanil	
Secobarbital‡	Sufentanil	
Pentobarbital*	Pentazocine	
	Butorphanol	
	Nalbuphine	

*May irritate tissues at injection site unless deposited deep into tissues.
†Long duration of action limits outpatient use.
‡Must be prepared immediately before administration.
§No longer available in the United States.

Intramuscular Techniques

The drugs discussed in this chapter are those most often used intramuscularly for sedation. Box 10-5 classifies them into therapeutic categories. Group A includes the most effective IM drugs when lesser degrees of anxiety are present.

Used alone, group A drugs provide light to moderate levels of conscious sedation in most patients. The benzodiazepines diazepam, lorazepam, and midazolam are preferred over the barbiturates secobarbital and pentobarbital, while promethazine and hydroxyzine are less often used intramuscularly.

Lorazepam is long acting and thus rarely indicated for IM administration in the outpatient environment. Diazepam should be injected deeply into muscle to decrease tissue irritation and to maximize its absorption, which might still be inconsistent. Water-soluble midazolam has proved to be a highly effective rapid-onset IM agent in the benzodiazepine class. Midazolam is extremely effective in the initial management of both patients with disabilities and pediatric patients who are precooperative or uncooperative and will not voluntarily be seated in the dental chair. The use of midazolam in these situations is discussed fully in Chapters 35 and 38.

The IM administration of barbiturates can no longer be recommended because of the greater degree of respiratory depression accompanying therapeutic doses and the presence of more effective and safer drugs (e.g., benzodiazepines). Pentobarbital may irritate tissues into which it is deposited and should therefore be injected deep into muscle.

Promethazine is a reliable drug for IM administration, providing slightly longer durations than midazolam or diazepam. Hydroxyzine must be injected deep into muscle to avoid tissue irritation.

When administered as discussed, group A drugs usually provide a level of conscious sedation adequate to permit treatment of adult patients with milder degrees of anxiety or to place the fearful pediatric or handicapped patient into the dental chair, where other, more controllable techniques of drug administration may be employed (i.e., IV and/or inhalation).

Group B drugs are the OAs and agonist/antagonists. Their most rational use is for pain control in the posttreatment period. Although they will also provide a variable degree of sedation, their primary use for this indication cannot be recommended. Group A drugs are more specific and effective in managing fear and anxiety and have the additional benefit of producing fewer adverse effects (specifically, respiratory depression).

Group B drugs are frequently administered in combination with a group A drug in the management of patients with greater degrees of dental or surgical fear. When combined, the dose of the group B drug must be decreased from its "normal" level (when they are administered alone) because of the very real possibility of additive or potentiating actions, especially CNS and respiratory depression. Combinations of group A and B drugs are most often used to provide deep sedation in pediatric patients (see Chapter 35) and patients with disabilities (see Chapter 38) and in the management of the overtly disruptive or uncooperative patient. Use of any group B drug for sedation or analgesia requires that the doctor and staff closely monitor the patient and quickly recognize and manage any adverse reactions.

Group C drugs, the anticholinergics, may be administered alone or in combination with group A or B drugs. They function not to provide CNS sedation (although scopolamine, to a minor degree, may do so), but rather to provide a vagolytic action (glycopyrrolate does this to a lesser degree) and to reduce secretions in the oral cavity and respiratory tract. Doses of group C agents need not be reduced when they are used in combination with group A and/or B drugs.

For decreasing salivary flow only, atropine is most commonly recommended. Glycopyrrolate maintains this action for too long a period for most dental procedures. Scopolamine may produce CNS depression and emergence delirium, the latter occurring more commonly in patients younger than 6 years and older than 65 years of age.

The IM administration of two drugs from the same therapeutic category (i.e., meperidine and fentanyl or diazepam and midazolam) is only rarely recommended. Table 10-7 summarizes the recommended use of the drug groups listed.

Commonly Used Intramuscular Drug Combinations

Diazepam or Midazolam and Opioid Agonist. The combination of benzodiazepine and opioid is used in both medicine and dentistry in both adult and pediatric patients. Because the clinical effect of both diazepam and midazolam lasts 3 to 4 hours following IM administration, the selection of an appropriate opioid is important. IM morphine, with a duration of up to 7 hours, is too long acting for most medical and dental procedures. Where a patient may be kept under continual observation for several hours immediately posttreatment, and where posttreatment pain is a significant factor, IM morphine may be indicated. Shorter-acting opioids, such as meperidine and fentanyl, are more appropriate for administration with midazolam or diazepam. Another problem arises where diazepam is to be used. Being lipid soluble, diazepam cannot be mixed in the same syringe with any of the opioids (which are water soluble). Two IM injections must therefore be administered. Water-soluble midazolam, on the other hand, which may be combined in the same syringe with the opioids, usually represents the most reasonable choice for an intramuscularly administered benzodiazepine.

TABLE 10-7 Recommended Use of Drug Groups

Drug Group	Recommendation	Level of Sedation*
A alone (benzodiazepines)	High	Light to moderate
A alone (nonbenzodiazepines)	Low (but better than B alone)	Moderate to deep
B alone	Low	Moderate to deep
C alone	High	For ↓ secretions
A and B	High	Moderate to deep
A and C	High	Light to moderate and ↓ secretions
B and C	Low	Moderate to deep and ↓ secretions
A, B, and C	High	Moderate to deep and ↓ secretions

*Level of sedation may vary considerably with the same milligram-per-kilogram dose from patient to patient. Level indicated is *usual* level sought. The training and ability of the sedation team to safely manage the patient ultimately determine the level of sedation that should be employed.

Promethazine Plus Opioid. Because of the moderate duration (2 to 4 hours) of promethazine, it may be combined with meperidine, fentanyl, and its congeners in the same syringe. Promethazine and meperidine are marketed in a premixed form, Mepergan. This combination is rather popular in pediatric medicine and dentistry for management of the overtly disruptive patient. Promethazine functions both as an antiemetic to counter this action of the opioid and to provide an added degree of sedation. Each milliliter of Mepergan contains 25 mg promethazine and 25 mg meperidine. Giovannitti and Trapp[18] consider this combination to be the most ideal choice for IM sedation. Suggested doses are 0.7 mg/kg promethazine and 1.0 mg/kg meperidine. Each drug is drawn up individually into the same syringe and administered intramuscularly. If, after 45 minutes, sedation is inadequate, N_2O-O_2 sedation may be added.[18]

Hydroxyzine Plus Opioid. Similar to promethazine and opioid in depth and duration, hydroxyzine may be combined with meperidine or fentanyl. Hydroxyzine serves to minimize opioid-induced nausea and vomiting and to provide a degree of sedation. It is used primarily in management of the acutely disruptive or uncooperative child. This technique, as well as promethazine plus opioid, may also be used in adults.

Barbiturate Plus Opioid. Providing a slightly longer duration and a slightly greater depth of sedation than the preceding combinations, the combination of either pentobarbital or secobarbital and an opioid is more likely to produce significant respiratory depression. Respiratory monitoring is more essential when this combination is used. IM administration of barbiturates is no longer recommended.

Pentobarbital, Meperidine, and Scopolamine. Commonly called *twilight sleep*, this combination is similar to the preceding one with the added effects of the scopolamine providing for a slightly greater depth of sedation and the production of a degree of amnesia in some patients. This technique was used for many years as preoperative sedation before the induction of general anesthesia. Used intravenously, this combination of drugs is called the *Jorgensen technique.*

Meperidine, Promethazine, and Chlorpromazine. This combination is probably more familiar by the name *lytic cocktail* or by its abbreviation, DPT, taken from the proprietary names of the three agents Demerol, Phenergan, and Thorazine. DPT is rarely used today for sedation, primarily because of the chlorpromazine and its potentially significant side effects. It provides a long duration and a moderately deep level of sedation. Administration of this technique for IM sedation is actively discouraged.[84,85]

Monitoring during Intramuscular Sedation

A significant change in the use of IM/SM sedation since the initial publication of this book in 1985 has been the increased importance of monitoring whenever IM/SM agents are used. The greater the depth of sedation (CNS depression) obtained, the greater is the level of monitoring required to ensure patient safety.

When conscious sedation is the goal, direct communication with the sedated patient is the most important monitor (CNS), although respiratory and cardiovascular monitoring are also necessary. However, patient responsiveness is diminished when deep sedation is the goal, and monitoring of other systems must be intensified.

Vital signs (blood pressure, heart rate and rhythm, respiratory rate) must be checked continuously or at regular intervals (every 5 minutes) throughout the period of sedation (which always starts before the actual dental or surgical treatment and extends into the posttreatment period). The use of the pretracheal stethoscope has become a standard of care for IM/SM techniques. In pediatrics, placement of the stethoscope over the precordium is acceptable, although its placement over the trachea, immediately superior to the sternal notch, is preferred. In adults, pretracheal placement is preferred.

The use of pulse oximetry is also considered standard of care for IM/SM conscious and deep sedation. The combination of a pretracheal stethoscope and pulse oximetry provides the doctor with an immediate and continuous "feel" as to the respiratory status of the sedated patient, which is important because the respiratory system is the system most readily influenced (after the CNS) by the IM/SM agents used for sedation.

Additional monitoring techniques, such as capnography and electrocardiography, are rarely used at present and are not considered essential monitors during IM/SM conscious sedation, although the use of the capnograph during deep sedation has become increasingly popular. I do not consider monitoring of the electrical activity of the myocardium (ECG) during conscious sedation to be of as critical importance as respiratory monitoring.

SUMMARY

The IM route of drug administration has definite advantages when compared with oral administration;

however, compared with the inhalation and IV routes, IM fares poorly. In adults the only rationale for the IM route is a lack of success with other, more controllable routes. In pediatrics or with patients with disabilities, however, the IM (or SM) route may prove to be the only effective patient management technique available aside from general anesthesia.

Drugs administered intramuscularly must have their dosages carefully calculated. Once administered IM, it is difficult, if not impossible, to reverse the actions of most drugs. Basic management of overly sedated patients must consist primarily of basic life support: airway maintenance, breathing (spontaneous, assisted, or controlled), and circulation. Doctors using the IM route must be adept at patient monitoring and be trained in management of the unconscious airway.

REFERENCES

1. Hine CH, Pasi A: Fatality after use of alphaprodine in analgesia for dental surgery: report of a case, *JADA* 84:858, 1972.
2. Okuji DM: Hypoxic encephalopathy after the administration of alphaprodine hydrochloride, *JADA* 103:50, 1981.
3. Goodson JM, Moore PA: Life-threatening reactions following pedodontic sedation: an assessment of narcotic, local anesthetic and antiemetic drug interaction, *JADA* 107:239, 1983.
4. Moore PA, Goodson JM: Risk appraisal of narcotic sedation for children, *Anesth Prog* 32:129, 1985.
5. Council on Governmental Affairs, American Dental Association, Chicago, June 2002.
6. Alphaprodine, *Pediatr Dent* 4 (special issue 1), 1982.
7. Trapp L, Goodson JM, Price DC: Evaluation of oral submucosal blood flow at dental injection sites by radioactive xenon clearance in beagle dogs, *J Dent Res* 56:889, 1977.
8. Hine CH, Pasi A: Fatality after use of alphaprodine in analgesia for dental surgery: report of a case, *J Am Dent Assoc* 84:858, 1972.
9. Metroka DC, Marchesani JR, Carrel R: A submucous technique utilizing a narcotic and a potentiator, *J Pedodont* 4:124, 1980.
10. Jensen ST, Coke JM, Cohen L: Intramuscular injection technique, *JADA* 100:700, 1980.
11. Zelman S: Notes on techniques of intramuscular injection: the avoidance of needless pain and morbidity, *Am J Med Sci* 241:563, 1961.
12. Evans E, Proctor J, Fratkin M et al: Blood flow in muscle groups and drug absorption, *Clin Pharmacol Ther* 17:44, 1975.
13. Ceravolo FJ, Meyers HE, Michael JJ et al: Full dentition periodontal surgery using intravenous conscious sedation: a report of 10,000 cases, *J Periodontol* 57:383, 1986.
14. Greenblatt D, Koch-Weser J: Intramuscular injection of drugs, *N Engl J Med* 295:542, 1976.
15. Grohar ME: *How to give an intramuscular injection,* New York, 1980, Pfizer Laboratories.
16. Greenblatt D, Shader R, Koch-Weser J: Serum creatinine phosphokinase concentration after intramuscular chlordiazepoxide and its solvent, *J Clin Pharmacol* 16:118, 1976.
17. Beyea SC, Nicoll LH: Administration of medications via the intramuscular route: an integrative review of the literature and research-based protocol for the procedure, *Appl Nurs Res* 8:23, 1995.
18. Giovannitti JA, Trapp LD: Adult sedation: oral, rectal, IM, IV. In Dionne RA, Phero JC, eds: *Management of pain and anxiety in dental practice,* New York, 1991, Elsevier.
19. Siew C, Chang SB, Gruninger SE et al: Self-reported percutaneous injuries in dentists: implications for HBV, HIV, transmission risk, *JADA* 123:36, 1992.
20. McCray E, Cooperative Needlestick Surveillance Group: Occupational risk of acquired immunodeficiency syndrome among health care workers, *N Engl J Med* 314:1127, 1986.
21. Jagger J, Hunt EH, Brand-Elnaggar J et al: Rates of needle-stick injury caused by various devices in a university hospital, *N Engl J Med* 319:284, 1988.
22. Stricof RL, Morse DL: HTLV-III/LAV seroconversion following deep intramuscular needlestick injury, *N Engl J Med* 314:1115, 1986.
23. Kerr D: New product to protect nurses from needlesticks, *Calif Nurs Rev* 39, May/June 1990.
24. Ribner BS, Landry MN, Gholson GL et al: Impact of a rigid, puncture resistant container system upon needlestick injuries, *Infect Control Hosp Epidemiol* 8:63, 1987.
25. Edmond M, Khakoo R, McTaggart B et al: Effect of bedside needle disposal units on needle recapping frequency and needlestick injury, *Infect Control Hosp Epidemiol* 9:114, 1988.
26. Rodger MA, King L: Drawing up and administering intramuscular injections: a review of the literature, *J Adv Nurs* 31:574, 2000.
27. Hanson DJ: Intramuscular injection injuries and complications, *Gen Pract* 27:109, 1963.
28. Tsokos M, Puschel K: Iatrogenic *Staphylococcus aureus* septicaemia following intravenous and intramuscular injections: clinical course and pathomorphological findings. *Int J Legal Med* 112:303, 1999.
29. Librium injectable, drug product insert, Roche Laboratory, 1996.
30. Greenblatt DJ, Shader RI, Koch-Weser J: Slow absorption of intramuscular chlordiazepoxide, *N Engl J Med* 291:1116, 1974.
31. McCaughey W, Dundee JW: Comparison of the sedative effects of diazepam given by the oral and intramuscular routes, *Br J Anaesth* 44:901, 1972.
32. Gamble JAS: Plasma levels of diazepam, *Br J Anaesth* 45:1085, 1973.
33. Kortilla K, Linnoila M: Absorption and sedative effects of diazepam after oral administration and intramuscular administration into the vastus lateralis muscle and the deltoid muscle, *Br J Anaesth* 47:857, 1975.
34. Moolenaar F, Bakker S, Visser J et al: Biopharmaceutics of rectal administration of drugs in man. IX: Comparative biopharmaceutics of diazepam after single

rectal, oral, intramuscular and intravenous administration in man, *Int J Pharmaceut* 5:127, 1980.
35. Divoll M, Greenblatt DJ, Ochs HR et al: Absolute bioavailability of oral and intramuscular diazepam: effect of age and sex, *Anesth Analg* 62:1, 1983.
36. Ativan, drug product insert, Wyeth-Ayerst Labs, 1997.
37. Odugbesan CO, Magbagbeola JA: Parenteral premedication with lorazepam: a dose/response study, *Afr J Med Sci* 14:65, 1985.
38. Malamed SF, Quinn CL, Hatch HG: Pediatric sedation with intramuscular and intravenous midazolam. *Anesth Prog* 36:155, 1989.
39. Malamed SF, Gottschalk HW, Mulligan R et al: Intravenous sedation for conservative dentistry for disabled patients, *Anesth Prog* 36:140, 1989.
40. Theissen O, Boileua S, Wahl D et al: Sedation with intranasal midazolam for endoscopy of the upper digestive tract, *Ann Fr Anesth Reanim* 10:450, 1990.
41. Phenergan, drug product insert, Wyeth-Ayerst Labs, 1995.
42. Allen GD: *Dental anesthesia and analgesia,* ed 2, Baltimore, 1979, Williams & Wilkins.
43. Vistaril, drug product insert, Pfizer Inc, 1995.
44. Harvey SC: Hypnotics and sedatives: the barbiturates. In Goodman IS, Gilman A, Rall TW et al, eds: *Pharmacological basis of therapeutics,* ed 7, New York, 1985, Macmillan.
45. Nembutal, drug product insert, Abbott Labs, 1991.
46. Chang KJ, Cuatrecasas P: Heterogeneity and properties of opiate receptors, *Fed Proc* 40:2729, 1981.
47. Gebhart GF: Opioid analgesics and antagonists. In Neidle EA, Yagiela JA, Dowd FJ, eds: *Pharmacology and therapeutics for dentistry,* ed 5, St Louis, 2003, Mosby.
48. Phillips WJ: Central nervous system pain receptors. In Faust RJ, ed: *Anesthesiology review,* New York, 2002, Churchill Livingstone.
49. Shields SE: Pharmacokinetics of epidural narcotics. In Faust RJ, ed: *Anesthesiology review,* New York, 2002, Churchill Livingstone.
50. Way EL: Sites and mechanisms of basic narcotic function based on current research, *Ann Emerg Med* 15:1021, 1986.
51. Jaffe JH, Martin WR: Opioid analgesics and antagonists. In Gilman AG, Goodman LS, Rall TW et al, eds: *The pharmacological basis of therapeutics,* ed 7, New York, 1985, Macmillan.
52. Manzini JL, Somoza EJ, Fridlender HI: Oral morphine in the treatment of patients with terminal disease, *Medicina* 50:532, 1990.
53. Roberts SM, Wilson CF, Seale NS et al: Evaluation of morphine as compared to meperidine when administered to the moderately anxious pediatric dental patient, *Pediatr Dent* 14:306, 1992.
54. Mepergan, drug product insert, Wyeth-Ayerst Labs, 1991.
55. Wright GZ: Pharmacotherapeutic approaches to behavior management. In Wright GZ, ed: *Behavior management in dentistry for children,* Philadelphia, 1975, WB Saunders.
56. Wilson S, Vann WF Jr, Dilley DC, Anderson JA: Pain and anxiety control, Section II: pain reaction control—conscious sedation. In Pinkham JR, ed: *Pediatric dentistry: infancy through adolescence,* ed 3, Philadelphia, 1999, WB Saunders.
57. Troutman KC: Use of alphaprodine in pediatric dentistry. Symposium, Los Angeles, December 14 and 15, 1981. *Pediatr Dent* 4(special edition):156, 1982.
58. Chen DT: Alphaprodine HCl: characteristics, *Pediatr Dent* 4:158, 1982.
59. Del Vecchio PJ Jr: 20/20, *Am Dent Assoc News* 14:4, 1983 (letter).
60. Wiullens JS, Myslinski NR: Pharmacodynamics, pharmacokinetics, and clinical uses of fentanyl, sufentanil, and alfentanil, *Heart Lung* 22:239, 1993.
61. Ackerman WE, Phero JC, Theodore GT: Ineffective ventilation during conscious sedation due to chest wall rigidity after intravenous midazolam and fentanyl, *Anesth Prog* 37:46, 1990.
62. Sublimaze, drug product information, Janssen Pharmaceutica, 1989.
63. Hsu JY, Lian JD, Shu KH et al: Pentazocine addict nephropathy: a case report, *Chung-hua I Hsueh Tsa Chih (Chin Med J)* 49:207, 1992.
64. Houde RW: Analgesic effectiveness of the narcotic agonist-antagonists, *Br J Clin Pharmacol* 7:297S, 1979.
65. Talwin, drug product information, Winthrop Pharmaceuticals, 1992.
66. Vandam LD: Butorphanol, *N Engl J Med* 302:381, 1980.
67. Laffey DA, Kay NH: Premedication with butorphanol: a comparison with morphine, *Br J Anaesth* 56:363, 1984.
68. Pinnock CA, Bell A, Smith G: A comparison of nalbuphine and morphine as premedication agents for minor gynaecological surgery, *Anaesthesia* 40:1078, 1985.
69. Nubain, drug product information, DuPont, 1997.
70. Cataldo PA, Senagore AJ, Kilbride MJ: Ketorolac and patient controlled analgesia in the treatment of postoperative pain, *Surg Gynecol Obstet* 176:435, 1993.
71. Buckley MMT, Brogden RN: Ketorolac: a review, *Drugs* 39:86, 1990.
72. Lassen K, Epstein-Stiles M, Olsson GL: Ketorolac: a new parenteral nonsteroidal anti-inflammatory drug for postoperative pain management, *J Post Anesth Nurs* 7:238, 1992.
73. Acute Pain Management Guideline Panel: *Acute pain management operative or medical procedures and trauma,* Clinical Practice Guideline. AHCPR Publication No. 92-2, Rockville, Md, 1992, Agency for Health Care Policy and Research, Public Health Service, U.S. Department of Health and Human Services.
74. *Drug facts and comparisons*, pocket version 2002, ed 6, Philadelphia, 2002, Lippincott Williams & Wilkins.
75. Reich DL, Silvay G: Ketamine: an update on the first twenty-five years of clinical experience, *Can J Anesth* 36:186, 1989.
76. White PF, Ham J, Way WL et al: Pharmacology of ketamine isomers in surgical patients, *Anesthesiology* 52:231, 1980.
77. Ketalar, drug product information, Parke-Davis, 1996.
78. Roelofse JA, Vander-Bijl P: Adverse reactions to midazolam and ketamine premedication in children, *Anesth Prog* 38:73, 1992.
79. Greenblatt DJ, Shader RI: Anticholinergics, *N Engl J Med* 288:1215, 1973.
80. Atropine, drug product information, Elkins-Sinn, 1997.

81. Holzgrafe RE, Vondrell JJ, Mintz SM: Reversal of postoperative reactions to scopolamine with physostigmine, *Anesth Analg* 52:921, 1973.
82. Scopolamine hydrobromide, drug product information, CIBA Pharmaceuticals, 1992.
83. Robinul, drug product information, AH Robins, 1995.
84. US Department Health Human Services: Management of postoperative and procedural pain in infants, children and adolescents. In *Clinical practice guideline: acute pain management: operative or medical procedures and trauma,* Rockville, Md, 1992, USDHHS.
85. Nahata M, Clotz M, Krogg E: Adverse effects of meperidine, promethazine, and chlorpromazine for sedation in pediatric patients, *Clin Pediatr* 24:558, 1985.

SECTION IV

INHALATION SEDATION

In the technique of inhalation sedation, gaseous agents are absorbed from the lungs into the cardiovascular system. Although any number of inhalation anesthetics may be administered by this route for the production of sedation (see Section VI), only one, nitrous oxide, is used by any appreciable number of health professionals (including, but not limited to, dentists, physicians, and podiatrists). This section is therefore devoted to a discussion of the use of nitrous oxide–oxygen (N_2O-O_2) inhalation sedation.

Inhalation sedation with nitrous oxide (N_2O) and oxygen (O_2) has significant advantages over other techniques of sedation, yet it possesses no disadvantages of importance. This technique is an important part of the armamentarium for the management of fear and anxiety; indeed, the number of health professionals using N_2O-O_2 has risen steadily during the past decade. In the United States it is estimated that approximately 40% of practicing dentists currently use N_2O-O_2,[1] and virtually all dental graduates today enter into dental practice proficient in its safe and effective use.[2] In addition, a growing number of states have modified their dental practice acts to permit the registered dental hygienist to administer N_2O-O_2.[3] In fields other than dentistry, health professionals are beginning to use this valuable technique of sedation to their patients' benefit. In anesthesia, N_2O-O_2 has been used for more than 100 years as an important component of most general anesthetics, primarily as a means of permitting other, more potent and potentially dangerous general anesthetics to be used effectively in smaller doses and consequently in a safer manner. In the past 20 years, N_2O-O_2 has been used by emergency medical personnel, both in the hospital and in mobile coronary care units, to decrease or to eliminate pain caused by an acute myocardial infarction.[4] Many dermatologists, plastic and reconstructive surgeons, urologists, radiologists, and ophthalmologists have begun to use N_2O-O_2 as an aid in patient management during minor surgical or diagnostic procedures.[5,6] In the practice of podiatric medicine, there has been a significant increase in interest in this technique in recent years.[7]

Much of the current interest in inhalation sedation has occurred following a change in the basic concept concerning the goals sought in the use of N_2O-O_2. Once used solely as a general anesthetic (1800s) and later as an analgesic (1940s to 1950s), N_2O-O_2 is now employed to produce conscious sedation. Safety to the patient is significantly increased because the sedated patient remains conscious (and responsive) throughout the procedure. In addition, there have been important changes in the design of the inhalation sedation unit used to deliver these gases. Derived from the operating room general anesthesia machine, today's inhalation sedation unit has incorporated into it safety features that make the technique of inhalation sedation one that is virtually free of significant risk to the patient.

This section consists of a series of smaller chapters than the preceding section. It is hoped that this will enable the reader to more effectively locate material that is of importance to him or her. Subsequent chapters in this section will provide in-depth discussions of the development of inhalation sedation; the advantages, disadvantages, and indications for inhalation sedation; the pharmacology of the gases used and the mechanisms by which gaseous anesthetics produce their effect; the armamentarium for inhalation sedation; techniques for administration of N_2O-O_2; complications associated with its administration; and current concerns about N_2O, including chronic exposure, recreational abuse, and the occurrence of sexual phenomena. Concluding chapters discuss practical considerations concerning the use of inhalation sedation and educational guidelines established that relate to this important technique. Nitrous oxide was the first drug employed to achieve this magical state that enables surgeons to successfully complete surgical procedures on patients without the dreaded presence of pain.

ACKNOWLEDGMENTS

To my family for their sacrifices that allowed this endeavor: Angela, Gregory, and Maureen. Special acknowledgments to Drs. Don Kleier, Michael Savage, and Homer L. Ash for their encouragement. Tom Kramkowski receives special acknowledgment for his assistance and hard work in bringing this project together. Last, thanks to Amy Ash and Deborah Malley for their assistance.

—Morris S. Clark

REFERENCES

1. Jones TW, Greenfield W: Position paper of the ADA ad hoc committee on trace anesthetics as a potential health hazard in dentistry, *J Am Dent Assoc* 95:751, 1977.
2. Commission on Dental Accreditation: *Accreditation standards for advanced education programs in general dentistry,* Chicago, 1998, American Dental Association.
3. Department of Educational Surveys: *Legal provisions for delegating functions to dental assistants and dental hygienists,* Chicago, 1993, American Dental Association.
4. Kerr F, Brown MG, Irving JB et al: A double-blind trial of patient-controlled nitrous-oxide/oxygen analgesia in myocardial infarction. LANCET 1(7922): 1397-1400, 1975.
5. Corboy JM: Nitrous oxide analgesia for outpatient surgery, *J Am Intra-ocular Implant Soc* 10:232, 1984.
6. Cruickshank JC, Sykes SH: Office sedation, *Adv Dermatol* 7:291, 1992.
7. Harris WC Jr, Alpert WJ, Gill JJ, Marcinko DE: Nitrous oxide and Valium use in podiatric surgery for production of conscious sedation, *J Am Podiatr Assoc* 72:505, 1982.

CHAPTER 11

Inhalation Sedation: Historical Perspective

CHAPTER OUTLINE

The story of the development of inhalation sedation as used today in medicine and dentistry is a fascinating one, for it is also the story of the development of the art and science of anesthesiology. Nitrous oxide (N_2O), the most commonly used inhalation anesthetic agent in dentistry and indeed in all of medicine, is credited as being the first anesthetic to be administered clinically for the elimination of surgical pain. The story of the discovery of this agent and of its subsequent trials and tribulations, as well as those of the persons involved in its discovery, is presented so that the reader may be better able to appreciate the agent, the equipment, and the technique that we take so much for granted today—more than 200 years since the discovery of N_2O and more than 150 years since it was first used as a pharmacosedative agent.

BEGINNINGS (PRE-1844)

As difficult as it is to imagine, the gases oxygen (O_2) and N_2O were once unknown. It was not until 1771 that the German scientist Karl Scheele and the Englishman Joseph Priestley (1733-1804), working independently, discovered O_2. In 1727 O_2 had been prepared by Stephen Hales; however, he did not recognize that it was an element, and credit for the discovery of O_2 is given to Scheele and Priestley. The year following the discovery of O_2 Priestley discovered N_2O.[1]

During the late 1700s a branch of science known as *pneumatic medicine* came into being. Thomas Beddoes's Pneumatic Institute in Bristol, England, became one of the major centers of investigation of the newly discovered gaseous "vapors." It was at this time that Sir Humphrey Davy (1778-1829) became interested in the study of these gaseous agents. In 1795, at the age of 17, Davy had become an apprentice to the surgeon J. B. Borlase and, during his stay with Borlase, had experimented with N_2O and the effects of its inhalation. Davy became the superintendent of the Pneumatic Institute in 1798 and a year later published his book *Researches, Chemical and Philosophical; Chiefly Concerning Nitrous Oxide.* In this book Davy hinted that the inhalation of N_2O might be used to diminish pain during surgical procedures. He also provided the still commonly used nickname "laughing gas" (Figure 11-1). The following is an excerpt from Davy's work on N_2O in which he explains the effects of the agent on himself following self-administration for a toothache and gingival inflammation:

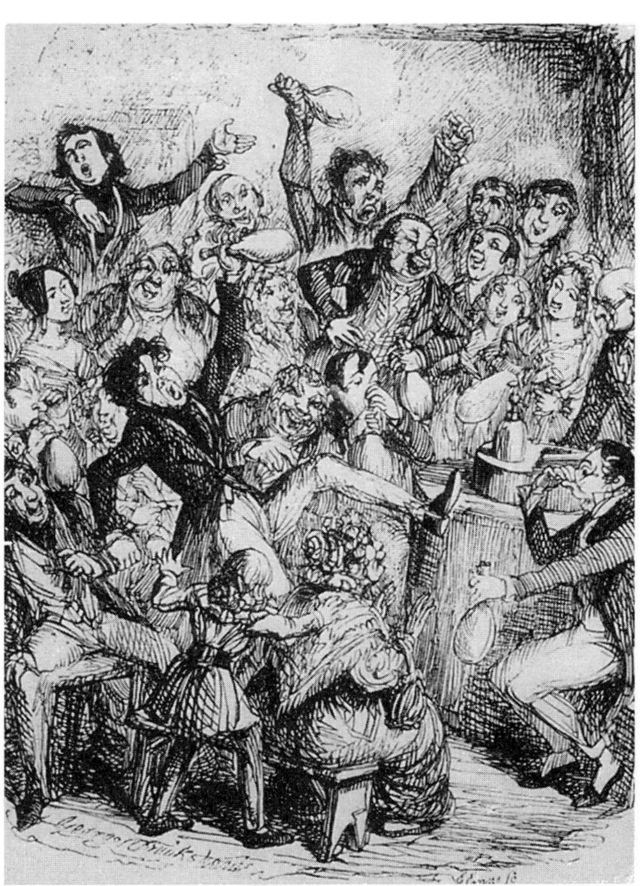

Figure 11-1 "Laughing gas." (From Scoffern: *Chemistry No Mystery,* 1839.)

> On the day when the inflammation was the most troublesome, I breathed three large doses of nitrous oxide. The pain always diminished after the first four or five inspirations; the thrilling came on as usual, and uneasiness was for a few minutes swallowed up in pleasure. As the former state of mind returned, the state of organ returned with it; and I once imagined that the pain was more severe after the experiment than before. . . . As nitrous oxide in its extensive operation appears capable of destroying physical pain, it may probably be used with advantage during surgical operations in which no great effusion of blood takes place.[2]

Unfortunately, both Davy and the rest of the medical profession failed to take serious notice of N_2O and to administer it for the relief of pain during surgery. One of the reasons for this failure to even try these newer gaseous agents was the fact that during the late 1700s and early 1800s, "ether frolics" and "laughing gas demonstrations" were a popular source of entertainment and enjoyment among younger people (Figure 11-2). Ether (ethyl ether) had been first described by Valerius Cordus in Germany in 1540, who called it *sweet vitriol.*[1] In 1794 Beddoes[3] reported that ether produced a deep sleep. As with N_2O, however, ether had also been used as a source of entertainment in the late eighteenth and early nineteenth centuries. The thought that agents such as ether and N_2O, which were commonly used to produce intoxication, could ever be employed during surgery as a means of abolishing pain was offered serious consideration by very few persons.

One of these persons, Henry Hill Hickman (1800-1830), an English physician, experimented with the use of carbon dioxide (CO_2) for the creation of "suspended animation." Hickman successfully performed surgical procedures on animals utilizing the inhalation of CO_2 to abolish pain during the procedure. In 1824 Hickman's paper, "A Letter on Suspended Animation," was published.[4] Unfortunately, the medical profession did not take notice, and Hickman's potentially important research was ignored and forgotten.

In 1831 yet another volatile agent, chloroform, was discovered. Working independently, Von Liebig (1803-1873) in Germany, Guthrie (1782-1848) in New York, and Soubeiran (1793-1858) in France are credited with its discovery.

In 1842 two other ambitious men took the great step forward and successfully administered ether to a patient during a surgical procedure. In Rochester, New York, Dr. W.E. Clark administered ether to a patient having a tooth extracted by a dentist, Dr. Elijah Pope. In Georgia, Dr. Crawford W. Long administered ether to John Venable for the removal of a tumor from his neck. It is interesting that neither of these persons thought this discovery important enough to write about it in the scientific journals. Dr. Long finally wrote about his use of the agent, stating that he had used it on three occasions in 1842 and on at least one occasion annually since that time.[5] The date of Long's paper was 1849, years after he had originally used ether clinically. The purpose of the paper was to lay claim to the title of the "Founder of General Anesthesia," which was at that time being contested among Morton, Wells, and Jackson, three men who are discussed shortly.

Thus for several more years patients requiring surgery were left with the same two options they had faced for centuries: endure the surgical procedure without benefit of any means of abolishing pain or elect not to have the surgery and face probable death.

However, as the 1840s progressed, things were about to change. It is interesting that one of these great changes occurred in a most unusual setting—a popular science lecture during which volunteers from the audience were permitted to experience the effects of N_2O.

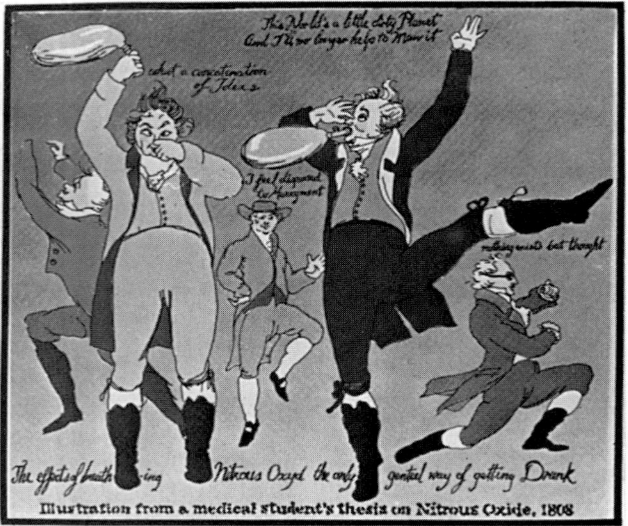
Illustration from a medical student's thesis on Nitrous Oxide, 1808

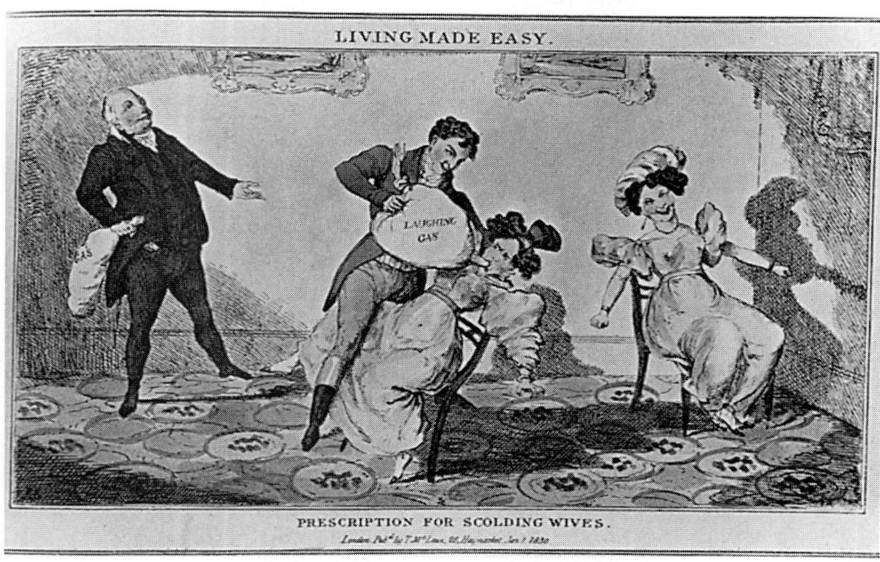
LIVING MADE EASY.
LAUGHING GAS
PRESCRIPTION FOR SCOLDING WIVES.

Figure 11-2 Nitrous oxide was used exclusively in a social setting in the early 1800s, as illustrated by these drawings from publications of that era. (From Shelden M, Wallechinsky D: *Laughing gas, nitrous oxide*, Berkeley, Calif, 1973, And/Or Press.)

THE EARLY DAYS (1844-1862)

On December 10, 1844, in the town of Hartford, Connecticut, Professor Gardner Quincy Colton presented a popular science lecture. Professor Colton was an itinerant medical school dropout from Columbia University, traveling around the countryside presenting his show of new scientific and quasi-scientific discoveries to eager audiences. In his show, N_2O gas was discussed and demonstrated, and as a part of the demonstration, male volunteers were invited from the audience to partake of the effects of N_2O (Figure 11-3). Women were also permitted to try N_2O, but not in the presence of the men. A private session was held for the women.

A Hartford dentist, Dr. Horace Wells (1815-1848), was in the audience on this particular evening (Figure 11-4). Wells had a productive dental practice but, being an especially sensitive person, had difficulty in dealing with the terrible anguish and suffering of his patients. In the early 1840s, in dentistry as in medicine, medications for the prevention and relief of pain were nonexistent. At the demonstration a store clerk by the name of Samuel Cooley volunteered to receive N_2O. Breathing 100% N_2O from a spigot attached to a bladder bag filled with the gas, Cooley quickly became intoxicated, running about the stage. During his running about, Cooley's leg hit the side of a table quite hard, yet Cooley continued to carry on as before, apparently oblivious of his injury. The skin had been broken, the wound bleeding, but there was no indication that Cooley either felt discomfort or was even aware of the injury. Wells spoke with Cooley after the incident and confirmed that he had been unaware of the injury.

Wells discussed this occurrence with Professor Colton and arranged for a demonstration of N_2O at Wells' dental office the next day. At the office, on December 11, 1844, a reluctant Colton served as the anesthesiologist as another dentist, Dr. John Riggs, extracted a wisdom tooth from Dr. Wells. After recovering from the effects of the N_2O, Wells stated that he had been totally unaware of the procedure and that there had been absolutely no pain associated with it.[6] Wells was taught the process of manufacturing N_2O by Professor Colton and shortly thereafter began using N_2O in his dental practice with great success.

Through his association with William T. G. Morton, Wells was able to gain permission to demonstrate his newly found technique to the medical students and faculty at the prestigious Harvard Medical School. Morton, a dentist who became a student and later a partner of Dr. Wells in Hartford, eventually left dentistry, becoming a medical student at Harvard. Morton was present in the audience on this fateful day. Using a medical student volunteer as a patient, Dr. Wells administered N_2O to the patient through a newly developed inhaler. As the patient lapsed into unconsciousness, Wells had to remove the inhaler, pick up his instruments, and attempt to extract the volunteer's infected tooth. During the extraction attempt the patient cried out. The audience, assuming that the procedure had failed, proceeded to boo and hiss Wells until he was forced to leave the demonstration hall, thoroughly humiliated and his demonstration a failure.[7]

On awakening, the patient stated that he was unaware that anything had happened, did not remember crying out, and had no memory of the attempted extraction. Unfortunately for Wells, this admission came too late. Wells returned to Hartford and continued his practice of dentistry, as well as the use of N_2O.

There are several possible explanations for the "failure" of the demonstration given by Wells. The first and most likely reason is that Wells had to function in the dual capacity of both the anesthesiologist and surgeon. Today it is quite apparent that the performance of two such important tasks by one person is not only extremely difficult but also increases risk to the patient during the procedure. However, at the time of Wells' demonstration there was no experience to judge from, for this was the first time such a procedure had been attempted. Although the patient was anesthetized by the N_2O initially, at the point at which Wells began the extraction of the tooth he had to stop the administration of the gas to the patient. Breathing only room air, the patient would naturally begin to recover from the

EXHIBITION
OF THE EFFECTS PRODUCED BY INHALING
NITROUS OXIDE, EXHILERATING OR
LAUGHING GAS
WILL BE GIVEN AT The Masonic Hall
Saturday EVENING 15 April 1845

30 GALLONS OF GAS will be prepared and administered to all in the audience who desire to inhale it.
MEN will be invited from the audience to protect those under the influence of the Gas from injuring themselves or others. This course is adopted that no apprehension of danger may be entertained. Probably no one will attempt to fight.
THE EFFECT OF THE GAS is to make those who inhale it either
LAUGH, SING, DANCE, SPEAK OR FIGHT, &c. &c.
according to the leading trait of their character. They seem to retain consciousness enough not to say or do that which they would have occasion to regret.

N.B. The Gas will be administered only to gentlemen of the first respectability. The object is to make the entertainment in every respect, a genteel affair.

Those who inhale the Gas once, are always anxious to inhale it the second time. There is not an exception to this rule.

No language can describe the delightful sensation produced. Robert Southey, (poet) once said that "the atmosphere of the highest of all possible heavens must be composed of this Gas."

For a full account of the effect produced upon some of the most distinguished men of Europe, see Hooper's Medical Dictionary, under the head of Nitrogen.

The History and properties of the Gas will be explained at the commencement of the entertainment.

The entertainment will be accompanied by experiments in
ELECTRICITY

ENTERTAINMENT TO COMMENCE AT 7 O'CLOCK.
TICKETS 12½ CENTS,
For sale at the principal Bookstores, and at the Door

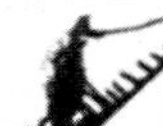

Figure 11-3 Nitrous oxide was discussed and demonstrated through exhibitions and shows that traveled around the countryside.

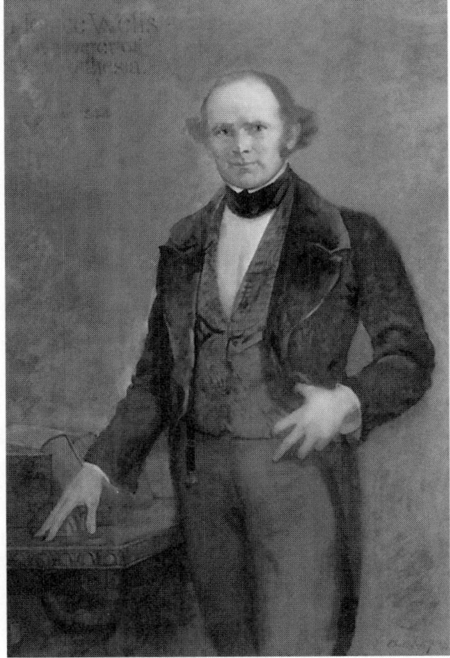

Figure 11-4 Horace Wells (1815-1848). (Courtesy Wadsworth Atheneum, Hartford, Conn. Gift of Charles Nöel Flagg. Endowed by C. N. Flagg and Company.)

effects of the N_2O, regaining consciousness. The pharmacokinetics of N_2O are such that the gas maintains a rapid onset of action and an equally rapid termination of action when its administration is discontinued.

A second possible explanation is the concept of biologic variability. As is well known today and has been stressed throughout this text, people respond differently when given the same dose of a drug. This concept is illustrated with the so-called bell-shaped, or normal distribution, curve. Unfortunately for Wells, in 1844 this concept was unknown. The patient may have been what would today be called a hyporesponder, a patient requiring a larger dose of a medication to achieve a desired clinical action.

The third possible explanation for the so-called failure is the lack of knowledge of the various levels of anesthesia. After the patient recovered, he stated that he had been unaware of any discomfort or of his crying out. These responses of Wells' patient are associated with the type of anesthesia commonly known as *ultralight general anesthesia.* At this level the patient is indeed unconscious, although minimally. He is quite able to react to pain and move about in response to it; however, because of the level of central nervous system (CNS) depression, he is unable to remember anything occurring at this time.

Unfortunately for Wells, the medical profession, and the many patients requiring surgery at that time, this information was unknown. Surgery continued for a short while longer without the benefit of pain-relieving medications.

Within a year or so of his ill-fated demonstration of N_2O, a discouraged Wells abandoned the practice of dentistry. He ceased to publicize N_2O and to attempt to introduce it into clinical use, although he personally knew that it could be used successfully. He was able to earn a living by partaking in several strange occupations—buying pictures in Paris, France, to sell in the United States and traveling around the countryside with a troupe of singing canaries. Wells continued to experiment with newer inhalation agents and soon became addicted to chloroform. Many of the founders of anesthesia became addicted to the chemicals they discovered, for they had no one to experiment on but themselves. The concept of addiction was unknown at the time and proved to be a terrible personal price to pay for the introduction of newer drugs and chemicals.[8]

In May 1848 a friend of Wells asked him to provide a vial of sulfuric acid so that he could throw it at a prostitute who earlier had damaged his clothes. Several days later, after Wells had inhaled some chloroform, he returned alone to Broadway in New York and while under the influence of the chloroform threw sulfuric acid at two other prostitutes. Arrested and placed in jail for these acts, Wells took his own life. The following are excerpts from the last letters written by Wells.[9]

> Sunday, 7 o'clock P.M.
>
> . . . I again take up this pen to finish what I have to say. . . . Before 12 tonight to pay the debt of Nature; yes, if I were free to go tomorrow I could not live and be called a villain. God knows I am not one. . . . Oh, what misery I shall bring on all my near relatives, and what still more distresses me is the fact that my name is familiar to the whole scientific world as being connected with an important discovery. And now, while I am scarcely able to hold my pen, I must to all say farewell! . . . Did I live I should become a maniac. The instrument of my destruction was obtained when the officer who had me in charge permitted me to go to my room yesterday.
>
> Horace Wells
>
> To my dear wife
>
> I feel that I am fast becoming a deranged man, or I would desist from this act. I can't live and keep my reason, and on this account God will forgive the deed. I can say no more.
>
> Horace Wells

On May 30, 1848, Horace Wells, later acknowledged as the founder of anesthesia, committed suicide while in jail by cutting the femoral artery in his left thigh with a razor. Prior to this act, Wells had inhaled some chloroform to produce insensibility to the pain.

Interestingly, N_2O was reintroduced in 1863 by Professor Colton in New Haven, Connecticut. The Colton Dental Association devoted the next 33 years to extracting teeth under N_2O. With 193,800 patients and no recorded fatalities, N_2O became the most commonly used inhalation anesthetic, a position it still maintains today.

William T.G. Morton (1819-1868) is the next major character in the story of the development of anesthesia. Morton learned of the idea of inhalation anesthesia from Wells, under whom he was a student of dentistry and then an associate in dental practice in Hartford. Morton later entered into medical school at Harvard, and it was through Morton's connections that Wells obtained the invitation to his ill-fated demonstration of N_2O anesthesia. Morton was a member of the audience at that demonstration. A more effective anesthetic gas was required, and Morton began to experiment with ether. How Morton came to work with ether became a topic of considerable discussion and controversy as the years passed. It is possible that he learned of ether through "ether parties" that were at the time a frequent entertainment of the medical students or that he was pushed into its use through a professor of his at Harvard, Charles Thomas Jackson (1805-1880), a physician and chemist.

Morton experimented to a small degree on animals (his family dog) and on himself before his first use of ether on a patient. That patient, Mr. Eben Frost, received ether for the extraction of a tooth on September 30, 1846. Morton recorded the incident as follows:

> Toward evening a man residing in Boston came in, suffering great pain, and wishing to have a tooth extracted. He was afraid of the operation, and asked if he could be mesmerized. I told him I had something better, and saturating my handkerchief, gave it to him to inhale. He became unconscious almost immediately. It was dark, and Dr. Hayden held the lamp while I extracted a firmly-rooted bicuspid tooth. There was not much alteration in the pulse and no relaxing of the muscles. He recovered in a minute and knew nothing of what had been done for him. He remained for some time talking about the experiment. This was the 30th of September 1846.[8]

Morton continued to experiment with ether, both on his own and with Dr. Henry J. Bigelow, for whom Morton administered ether for more than 37 operations. All of these cases were done prior to the famous demonstration of ether at the Massachusetts General Hospital in 1846.[10]

On October 16, 1846 (now called Ether Day), Morton administered ether to Gilbert Abbott (Figure 11-5). The famous surgeon John Collins Warren excised a tumor from the jaw of Mr. Abbott. Although considered an absolute success, Morton's demonstration was actually little more successful than Wells' had been. Abbott later mentioned that when the incision was first made it felt as though his neck had been scratched by a hoe. However, unlike Wells, Morton was not hissed out of the operating theater. The reason for this is twofold: first, Dr. Bigelow had attested to Dr. Warren the success of ether; therefore Warren was more inclined to believe that this new agent was not a fraud but in fact the real thing. Second, and of considerable importance, is the fact that Morton was a physician and not a dentist. At the time, dentistry was looked down on by the medical profession as a mere trade. That Wells should have even attempted to demonstrate his new technique to such an august group, including Warren, was, sad to say, quite laughable. His audience was filled with cynics and disbelievers. Morton, on the other hand, being a member of the "club," was more readily accepted. When the endorsement of Bigelow is added, it is readily seen why the less than absolutely successful procedure was proclaimed as the great event it truly was. In the words of John Collins Warren, "Gentlemen, you have witnessed a miracle. This is no humbug!"[10-12]

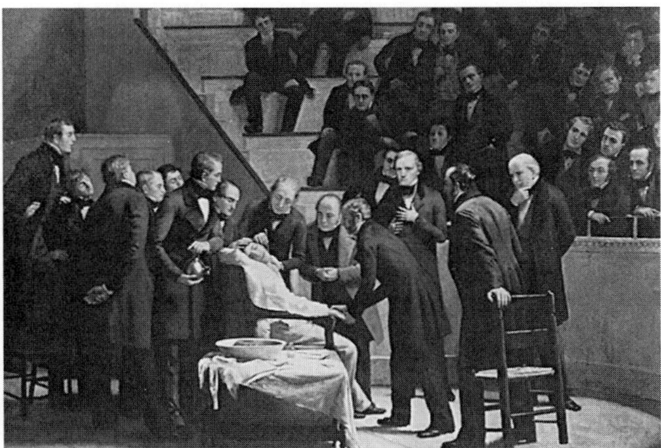

Figure 11-5 William T. G. Morton administering ether to Gilbert Abbott as John Collins Warren removes tumor from neck of Abbott in the famed Ether Dome at the Massachusetts General Hospital, October 16, 1846. (Courtesy Boston Medical Library in the F. A. Countway Library of Medicine, Boston.)

Ether had been for many years a popular agent for enjoyment. Ether follies were a popular form of entertainment, especially among medical students. Morton, acutely aware that if he were to suggest that this same agent be used for a serious purpose he might also be laughed at, modified the agent. He added a dye to it and called it *Letheon,* thus gaining acceptance for it among his colleagues.[13] The surgical amphitheater at the Massachusetts General Hospital in which this famed event took place has been preserved and is today known as the Ether Dome.

News of Morton's "etherization" spread rapidly throughout the United States and Europe, creating a degree of celebrity for Morton. On December 21, 1846, Dr. Robert Liston performed the first surgical procedure under "etherization" in England. Almost immediately following the introduction of etherization into surgery by Morton, Dr. Charles T. Jackson came forward to lay claim to its discovery, stating that it was he who had suggested its use to Morton, had advised him about the nature of the agent, and had advised him of the best manner in which to administer it. The controversy was only beginning. Soon Morton, Wells, and Jackson were engaging in bitter accusations and secret deals, each in an effort to prove that it was he in fact who was the sole founder of anesthesia. To complicate the matter still further, Crawford W. Long, who had first administered ether in 1842, came forward in 1849 to lay claim to this title.[14]

The name *etherization* was used for only a short time, and a more acceptable name for this new technique was being sought. Among the terms offered for this process were the following: *aethereal influence, aethereal inhalation, aetherealization, aetherization, anaestheticization, anaesthism, anodyne process, apathisation, ethereal state, etherification, hebetization, lethargic state, letheonization, narcotism, somniferous agent, sopor, soporization, soporized state,* and *stupefaction.*[10]

It was Dr. Oliver Wendell Holmes, the physician, author, and father of a Supreme Court justice, who suggested the name *anesthesia.* At the height of the controversy over the founding of anesthesia, Holmes wrote to Morton:

> Everybody wants to have a hand in the great discovery. All I will do is to give you a hint or two as to the names to be applied to the state produced and to the agent. The state should, I think, be called anesthesia. The adjective will be anesthetic. Thus we might say the "state of anesthesia" or the "anesthetic state."[6]

The name *anesthesia,* as suggested by Holmes, had been used by Plato in 400 BC to describe the absence of feelings in a philosophical sense. In the first century AD, Dioscorides also used the term to denote the absence of physical sensation.

Morton shortly gave up the practice of dentistry, devoting his time to the practice of anesthesia. He was thus the first person to specialize full-time in the field of anesthesiology (Figure 11-6). In addition, he was also involved in the manufacture of anesthetic inhalers and other devices for the administration of anesthetic gases.

Morton fought bitterly seeking to obtain recognition as the founder of anesthesia. Three times he petitioned the Congress of the United States for such recognition, and he spoke personally with President James Knox Polk, but during his lifetime Morton was never granted recognition as the father of ether anesthesia. Morton died of a cerebral hemorrhage in 1868, a discouraged and disappointed man. His tombstone reads: "Inventor and Revealer of Inhalation Anesthesia: Before Whom, in All Time, Surgery was Agony; By Whom, Pain in Surgery was Averted and Annulled; Since Whom, Science has Control of Pain."

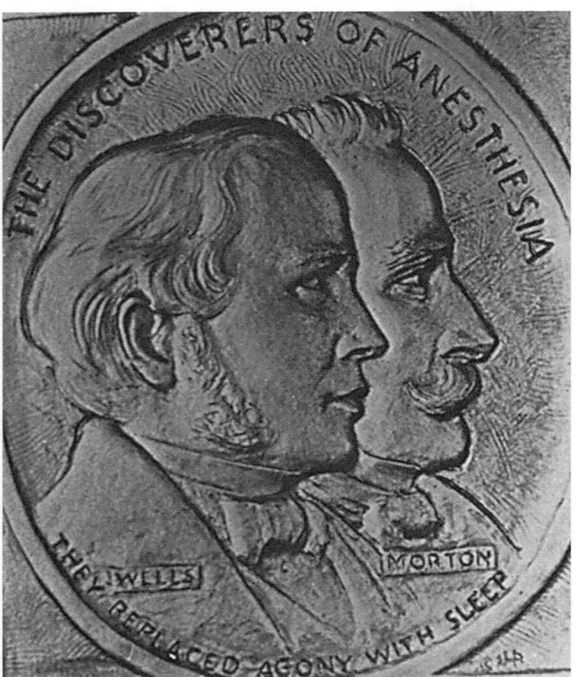

Figure 11-6 William T. G. Morton and Horace Wells, the discoverers of anesthesia.

As to the matter of who was the discoverer of anesthesia, the question is still debated. However, in 1864 the American Dental Association passed the following resolution:

> Therefore Be It Resolved, by the American Dental Association, that to Horace Wells, of Hartford, Connecticut (now deceased), belongs the credit and honor of the introduction of anesthesia in the United States of America, and we do firmly protest against the injustice done to truth and the memory of Dr. Horace Wells, in the effort made during a series of years and especially at the last session of Congress, to award the credit to other persons or person.[14]

In 1870 the American Medical Association followed suit, and a resolution, introduced by Dr. H. R. Storer of Massachusetts, was passed recognizing the discovery of anesthesia by Horace Wells: "Resolved, that the honor of the discovery of practical anesthesia is due to the late Dr. Horace Wells of Connecticut."[15]

Despite the controversy surrounding the discovery of anesthesia, the use of both N_2O and Letheon, as Morton's ether was known, was quite slow in developing. Bitter opposition to these new drugs was found within both the medical and dental professions in the United States in the late 1840s. In 1848 the American Society of Dental Surgeons stated in regard to the use of ether and chloroform: "Hence, in all minor operations in surgery their administration is forbidden; and that their demand in the practice of dental surgery is small."[16] The *Dental News Letter* of July 1849, which was published in Philadelphia, stated "The Letheon is still used to considerable extent in Boston, for extraction of teeth; while in this city and in most other places, so far as we have been able to learn, it has been generally abandoned."[17] It was claimed that the use of ether encouraged charlatanism.

Meanwhile, in England in the late 1840s and early 1850s, the discoveries of Wells and Morton were well received. In addition, chloroform, which had been introduced in 1831, became widely used.[11] Two names—John Snow and James Young Simpson—must be mentioned. John Snow (1813-1858) became the first physician after Morton to specialize in anesthesia. During his career he designed new inhalers for the delivery of anesthetics, primarily ether, which he used for extractions. In 1847 Snow published his classic textbook *On the Inhalation of Ether,* and in 1858, he published *On Chloroform and Other Anaesthetics.*[18,19]

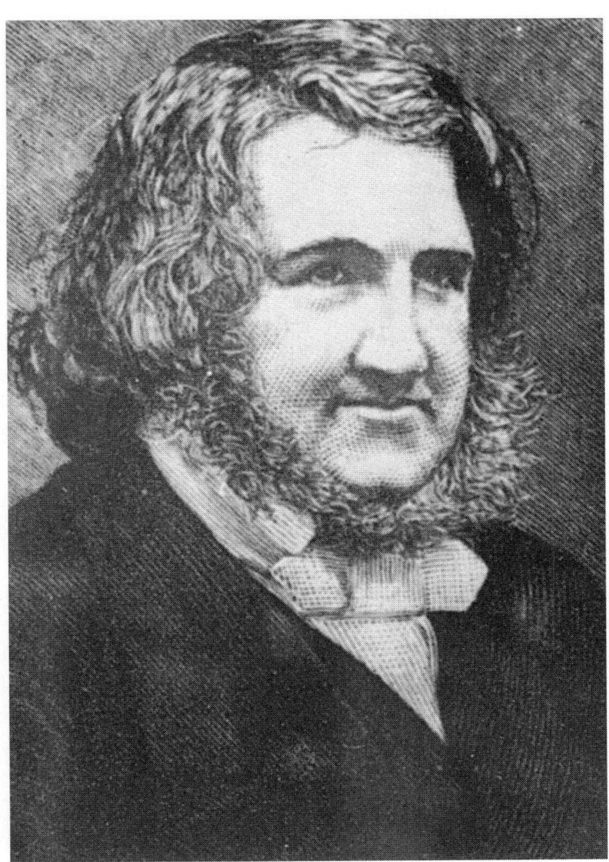

Figure 11-7 James Young Simpson (1811-1870).

James Young Simpson (1811-1870) was an English obstetrician (Figure 11-7). On January 19, 1847, Simpson introduced the use of ether into his obstetric practice. Although he liked the drug and the lessening of discomfort it brought his patients, Simpson disliked the disagreeable odor and the potential for nausea and vomiting associated with ether. He began to search for a better agent.

Simpson and his assistants, Keith and Matthew Duncan, began to experiment on themselves by inhaling various chemicals. Although their research was not extensive, it did produce a very valuable clinical agent. In November 1847, at the suggestion of David Waldie, a pharmacist from Liverpool, Simpson and his assistants experimented with perchloride of formyl, or chloroform, as it is known today. They found that chloroform worked quite well, and Simpson almost immediately began to use it as a means of alleviating the pains of childbirth.

Immediately, Simpson found himself embroiled in controversy with the Church of England. The propriety of abolishing pain during childbirth was the major point of contention. The argument used by the anti-Simpson clergy came from the Bible (*Genesis* 3:16):

> Unto the woman he said, I will greatly multiply thy sorrow and thy conception; in sorrow thou shalt bring forth children, and thy desire shall be to thy husband, and he shall rule over thee.

Simpson was quite able to cope with the controversy and continued to use chloroform as an analgesic to diminish labor pains. However, because of the controversy, other physicians were very slow to use chloroform. On April 7, 1853, John Snow administered chloroform analgesia to Queen Victoria at the birth of Prince Leopold, however, despite the fact that *The Lancet* had stated in no uncertain terms that the use of chloroform in normal labor is *never* justified. Nevertheless, Queen Victoria received chloroform analgesia for 53 minutes, the chloroform administered by a handkerchief. As mentioned by Snow in his subsequent book on chloroform, Queen Victoria expressed herself as greatly relieved by the administration.[19] Indeed, on April 14, 1857, Snow again administered chloroform analgesia to the queen at the birth of Princess Beatrice.

The use of chloroform as an analgesic and the administration of anesthetics for the relief of pain during childbirth received a great boost by the actions of Queen Victoria. The field of anesthesia began to grow, as did its problems.

On November 10, 1847, Simpson published an account of his experiences with chloroform. This report was published only 6 days after Simpson first began to use chloroform and contained a glowing account of its anesthetic capabilities. Unfortunately, as is known today, all drugs possess undesirable as well as desirable effects. At the time of publication of Simpson's report, the undesirable effects of chloroform were unknown (or unreported). Its ability to produce sudden cardiac arrest remained unknown for approximately 11 weeks, until January 28, 1848, when Dr. Meggison, an untrained country doctor, administered chloroform to a 15-year-old patient, Hannah Greener, who "died like a shot rabbit" upon receiving chloroform.[20] Today it is known that the effects of epinephrine on the myocardium and heart rhythm are exaggerated by chloroform, producing possibly fatal ventricular fibrillation.[21] Hannah Greener was, in the words of Dr. Meggison, "fretting all the day before 'crying continually and wishing she were dead rather than submit to it'."[22]

Simpson could not believe that chloroform could have been responsible for the death of Hannah Greener. He stated, in defense of chloroform, that the death of Hannah Greener had been caused by the brandy and water that had been poured into her mouth while she was unconscious (done in an attempt at resuscitation). He said that Greener had drowned from this fluid. The fact is, we will never know what killed Hannah

Greener. Deaths from light chloroform anesthesia continued to be reported, but the older generation of doctors and chloroform advocates refused to believe that a very small dose of chloroform could possibly kill a patient. It was not until 1911, when A. Goodman Levy published the results of his experiments on epinephrine and light chloroform anesthesia, that a possible mechanism of Hannah Greener's death was finally and satisfactorily explained—the propensity of chloroform to induce cardiac dysrhythmias, especially in the presence of elevated plasma epinephrine.[21]

During the ensuing 10 years (1850 to 1860), the use of ether and chloroform in dentistry became quite widespread and deaths continued to be reported. Controversy developed over the use of these agents within both medicine and dentistry. Thomas, in his interesting paper, "Some Early Papers on Dental Anaesthesia,"[23] cites two authors, Fowell[24] and Tomes,[25] regarding these agents. Fowell is quoted:

> Some persons, I am sorry to say, have become so enamored of chloroform or ether . . . as to refuse to permit the operation (of dental extraction) without its assistance . . . but when it comes to the removal of a tooth, which is an act simple in its execution and quick in its effect, I must confess that I think it is indiscreet.

Tomes stated: "We surely use a great power to overcome a very trifling difficulty, when we give chloroform preparatory to extracting an ordinary tooth." Tomes was also aware of the advantages of analgesia as opposed to general anesthesia: "On many occasions the patient has been perfectly aware of the steps of the operation, has felt the instrument grasp the tooth . . . and yet has felt little or no pain."

At the beginning of the 1860s, ether and chloroform were the dominant forms of anesthesia being used in the medical and dental professions. N_2O was used, but not as extensively, primarily because of the difficulties in its manufacture and storage.

ANESTHESIA DEVELOPS (1863-1898)

In July 1863 Gardner Quincy Colton, the man who had given Horace Wells the idea of using N_2O as an anesthetic in 1844, reintroduced N_2O to the dental profession. N_2O had not been in very common use since the death of Wells and the introduction of ether and chloroform. Colton established "dental institutes" in cities throughout the United States. These institutes specialized in tooth extractions under N_2O general anesthesia. One hundred percent N_2O was administered with the patient's nose held closed by the administrator as the patient inhaled through his or her mouth. Colton soon became the most renowned figure in the world of N_2O. By the year 1881, 18 years after his reintroduction of N_2O, Colton had administered N_2O to 121,709 persons without a death. Each of these cases has subsequently been documented.[26] That Colton was able to obtain such an outstanding record using an anesthetic gas without supplemental O_2 is truly outstanding. Yet Colton would have argued that the use of 100% N_2O was perfectly safe because the oxygen molecule attached to the nitrogen (N_2) would provide the cells of the body with whatever oxygen they required. It is now known that this oxygen is not available for use by the body. Fortunately, the vast majority of cases reported by Colton were of only 1 or 2 minutes in duration (tooth extraction); however, some did last for as long as 16 minutes without adverse effect, according to Colton. In addition, such was the clinical experience and technical excellence of Colton that he was able to administer this drug to more than 120,000 persons without a single death, despite the fact that his entire practice was based on an incorrect principle!

Dr. Edmund W. Andrews (1824-1904), a physician born in Vermont, was one of the founders of the Chicago Medical College, the forerunner of the Northwestern School of Medicine. However, Andrews's major claim to fame, and indeed a most significant one in the history of anesthesia, was the addition of 20% O_2 to N_2O. Andrews published his findings in an 1868 article in the *Chicago Medical Examiner,* titled "The Oxygen Mixture; A New Anesthetic Combination."[27] Andrews claimed this combination to be safer and more pleasant than any anesthetic mixture then known. In 1862 Joseph T. Clover (1825-1882) had introduced the mixture of chloroform and air. Clover also sought to make ether anesthesia safer by inducing anesthesia with N_2O and then maintaining anesthesia by adding ether to the N_2O. Indeed, Andrews was right in his thoughts about the combination of 20% O_2 and 80% N_2O. His concept of the use of this agent, as well as all other anesthetics, still holds true today, 126 years later.

In 1868 Paul Bert, a student of the great Claude Bernard, wrote that the use of 100% N_2O for more than 2 minutes would bring about signs and symptoms of asphyxia. Bert designed an apparatus capable of delivering 25% O_2 and 75% N_2O.[28]

Shortly thereafter, in 1872 in England, liquid N_2O became commercially available to the dental and medical professions, making its use much more practical and considerably safer. No longer did physicians and dentists have to manufacture their own N_2O with the risk of including impurities in the gas.

In 1881 two developments that had profound effects on the use of N_2O occurred in widely separate parts of the world. In St. Petersburg, Russia, an obstetrician, S. Klikovitsch, first used N_2O as an analgesic to relieve the pains of labor. As the years passed, the production of analgesia was to become a primary indication for the use of N_2O.

In the same year in Philadelphia, the S. S. White Manufacturing Company began to supply liquefied N_2O to the medical and dental professions. It also introduced an apparatus that permitted the delivery of the gas from the cylinder to the patient. This device revolutionized and simplified the administration of N_2O and provided a great boost to its use.

Sir Frederick Hewitt (1857-1916) invented the first practical anesthesia machine for administering N_2O and O_2 in fixed proportions in 1887. By 1889, N_2O-O_2 analgesia was being used in dentistry during cavity preparation in Liverpool, England. Several problems were associated with the use of N_2O-O_2 analgesia at that time. The use of very-low-speed handpieces, with no local anesthesia (by 1890 cocaine injection into the gums was becoming an accepted method of pain control) or poor local anesthesia, plus the fact that much of the N_2O and O_2 being used was impure, led to a significant number of side effects (e.g., nausea, vomiting, and excitement). As the 1890s continued, the use of N_2O-O_2 analgesia gradually declined.

THE TWENTIETH CENTURY

By 1898 both Hewitt in England and White in the United States had developed new devices for the administration of N_2O-O_2. In 1902 the Cleveland Dental Manufacturing Company introduced a machine designed by Charles K. Teter, DDS. This machine could deliver O_2, N_2O, and other anesthetic gases. Eight years later (in 1910), two of the major manufacturers of anesthesia equipment entered into the marketplace. J. A. Heidbrink, of Minneapolis, Minnesota, modified the 1902 Teter machine and introduced a new model for the administration of N_2O and O_2. Heidbrink's interest in anesthesia began while he was a dental student. He had suffered such excruciating pain during the extraction of his third molars without the benefit of anesthesia that he decided to correct the situation. Also in 1910, E. I. McKesson, MD, introduced the first intermittent-flow machine with accurate percentage control for N_2O-O_2. McKesson soon became the undisputed international authority on N_2O anesthesia and a leader in its development.

Teter, Heidbrink, and McKesson, by virtue of the many papers they wrote and lectures and clinical demonstrations they presented, were largely responsible for the increased use of N_2O-O_2 anesthesia for surgical operations throughout the United States.[29,30]

Periods of interest in N_2O were invariably followed by periods of almost total neglect. Two such periods of heightened interest occurred between 1913 and 1918 and between 1932 and 1938. Failures and side effects with the technique were not uncommon, even with the advent of newer machines and the increasing purity of the gases. The technique of N_2O anesthesia was not taught at any dental school or in any postgraduate program during this time; thus it was difficult for a dentist to learn the technique. The manufacturers of the anesthesia machines provided courses for doctors, but the quality of these courses was uniformly poor by modern standards.

A good description of the use of N_2O-O_2 analgesia in dentistry in 1923 is provided by Nevin and Puterbaugh:

> For its administration the patient is seated comfortably in the dental chair and the nasal inhaler adjusted carefully in order to avoid leakage about its margin and waste of the anesthetic. Since the patient does not lose consciousness at any time the mouth is left uncovered, no prop between the teeth being required. Before the anesthetic is started it is explained to the patient that he is to administer his own anesthetic. He is directed to breathe through his nose until a sense of numbness and stiffness comes over him which is felt extending to his finger tips, at which time his teeth, when snapped sharply together, will feel like wooden pegs set in wooden jaws. He is told that in this state he will feel no pain; that he need not go to sleep but that when he feels he is about to lose consciousness he is then to breathe through his mouth and by so doing he will remain awake. He is repeatedly reminded that while he will feel the vibration of the bur and be conscious of everything that is going on, the sense of pain will be entirely obtunded; that should he feel the slightest indication of pain he is to breathe entirely through his nose until the pain disappears. Nitrous oxid [sic] and oxygen are then turned on in proportion of twenty per cent oxygen and eighty per cent nitrous oxid. This mixture is administered throughout and, being of the same oxygen percentage as atmospheric air, there are no asphyxial symptoms exhibited at any time during the administration. Patients take quite an interest in this type of anesthesia for they feel that they are a part of its administration and willingly endeavor to cooperate for its success. This method may be safely employed for periods up to one half hour; if continued longer it is occasionally followed by nausea and slight headache, which, of course, should be avoided by arranging for a greater number of sittings of shorter periods each.
>
> The types of operations best suited to analgesia are the excavation of hypersensitive dentin, the preparing of roots for the adaptation of crowns and bridges, the scaling of deep pyorrhea pockets, etc. It will not obtund pain sufficiently to permit of the removal of vital pulps or the extraction of teeth or the lancing of abscesses, all of which require complete anesthesia for their performance.[31]

Throughout the 1930s and into the 1940s, most dentists who used N_2O worked with N_2O-O_2 in a ratio of 80% to 20% described previously, although many still employed 100% N_2O general anesthesia. The number of dentists using N_2O increased as the 1940s passed, the purity of the gases improved, and the quality of the machines for gas delivery increased, yet the success rate of N_2O-O_2 analgesia still remained low.[32]

During the 1940s fundamental changes in pain control in dentistry occurred. The use of local anesthesia as the primary means of pain control became more accepted. In 1945 lidocaine, the first of the newer, more effective amide-type local anesthetics, was introduced into clinical use. N_2O, which had been introduced in 1844 as a means of eliminating pain, was no longer the "ideal" drug for this task. Over the next few years the manner in which N_2O was used was modified. Rather than seeking the elimination of pain as its primary goal, N_2O could now be used for the management of anxiety and the production of relaxation (sedation). With this change in the goal being sought came changes in technique, dosage, and the approach to the patient.

In 1947 the third edition of Dr. Harry M. Seldin's classic textbook, *Practical Anesthesia for Dental and Oral Surgery: Local and General,* was published. In Chapter 22, The Administration of Nitrous Oxide and Its Mixtures, Dr. Seldin describes the ways in which the drug was used in the 1940s:

> The administration of nitrous oxide is no longer limited to the use of the gas by itself. In order to obviate the haphazard technique of "straight" nitrous oxide anesthesia, to reduce the possibility of unfavorable sequelae, and to extend the operating time, oxygen has been added. . . . Nitrous oxide is given in one of three ways:
>
> 1. Pure nitrous oxide, with the exclusion of air or oxygen, usually referred to as "straight nitrous oxide."
> 2. Nitrous oxide with air.
> 3. Nitrous oxide with oxygen.
>
> *Straight nitrous oxide.* Pure nitrous oxide without the addition of air or oxygen was the first form in which the gas was employed for the purpose of producing unconsciousness. Today, in spite of the tremendous advances in the art of anesthesia, some practitioners still persist in the use of so-called "straight nitrous oxide."
>
> The technique is simplicity itself. The pure gas is delivered to the patient from . . . the tank. . . . As soon as the patient shows the classical signs of asphyxia (thirty to sixty seconds): dilated pupils, absence of all reflexes, cyanosis, clonic muscular spasms, and jactitation, the inhaler is removed, a gauze pack forced into the posterior part of the mouth, and the operation commenced. The exodontist must work at top speed, usually with little regard for the oral tissues. It is evident that lacerations and sharp bony processes are inevitable when extensive exodontia must be completed in the two minutes or so available before consciousness returns. . . . Many of the pioneers in dental anesthetics developed unusual speed and dexterity, and could accomplish an unbelievable amount of work with a single administration. . . .
>
> There are certain limitations to this method. The period of anesthesia is very short, being frequently less than thirty seconds and rarely longer than one minute. . . . When the operation requires more time, the patient often recovers sufficiently to interfere with the procedure.
>
> However, in light of the present knowledge of anesthetic gases, there is very little justification for the rather crude method described. The addition of oxygen to the nitrous oxide has immeasurably improved operative technique under anesthesia. Speed ceases to be the prime factor.[33]

The term *blue gassing* refers to this technique of administration of pure N_2O. Blue gassing was employed in dentistry for many years, even well into the 1950s and early 1960s. Seldin goes on to describe two other techniques of N_2O anesthesia:

> *Nitrous oxide–air mixtures.* Although narcosis with gas and air has been employed, it can hardly be recommended. This method is extremely trying for the anesthetist, and the end result is not particularly gratifying. In addition to the prevalence of asphyxial symptoms . . . anesthesia is not smooth, and nausea appears almost routinely after anesthesias of more than five minutes' duration; the recovery of the patient is uncomfortably retarded. Most of these deleterious effects may be attributed to the high percentage of nitrogen included in the anesthetic mixture.
>
> *Nitrous oxide–oxygen mixtures.* Mixtures of nitrous oxide with oxygen have held and still hold a paramount and proved position in dental anesthesia.

Seldin describes two induction techniques. The first is the slow induction technique in which the patient is administered a N_2O-O_2 ratio of 93% to 7% for 1 minute. As signs of excitement develop, 100% N_2O is administered until the patient reaches the third stage of anesthesia. Sufficient O_2 is then added to maintain the desired plane of anesthesia. In the rapid induction technique, 100% N_2O is given for 45 to 60 seconds until the patient reaches the third stage of anesthesia, at which point 10% O_2 is added. The percentage of O_2 is changed to meet the needs of the patient:

> The anesthetic level is a variable depending upon the type of individual and may differ within the limits of 5 to 80 percent of oxygen and 20 to 95 percent of nitrous oxide. Any point within these rather widely-divergent extremes may be required to maintain different subjects at an even keel in the normal plane in the third stage.

Seldin then recommends "setting the dial at 100% oxygen for several inhalations" at the end of the procedure." In discussing analgesia with N_2O, he states:

> It is evident that analgesia with nitrous oxide and oxygen is an exceedingly safe procedure, because nitrous oxide is in itself the least harmful anesthetic known to the profession. . . . Analgesia may be maintained without the slightest danger for periods of thirty minutes and longer on any patient, regardless of age. As a matter of fact, elderly patients frequently make the best cases.

The concepts of individual variation and titration are discussed by Seldin:

> After the first few inhalations, each subject becomes a law unto himself, and his personal needs in respect to the proper mixture of these gases must be determined by the various symptoms of analgesia manifested by him from one minute to the next. In fact, considerable variations in the dial settings may be detected for the same person from day to day. This proves the falsity and irrationality of the recommendations made by gas-machine demonstrators that a standard percentage setting, consistently maintained, will induce and sustain perfect analgesia on all patients, irrespective of age or physical condition.

Many of the so-called modern concepts underlying the use of inhalation anesthetics and other parenterally administered drugs were discussed in Seldin's textbook. Much of the impetus for the use of N_2O-O_2 analgesia and sedation stems from his writings and lectures.

MODERN TIMES (1950-PRESENT)

The Development of Courses and Guidelines

In the 1950s and 1960s N_2O was becoming more frequently used in dentistry. The use of 100% N_2O was decreasing rapidly, and with the advent of newer local anesthetics for operative pain control, N_2O-O_2 became a very popular agent for the management of the apprehensive dental patient. Interest in the field of anesthesiology in dentistry grew, and in 1953 the American Dental Society of Anesthesiology was formed. In the years that have followed, this organization has led the way in advancing the standards and practices in the use of anesthesia (general, local, and sedation) within dentistry in the United States.[34,35]

A few dental schools added courses in inhalation sedation to the dental curriculum as the 1950s gave way to the 1960s. Postgraduate programs in inhalation sedation increased in number; however, with but few exceptions, their quality remained low. One man, however, Dr. Harry Langa, presented postgraduate programs of quality throughout these years. Dr. Langa began using N_2O in 1936 and presented his first course in 1949. Between that time and the publication of the second edition of his classic textbook, *Relative Analgesia in Dental Practice: Inhalation Analgesia and Sedation with Nitrous Oxide,* in 1976, he had trained more than 6000 dentists to use this technique safely.[36] *A Handbook of Nitrous Oxide and Oxygen Sedation,* coauthored by Morris Clark and Ann Brunick, published in 1999,[37] is the most comprehensive textbook devoted solely to inhalation sedation with N_2O. This text was written to be an updated and contemporary work in the use of N_2O-O_2 sedation. Its authors have trained more than 3500 dentists and hygienists in inhalation sedation (Figure 11-8).

As schools and other organizations began to present courses in inhalation sedation, it became obvious that the level of training being offered and its quality varied considerably. It was decided that standards ought to be established for the teaching of the various techniques of pain and anxiety control in dentistry. In 1964 the American Dental Society of Anesthesiology held the first of four workshops, attended by representatives of 43 dental schools, out of which came the *Guidelines for Teaching the Comprehensive Control of Pain*

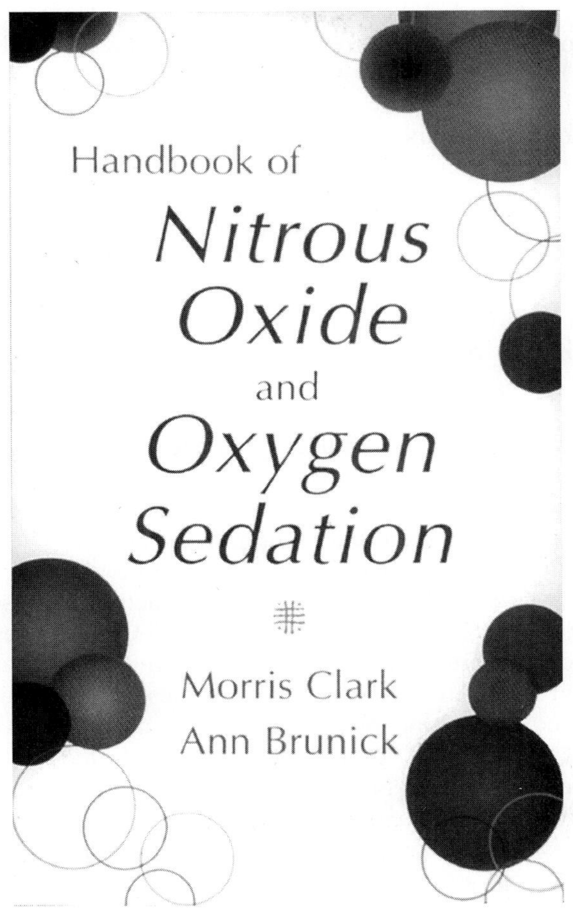

Figure 11-8 *Handbook of Nitrous Oxide and Oxygen Sedation,* by Morris Clark and Ann Brunick, published in 1999.

and Anxiety in Dentistry. Included within these guidelines is an outline for inhalation sedation courses.[38] The most recent version of these recommendations is presented in Chapter 19.[39] With the adoption of these guidelines, the overall quality of training in inhalation sedation was significantly improved. Three primary areas—the undergraduate dental student, the graduate dental student, and continuing education for the postgraduate student—were addressed by the guidelines. There remains a growing trend to learn more about the use of N_2O and how it can be more useful in today's dental and medical practice. The topic of teaching inhalation sedation is discussed in detail in Chapter 19.

The Anesthesia Machine

Another area requiring improvement was the inhalation sedation unit itself. Significant changes had been made in the method of delivering N_2O-O_2 to the patient since the first clinical use of the agent in 1844. Early in the history of inhalation anesthesia, a bladder bag filled with 100% N_2O was used. A spigot attached to the bag was placed into the patient's mouth, the patient inhaled the gas and lost consciousness, and the procedure was carried out as quickly as was possible.

By 1846 Morton had improved on this method of delivering inhalation anesthetics to the patient. John Snow, in England, devised and first used an inhaler in 1847 that was quite similar to the full-face masks used today in anesthesia.[18]

As has been mentioned in this chapter, one of the major drawbacks to the use of N_2O was the need for the doctor to manufacture the agent himself. The process was cumbersome, and storage of the gas difficult. However, in 1872 the Johnson Brothers, in England, began to produce liquefied N_2O on a commercial basis. Approximately 5 years later, the S.S. White Company of Philadelphia began the marketing of liquefied N_2O cylinders in the United States. They also manufactured an anesthesia device that administered N_2O gas from the cylinder to the patient. The use of N_2O was greatly enhanced by this innovation.

In 1898 Sir Frederick Hewitt manufactured and sold the first devices for delivering N_2O-O_2 anesthesia. Shortly thereafter, the S.S. White Company patented their own similar device. Dr. Charles K. Teter introduced the second N_2O-O_2 anesthesia machine in the United States in 1902. E. I. McKesson perfected the first intermittent-flow N_2O-O_2 anesthesia machine with an accurate means of controlling the percentages of both gases and marketed it in 1910. Also in 1910, the third of the pioneers in the manufacture of anesthesia devices, J. A. Heidbrink, DDS, entered the marketplace. His model "OO" appeared, later followed by the model "T." This device included a reducing valve that served as a flowmeter. By 1918 the four major manufacturers of anesthesia devices in the United States were McKesson, Connell, von Foregger, and Heidbrink.

From the designs of these and other pioneers, the modern anesthesia machine has developed. The inhalation sedation apparatus used today for the administration of N_2O-O_2 is modified from this device (Figure 11-9). The major change required to adapt the anesthesia machine for inhalation sedation was the removal from the unit of all but the O_2 and N_2O gas supplies and flowmeters. However, situations developed in which the cylinder of O_2 became depleted during a procedure, resulting in the delivery of 100% N_2O to the patient. In too many situations serious morbidity and in some cases mortality occurred. In 1976 the American Dental Association's Council on Dental Materials, Instruments, and Equipment adopted standards for the manufacture of inhalation sedation units in the United States.[40] These standards required inhalation sedation devices to incorporate a series of fail-safe devices into the unit. The primary goal of these devices was to prevent the administration of O_2 in a less than atmospheric concentration.

With more and more scientific information being gathered about the effects of the gases used in inhalation sedation, further modification of these units has

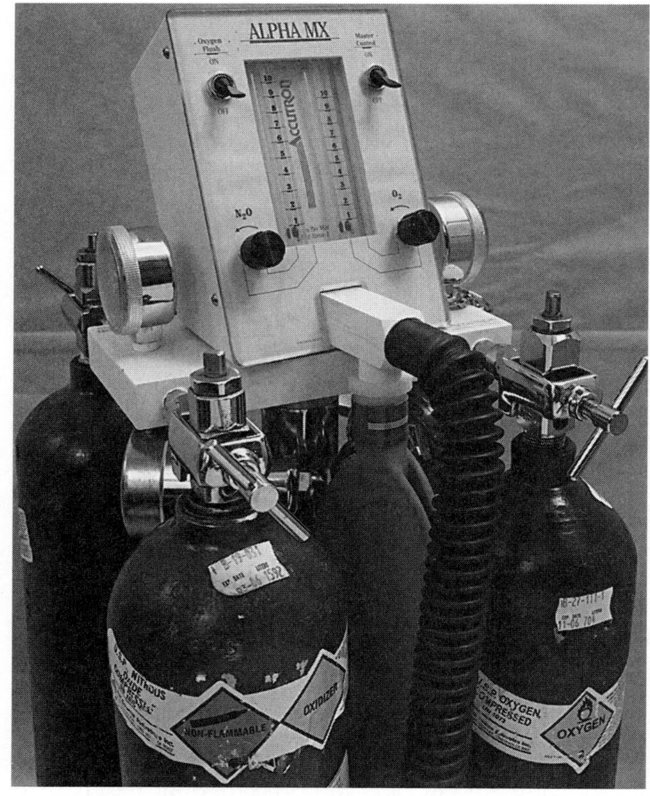

Figure 11-9 Modern inhalation sedation unit.

occurred. For example, in recent years the nasal inhaler has undergone a change in design because of a potential problem associated with the chronic inhalation of trace amounts of N_2O by dental personnel.[41] The scavenging nasal hood has been introduced. Other refinements in the apparatus for the delivery of N_2O-O_2 may be forthcoming as knowledge of the technique and drugs increases.

Since the first edition of this book was published in 1985, I have noticed a significant change in the composition of enrollees in continuing education courses in inhalation sedation. Throughout the 1970s and early 1980s, course participants were almost exclusively dentists and other dental personnel. Only occasionally did other health professionals (physicians, podiatrists) enroll in these programs. Indeed, review of course rosters through 1984 reveals but three nondental health professionals (one physician, two podiatrists) of a total course enrollment of more than 800 "offices."

As mentioned, there is a tremendous growing interest among practitioners across all lines and disciplines of medicine and dentistry about N_2O inhalation sedation. The use of inhalation sedation in dental hygiene has continuously grown in popularity. N_2O is currently being used by dental hygienists in 17 states with the physical presence of a dentist. Hygienists are capitalizing on the comfort afforded patients with use of N_2O for procedures such as scaling and root planing. As we progress through these chapters on inhalation sedation, we review various aspects of nitrous oxide delivery. These include tangential information that will be offered to help the practitioner problem solve and apply inhalation sedation even more creatively. The history of N_2O-O_2 sedation is colorful, interesting, insightful, and potentially helpful inasmuch as we can gain an appreciation for the sacrifices made to make this first anesthetic available to humankind. It has been said, "the only thing new under the sun is the history we have not read."

In the succeeding chapters in this section, we review the indications for inhalation sedation, the pharmacology of N_2O and O_2, techniques of their delivery to patients, and complications associated with its use, as well as the components of the armamentarium. All of the material contained in these chapters was in large part first discovered or developed by the men discussed in this chapter. The history of anesthesia to a very large degree is the history of N_2O.

REFERENCES

1. Lee JA, Atkinson RS: *A synopsis of anesthesia,* ed 5, Baltimore, 1964, Williams & Wilkins.
2. Davy H: Researches, chemical and philosophical; chiefly concerning nitrous oxide, 1800. In Fullmer JZ, ed: *Sir Humphry Davy's published works,* Cambridge, Mass, 1969, Harvard University Press.
3. Cartwright FF: *The English pioneers of anaesthesia (Beddoes, Davy, and Hickman),* Bristol, 1952, J Wright.
4. Hickman HH: A letter on suspended animation, 1824 (pamphlet).
5. Long C: An account of the first use of sulphuric ether by inhalation as an anaesthetic in surgical operations, *South Med Surg J* 1849.
6. Raper HR: *Man against pain,* New York, 1945, Prentice Hall.
7. Fenster JM: *Ether day: the strange tale of America's greatest medical discovery and the haunted man who made it,* New York, 2001, HarperCollins.
8. Archer WH: Chronological history of Horace Wells, discoverer of anesthesia, *Bull Hist Med* 7:1140, 1939.
9. Wells H: Letter, *Br Med J,* May 31:305, 1848.
10. Bankoff G: *The conquest of pain: the story of anesthesia,* London, 1946, MacDonald.
11. Sykes WS: *Essays on the first hundred years of anaesthesia,* vols I and II, Edinburgh, 1961, E & S Livingstone.
12. Driscoll EJ: Dental anesthesiology: its history and continuing evolution, *Anesth Prog* 25:143, 1978.
13. Smith WDA: *Under the influence: a history of nitrous oxide and oxygen anaesthesia,* Park Ridge, Ill, 1982, Wood Library, Museum of Anesthesiology.
14. American Dental Association: Transactions of the fourth annual meeting at Niagara Falls, NY, 1864.
15. Archer WH: Life and letters of Horace Wells, discoverer of anesthesia, *J Am Coll Dent* 11:81, 1944.
16. American Society of Dental Surgeons: Resolutions adopted at Eighth Annual Meeting, *Am J Dent Sci* 9:1848.
17. Greenfield W: Anesthesiology in dentistry: past, present and future, *Anesth Prog* 23:104, 1976.
18. Snow J: *On the inhalation of ether,* London, 1858, J Churchill.
19. Snow J: *On chloroform and other anaesthetics,* London, 1858, J Churchill.
20. Sykes WS, Ellis RH, ed: *Essays on the first hundred years of anaesthesia,* vol III, Edinburgh, 1982, Churchill Livingstone.
21. Levy AG: Sudden death under light chloroform anaesthesia, *J Physiol* 42:3, 1911.
22. *Medical Times,* February 5, 1848, p 317.
23. Thomas KB: Some early papers on dental anaesthesia, *Br Dent J* 116:139, 1964.
24. Fowell S: *A treatise on dentistry,* ed 2, London, 1859, J Mitchell.
25. Tomes J: *A course of lecture notes on dental physiology and surgery,* London, 1848, John Parker.
26. Archer WH: *A manual of dental anesthesia: an illustrated guide for student and practitioner,* Philadelphia, 1952, WB Saunders.
27. Andrews E: The oxygen mixture: a new anesthetic combination, *Chic Med Exam* 9:656, 1868.

28. Bert P: Sur la possibilité d'obtenir, a l'aide du protoxyde de d'azote, une insensibilité de longue durée, et sur l'innocuité de cet anesthétique [Concerning the possibility of obtaining, by the aid of the protoxide of nitrogen, an insensibility of long duration and concerning the innocuousness of that anesthetic], *C R Acad Sci (Paris)* 87:728, 1878.
29. Archer WH: *The history of anesthesia,* Proceedings of the dental centenary celebration, Baltimore, 1940, Waverly Press.
30. Archer WH: The history of anesthesia. In Archer WH, ed: *A manual of dental anesthesia,* Philadelphia, 1958, WB Saunders.
31. Nevin M, Puterbaugh PG: *Conduction, infiltration and general anesthesia in dentistry,* New York, 1923, Dental Items of Interest Publishing.
32. Lippe HT: Nitrous oxide analgesia in cavity preparation, *Temple Dent Rev* 14:7, 1944.
33. Seldin HM: *Practical anesthesia for dental and oral surgery,* ed 3, Philadelphia, 1947, Lea & Febiger.
34. Allison ML, Kinney W, Lynch DF et al: The American Dental Society of Anesthesiology: 1953-1978, *Anesth Prog* 25:9, 1978.
35. Greenfield W: Anesthesiology in dentistry: past, present and future, *Anesth Prog* 23:104, 1976.
36. Langa H: *Relative analgesia in dental practice,* ed 2, Philadelphia, 1976, WB Saunders.
37. Clark MS, Brunick A: *Handbook of nitrous oxide and oxygen sedation,* St Louis, 1999, Mosby.
38. American Dental Association Council on Dental Education: Guidelines for teaching the comprehensive control of pain and anxiety in dentistry, *J Dent Educ* 36:62, 1972.
39. American Dental Association Council on Dental Education: *Guidelines for teaching the comprehensive control of pain and anxiety in dentistry,* section I, Chicago, 1992, The Association.
40. American Dental Association, Council on Dental Materials, Instruments and Equipment: *Revised guidelines for the acceptance program for nitrous oxide-oxygen sedation machines and devices,* Chicago, 1986, The Association.
41. Whitcher C, Zimmerman DC, Piziali RL: Control of occupational exposure to nitrous oxide in the oral surgery office, *J Oral Surg* 36:431, 1978.

CHAPTER 12

Pharmacosedation: Rationale

CHAPTER OUTLINE

The technique of inhalation sedation with nitrous oxide (N_2O) and oxygen (O_2) possesses many significant advantages over other techniques of pharmacosedation. It is my belief that inhalation sedation represents the most nearly "ideal" clinical sedative circumstance. This chapter discusses and demonstrates the indications for use of N_2O-O_2 in dentistry, as well as other constantly expanding branches of medicine (Figure 12-1).

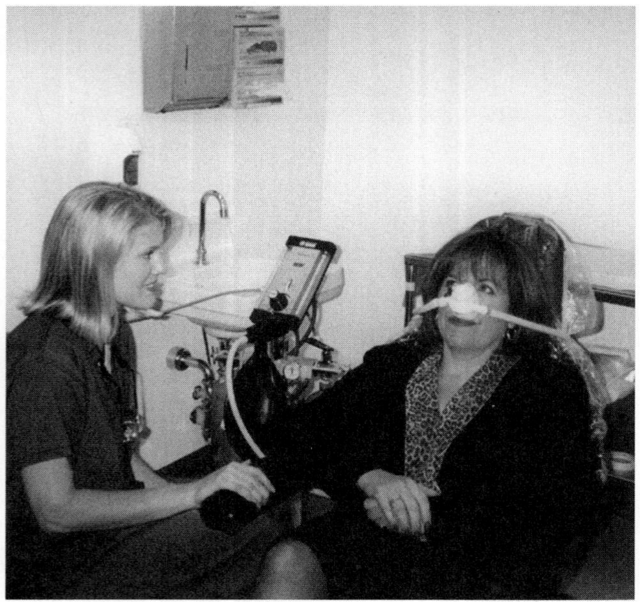

Figure 12-1 Patient receiving inhalation sedation with nitrous oxide and oxygen.

ADVANTAGES

1. The onset of action of inhalation sedation is more rapid than that of oral, rectal, or intramuscular (IM) sedation. The onset of action of intravenous (IV) medications is approximately equal to that of inhalation sedation.

Oral	30-minute onset
Rectal	30-minute onset
IM	10- to 15-minute onset
IV	20-second onset (approximate arm-to-brain circulation time); 1 to 2 minutes for clinical actions to develop
Inhalation	<20 second pulmonary circulation to brain time; 2- to 3-minute onset for clinical actions to develop

2. Peak clinical effect does not develop in most techniques for a considerable time. Although variations do exist, peak clinical actions do not develop for most orally, rectally, and intramuscularly administered drugs for a period of time that makes titration absolutely impossible. Only inhalation and IV drug administration provide peak clinical actions in a time span permitting titration. For the IV route this time-to-peak effect varies with the drug administered, ranging from 1 minute to approximately 20 minutes (e.g., lorazepam).

Oral	60-minute peak action
Rectal	60-minute peak action
IM	30-minute peak action
IV	60-second to 20-minute peak action
Inhalation	3- to 5-minute peak action

3. The depth of sedation achieved with inhalation sedation may be altered from moment to moment, permitting the drug administrator to increase or decrease the depth of sedation. With no other technique of sedation does the administrator have as much control over the clinical actions of the drugs. This degree of control represents a significant safety feature of inhalation sedation.

Oral	Cannot easily deepen or lighten sedation
Rectal	Cannot easily deepen or lighten sedation
IM	Cannot easily deepen or lighten sedation
IV	Sedation level may easily be deepened; however, lessening of sedation is difficult to achieve
Inhalation	Sedation levels *easily* changed either way

4. The duration of action is an important consideration in the selection of a pharmacosedative technique in an outpatient. In situations in which a sedation technique has a relatively fixed duration of clinical activity, dental treatment must be tailored to this, whereas in those techniques with a flexible duration of action, the planned procedure may be of any length, for example, a minute or so for the taking of radiographs or 3 to 4 hours for preparation and impression of multiple abutments for fixed bridgework.

Oral	Fixed duration of action, approximately 2 to 3 hours
Rectal	Fixed duration of action, approximately 2 to 3 hours
IM	Fixed duration of action, approximately 2 to 4 hours, with significant variation by drug
IV	Fixed duration of action, with signifi cant variation by drug Diazepam, midazolam, 45 minutes Promethazine, 90 minutes Pentobarbital, 2 to 4 hours
Inhalation	Duration variable, at discretion of administrator

5. Recovery time from inhalation sedation is rapid and is the most complete of any pharmacosedation technique. Because N_2O is not metabolized by the body, the gas is rapidly and virtually completely eliminated from the body within 3 to 5 minutes. In all other techniques the recovery from sedation is considerably slower.

Oral	Recovery not entirely complete even after 2 to 3 hours
Rectal	Recovery not entirely complete even after 2 to 3 hours
IM	Recovery not entirely complete even after 2 to 3 hours
IV	Recovery not entirely complete even after 2 to 3 hours
Inhalation	Recovery usually complete following 3 to 5 minutes of inhalation of 100% O_2

6. As discussed, titration is the ability to administer small, incremental doses of a drug until a desired clinical action is obtained. In my opinion the ability to titrate a drug represents the greatest safety feature a technique can possess because it permits the drug administrator virtually absolute control over the actions of the drug. Significant drug overdose will not develop in techniques in which titration is possible as long as the administrator does indeed titrate the drug.

Oral	Titration not possible
Rectal	Titration not possible
IM	Titration not possible
IV	Titration possible
Inhalation	Titration possible

7. In an outpatient setting it is advantageous for the patient to be discharged from the office following a procedure with no prohibitions on activities. Unfortunately, because all of the drugs administered for the reduction of fear and anxiety are central nervous system (CNS) depressants, the patient may not be permitted to leave the office unescorted to operate an automobile or to perform tasks requiring mental alertness for a number of hours following the administration of these drugs. To do so is to increase the potential risk to both the patient (physical risk) and the doctor (legal risk). Recovery must be complete, with absolutely no doubt in the mind of the doctor that the patient is able to function normally; if not, the patient should not be permitted to leave the office unescorted.

Oral	Recovery not complete; patient requires escort if less than 3 hours since drug administration
Rectal	Recovery not complete; as usually used in pediatric dentistry, patient will be escorted by parent or guardian
IM	Recovery not complete; patient always requires escort
IV	Recovery not complete; patient always requires escort
Inhalation	Recovery almost always complete; patient usually may be discharged from office alone, with no admonitions about activities

8. No injection is required with inhalation sedation.
9. Inhalation sedation with N_2O-O_2 is safe. Very few side effects are associated with its use, as described in the following chapters.
10. The drugs used in this technique have no adverse effects on the liver, kidneys, brain, or cardiovascular and respiratory systems.
11. Inhalation sedation with N_2O-O_2 can be used instead of local anesthesia in certain procedures. N_2O does possess analgesic properties when given in the usual sedative concentrations. The analgesia produced by a 20% concentration of N_2O is equivalent to that of 10 to 15 mg of morphine. However, the degree of analgesia is quite variable from patient to patient and therefore cannot be relied on to provide all of the pain control required for a procedure. Certain procedures, such as those involving soft tissues (scaling, curettage), may be performed in many instances without using local anesthesia.

DISADVANTAGES

The following are disadvantages associated with N_2O-O_2 inhalation sedation.

1. The initial cost of the equipment required for inhalation sedation is high.
2. The continuing cost of the gases (O_2 and N_2O) used in inhalation sedation is high.
3. The equipment required for inhalation sedation occupies considerable space within the dental surgery suite. Placed in the usual small dental surgery office, a portable N_2O-O_2 unit can be quite cumbersome.
4. N_2O is not a potent agent. When it is used in combination with at least 20% O_2, there will be a small percentage of patients in whom the technique will fail to produce the desired clinical actions. In no circumstance should N_2O ever be

administered with less than 20% O_2. Inhalation sedation with N_2O-O_2 is not a panacea. Failures will occur, primarily because of the lack of potency of the agent.

5. A degree of cooperation is required from the patient. For inhalation sedation to be effective, the patient must be able to inhale the gases through either the nose or the mouth. Should the patient be unable or unwilling to do so, clinical failure will result.
6. All members of the dental staff employing N_2O-O_2 must receive training in its safe and effective use. Ideally, this training is acquired in dental, dental hygiene, or dental assisting school. Postgraduate continuing education courses are also available, but quality varies tremendously in these programs. The guidelines established by the American Dental Association (ADA), the American Dental Society of Anesthesiology (ADSA), and the American Dental Education Association (ADEA) recommend not less than 14 hours of training, to include treatment of dental patients receiving inhalation sedation (see Chapter 19).[1]
7. There is a possibility that chronic exposure to trace amounts of N_2O is deleterious to the health of dental personnel.

INDICATIONS

The primary indications for the use of inhalation sedation are the same as those for other sedative techniques: the management of fear and anxiety, the medically compromised patient, and the management of gagging. Over and above these usual indications, the fact that N_2O-O_2 is as readily controllable as it is permits it to be used for aspects of dental care in which the use of conscious sedation might not usually be considered.

Many procedures that are generally considered nonthreatening or even innocuous might however prove to be extremely traumatic to some patients. Many of these procedures lend themselves quite readily to the use of N_2O-O_2.

Anxiety

The major indication for the use of N_2O-O_2 inhalation sedation in dentistry is, of course, the management of fear and anxiety related to the dental experience. As discussed in the preceding section on the advantages of inhalation sedation, N_2O-O_2 represents the most nearly ideal sedation technique. Were it not for the fact that some persons are not comfortable with the effects of N_2O-O_2, that some others will not achieve clinically adequate sedation at permissible percentages, and that still others are unable to breathe through their noses, inhalation sedation would be the only technique of sedation required for the management of dental anxieties.

Medically Compromised Patients

In recent years the use of N_2O-O_2 has become increasingly important in the management of medically compromised patients. The general evaluation of these patients is discussed in Chapter 4; however, I believe that it is important to review some of these patients and discuss the relevance of their diseases to the use of N_2O-O_2.

Cardiovascular Disease. The use of N_2O-O_2 in patients with cardiovascular disease is one of the most valuable methods of minimizing risk to the patient during dental care. In most, if not all, significant cardiovascular disease states, one factor likely to produce an exacerbation of clinical signs and symptoms is an oxygen deficit in the myocardium. Myocardial ischemia is produced in many patients by an increased cardiovascular workload—an increase in the heart rate and in the force of contraction of the heart. In the patient with an underlying cardiovascular disorder that may be asymptomatic while the patient is at rest (nonstressed), this increased workload of the myocardium, leading to ischemia, may precipitate an acute cardiovascular event.

Because oxygen deficit is responsible for the onset of most anginal episodes, an increased severity of heart failure, cardiac dysrhythmias, and possibly myocardial infarction, any sedative technique that decreases myocardial O_2 requirement will decrease the risk to the patient during dental treatment. Therefore any sedative procedure is appropriate for use in these patients. However, N_2O-O_2 inhalation sedation has several advantages over other techniques: in addition to providing a reduction of anxiety, it also produces an elevation in the pain reaction threshold, as well as providing the myocardium and entire body with a minimum of 30%, but more frequently 50% to 70%, O_2. Therefore, at its very worst, the patient is receiving approximately 50% more O_2 than he or she would from atmospheric air, which has an O_2 content of 20.9%.

I have employed N_2O-O_2 inhalation sedation as an emergency and preoperative agent with great success in patients with angina pectoris, congestive heart failure, severe cardiac dysrhythmias, status post–myocardial infarction, and high blood pressure, as well as other cardiovascular disorders.

The use of N_2O-O_2 in patients with severe cardiovascular disease has received considerable attention in the past 20 years. Emergency medical personnel in Wales and Great Britain have employed a premixed combination of N_2O and O_2 in a ratio of 40% to 60% (Entonox) for the management of pain during an acute myocardial infarction.[2] In the past, management of the pain of a myocardial infarction was achieved through the administration of opioid analgesics. The success of N_2O-O_2 in this life-threatening situation was such that paramedical units in a growing number of areas throughout the United States are today incorporating the use of N_2O-O_2 into their armamentarium (Figure 12-2).[3] In the United States the most commonly used concentration of N_2O to O_2 has been 35% to 65%. At this concentration (available under the proprietary name Dolonox), N_2O has analgesic properties, diminishing or eliminating pain; has sedative properties, helping the victim to relax and become more comfortable, thereby reducing the workload of the myocardium; and provides the patient with 65% O_2—more than three times the volume found in atmospheric air. In a study by Thompson and Lown[2] it was found that 75% of patients receiving 35% N_2O and 65% O_2 during acute myocardial infarction have either a distinct decrease in the severity of their pain (36%) or state that the pain was eliminated entirely (39%). Inhalation sedation with N_2O-O_2 has been found to be the most appropriate technique of sedation for the patient with preexisting cardiovascular disease.

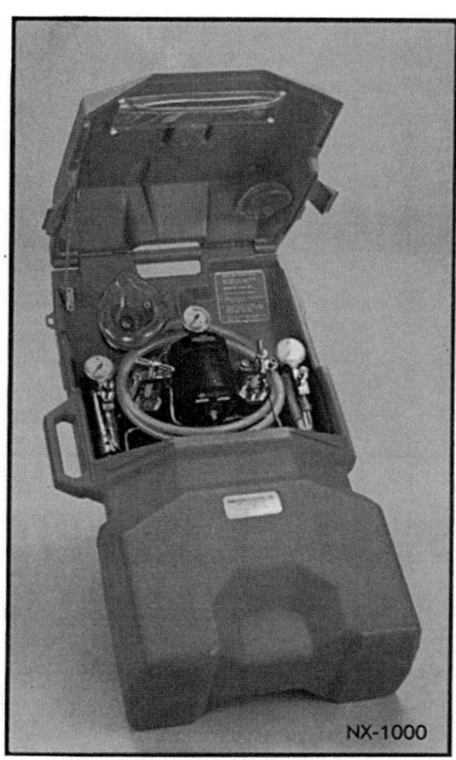

Figure 12-2 Portable nitrous oxide–oxygen unit employed by paramedical personnel.

Respiratory Disease. The use of inhalation anesthetics is frequently contraindicated in patients with acute or chronic respiratory disease. However, N_2O-O_2 is used quite successfully and without untoward incident in many patients with respiratory disease.

Chronic obstructive pulmonary disease (COPD) represents a relative contraindication to the successful use of N_2O-O_2. Although it is possible for the patient to become apneic during the procedure as a result of the elevation of the O_2 level in the blood, this is rarely a clinical finding. In my involvement with the administration of N_2O-O_2 inhalation sedation since 1972, including many patients with respiratory disorders, this situation has never developed. The primary concern with patients with respiratory disease is the potential lack of sedative effect of the N_2O-O_2.

Occasionally, the dentist will receive a medical consultation that states that the use of N_2O-O_2 is contraindicated in asthmatic patients. N_2O may be administered quite safety in patients such as these.[4] The reason behind this medical consultation is the fact that anesthetic gases that are irritating to the respiratory mucosa may precipitate an acute episode of bronchospasm. Many anesthetic gases are in fact contraindicated in asthmatic patients. However, N_2O is a nonirritating vapor that does not exacerbate asthma. The use of sedation in the asthmatic patient is frequently warranted because increased stress is a potential cause of acute exacerbation of their asthma. N_2O-O_2 represents a very effective and safe technique of sedation in these patients.

Patients with chronic nasal obstruction, either from anatomic abnormalities (deviated nasal septum) or pathologic conditions (allergy, upper respiratory tract infection), will be difficult to sedate adequately with gaseous agents. In addition, the potential for the infection of other patients through the use of a nasal hood that has become contaminated should be considered before N_2O-O_2 is administered to patients who are ill.

Cerebrovascular Disease. The post–cerebrovascular accident ("stroke") patient is unable to tolerate levels of O_2 below normal without an increased risk of developing seizure activity or additional neuronal damage. Deep sedation is contraindicated because of the increased (although unlikely) possibility of hypoxia. Whereas other techniques of sedation may be considered for these patients, the one most highly recommended for the status post–cerebrovascular accident patient is N_2O-O_2 inhalation sedation. The major recommendation for this technique is the elevated level of O_2 that is routinely provided to the patient. As it is used in dentistry today, there is little or no likelihood of a hypoxic episode developing.

Hepatic Disease. Hepatic disease, such as cirrhosis or hepatitis, represents a contraindication (either relative or absolute) to the use of many of the drugs discussed in this text because most of them undergo biotransformation in the liver. In the presence of significant hepatic dysfunction, the rate of biotransformation (half-life) of a drug is slowed, potentially resulting in higher plasma levels, which in turn leads to an increase in the drug effect, as well as a prolongation of its clinical activity. However, N_2O does not undergo biotransformation anywhere within the body (see Chapter 13) and may therefore be used without additional risk and with a high probability of success in the patient with hepatic dysfunction.

Epilepsy and Seizure Disorders. As with status post–cerebrovascular accident patients, patients with a history of chronic seizure activity (epilepsy) are more sensitive to hypoxia than are healthy patients. Seizure activity is precipitated more readily in these patients; therefore hypoxia must be guarded against much more scrupulously. N_2O is not epileptogenic (it does not increase the risk of seizures developing) and therefore may be administered to these patients as long as hypoxia is avoided. Increased stress and anxiety have been demonstrated to be precipitating causes of seizures. With the sedation machines available today and adherence to the technique of administering N_2O-O_2 presented in Chapter 15, epilepsy does not represent a contraindication to the use of inhalation sedation.

Pregnancy. N_2O does cross the placenta to the fetus, producing the same degree of CNS depression as in the mother. If delivered in combination with adequate levels of O_2 (greater than 20%), N_2O-O_2 inhalation sedation represents the recommended sedation technique for use during pregnancy. Medical consultation with the patient's physician before its use is suggested.

Allergy. No allergies to N_2O have ever been reported.

Diabetes. Diabetes mellitus does not represent a contraindication to the use of N_2O-O_2.

Gagging

Gagging is a potential problem during many dental procedures, especially in the maxillary palatal and mandibular lingual regions. Although there is no absolute solution to this problem, inhalation sedation with N_2O-O_2 has proved to be highly effective in eliminating or at least minimizing severe gagging. Patients are titrated with N_2O-O_2 to their sedation level, at which point impressions, radiographs, or other procedures may be completed. The use of N_2O-O_2 to diminish the gag reflex may require placing the patient in an upright position for some or all of the procedure. Although this position is not usually recommended during sedation (supine is preferred), some procedures, such as impressions in the maxilla, may require modification of position for increased patient safety. Where other sedation techniques (especially IV sedation) are also effective in decreasing gagging, only N_2O is practical to use for extremely short procedures such as radiographs or impressions.

CONTRAINDICATIONS

There are no absolute contraindications to the administration of N_2O-O_2 inhalation sedation as long as the percentage of O_2 administered with the N_2O is greater than 20% (atmospheric concentration). However, there are several relative contraindications to this technique. A relative contraindication implies that there is an increased potential for an adverse reaction to develop in a certain patient. Although the technique in question may be used, if there exists another technique without this contraindication that would prove to be equally successful, it should be used in place of the contraindicated technique. The following are relative contraindications to N_2O-O_2 inhalation sedation.

Patients with a Compulsive Personality

The use of N_2O-O_2 sedation (or for that matter, any sedation technique) in a person with a compulsive personality would result in a very low probability of success. Persons with compulsive personalities or "take-charge" people are ones who would not like the feeling of "losing control" associated with the use of sedation. These patients will consciously, or more likely subconsciously, "fight" the effects of the drug(s).

Claustrophobic Patients

Inhalation sedation will have a very low success rate in patients who are unable to tolerate the nasal hood or face mask used in the administration of gaseous agents. This is not a problem in patients undergoing general anesthesia because anesthesia may be induced by IV drugs with the face mask applied after unconsciousness is induced; however, sedated patients are, of course, conscious throughout the procedure and, if fearful of the mask, will be unable to become comfortable. The nasal cannula is a possible alternative to the nasal hood in these patients; however, with the increased concern over the inhalation of trace levels of N_2O by dental personnel, the nasal cannula has fallen out of favor (see Chapters 13 and 17).

Children with Severe Behavior Problems

The use of N_2O-O_2 in children who are severely disruptive will usually prove to be futile. A degree of patient cooperation is required for this technique to be successful. Patients must accept the nasal hood and be willing and able to breathe through their noses. Precooperative or noncooperative children (or adult patients with disabilities) will breathe through their mouths, crying, screaming, or moving about in the chair, thus negating the effects of any N_2O they may inhale. Management of these patients is discussed in Chapter 35.

Patients with Severe Personality Disorders

Patients who are under psychiatric care and are receiving psychotropic drugs, usually mood-elevating antidepressants, should be evaluated carefully before the administration of any form of sedation. Although no serious drug-drug interactions develop between N_2O-O_2 and these psychotropic drugs, it may be prudent to avoid altering the consciousness of persons who have but a tenuous grip on reality. Medical consultation before the use of any sedative technique is strongly indicated.

Upper Respiratory Tract Infection or Other Acute Respiratory Conditions

Because N_2O-O_2 must be inhaled through the nose during dental treatment, any respiratory problem preventing the use of the nose as a route of entry for the anesthetic gases represents a relative contraindication to using this technique. The common cold, acute or chronic sinus problems, chronic mouth breathing, allergy, tuberculosis, bronchitis, and cough all represent situations in which the technique of inhalation sedation would best be avoided if possible. Other techniques may be substituted effectively. Aside from the difficulty in achieving sedation when the patient is unable to inhale through the nose, there is the distinct possibility of contaminating the rubber goods of the inhalation sedation unit.

Patients with chronic respiratory or other potentially contagious diseases (tuberculosis, human immunodeficiency virus/acquired immunodeficiency syndrome) who require inhalation sedation may be provided (at cost, of course) with their own "disposable" rubber goods for inhalation sedation. Such disposable systems, consisting of nasal hood, tubing, and reservoir bag, are available at relatively modest cost and will minimize the risk of cross-contamination.

Chronic Obstructive Pulmonary Disease

COPD (e.g., emphysema, chronic bronchitis) represents a relative contraindication to inhalation sedation because of the potential effect of administering a gas mixture enriched with O_2 to these patients, many of whom have chronically elevated CO_2 blood levels. Whereas the usual stimulus for breathing in a healthy person is an increase in the blood CO_2 level, patients with COPD have a diminished or absent ability to respond to this stimulus. In its place the stimulus for breathing in these patients is a lowered blood O_2 content. In the administration of inhalation sedation, an O_2-enriched mixture of gases is always provided, raising the O_2 saturation of the blood. The stimulus for involuntary breathing has now been removed, and the patient should be watched for apnea. In the unconscious patient during general anesthesia, the patient will be closely observed; however, in the conscious patient (e.g., during inhalation sedation), where voluntary control over breathing is maintained, prolonged apnea does not develop. These patients should be evaluated quite carefully before the planned dental treatment to assess their ability to tolerate dental therapy in general. Most of these patients represent American Society of Anesthesiologists (ASA) III or IV risks during dental treatment.

The Patient Who Does Not Want N_2O-O_2

The nasal hood should never be forced onto a patient. Should the adult patient be uncomfortable with the nasal hood, it is often best to remove it. Discuss the reason for the discomfort and, if needed, employ a different sedation technique. Because of the light level of conscious sedation produced by N_2O-O_2, it is impossible to overwhelm a patient with the drug against his or her will.

Pregnancy

The use of sedation in the pregnant patient has been discussed in Chapter 4. It is desirable to avoid the use of any drugs (if possible) during the first trimester to avoid increasing the slight possibility of spontaneous abortion or the development of a fetal malformation that might be related to a drug administered at this time. Drugs may be employed in the second trimester if necessary but, as always, with caution, especially CNS depressants. Of the techniques that might be used for the reduction of anxiety in the pregnant patient, the safest and most recommended is inhalation sedation with N_2O-O_2. N_2O is not metabolized in the body and has virtually no effect on most organ systems, and it is rapidly and almost totally removed from the body within 3 to 5 minutes; these facts provide ample evidence of its superiority over other techniques. In the third trimester of pregnancy the major consideration in determining whether to treat the patient must be the possibility of the patient giving birth during the dental appointment. As the patient nears term, it might be prudent to postpone any nonemergency treatment. However, should emergency care be necessary and if the patient requires sedation, the use of inhalation sedation is suggested. Prior consultation with the patient's obstetrician is advisable whenever sedation is being considered for a pregnant patient.

Besides the three major indications for the use of inhalation sedation—anxiety, medically compromised patient, and gagging—there are a multitude of uses for this technique in other areas of dentistry, including procedures that are usually considered too minor or too short to employ sedation. Very often, the doctor or hygienist will advise a patient that the procedure will "hurt just a little." It is this type of procedure that is appropriate for the use of inhalation sedation.

RESTORATIVE DENTISTRY

Initial Dental Examination

Patients who have come to the dental office in pain may be extremely uncomfortable during the initial examination because of the sensitivity of their soft tissues or teeth. Sedation with N_2O-O_2 and the elevation in pain threshold accompanying it will make this potentially traumatic procedure more tolerable for the patient.

Removal of Provisional Crowns or Bridges

The removal of provisional crowns or bridges from vital teeth is often done without the benefit of local anesthesia because the procedure is short and associated with a minimum of discomfort. This discomfort may be eliminated or minimized through the use of N_2O-O_2. The drying and cleansing of the prepared vital teeth for the cementation of crowns or bridges is also an appropriate area for the use of N_2O-O_2 sedation.

Occlusal Adjustment

Occlusal adjustment of crowns, bridges, or natural teeth rarely requires the use of local anesthesia. There are many patients, however, who are quite uncomfortable during this procedure. The sound of the drill or the vibration of the bur on the tooth makes some patients extremely tense. Sedation with N_2O-O_2 can eliminate this response in most patients.

Insertion of Matrix Bands or Wedges

The insertion of matrix bands or wedges between teeth prior to the placement of a restoration may be uncomfortable for the patient if soft tissue anesthesia is not present. Sedation with N_2O-O_2 provides soft tissue anesthesia in many patients, thus making this procedure less traumatic.

PERIODONTICS AND DENTAL HYGIENE

Within the specialty of periodontology there is a need for sedation. Surgical procedures in general are more anxiety producing than more routine nonsurgical procedures. The use of inhalation sedation with N_2O-O_2 is especially recommended in periodontics, primarily in its nonsurgical aspect, for in a significant percentage of patients a degree of soft tissue analgesia will be noted, helping make the procedure less traumatic.

Initial Periodontal Examination

The initial periodontal examination and probing can be quite traumatic to patients, especially patients in whom significant periodontal disease is present. Inflamed, sensitive soft tissues and teeth with deep periodontal pockets will be extremely sensitive during this examination. Inhalation sedation provides both a relaxed patient and a degree of soft tissue analgesia, which ranges from the total loss of sensation in these tissues to decreased sensitivity so that, although the patient still feels the pain, it no longer bothers her or him.

Scaling, Curettage, and Root Planing

One of the most important uses of N_2O-O_2 within periodontics is for scaling, curettage, and root planing. As mentioned, most patients receiving N_2O-O_2 at sedative levels will develop a degree of soft tissue analgesia. Scaling, curettage, and root planing are three procedures that, although not normally traumatic, may be so on occasion. The administration of local anesthesia is one means of alleviating this discomfort; however, N_2O-O_2 offers the patient and doctor or hygienist a more pleasant means of achieving essentially the same goal with a technique that is almost immediately reversible on completion of the procedure. A growing number of states in the United States permit trained registered dental hygienists to administer N_2O-O_2 to their patients. The response from hygienists, doctors, and patients has been almost universally positive.

Emergency Management of Necrotizing Ulcerative Gingivitis

The management of necrotizing ulcerative gingivitis (NUG) requires debridement of periodontal soft tissues that are extremely sensitive, a situation that can be greatly altered to the benefit of the patient and doctor through the use of N_2O-O_2.

Use of Ultrasonic Instruments

Ultrasonic instruments are commonly used during periodontal procedures to aid in the removal of calculus from teeth. Some patients may find the use of these devices threatening and uncomfortable. Sedation with N_2O-O_2 is a means of eliminating this fear for most patients.

Periodontal Surgery

Patients facing periodontal surgery often request the use of sedation because of the nature and length of the surgical procedure. Inhalation sedation with N_2O-O_2 is an appropriate procedure for many of these patients, although IV sedation is also commonly used during periodontal surgery.

ORAL AND MAXILLOFACIAL SURGERY

Lengthy Surgical Procedures

As discussed in the preceding paragraph, N_2O-O_2 sedation is an acceptable technique for use in the patient undergoing any lengthy procedure as a means of helping make the procedure more tolerable and for providing analgesia.

Management of Abscesses

When an incision and drainage (I & D) procedure is planned to help relieve the discomfort of an abscess, it is often difficult to achieve adequate pain control through the administration of local anesthetics, primarily because of the change in tissue pH brought about by the formation of purulent material within the infected area. Inhalation sedation with N_2O-O_2 may be used to advantage in this situation because of its tendency to provide a degree of soft tissue analgesia. Titration of the patient to the usual sedative level will almost always provide a degree of soft tissue analgesia sufficient to permit the I & D procedure to be completed in comfort or with a minimum of discomfort.

Management of Postoperative Complications

Inhalation sedation can be of great benefit in the management of localized osteitis (dry socket). Localized osteitis most commonly occurs following extraction of third molars, and its management requires irrigation of the socket and placement of medicated packs into the socket to cover the exposed bone. Local anesthesia is not always used for this procedure, which may produce some patient discomfort. Inhalation sedation can provide a degree of sedation and analgesia for the brief period necessary to complete the irrigation and packing of the extraction site.

Suture Removal

Another potential postoperative use for N_2O-O_2 is as an aid in the removal of sutures, although it is not normally required for this procedure. However, there are occasions when sutures are difficult to locate, and there also is a potential for the scissors to irritate the soft tissues as the sutures are being sought. Inhalation sedation is an excellent means of minimizing potential discomfort.

ENDODONTICS

Clinically, adequate pain control in endodontically involved teeth, although not usually a problem, may occasionally prove to be difficult to achieve. Unfortunately, there are no panaceas. An aid to achieving adequate pain control in such cases, however, is N_2O-O_2 sedation. Although the discomfort involved in the opening of a "hot" tooth may not be entirely eliminated, N_2O will raise the pain reaction threshold, thereby modifying the patient's response to it so that the patient, although still aware of her or his pain, is no longer bothered by it.

Rubber Dam Clamps

The placement of a rubber dam clamp on the neck of an endodontically involved tooth is almost always entirely atraumatic. However, when the clinical crown of a tooth is inadequate to support the clamp, tissue clamping may be required. Either local anesthesia or N_2O-O_2 inhalation sedation may be employed to alleviate patient discomfort in this procedure.

Gaining Access to the Pulp Chamber

It may be difficult to achieve adequate pulpal anesthesia in the vital tooth about to undergo pulpal therapy. As the endodontic access preparation nears the pulp chamber, the patient experiences greater and greater discomfort. Once the pulp chamber has been entered, an intrapulpal injection may be administered that will usually eliminate, once and for all, any further discomfort. However, the greatest problem may be in reaching the point at which an intrapulpal injection can be administered. Should the patient experience great discomfort as the preparation approaches the pulp chamber, N_2O-O_2 inhalation sedation may be administered to raise the pain reaction threshold, thereby modifying (although not usually eliminating) the discomfort experienced by the patient.

Instrumenting Canals

Following extirpation of pulpal tissues, the endodontically involved tooth must be prepared for filling. During instrumentation, local anesthetics might not be used because there should be no discomfort, or at the very most minimal discomfort. Some patients, however, may be quite uncomfortable, and for them the administration of local anesthesia and/or N_2O-O_2 is recommended.

Filling of Root Canals

As in the instrumentation of the root canal, discomfort is usually nonexistent or at most only minimal during the filling of root canals; therefore local anesthesia is rarely used. Should patient discomfort or anxiety be present, N_2O-O_2 administration is recommended.

FIXED PROSTHODONTICS

Impression Taking

Inhalation sedation may be valuable in two parts of the impression-taking process. First, if local anesthesia has not been administered, N_2O-O_2, through its ability to elevate the pain reaction threshold, will enable the patient to tolerate better any discomfort associated with the procedure. Second, N_2O-O_2 will aid in diminishing the gag reflex, so there will be little or no difficulty in placing the impression materials and trays.

The gingival retraction cord is placed into the sulcus of abutment teeth before taking impressions to aid in visualizing and gaining access to the margins of the impression. In the absence of local anesthesia, packing of retraction cord may prove to be uncomfortable for the patient, a situation that can be minimized or eliminated by N_2O-O_2.

Removal of Provisional Crowns and Bridges

It is not uncommon for provisional crowns and bridges to be removed without local anesthesia. This will precede the taking of impressions, the trying-in of crowns and bridges, and their cementation. The removal of excess cement from a vital tooth, as well as its drying before impressions or cementation, may be associated with a degree of discomfort. This sensitivity may be decreased or eliminated with N_2O-O_2.

Adjustment of Castings

After provisional crowns and bridges are removed, the cast crowns and bridges will be tried in and, if necessary, adjusted. This process may be uncomfortable for some patients, especially if the abutment teeth are vital and if local anesthesia has not been administered (as is often the case). Occlusal adjustment of these castings may produce intense vibration and noise, which may bother the patient. Sedation with N_2O-O_2 is recommended in these situations.

REMOVABLE PROSTHODONTICS

Preparation of Abutment Teeth

Unlike fixed prosthodontics, in which pain control with local anesthetics is normally required for the preparation of abutment teeth, there is usually a minimum of discomfort associated with the preparation of teeth for removable prostheses. Local anesthesia is rarely required for this process, yet some patients will experience a degree of tooth sensitivity or anxiety related to this procedure. Inhalation sedation with N_2O-O_2 is an appropriate means of managing any anxiety or discomfort associated with preparing teeth for the removal of prosthodontic appliances.

Determination of Centric Relationships

Although it is not a muscle-relaxing drug combination, N_2O-O_2 can aid in determining centric relationship in a patient having difficulty relaxing his or her muscles by helping the patient relax psychologically, thereby taking his or her mind off the procedure and permitting a more accurate tracing of centric relationship.

Occlusal Adjustments and Impression Taking

As in fixed prosthodontics, N_2O-O_2 inhalation sedation may prove to be a valuable help in adjusting occlusion and taking impressions for removable prostheses.

Fitting of Immediate Dentures

Immediate dentures are placed into the patient's mouth immediately after the extraction of teeth. The tissues in the oral cavity at that time are usually well anesthetized, and there is no discomfort during this procedure. However, at subsequent visits the removal of the immediate full denture may prove to be quite uncomfortable because the underlying soft tissues may have not yet fully healed and there may be areas of tissue irritation from the denture itself. When used at this time, N_2O-O_2 sedation can benefit both the patient and the doctor.

ORAL RADIOLOGY

Although N_2O-O_2 is not historically used in oral radiology, there are some scenarios during which its use may prove beneficial. The use of N_2O with the placement of intraoral films can be highly effective in eliminating or at least minimizing the gag reflex. Patients with limiting anatomy such as shallow palates, exostosis, or trauma can also benefit from reduced pain. The previously mentioned indications such as anxiety and managing appropriate medically compromised patients also apply to oral radiology. It is worth noting that proper film placement and tubing adjustment must be monitored to prevent shadowing in radiographs.

ORTHODONTICS

The need for sedation and pain control is minimal in most orthodontic procedures, so much so that many orthodontists rarely, if ever, administer local anesthetics. However, there are occasions when the use of sedation for a brief time may prove to be quite beneficial. These include impression taking, in which excessive gagging can be minimized, and the placement or removal of bands and wires, in which soft tissue analgesia produced by the N_2O-O_2 can eliminate or modify any discomfort.

PEDIATRIC DENTISTRY

Inhalation sedation with N_2O-O_2 is one of the most valuable sedative techniques available for use in children. The range of procedures in which the use of this technique is appropriate is unlimited. The indications for inhalation sedation in children are the same as those for adults. One complicating factor to be considered is that in order for inhalation sedation to be effective, the patient must be willing to accept the nasal hood and to breathe through his or her nose. Unfortunately, the patient who presents a more severe management problem may be unwilling to accept the nasal hood, condemning the technique to failure. The use of N_2O-O_2 inhalation sedation in pediatric dentistry is discussed in greater detail in Chapters 15 and 35.

As new demands and treatment emphasis change within the dental profession, there will most certainly be broader applications for using inhalation sedation to reduce anxiety and provide pain relief to our patients. As the population ages, there will be a larger pool of potential patients who will benefit from a noninvasive fully reversible agent such as N_2O. We are limited only by our imagination. As we have seen comparatively, N_2O has unique and distinct advantages that are not easily matched. Surely with consideration of patient escort, cost, recovery time, training, and ease of administration, N_2O is superior to other techniques of pharmacosedation.

REFERENCES

1. American Dental Association, Council on Dental Education: *Guidelines for teaching the comprehensive control of pain and anxiety in dentistry,* part III, Chicago, 1992, The Association.
2. Thompson PL, Lown B: Nitrous oxide as an analgesic in acute myocardial infarction, *JAMA* 235:924, 1976.
3. O'Leary U, Puglia C, Friehling TD et al: Nitrous oxide anesthesia in patients with ischemic chest discomfort: effect on beta-endorphins, *J Clin Pharmacol* 27:957, 1987.
4. Rogers MC, Tinker JH, Covino BG et al: *Principles and practice of anesthesiology,* St Louis, 1993, Mosby.

CHAPTER 13

Pharmacology, Anatomy, and Physiology

CHAPTER OUTLINE

PHARMACOLOGY

NITROUS OXIDE

Preparation

Nitrous oxide (N_2O, nitrogen monoxide) is prepared commercially through the heating of ammonium nitrate crystals to 240° C, at which point the ammonium nitrate decomposes into N_2O and H_2O.

The gas is then chemically scrubbed to remove any alkaline and acid substances and is then compressed in stages so that the less easily liquefied gases such as N_2 and O_2 are separated out. Finally, it is compressed and stored in metal cylinders, in which approximately 30% of the N_2O in the full cylinder is liquefied. According to the *U.S. Pharmacopeia*, N_2O must be 97% pure; however, with the manufacturing processes in use today, the gas usually approaches a purity of 99.5% (Figure 13-1).[1]

$$NH_4NO_3 \xrightarrow[240°C]{heat} N_2O + 2H_2O$$

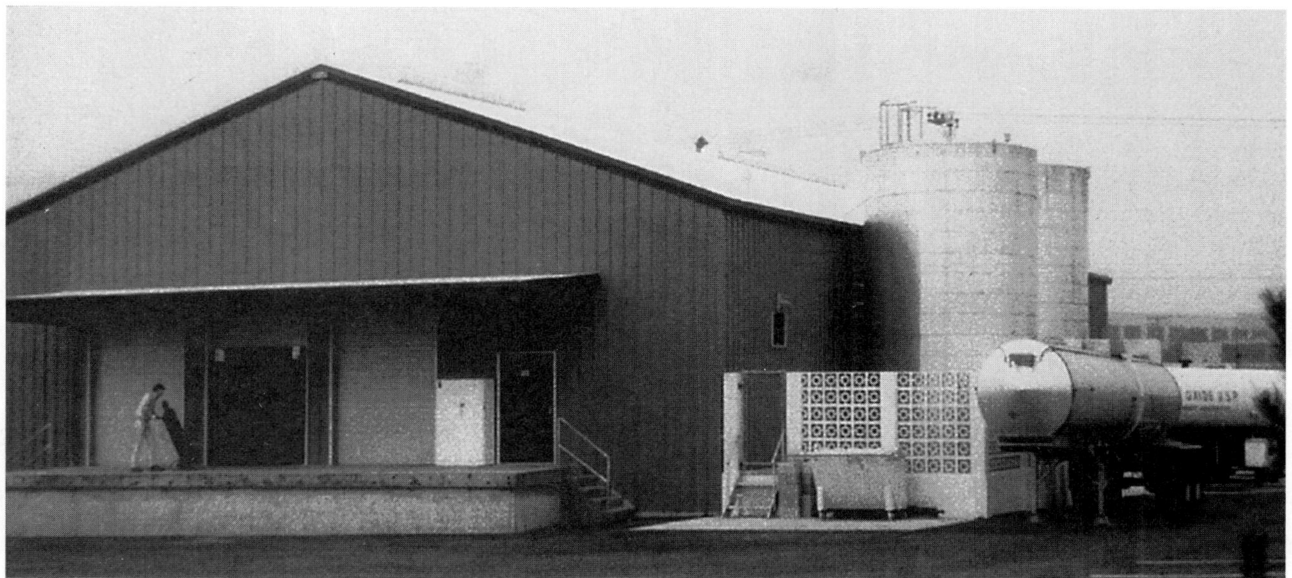

Figure 13-1 A typical manufacturing plant in which nitrous oxide is prepared.

The most common impurities associated with the manufacture of N_2O are nitrogen (N_2), nitric oxide (NO), nitrogen dioxide (NO_2), ammonia (NH_4), water vapor, and carbon monoxide (CO). NO is the most dangerous impurity because, like CO, it may combine with hemoglobin and prevent the absorption of O_2, or it may react with water vapor to form acids that may damage the pulmonary epithelium and produce pulmonary edema. NO is formed when N_2O is heated above 450° C.

As prepared, N_2O is anhydrous. The absence of water in the gas is of importance because water vapor would freeze as it passes through the reducing valve (see Chapter 14), leading to a drop in the gas pressure.

Properties

Physical Properties. N_2O is a nonirritating, sweet-smelling, colorless gas. It is the only nonorganic compound other than CO_2 that has any central nervous system (CNS) depressant properties and is the only inorganic gas used to produce anesthesia in humans. The molecular weight of N_2O is 44, and its specific gravity is 1.53, compared with that of air, which is 1.

N_2O gas is converted to a clear and colorless liquid at 28° C at 50 atm of pressure. The boiling point of N_2O is –89° C. Its oil-water solubility coefficient is 3.2, and the blood-gas solubility coefficient is 0.47.

Chemical Properties. N_2O is stable under pressure at usual temperatures. However, NO is formed when N_2O is heated above 450° C. Marketed in cylinders as a liquid under pressure (vapor pressure at room temperature is 50 atm), N_2O returns to the gaseous state as it is released from the cylinder. An interesting phenomenon occurs as the N_2O exits the cylinder. The walls of the cylinder become cold, and in some instances frost may be evident around the exit portal of the gas. This occurs because the liquid N_2O requires heat for vaporization into the gaseous state. The heat required for vaporization is obtained from the walls of the metal cylinder and from the surrounding air, with the result that the cylinder becomes cool to the touch.

Solubility. N_2O is relatively insoluble in the blood (its blood-gas solubility coefficient is 0.47 at 37° C) and is carried in the blood in physical solution only, not combining with any blood elements. The oxygen in the N_2O molecule is not available for use by the tissues because N_2O does not break down in the body.

Solubility is a term used to describe how a gas is distributed between two media, for example, gas and blood. If the concentration of an anesthetic gas in blood is 2 volumes percent, and this is in equilibrium with a concentration in the alveolus of 1 volume percent, the blood-gas solubility would be 2.

When an anesthetic gas is first inspired, blood entering the alveolus by the pulmonary artery contains none of it. When reaching the pulmonary capillary, the blood is suddenly exposed to the tension of the gas present in the alveolus. If the gas is totally insoluble in the blood (blood/gas partition coefficient of 0), then none of the agent will be taken up by the circulation and the alveolar concentration will rise rapidly and will soon equal the inspired concentration (Figure 13-2).

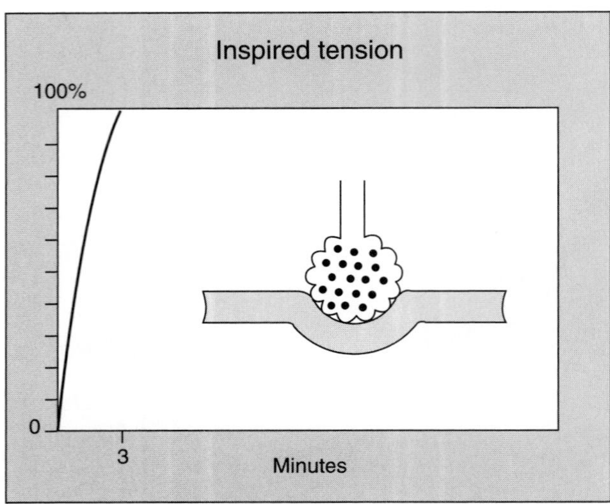

Figure 13-2 Primary saturation of a gaseous agent with a blood-gas solubility coefficient of 0.00 (totally insoluble) occurs within a very brief period. Both onset and recovery are extremely rapid.

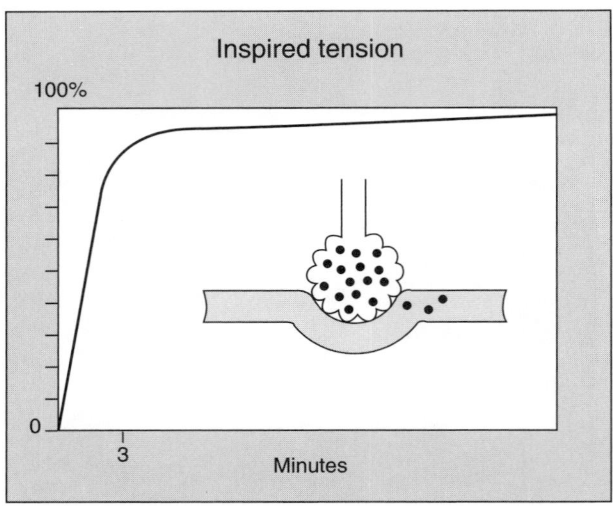

Figure 13-3 Nitrous oxide, with a blood-gas solubility coefficient of 0.47 (relatively insoluble), demonstrates both rapid onset and rapid recovery. Primary saturation of blood occurs within 3 to 5 minutes.

If, on the other hand, the anesthetic is slightly soluble in blood, then only small quantities will be carried by the bloodstream. Alveolar concentration will again rise rapidly (Figure 13-3). Because alveolar concentration determines the tension of the anesthetic in the arterial circulation, the tension will also rise rapidly, even though only a small volume of the agent is present in the blood. As the blood travels through the various tissues of the body, the anesthetic is given up and the venous blood returns to the lungs with a decreased anesthetic gas tension.

N_2O and cyclopropane are examples of anesthetic gases with low blood solubility (Table 13-1). On inhalation, these gases rapidly diffuse across the alveolar membrane into the blood. Because of their poor blood solubility, only a small quantity is absorbed and the alveolar tension rises rapidly so that the tension of the gas in the blood is also increased quickly (see Figure 13-3). Because of the rich cerebral blood supply, the tension of these gases within the brain also rises rapidly and the onset of clinical actions is quickly apparent. Likewise, the rate of recovery from sedation or anesthesia produced by these gases is equally rapid once delivery of the anesthetic ceases.[2,3]

TABLE 13-1 Blood-Gas Partition Coefficients of Inhalation Anesthetics

Agent	Blood-Gas Solubility Coefficient
Cyclopropane	0.42
Nitrous oxide	0.47
Fluroxene	1.37
Isoflurane	1.40
Enflurane	1.91
Halothane	2.36
Trichloroethylene	9.15
Chloroform	10.30
Diethyl ether	12.10
Methoxyflurane	13.00

Conversely, gases with high blood solubility require longer periods of time for the onset of action to develop. Large volumes of the gas are absorbed by the blood (as by a piece of absorbent paper) so that the alveolar tension rises quite slowly (Figure 13-4). Tension of the gas within the blood also rises slowly in this case, and the induction of sedation or anesthesia is noticeably slower, as is the return to the preanesthetic state after termination of drug administration.

N_2O is neither flammable nor explosive. However, it will support combustion of other agents, even in the absence of oxygen, because at temperatures above 450° C N_2O breaks down into N_2 and O_2.

Potency

N_2O is the least potent of the anesthetic gases; however, it remains the most frequently administered inhalation anesthetic. At one time it was thought that any anesthetic effects of N_2O were a result of the exclusion of O_2 from cells in the brain because N_2O is 35 times more soluble in plasma than N_2 and 100 times more soluble than O_2.[4] It has since been demonstrated that N_2O can, in the presence of adequate O_2, produce CNS depression. Stage II anesthesia (delirium) is often produced if the patient is not monitored properly.

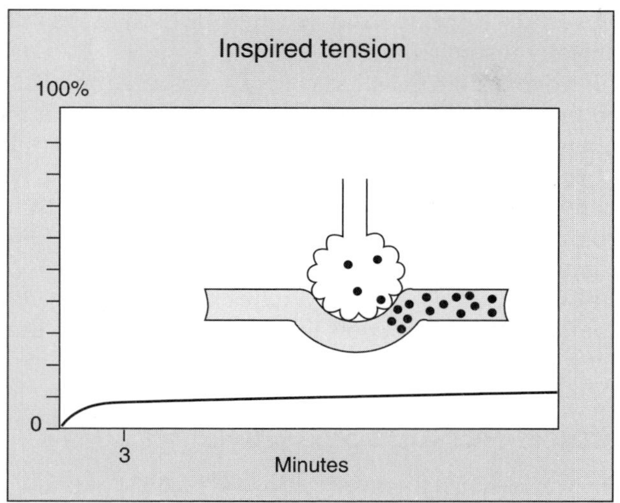

Figure 13-4 Primary saturation of a gaseous agent with a high blood-gas solubility coefficient (quite soluble) occurs quite slowly. Both onset and clinical recovery are prolonged. Methoxyflurane is an example of a very soluble agent.

With a MAC (the minimal alveolar concentration of anesthetic that prevents movement in 50% of subjects in response to a standard surgical incision) of 105%, N_2O is unable to produce adequate anesthesia unless it is administered under hyperbaric conditions. More realistically, surgical-depth anesthesia is usually not obtainable unless a more potent inhalation or intravenous (IV) anesthetic is combined with N_2O. Such IV agents include the barbiturates and opioids, and inhalation anesthetics include halothane, isoflurane, and enflurane. These are discussed in Section VI.

That N_2O in subanesthetic doses produces analgesia, a change in the patient's perception of pain, is no longer doubted. It is estimated that a 20% : 80% mixture of N_2O-O_2 produces the analgesic effectiveness of 10 to 15 mg of morphine.[5] The optimal concentration of N_2O for the production of analgesia while still maintaining patient cooperation is approximately 35%. However, biologic variability can significantly alter these figures in individual patients.

Pharmacology

After N_2O is inspired through the mouth and/or nose, the gas is transported through the respiratory tract into alveolar sacs, where it is rapidly absorbed into the pulmonary circulation. Because of the high inspired concentration of N_2O and the large gradient of N_2O between the alveolar sacs and the blood, up to 1000 ml of N_2O may be absorbed every minute. N_2O replaces N_2 in the blood, the N_2 being eliminated as the N_2O-O_2 mixture is inhaled. Because N_2O is 35 times as soluble in the blood as the N_2 it replaces, large volumes of N_2O may be absorbed over prolonged periods of administration.[4,6]

Potential changes may occur within air-filled body cavities during the administration of N_2O because of the extent of its absorption. During the induction of N_2O-O_2 sedation or anesthesia and during long procedures, N_2O enters a closed air-filled space 35 times more rapidly than N_2 leaves the cavity. This produces an increase in the pressure or volume of that cavity or space. Specific examples of this include increased intestinal distention if bowel obstruction is present, increased pressure in the pleural space aggravating a pneumothorax, and expansion of the middle ear airspace to the point of actually displacing a tympanoplasty graft.[7]

Because of its rapid uptake, two interesting phenomena—the so-called concentration effect and the second-gas effect—are seen when N_2O is administered. The *concentration effect* occurs when high concentrations of a gas are administered. The higher the concentration of the gas inhaled, the more rapidly arterial tension of the gas increases. For example, a patient receiving N_2O-O_2 in a ratio of 75% : 25% will absorb up to 1000 ml/min of N_2O during the initial stages of induction. As the volume of N_2O is removed from the lungs into the blood, fresh gas is literally sucked up into the lung from the anesthesia machine, thereby increasing the rate at which the N_2O arterial tension increases. If, however, a patient receives only 10% N_2O (a figure more appropriate in dentistry than 75%), the uptake of N_2O by the blood will be only 150 ml/min, which results in no significant change in the rate at which the agent is absorbed or the rate of rise of N_2O arterial tension.[8]

The *second-gas effect* occurs when a second inhalation anesthetic is administered along with N_2O-O_2. The second-gas effect is also related to the rapid uptake of as much as 1000 ml/min of N_2O-O_2 during the induction of anesthesia. Because of the extremely rapid uptake of a large volume of N_2O, a form of vacuum develops in the alveoli that forces even more fresh gas (N_2O-O_2 plus other inhalation anesthetics) into the lungs. For example, if halothane (1%) is administered along with N_2O-O_2 in a ratio of 75% : 25%, its uptake will be more rapid than predicted. This is the second-gas effect.[9]

N_2O is absorbed rapidly from the alveolar sacs into the pulmonary circulation. Primary saturation of the blood and brain with N_2O is accomplished by the displacement of N_2 from the alveoli and the blood and occurs within 3 to 5 minutes of the onset of N_2O-O_2 administration.[10] Clinically, this is significant because the patient should be permitted to remain (ideally) at a given level of N_2O for 3 to 5 minutes before the inspired N_2O concentration is increased. This permits the full clinical effect of the given concentration of N_2O to develop before additional gas is added. In actual clinical practice, the 3- to 5-minute wait is not necessary. A thorough discussion is presented in Chapter 15. Tissues with a greater blood flow, including the brain, heart, liver, and kidneys, will receive more N_2O and consequently absorb greater volumes of the gas. The remaining tissues, with a relatively poor blood supply, fat, muscle, and connective tissues, absorb only a small portion of N_2O until primary saturation is completed. At this time these tissues play a predominant role in N_2O absorption. Because the uptake and absorption of N_2O by these tissues is slow (denitrogenation may require 6 to 7 hours), there is no reservoir of N_2O present in them to impede recovery when N_2O delivery is terminated.

For years it was believed that N_2O did not undergo biotransformation in the body. However, it is demonstrated that anaerobic bacteria in the bowel metabolize N_2O through a reductive pathway with the production of free radicals. There is no convincing evidence that these free radicals cause any specific organ damage.[11] Despite this, the vast majority of inhaled N_2O is exhaled through the lungs within 3 to 5 minutes after termination of its delivery. Approximately 1% of the inhaled N_2O will be eliminated more slowly (over 24 hours) through the lungs and skin.[12]

At the completion of the procedure, the N_2O flow is terminated. N_2O diffuses out of the blood and into the alveoli as rapidly as it diffused into the blood during induction. If the patient is allowed to breathe atmospheric air at this time, a phenomenon known as *diffusion hypoxia* (and the Fick principle) may develop.[13] Diffusion hypoxia is responsible for most reports of headache, nausea, and lethargy occurring after N_2O administration—a hangover effect. The alveoli of the patient breathing atmospheric air become filled with a mixture of N_2, O_2, CO_2, water vapor, and N_2O. During the first few minutes the patient breathes atmospheric air, large volumes of N_2O diffuse through the blood into the lungs and are exhaled. As much as 1500 ml of N_2O may be exhaled in the first minute by a patient having breathed N_2O-O_2 in a ratio of 75% : 25%. This figure falls to 1200 ml in the second minute and 1000 ml in the third. The concentration effect, discussed previously, is now reversed, and gases rush out of the lungs. More CO_2 is removed from the blood than usual because of this effect, lowering the CO_2 tension of the blood. Decreased CO_2 tension of the blood reduces the stimulus for breathing and produces a depression of respiration.

More important, the rapid diffusion of large volumes of N_2O into the alveoli produces a significant dilution of the O_2 present. In the normal alveolus approximately 14% O_2 is present. This may be reduced to as little as 10% during the first few minutes after termination of N_2O flow. Hypoxia results, producing headache, nausea, and lethargy.

The adverse effects of diffusion hypoxia may be prevented through the routine administration of 100% O_2 for a minimum of 3 to 5 minutes at the termination of the procedure.[14] After N_2O-O_2 inhalation sedation as usually employed in dentistry, diffusion hypoxia is unlikely to develop, and when it does, it is usually clinically insignificant.

Recovery from the effects of N_2O is usually rapid and complete. If in the opinion of the drug administrator the patient has fully recovered, the patient may be permitted to leave the office unescorted, to drive his or her automobile, and to return to normal activities with no prohibitions. This vitally important aspect of N_2O-O_2 sedation is discussed thoroughly in Chapter 15.

N_2O is nonallergenic. There has never been a reported allergic reaction to N_2O. It is less toxic than any other inhalation anesthetic.

Central Nervous System

The actual mechanism of action of N_2O is unknown, but almost all forms of sensation are depressed (sight, hearing, touch, and pain). Memory is affected to a minimal degree, as is the ability to concentrate or perform acts requiring intelligence.[15] When administered in conjunction with physiologic levels of oxygen (greater than 20%), N_2O produces a mild depression of the CNS, primarily the cerebral cortex. At therapeutic levels, N_2O does not exert any other actions on the CNS. The area postrema (the vomiting center) of the medulla is not affected by N_2O unless hypoxia or anoxia is present. Nausea and vomiting occurring after the administration of N_2O are uncommon in the absence of anoxia or hypoxia.[16]

Cardiovascular System

A slight depression of myocardial contraction is produced at a ratio of 80% N_2O : 20% O_2 through a direct action of the drug on the heart.[17] The response of vascular smooth muscle to norepinephrine is slightly increased at this level. At levels below this ratio, there is no clinically significant effect on the cardiovascular system.

No changes in the heart rate or cardiac output are directly attributable to N_2O. In the absence of hypoxia or hypercarbia, blood pressure remains stable with an insignificant drop as sedation continues.[18] Cutaneous vasodilation is observed, which produces a degree of flushing and perspiration.[19] The vasodilation can be used to clinical advantage to facilitate venipuncture in patients who are apprehensive or in whom superficial veins are difficult to locate.

Respiratory System

N_2O is not irritating to the pulmonary epithelium; it may therefore be administered to patients with asthma with no increased risk of bronchospasm.[20] Changes in respiratory rate or depth are more likely to result from the sedative relief of anxiety (slower, deeper) or the approach of the excitement stage (rapid, shallow) rather than through a direct action of N_2O on the respiratory system. The resting respiratory minute volume is slightly elevated at a ratio of N_2O-O_2 of 50% : 50% with no effect on the respiratory response to CO_2.[21]

Gastrointestinal Tract

N_2O has no clinically significant actions on the gastrointestinal tract or any organs. In the presence of hepatic dysfunction, N_2O may still be used to effect with no increased risk of overdosage or adverse reaction.[22]

Kidneys

N_2O exerts no significant effects on the kidneys or on the volume and composition of urine.[23]

Hematopoiesis

N_2O inhibits the actions of methionine synthetase, an enzyme involved in vitamin B_{12} metabolism, leading to impaired bone marrow function.[24] This can affect deoxyribonucleic acid (DNA) synthesis, producing a picture similar to pernicious anemia in laboratory animals exposed to N_2O for prolonged periods. Long-term exposure to N_2O (as in the management of tetanus) can produce transient bone marrow depression. All reported cases have involved exposure to N_2O for more than 24 hours.[25,26]

The effects of repeated short-term exposure to N_2O are of greater concern. A neuropathy resembling vitamin B_{12} deficiency has been reported in dentists using N_2O regularly in their practices and in persons abusing the drug.[27] It is thought that this is a result of the combination of N_2O's actions on methionine synthetase and of the long-term exposure to unusually high N_2O concentrations as the dental team operates in the oral cavity.[28] In addition, there is a consistent finding in retrospective epidemiologic studies that the incidence of spontaneous abortion is increased among women working in operating rooms.[29] To date, no cause-and-effect relationship has been proved. A recent study has indicated that fertility is decreased in women exposed to N_2O for long periods.[30] The important subject of the safety of N_2O use in a dental office, to the dental staff, is discussed in depth in Chapter 17.

Skeletal Muscle

N_2O does not produce relaxation of skeletal muscles. Any observed effect of this nature during inhalation sedation is attributable to the relief of anxiety rather than to a direct action of N_2O.

Uterus and Pregnancy

N_2O and O_2 are commonly used as an aid in the management of discomfort during labor and delivery.[31] Uterine contractions are not inhibited in either amplitude or frequency.[32] N_2O passes easily across the placenta into the fetus, where the O_2 concentration of fetal blood may fall dramatically if less than 20% O_2 is being delivered with the N_2O.[33] Pregnancy does not pose a contraindication to the use of N_2O-O_2 inhalation sedation (see Chapters 4 and 12 for a more complete discussion of the use of sedation during pregnancy).

Physiologic Contraindications

"There are no contraindications to the use of nitrous oxide in combination with an adequate percentage of oxygen."[34]

"If administered with a minimum of 25% oxygen, it is a safe agent."[35]

"Nitrous oxide is a very safe anesthetic if oxygen is supplied in sufficient concentration."[36]

In the past few years it has become apparent that N_2O is not an innocuous vapor, as it was once considered. Chronic exposure of dental personnel to low levels of N_2O has been associated (though not definitively proved) with increased risk of spontaneous abortion, fetal malformation, and other types of disease.[37-39] On the other hand, chronic exposure of dental personnel (or others) to high levels of N_2O has been demonstrated beyond doubt to be capable of producing a sensory neuropathy that is extremely debilitating to the professional.[40,41] The occurrence of N_2O neuropathy is usually limited to persons who have purposefully abused the drug. These two very important subjects are discussed in depth in Chapter 17.

OXYGEN

O_2 is the second component of the inhalation sedation technique. First prepared in 1727 by Stephen Hales (who did not recognize it as an element), it was discovered as an element in 1771 by Joseph Priestley (the same man who discovered N_2O 5 years later) and almost simultaneously by Karl Scheele (1771).[42]

Preparation

O_2 is most commonly prepared by the fractional distillation of liquid air. N_2 is the first gas to boil off, with O_2 remaining as a liquid. This method of preparation was first employed in 1895 by Linde. Other methods of preparation of O_2 include the following:

1. Heating of barium peroxide (BaO_2) to 800° C, at which point it forms $BaO + O_2$

2. The electrolysis of water $2\ H_2O \rightarrow 2\ H_2 + O_2$
3. The reaction between sodium peroxide and water $2\ Na_2O_2 + 2\ H_2O \rightarrow 4\ NaOH + O_2$

Properties

O_2 is a clear, colorless, odorless gas with a molecular weight of 32. It comprises 20.9% of atmospheric air. Its specific gravity is 1.105, whereas that of air is 1. It is stored in compressed gas cylinders in a gaseous state. A full cylinder has 2000 pounds of pressure per square inch (psi) at room temperature. Its solubility in water is 2.4 volumes percent at 37° C and 4.9 volumes percent at 0° C. The cylinder of O_2 is green in the United States and white internationally, as per World Health Organization standards.[43]

O_2 is not flammable (cannot be ignited) but will support combustion. Under high pressure in the presence of oil or grease, O_2 may cause an explosion. Therefore the use of oil and grease should be strictly avoided in and around O_2 cylinders, reducing valves, wall outlets, and cylinder outlets.

Effects of 100% Oxygen

Central Nervous System. The inhalation of 100% O_2 has no effect on the cerebral cortex. Electroencephalographic (EEG) tracings are unchanged.[44] Cerebral blood flow may be decreased by as much as 10% as a result of constriction of the cerebral blood vessels occurring with 100% O_2 inhalation.[45]

Cardiovascular System. The inhalation of 100% oxygen is associated with a slight fall in both the heart rate (3 to 4 beats/min) and cardiac output (10% to 20%).[46] Coronary artery blood flow may be decreased up to 10% at this time. There is a slight increase in diastolic, but no change in the systolic, blood pressure with inhalation of 100% O_2.[47] This is a result of increased peripheral resistance secondary to a generalized vasoconstriction that occurs in the systemic, cerebral, renal, and retinal vessels on inhalation of 100% O_2.[48]

The inhalation of more than 40% O_2 in premature infants may produce retrolental fibroplasia many months later.[49]

Respiratory System. After 2 minutes of inhaling 100% O_2, minute volume is slightly depressed (3%). This occurs because ambient air (20.93% O_2) produces a continuous tonic stimulation of respiration through the chemoreceptors that are located in the carotid and aortic bodies. Inhalation of 100% O_2 abolishes this reflex stimulation, resulting in a decrease in minute volume. Following 6 to 8 minutes of 100% O_2, minute volume exchange actually increases by 7.6%. This increase is produced through stimulation of the lower respiratory passages by O_2, which acts as an irritant, or by dilation of the pulmonary capillaries by O_2 with the production of reflex respiratory stimulation from mild pulmonary congestion.

ANATOMY

RESPIRATORY SYSTEM

The anatomy of the respiratory system is reviewed here so that those involved in the use of inhalation sedation will possess a better knowledge of the processes involved in producing the observed state of relaxation.

The respiratory system is composed of a number of parts. These may be divided into two groups: (1) those parts of the respiratory system involved in the transport of gases to and from the outside of the body to and from the respiratory zone of the lungs and (2) those parts involved with the exchange of gases between the blood and the air, variously called the *exchange portion of the lung* and the *respiratory zone*. The portion of the respiratory system involved in conduction of gases is termed *anatomic dead space* because there is no exchange of O_2 and CO_2 between the air and the blood.

Structures included in the conducting portion of the respiratory system are as follows (Figure 13-5):

Nose
Pharynx
- Nasopharynx
- Oropharynx
- Hypopharynx

Larynx
Trachea
Bronchi
Bronchioles

The mouth is considered to be an accessory respiratory passage. Structures included in the respiratory zone are as follows (Figure 13-6):

Respiratory bronchioles
Alveolar ducts
Alveolar sacs
Alveoli

Nose

The nose, or nasal cavity, is anatomically the most superior part of the respiratory system. It starts as two flexible, flared, rubbery entryways termed *wings* or *alae*, enclosing a space on either side called the *vestibule*. The nasal cavities continue posteriorly as paired air spaces. The right and left sides are separated

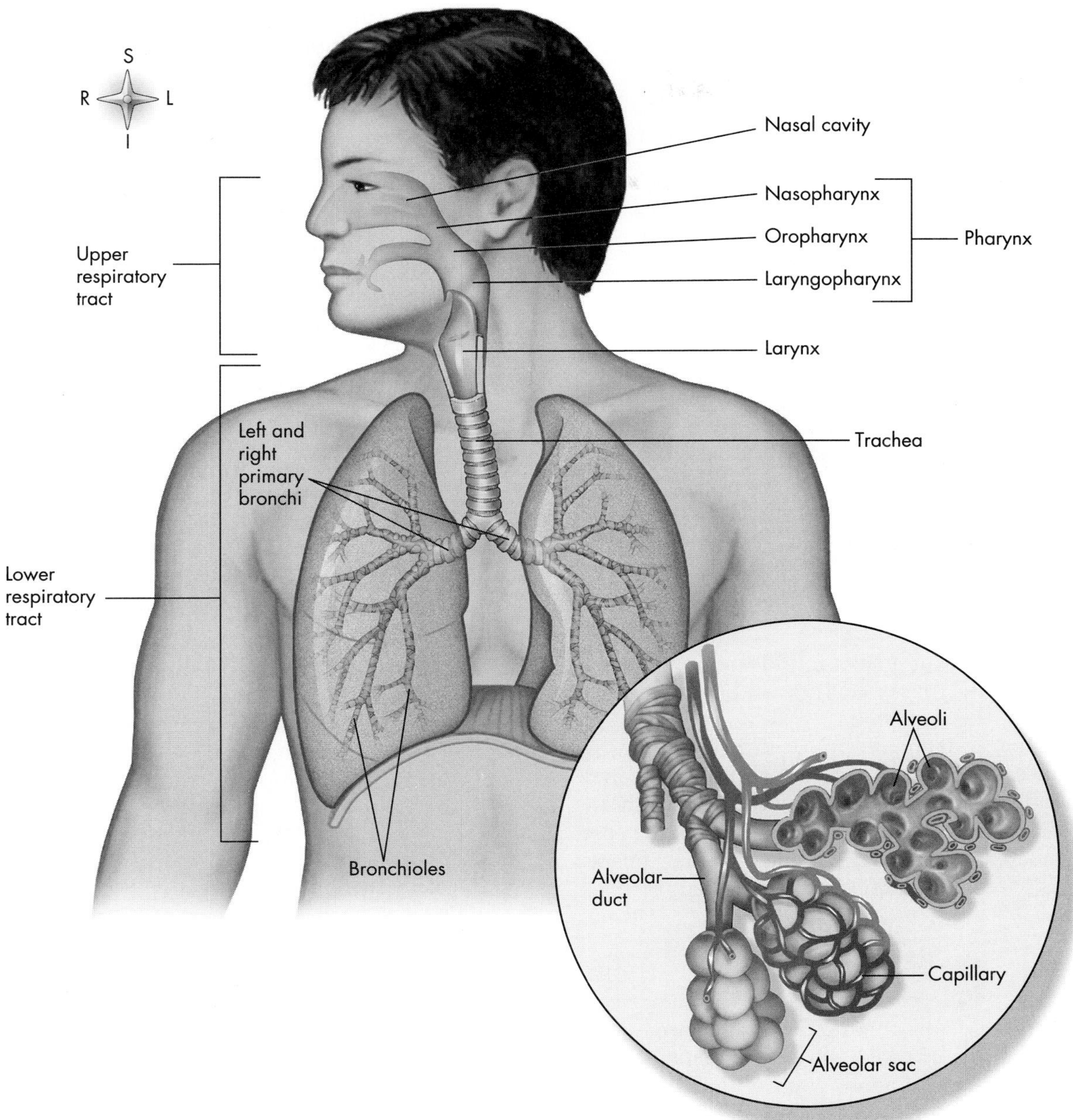

Figure 13-5 Structures forming the conducting portion of the respiratory system. The inset shows the alveolar sacs where the interchange of oxygen and carbon dioxide takes place through the walls of the grapelike alveoli. Capillaries surround the alveoli. (From Thibodeau GA, Patton KT: *The human body in health & disease*, ed 3, St Louis, 2002, Mosby.)

by the bony nasal septum. At its posterior aspect above and behind the soft palate the septum ends and the right and left nasal cavities unite to form the uppermost portion of the pharynx, the nasopharynx.

The nose has several functions in respiration.[50,51] Its primary function is to warm and humidify air. The process of warming air is readily accomplished by the mucous membranes of the nose, which are well endowed with an excellent blood supply. This large blood flow through the mucous membranes of the nose is responsible for warming of the air, a process that continues throughout the respiratory tract.

The nose also serves as (1) a defense against organisms and foreign materials, a function carried out by cilia found throughout the nose and by the mucous film found throughout the respiratory tract—submucosal glands and goblet cells are responsible for the formation of this mucinous lining; (2) a conduit for air to travel to and from the external environment to the lungs; (3) vocal resonance, a function of both the nose

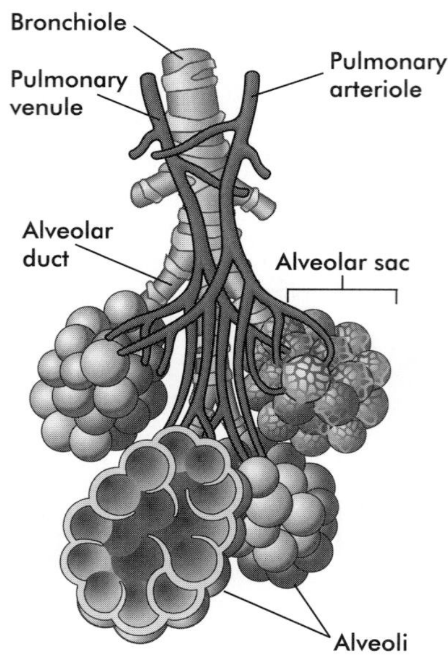

Figaure 13-6 Structures forming the respiratory zone of the respiratory system. (From Thibodeau GA, Patton KT: *The human body in health & disease*, ed 3, St Louis, 2002, Mosby.)

and sinuses (empty air spaces found within the skull, emptying into the nasal cavity); and (4) an organ involved in the sense of smell.

In inhalation sedation as practiced in dentistry, the nose is, of necessity, the prime route of entry of the anesthetic gases into the patient. Situations in which the patient becomes unable to breathe well through the nose, such as deviated septum and chronic or acute sinusitis, will complicate the inhalation sedation procedure.

Mouth

The mouth is considered an accessory respiratory passage. Most people will breathe through the mouth at times, especially during speech and whenever their nasal passages are occluded, such as in respiratory infections. As with the nose, the mouth, because of its mucosal surface and its rich blood supply, serves to warm and humidify the air as it enters the body. The mouth ends at the posterior palatine pillars. These pillars extend superiorly to meet the uvula, a fleshy tab of soft tissue located in the midline at the posterior border of the soft palate.

The base of the tongue rises out of the hypopharynx to occupy the floor of the mouth. Using the other passive structures of the oral cavity for support, the tongue and the oropharyngeal reflexes actively protect against threats to the airway.[52]

Because the mouth is the region in which dentistry is performed, this area is not involved in the routine administration of N_2O and O_2; however, the mouth is available for the administration of gases, especially O_2, during emergencies. In such cases both the mouth and nose may be used for the purposes of ventilation.

Pharynx

The pharynx extends from the posterior portion of the nose to the level of the lower border of the cricoid cartilage, where it becomes continuous with the esophagus and the respiratory tract through the larynx.[51] The word *pharynx* is derived from the Greek word for "throat." For anatomic purposes, the pharynx is divided into three regions: the *nasopharynx, oropharynx,* and *hypopharynx*. The nasopharynx extends from the back of the nasal cavity to the level of the soft palate. The eustachian tubes open into the nasopharynx and connect with the middle ear. The oropharynx starts superiorly at the level of the soft palate to the level of the cricoid cartilage and the base of the tongue inferiorly. The hypopharynx, also known as the *laryngopharynx*, starts superiorly at the epiglottis to the division of the esophagus and larynx. It is the shortest of the three divisions. The major functions of the pharynx are the conduction, warming, and humidification of air and the removal of foreign materials. The junction of the pharynx and the esophagus represents the narrowest part of the alimentary canal. Foreign bodies trapped at this level may produce aspiration or significant decreases in airflow.[53,54]

Epiglottis

Although not an integral part of the respiratory system, the epiglottis, a platelike structure extending from the base of the tongue backward and upward, must be mentioned. It functions as a flaplike covering over the larynx that closes during swallowing, covering the airway so that swallowed materials enter the esophagus.[50]

Larynx

In the adult the larynx is found at the level of the first through the fifth cervical vertebrae, consisting of a number of articulated cartilages surrounding the upper end of the trachea (Figure 13-7).[55] *Adam's apple* is another common name for the larynx (more accurately, *Adam's apple* denotes the thyroid cartilage). The laryngeal cavity extends from just below the epiglottis to the lower level of the cricoid cartilage, where it becomes continuous with the trachea.

The primary function of the larynx is phonation, but it also has a protective function because the airway becomes quite narrow at this point. Structures found within the laryngeal cavity include the vestibular folds (i.e., the false vocal cords) and the vocal cords (i.e. the

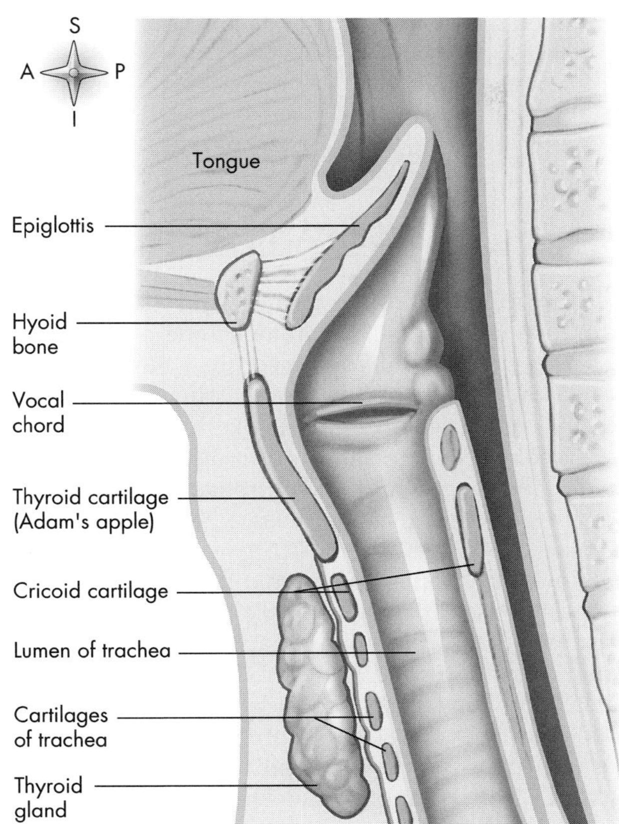

Figure 13-7 Sagittal section of the larynx. (From Thibodeau GA, Patton KT: *The human body in health & disease*, ed 3, St Louis, 2002, Mosby.)

true vocal cords), which are two pearly white folds of mucous membrane.

The narrowest portion of the larynx in the adult is located at the true vocal cords.[50] Larger aspirated objects will become lodged at this site. They can usually be dislodged by the abdominal thrust or chest thrust. In the child younger than 10 years, the narrowest portion of the larynx occurs at the level of cricoid cartilage.[50,51] Should material be small enough to pass between the vocal cords, in the adult and in most children it will usually enter either the right or left mainstem bronchus, a situation that is serious but not acutely life-threatening.

Trachea

The trachea is a tubular structure that begins at the cricoid cartilage. The tube of the trachea is formed of approximately 16 to 22 C-shaped cartilaginous rings that are incomplete on their posterior surface. A thin muscle band extends between the incomplete posterior ends of the U-shaped cartilages. The trachea extends through the neck into the mediastinum to a point behind the junction of the upper and middle thirds of the sternum, where it divides into the right and left mainstem bronchi. The carina is the name given to the cartilage that is located at the point of bifurcation. The carina is located approximately 5 cm below the suprasternal notch.[50] The trachea is about 10 to 13 cm long and has an outer diameter of 2.5 cm and an inner diameter of 1.0 to 1.5 cm. This dimension is enlarged in elderly persons and decreased during pregnancy (because of edema).

Bronchi

At the level of the carina the right and left mainstem bronchi branch off from the trachea. Because of the position of the heart in the left side of the mediastinum, the angle formed by the left mainstem bronchus (45 to 55 degrees) is somewhat greater than that formed by the right mainstem bronchus (20 to 30 degrees). This is of importance because aspirated objects will have a greater tendency to enter into the right lung than the left.[50,51]

Each of the mainstem bronchi divides into branches that supply each of the lobes of the lung. The right mainstem bronchus is wider and shorter than the left, giving branches to the upper and middle lobes and then continuing to become the branch to the right lower lobe. The right upper lobe bronchus has its origin about 2 cm from the carina, whereas the left arises about 5 cm from the carina.[51] Each of these bronchi in turn gives off branches.[56] The right upper lobe bronchus gives rise to three main divisions, the right middle lobe bronchus to two divisions, and the right lower lobe bronchus to five or six divisions. The left mainstem bronchus is somewhat longer and narrower than the right. It ends at the origin of the left upper lobe bronchus and continues to become the main bronchus to the left lower lobe. The left upper lobe main bronchus originates at the bifurcation of the left mainstem bronchus and gives off three branches. The left lower lobe main bronchus, the direct continuation of the left mainstem bronchus, gives rise to four branches.[57]

Bronchioles

The bronchi continue to bifurcate and trifurcate well into the periphery of each lung. As these divisions occur the number of bronchi increases significantly, as does the total surface area of the lung. As the bronchi continue to divide, they become smaller, and their cartilaginous rings gradually recede, becoming irregular plates. Cartilage is found in bronchioles until their diameter is approximately 0.66 to 1 mm, at which point cartilage disappears entirely.[58]

The first 17 divisions of the tracheobronchial tree comprise the conducting zone because the exchange of O_2 and CO_2—the primary function of the lungs—cannot occur here. This is also termed *dead space.*

Approximately 150 ml of air is found in the conducting zone in the average-sized adult.[59] From divisions 17 to 23, changes occur in the walls and linings of the airway that dramatically increase their surface area. These airways comprise what is called the *respiratory zone* and include respiratory bronchioles, alveolar ducts, alveolar sacs, and alveoli (see Figure 13-6). The alveolus represents the final air space and is the unit in which the exchange of gases occurs.

Alveolus

The alveolus is essentially a pocket of air surrounded by a thin membrane containing capillaries (Figure 13-8). The distance between the air within the alveolus and the capillary is approximately 0.35 to 2.5 μm. This thin wall is essential for the rapid exchange of gases between air and blood. Gases within the alveoli are separated from blood by four thin layers:

1. Mucinous covering
2. Alveolar epithelium (incomplete)
3. Interstitial layer
4. Endothelial cells lining pulmonary capillaries

Blood remains within the pulmonary capillaries for approximately 0.5 second, yet gas exchange is so swift that it is completed by the time the blood has completed only one fourth of its journey through the capillary.

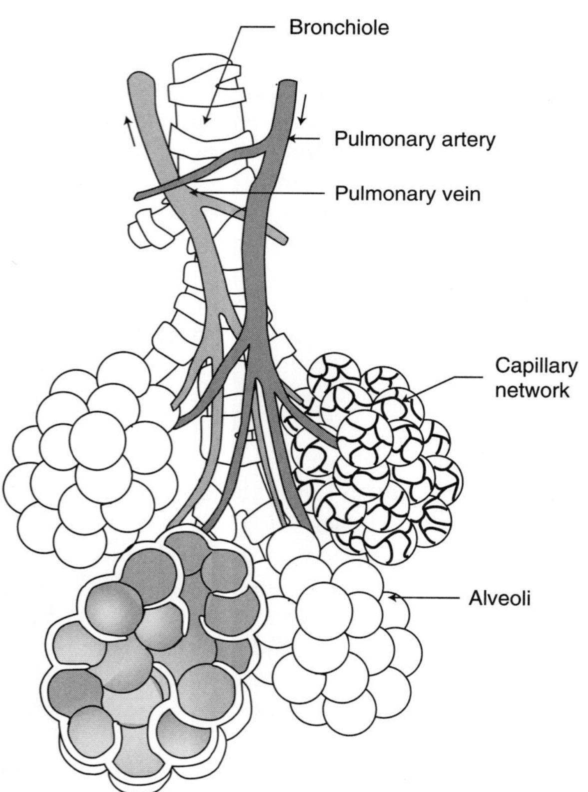

Figure 13-8 Alveoli and surrounding vasculature. The capillary bed in this area is the densest vascular network in the entire body.

PHYSIOLOGY

RESPIRATION

Gases are inhaled through the nose and/or mouth and are transported to the respiratory zone of the lungs, the more than 300 million alveoli in which the interchange of gases between the alveolus and the pulmonary capillaries occurs. The exchange of gases in the alveoli depends entirely on diffusion of gases across membranes and is controlled by the partial pressures of the respective gases on either side of the alveolar membrane.

Pulmonary capillaries are unique in that they form the most dense capillary network in the entire body. It is estimated that pulmonary capillaries are approximately 10 μm long and 7 μm wide. So finely interlaced are they that they may be considered more of a pool of blood vessels than a series of pipes. In adults the surface area of the pulmonary capillary-alveolar interface is about 70 m^2, or approximately 40 times the surface area of the body.[60] At any given moment, there is approximately 100 to 300 ml of blood within these pulmonary capillaries. Dail has compared this to the spreading of a teaspoon of blood over 1 m^2 of surface area.[58]

The gases within the alveoli are separated from the capillaries by approximately 1 to 2 μm of tissue: the mucinous covering of the alveolus; the alveolar epithelium, which in some places is incomplete; an interstitial layer; and the endothelium covering the pulmonary capillary.

Mechanics of Respiration

How do gases get into the alveolus from outside the body? Air moves from the external environment to the level of the alveolar capillary membrane because of differences of pressure within the respiratory system. Gases move from a zone of higher pressure to one of lower pressure.

The typical respiratory cycle can be divided into five phases: preinspiration, peak inspiration, end inspiration, peak expiration, and end expiration.

At preinspiration the pressure within the pleural cavity is negative: –5 cm H_2O, the pressure of the normal resting lung. This negative pressure is produced by the natural tendency of the lung to recoil inward and of the chest wall to recoil outward.

As inspiration begins, the muscles of inspiration contract and the chest cavity (thorax) expands, increasing the negative pressure within the thorax to even more than it was at rest. This results in an expansion of the alveoli as well as the development of negative pressure within them.

With the development of negative pressure within the alveoli—a pressure negative to atmospheric pressure—air begins to flow into the respiratory system through the nose and mouth. As air enters the system, a tidal volume develops, resulting in the end of inspiration. Pleural pressure reaches its most negative point, alveolar pressure returns to zero as gases enter the alveoli, airflow into the lung ceases, and the maximum inspiratory volume is reached. Expiration now begins.

Pleural pressure begins to return to its original value (–5 cm H_2O), resulting in the creation of positive pressure within the alveoli during expiration and maximal expiratory flow out of the respiratory system. At the end of expiration, pleural pressure has returned to baseline, alveolar pressure has returned to zero, flow has ceased, and the expiratory volume has been delivered, returning the lung to its resting lung capacity. Under normal respiratory conditions (quiet breathing), most of the pressure that is generated occurs as a result of the elastic characteristics of the lungs.

Muscles are involved in the process of breathing, helping produce the increases in negative pressures that draw air into the respiratory system. These muscles are as follows:

1. Diaphragm (primary)
2. Intercostals (primary)
3. Abdominals (accessory)
4. Scalenes (accessory)
5. Sternocleidomastoid (accessory)
6. Some back muscles (accessory)

The *diaphragm* is the primary muscle involved in quiet breathing. In normal breathing a 1-cm downward movement of the diaphragm causes 350 ml of air to enter the lung. The normal 500-ml tidal volume will therefore require approximately a 1.5-cm downward movement of the diaphragm. In quiet breathing the diaphragm is probably the only muscle of respiration working. *Intercostal muscles* do not participate in quiet breathing. *Abdominal muscles* do not participate in quiet breathing or in ventilation up to about 40 L/min (lpm). The abdominal muscles take a more active part as the volume of air inspired increases, and above 90 lpm (as seen in strenuous exercise), the abdominals are actively contributing by forceful contraction. The *scalenes* do contract during quiet breathing; however, their contribution to the total volume of air inspired is not great. The *sternocleidomastoids* do not participate in quiet respiration; however, their actions do become more forceful as ventilation increases. All of the muscles that participate in respiration are attached to the thoracic cage.

Composition of Respiratory Gases

The composition of the major gases found in the respiratory system is shown in Table 13-2. Water vapor constitutes less than 1% of atmospheric air, whereas alveolar air, fully saturated with water vapor, contains 6.2%. The pressure exerted by the water vapor is 47 mm Hg and must be taken into account in determining the partial pressures of the gases within the alveoli.

Barometric pressure – Water vapor pressure
= Alveolar partial pressure

760 mm Hg – 47 mm Hg = 713 mm Hg

The partial pressure of gases within the alveolus is determined as follows:

Alveolar O_2 tension	= 713 × 14.2/100	= 103 mm Hg
Alveolar CO_2 tension	= 713 × 5.5/100	= 40 mm Hg
Alveolar N_2 tension	= 713 × 80.3/100	= 570 mm Hg
Water vapor		47 mm Hg
Total pressures		= 760 mm Hg

The speed at which gases diffuse across membranes is controlled by several factors, the most important of which is their partial pressure in each compartment (Table 13-3). For example, the partial pressure of O_2 within the alveolus is 103 mm Hg, whereas in the pulmonary capillary its tension is only 40 mm Hg. O_2 is therefore forced into the capillary from the alveolus.

When arterial blood arrives at the tissues in the body, it still has an O_2 tension of 100 mm Hg, whereas

TABLE 13-2 Composition of the Major Gases Found in the Respiratory System (Percentages)

Gas	Inspired Air	Alveolar Air	Expired Air
O_2	20.94	14.2	16.3
CO_2	0.04	5.5	4.0
N_2	79.02	80.3	79.7

TABLE 13-3 Partial Pressures of Gases

Gas (mm Hg)	Air (mm Hg)	Alveolus (mm Hg)	Arterial Blood (mm Hg)	Venous Blood (mm Hg)
O_2	158.2	103	100	40
CO_2	0.3	40	40	46
N_2	596.5	570	573	573
H_2O vapor	5.0	47	47	47

the O_2 tension within the tissues is only 40 mm Hg. The O_2 therefore travels from the plasma into the tissues because of this pressure gradient. The O_2 tension within the plasma falls. In a resting state the tissues remove approximately 30% of the available O_2. Venous blood leaving the tissues still contains quite a bit of O_2; however, during violent exercise the tissues may remove almost all of the available O_2. On returning to the lungs, venous blood quickly surrenders its CO_2 (partial pressure 46 mm Hg) to the alveolus (partial pressure 40 mm Hg), and O_2 diffuses from the alveolus into the capillary blood (capillary PO_2 40 mm Hg; alveolar PO_2 103 mm Hg).

Disease states may alter the rate at which the exchange of gases occurs within the lungs. For example, in emphysema the total surface area of the alveolar membranes is decreased; in pneumonia the alveolar walls become thickened, thereby inhibiting diffusion; and in asthma the increase in bronchial secretions also acts to impede the exchange of gases. In methemoglobinemia the oxygen-carrying capacity of the blood is decreased.

N_2O when inhaled into the lungs will act in the same manner as the gases described previously. When N_2O is first inhaled, its partial pressure within the alveolus will be quite high, whereas that within the capillary will be zero. N_2O flow will occur rapidly from the alveolus to the capillary, and the same response will develop within tissues. As the blood becomes saturated with N_2O (3 to 5 minutes), the rate of diffusion into the cardiovascular system decreases. At the termination of the procedure, the patient is administered 100% O_2, and N_2O is eliminated. The alveolus now contains little or no N_2O, whereas venous blood returning to the lung is rich in N_2O, so N_2O now diffuses out of the blood into the alveolus and out of the body through the respiratory tract.

REFERENCES

1. The National Formulary: *The US pharmacopeia*, Rockville, Md, 1990, US Pharmacopeial Convention.
2. Wood M, Wood AJJ: *Drugs and anesthesia: pharmacology for anesthesiologists*, Baltimore, 1982, Williams & Wilkins.
3. Wollman H, Smith TC: Uptake, distribution, elimination, and administration of inhalational anesthetics. In Goodman LS, Gilman A, eds: *Pharmacological basis of therapeutics*, ed 5, New York, 1975, Macmillan.
4. Gould DB, Lampert BA, MacKrell TN: Effect of nitrous oxide solubility on vaporizer aberrance, *Anesth Analg* 61:938, 1982.
5. Gillman MA: Analgesic (sub anesthetic) nitrous oxide interacts with the endogenous opioid system: a review of the evidence, *Life Sci* 39:1209, 1986.
6. Longnecker DE, Miller FL: Pharmacology of inhalational anesthetics. In Rogers MC, Tinker JH, Covino BG et al, eds: *Principles and practice of anesthesiology*, St Louis, 1993, Mosby.
7. Taylor E, Feinstein R, White PF et al: Anesthesia for laparoscopic cholecystectomy: is nitrous oxide contraindicated? *Anesthesiology* 76:541, 1992.
8. Severinghaus JW: The rate of uptake of nitrous oxide in man, *J Clin Invest* 33:1183, 1954.
9. Epstein RM, Rackow H, Salanitre E et al: Influence of the concentration effect on the uptake of anesthetic mixtures, *Anesthesiology* 25:364, 1964.
10. Longnecker DE, Miller FL: Pharmacology of inhalational anesthetics. In Rogers MC, Tinker JH, Covino BG et al, eds: *Principles and practice of anesthesiology*, St Louis, 1993, Mosby.
11. Eger EI II: *Nitrous oxide*, New York, 1985, Elsevier.
12. Longnecker DE, Miller FL: Pharmacology of inhalational agents. In Rogers MC, Tinker JH, Covino BG et al, eds: *Principles and practice of anesthesiology*, St Louis, 1993, Mosby.
13. Stewart RD, Gorayeb MJ, Pelton GH: Arterial blood gases before, during, and after nitrous oxide: oxygen administration, *Ann Emerg Med* 15:1177, 1986.
14. Quarnstrom FC, Milgrom P, Bishop MJ et al: Clinical study of diffusion hypoxia after nitrous oxide analgesia, *Anesth Prog* 38:21, 1991.
15. Ramsey DS, Leonesio RJ, Whitney CW et al: Paradoxical effects of nitrous oxide on human memory, *Psychopharmacology* 106:370, 1992.
16. Smiley BA, Paradise NF: Does the duration of N_2O administration affect postoperative nausea and vomiting? *Nurse Anesth* 2:13, 1991.

17. Stowe DF, Monroe SM, Marijic J et al: Effects of nitrous oxide on contractile function and metabolism of the isolated heart, *Anesthesiology* 73:1220, 1990.
18. Hornbein TF, Martin WE, Bonica JJ et al: Nitrous oxide effects on the circulatory and ventilatory responses to halothane, *Anesthesiology* 31:250, 1969.
19. Moore PA: Nitrous oxide: oxygen sedation: induction and recovery, *Curr Rev Nurse Anesth* 4:35, 1981.
20. Pasternak LR: Outpatient anesthesia. In Rogers MC, Tinker JH, Covino BG et al, eds: *Principles and practice of anesthesiology*, St Louis, 1993, Mosby.
21. Yacoub O, Doell D, Kryger MH, et al: Depression of hypoxic ventilatory response by nitrous oxide, *Anesthesiology* 45:385, 1976.
22. Ross JA, Monk SJ, Duffy SW: Effect of nitrous oxide on halothane-induced hepatotoxicity in hypoxic, enzyme-induced rats, *Br J Anaesth* 56:527, 1984.
23. Eckenhoff RG, Longnecker DE: The therapeutic gases: oxygen, carbon dioxide, helium, and water vapor. In Gilman AG, Rall TW, Nies AS et al, eds: *Goodman and Gilman's the pharmacological basis of therapeutics*, ed 8, New York, 1990, Pergamon.
24. Deacon R, Lumb M, Perry J et al: Selective inactivation of vitamin B_{12} in rats by nitrous oxide, *Lancet* 2:1023, 1978.
25. Henry RJ: Assessing environmental health concerns associated with nitrous oxide, *JADA* 123:41, 1992.
26. Franco G: Occupational exposure to anaesthetics: liver injury, microsomal enzyme induction and preventive aspects, *Ital Med Lavoro* 11:205, 1989.
27. Layzer RB: Myeloneuropathy after prolonged exposure to nitrous oxide, *Lancet* 2:1227, 1978.
28. Longnecker DE, Miller FL: Pharmacology of inhalational anesthetics. In Rogers MC, Tinker JH, Covino BG et al, eds: *Principles and practice of anesthesiology*, St Louis, 1993, Mosby.
29. Eger EI II: Fetal injury and abortion associated with occupational exposure to inhaled anesthetics, *AANA J* 59:309, 1991.
30. Wynn RL: Nitrous oxide and fertility, part I, *Gen Dent* 41:122, 1993.
31. Marx GF, Katsnelson T: The introduction of nitrous oxide analgesia into obstetrics, *Obstet Gynecol* 80:715, 1992.
32. Arai M, Nishijima M, Tatsuma H: Analgesia and anesthesia during labor in Japan and developed countries, *Asia-Oceania J Obstet Gynaecol* 15:213, 1989.
33. Landon MJ, Toothill VJ: Effect of nitrous oxide on placental methionine synthase activity, *Br J Anaesth* 58:524, 1986.
34. Wylie WD, Churchill-Davidson HC: *A practice of anesthesia*, ed 4, Philadelphia, 1978, WB Saunders.
35. Lichtiger M, Moya F: *Introduction to the practice of anesthesia*, New York, 1974, Harper & Row.
36. Snow JC: *Manual of anesthesia*, Boston, 1977, Little, Brown.
37. Baden JM, Fujinaga M: Effects of nitrous oxide on day 9 rat embryos grown in culture, *Br J Anaesth* 66:500, 1991.
38. Schumann D: Nitrous oxide anaesthesia: risks to health personnel, *Int Nurs Rev* 37:214, 1990.
39. Littner MM, Kaffe I, Tamse A: Occupational hazards in the dental office and their control. IV. Measures for controlling contamination of anesthetic gas: nitrous oxide, *Quintess Intern* 14:461, 1983.
40. Stacy CB, DiRocco A, Gould RJ: Methionine in the treatment of nitrous oxide-induced neuropathy and myeloneuropathy, *J Neurol* 239:401, 1992.
41. Chanarin I: The effects of nitrous oxide on cobalamins, folates, and on related events, *Crit Rev Toxicol* 10:179, 1982.
42. Eckenhoff, Longnecker DE: The therapeutic gases: oxygen, carbon dioxide, helium, and water vapor. In Gilman AG, Rall TW, Nies AS et al, eds: *Goodman and Gilman's the pharmacological basis of therapeutics*, ed 8, New York, 1990, Pergamon.
43. Robiolio M, Rumsey WL, Wilson OF: Oxygen diffusion and mitochondrial respiration in neuroblastic cells, *Am J Physiol* 256:C1207, 1989.
44. Bleiberg B, Kerem D: Central nervous system oxygen toxicity in the resting rat: postponement by intermittent oxygen exposure, *Undersea Biomed Res* 15:337, 1988.
45. Bryan RM Jr: Cerebral blood flow and energy metabolism during stress, *Am J Physiol* 259:H269, 1990.
46. Voelkel NF: Mechanisms of hypoxic pulmonary vasoconstriction, *Am Rev Respir Dis* 133:1186, 1986.
47. Martindale W: *Extra pharmacopoeia*, ed 29, London, 1989, Pharmaceutical Press.
48. Rothe CF, Maass-Moreno R, Flanagan AD: Effects of hypercapnia and hypoxia on the cardiovascular system: vascular capacitance and aortic chemoreceptors, *Am J Physiol* 259:H932, 1990.
49. Weiss NS: Oxygen and retrolental fibrodysplasia: did epidemiology help or hinder? *Epidemiology* 2:60, 1991.
50. Morris IR: Functional anatomy of the upper airway, *Emerg Med Clin North Am* 6:639, 1988.
51. Young GP: Clinical airway anatomy. In Dailey RH, Simon B, Young GP et al, eds: *The airway: emergency management*, St Louis, 1992, Mosby.
52. Block C, Vrechner V: Unusual problems in airway management. II. The influence of the temporomandibular joint, the mandible, and associated structures on endotracheal intubation, *Anesth Analg* 50:115, 1971.
53. Daniilidis J, Symeonidis B, Triaridis K et al: Foreign body in the airways, *Arch Otolaryngol* 103:570, 1977.
54. Kim IN, Brummitt WM, Humphry A et al: Foreign body in the airway: a review of 202 cases, *Laryngoscope* 83:347, 1973.
55. Meller SM: Functional anatomy of the larynx, *Otolaryngol Clin North Am* 17:1, 1984.
56. Ellis H, Feldman S: *Anatomy for anesthetists*, ed 4, Oxford, 1983, Blackwell Scientific.
57. Clemente CD, ed: *Gray's anatomy of the human body*, ed 30, Philadelphia, 1984, Lea & Febiger.
58. Dail DH: Anatomy of the respiratory system. In Moser KM, Spragg RG, eds: *Respiratory emergencies*, ed 2, St Louis, 1982, Mosby.
59. Benumof JL: The respiratory physiology and respiratory function during anesthesia. In Miller RD, eds: *Anesthesia*, ed 3, New York, 1990, Churchill-Livingstone.
60. Levine S, Kuna ST: Introduction to the respiratory system. In Rose LF, Kaye D, eds: *Internal medicine for dentistry*, St Louis, 1983, Mosby.

CHAPTER 14

Armamentarium

CHAPTER OUTLINE

The armamentarium for the delivery of nitrous oxide–oxygen (N_2O-O_2) inhalation sedation is quite simple. Primary equipment consists of a supply of the gases and an apparatus for their delivery to the patient. The modern inhalation sedation unit is a compact, continuous-flow machine used for the administration of compressed gases under controlled conditions. This sedation unit is a modification of the machines used to administer inhalation general anesthesia. These machines (Figure 14-1) are capable of delivering a number of inhalation anesthetics, whereas the inhalation sedation unit has been altered to deliver only two gases: N_2O and O_2.

TYPES OF INHALATION SEDATION UNITS

Although two basic types of inhalation sedation units are available, only one is recommended for use. These are the continuous-flow machine and the intermittent- or demand-flow unit. Although these devices are similar in design, there are some very significant differences in their operation. Even though the demand-flow unit is not in popular use for dentistry in the United States, it is mentioned here for the sake of completeness. The reader will be better able to understand

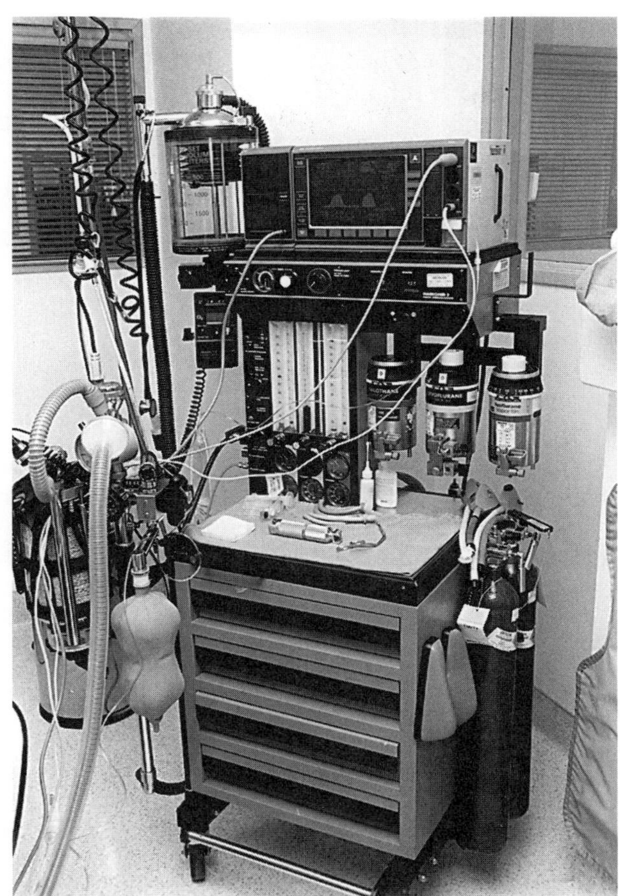

Figure 14-1 General anesthesia machines can deliver multiple anesthetic gases and contain multiple monitoring devices.

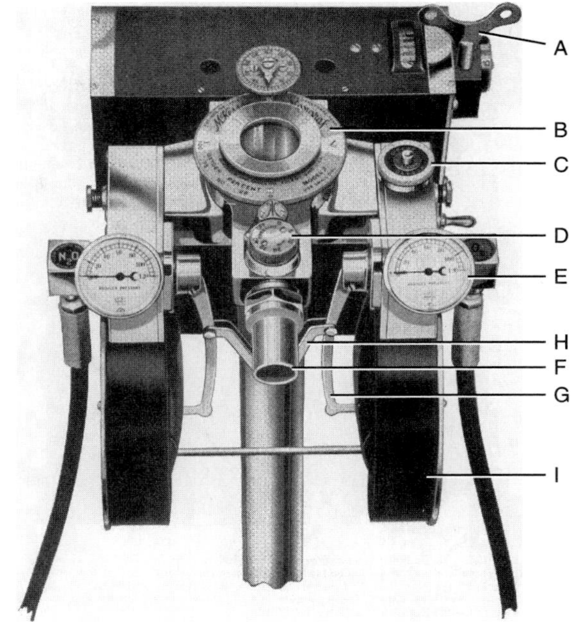

Figure 14-2 Demand-flow N_2O-O_2 unit. Front view of Nargraf machine. *A*, Pressure adjuster for rebreathing device; *B*, mixing top; *C*, oxygen flush valve; *D*, pressure control; *E*, pressure gauge; *F*, outlet; *G*, lever arm; *H*, toggle arm; and *I*, metal drum. (Courtesy McKesson Company, a division of Narco Medical Company.)

the mechanism and reasons why the continuous-flow unit is more popular and recommended for use in dentistry.

Demand-Flow Units

The demand-flow type of N_2O-O_2 inhalation sedation unit (Figure 14-2) does not deliver gas continuously to the patient but instead varies the rate and volume of delivered gas according to the patient's respiratory demands and requirements. In this sense the demand-flow type of inhalation sedation unit may be compared to the face mask employed by SCUBA (self-contained underwater breathing apparatus) divers, which operates on the same principle. A major advantage of the demand-flow type unit is the economy obtained from the decreased volume of compressed gases used.

In operation the gases delivered are proportioned by the machine. Only one dial, which changes the percentages of gases being delivered, need be adjusted. This dial provides a direct indication of the percentage of O_2 being delivered in the mixture (the remainder of gas is N_2O). The mechanism involved in the demand-flow unit is much more complex than the flowmeter and in clinical practice has been subject to a greater percentage of error. Demand-flow units show only what was set, not what is actually delivered. If a discrepancy develops between the dial and the actual gas flow, there is no warning while the unit is in operation.[1]

Several disadvantages are associated with demand-flow units. One is that the volume flow of anesthetic gases per minute is not visible or registered anywhere on the machine. In place of this there is a dial on which the percentages of the gases being delivered are recorded and another on which the pressure at which they are being delivered is visible. The lack of ability to visually monitor the flow of gases to the patient is a major disadvantage of the demand-flow unit.

A second disadvantage of the demand-flow unit is the lack of accuracy of the mixer valve. The percentage of gas being delivered is not accurate over the full range of delivery (0% to 100% N_2O). Gauert and Hustead[2] and Allen[3] demonstrated the lack of accuracy of two demand-flow units, the McKesson Nargraph and Narmatic. At an indicated O_2 percentage of 75% the actual delivered O_2 percentage ranged from 80% to 45%, whereas at 50% indicated O_2 the actual delivered percentage ranged from 75% to 22%. Having to rely on a mixer valve that is inaccurate in a machine in which the flow of the individual gases cannot be visualized provides two significant disadvantages to the use of demand-flow units.

The gas circuit followed by the N_2O and O_2 in the demand-flow machine is as follows:

1. Compressed-gas cylinders
2. Pressure-reducing valves
3. Mixing valve with percentage of N_2O or O_2
4. Pressure regulator (to vary flow of gases)
5. Demand valve
6. Conducting tubes
7. Nasal hood
8. Expiratory valve

Clinical examples of demand-flow inhalation sedation/anesthesia units include the following:

1. Jectaflow
2. Walton (primarily used in United Kingdom)
3. McKesson Euthesor
4. McKesson Nargraph
5. McKesson Narmatic

Allen has stated that fatalities have resulted from misunderstanding the use of the demand-flow machine.[3] In light of this and the distinct advantages of the continuous-flow machines, primarily their greater accuracy and the fact that the flow of gases can be visualized, use of demand-flow inhalation sedation units cannot be recommended. A demand-flow unit known as Nitronox is used in the hospital and ambulatory setting. This demand-flow unit is unique in that the percentage is not adjustable (fixed at 50/50, O_2 and N_2O) and extremely accurate. This type of unit is not recommended for dentistry in that it prevents the important practice of titration from occurring.

Continuous-Flow Units

In contrast to demand-flow units are the continuous-flow units. These units contain flowmeters and are characterized by the continuous flow of gases, regardless of the respiratory pattern of the patient. Gas continues to be delivered through the machine even as the patient exhales. Whereas continuous-flow machines use a greater volume of gas over a given period of time than the demand-flow unit, this minor disadvantage is more than compensated for by the significantly greater accuracy and safety of continuous-flow units. The two major disadvantages of the demand-flow unit are eliminated in continuous-flow machines. The inability to visualize the flow of gases and the inaccuracy of the mixer valve are eliminated through the incorporation of a flowmeter. Accuracies to within plus or minus 2% can be achieved in gas flow with the flowmeters available today.

The gas circuit utilized in the typical continuous-flow unit consists of the following:

1. Gas cylinders
2. Reducing valves
3. Flowmeters
4. Reservoir bag
5. Conducting tubing
6. Nasal hood

All inhalation sedation units contain the same basic components. These are (Figures 14-3 to 14-5) the following:

1. Compressed-gas cylinders
2. Reducing valves (regulators)
3. Pressure gauges
4. Flowmeters
5. Reservoir bag
6. Conducting tubing
7. Full face mask/nasal hood/nasal cannula

In addition to these, the central storage systems contain manifolds and wall outlets. Modern inhalation sedation equipment is also equipped with safety features, all of which are designed to prevent the inadvertent or accidental administration of less than 20% O_2. These safety features are discussed in the following paragraphs.

Among the continuous-flow inhalation sedation units, there are three subgroupings. Although each is

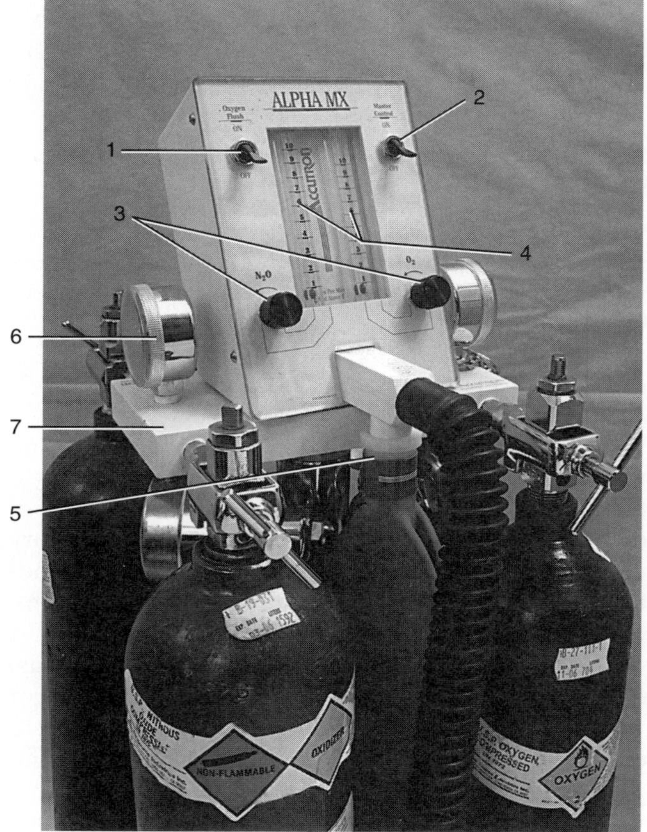

Figure 14-3 Continuous-flow inhalation sedation unit (portable, front view). *1*, Oxygen flush button; *2*, master control (on/off); *3*, control knobs for N_2O and O_2; *4*, flowmeters; *5*, reservoir bag/tee; *6*, pressure gauge; and *7*, yoke assembly.

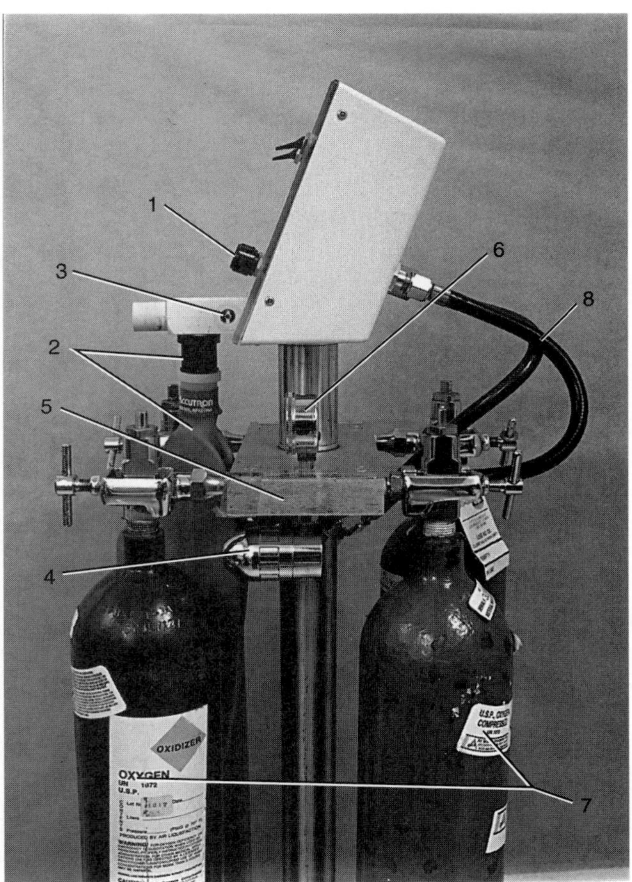

Figure 14-4 Continuous-flow inhalation sedation unit (portable, side view). *1*, Control knobs for gas flow; *2*, reservoir bag/tee; *3*, emergency air intake valve; *4*, regulator (O_2); *5*, yoke assembly; *6*, pressure gauge; *7*, compressed-gas cylinders; and *8*, low-pressure tubing. Note angle of incline of head and flowmeters.

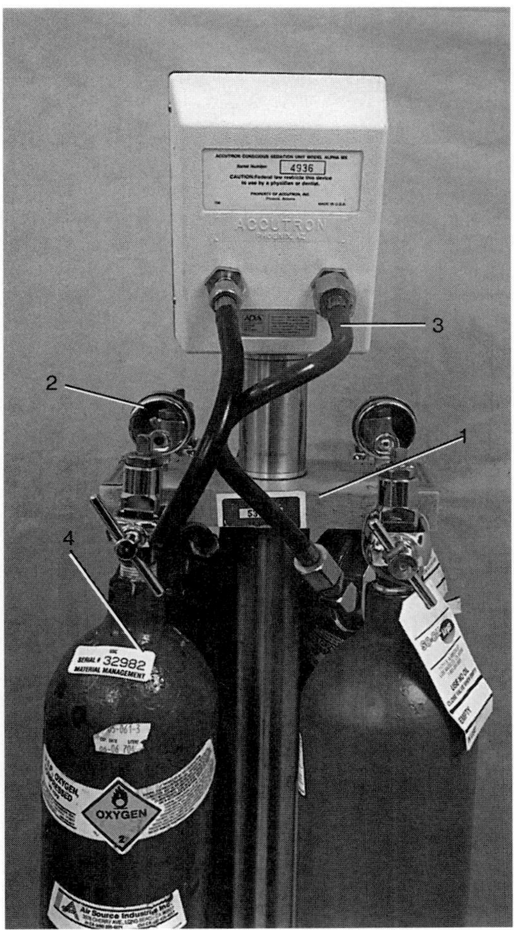

Figure 14-5 Continuous-flow inhalation sedation unit (portable, from behind). *1*, Yoke assembly; *2*, pressure gauge; *3*, low-pressure tubing; and *4*, compressed-gas cylinders.

the same basic unit, the differences among them are the manner in which compressed gases are delivered to the unit and their portability.

Portable System

In the portable system (Figure 14-6), compressed-gas cylinders are attached to the inhalation sedation unit at the yoke assembly. This system is used in offices where the frequency of N_2O-O_2 use is low or in situations in which the expense of a central storage system is prohibitive.

The primary drawback to long-term use of a portable system lies in its economics. Portable systems require use of smaller compressed-gas cylinders ("E"), which consequently require replacement more frequently than the larger "G" and "H" cylinders used in central systems. The lower cost of larger, nonportable cylinders more than justifies their use, especially where N_2O-O_2 is used more frequently.

Central Storage System

In the central storage system (Figure 14-7), the supply of N_2O and O_2 is located at a distance from the area in which the gases are delivered to patients. In the treatment area the inhalation sedation unit (also called the *head*) will be present along with the accessory equipment required for the delivery of the gases. The head is usually mounted on a wall or bracket. Heads are available in numerous versions from entry level, pneumatic type systems to modern digital gas delivery systems. Gas cylinders are maintained in a storage area, and gases are delivered to the treatment area through copper pipes. Because these cylinders are stored in a separate location at a distance from the treatment area, larger cylinders are used in the central storage systems. These cylinders are not portable, but they contain significantly more compressed gas than do the smaller cylinders used on portable systems. Multiple treatment areas may be connected through copper

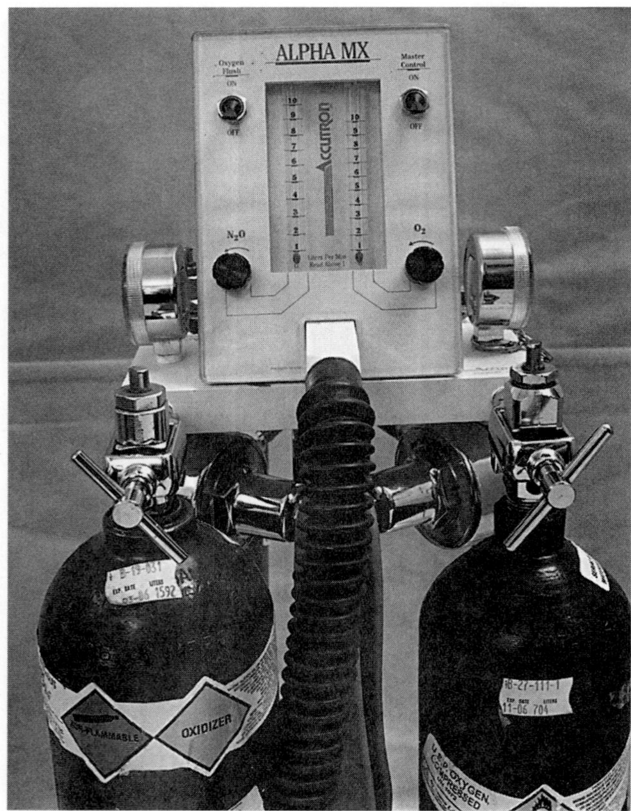

Figure 14-6 Portable inhalation sedation system. Compressed gases are attached to the unit at the yoke assembly.

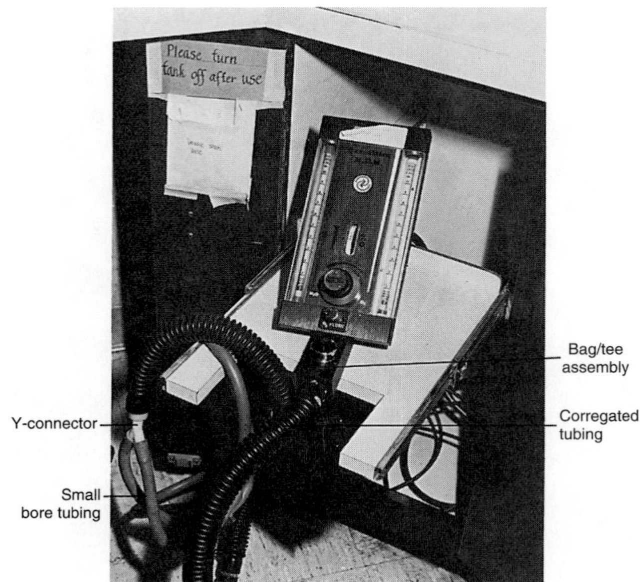

Figure 14-7 Central storage system. Inhalation sedation unit is contained within a cabinet, and compressed-gas cylinders are stored at a distant site.

piping to this storage area and operated from this bank of cylinders.

The central system is most advantageous in offices that use inhalation sedation on a more regular basis. The greater initial cost of a central storage system is quickly made up in savings obtained from use of the larger gas cylinders.

Central Storage System with Mobile Heads

Representing a compromise between the portable and central storage systems, the central storage system with mobile heads permits the use of larger compressed-gas cylinders while the inhalation sedation unit sits on a portable stand (without the yoke apparatus), which may be moved from treatment area to treatment area as the need for inhalation sedation arises. Quick-connect tubing attaches the unit to the oxygen and N_2O outlets on the wall in each treatment area.

This system is recommended for offices in which the economics of central storage warrant its installation but the frequency of use of inhalation sedation does not justify the purchase of heads for all treatment areas. One head may be used throughout the office, with others being added to the system as increased demand dictates.

Only the continuous-flow unit is considered in our discussions of inhalation sedation. Major components of these systems are discussed in depth so that the administrator of inhalation sedation will become knowledgeable about this equipment and comfortable in its clinical use.

Compressed-Gas Cylinders

Gases dispensed at a pressure greater than 25 pounds per square inch (25 psig [pounds per square inch gauge pressure]) at 25° C (70° F) are considered compressed gases, according to the Hazardous Materials regulations of the U.S. Department of Transportation (DOT). Such gases are used in the health professions and in nonhealth professions (e.g., construction, automobile racing). Because of the potential for serious injury from improper handling of these cylinders, the DOT has promulgated regulations for these gases, some of which are discussed in the following paragraphs.[4]

Cylinders that are used to store and transport compressed gases are manufactured from 3/8-inch-thick steel. Some cylinders of N_2O have been made from aluminum.

All compressed-gas cylinders are tested in accordance with DOT regulations every 5 years to ensure their integrity. Testing is performed by internal hydrostatic pressure, the pressure to which the cylinder is tested being based on the size of the cylinder. The shoulder of the cylinder is marked with a metal stamp indicating the date the cylinder was commissioned, dates of testing in accordance with DOT regulations, the pressure for which the cylinder is designed, the insignia of the testing facility, and the identification of the manufacturer of the cylinder (Figure 14-8). Cylinders are designed to handle 1.66 times the usual pressure. For example, an O_2 cylinder usually under 2000 psig is designed to hold up to 3400 psig.

In addition, the American Society of Anesthesiologists, the American Hospital Association, and the medical gas industry have adopted a uniform color code that is used on all compressed-gas cylinders (Table 14-1). The agents used in inhalation sedation, N_2O and O_2, are color coded light blue and green, respectively.

The following are important considerations for handling compressed-gas cylinders:

1. Use no grease, oil, or lubricant of any type to lubricate cylinder valves, gauges, regulators, or other fittings that may come into contact with gases. This is extremely dangerous!
2. Store full cylinders in the vertical position.
3. Store cylinders in an area in which the temperature does not fluctuate; heat in particular should be avoided.
4. Handle cylinders with care: especially avoid dropping them.
5. Open cylinder valves slowly in a counterclockwise direction. Valves must be fully opened to prevent gas leakage from the valve stems.
6. Close all cylinder valves tightly when not in use. This is important to prevent contamination from water or dirt, regardless of whether the cylinder contains gas or is empty.
7. Cylinders should be "cracked" before being attached to the sedation or anesthesia machine. The term *cracked* signifies opening the cylinder just slightly, allowing some gas to escape, thereby blowing out any particles of dust that may have lodged in the orifice of the cylinder.

TABLE 14-1 Color Coding of Compressed Gases

Gas	Coding Color
O_2	Green (white—international)
N_2O	Light blue
N_2	Gray bottom, orange shoulder
CO_2	Gray
Cyclopropane	Orange
Helium	Brown
Ethylene	Red (violet—international)

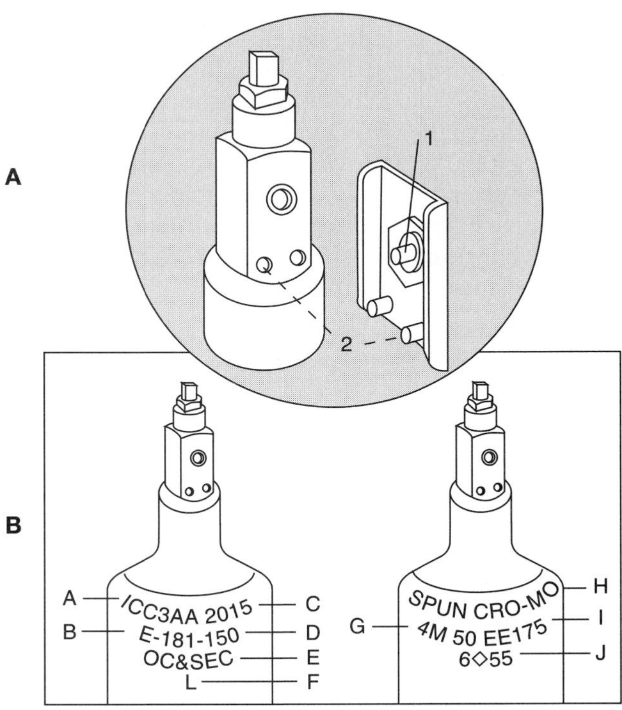

Figure 14-8 **A,** Pin index safety system prevents accidental crossing of anesthetic gases (see Figures 14-10 and 14-11). **B,** Compressed-gas cylinders contain much information: *A,* Interstate Commerce Commission specifications; *B,* cylinder size; *C,* maximum working pressure (psi); *D,* manufacturer's serial number; *E,* ownership; *F,* inspector's mark; *G,* manufacturer's mark and date of original test; *H,* composition: chrome-molybdenum (steel); *I,* elastic expansion (ml at 3360 psi); and *J,* retest dates. (Redrawn from Dripps RD, Eckenhoff JE, Vandam LD: *Introduction to anesthesia,* ed 6, Philadelphia, 1982, WB Saunders.)

The importance of keeping grease and oil away from compressed gases is so important that additional comment is required. Grease or oil in the presence of a compressed gas forms a potentially explosive mixture. When a cylinder is opened, high-pressure gas (for example O_2 at 2000 psig) is reduced suddenly to approximately 50 psig and to atmospheric pressure by the reducing valve (regulator; see p. 218). Sudden expansion of the compressed gas as it exits the cylinder cools the gas to subzero temperatures. The cylinder valve will become cool, with frost possibly forming. However, almost immediately, as more gas rushes from the cylinder into the restricted space of the reducing valve, both the pressure and temperature are increased. The temperature may increase sufficiently, although only for a few seconds, to ignite any combustible materials that may be present (e.g., grease or oil). Temperatures in excess of 1500° F—well above the ignition temperature of grease or oil—can be produced at this time.

Once the grease or oil ignites, either N_2O or O_2, although nonflammable, will support combustion. Temperature and pressure within the cylinder increase even further, producing two grave problems: (1) the rapid increase in pressure will soon exceed the limits of the cylinder, leading to an explosion, and (2) as the temperature within the cylinder increases, the valve stem of the cylinder, comprised of an alloy with a melting point of 93° C, will melt, thereby releasing the contents of the cylinder. These processes may occur within 1 to 2 seconds. Death and serious injuries to doctor, staff, and patients have occurred in this manner.[5]

Compressed-gas cylinders are manufactured in a variety of sizes. They are classified by letter, the "A" cylinder being the smallest and the "HH" the largest (Figure 14-9). In inhalation sedation with N_2O-O_2, the cylinder sizes used are the "E," "G," and "H." E cylinders are used for both N_2O and O_2 in portable units, whereas larger cylinders are used in central storage systems—G cylinders for N_2O and H cylinders for O_2. The physical characteristics of these and other compressed-gas cylinders are compared in Table 14-2, and the gas capacities of the E, G, and H cylinders are compared in Table 14-3.

Safety features incorporated in the compressed-gas cylinders include color coding (N_2O, blue; O_2, green) and the pin index safety system (see Figure 14-33). The pin index safety system is designed so that it becomes physically impossible for an N_2O cylinder to be inadvertently attached to the O_2 portion of the delivery system and vice versa. This is achieved through a series of holes in the stem of the cylinder that have a unique configuration permitting attachment only to the correct yoke on the sedation unit. Figure 14-10 illustrates the pin index safety system for N_2O and O_2.

TABLE 14-2 Characteristics of Compressed-Gas Cylinders

Cylinder	Dimensions (inches)	Weight of Empty Cylinder (lb)
A	3.0 × 10	2.75
B	3.5 × 17	8
D	4.25 × 20	12
E	4.25 × 29.5	21
M	7.12 × 46	74
G	8.5 × 55	130
H	9.0 × 55	130
HH	9.25 × 59	136

The large hole on the top of the stem is the orifice through which the compressed gas exits the cylinder. The two holes beneath the orifice accept pins found on the yoke of the sedation machine. They are countersunk approximately 0.25 inch. On the appropriate yoke of the inhalation sedation unit are found pins that will permit the attachment of the appropriate compressed-gas cylinder (Figure 14-11). These pins are welded into the unit. The pin index safety system is designed to prevent the inadvertent attachment of a gas cylinder to the wrong yoke and thus the accidental delivery of 100% N_2O when 100% O_2 is desired, a situation with potentially catastrophic consequences. Errors have been noted in pin indexing of cylinders.[6,7] Careful checking of all compressed-gas cylinders before their use is essential to safety.

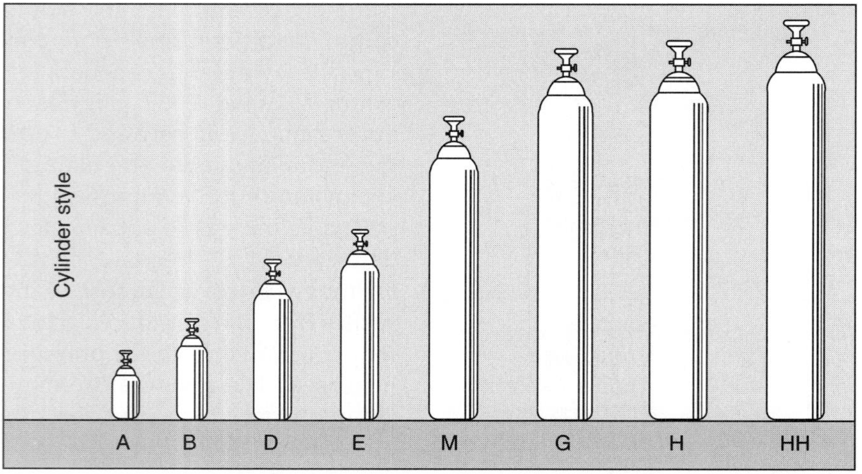

Figure 14-9 Various sizes of compressed-gas cylinders. (Redrawn from Williams RH: *Textbook of endocrinology*, ed 6, Philadelphia, 1982, WB Saunders.)

TABLE 14-3 Comparison of E, G, and H Cylinders

N_2O (Nitrous Oxide)		
Cylinder size	E	G
Dimensions	4.5″ wide 29.5″ high 21 pounds weight	8.5″ wide 55″ high 130 pounds weight
Color of cylinder	Blue	Blue
psi—full	750-800	750-800
Capacity (liters)	159	13,839
(gallons)	420	3200
Physical state of contents	Gas and liquid	Gas and liquid
O_2 (Oxygen)		
Cylinder size	E	H
Dimensions	4.5″ wide 29.5″ high 21 pounds weight	9″ wide 55″ high 130 pounds weight
Color of cylinder	Green	Green
psi—full	2000	2200
Capacity (liters)	625	6909
(gallons)	165	1400
Physical state of contents	Gas	Gas

Oxygen Cylinder and Contents

O_2 in a compressed-gas cylinder is present in a gaseous state. The gas pressure in a full E cylinder is approximately 1900 psig[8] at 70° F (25° C) (Figure 14-12, *A*), whereas the pressure within the larger H cylinder is approximately 2200 psig.[9] Oxygen cylinders are color coded green in the United States and white internationally. One ounce of O_2 liquid is equivalent to 5.22 gallons of O_2 gas.

Because the O_2 cylinder contains only gas, the pressure gauge on the machine yoke reflects the actual contents of the cylinder. In other words, as oxygen leaves the cylinder, the pressure within the cylinder will drop accordingly. Therefore, if an O_2 cylinder records a pressure of 1000 psig (Figure 14-13), the

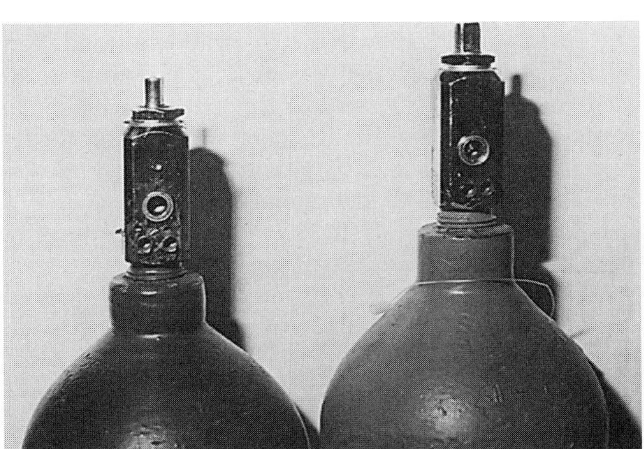

Figure 14-10 Pin index safety system for O_2 *(left)* and N_2O *(right)*. Large orifice on top of cylinder permits gas to exit cylinder. Smaller holes below are pin-indexed for specific compressed gas.

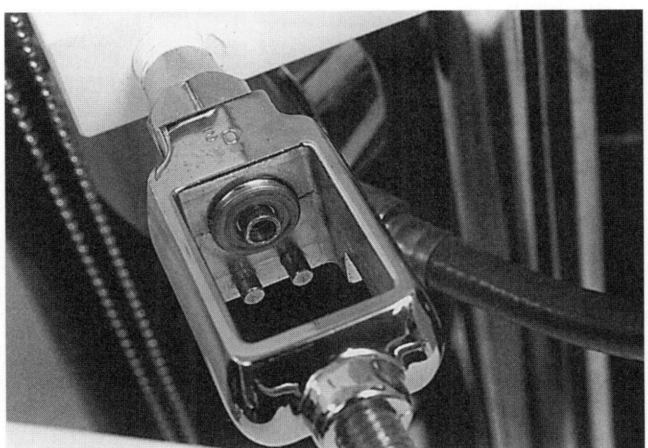

Figure 14-11 Pins, which are located on yoke of inhalation sedation unit, are aligned to permit attachment of only one compressed gas.

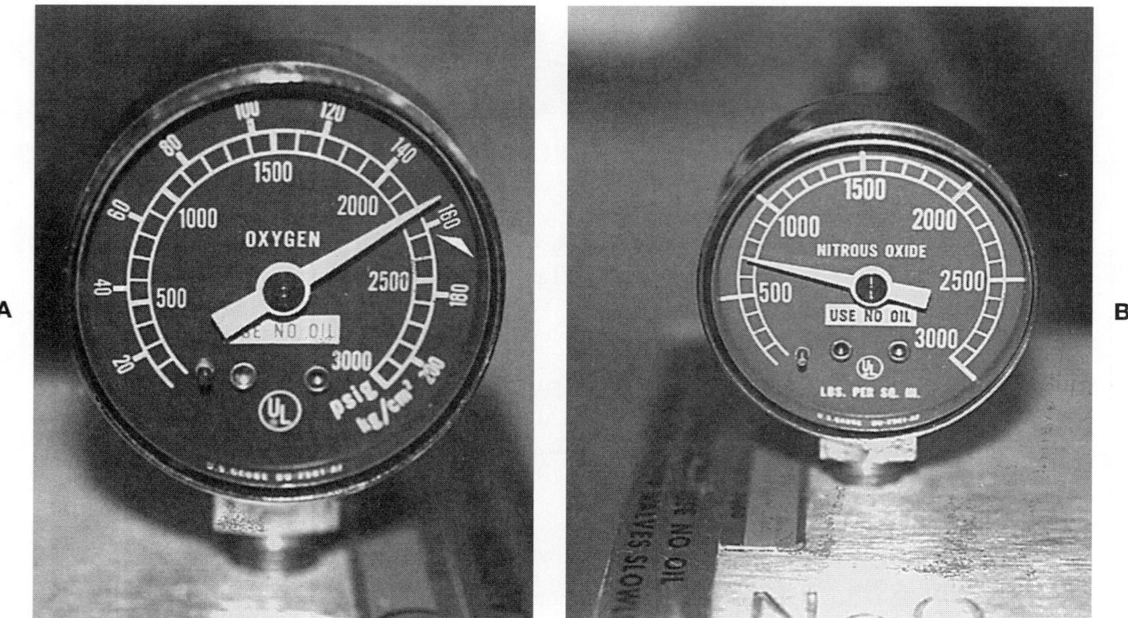

Figure 14-12 Pressure gauges on inhalation sedation unit. **A,** O_2 pressure gauge. **B,** N_2O pressure gauge.

cylinder is 1000/1900, or 52% full. A full E cylinder of O_2 will produce 660 L of gaseous oxygen. At a flow rate of 6 L/min this tank would empty in 110 minutes (660/6 = 110 minutes). This is an important factor in the safety of inhalation sedation because if an O_2 cylinder became empty during a procedure while the N_2O cylinder still contained gas, it would be potentially possible to administer 100% N_2O. Although there are additional safety features designed to prevent this occurrence, the fact that the administrator of the N_2O-O_2 can see the "fuel gauge" for the O_2 permits a new cylinder to be opened before the nearly empty cylinder is depleted. If the sedation machine is equipped with two E cylinders of O_2, only one should be open and in use at any one time so that both tanks are not emptied simultaneously.[10]

Nitrous Oxide Cylinder and Contents

N_2O in compressed-gas cylinders is present in both the liquid and gaseous states. N_2O cylinders are factory filled to 90% to 95% capacity with liquid N_2O.[9] Above the liquid in the tank is N_2O vapor. The gas pressure within the cylinder of N_2O is approximately 750 psig at 70° F (25° C) (see Figure 14-12, *B*) within both the E and G cylinders. N_2O compressed-gas cylinders are color coded light blue in the United States and blue internationally. One ounce of N_2O liquid provides 3.88 gallons of N_2O gas. A full E cylinder of N_2O produces approximately 1600 L of gaseous N_2O at sea level and room temperature, whereas the larger H cylinder provides approximately 16,000 L of N_2O gas.[9]

Because of the presence of liquid in the N_2O cylinder, the gas pressure gauge on the cylinder will record "full" (approximately 750 psig) as long as any liquid remains in the cylinder. The pressure of the N_2O vapor floating above the liquid N_2O is 750 psig (see Figure 14-13). As the gaseous N_2O exits from the cylinder, liquid N_2O vaporizes to replace it. The pressure of this "new" gas is 750 psig. This process continues, liquid N_2O becoming converted to gaseous N_2O, with the gas pressure remaining at 750 psig, until no more liquid remains to replace the gas. The pressure gauge for N_2O therefore cannot be used as an accurate measurement of the contents of the cylinder. Once all of the liquid N_2O is gone and only gaseous N_2O remains, the pressure gauge will fall in relation to the pressure of gas now remaining (acting now like an O_2 pressure gauge). In normal clinical usage of inhalation sedation, it has been our experience that 2.5 O_2 cylinders are used for every N_2O cylinder of the same size. The presence of N_2O in a liquid state is the reason for the increased volume of gas within the N_2O cylinder as compared with the O_2 cylinders.

In central storage systems it is recommended that there be not less than two H O_2 cylinders and one G N_2O cylinder. In portable systems, on the other hand, one or two E cylinders of N_2O and two O_2 cylinders are recommended.

Regulators

Regulators, also called *reducing valves*, are located between the compressed-gas cylinder and the flowmeter. In central storage systems, regulators are

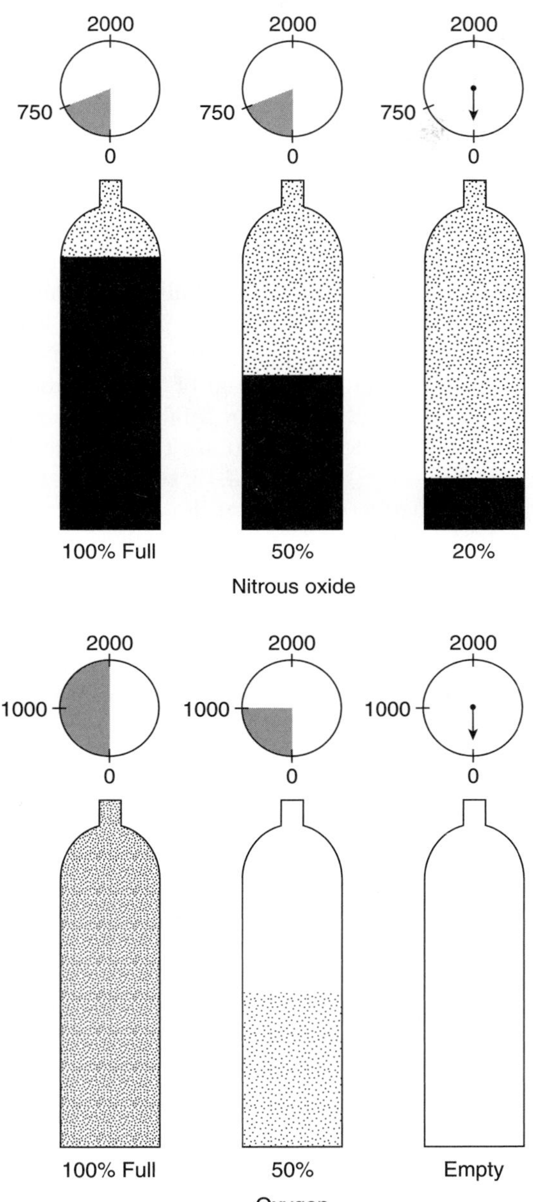

Figure 14-13 Pressure gauge readings for nitrous oxide and oxygen cylinders. (From Clark MS, Brunick AL: *Handbook of nitrous oxide and oxygen sedation*, St Louis, 1999, Mosby.)

commonly placed on the cylinder itself. The regulator functions to reduce the high-pressure gas coming from the cylinder (750 to 2200 psig) to a pressure that is safe for both the patient and the sedation unit. Regulators function to maintain a constant gas pressure to flowmeters and the patient regardless of the pressure of gas contained within the cylinder. Maintaining a constant, relatively low pressure within the body of the N_2O unit minimizes the potential for damage to the machine produced by high-pressure gases. The actual delivery pressure is set by the manufacturer of the equipment at 45 to 55 psig. When gases enter directly from cylinders, the pressure is reduced to 45 psig, whereas gases entering through a pipeline (central systems) maintain a pressure of 50 to 55 psig.

Regulators on portable units are located between the cylinders of gas and the flowmeters on the yoke (see Figure 14-4). Central systems commonly have a regulator attached directly to the cylinder, in which case it often has a gas pressure gauge combined with it. This type of system, with individual regulators for each cylinder of compressed gas, requires that the cylinders be switched on and off each day. In addition, when a cylinder of gas empties, there is no automatic system for switching to a reserve tank (as is present with the more expensive manifold system; see next section).

It is within the reducing valve that the recompression of gases produces a tremendous increase in temperature to about 1500° to 2000° F. This happens when a cylinder of O_2 at 1900 psig is quickly opened and the high-pressure gas is forced into a reducing valve. Although the reducing valve lowers this pressure to approximately 50 psig, gas backs up in the reducing valve, producing a recompression of gas that leads to a temperature increase. Temperature increases can ignite oil, grease, or Teflon that might be found in this area, leading to explosion and fire. Proper care and handling of cylinders (see previous discussion) will prevent this potentially disastrous consequence.

Manifolds (Central System Only)

A manifold joins multiple compressed-gas cylinders (Figure 14-14). For example, 12 N_2O cylinders may be attached to a single manifold. Twelve hoses will enter into the manifold, one from each regulator on the cylinder; but only one hose will exit the manifold, carrying the gas under low pressure (50 psig) to each station outlet in the individual operatories. The National Fire Protection Agency (NFPA) allows for only a level 3 system in dental offices. This allows for the equivalent of two (H size) oxygen cylinders and two (G size) N_2O cylinders in use and an additional two of each cylinder to be in storage.

A nonautomatic manifold is most commonly used. When a cylinder is empty, it must physically be turned off and a new cylinder opened by a staff member. Automatic manifolds are also available. The advantage of these more expensive devices is that they automatically activate a full reserve cylinder of gas when the cylinder in use empties. Other items found on all manifolds include a safety pressure relief valve and an alarm monitor gauge. The latter monitors the pressure of gas in the line (50 psig) and activates a high/low alarm should the pressure exceed 75 psig or fall below 40 psig. A typical manifold in a dental office will operate two O_2 cylinders, and a second manifold operates either one or two N_2O cylinders.

Yokes (Portable System Only)

The yoke assembly holds the cylinder of compressed gas tightly in contact with the nipples of the portable sedation unit (see Figure 14-8, *A*). Metal pins below the collar of the nipple are situated in such a way that they will accept only one specific type of compressed gas (see Figure 14-11). This constitutes the pin index safety system.

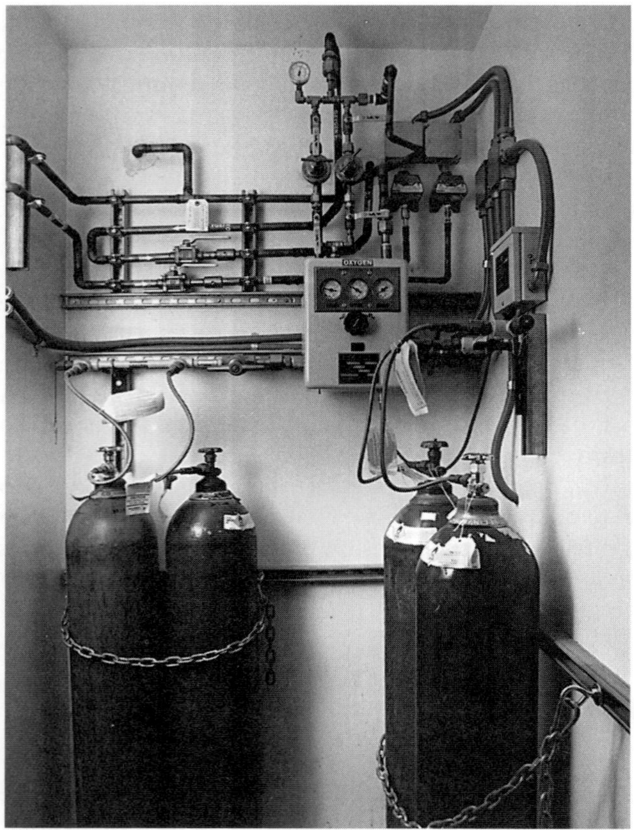

Figure 14-14 Manifold connecting a series of nitrous oxide and oxygen cylinders for use in a central system. Manifold provides automatic switch-over from the cylinder in use.

In the portable inhalation sedation unit, the circuit of gases to this point has been from the cylinder through the yoke and into the reducing valve, a portion of the circuit termed the *high-pressure system;* the circuit from the reducing valve to the patient is called the *low-pressure system*. From the reducing valve the gas enters low-pressure tubing (color coded for specific gases) that conducts the gas to attachments at the rear of the inhalation sedation unit. It is here that another safety feature of inhalation anesthetic systems is found. The diameter index safety system (DISS) (Figure 14-15; see also Figure 14-34 later) is designed to ensure that the correct medical gas enters the correct part of the anesthesia (sedation) machine.[11,12] Accidental attachment is prevented in two ways: First, the diameter of the attachments differs considerably, and second, the threading of the attachments differs, making it physically impossible to inadvertently attach tubing to the wrong inlet on the sedation or anesthesia machine. Once in the machine the gases are directed to the appropriate flowmeters, where precise volumes may be delivered to the patient.

The circuit thus far in the central system is similar, with a few important differences. Gas leaving the cylinder enters the reducing valve and the manifold directly, from which it is directed from the storage area through specially prepared copper tubing to the individual treatment areas in the dental office. This tubing may be found in the walls, ceilings, or floors and leads to outlets in the individual treatment rooms. The outlet station possesses attachments for N_2O and O_2 hoses that are quick-connects, permitting rapid attachment and disconnection of the hoses.[9] To prevent accidental

A

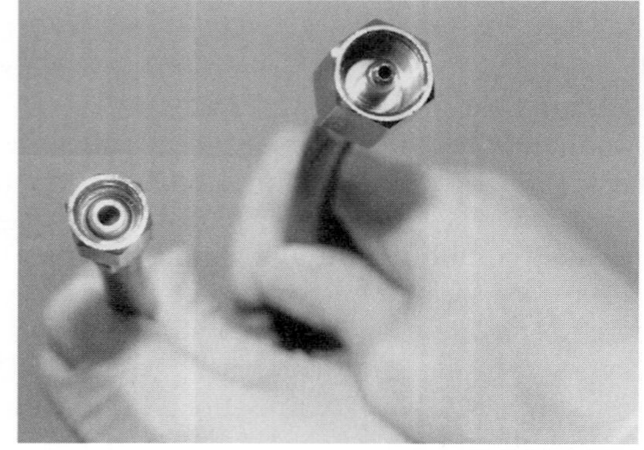

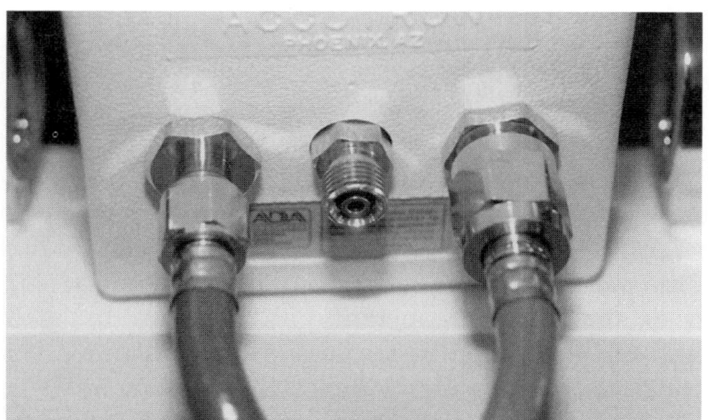

B

Figure 14-15 **A** and **B,** Diameter index safety system. Connectors attaching low-pressure tubing to inhalation sedation unit are of different diameters. Oxygen *(left)* is of smaller diameter than nitrous oxide *(right)*, thus preventing accidental crossing of attachments. (From Clark MS, Brunick AL: *Handbook of nitrous oxide and oxygen sedation*, St Louis, 1999, Mosby.)

crossing of these hoses, the DISS is incorporated into the quick-connect for N_2O and O_2.

Flowmeters

From the reducing valves, the individual gases are carried through low-pressure tubing into the back of the unit. The gases are then directed to the flowmeters (see Figure 14-3), which permit the administrator to deliver a precise volume of either gas to the patient. Flowmeters are calibrated only for the gas that will flow through it (N_2O or O_2).[10] Gas flows are calibrated to be read at 25° C at 76 cm Hg (atmospheric pressure). Flowmeters measure the actual quantity of gas in motion rather than static cylinder pressure (as measured by the pressure gauges). If the flow of gas is interrupted, the flowmeter will read zero.

The flowmeter is actually a very simple device. Gas enters a tube formed with a tapering lumen that grows wider from the gas inlet at the bottom to the outlet at its top. A float used for measuring the volume is found inside the flowmeter. The float is either a ball or a rotameter. When a ball is used, the precise flow volume of gas is read using the middle of the ball, whereas with the rotameter the flow is read at the top of the bobbin.

Once the flow of gas is started, gas enters the bottom of the flowmeter. The gas forces the float up into the flowmeter tube. Because the flowmeter is tapered, the area surrounding the float increases in size as the increased flow of gas causes the float to bob at a higher level; the flow rate is proportional to the size of the space surrounding the float.

The calibrations on the flowmeter tubes indicate the flow of gas in liters per minute (L/min). Adjustment of the gas flow is accomplished by means of a fine-needle valve for each flowmeter. The knobs that control the gases are both touch coded and color coded. In the United States the O_2 control knob is green in color and fluted, whereas the N_2O control knob is blue and not fluted (Figure 14-16).[13] The characteristics of the knobs may vary with dental mixers. In North America the oxygen flowmeter is positioned on the right side of the bank of flowmeters.[14]

The three types of devices—the rotameter, ball, and rod—are used inside the flowmeter to measure gas flow. The rod-type flowmeter is seldom used any longer primarily because its accuracy is not as great as that of the ball or rotameter. Accuracy for the rod-type flowmeter is ± 7%.

In the ball-type flowmeter a ball is forced up into the flowmeter by the gas entering the meter. For best accuracy this type of flowmeter is placed on an inclined plane (Figure 14-17). The ball-type flowmeter is the most commonly used today. Its accuracy is ± 5%, and it is least accurate at very low flow rates.

The rotameter-type flowmeter is the most accurate, with an accuracy of ± 2%. A metal bobbin, usually aluminum, is pushed upward in the flowmeter by the force of the gas passing through the meter. This stream of gas also causes the rotameter to rotate. Flowmeters in this type of unit must be vertical (Figure 14-18). The three types of flowmeters are compared in Table 14-4.

As the anesthetic gases leave through the top of their respective flowmeters, they are combined in the mixing chamber, which is found within the head of the sedation unit. From this point a combination of the gases flows through the machine. These gases now exit the sedation unit through the outflow tube, which is also known as a *bag/tee* (see Figures 14-3 and 14-4), and are carried to the patient.

Flowmeter Advancements. Although the old flow tube flowmeter technology is still available today, it is being replaced by state-of-the-art digital electronic flow control devices, most notably the Centurion Mixer and Digital MDM (Figure 14-19). Both of these devices are percentage devices and overcome the limitations of the older flow tube technology. The devices have resolution of the gas flow in increments of 0.1 L/min, and the total flow and percentage oxygen are displayed digitally, eliminating the guesswork or calculations required with simple flow tube devices. The ability to clean the front panel with just a "wipe" reduces the potential of cross-infection among patients, an issue associated with crevasses created by knobs and levers. Patient safety is ensured with built in alarms for all gas depletion conditions along with servo control of the gas delivery (what you see is what you get). Continuous internal self-monitoring of all operational parameters by the device frees the practitioner to concentrate on the patient's needs. The device alerts the practitioner or staff to unusual parameters requiring attention, similar to those seen in larger hospital-based systems.

The digital units deliver pure oxygen during the "flush" function by electronically shutting off the N_2O flow, as opposed to the flow tube units, which only dilute the N_2O delivered. Again, the removal of extra steps in shutting down the N_2O supply before pressing the "flush" button greatly simplifies the practitioner's tasks.

The units contain flashing light-emitting diodes (LEDs) to afford the practitioner a simple method of ensuring that the individual component gas is flowing and that the relative ratio and amount of flow are correct. In addition, the digital unit provides the capability of displaying the flow rate of either of the

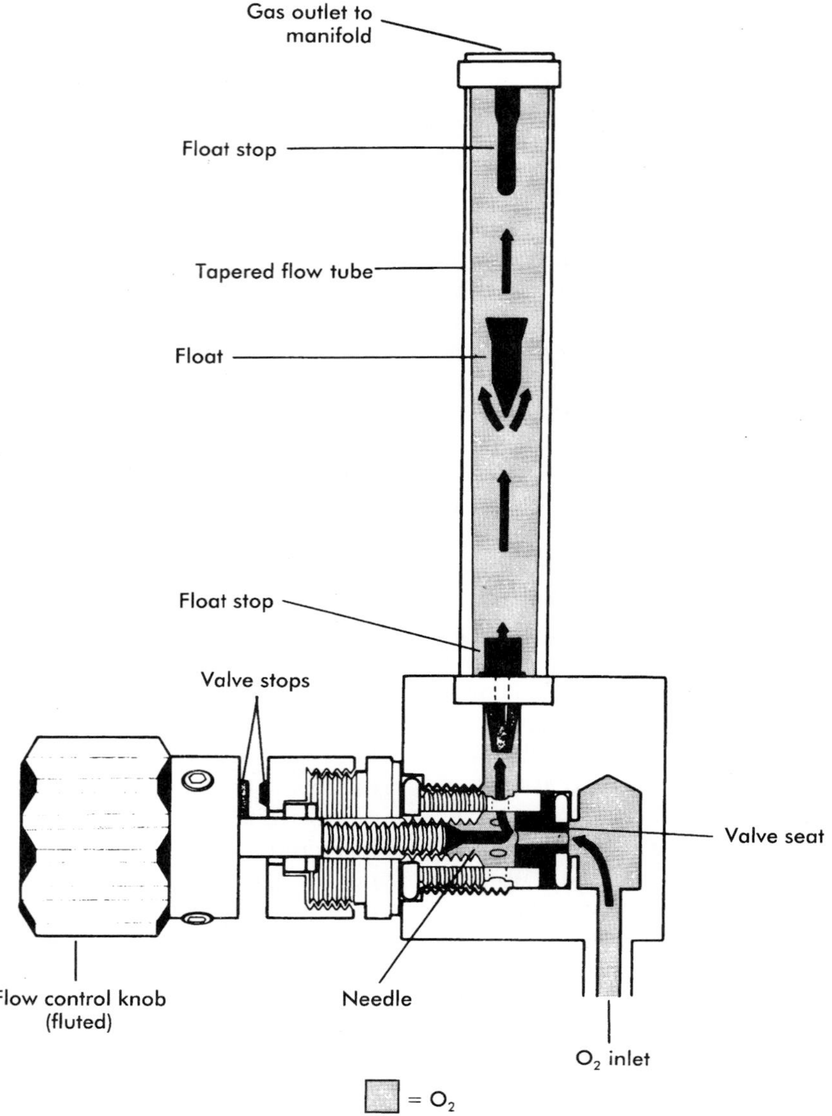

Figure 14-16 Oxygen flowmeter and flow control valve. (Modified from Bowie E, Huffman LM: *The anesthesia machine: essentials for understanding,* Madison, Wisc, 1985, Ohmeda, BOC Health Care.)

constituent gasses. The nonsilenceable alarm function for oxygen depletion ensures adequate patient safety. The air intake valve located on the bag/tee provides room air to the patient whenever the patient's breathing demand is greater than the combined output of the mixer head's settings and reservoir bag volume.

Various models of the electronic gas-mixing head allow mounting as a wall unit, portable unit, countertop unit, or as a flush mount unit in modern cabinetry. Digital heads have the most flexibility, especially when combined with various remote bag/tee options provided by the manufacturer. The units are fully compatible with central gas supply systems such as the popular Flo-Safe Manifold, Centurion Gas Manifold, and all existing scavenging systems. It is available with the American Dental Association (ADA) recommended 45 L/min[15] scavenging control valve in various mounting configurations.

Electronic digital administration heads for delivery of conscious sedation advance the art of dentistry. The digital heads, once considered the wave of the future, are the de facto "standard" today. The digital accuracy and exacting control are highly recommended for patient comfort and safety.

Emergency Air Intake Valve

On the bag/tee, above the reservoir bag, an emergency air valve is located (see Figure 14-4). It provides the patient with a supply of atmospheric air in the event

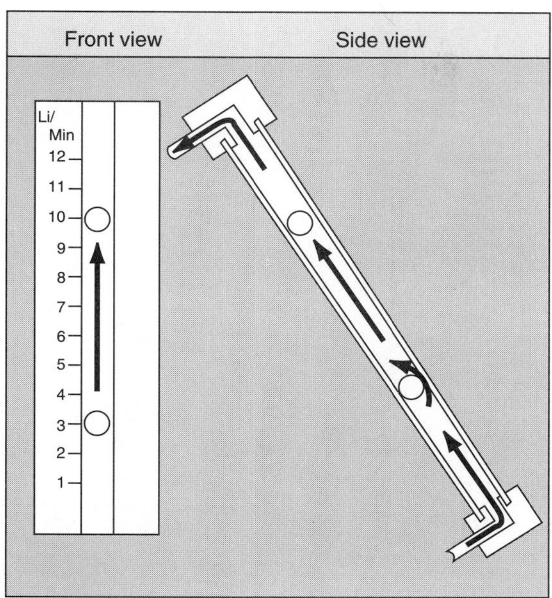

Figure 14-17 Ball-type flowmeter. (Redrawn from Allen GD: *Dental anesthesia and analgesia*, ed 2, Baltimore, 1979, Williams & Wilkins.)

that the sedation unit ceases to function and gas flow from the machine is terminated. During normal use, the emergency air valve remains shut, but it opens automatically once gas flow through the machine is terminated. This prevents the patient from experiencing a feeling of discomfort or suffocation as he or she attempts to breathe through the nasal hood when the unit is not working and the reservoir bag is deflated.

Rubber Goods

From the outlet tube the anesthetic gases are carried to the patient. In addition to the reservoir bag, the rubber goods consist of conducting tubes and a face mask, nasal hood, or nasal cannula.

Reservoir Bag. Reservoir bags are bladder-type bags, made of rubber or silicone, ranging in size from 1 to 8 L. The 3-L reservoir bag is the most frequently used in dentistry. Although commonly used, rubber bags deteriorate more rapidly than silicone bags, especially in areas in which high levels of atmospheric pollutants are found (the planet Earth).

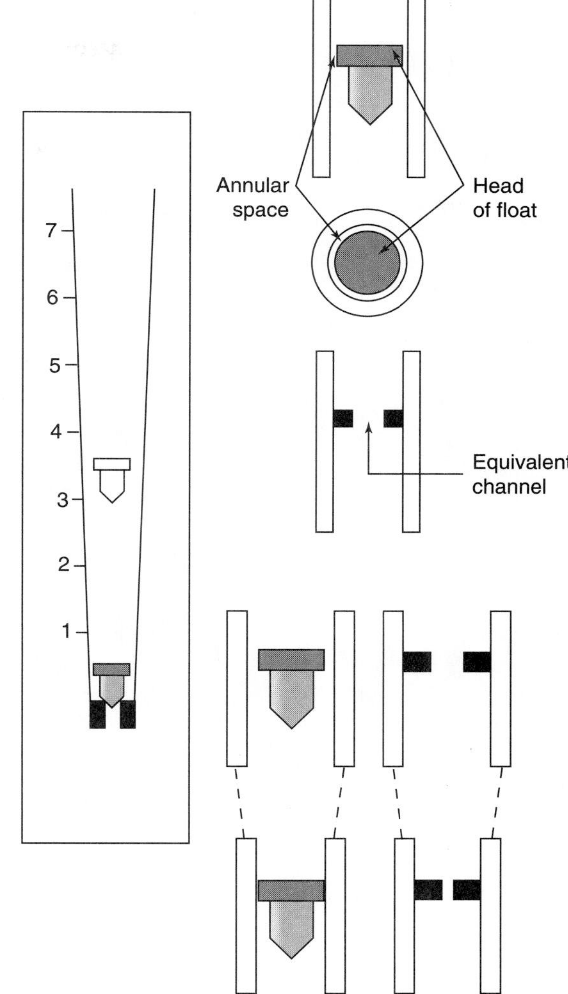

Figure 14-18 Rotameter-type flowmeter. (Redrawn from Allen GD: *Dental anesthesia and analgesia*, ed 2, Baltimore, 1979, Williams & Wilkins.)

The reservoir bag attaches to the base of the bag/tee, usually immediately below the emergency air inlet valve (see Figures 14-3 and 14-4). A portion of the

TABLE 14-4 Characteristics of Flowmeters

	Rotameter	Ball	Rod
Accuracy	± 2%	± 5%	± 7%
Current use	Intermediate use	Most common	Least common
Flowmeter angle	Vertical	Inclined	Vertical
Material	Aluminum	Plastic	Metal

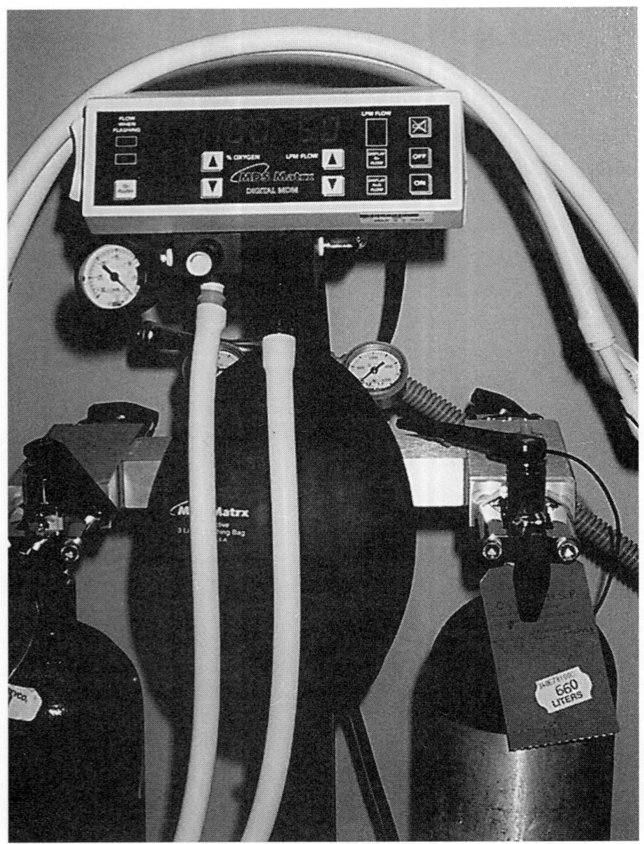

Figure 14-19 MDS Matrix digital electronic flow control device.

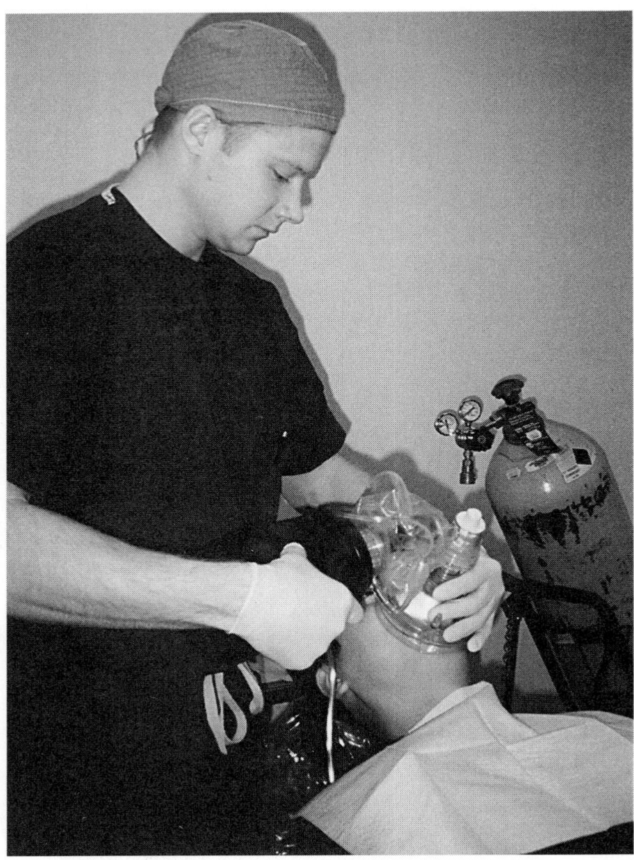

Figure 14-20 One can use the reservoir bag to provide oxygen during assisted or controlled ventilation by squeezing the contents and forcing them into the patient's lungs.

gas(es) being delivered through the unit to the patient is diverted into the reservoir bag, where it may be used for any of several purposes.

The primary function of the reservoir bag during inhalation sedation is to provide a reservoir from which additional gas may be drawn should the respiratory demands of the patient exceed the gas flow being delivered from the machine. During normal (quiet) respiration the patient receives only fresh gases delivered from the sedation unit, with little or none being taken from the reservoir bag. However, should the patient take an especially deep breath, the machine will be unable to accommodate the necessary volume; in the absence of the reservoir bag, the patient will experience a feeling of suffocation. The reservoir bag prevents or minimizes this occurrence.

A second use of the reservoir bag during conscious sedation is to serve as a monitoring device for respiration. Assuming an airtight seal of the nasal hood and no mouth breathing, the reservoir bag will inflate slightly with every exhalation and deflate slightly with each inspiration, permitting the operator to easily determine respiratory rate.

A third potential use for the reservoir bag is its use as a means of providing O_2 during assisted or controlled ventilation. Provided that a full face mask is properly positioned with an airtight seal and a patent airway, the reservoir bag is squeezed, and its contents are forced into the patient's lungs (Figure 14-20). It is quite a bit more difficult to ventilate the patient with the reservoir bag when the nasal hood is used. Adequate ventilation can be accomplished with the nasal hood, but this is not likely to be effective in the hands of an inexperienced person (a person who is not trained in anesthesiology). Controlled and assisted ventilation are impossible with a nasal cannula because the reservoir bag is removed from the sedation machine when a cannula is used.

The reservoir bag is of considerable importance in general anesthesia, for during this time the patient is unconscious and unable to respond to the commands of the anesthesiologist. Other means of determining the physical status of the patient must be used. Monitoring vital signs becomes quite important. Respiratory rate and depth can be monitored easily by observing and feeling the reservoir bag. Should respiratory depth become shallow, the anesthesiologist can assist a patient's breathing by gently squeezing the bag as the patient begins to breathe spontaneously. Should spontaneous respiration cease, controlled respiration can be started, with the anesthesiologist squeezing the reservoir bag once every 5 seconds for an adult, every 4 seconds for a child, and every 3 seconds for an infant.

The reservoir bag was, in the past, called a *rebreathing bag*. Not too many years ago it was possible for the patient to exhale into the nasal hood, and if the total flow of gas from the sedation unit was low, the exhaled gases could be forced backward through the conducting tubing to reach the reservoir bag. On inhalation these same gases, now containing elevated concentrations of carbon dioxide (CO_2), would be rebreathed. Rebreathing gas containing elevated CO_2 levels can lead to unpleasant consequences if permitted to continue for extended periods. One-way valves have been placed into the bag/tee of contemporary machines to prevent the possibility of rebreathing.

For the adult patient receiving conscious sedation, the 3- or 5-L reservoir bag is used. In pediatric procedures, smaller (1-, 2-, or 3-L) reservoir bags are used.

Conducting Tubes. A variable length of hose, called either *conducting tubing* or a *breathing tube* (Figure 14-21, *A*), connects the bag/tee to the nasal hood. The hose is of large diameter, is corrugated, and is usually made of black rubber. The large diameter minimizes any resistance to the flow of gases from the machine through the tubes to the patient, and the corrugation prevents inadvertent kinking or occlusion of its lumen. In conscious sedation procedures, the corrugated tubing is less essential than it is during general anesthesia. During N_2O-O_2 sedation, should a hose conducting gas to the patient become occluded by some means, the patient, still conscious, would comment on the increased difficulty of obtaining an adequate gas supply through the nosepiece. During general anesthesia, however, with the patient unconscious and unable to reply, occlusion of the tube carrying gas from the anesthesia machine would produce little or no immediate outward change in appearance, the lack of O_2 producing a deeper level of "general anesthesia." Only after possibly irreversible brain damage has occurred will changes be noticed by the less than expert observer. Thus the corrugated tubing present on all sedation units is a remnant of the general anesthesia machine from which the modern sedation unit evolved.

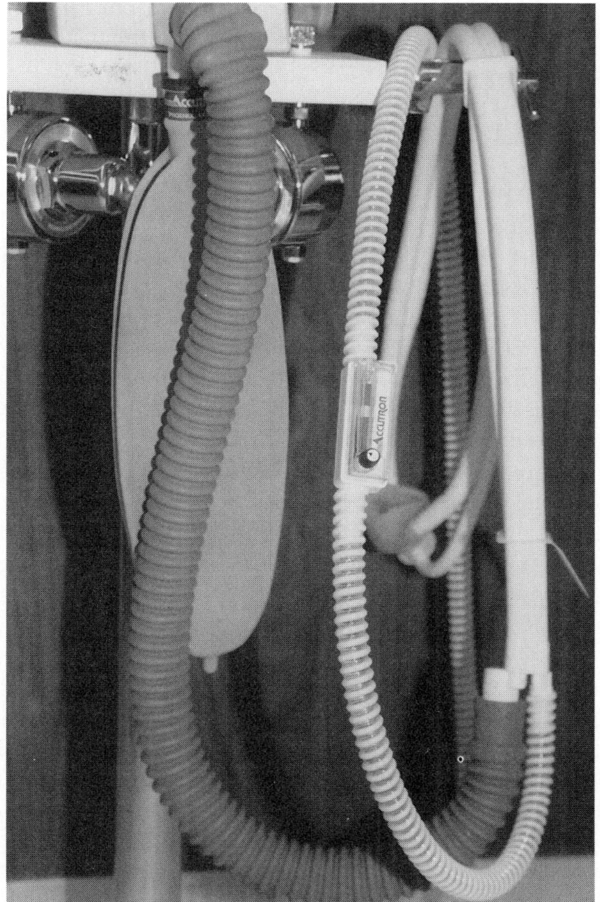

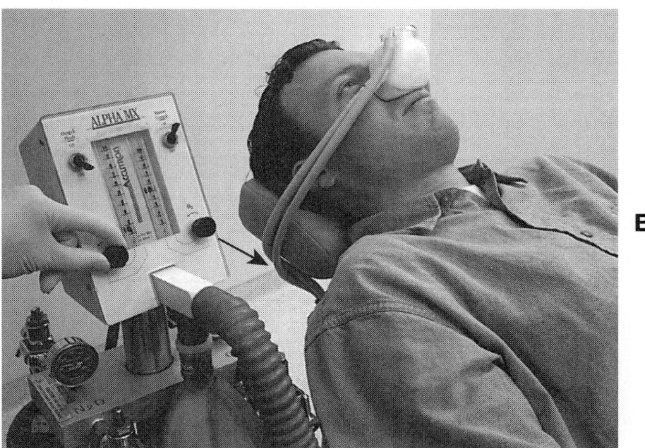

Figure 14-21 **A,** Conducting tubing connects the bag/tee to the nasal hood. **B,** Noncorrugated tubing can become occluded as it bends around the sides of the dental chair *(arrow)*. (**A** from Clark MS, Brunick AL: *Handbook of nitrous oxide and oxygen sedation*, St Louis, 1999, Mosby.)

The corrugated tubing is attached to one or two noncorrugated tubes that attach directly to the breathing apparatus on the patient (Figure 14-21, *B*). These tubes are of smaller diameter than the corrugated tubing; however, they do not add significantly to the resistance to gas flow to the patient. In units with one larger-diameter tube flowing to the breathing apparatus, the tube is carried over the top of the patient's head and forehead and then to the breathing apparatus on the patient's nose. More commonly, two tubes are attached to the corrugated tubing. These tubes come around the sides of the dental chair and are attached to the breathing apparatus. In both cases the tubing must be secured so that the patient remains comfortable and so that leakage will not occur around the sides of the breathing apparatus. With double tubing, there is the possibility that the tubing will be kinked as it comes around the side of the dental chair (see Figure 14-21, *B*). Care is required when securing the tubing to prevent this from occurring.

Breathing Apparatus

Full Face Mask. Three types of breathing apparatus may be used to deliver N_2O-O_2 to the patient. The full face mask covers both the mouth and nose of the patient (Figure 14-22; see also Figure 14-20). Although the face mask is the most effective method of delivering gases to the patient, in dentistry the full face mask is impractical because the mouth must remain available for the dental procedure to be completed. However, the presence of a face mask in the dental office is important in emergency situations because the full face mask provides the optimal means of delivering O_2 to the patient (provided the person delivering the O_2 has received training in emergency airway management).

Nasal Cannula. The nasal cannula (Figure 14-23) is quite different from the face mask. Made from a softened plastic, the two short (1/8-inch-long) prongs are placed into the nostrils of the patient, and the device is used primarily to provide hospitalized patients with supplemental O_2. It is impossible to obtain an airtight seal with the nasal cannula, a fact that is detrimental to its use during N_2O-O_2 sedation because it leads to a significant degree of dilution of the gases being delivered from the machine. To compensate for this air dilution, greater volumes of gases must be delivered to the patient. This is especially relevant for N_2O because significantly greater volumes of N_2O will be needed to produce a desired sedation level. In fact, it is often impossible to obtain clinically adequate sedation with the cannula even when maximal volumes of N_2O are being delivered. Because of air dilution and the greater volumes of gases being used, there is considerably greater contamination of the clinical environment with N_2O than is present when a nasal hood is used.

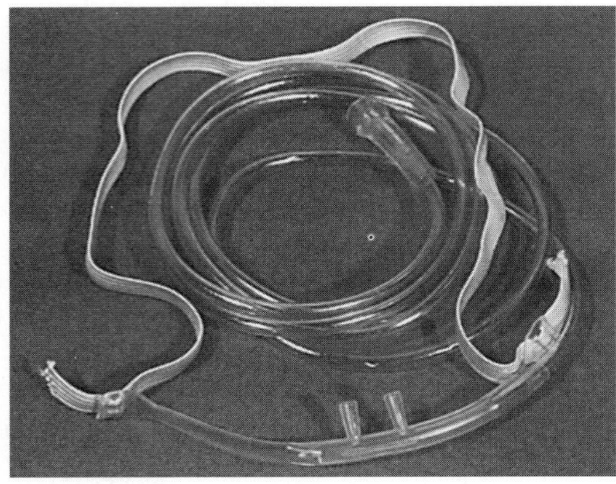

Figure 14-23 Nasal cannula. Two short plastic prongs are placed in nares of the patient.

The primary advantages of the nasal cannula include its usefulness in patients with a fear of the full face mask or the nasal hood and in claustrophobic patients. These persons are unable to tolerate the full face mask or nasal hood comfortably, whereas the nasal cannula invariably proves satisfactory to them. A second advantage of the cannula is during treatment of maxillary anterior teeth. With a traditional nasal hood that rests over the patient's upper lip and against his or her maxillary anterior teeth, treatment involving the labial soft tissues or the teeth themselves may prove difficult because the nasal hood compresses the upper lip against the soft and hard tissues in this region. One way to minimize this potential difficulty is to place cotton rolls under the patient's upper lip before placing the nasal hood. The cannula, however, does not interfere with dental treatment in this area (Figure 14-24).

A disadvantage of the nasal cannula is the necessity to remove the reservoir bag from the sedation unit,

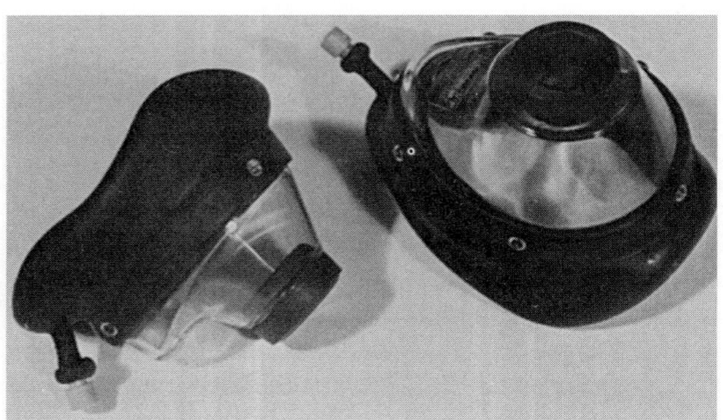

Figure 14-22 Full face mask covers both nose and mouth of patient. Although inconvenient during dental care, it is appropriate for use in emergency situations (see also Figure 14-20).

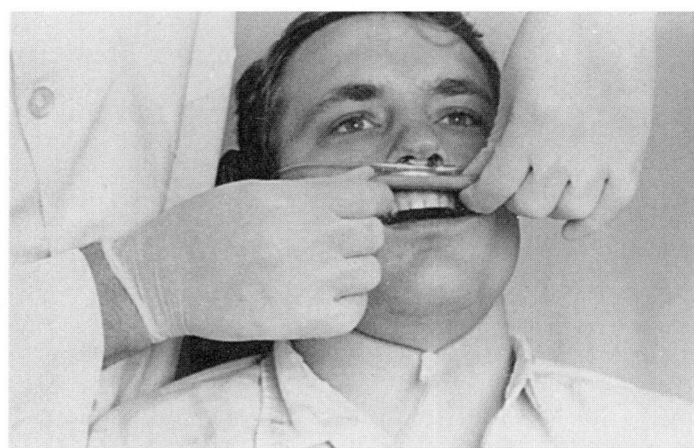

Figure 14-24 Nasal cannula does not interfere with dental treatment in maxillary anterior region.

thereby negating its usefulness as a monitoring or ventilatory device. In its place is a plug, directing all gases from the machine into the cannula.

Because the gases delivered from the sedation unit (O_2 and N_2O) are both anhydrous, they are directed through a humidifier before being sent to the patient (Figure 14-25). The humidifier is placed on the end of the outlet tube, to which is attached the nasal cannula.

The tubing of the nasal cannula is narrow. Gases being delivered to the cannula through the outlet tube and humidifier will therefore gain considerable velocity as they pass from the wider bore of the outlet tube to the narrower space of the cannula. The force of the gas exiting the cannula may in fact prove uncomfortable for the patient. With today's concern about the potential hazards of trace contamination of the environment with N_2O, the use of the nasal cannula cannot be recommended except in very few cases in which inhalation sedation must be used and other methods of delivering the gases to the patient are unacceptable.

Nasal Hood. The nasal hood, a device designed to fit comfortably and securely over the patient's nose, comes in two types. The traditional nasal hood (commonly called a *nosepiece*) has one or two tubes entering into it (Figure 14-26). These tubes deliver gases from

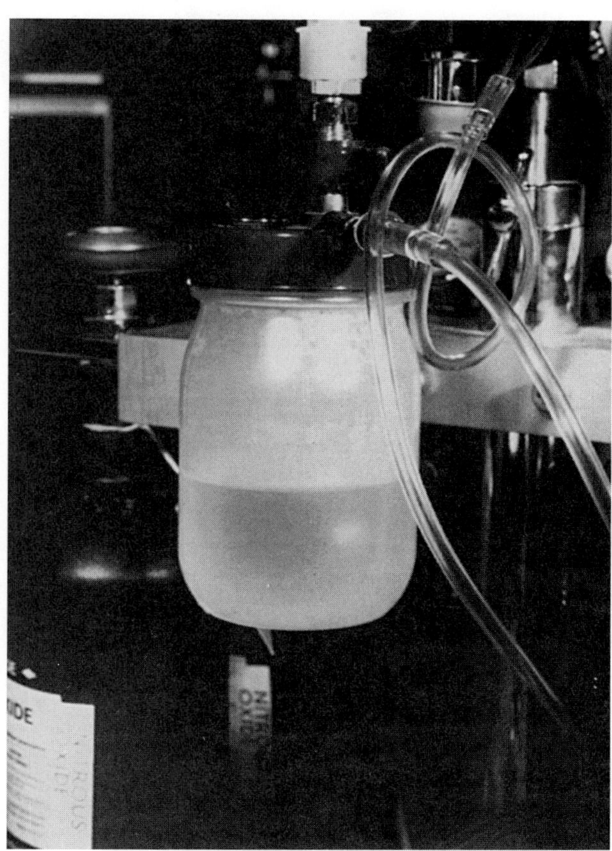

Figure 14-25 Nasal cannula with humidifier.

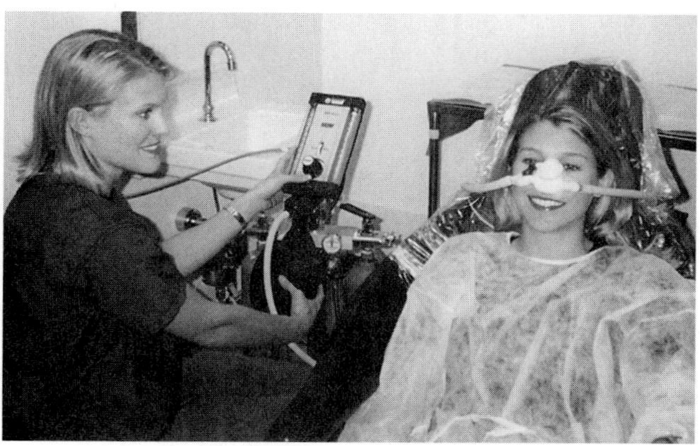

Figure 14-26 Traditional nasal hood.

the inhalation sedation unit. Exhaled gases are eliminated into the surrounding environment through an exhaling valve located on top of the nasal hood. Along with the exhaling valve, the nasal hood may also possess an air-dilution valve.

The second type of delivery system is the more recently introduced scavenging nasal hood. The prototypical scavenging nasal hood has four tubes entering it. Two tubes deliver fresh gases from the sedation unit, the other tubes carrying exhaled gases away from the treatment area to a safe repository (Figure 14-27). With concern increasing about the possible deleterious effects on dental staff of prolonged exposure to low levels of N_2O, the scavenging nasal hood is mandatory.

The nasal hood is made of rubber or silicone, which readily adapts to the contours of the patient's face, providing an airtight seal (Figure 14-28). Nasal hoods are designed in a variety of sizes, and it is important that several sizes be available.

The traditional nasal hood contains one or two inlets through which fresh gases are delivered from the sedation unit to the patient. On the top of the mask is an opening into which has been placed one or more valves. When only one valve is present, it is an exhaling or one-way valve, permitting the patient to eliminate all exhaled gases into the environment and to inhale only fresh gases from the machine. The exhaling valve contains a thin wafer (Figure 14-29, *A*) that sits over the opening in the valve. On exhalation, the wafer is lifted by the force of the gases and the gases are eliminated. On inhalation, the negative pressure created within the nosepiece forces the wafer down into the hole, sealing it shut and thus allowing the patient to inhale only the gases from the machine.

A second valve, present on some nasal hoods, is called the *inhaling* or *air-dilution valve.* It consists of an opening from the inside of the nasal hood directly to the atmosphere (Figure 14-29, *B*). As the patient exhales, gases escape from this valve (as in the exhaling

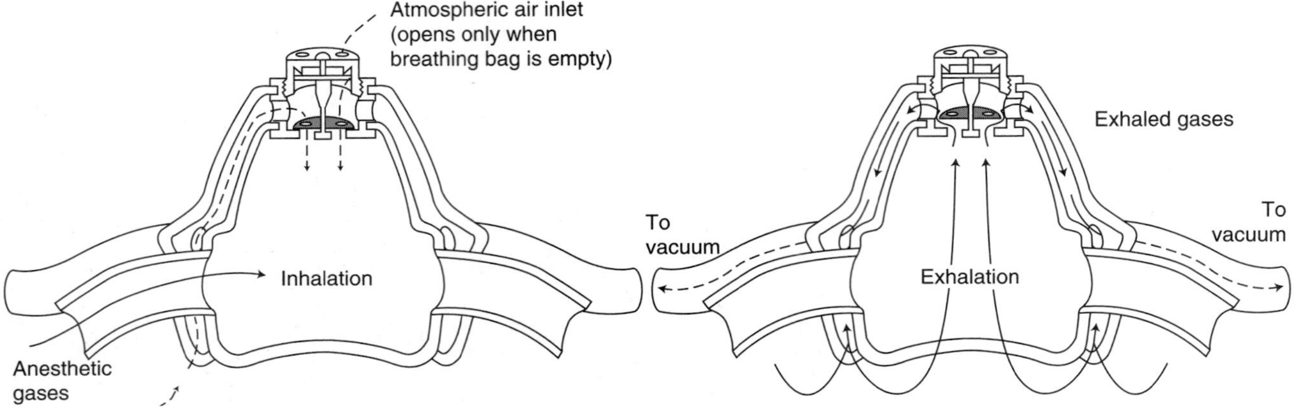

Figure 14-27 Diagram of scavenging nasal hood.

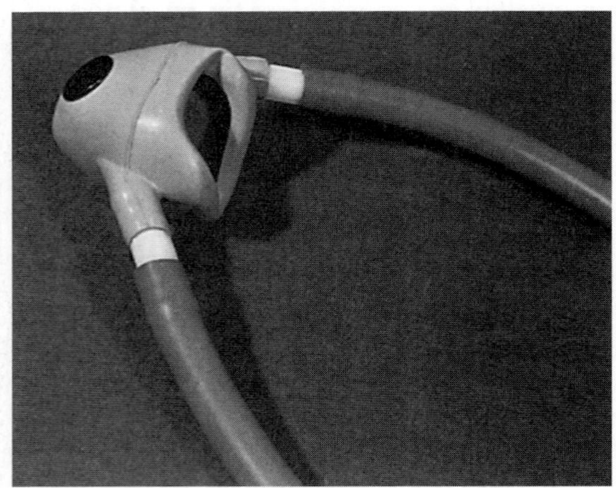

Figure 14-28 Nasal hood with connecting tubes.

valve); however, on inhalation this valve remains open, permitting the patient to breathe in an unknown quantity of ambient air along with the fresh gases from the sedation unit. It has been estimated that the inspired percentage of N_2O may be diluted by 50% if the air-dilution valve is fully opened. The value of the air-dilution valve is that it permits the patient to breathe comfortably regardless of the volume of gas being delivered from the machine; however, because of dilution, the volume of N_2O must be increased significantly, producing considerably higher concentrations of N_2O in the ambient air, which is undesirable.

The air-dilution valve is capable of being opened or closed, whereas the exhaling valve cannot be closed. If two valves are present on the nasal hood, it is recommended that the air-dilution valve be kept closed. There are virtually no indications for the use of an opened air-dilution valve; in fact, many newer nasal hoods are being manufactured without the air-dilution valve.

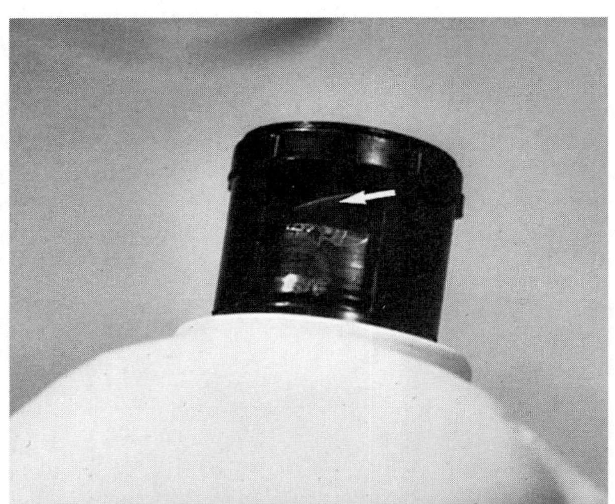

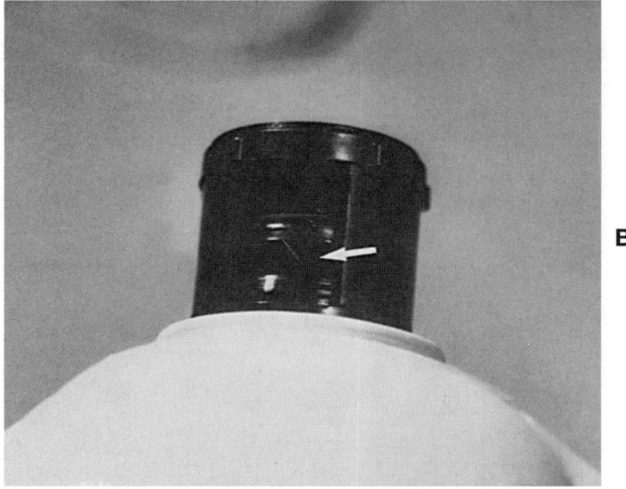

Figure 14-29 **A,** Exhaling valve on nasal hood. Thin wafer *(arrow)* seals orifice while patient inhales but is forced off orifice when patient exhales. **B,** Air dilution valve is opening below exhaling valve *(arrow)*, which permits entry of atmospheric air during inhalation.

The conventional nasal hood is no longer recommended for use with inhalation sedation. Although the absolute risk of chronic inhalation of low concentrations of N_2O is as yet undetermined, evidence indicates that there are no desirable attributes to its being inhaled by health professionals. The scavenging nasal hood should be used whenever N_2O is administered.

Scavenging Nasal Hood. With recent concern over the possible long-term effects of trace levels of N_2O on chairside personnel (see Chapter 17), it has become expedient to attempt to eliminate exhaled N_2O from the ambient air: To this end the scavenging nasal hood has been developed (see Figure 14-27). A number of such devices are currently available, but the principle behind their effectiveness is essentially the same. The Brown nosepiece was one of the earliest scavenging devices and will serve as the prototypical scavenging nasal hood (Figure 14-30).

Scavenging nasal hoods are, quite simply, double nosepieces: a smaller inner mask receiving anesthetic gases from the machine and a slightly larger outer mask that sits directly over the first, which removes exhaled gases from the treatment area. The outer nosepiece is connected to the suction device in the dental operatory, permitting exhaust gases to be vented from the dental operatory through the vacuum system. The effectiveness of this system is in part responsible for the 50 ppm standard for ambient levels of N_2O currently in use today. The scavenging system is discussed in Chapter 17, but at present, the scavenging mask represents the most effective means of minimizing N_2O contamination in the dental or surgical environment.

Other scavenging systems incorporate dual exhaust tubes with a single fresh gas inlet (Allen scavenging mask, Figure 14-31), and still others include a scavenging cone that sits atop the nasal hood (Matrix scavenging nasal hood, Figure 14-32). This type of mask has the additional advantage of scavenging the treatment room when not scavenging the patient's exhalation. As suggested, it is recommended that scavenging nasal hoods be employed during the administration of N_2O-O_2 inhalation sedation.

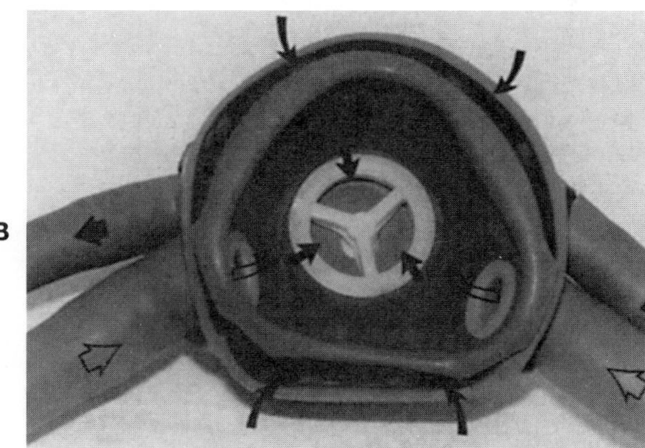

Figure 14-30 **A,** An exterior view of a Brown mask. Gas intake *(open arrows),* waste gas removal *(solid arrows),* and suction intake holes *(smaller solid arrows).* **B,** An interior view of a Brown mask revealing the double-mask construction and gas flow. (From Dionne RA, Phero JC: *Management of pain and anxiety in dental practice,* New York, 1991, Elsevier.)

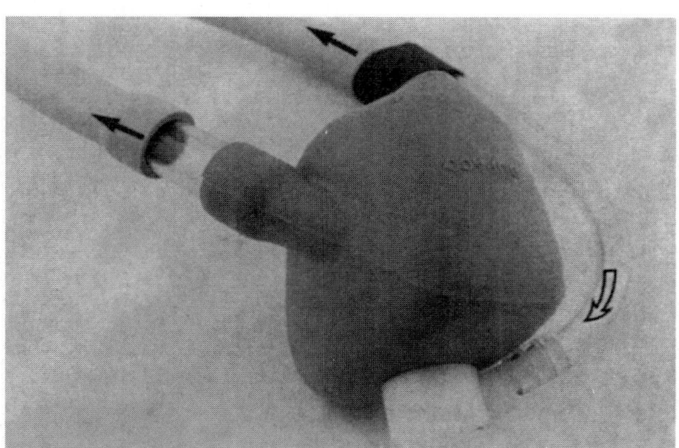

Figure 14-31 A Dupaco (Allen) scavenging mask with fresh gas inlet *(open arrow)* and waste gas removal *(solid arrows).* (From Dionne RA, Phero JC: *Management of pain and anxiety in dental practice,* New York, 1991, Elsevier.)

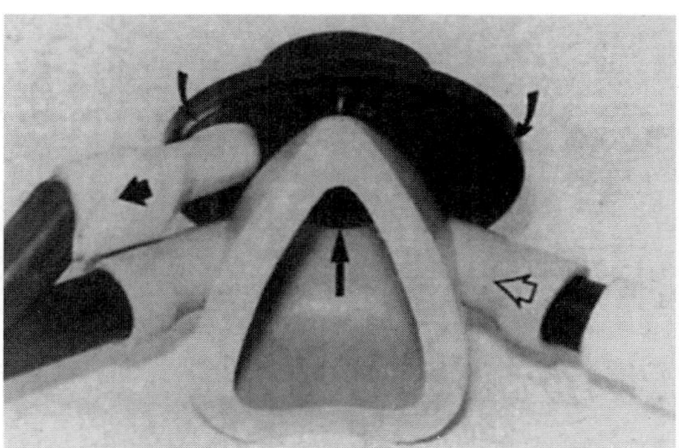

Figure 14-32 Internal view of Matrix nosepiece demonstrating fresh gas inlet *(open arrow)* and waste gas outflow through the plastic scavenging cone *(solid arrows).* (From Dionne RA, Phero JC: *Management of pain and anxiety in dental practice,* New York, 1991, Elsevier.)

Modern nasal hoods do not contain any metal. This contrasts dramatically with older nasal hoods in which the valves very often contained metal springs or clips. The disadvantage of nasal hoods containing metal became apparent whenever radiographs were taken. Invariably, the metal would be superimposed directly above a critical portion of the film. With modern nasal hoods, radiographs may be taken without removing the nasal hood.

SAFETY FEATURES

All inhalation sedation units available in the United States incorporate a series of safety features. The primary purpose of these features is to prevent the delivery, either accidental or intentional, of less than atmospheric levels of oxygen (20.9%).

The Council on Dental Materials, Instruments and Equipment of the American Dental Association has issued guidelines for inhalation sedation units.[16] Although these safety features work well to minimize the occurrence of accidents, it must be emphasized that all mechanical devices are capable of failing, so the administrator of inhalation sedation should never rely entirely on them for a patient's safety.[5-7] Visual and verbal monitoring of the patient and visual monitoring of the sedation unit are essential at all times.

Pin Index Safety System

The pin index safety system makes it physically impossible to attach an N_2O-compressed-gas cylinder to the yoke attachment for O_2 (or any other compressed-gas yoke except N_2O), which could result in the inadvertent administration of 100% N_2O instead of 100% O_2. The pin index safety system consists of a series of pins, the configuration of which differs for each compressed gas (Figure 14-33), on the yoke of the sedation unit and a matching series of holes on the compressed-gas cylinders. However, I have seen a blue cylinder (presumably N_2O) with the pin index system for O_2! Beware!

Diameter Index Safety System

The diameter index safety system makes it impossible to attach a low-pressure hose to the wrong outlet on the sedation unit (Figure 14-34).[17] The diameter of the couplings differs significantly (the coupling for N_2O being larger than that for O_2). In addition, the threading of the attachments differs. It becomes physically impossible to accidentally cross the low-pressure hoses and deliver the wrong gas to the patient. This system also exists as a safeguard on the larger G and H cylinders.

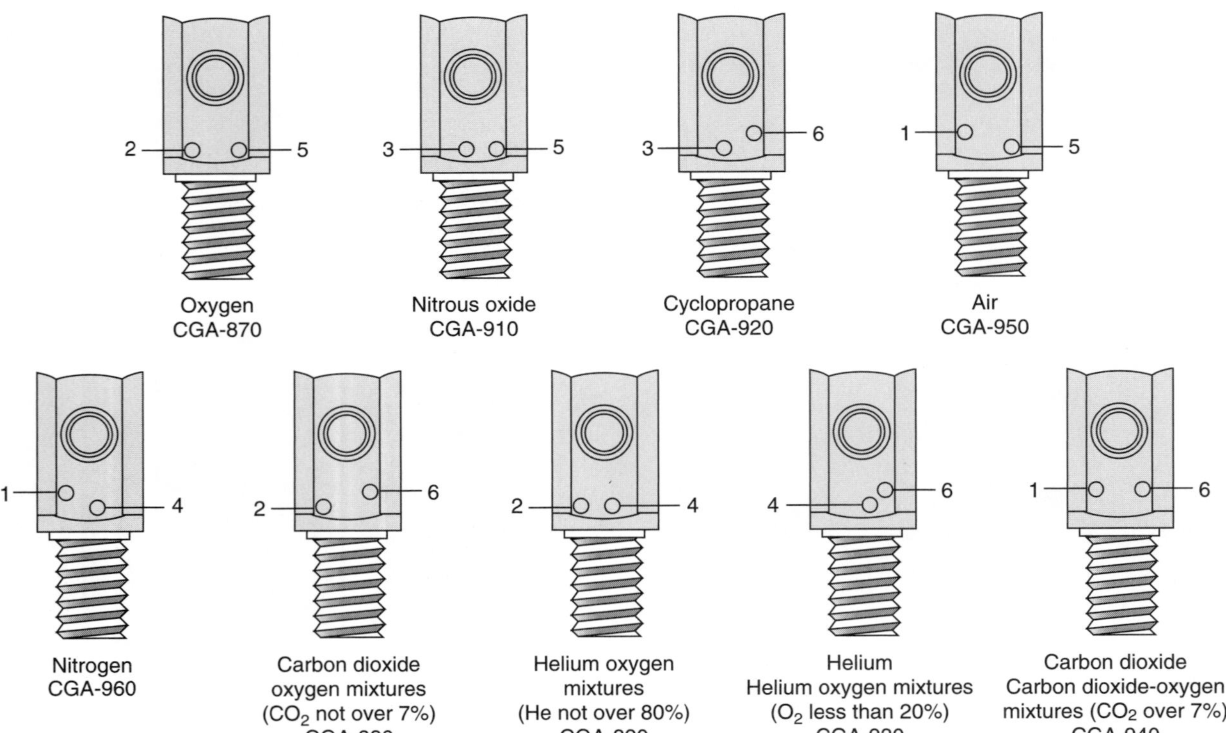

Figure 14-33 Pin index safety system for compressed-gas cylinders.

Minimum Oxygen Liter Flow

Inhalation sedation units are designed so that once turned on the unit delivers a preset minimum liter flow of O_2 through the flowmeter. In most units this minimum flow is 2.5 or 3.0 L/min of O_2. The flow of N_2O cannot start until a flow of O_2 has been established.

Minimum Oxygen Percentage

Similar to the minimum O_2 liter flow, this safety feature sets a minimum percentage of O_2 that may be delivered to the patient. This minimum O_2 percentage is 30% (some units provide 25%). This allows for a possible error in calibration of the flowmeters of approximately ± 5% while still delivering more than 20% O_2 to the patient. The ball-type flowmeter has a ± 5% accuracy rating, and the rotameter has a ± 2% accuracy rating.

In a sedation unit in which a minimum O_2 flow of 2.5 L/min is delivered, the N_2O control knob may be turned up as high as the administrator desires, but the flow of N_2O gas will not exceed 5.5 L/min. This provides a 31% oxygen concentration (2.5 L/min per 8.0 L/min). If, however, the flow of O_2 is increased above the minimum flow rate, the N_2O flow may also be increased.

Oxygen Fail-Safe

In either the portable or central systems, the cylinder of O_2 will become depleted before the cylinder of N_2O. In fact, approximately 2.5 O_2 cylinders will be used for each N_2O cylinder of comparable size. It is obvious that a potentially dangerous situation exists because if the O_2 cylinder becomes depleted during a procedure, the patient might conceivably receive 100% N_2O.

The O_2 fail-safe system is designed to prevent this from happening by automatically terminating the flow of N_2O whenever the delivery pressure of O_2 falls below a predetermined level. For example, both N_2O and O_2 are delivered to the patient at a pressure of approximately 50 psig. When the pressure in the O_2-compressed-gas cylinder nears zero (but is not quite at zero), the delivery pressure of O_2 through the reducing valve can no longer be maintained at 50 psig. As this pressure falls, to 40 psig, for example, the oxygen fail-safe mechanism is activated and the flow of N_2O gas (from a cylinder that may in fact be almost full) is terminated. The patient at no time receives 100% N_2O. Several other safety devices are activated once the oxygen fail-safe is brought into use. These are discussed in the following paragraphs.

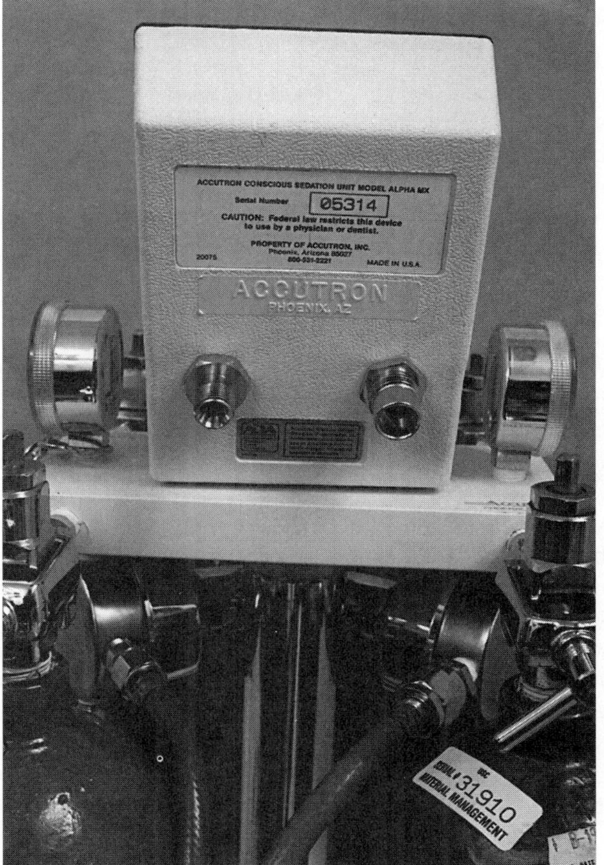

A

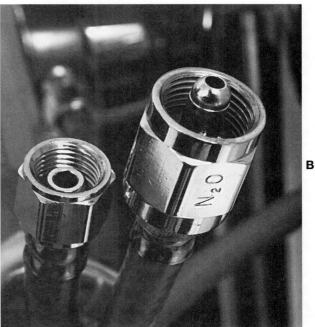

B

Figure 14-34 **A,** Back of inhalation sedation unit. Note different diameters of N_2O *(right)* and O_2 *(left)* connectors. **B,** Diameter index safety system. Diameter and threading of N_2O coupling *(right)* differ from those of O_2 coupling *(left)*, thus preventing accidental attachments to wrong side of inhalation sedation unit.

Emergency Air Inlet

Located on top of the bag/tee outlet, the emergency air inlet is maintained in a closed position as long as O_2 or N_2O-O_2 is delivered through the sedation unit. When the flow of gas ceases, as in the preceding example in which the O_2 fail-safe is activated, the emergency air inlet valve opens, permitting the patient to continue to breathe comfortably, although the gas being inhaled now is atmospheric air (see Figure 14-4). Should the termination of gas flow through the machine fail to be noticed by the administrator and assistant, the patient will gradually become less and less sedated or may mention an increasing resistance to inhalation.

Alarm

An alarm may be attached to the O_2 fail-safe system that is audible when this system is activated. This will prevent a situation in which the administrator, being so involved in the dental procedure at hand, fails to notice the shutting off of the gas flows on the unit. In central systems an alarm system is placed in an area (e.g., the reception desk) where personnel are frequently located (Figure 14-35).

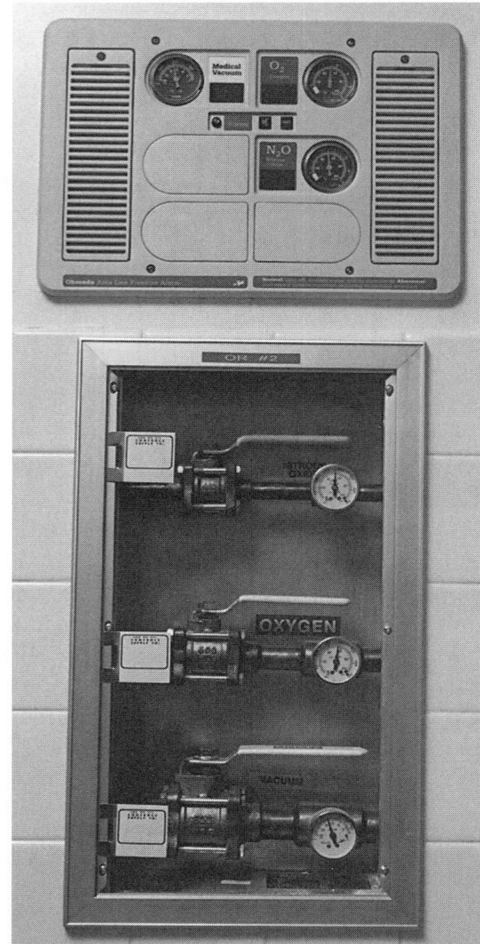

Figure 14-35 Alarm system for central system. Alarm is activated when O_2 or N_2O pressures are low or high and when reserve tanks are in use.

Oxygen Flush Button

The O_2 flush button permits the rapid delivery of high flows of O_2 to the patient. With the older pneumatic mixers, the N_2O had to be manually turned off to be able to deliver 100% O_2. With the newer electronic devices, 100% O_2 delivery is ensured by the unit automatically stopping the N_2O delivery when the O_2 flush button is pressed. All of this can be accomplished without user intervention. This automation of pure oxygen delivery is a distinct advantage during emergency situations. The button is ideally located on the front of the sedation unit in easy view (see Figure 14-3). Most O_2 flush buttons permit the delivery of at least 35 L/min of O_2. This is intended for use in emergency situations. This one feature alone is reason enough to purchase an inhalation sedation unit. Positive-pressure oxygen can also be delivered with this system.

Reservoir Bag

The reservoir bag may be considered a safety feature because it may be used to assist or control respiration in emergency situations (see Figure 14-3). All inhalation sedation units should have a reservoir bag.

Color Coding

Although simple, color coding is an important safety feature of all inhalation sedation units. All parts of the unit that carry or operate O_2 are colored green, whereas tubes, knobs, and other parts handling N_2O are colored light blue.

Lock

Locks may be included in the inhalation sedation unit and on protective caps found on the larger cylinders. As discussed in Chapter 17, abuse of N_2O is not uncommon. Although persons in the dental profession are prime candidates for abuse of this technique, there are instances in which nondental persons have gained access to dental systems. The use of a lock on the cylinders makes it less likely that this situation will develop.

Quick-Connect for Positive-Pressure Oxygen

All inhalation sedation units have a quick-connect attachment for positive-pressure O_2 located on the head. If it is not present, the units must be adaptable to this device.

AVAILABLE INHALATION SEDATION UNITS

Many inhalation sedation units are currently available for use in the dental or medical office. The underlying mechanism in all is quite similar; however, there are significant differences in appearance. Some units have a wooden veneer, whereas others are made of molded plastic; some are quite large, and others are more compact. Several machines are being advertised with unique features relating to safety, appearance, or operation. Three examples of inhalation sedation units are the latest models for Accutron Inc., Porter, and MDS Matrix Nitrous Oxide Sedation Systems (Figures 14-36 and 14-37; see also Figure 14-19).

One factor that I believe must be present regarding the inhalation sedation unit is that the unit should have received an acceptable rating from the American Dental Association's Council on Scientific Affairs.[16] The American Dental Association has adopted an Acceptance Program for inhalation sedation units that permits the doctor to better evaluate those units being considered for purchase. The primary emphasis of this program in recent years has been the addition of safety features to these units, which are aimed at making it difficult, if not impossible, to administer less than 20% oxygen to the patient. To receive a satisfactory classification, the manufacturer must submit its devices to the Council on Scientific Affairs for evaluation. The guidelines of the Council are shown in Box 14-1. The

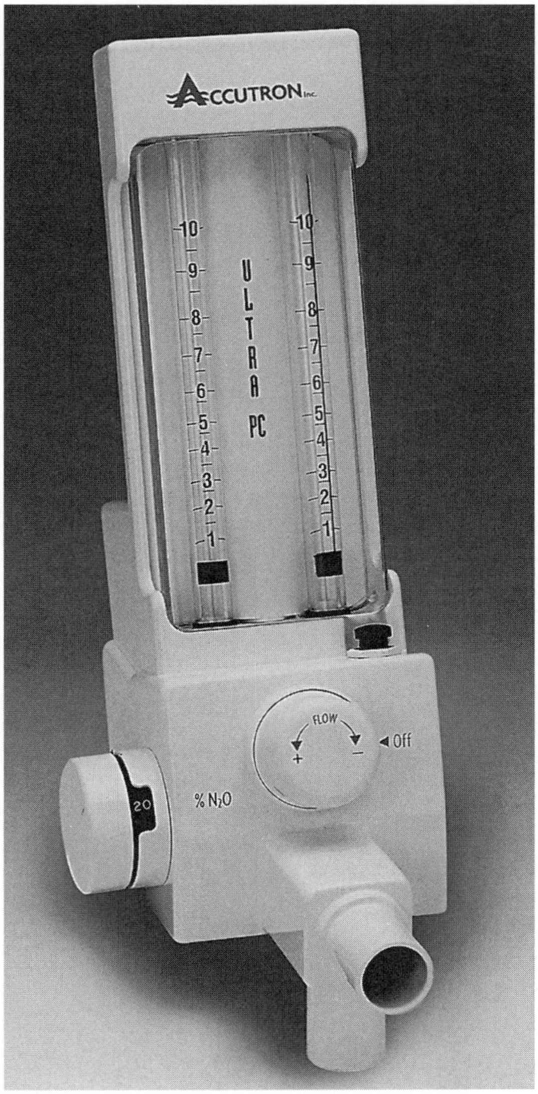

Figure 14-36 Accutron Inc. ultra PC % Flowmeter. Features an N_2O Lock, which prevents unauthorized use of N_2O.

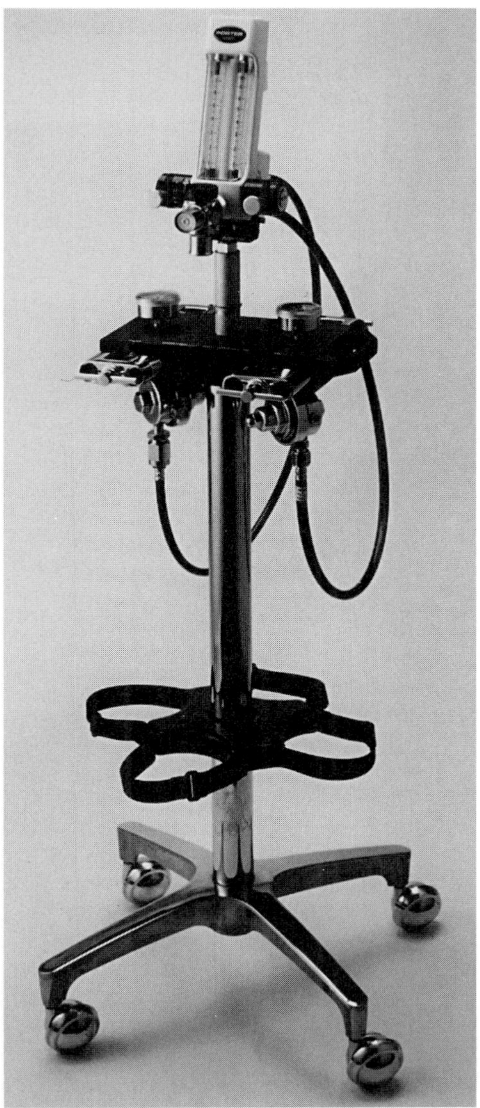

Figure 14-37 Porter MXR. Features an automatic vacuum system for the breathing circuit creating an interlock between the gas flow and vacuum. This prevents N_2O-O_2 from being administered without scavenging.

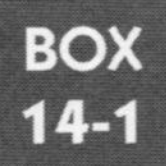

BOX 14-1 Acceptance Program Guidelines: Nitrous Oxide–Oxygen Conscious Sedation Systems

These guidelines apply to nitrous oxide–oxygen conscious sedation systems used in dentistry.

I. SUBMISSION DIRECTIONS
  1. General Information
    A. Submissions are to be sent to the Council Office:
       Director, Product Evaluations; Council on Scientific Affairs; American Dental Association; 211 East Chicago Avenue; Chicago, IL 60611-2678
    B. Submissions are to be sent in triplicate along with a market sample of the product (i.e., packaged as marketed). In addition, one single-sided copy shall be provided for internal duplicating. The Council agrees to return the product sample within 6 months if requested. If possible, the submission should be less than 200 pages exclusive of appendices.
    C. A manufacturer is advised that the review process is complex. Typically, notification of Council action may be expected 90 to 150 days from the receipt of a complete submission by the Council. More time may be required if additional information or clarification is needed from the manufacturer.
    D. When a product is classified as "Accepted," the classification is for 3 years. Renewal of the classification will be considered by the Council upon request by the manufacturer.
    E. Classification of a product under the Acceptance Program is subject to the conditions stated in the contract entitled "Agreement Governing Use of ADA Seal of Acceptance."
  2. Arrangement of a Submission
     The submission is to be divided into sections and arranged in order as indicated in Part II. Sections to be identified by tabs are designated by an asterisk (*).

II. INFORMATION TO BE SUBMITTED
  1. Cover Page
    A. Name of company
    B. Product name
  *2. Table of Contents
  *3. Company Information
    A. Name of company (to be used in official list of ADA Accepted Products)
    B. Address (to be used in listing)
    C. Phone number (to be used in listing)
    D. Fax number and e-mail address
    E. Names of owners, officers, and other individuals authorized to furnish information to the Council and represent the firm in dealing with the Council (foreign manufacturers must have an office or branch located in the United States, and the product must be available for purchase in the United States)
    F. Names and qualifications of scientific personnel responsible for formulation and testing of the product in its manufacturing process
  *4. Summary of Submission
     Comprehensive summary of the information submitted on safety and effectiveness of the conscious sedation system
  *5. Product Information
    A. Name of product (to be used in listing)
    B. Evidence of FDA approval to market (e.g., 510[k] letter or premarket approval [PMA] letter), including approved indications for use
    C. Claims of efficacy
      (i) List claims of efficacy. All claims of efficacy listed must be documented (see following), including all claims in advertising and promotional materials.
      (ii) The studies (or parts of studies) that provide documentation for each claim must be identified.
      (iii) The FDA clearance to market must encompass all of the claims of efficacy.
    D. Patent title(s) and patent number(s) relating to the product
    E. Product description
      (i) Materials of construction, including composition
      (ii) Principles of design
    F. Instructions, installation, and maintenance
       The following shall be incorporated in the product instructions:
      (i) "The installation of the gas storage and piping systems should be in accordance with applicable building codes, i.e., National Fire Protection Association (NFPA) Standards or other fire safety standards."

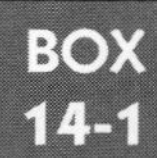

BOX 14-1 Acceptance Program Guidelines: Nitrous Oxide–Oxygen Conscious Sedation Systems—cont'd

(ii) "The nitrous oxide–oxygen conscious sedation systems shall be used in conjunction with a nitrous oxide scavenging system."
(iii) Methods for maintaining components that regulate proper gas delivery shall be described.

G. Labeling
A label shall be attached to the machine that reads: "CAUTION, Federal law prohibits this device to sale by or on the order of a physician or dentist."

H. Packaging

I. Promotional materials

*6. Quality Control Procedures for the Manufacturing of the Product

*7. Properties

A. Fittings
(i) The gas cylinders, hoses, and flow measuring devices shall be color coded in accordance with U.S. standards: green for oxygen and blue for nitrous oxide.
(ii) Both pin index safety systems and diameter index safety systems are to be used, as appropriate.

B. Dispensing unit
(i) The maximum percentage of nitrous oxide that can be given will be 70%.
(ii) A quick connector or DISS fitting shall be provided for oxygen with a minimum flow specification greater than 100 L/min to allow for fitting of resuscitation.
(iii) A protective housing shall completely enclose the glass tube flowmeters, if used, and will be fronted by a transparent safety shield.
(iv) A reservoir bag shall be provided for delivery of nitrous oxide and oxygen. The reservoir bag should be located downstream of the flowmeters but upstream of the common outlet. The mount for this bag should be a 22 mm (7/8") connection. The reservoir bag should be mounted to allow unrestricted visual monitoring.
(v) Flow-measuring devices should be accurate to ± 5% of full-scale reading. Where independent flow indicators are used, the oxygen indicator should be located on the right side of the machine as viewed from the front. The flow-measuring devices should provide for visual monitoring of the gas flow.
(vi) An on-demand valve shall be available to allow the automatic admission of room air to the system if gas flows are inadequate for the patient's needs.
(vii) A check valve shall be an integral part of the dispensing unit, mounted between the reservoir bag and the common outlet to prevent exhaled gases from reentering the reservoir bag.
(viii) A fail-safe device shall be installed to close off the nitrous oxide if the oxygen supply fails.

C. Central gas supply
(i) Piping systems shall conform to NFPA 99, Chapter 4, Type II.

D. Portable gas supply unit
(i) If an audible alarm is not provided on the dispensing unit, then it shall be provided in the portable gas supply to warn of the loss of oxygen-supply pressure.

*8. Safety Data
Provide evidence of safety.

*9. Efficacy Data
Provide evidence of efficacy.

*10. Appendices
Detailed description of evaluation methods and any other defined areas

III. REQUIREMENTS (PERFORMANCE CRITERIA) FOR CLASSIFICATION OF "ACCEPTED"
The nitrous oxide–oxygen conscious sedation system must meet all the properties requirements as specified.

IV. STATEMENT TO BE USED FOR PRODUCTS CLASSIFIED UNDER THESE GUIDELINES, INCLUDING QUALIFIERS
"[Product Name] is Accepted for the delivery of nitrous oxide–oxygen conscious sedation in the practice of dentistry."
Council on Scientific Affairs—American Dental Association.

From American Dental Association Council on Scientific Affairs, Chicago, 2000.

Council publishes a listing of acceptable devices in the *Journal of the American Dental Association*, the *Dentist's Desk Reference*,[18] and on the ADA web site (www.ada.org). All of the devices listed have been accepted by the Council on Scientific Affairs of the American Dental Association. The decision as to the most appropriate unit for your dental or medical office should be made after careful consideration of your needs and available space.

Effective in September 1994, the American Dental Association discontinued the Acceptance Program for N_2O-O_2 scavenging devices after rescinding the then-current American Dental Association guidelines used in evaluation of N_2O scavenging systems.[19]

REFERENCES

1. McCarthy FM, Shuken RA: Appraisal of the demand flow anesthetic machine and review of the literature, *J Oral Surg* 27:624, 1969.
2. Gauert WB, Husted RF: Differences in metered and measured oxygen concentrations during nitrous oxide analgesia, *Anesth Analg* 47:441, 1968.
3. Allen GD: *Dental anesthesia and analgesia*, ed 2, Baltimore, 1979, Williams & Wilkins.
4. Department of Transportation, Office of Federal Regulations, National Archives Administration: Code of Federal Regulations, title 49, section 178, Washington, DC, 1986.
5. Follmer KE: Anesthetic gas fires are preventable, *Anesth Prog* 19:2, 1972.
6. Hogg CF: Pin-indexing failures, *Anesthesiology* 38:85, 1973.
7. Sawhney KK, Yoon YK: Erroneous labeling of a nitrous oxide cylinder, *Anesthesiology* 59:260, 1983.
8. Parbrook GD, Davis PD, Parbrook EO: *Basic physics and measurement in anesthesia*, ed 2, Norwalk, Conn, 1986, Appleton-Century-Crofts.
9. Dorsch JA, Dorsch SE: *Understanding anesthesia equipment*, ed 2, Baltimore, 1984, Williams & Wilkins.
10. Eisenkraft JB: Anesthesia delivery system. In Rogers MC, Tinker JH, Covino BG et al, eds: *Principles and practice of anesthesiology*, St Louis, 1993, Mosby.
11. Compressed Gas Association: *Compressed gas cylinder valve outlet and inlet connections*, vol 1, New York, 1977, The Association.
12. Compressed Gas Association: *Diameter-index safety system*, New York, 1978, The Association.
13. Bowie E, Huffman LM: *The anesthesia machine: essentials for understanding*, Madison, Wis, 1985, Ohmeda, BOC Health Care.
14. American Society for Testing and Materials: *Standard specification for minimum performance and safety requirements for components and systems of anesthesia gas machines*, Philadelphia, 1989, The Society.
15. ADA Council of Scientific Affairs: Nitrous oxide in the dental office, *JADA* 128:364, 1997.
16. Council on Scientific Affairs: *Acceptance Program guidelines: nitrous oxide-oxygen conscious sedation systems*, Chicago, 2000, American Dental Association.
17. National Fire Protection Association: *Standard for health care facilities*, Quincy, Mass, 1990, The Association.
18. *Dentist's desk reference: materials, instruments and equipment*, Chicago, 1983, American Dental Association.
19. Fan PL: Letter to manufacturers of nitrous oxide scavenging systems and other interested parties, Sept 1, 1994. In *ADA guidelines for nitrous oxide scavenging systems*, Chicago, 1994, American Dental Association.

CHAPTER 15

Inhalation Sedation: Techniques of Administration

CHAPTER OUTLINE

The administration of nitrous oxide–oxygen (N_2O-O_2) for pharmacosedation is a very easy and straightforward procedure. It requires an approved sedation unit, a trained administrator, and a patient desiring sedation. Proper training conveys confidence to the patient and, as a result, an expectation of a successful outcome. Training, as defined by the American Dental Association guidelines, requires instruction in pain and anxiety control consisting of 16 hours of course content, with 4 of those hours being laboratory or clinical experience. Even though N_2O-O_2 is considered a very safe drug, a number of unpleasant and potentially dangerous complications can still develop. Therefore the person responsible for the administration of N_2O-O_2 must be aware of these potential problems and know how to prevent them from occurring and how to recognize and manage them.

Some operators insist in turning on a sedation unit to a fixed percentage of N_2O. This fixed percentage is either arbitrary or the one that was used at a previous appointment. This concept clearly violates the principle of titration, which allows for the correct amount (percentage) of N_2O-O_2 for the desired level of sedation. Titration, an important concept in the administration of any drug to a patient, is the primary guiding principle along with monitoring the patient for depth of sedation. Titration for each appointment is necessary both to compensate for individual variation in patient response to N_2O and because patients may respond differently at each appointment and may not require the same level of sedation for different procedures. The ability to quickly increase or decrease flow of N_2O permits every patient to achieve the level of sedation that he or she and the administrator are seeking. It allows for comfortable sedation for those who are difficult to sedate and those who are easily affected by the gas.

The techniques described emphasize titration as the guiding principle to successful N_2O-O_2 administration for both the patient and the administrator. This will result in fewer adverse side effects (e.g., nausea, vomiting, or poor behavioral reactions) and an overall normal pleasant experience.

GENERAL DESCRIPTION

The technique of inhalation sedation for the cooperative adult patient (the patient who willingly accepts the nasal hood) is as follows. Management of the more difficult patient, such as the child or adult with a disability or the pediatric patient, is described in Chapters 35 and 38.

1. A flow rate (liter per minute) of 100% oxygen is established, and the nasal hood is placed on the patient's nose. The patient is instructed to self-adjust the hood as needed for comfort.
2. The appropriate flow rate is established while the patient is breathing 100% O_2. The bag is neither expanding nor shrinking in size but remains uniform during breathing.
3. The percentage of N_2O is started, usually 20% initially. Then N_2O is titrated in 10% increments every 60 seconds.
4. When the patient states that he or she feels pleasant and more relaxed, the ideal level of clinical sedation has been achieved.
5. Once the ideal level of sedation is achieved, local anesthetic may be given and the planned dental/surgical procedure completed.
6. N_2O flow is terminated, and the patient is given 100% (pure) O_2 at a flow rate equivalent to the established rate for this patient. This may be started earlier than the absolute completion of the procedure to ensure an expedient recovery. Oxygen is given for 3 to 5 minutes or longer if clinical signs of sedation persist.
7. The patient may leave the dental office unescorted if he or she is completely recovered from sedation.

The approach to the N_2O-O_2 sedation technique is divided into three phases: the induction phase (steps 1 to 4), the injection and treatment phase (step 5), and the recovery phase (steps 6 and 7).

ADMINISTRATION

The following description of the administration of N_2O-O_2 applies to the adult patient (teenager included) who willingly accepts the nasal hood, is able to breathe through the nose, and is able to sit in the dental chair without involuntary muscular movements interfering with the procedure. The technique of administration will differ slightly for a patient who has never before received N_2O-O_2. At appropriate points in the technique, these differences are explained.

Pretreatment Visit and Instructions

A patient who has a deep fear or phobia may not be a candidate for N_2O-O_2 administration. N_2O-O_2 is not effective in patients with severe fear and/or phobias. Whether the patient has a deep fear or phobia is best determined through an appointment for discussion and possible demonstration of the use of N_2O-O_2. Because fear of the unknown often leads to phobias, an appointment to discuss N_2O-O_2 procedures in advance can help identify potential candidates for its use. The ideal time to introduce an apprehensive patient to inhalation sedation for the first time is not at an appointment at which actual dental or surgical treatment is scheduled. A further increase in anxiety can occur if the doctor or hygienist attempts to use N_2O-O_2 without having previously described the technique. Even the first sight of the nasal hood might remind the patient of unpleasant experiences that have occurred in the past, such as nausea and vomiting following general anesthesia or a sense of suffocation produced by the nasal hood.

In the ideal situation the doctor, recognizing the patient's need for N_2O-O_2 sedation (e.g., anxiety, medically compromised states, gagging), will discuss with the patient the reasons for selecting this technique and the benefits to be gained from its use both for the doctor and for the patient. This appointment can be used for a "demonstration" of the N_2O-O_2 equipment and to allow the patient the opportunity to ask questions about the upcoming procedure. It is remarkable how this familiarization can help relieve fear and promote a positive interaction between the clinician and the patient.

It is unusual to find an adult patient who has not heard of or been given N_2O-O_2. *Laughing gas,* or so-called sweet air, is a common term to the lay public. Some may have had a previous unpleasant experience with it. It is important for these patients to know that they are not obligated to experience it again, but it may be worthwhile to explain that they could have been easily overdosed (not titrated!) and that you are confident you can provide a better experience. In any event, this time spent with the patient without the concern of an actual procedure is often all that is needed to get the partnership with the patient that you are seeking. These patients can be and often are your best practice ambassadors.

In discussing with the patient what he or she can expect from the experience, it is crucial to present honesty and clarity in the preoperative and the operative appointment. Do not tell the patient what he or she will or will not feel during this experience because each patient may respond differently. Instead of informing the patient that "you will feel tingling in your fingers or toes," use a more open-ended statement such as "you should feel more relaxed and at ease." Some patients who do not experience the suggested signs, such as tingling, will think that the N_2O-O_2 is not working for them or that something is wrong. Being more vague and general here is better. In a patient who, for religious, medical, or other personal reasons, does not use or like the effects of alcohol, comparing the actions of N_2O to those of alcohol or other drugs will make the patient less willing to try and accept it. For the sake of these patients and the patient who has had a personal negative experience with substance abuse, the comparison of N_2O and alcohol should be avoided.

At the conclusion of this initial visit, preoperative medications such as prophylactic antibiotics, antianxiety drugs, or sleeping medication may be prescribed. Oral antianxiety drugs are useful in the patient who becomes increasingly fearful as the dental appointment nears. Oral drugs help reduce these fears. Once in the dental office, the patient may then receive N_2O-O_2 for any additional sedation required during the dental treatment. Also, postoperative instructions can be given and financial matters handled before the patient is released.

Patients may have a light meal a few hours before an appointment for N_2O-O_2 administration. A heavy meal, particularly with children, should be avoided because this can often lead to nausea and vomiting. Conversely, a patient who has had nothing to eat can also become nauseous.

Day of Appointment

Monitoring during Inhalation Sedation. The following is the recommended monitoring for inhalation sedation procedures:

1. Baseline vital signs, preoperatively
2. Verbal communication with patient
3. Vital signs recorded periodically during the procedure
4. Postoperative vital signs

Other monitors, such as the pretracheal stethoscope and the electrocardiogram (ECG), are considered optional in both the adult and pediatric patient whenever inhalation sedation is used as a sole technique. Pulse oximetry, although not mandatory or required, is relatively inexpensive and an excellent way to ensure that the patient is in fact adequately O_2 saturated. This is the surest way to confirm that all N_2O-O_2 equipment and anatomic systems are functioning properly.

Preparation of the Equipment. Experts in the use of N_2O-O_2 met in 1995 at the request of the American Dental Association to consider the then-current use of N_2O-O_2 in the dental office. One outgrowth of that meeting was the development of guidelines for equipment inspection and use. They are as follows.

On the day of the scheduled appointment, the dental assistant prepares the unit by opening one O_2 and one N_2O cylinder. The cylinders are opened by turning the knob on the top of the cylinder in a counterclockwise direction. Start by turning the knob only slightly, just barely opening the cylinder, permitting the pressure gauge to rise slowly. Once the pressure reaches its maximal level, the knob may be turned freely until fully open. The purpose of slowly opening the cylinder is to minimize any increase in internal temperature within the reducing valve as gas under high pressure rushes from the cylinder into the reducing valve.

After the cylinders have been prepared, the nasal hood is checked to be certain that it is clean and the other rubber goods (tubes and reservoir bag) are checked for leaks.

Preparation of the Patient

1. Request That the Patient Visit the Restroom and Void if Necessary before the Start of the Sedative Procedure

COMMENT: Patients receiving N_2O-O_2 sedation do not urinate any more frequently than other persons; however, more urine is produced when a person is in the supine position than when standing. In addition, the patient who has to urinate while receiving N_2O-O_2 must be unsedated (given 100% O_2), permitted to visit the restroom, and then resedated, a process requiring approximately 10 minutes. This time may be saved by requesting the patient to void, if necessary, before treatment.

2. Review the Medical History Questionnaire and Record Preoperative Vital Signs before the Start of the N_2O-O_2

COMMENT: Vital signs to be recorded include blood pressure, heart rate and rhythm, and respiratory rate. Vital signs may be recorded by the doctor, the dental hygienist, the dental assistant, or a nurse.

3. If the Patient Wears Contact Lenses, the Lenses Should Be Removed before the Start of Inhalation Sedation

COMMENT: Gas leaks from the mask around the bridge of the nose may produce drying of the eyes with potential irritation of the patient.

Technique of Administration

1. Position Patient in Comfortable, Reclined Position in Dental Chair

COMMENT: The preferred position (Figure 15-1) is first a consideration of patient comfort. The partially reclined position may be used if necessary for the patient's comfort or the convenience of the doctor during the procedure. The upright position is not recommended unless essential for the procedure, such as when taking impressions or radiographs.

2. *Position the Inhalation Sedation Unit*

COMMENT: This procedure applies only to the use of the portable inhalation sedation unit (Figure 15-2), as opposed to the fixed, central systems commonly found in dental offices. The N_2O-O_2 unit should always be placed behind the patient, out of his or her line of sight. A positive placebo response will occur in a percentage of patients receiving N_2O-O_2, but if the patient can see the unit and watch as the administrator adjusts the controls, this response can be negated.

3. *Start the Flow of O_2 at 6 L/min, Place the Nasal Hood over the Patient's Nose, and Remind the Patient to Breathe through the Nose*

COMMENT: Placing the nasal hood on the patient (Figure 15-3) after starting the flow of O_2 will prevent the patient from feeling suffocated when breathing through the nose if the O_2 flow is not begun before placement of the nasal hood.

Although it may appear ridiculous to remind a patient to breathe through the nose once the nasal hood has been positioned, this is a very important part of the procedure. Many persons will continue to breathe through their mouths unless they are specifically reminded not to do so, and this contaminates the environment.

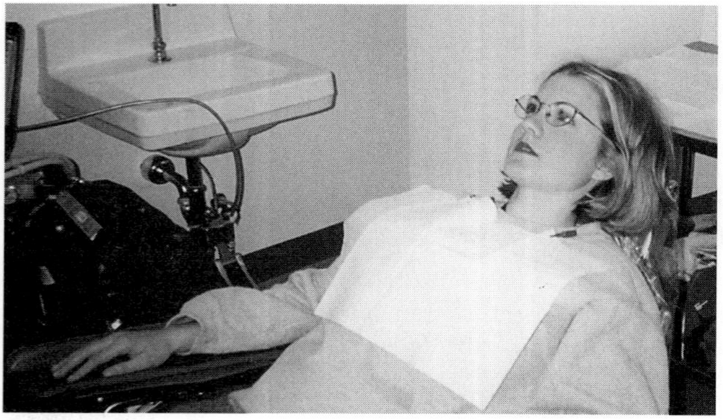

Figure 15-1 Patient is positioned in a comfortable, reclined position.

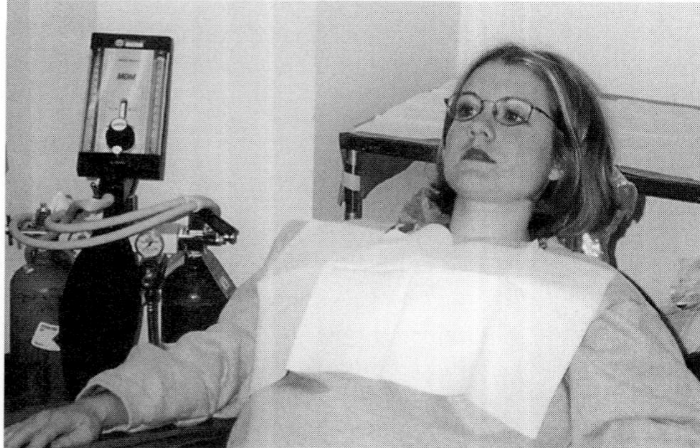

Figure 15-2 Inhalation sedation unit is best placed behind the patient, out of line of sight.

4. *Secure the Nasal Hood*

COMMENT: The nasal hood usually has two hoses coming from the N_2O-O_2 unit. These are placed around the sides of the dental chair, and the nasal hood is secured by adjusting the slip ring behind the headrest (Figure 15-4). The patient is asked to hold the nasal hood in a comfortable position as this is being done. Care must be taken in adjusting the nasal hood because one of the tubes is often pulled more than the other, making the nasal hood tilt to one side.

If the nasal hood has only one hose, it is placed over the patient's forehead and secured. The nasal hood should not

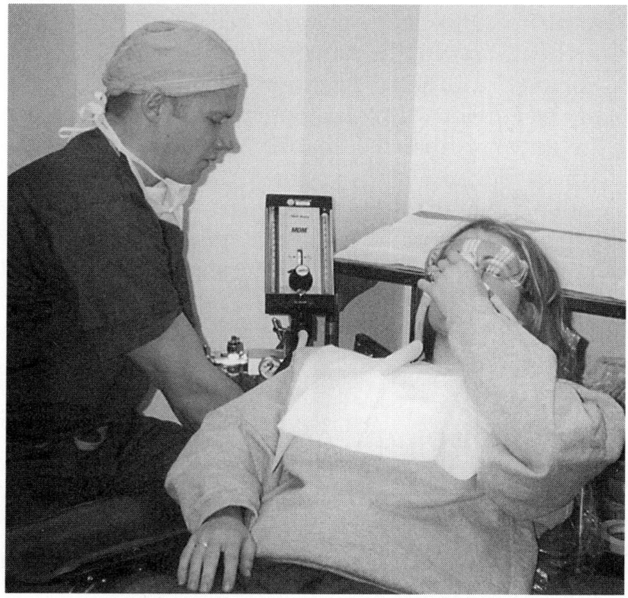

Figure 15-3 Nasal hood is placed on patient. Note 6 L/min flow of oxygen.

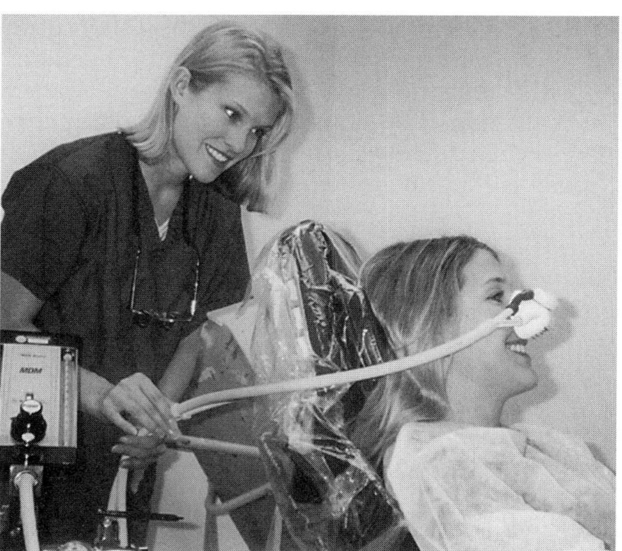

Figure 15-4 Nasal hood is secured by adjusting slip ring behind back of chair.

be too tight or too loose. The patient should have some lateral and up-and-down movement of the head. The *patient* serves as the final check as to whether the nasal hood is secure.

Leaks develop on occasion around an ill-fitting mask. Nasal hoods are available in a variety of sizes. The size is checked before the start of the procedure. The nasal hood being used should fit the patient's nose. An overly small or overly large mask will leak. Leaks may also develop with masks of the appropriate size. Most often, these leaks occur around the bridge of the nose, with the patient complaining of "air" being exhaled into his or her eyes. Permitting the patient to adjust the nasal hood is often all that is needed to correct this situation. If this simple solution is ineffective, the hood is removed, a folded 2-inch square gauze pad is placed over the bridge of the nose, and the nasal hood is replaced. This usually seals the leak (Figure 15-5).

When a scavenging nasal hood is used, the exhalation tubes must be connected to the vacuum system. It is important to adjust the vacuum so that the patient is able to exhale and inhale comfortably. If the vacuum is too weak, the patient may experience difficulty in breathing out, and if the vacuum is too forceful, the patient may not receive any N_2O-O_2 as the gases are rapidly sucked from the nasal hood into the overly efficient vacuum system.

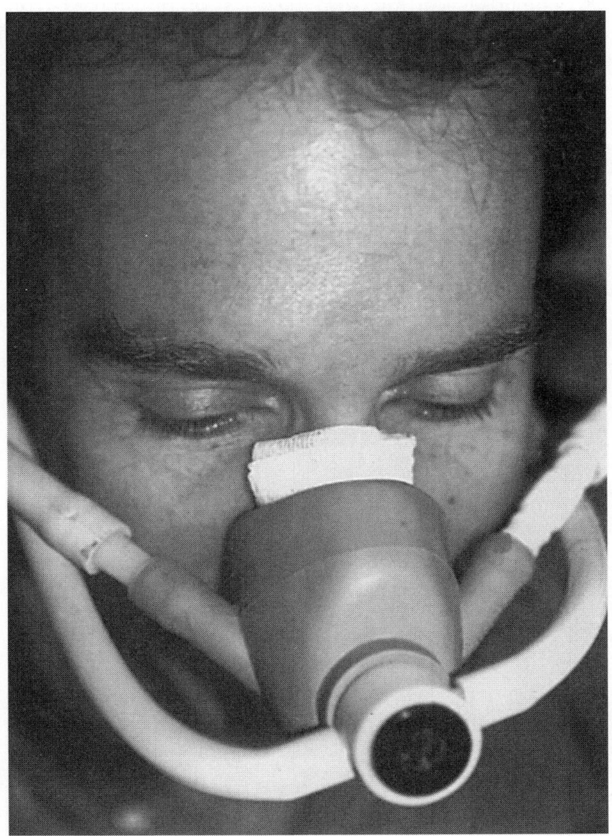

Figure 15-5 Folded 2-x-2-inch gauze on bridge of nose prevents leaks.

5. Determine Proper Flow Rate for the Patient

COMMENT: This is one of the most important steps in the successful use of N_2O-O_2 sedation. The patient must be able to breathe comfortably at this point, before the start of N_2O flow, in order to be comfortable throughout the procedure.

At the onset of the procedure, a 6-L/min flow of 100% O_2 is initiated for the adult (3 or 4 L/min for smaller pediatric patients), the nasal hood is placed on the patient, and the patient is instructed to breathe only through the nose. In most adult patients (and virtually all children), this minute volume will be more than adequate for the patient to breathe comfortably. Breathing comfortably implies that the patient is able to take a normal breath and feel as though the volume of "air" is adequate, as opposed to the patient who states that the machine is not delivering enough "air," causing him or her difficulty in breathing. I have never seen the opposite situation, in which the patient states that there is too much "air" being delivered.

It is impossible to predict which patient will require a minute volume greater than 6 L/min. Larger patients may be quite comfortable at 6 L/min, whereas petite patients may require higher flow rates. Persons who participate in endurance sports, such as marathon running, swimming, and bicycle racing, are more likely to require larger minute volumes. In addition, persons with chronic obstructive pulmonary disease (COPD), congestive heart failure (CHF), or partial nasal obstruction may also require larger volumes.

The patient is asked, "Can you breathe normally?" or "Are you comfortable?" If the answer is yes, the flow rate is left at 6 L/min; if the patient requests a greater volume, the O_2 flow rate is increased to 7 L/min and allowed to remain there for a minute, and the same question is asked. This process is repeated until the patient becomes comfortable. The appearance of the reservoir bag is a reliable indicator of appropriate flow rate.

It is not uncommon for a patient to require a higher flow rate at the beginning of N_2O-O_2 sedation. This is especially so for the patient receiving N_2O-O_2 sedation for the first time. Placing the nasal hood on the patient's nose may pose a subconscious threat, and the individual may overcompensate by breathing more deeply and/or rapidly until satisfied that he or she will not suffocate. This same phenomenon is seen in early training of SCUBA (self-contained underwater breathing apparatus) divers. After the N_2O-O_2 provides sedation at this elevated flow rate, the doctor might return the flow rate to the original 6 L/min (without telling the patient). In almost all cases the patient will be unable to detect the change.

Establishing the minimal flow rate is important, for if it is assumed that the patient can tolerate 6 L/min comfortably but actually cannot, then the individual will probably never become comfortably sedated with N_2O-O_2 during the procedure. This step is always carried out with the patient receiving 100% O_2 (Figure 15-6).

6. Observe the Reservoir Bag

COMMENT: The appearance of the reservoir bag indicates the respiratory depth and rate. The reservoir bag on the sedation unit will provide an indication of the seal on the

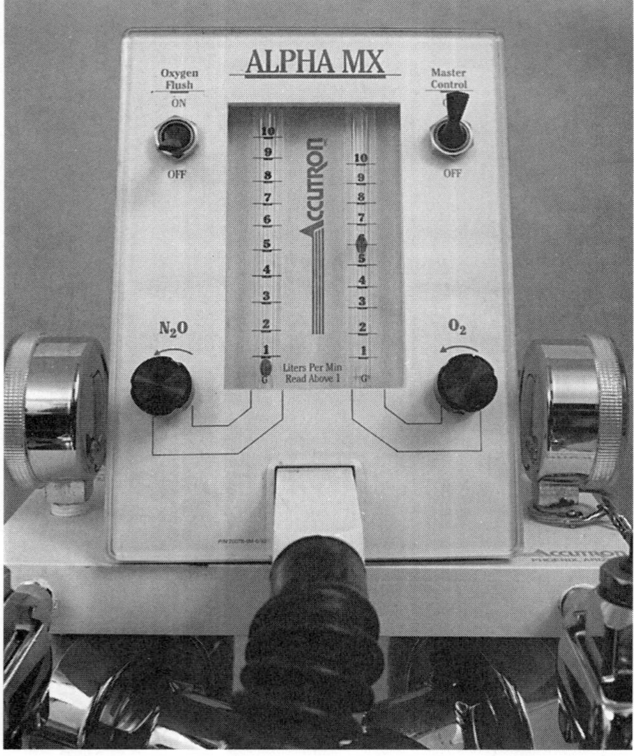

Figure 15-6 Establishing minimum O_2 flow before the start of titration.

nasal hood, in addition to allowing a determination of the adequacy of the minute volume of gas being delivered to the patient. However, the patient is always the most reliable indicator of the signs and symptoms of inhalation sedation, including the seal of the hood and the adequacy of minute volume.

The reservoir bag that remains partially inflated (deflated) (Figure 15-7, *A*) and deflates and inflates partially with each breath usually indicates that the minute volume is adequate (the bag remains partially inflated throughout the procedure) and that the seal of the nasal hood is tight (inflates and deflates with each breath).

A bag that remains totally deflated (Figure 15-7, *B*) may indicate one of the following:

- The minute volume of gas is inadequate; in this situation the patient will usually complain of not receiving enough "air."
- The nasal hood has relatively large leaks; in this case the patient will have no difficulty breathing because any lack of gas from the N_2O-O_2 unit is compensated for by ambient air entering through the leaks. The patient may also say, "Air is blowing into my eyes every time I breathe."
- The vacuum on the scavenging system is too high, forcing gases directly out of the nasal hood into the vacuum system. The patient will usually complain of not receiving enough "air."

A bag that is overly inflated (Figure 15-7, *C*), looking like a balloon about to burst, may indicate one of the following:

- The minute volume is too great for the patient. Although an unlikely occurrence, the patient might complain about being unable to breathe against the rapid flow of air into the nasal hood.
- The hoses leading from the sedation unit have become kinked (occluded). In this case the patient will complain about being unable to breathe comfortably through the nasal hood.

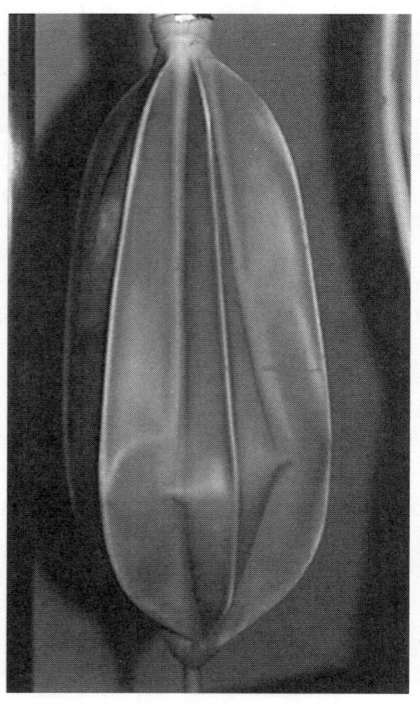

A

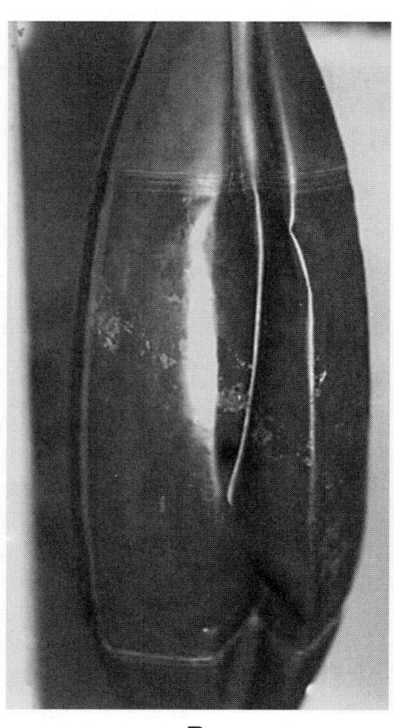

B

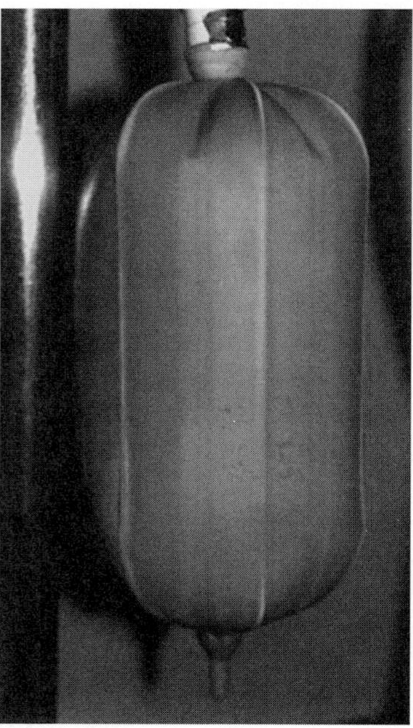

C

Figure 15-7 **A,** Partially inflated reservoir bag usually indicates adequate seal and minute volume. **B,** Deflated reservoir bag usually indicates either a leak around the nasal hood or a deficient minute volume. **C,** Distended reservoir bag indicates either an overly large minute volume or occluded breathing tubes.

Of these two situations involving an overly inflated bag, the second—occluded tubes—is the more likely to occur.

7. Begin Titration of N_2O

COMMENT: Once an adequate minute volume of gas flow for the patient has been determined, the administration of N_2O may begin. Two methods of administering N_2O to the patient are presented, both of which are quite acceptable. In the first, the total liter flow of gases (N_2O and O_2) per minute is kept constant throughout the procedure (the *constant liter flow technique*). In the second method, the liter flow of oxygen remains constant (the *constant O_2 flow technique*), and the volume of N_2O is adjusted. Advantages and disadvantages of both techniques are discussed. These techniques are used with inhalation sedation units that possess separate control knobs for the N_2O and the O_2 flows. On inhalation sedation units with a mixing dial, the operator needs only to adjust the dial to the desired concentration of N_2O or O_2. These units operate by keeping the total volume of gas flow constant throughout the procedure (constant liter flow technique).

In all situations, regardless of the type of unit or the technique used, the initial percentage of N_2O should be approximately 20%. With the mixing dial units, the administrator needs merely to adjust the percentage dial to either 20% N_2O or 80% O_2. Flows of the individual gases are automatically adjusted. If a 6-L/min O_2 flow is adequate for the patient, when the dial is adjusted to 20% N_2O, the N_2O flowmeter will read 1.2 L/min and the O_2 flowmeter will decrease from 6 to 4.8 L/min.

When operating a unit with individual control knobs for N_2O and O_2 and using the constant liter flow technique, the administrator increases the N_2O flow to 1 L/min and then decreases the O_2 flow rate to 5 L/min (Figure 15-8). This produces an N_2O percentage of 16.6% (1 L/min N_2O/6 L/min total gas flow). In the constant O_2 flow technique, the O_2 flow is left at its initial rate (6 L/min in this case) and the N_2O flow is increased to 1 L/min. The N_2O concentration is 14.3% (Figure 15-9).

In my experience, many persons learning to use N_2O-O_2 inhalation sedation have difficulty determining the concentrations of the gases being delivered. One of the most common misconceptions is that the liter flow of the N_2O is equal to the percentage of the gas being delivered. For example, a 2-L/min flow of N_2O actually does not equal 20%. The only situation in which this would be the case is when the total gas flow (O_2 + N_2O) is 10 L/min. The percentage of a gas being delivered through the N_2O-O_2 unit can readily be determined by dividing the liter flow per minute of the gas by the total volume of both gases being delivered:

$$\text{Percentage } N_2O = \frac{\text{L/min } N_2O}{\text{L/min } O_2 + \text{L/min } N_2O}$$

$$\text{Percentage } O_2 = \frac{\text{L/min } O_2}{\text{L/min } O_2 + \text{L/min } N_2O}$$

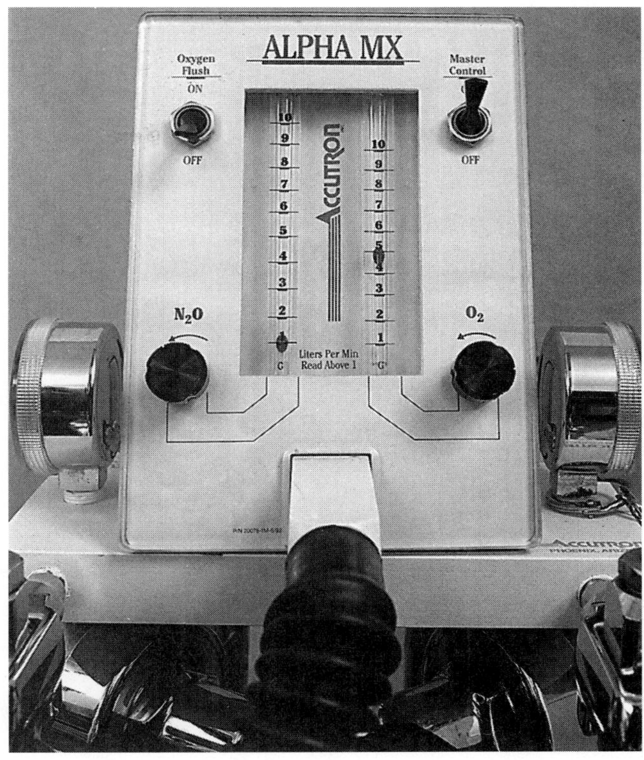

Figure 15-8 Constant liter flow technique: O_2 flow decreases 1 L/min to 5 L/min, N_2O flow increases 1 L/min to 1 L/min, and N_2O percentage = 16.6%.

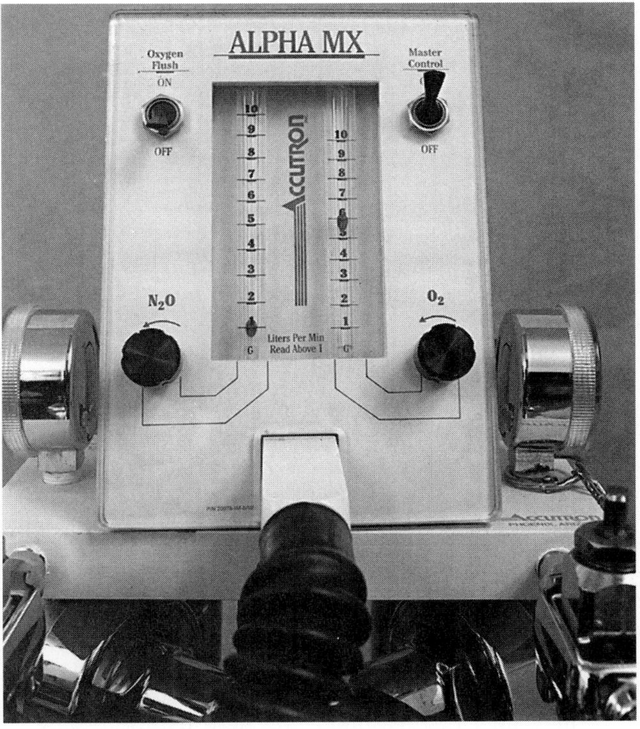

Figure 15-9 Constant O_2 flow technique: O_2 flow remains constant at 6 L/min, N_2O flow is raised 1 L/min, and N_2O percentage = 14.4%.

TABLE 15-1 N_2O Percentage Chart

	L/min N_2O									
L/min O_2	1	2	3	4	5	6	7	8	9	10
10	9	17	23	29	33	38	41	44	47	50
9	10	18	25	31	36	40	44	47	50	53
8	11	20	27	33	38	43	47	50	53	56
7	13	22	30	36	42	46	50	53	56	59
6	14	25	33	40	45	50	54	57	60	63
5	17	19	38	44	50	55	58	62	64	67
4	20	33	43	50	56	60	64	67	69	71
3	25	40	50	57	63	67	70	73	75	77
2	33	50	60	67	71	75	78	80	82	83
1	50	67	75	80	83	86	88	89	90	91

Table 15-1 provides an easy method of determining the percentage of N_2O being delivered at common flow rates.

8. *Observe the Patient*

COMMENT: The patient breathes this concentration of N_2O for approximately 60 to 90 seconds. During this time the administrator should observe the patient, looking for signs or symptoms of sedation. At the end of the 60- to 90-second period, the patient is asked, "What are you feeling?" It is important to ask open-ended questions that require the patient to respond with more than a simple yes or no. "What are you feeling?" requires the patient to answer in sentences, stating "I feel no different from before," or "I feel a little lightheaded." The question, "Do you feel good?" brings responses of only "yes" or "no."

The typical patient receiving approximately 20% N_2O will have little or no effect after 1 to 2 minutes. In this case the titration of the N_2O continues.

Two points that may appear minor must be mentioned:

1. *During the titration of N_2O to a patient, the administrator or assistant must remain by the patient at all times, either in visual, physical, or verbal contact.* Otherwise, the patient may think that he or she has been left alone during the procedure and may panic, remove the nasal hood, and become agitated. Contact with the patient prevents this.
2. *The patient's legs should be uncrossed during sedation.* The significance of this lies in the fact that once sedated, the patient rarely moves at all. Should the legs be crossed for prolonged periods, circulation of blood to the periphery may be compromised and paresthesia may develop. As blood flow returns, the feeling of hyperesthesia will be quite uncomfortable.

9. *Continue Titration of N_2O*

COMMENT: If the initial concentration of N_2O proves inadequate, the level of N_2O is increased. Following the initial level of 20% N_2O, all subsequent increases will be smaller, approximately 10%.

With the *mixing dial units,* the administrator simply turns the percentage dial to 30% N_2O (or 70% O_2). The machine will automatically adjust the individual gas flows.

In the *constant liter flow technique,* all subsequent increases in N_2O and decreases in O_2 will be 0.5-L/min changes. Thus with a 6-L/min flow, the N_2O is increased to 1.5 L/min, and the O_2 is decreased to 4.5 L/min, giving a concentration of 33% N_2O (Figure 15-10).

With the *constant O_2 flow technique,* the O_2 remains at 6 L/min and the N_2O is increased to 2 L/min, a N_2O concentration of 28.6% (Figure 15-11).

10. *Observe the Patient*

COMMENT: Questioning the patient after 60 to 90 seconds at approximately 30% N_2O is more likely to provide positive responses about the clinical effects of N_2O. Table 15-2 lists the usual sequence of signs and symptoms of N_2O-O_2 inhalation sedation. Following are the more common signs and symptoms:

- *Lightheadedness:* The first clinical evidence of the effect of N_2O is usually the feeling of lightheadedness. Many patients, having never before received N_2O, may describe this as dizziness, which they may find uncomfortable. The administrator should immediately tell the patient that this feeling is transient and will pass as the concentration of N_2O is increased. The feeling of lightheadedness develops at a level that is clinically inadequate for the management of most patients.

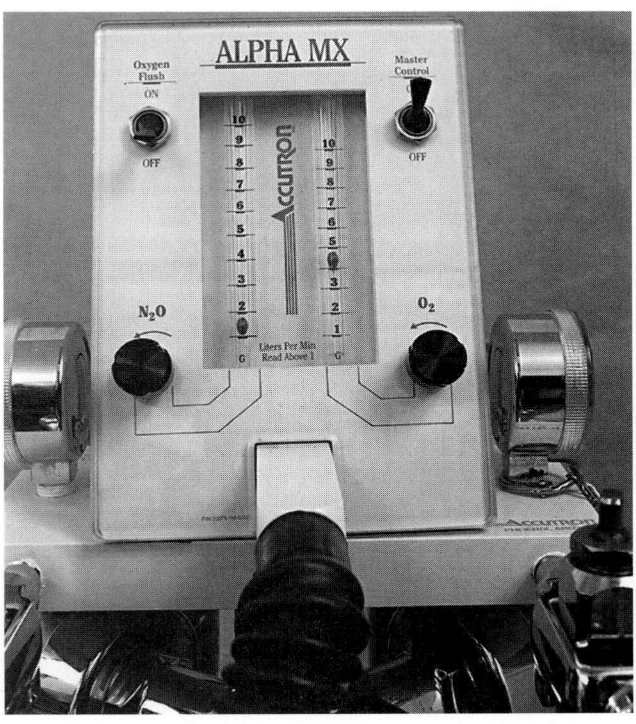

Figure 15-10 Constant liter flow technique; subsequent changes in gas flow every 60 to 90 seconds are an 0.5-L/min O_2 decrease and 0.5-L/min N_2O increase.

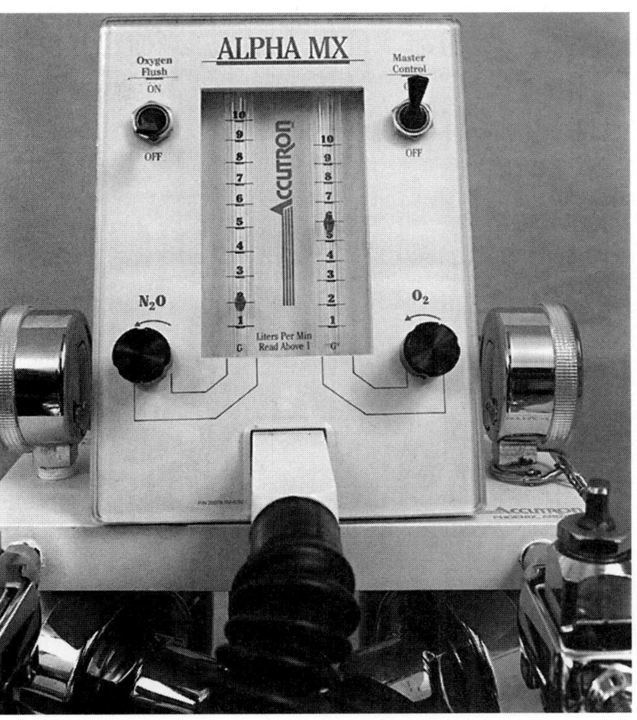

Figure 15-11 In constant O_2 flow technique, subsequent changes in gas flow are a 1-L/min increase in N_2O every 60 to 90 seconds.

TABLE 15-2 Signs and Symptoms of N_2O-O_2 Sedation

Phase	Symptoms	Signs
1. Early to ideal sedation	Lightheadedness (dizziness) Tingling of hands and feet Wave of warmth Feeling of vibration throughout body Numbness of hands and feet Numbness of soft tissues of oral cavity Feeling of euphoria Feeling of lightness or heaviness of extremities Analgesia	Blood pressure, heart rate elevated slightly early in procedure, then return to baseline values Respirations are normal, smooth Peripheral vasodilation Flushing of extremities, face Decreased muscle tone as anxiety decreases (arms and legs relax)
2. Heavier sedation/ slight oversedation	Hearing, especially of distant sounds, becomes more acute Visual images become confused (patterns on ceiling begin to move) Sleepiness Sweating increases Laughing, crying Dreaming Nausea	Increased movement Increased heart rate, blood pressure Increased rate of respiration Increased sweating Possibly lacrimation
3. Oversedation	Nausea	Vomiting Loss of consciousness

- *Tingling (paresthesia) sensation of arms, legs, or oral cavity:* Following the sensation of lightheadedness, the typical patient will describe a sensation of tingling in the arms, legs, or oral cavity. This symptom also develops at a level that is still inadequate to permit the ideal management of the fearful patient. However, advantage may be taken of the paresthesia that develops. Dental procedures involving soft tissues (i.e., scaling, curettage) can usually be completed without the use of local anesthesia and with minimal, if any, discomfort. The patient receiving N_2O-O_2 may state that the "pain" is still felt but that it no longer hurts. In other words, the nature of the discomfort has been altered from a sharp, knifelike pain to a duller, much more tolerable one.

  Advantage may also be taken of the paresthesia developing in the patient's arms during intravenous sedation. N_2O-induced paresthesia will make venipuncture more tolerable for the patient fearful of injections.

  Another area of medicine in which peripheral paresthesia is of value is in surgery of the foot. Injections of local anesthetic into the sole of the foot are extremely painful. The use of N_2O-O_2 sedation and the ensuing paresthesia will make this procedure significantly more tolerable.
- *Feeling of warmth, floating, or heaviness:* The next symptoms that develop usually indicate entry into a level of sedation at which the patient is either at or near the ideal for treatment. The ideal sedation level was described as a stage at which the patient is relaxed and comfortable and at which the administrator is also relaxed and able to treat the patient without compromising the quality of care. This ideal level varies from doctor to doctor according to the patient's needs, the training and experience of the doctor and the staff, and the desires of the doctor.

  The clinical sensations of heaviness, warmth, and floating usually indicate that the patient is approaching the desired level. Warmth develops first in most cases, the patient stating that he or she feels warmer. Observation will show the patient to be more flushed, a finding most noticeable on the patient's forehead, where perspiration may be observed. The patient's hands and arms may also feel warmer. A few patients may begin to perspire heavily, a situation that may be uncomfortable. If this occurs, the percentage of N_2O should be lowered by approximately 5% (a 0.5-L/min decrease in N_2O and a 0.5-L/min increase in O_2) to attempt to decrease perspiration without significantly altering the sedative action of the N_2O. A feeling of heaviness or floating may also be noted. The patient may state that his or her arms and legs feel either quite heavy (so heavy that they cannot be moved) or extremely light (so light that they float).

Because clinical signs and symptoms may vary considerably from patient to patient, I rarely describe these symptoms in detail to patients before the procedure. Rather, I have found it useful to be purposefully vague, describing the effects of N_2O-O_2 sedation in general terms. Patients are told only that they will feel more relaxed and comfortable. When patients have been told specifically that they will experience lightheadedness, tingling, numbness, warmth, and heaviness, it has sometimes been observed that they become upset if any of these symptoms fail to develop, as indeed may be the case.

The administrator always observes the patient throughout the sedative technique. Watching the apprehensive patient begin to experience the effects of N_2O-O_2 is of great benefit in determining the proper level of sedation. As mentioned, a patient who has never before received N_2O-O_2 sedation will prove a little more difficult to sedate than one who has. Patients who have previously achieved ideal sedation (have "been there") can simply tell the administrator when they are "there" again. The patient for whom N_2O-O_2 is being used for the first time finds it somewhat more difficult to gauge the proper level of sedation.

Careful observation of the patient aids in determining this. The appearance of apprehensive patients is described in Chapter 4. They do not appear comfortable when seated in the dental chair. Hands may firmly clench the armrest in the so-called white-knuckle syndrome, and their legs may seem quite stiff (Figure 15-12, *A*). As sedation develops, the patient's arms and legs relax and he or she eventually achieves a "sedated look" (Figure 15-12, *B*).

The verbal response of the patient will also change as the effect of N_2O increases. Early in the procedure the patient may state that he or she feels relaxed; however, this may be said in a very rapid, unrelaxed manner. In fact, the patient does feel somewhat relaxed (compared with the feeling on first entering the dental office). However, should the administrator mistake this level of relaxation for the ideal sedative state and attempt to treat the patient, the result would most likely prove to be less than adequate. As sedation increases, the patient's responses become slower, with an increasing lag time observed between questions and the patient's response to them. It appears almost as though the patient experiences difficulty in phrasing replies. The patient's state is now more near the ideal.

The state produced by N_2O-O_2 should not be compared with that of alcohol unless the patient volunteers the comparison spontaneously. To compare the effects of N_2O-O_2 to alcohol to patients who do not consume alcohol for religious, medical, or other personal reasons will probably make them less likely to want to try the technique.

11. Begin Dental Treatment

COMMENT: The patient appears quite relaxed at this point. Titration has continued, with approximately 10% increases in the level of N_2O until the signs and symptoms associated with adequate sedation have been noted. Despite this, the only way of determining with absolute accuracy whether the proper sedative level has been achieved is to begin the planned treatment and observe the patient's response.

If the planned treatment proceeds without any overt signs of discomfort from the patient, it can be assumed that sedation is successful. However, once the procedure begins, it is not unusual for the patient to make movements, espe-

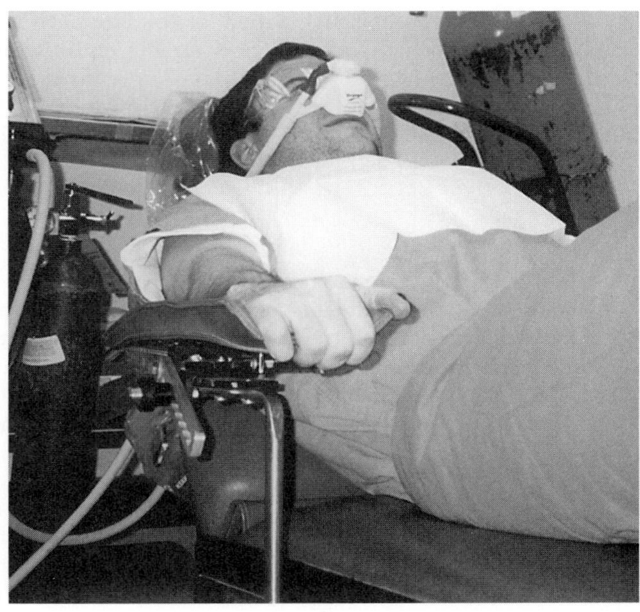

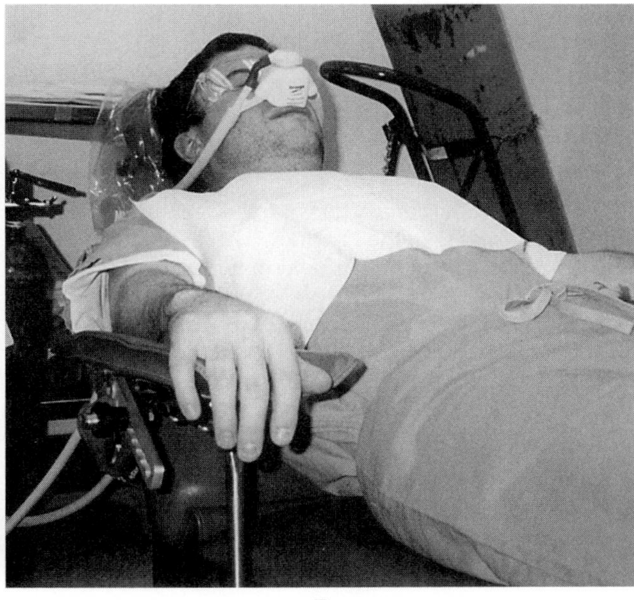

Figure 15-12 **A,** White-knuckle syndrome exhibited by apprehensive patient at start of procedure. **B,** Relaxation of hands is commonly observed when patient becomes sedated.

cially when potentially traumatic procedures, such as the administration of local anesthetics, are carried out. If the movements are significant or disruptive, the procedure should be halted and the level of sedation increased by approximately 5% N_2O. This apparent lack of adequate sedation can easily be explained when it is realized that the signs and symptoms of ideal sedation observed earlier were produced while N_2O-O_2 was being administered to a patient who was merely sitting in the dental chair. Placing a local anesthetic syringe into a fearful patient's mouth raises his or her anxiety level considerably, potentially to a point beyond which the concentration of N_2O-O_2 being inhaled can effectively manage the patient's fears. Halting the procedure and increasing the percentage of N_2O slightly (5%) usually eliminates this problem.

Once pain control (via local anesthesia) has been obtained, the procedure usually proceeds with little difficulty. However, the patient may experience periods when the level of sedation may lessen and, conversely, when the level becomes too intense. N_2O, because of its analgesic and sedative qualities, is excellent in combination with local anesthetic to achieve cooperation for most patients in a dental/surgical environment.

One of the prime benefits of inhalation sedation with N_2O-O_2 is the ability to tailor the sedation to the needs of the patient. The administrator and assistant must continually observe the patient for any indication of changes in level of sedation. The level of sedation may become too light when a particularly traumatic part of the procedure is started. For example, the patient may be relaxed until the handpiece is placed in the mouth and turned on. In some patients the sound of the handpiece is quite anxiety provoking. At this point the patient may tell the administrator that the effect of the N_2O is gone, as though the machine were turned off. As before, the procedure should be temporarily halted, the percentage of N_2O increased by approximately 5% (or more, if needed), the patient resedated, and the procedure resumed.

A sedative level that has been particularly effective during therapy will become too intense when the procedure is finished and the patient's anxiety level lessens. The percentage of N_2O being inhaled by the patient is too great for the now-diminished anxiety level, and the patient becomes overly sedated. Management of this situation simply requires a decrease of the N_2O flow by approximately 5%. Within 30 to 60 seconds the patient will become less sedated.

12. Observe the Patient and Inhalation Sedation Unit during the Procedure

Comment: Throughout the procedure the patient and the inhalation sedation unit must be observed by the doctor, hygienist, or assistant. The level of sedation sought with N_2O-O_2 is such that communication between the administrator or assistant and the patient are readily achieved. The patient should be able to respond to any requests or questions posed. Lack of response to any command should indicate to the staff that treatment be terminated immediately and the patient evaluated. In most cases a decrease in the N_2O by 5% to 10% quickly brings about a response from the patient. The assistant or doctor should also observe the N_2O-O_2 unit periodically to reconfirm that the gases are indeed still flowing. All units have fail-safe devices designed to prevent the inadvertent administration of 100% N_2O, and these devices are usually quite effective. However, situations have occurred in which these devices have failed and patients have received 100% N_2O, often with serious consequences. Visual observation of the N_2O-O_2 unit will prevent this from occurring.

13. Terminate the Flow of N_2O

COMMENT: At the completion of treatment or of that part of it requiring sedation, the N_2O flow will be terminated. In all instances the O_2 will be returned to the original flow rate determined at the start of the procedure. (This will not be necessary, of course, in the constant O_2 flow technique.) The patient is permitted to breathe 100% O_2 for not less than 3 to 5 minutes. Longer periods may be necessary should the patient exhibit any clinical signs or symptoms of sedation at the end of this period. There is no formula for determining the length of time to breathe 100% O_2, but for most patients, the longer the N_2O-O_2 sedation procedure was, the greater the length of time is required to reverse the sedative effects.

N_2O is not titrated "out of the patient" at the end of the procedure the way it must be done at the start. The N_2O flow is simply turned to 0 L/min (0%) and O_2 increased to its original level. It is suggested that the reservoir bag not be emptied of any residual gas when the N_2O flow is terminated, the thought being that the reservoir bag contains some N_2O that will contaminate the atmosphere.

The proper time to terminate the flow of N_2O varies from patient to patient. For example, in the extremely fearful patient, whose anxieties relate to all aspects of dental or surgical treatment, it is advisable to continue the N_2O flow until the entire procedure is completed. However, in the more typical patient, whose apprehensions about dentistry are more specific, such as the administration of local anesthesia or the sound or feel of the handpiece, it is possible to terminate the N_2O flow after the traumatic element of treatment is completed but before the end of the entire procedure. There are several benefits to the early termination of the N_2O flow, especially when the duration of treatment has been prolonged.

When the N_2O flow is terminated before the end of a long procedure (in excess of 1 hour), discharge of the patient from the office is hastened. Rather than waiting until completion of the procedure to remove the N_2O and start the 100% O_2 flow, the doctor elects to administer 100% O_2 after completing the preparation of the teeth but before placing the restorations. The doctor or assistant will increase the O_2 flow to its original value and turn off the N_2O. This can be done without the patient being aware of it, if possible. The reason for this apparent subterfuge is that when asked how they feel, many patients, unaware that the N_2O has been turned off and that they have been breathing 100% O_2 for many minutes, will state that they are still as relaxed as they were before N_2O was terminated. There is a 30% positive placebo response for most drugs, and if approached carefully, this response may be used to advantage in many N_2O-O_2 patients. In the event that the placebo response does not occur in a patient, the patient will simply state that the effect of the N_2O is no longer felt, to which the doctor will reply that it has been turned off because the procedure is almost completed.

For the more apprehensive patient or for shorter procedures, N_2O-O_2 may be administered for the entire treatment. On completion, the same procedure of returning the O_2 flow to its original levels and of turning off the N_2O is carried out. The patient inhales 100% O_2 for not less than 3 to 5 minutes.

14. Discharge the Patient

COMMENT: Determination of recovery from the effects of inhalation sedation is quite important, for in many cases the patients will be dismissed from the office and be allowed to resume their normal activities without any prohibitions. For this reason the doctor must be absolutely certain that recovery is complete before considering discharge of the patient. *Not all patients receiving inhalation sedation with N_2O-O_2 will recover adequately enough to permit their discharge from the office without an escort.*

Because it is common practice to permit most patients to leave the office unescorted after inhalation sedation and to operate a motor vehicle or other potentially dangerous machinery, valid criteria must be used to determine the degree of recovery. Several factors are used in evaluating the recovery process: response of the patient to questioning, vital signs, and a test for motor coordination.

The response of the patient to questioning is, in fact, the primary determinant of recovery from sedation. However, because this is a purely subjective response, other, more valid (from a medicolegal standpoint), objective criteria must also be used. The patient has, at this point in the procedure, received 100% O_2 for at least 3 to 5 minutes. This is adequate to bring about an almost total reversal of symptoms in most patients. Longer periods may be necessary in some patients, particularly those who received N_2O-O_2 for a longer duration. The reason for insisting on a minimum of 3 to 5 minutes of 100% O_2 at the end of the procedure is to decrease the possibility of diffusion hypoxia. Diffusion hypoxia can occur when the N_2O exits through the lungs at a much faster rate than the N_2 that replaces it, thereby diluting and reducing the oxygen supply and blood saturation. Diffusion hypoxia is discussed further in Chapter 18.

The position of the patient is altered from the supine or semisupine (during treatment) to a more upright one as recovery continues. The nasal hood remains in position at this time. The patient is asked what he or she is feeling. Any reply other than "I feel perfectly normal" or "I feel the way I did when I arrived in the office" indicates the need for additional O_2. The nasal hood, providing O_2, should be left on the patient for an additional 2 to 3 minutes and the question then repeated. The patient should not be discharged while any signs or symptoms of sedation remain. In those cases in which N_2O-O_2 was used in combination with other sedation techniques (oral, rectal, intranasal, intramuscular, or intravenous), the patients should have an adult in attendance to escort him or her from the office.

Vital signs are valuable adjuncts in the evaluation of recovery from sedation (Figure 15-13). They are objective parameters that indicate the state of function of the patient's cardiorespiratory systems. Vital signs to be meas-

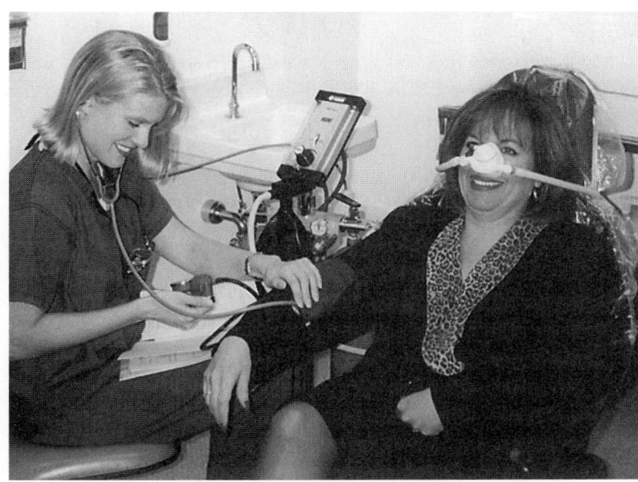

Figure 15-13 Vital signs are valuable adjuncts in the evaluation of recovery from sedation.

ured and recorded on the sedation record include blood pressure, heart rate and rhythm, and respiratory rate. It must be understood that vital signs recorded after the procedure will not be exactly the same as those recorded preoperatively or even those obtained at the patient's preliminary visit to the office. Fluctuation in either direction is normal. Parameters that may be useful in determining the degree of recovery following sedation are the following:

- Blood pressure: ±20 mm Hg/10 mm Hg from baseline
- Heart rate and rhythm: ±15 beats/min from baseline; same rhythm as baseline
- Respirations: ±3 breaths/min from baseline

Variations in vital signs beyond these parameters are normal, or they may indicate a residual effect of the drugs. There may be no correlation between the changed vital signs and the use of inhalation sedation. Significant alteration in one or more of the vital signs should be evaluated before the patient is discharged.

Another modified neurologic test such as touching the tip of the nose with the little finger can indicate recovery. A most valuable criterion in determining recovery from inhalation sedation will be an evaluation of the patient's motor coordination called the *Trieger test*. This test is an objective measurement of the patient's ability to perform fine motor movements. The Trieger test was originally introduced in 1941 as the Bender Motor Gestalt test and was used as an adjunct in the diagnosis and psychotherapy of organic brain damage in children.[1] In 1967, Dr. Norman Trieger modified the original test by selecting one figure and replacing its solid lines with dots (Figures 15-14 and 15-15). The adaptation of this test for measuring recovery from anesthesia and sedation is based on the fact that fatigue and central nervous system (CNS) depressant drugs exaggerate psychomotor dysfunction.[2] Disturbance in motor coordination is determined by successive trials on the test by the same individual.

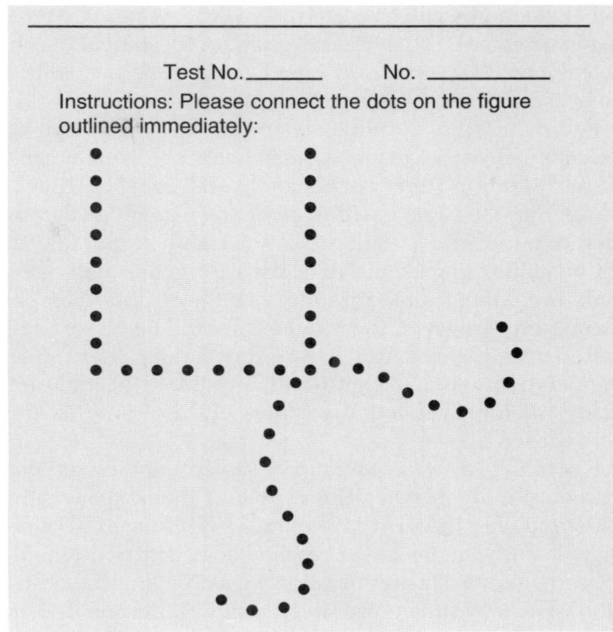
Test No.______ No. ________
Instructions: Please connect the dots on the figure outlined immediately:

Figure 15-14 Trieger test for motor coordination.

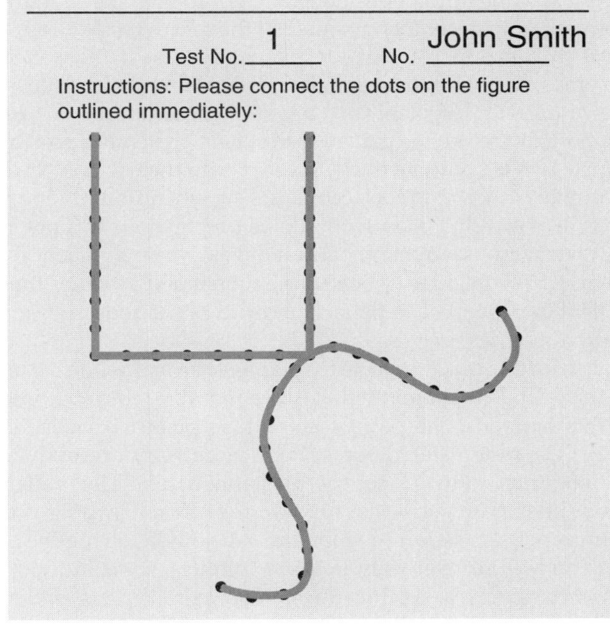
Test No. 1 No. John Smith
Instructions: Please connect the dots on the figure outlined immediately:

Figure 15-15 Baseline Trieger test. All dots connected and quality of lines good.

The patient is requested to complete the test preoperatively. This test provides a baseline with which subsequent tests are compared. The test is supported on a firm surface (e.g., clipboard), and the patient is asked to carefully connect all of the dots. Scoring of the test is based on the number of dots that are missed completely. Two other factors that may be evaluated are (1) the time required for the patient to complete the test (e.g., 10 seconds) and (2) the general quality of the lines (i.e., straight, wavy, or erratic).

Following the administration of 100% O_2 and the patient's subjective response that he or she feels normal, the postsedation Trieger test is administered. The patient is returned to the same position he or she was in for the preoperative test and is reminded to carefully complete the test by connecting all the dots; the results are then evaluated. The patient may miss more or fewer dots than preoperatively; however, the numbers should be close. Seven missed dots after sedation, with 5 dots having been missed preoperatively, is not significant, provided the time and quality of the lines are approximately the same as they were earlier.

Use of the Trieger test with patients during their sedation procedure is interesting. The degree of motor dysfunction evident at this time is often quite significant. In Trieger's original study, return to the baseline level occurred within 2 to 4 minutes after the termination of the N_2O.[3] If the postsedation Trieger test demonstrates a residual effect of N_2O, the patient should recover for several more minutes and then retake the Trieger test.

When it has been determined to the administrator's satisfaction that the patient has fully recovered from the effects of the N_2O-O_2, the nasal hood is removed and the patient is returned to the upright position and permitted to stand. At this point it is important for a member of the office staff (e.g., assistant) to stand in front of the patient so that if the patient becomes dizzy or his or her legs feel weak on standing (possible orthostatic hypotension), the staff member can provide support and return the patient to the chair, preventing possible injury. This is not more likely to occur with the use of N_2O-O_2 than with other sedation techniques or when no sedation is used. It is merely good practice to be prepared for this potentially dangerous situation that can develop in any patient following prolonged recumbency (the time required varies from patient to patient) or in patients receiving certain drugs, especially antihypertensives.

It is not unusual for a patient to feel normal while seated in the dental chair and then lightheaded upon first standing. If this happens, the patient should be placed back in the chair, O_2 administered for several more minutes, and the patient then allowed to try to stand again. The patient should never be permitted to leave the office if any signs or symptoms of sedation remain. Although virtually all patients will recover fully in a few minutes, some individuals will require a significantly longer period. This patient and others with similar symptoms should neither be discharged from the office unescorted nor permitted to drive a car or return to work where mental alertness is required. Provisions must be made for a companion to escort the patient home. Although this negates a major advantage in the use of inhalation sedation, strict adherence to this provision will prevent potential injury to the patient and potential liability to the doctor.

In some situations it may prove prudent to insist on an escort for all patients receiving inhalation sedation. Standard operating procedure in the U.S. Navy for inhalation sedation includes the requirement of an escort for the patient.

Most patients recover completely following inhalation of 100% O_2 for at least 3 to 5 minutes. If the doctor is satisfied that this is the case, the patient may be permitted to leave the office unescorted. This is the only technique of sedation in which this may be considered.

The patient's ability to operate a motor vehicle after receiving inhalation sedation has been studied.[4] Several parameters were evaluated, including steering errors, speeding errors, and braking reaction time (Table 15-3). Subjects were evaluated before, during, and after the administration of N_2O-O_2. In all categories subjects demonstrated a deterioration of ability during the inhalation of N_2O-O_2 similar to that produced by alcohol. Following the administration of O_2 and then room air, all measured parameters had returned to baseline values or exceeded them. It was concluded that the typical patient may safely operate a motor vehicle following recovery from N_2O-O_2 inhalation sedation.

Postoperative instructions relevant to the dental or surgical procedure are given in written form to the patient. The patient is then dismissed from the office.

15. Record Data Concerning the Sedation Procedure

COMMENT: The assistant should record in the patient's chart that inhalation sedation was used (Figure 15-16). A sample entry in the chart follows.

> The patient received ____% N_2O- ____% O_2 at a total liter flow of ____ L/min. The procedure lasted approximately ____ minutes. At the termination of the procedure the patient received 100% O_2 for ____ minutes at a flow of ____ L/min. The patient tolerated the procedure well and was dismissed from the office in good condition.

Vital signs	**Baseline**	**After procedure**
Blood pressure (mm Hg)	112/76	118/78
Heart rate (beats/min)	88	82
Respirations (breaths/min)	18	16

In addition, any postoperative instructions should be indicated on the chart. A rubber stamp or preglued labels may be prepared with this information and included in the patient's chart, and the blanks filled in after the procedure.

16. Cleanse the Equipment

COMMENT: The rubber goods of the inhalation sedation unit are in contact with the patient's skin and exhaled breath and will naturally become contaminated with foreign material, bacteria, and viral agents. Serious respiratory infections have resulted from the use of contaminated anesthesia machines in operating rooms.[5-7] Nasal hoods for inhalation sedation have also been demonstrated to be contaminated with multiple human pathogens capable of

TABLE 15-3 Recovery from Nitrous Oxide

	Presedation	Sedation	Postsedation
Speeding errors Max possible = 11 Mean + s/d	4.33 ± 2.15	3.75 ± 2.05	2.58 ± 1.31
Steering errors Max = 16	9.73 ± 2.87	11.09 ± 3.33	9.09 ± 2.43
Braking errors Max = 35	24.25 ± 4.47	30.42 ± 2.16	23.42 ± 5.50
Signaling errors Max = 19	7.17 ± 1.85	10.42 ± 4.46	4.92 ± 1.93
Mean braking time (sec) (range)	0.486 (0.442-0.608)	0.578 (0.448-0.986)	0.474 (0.412-0.604)

From Jastak JT, Orendorff D: *Anesth Prog* 22:113, 1975.

Date: __________ Patient: ______________________________ Age: ____

ASA classification: I II III IV

Med consult needed: Yes/No Operative procedure: ____________

Procedural data:

	PREOPERATIVE		POSTOPERATIVE
BP:	__________		__________
Pulse/quality:	__________		__________
Respiration:	__________		__________
N_2O Start time:	__________	N_2O Finish time:	__________
Titrated % of N_2O: (for documentation purposes only)	__________	Postoperative O_2: (in minutes)	__________

Comments:

Clinician signature: ________________________________

Figure 15-16 Example of clinical record for conscious sedation. (From Clark MS, Brunick AL: *Handbook of nitrous oxide and oxygen sedation,* St Louis, 1999, Mosby.)

transmission from one patient to another.[8] In a study by Yagiela, Hunt, and Hunt,[9] 100% of nasal hoods used for 10-minute sedative procedures were inoculated with bacteria.

Cleansing of nasal hoods is mandatory. Simple washing of the nasal hood with soap and water has been shown merely to decrease the number of bacterial and viral contaminants.[10] Other techniques have been used, including using alcohol, glutaraldehyde, and iodophor; autoclaving; and microwaving.[7,10-12] All of these techniques have disadvantages when used on nasal masks.

Under the Spaulding classification of inanimate surfaces, nasal hoods are considered semicritical in terms of infection risk.[13] Items in this grouping come into contact with intact mucous membranes and are therefore resistant to infection by common bacterial spores.[7]

The following is the current recommended procedure for sterilization of nasal hoods.[7,9] After each use, the nasal hood is washed with soap and warm water and then immersed in glutaraldehyde solution for 10 minutes. It is then rinsed thoroughly with tap water to remove the disinfectant solution. At the end of each week, all tubing, reservoir bags, and nasal hoods are stored in glutaraldehyde for 10 hours to achieve complete sterilization. Following this 10-hour period the equipment is rinsed in warm tap water for 1 hour.

Subsequent Appointments

Once a patient has successfully received inhalation sedation, it is highly likely that the use of N_2O-O_2 will be desired for future treatment. At subsequent visits the same technique should be used. The experience and information gathered from the initial N_2O-O_2 experience will facilitate any such future procedures. The rate at which the sedation at these subsequent appointments is induced should not be increased. Increasing the speed of induction often leads to increased patient discomfort. Patients should be better able to tell the administrator when "they are there" (at ideal sedation), having been "there" before. The ultimate goal, however, is to have patient acceptance of dental treatment fearlessly without the need for N_2O-O_2.

It is important to note that the concentration of N_2O required for ideal sedation may vary somewhat from visit to visit. Ideally, this percentage will decrease over time as a patient's level of comfort with treatment increases; however, other, nondental or medical factors will come into play. Factors such as the patient's social life, working life, altered physical condition, and time of day may decrease or increase the percentage of N_2O required by the patient. Normally, variation from visit to visit is slight (35% today, 40% or 30% at the next visit). Only rarely will significant differences be noted over short periods (e.g., 35% to 65%). To use the same concentration of N_2O at each visit, or not to titrate as a means of "saving time" (see following discussion), is to increase the risk of discomfort to the patient.

COMPARISON OF TECHNIQUES OF ADMINISTRATION

Both the constant liter flow and the constant O_2 flow technique may be used in the delivery of N_2O-O_2. There is little clinical difference between these techniques. The few differences that do exist are presented. The selection of the technique to be used clinically is made at the discretion of the administrator.

Constant Liter Flow Technique

Summary of Technique

1. Establish O_2 flow rate.
2. Increase N_2O to 1 L/min, and decrease O_2 by 1 L/min.
3. Subsequently increase N_2O at 0.5 L/min, and decrease O_2 at 0.5 L/min, maintaining the same total flow rate during the procedure.

Advantages

1. Smaller volumes of gases used
2. Less costly
3. Decrease in exhaled N_2O contamination

Disadvantage. Percentage increments of N_2O are fixed; thus it is easier to oversedate the patient.

Examples of Technique. Most inhalation sedation units are incapable of delivering less than a 2.5- or 3-L/min flow of O_2. In this case the O_2 flow rate will not fall below 2.5 or 3 L/min even as the N_2O rate continues to be increased at its usual 0.5-L/min increment. Thus this becomes equivalent to the constant O_2 flow technique:

6.0-L/min Flow

N_2O L/min	O_2 L/min	Percentage of N_2O
0	6.0	0
1.0	5.0	16
1.5	4.5	25
2.0	4.0	33
2.5	3.5	41
3.0	3.0	50
3.5	2.5	58
4.0	2.5*	61
4.5	2.5*	64

*Unable to deliver less than 2.5 L/min.

Constant O_2 Flow Technique

Summary of Technique

1. Establish O_2 flow rate.
2. Increase N_2O flow rate to 1 L/min, and leave O_2 constant.
3. Subsequently increase N_2O in increments of 1 L/min.
4. Oxygen flow rate remains constant throughout procedure.

Advantages

1. Slightly easier to use; requires adjustment of one dial
2. Larger volumes of gases used; thus little difficulty in breathing adequately

7.0-L/min Flow

N_2O L/min	O_2 L/min	Percentage of N_2O
0	7.0	0
1.0	6.0	14
1.5	5.5	21
2.0	5.0	28
2.5	4.5	35
3.0	4.0	42
3.5	3.5	50
4.0	3.0	58
4.5	2.5	65
5.0	2.5*	67
5.5	2.5*	69

*Unable to deliver less than 2.5 L/min.

3. Percentage increments of N_2O decrease as the percentage of N_2O increases (see charts), minimizing inadvertent oversedation

Disadvantages

1. Larger volumes of gases used; thus more costly to administer
2. Larger volumes of N_2O used; thus greater contamination of environment with N_2O

Examples of Technique

6.0-L/min O_2

N_2O L/min	O_2 L/min	Percentage of N_2O
0	6.0	0
1.0	6.0	14
2.0	6.0	26
3.0	6.0	33
4.0	6.0	40
5.0	6.0	45
6.0	6.0	50
7.0	6.0	54

7.0-L/min O_2

N_2O L/min	O_2 L/min	Percentage of N_2O
0	7.0	0
1.0	7.0	12
2.0	7.0	22
3.0	7.0	30
4.0	7.0	36
5.0	7.0	41
6.0	7.0	46
7.0	7.0	50

NORMAL DISTRIBUTION CURVE

As has been stressed throughout this book, patients vary in their response to drugs. However, if the percentage of N_2O required to achieve ideal sedation is summarized for many hundreds or thousands of patients, then a normal distribution curve may be formulated. The following information is a compilation of more than 5000 N_2O-O_2 inhalation sedations administered at the University of Southern Carolina School of Dentistry from 1973 through September 1992.[14] Statistics were obtained at sea level. At higher altitudes (e.g., 5200 ft in Denver, Colorado, or 7200 ft in Mexico City, Mexico), greater percentages of N_2O will be required to achieve comparable sedation levels. An increase of approximately 5% is necessary at Denver's altitude.

Normal Distribution Curve for Adults Successfully Sedated with N_2O-O_2

Percentage of N_2O	Percentage of Patients Achieving Ideal Sedation
10	<1
15	1
20	4
25	7
30	22
35	24
40	24
45	10
50	4
55	1
60	2
65	<1
70	<1

When the patients are divided into larger groups, it can be seen that 70% of patients who achieve ideal sedation with inhalation sedation did so at a N_2O

percentage between 30% and 40%. Approximately 12% required concentrations of N_2O below 30%, whereas 18% required N_2O concentrations in excess of 40% to achieve the same level of sedation.

This chart includes only patients who reached ideal sedation with N_2O-O_2. Not included are the approximately 3% of patients receiving these agents who did not achieve clinically adequate sedation levels. For whatever reason (e.g., too fearful, required more than 70% N_2O, mouth breathing, claustrophobia), the technique failed to achieve its goals. This is to be expected with inhalation sedation, as well as with every other technique of sedation.

TITRATION AND TIME

One of the major problems that develops over time in the typical dental practice where inhalation sedation is used is that the doctor stops titrating. Fixed concentrations are delivered to all patients, the percentage of N_2O being approximately 40% or 50%. This technique of not titrating N_2O cannot be recommended for routine use and is reviewed in Chapters 16 and 18. The rationale presented for not titrating N_2O is that titration takes too long to be done properly and that in the typical dental office such time is not available. Table 15-4 demonstrates that when titrated according to the schedule presented in this chapter (every 60 to 90 seconds), the typical patient requiring approximately 30% to 40% N_2O will be sedated within 3 to 6 minutes.

The 3 to 6 minutes required for sedation to be achieved is compensated for by the fact that, once relaxed, the patient will move little, if at all, during the remainder of the procedure. This is in stark contrast to a fearful, unsedated patient who moves constantly, making treatment more difficult and stressful for both the staff and the patients. Achieving effective pain control is considerably more difficult (and potentially dangerous) as the patient moves during local anesthetic administration. Once treatment begins, the patient will often ask to have it stopped so that he or she may do any number of things that prevent the doctor from completing treatment (e.g., drinking water, going to the restroom). The few minutes required to achieve ideal sedation with inhalation sedation are worth the effort and time invested.

SIGNS AND SYMPTOMS OF OVERSEDATION

If titration is adhered to, it is unlikely that the patient will become uncomfortable or oversedated. However, it is possible that at various times during treatment, the depth of sedation will become greater without the N_2O percentage having been altered. This occurs most often when a part of the treatment is completed and there is a lull (a lack of stimulation of the patient) while additional equipment or materials are prepared for use. During tooth preparation, for example, there is a constant stimulus provided by the sound and vibration of the handpiece. The patient is receiving a concentration of N_2O adequate to produce a calming effect at this time. However, when the preparation is completed and the restorative material is being prepared and inserted, little or no stimulation of the patient occurs. This same level of N_2O will produce a deepening of the sedation at this time.

Following are some clinical indicators of oversedation.[15] Management of this situation is simply to decrease the level of N_2O by approximately 5% to 10%. There is no need to use the O_2 flush or to terminate the

TABLE 15-4 Titration Times According to Percentage of N_2O Required for Sedation

	Constant Liter Flow			*Constant O_2 Flow*		
Time (min)	N_2O (L/min)	O_2 (L/min)	Percentage of N_2O	N_2O (L/min)	O_2 (L/min)	Percentage of N_2O
0	0	6.0	0	0	6.0	0
1.0-1.5	1.0	5.0	16	1.0	6.0	14
2.0-3.0	1.5	4.5	25	2.0	6.0	25
3.0-4.5	2.0	4.0	33	3.0	6.0	33
4.0-6.0	2.5	3.5	41	4.0	6.0	40

flow of N_2O. Within 30 seconds of decreasing the N_2O flow (approximately 0.5 to 1 L/min), the patient will be more responsive.

Clinical Indicators of Oversedation

The Patient Persistently Closes the Mouth. Patients receiving N_2O-O_2 sedation should be capable of keeping their mouths open without use of mouth props during the entire procedure. The administrator will tell patients at the start of the sedation that they are to breathe through their nose but are to keep their mouth open. If the patient needs constant reminders to keep the mouth open during dental treatment, the percentage of N_2O should be decreased slightly.

Mouth props may be used but are not recommended for the inexperienced N_2O-O_2 administrator, for they take away one of the earliest signs of oversedation. With clinical experience other clinical clues of oversedation are recognizable to the doctor and assistant, and mouth props may again be recommended.

Most medical procedures in which N_2O-O_2 is used occur away from the mouth. The need for maintaining the mouth in an open position is, of course, nonexistent. In these cases the physician loses an important guide to early detection of oversedation. The doctor or surgical nurse must become more aware of the "other" aspects of patient monitoring.

The Patient Spontaneously Begins Mouth Breathing. Patients receiving N_2O-O_2 have been told by the administrator to breathe only through the nose. A possible sign of oversedation is a spontaneous reversion to mouth breathing, especially in adults (children are more likely to do this in the absence of oversedation). The first time this occurs, the patient is simply reminded to breathe through the nose; however, after several recurrences, the N_2O flow is decreased by 0.5 L/min.

Mouth breathing is easy for the dentist, hygienist, and dental assistant to detect. Mouth mirrors become fogged, and the exhalation of air through the mouth can be felt. A rubber dam effectively eliminates the potential for mouth breathing.

For physicians and other health professionals working at a distance from the mouth, the occurrence of mouth breathing will be more rare than in dentistry. Patients should be told at the start of the procedure to breathe solely through their nose and not to open their mouth.

The Patient Complains of Nausea and Effects of Sedation Felt as Too Intense or Uncomfortable. When a patient says that he or she is uncomfortable, the administrator should immediately decrease the flow of N_2O. Most patients tolerate a degree of discomfort in silence, so at any mention of discomfort, the N_2O flow should be decreased by 0.5 L/min.

If this plea is ignored by the administrator or if the patient does not volunteer the information, it is not unusual for the patient to suddenly and without warning remove the nasal hood. As patients begin to lose control (become oversedated), they respond by attempting to remove the cause of this feeling—the nasal hood. Listening to and watching the patient carefully can prevent these unpleasant situations from arising.

The Patient Fails to Respond Rationally or Gives Sluggish Responses. The sedated patient becomes distracted from the office environment. To a degree this is desirable; however, when a patient no longer responds to verbal command, the level of sedation should be decreased.

It is not uncommon for a patient to respond more slowly than usual to spoken commands during N_2O-O_2 sedation. However, when the command must be repeated more than twice, decrease the flow of N_2O by 0.5 L/min. The patient receiving N_2O-O_2 conscious sedation should be able to respond rationally and relatively quickly to command.

The Patient Becomes Sleepy. As mentioned, a level of sedation will develop at which the patient feels as though he or she is losing control. In the absence of the patient volunteering this information to the administrator, a sudden jerking movement by the patient will be noticed and the patient may remove the nasal hood. The N_2O flow should be decreased slightly, and within 30 seconds the patient will recover. When questioned about their experience, patients will say, "I felt as though I was falling into a bottomless, black hole." This is similar to the feeling that many people experience when lying down to sleep when quite tired. Commonly, the person will suddenly jerk his or her body upward. This is in response to the feeling of falling into the bottomless hole—an attempt to grab hold of something.

The Patient Speaks Incoherently or Dreams. Speaking incoherently indicates that the level of sedation is too great. The patient is probably dreaming, and the speaking is a part of the dream. In any case it becomes impossible for dental therapy to be continued at this time. The N_2O flow should be decreased and the patient carefully tended to.

The Patient Becomes Uncooperative. One of the goals of sedation is for the patient to become more cooperative. As with any technique, this goal will not always be obtainable. In this case the patient, as sedation progresses, becomes more outgoing and verbal and may even be somewhat physical (moving about in the chair more than before). Decreasing the level of N_2O may decrease this effect, yet still provide adequate sedation for the planned treatment to continue.

This effect on patients may be seen with any CNS depressant, including N_2O, but it is especially common with alcohol. Many persons become more outgoing and friendly after several drinks. Alcohol produces a generalized depression of the cerebral cortex, decreasing inhibitions and allowing the individual to act in an out-of-the-ordinary manner. Unlike the effect of alcohol, this effect of N_2O may be readily reversed by decreasing the flow of N_2O.

The Patient Laughs, Cries, or Becomes Giddy. N_2O is commonly known as *laughing gas* because of the propensity of many persons receiving it to begin uncontrollable laughing. Its administration can also lead to uncontrolled crying.

N_2O does not make a person happy or sad. N_2O decreases the inhibitions of the patient and increases the intensity of emotions. For example, a person in a very good, happy mood will feel even better when N_2O is administered. This person will be more likely to enjoy the sedative experience and to start laughing should humorous thoughts come to mind. Conversely, the patient coming to the appointment in a poor mood will be more apt to release these feelings when N_2O-O_2 is administered. Without N_2O-O_2 the person would not cry but does so quite readily once the N_2O is administered.

In either case, laughing or crying, the continuation of dental treatment becomes impossible. The concentration of N_2O must therefore be decreased to a more appropriate level.

The Patient Has Uncoordinated Movements. When a patient receiving N_2O-O_2 makes uncoordinated movements, the concentration of N_2O must be decreased. For example, a 20-year-old woman was receiving 40% N_2O for dental treatment because of her fears of dentistry. She was well sedated, but occasionally during the procedure she suddenly, without warning, lifted her legs upward as high as she could and then let them drop back onto the chair. After the N_2O flow was reduced by 0.5 L/min, the patient was asked about this reaction. She stated that she was unaware of lifting her legs but that she did remember that her legs had become extremely light and began to float upward by themselves. She then would "catch them" and bring them back down. Such uncoordinated movement is potentially injurious. Immediate reduction of the N_2O flow by 0.5 L/min is recommended.

In each of the situations presented, the patient has entered into a level of sedation that is just slightly beyond that which is deemed ideal. Management is not dramatic; the simple reduction of N_2O flow by approximately 5% to 10% corrects the situation. It is very rare indeed when the flow of N_2O must quickly be terminated. N_2O-O_2 has the unique ability to quickly allow for physiologic change by increasing or decreasing the concentration.

REFERENCES

1. Trieger N, Newman MG, Miller JG: An objective measure of recovery, *Anesth Prog* 16:4, 1969.
2. Trieger NT, Laskota WI, Jacobs AW et al: Nitrous oxide: a study of physiological and psychological effects, *J Am Dent Assoc* 82:142, 1971.
3. Newman MG, Trieger NT, Millar JC: Measuring recovery from anesthesia: a simple test, *Anesth Analg* 48:136, 1969.
4. Jastak JT, Orendorff D: Recovery from nitrous oxide sedation, *Anesth Prog* 22:113, 1975.
5. Joseph JM: Disease transmission by inefficiently sanitized anesthetizing apparatus, *JAMA* 149:1196, 1952.
6. Olds JW, Kisch AL, Eberle BJ et al: *Pseudomonas aeruginosa* respiratory tract infection acquired from a contaminated anesthesia machine, *Am Rev Respir Dis* 105:628, 1974.
7. Jastak JT, Donaldson D: Nitrous oxide. In Dionne RA, Phero JC, eds: *Management of pain and anxiety in dental practice,* New York, 1991, Elsevier.
8. Hunt LM, Yagiela JA: Bacterial contamination and transmission by nitrous oxide sedation apparatus, *Oral Surg Oral Med Oral Pathol* 44:367, 1977.
9. Yagiela JA, Hunt LM, Hunt DE: Disinfection of nitrous oxide inhalation equipment, *J Am Dent Assoc* 98:191, 1979.
10. Christensen RP, Robison RA, Robinson DF et al: Antimicrobial activity of environmental surface disinfectants in the absence and presence of bioburden, *J Am Dent Assoc* 119:493, 1989.
11. Rohrer MD, Bulard RA: Microwave sterilization, *J Am Dent Assoc* 110:194, 1985.
12. Young SK, Graves DC, Rorer MD et al: Microwave sterilization of nitrous oxide nasal hoods contaminated with virus, *Oral Surg Oral Med Oral Pathol* 60:581, 1985.
13. Favero MS: Chemical disinfection of medical and surgical materials. In Block SS, ed: *Disinfection, sterilization and preservation,* ed 3, Philadelphia, 1985, Lea & Febiger.
14. School of Dentistry, University of Southern California: *Statistics from Section of Anesthesia & Medicine,* Los Angeles, 1992, Unpublished.
15. Bennett CR: *Conscious sedation in dental practice,* ed 2, St Louis, 1978, Mosby.

CHAPTER 16

Inhalation Sedation: Complications

CHAPTER OUTLINE

As with any technique or procedure, potential complications can be associated with the use of inhalation sedation. Complications, however, can usually be avoided with training and preparation. Inhalation sedation is very safe, and one almost has to try intentionally to have a serious problem with its use. The potential complications include the following:

1. Inadequate/incomplete sedation
2. Poor patient experience
3. Equipment performance

INADEQUATE/INCOMPLETE SEDATION

First, inadequate or incomplete sedation usually involves poor patient selection for the use of nitrous oxide–oxygen (N_2O-O_2) sedation. An example would be the authoritarian-type personality who, when faced with the prospect of loss of control or the sense of this loss, becomes uncomfortable. The patient not wanting to lose control will consciously or subconsciously fight the effects of the agent (N_2O). Unfortunately, other similar sedative procedures produce the same effects, and the success rate of most will be poor in the authoritarian type of patient unless more potent agents are used.

Patients who are emotionally or psychologically unstable may not fare well with N_2O-O_2. Patients who use mind-altering drugs may also have residual conflicting or counterproductive effects from N_2O administration. These patients, particularly if chronic abusers, may be "resistant" to the effects of N_2O and/or expect or require a level of potency that is beyond the capacity of N_2O in therapeutic percentages. Hyporesponders, representing approximately 18% of the population, may not respond to the highest levels of N_2O that can be possibly given (70% concentration). N_2O-O_2 use is also not intended for severely fearful patients. Choose your patient carefully and be mindful that N_2O-O_2 works best in conjunction with local anesthetic.[1]

POOR PATIENT EXPERIENCE

The second classification of potential complications—poor patient experience—can be best managed by prevention. Prevention is most easily and best accomplished by titration of the N_2O during administration. Titration allows for enough N_2O to be given to achieve the desired clinical effect for a given patient for a particular procedure. *Most patients who have complications are oversedated.* Physical signs and symptoms such as excessive perspiration, nausea and vomiting, hallucinations, expectoration, and increased agitation rather than sedation, are all clear signs and symptoms of oversedation. If a patient exhibits any of these signs, the N_2O concentration should be decreased, and in a very short time, a reversal of these adverse reactions will be evident and the patient's status returned to normal. It is truly amazing to observe how quickly a patient will return to a level of cooperation and acceptance of treatment after this decrease in N_2O concentration. It is important to keep the O_2 flow unchanged. The built-in features of modern inhalation sedation units prevent a flow with more than 70% N_2O from occurring. This safety feature helps reduce the possibility of oversedation and possible hypoxia.

The primary reason to administer N_2O-O_2 is to provide a pleasant experience for the patient by altering his or her mood. Anything less is unacceptable. Some patients can have an inexplicable idiosyncratic reaction to a drug, but this is extremely rare with N_2O, and in fact, there are no true outright contraindications, only relative contraindications. The relative contraindications of N_2O-O_2 are discussed in Chapter 12.

EQUIPMENT PERFORMANCE

The last classification of potential complication is equipment performance. This has become much rarer as a result of the intense scrutiny placed on manufacturers by numerous professional agencies, as well as the extreme desire by the manufacturers to provide a safe and excellent product. The manufacturers have succeeded in providing a safe machine with backup systems that ensure adequate levels of O_2 are present to maintain operation. Even with a failure in the O_2 supply, the machine still allows the patient to receive room air without impediment. The possibility for machine or equipment failure usually revolves around purposeful alteration of the equipment as sold or the use of outdated equipment. The rubber parts of the sedation machine can tear, leak, or malfunction and should therefore be frequently inspected per the American Dental Association's protocol. The chance of equipment failure in today's environment is extremely small. Equipment failure can best be prevented by routine examination and inspection of the inhalation sedation unit.

POTENTIAL COMPLICATIONS

Potential complications, as mentioned, rarely occur. When a complication does arise, it is commonly the result of a high concentration of N_2O (greater than 50%) and long duration of use (greater than 1 hour).

Nausea and Vomiting

The incidence of nausea and vomiting with the administration of N_2O-O_2 inhalation sedation is very low. Nausea and vomiting occur in the sedation arena as a result of hypoxia or oversedation. N_2O was historically administered without the addition of supplemental oxygen. In fact, the "technique" was to create an intentionally hypoxic (cyanotic) patient and then work as rapidly as possible until the patient recovered. Some patients did not recover; some woke up very nauseated and vomiting. This history has in some areas persisted to the erroneous conclusion that N_2O-O_2 was the cause of the nausea and vomiting.[1] It has been shown in large studies that nausea and vomiting occur in fewer than 0.5% of patients.[2] When nausea does occur, it is usually associated with the following causes.

Presence of Food in the Stomach. Heavy meals preceding an inhalation sedation administration can easily cause nausea and vomiting, particularly in pediatric patients. The converse is also true. Patients being treated on an empty stomach also are more susceptible to nausea and vomiting. I ask patients to have a high-carbohydrate meal 4 to 6 hours before the appointment. This prevents starvation and yet allows for stomach contents to be minimized.

Oversedation. A reliable and consistent sign of oversedation is a response from the patient that he or she feels bad, "sick to the stomach," usually preceded by sweating and pallor. No matter the percentage of N_2O concentration, *the patient is oversedated!* The N_2O flow must be turned off, and the patient will quickly recover.

The "Roller Coaster Ride." Administration of N_2O-O_2 allows the best possible degree of titration of any drug route. However, this great advantage can be used to a disadvantage by increasing and decreasing the N_2O-O_2 flows, causing a so-called roller coaster ride. This can precipitate nausea and vomiting. Patient titration is encouraged, but wide swings in concentration can have a deleterious effect on the patient. Levels of sedation may also fluctuate if the patient is allowed to maintain conversation and breathe through his or her mouth.

Length of Sedation. The longer the patient has N_2O-O_2 sedation, the greater is the incidence of nausea and vomiting. Although this is not nearly as problematic as high concentrations and oversedation, length of sedation should be monitored.

Prior History of Nausea and Vomiting. Some patients are more prone to nausea and vomiting than are others. Although this is most likely related to their psychological profile, it is nonetheless a factor of predisposition. Serious consideration should be given to whether these patients should receive an antiemetic. This is especially true for children.[3] Antiemetics can be delivered orally or rectally to help prevent nausea in patients (Table 16-1).

Patient Positioning. Patient positioning should promote comfort. If a patient is moving a lot in the chair, make sure clothing is not ill fitting and encourage the patient to get comfortable, because this, to some degree, is thought to contribute to nausea and vomiting.

Management of Vomiting. Historically, before the development of fail-safe machines that ensure delivery of supplemental oxygen, hypoxia or anoxia would possibly result in nausea or vomiting. As a result, in the past, N_2O-O_2 administration was associated with nausea and vomiting. With the advent of the fail-safe machine in 1976, the incidence of vomiting in one study conducted at the University of Southern California was found to be 0.3% of the 5000 cases studied.[2] The most dangerous circumstance (although highly unlikely to occur), in my opinion, is for a patient to become unconscious while receiving N_2O-O_2 and have a secondary sequela of silent regurgitation with aspiration of vomitus. This life-threatening situation would most likely occur only with an unmonitored patient receiving a high level of N_2O. The greater the depth of sedation is, the more likely is the incidence of nausea and vomiting. Parkhouse et al.[4] demonstrated that the incidence of nausea rose with increasing concentration of N_2O. The duration of sedation is also of importance, but not as great as that of depth of sedation.

Patients who are about to vomit usually have a period of impending awareness of the event: hypersalivation, sweating, and nausea. If the patient expresses this awareness, the following should be carried out:

1. The clinician should turn off the N_2O flow and have the patient continue breathing 100% pure O_2.
2. As vomiting begins, remove the nasal hood or other delivery apparatus from the patient's face.
3. Remove the rubber dam, if present, and any other dental equipment from the oral cavity.
4. Turn the patient's head and body to the side away from the side on which the person treating the patient is stationed (Figure 16-1). This permits the vomitus to pool in the cheek instead of flowing back into the patient's pharynx, where airway obstruction may occur. A kidney or emesis basin and high-volume suction tip may be used to assist in removing the vomitus (Figure 16-2). A dry 4 × 4 piece of gauze can also quickly aid in removing vomitus.
5. Following the incident, replace the nasal hood on the patient's nose so that he or she may be permitted to breathe 100% O_2 for at least 3 to 5 minutes. The patient may be somewhat reluctant to have the nasal hood placed back on for fear of

TABLE 16-1 Antiemetics

Generic Name	Proprietary Name	Adult Oral Dose (mg)
Dimenhydrinate*	Dramamine	50-100
Cyclizine*†	Marezine	50
Meclizine*†	Bonine	25-50
Hyoscine, scopolamine	—	0.6-1
Hydroxyzine†	Vistaril	25-100
Diphenidol†	Vontrol	25-50
Trimethobenzamide	Tigan	100-300
Prochlorperazine	Compazine	5-10
Promethazine	Phenergan	12.5-25

*Nonprescription.
†Should be used with caution; can be teratogenic in pregnancy.

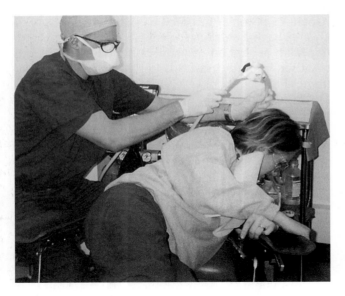

Figure 16-1 If vomiting occurs, turn the patient's head and body to the side away from the operator.

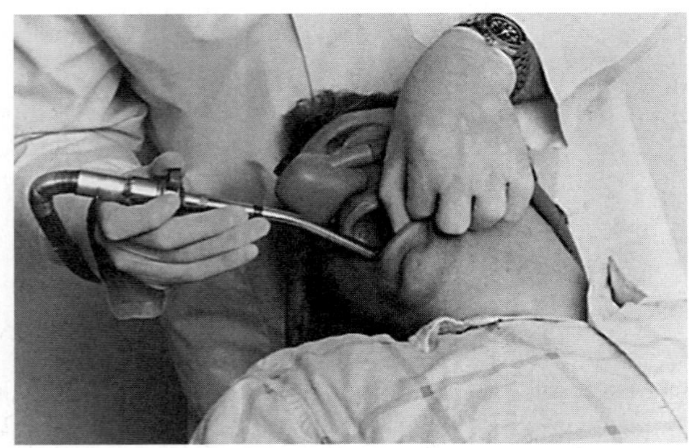

Figure 16-2 Vomitus is removed with suction or finger. The patient should receive 100% O_2.

becoming sick again. Explain to the patient that he or she will breathe only 100% O_2 and that the reason for so doing is to minimize the chance of becoming sick again.

If the patient does not wish to continue with N_2O-O_2 during treatment, it is best to adhere to these wishes. However, the door should not be closed on the future use of this important technique. It should be stressed to the patient that vomiting is a very unusual occurrence and that it is unlikely to occur again. If necessary, antiemetics may be prescribed preoperatively for this patient.

Tooth Pain Associated with Sinus Pressure

N_2O can displace air from the maxillary sinus. This complication is associated with prolonged use and noticed as discomfort, possibly presenting as a toothache. This is because the anterior, middle, and posterior alveolar nerves pass through the sinus membrane and are affected.

Vertigo

Prolonged exposure of the vestibulocochlear complex to N_2O can result in vertigo. This complication can cause increased tension on the tympanic membrane. This tension can result in an alteration in hearing acuity, and the patient may complain of this alteration in hearing.

Bowel Discomfort

Air spaces in the gut can be displaced by N_2O. This nonrigid potential space can have an enlargement to the extent that there are discomfort and flatulence as a result of high concentration and prolonged use of N_2O.

Claustrophobia

Claustrophobia is a disorder that is shared by many patients. The nasal hood and/or face mask of the sedation unit can precipitate a claustrophobic response. Patients will often pinpoint the mask coming into contact with their face as the most unpleasant part of a general anesthesia experience in the hospital. Allowing a patient with this concern to adjust the nasal hood can help improve the experience. Claustrophobia is a real fear that requires understanding on the part of the health-care provider.

Contact Lens Wearers

Large numbers of patients wear contact lenses today. People usually think of them as being part of their normal anatomy. The nasal mask, if not snugly in place over the nose, will potentially allow the dry gas to affect the lens and cause irritation to the eye. Patients should remove contact lenses before receiving inhalation sedation.

Anatomic Obstruction

Anatomic variations such as enlarged tonsils and/or adenoids can present a significant obstacle for the adequate administration of N_2O-O_2. A deviated nasal septum can also potentially decrease the ease of gas flow through the entirety of the airway. It is worth exploring these possible anatomic considerations with patients to anticipate possible interference.

Understanding of the Language

The continual change in demographics in the United States and the increase in cultural diversity have presented a potential complicating factor because of the increasing difficulty in verbal communication. Although simple instructions may seem to be clear and well understood, the doctor must try to anticipate the need for additional resources for the communication of more detailed instruction.

Esoteric Potential Complications

Pulmonary conditions such as chronic obstructive pulmonary disease (COPD), emphysema, decompression illness ("bends"), or pneumothorax are all pathophysiologic circumstances that can be initiated or exacerbated by the administration of N_2O. These "complications" can certainly be real, but practically, they are not recorded in the literature to be significant. The astute clinician should understand that the N_2O dynamics should apply to the clinical situation.

MANAGING COMPLICATIONS

As mentioned, these complications are generally very preventable through the use of titration and by being aware that high concentrations and, to a lesser degree, prolonged use can precipitate these events. Monitoring allows observation of the patient to assess his or her level of sedation and allows general assessment of the physiognomy. A preoperative evaluation of baseline vital signs is important. The use of a pulse oximeter while administering N_2O-O_2 has no parallel for detection of oxygen perfusion at the cellular level. A pulse oximeter reading will usually be at 100% O_2 saturation concentration during administration of N_2O-O_2. The instruments are inexpensive and, although not mandated or necessary, provide an added level of confidence to the clinician. Periodic recording of vital signs, most importantly postoperative vital signs, is highly recommended. A postoperative vital sign record is essential before the patient is discharged.

In conclusion, N_2O-O_2 as a technique for sedation is very useful and safe. As with all medications and procedures, we should be prepared to treat the unexpected. The complications that can and do present are easily managed or possibly prevented by the trained practitioner.

REFERENCES

1. Langa H: *Relative analgesia in dental practice: inhalation analgesia with nitrous oxide,* Philadelphia, 1968, WB Saunders.
2. School of Dentistry, University of Southern California: Statistics from Section of Anesthesia & Medicine, Los Angeles, 1992, unpublished.
3. Houck WR, Ripa LW: Vomiting frequency in children administered nitrous oxide-oxygen in analgesic doses, *J Dent Child* 38:404, 1971.
4. Parkhouse J, Henrie JR, Duncan GM et al: Nitrous oxide analgesia in relation to mental performance, *J Pharmacol Exp Ther* 128:44, 1960.

CHAPTER 17

Contemporary Issues Surrounding Nitrous Oxide

CHAPTER OUTLINE

Inhalation pharmacosedation with nitrous oxide–oxygen (N_2O-O_2) is steadily increasing in its use in medical, dental, and paraprofessional offices. The tremendous reduction of stress in the apprehensive and medically compromised patient is pushing its growth exponentially. The aging population that in years past would not have presented to the dental office because of systemic illness are now capable of undergoing extensive treatment because of advancing medical technology. These new patients not only are increasing in numbers but also have the affluence to pay for treatment and comfort.

The evolution of sedation should include advances in supportive medications and therapies in addition to the heightened awareness of the public to the possibility of increased therapeutic service with sedation; these factors have helped thrust N_2O-O_2 to the forefront. Professional education became more formalized and took a significant step forward approximately 30 years ago when the Council on Dental Education of the American Dental Association accepted standards for educational programs for inhalation sedation.

Along with the increased use of N_2O-O_2 has come a greater concern for the safety of personnel who are in contact with it for the greatest length of time—the dental office staff. The following three categories are addressed in this regard:

1. Potential biohazards from long-term exposure to trace anesthetic gas
2. Recreational abuse of N_2O
3. Sexual awareness regarding N_2O

POTENTIAL BIOHAZARDS FROM LONG-TERM EXPOSURE TO TRACE ANESTHETIC GAS

Throughout the history and evolution of N_2O, N_2O was widely recognized to exert an influence on the general physiognomy of humans. What was not understood was the concept of addiction. From Horace Wells to Sigmund Freud, we see through the pages of history the great scientists and many unknowns who have succumbed to experimentation, usually without thought of chemical consequence.

As times have passed, the fact that chemicals have biologic effects and are even capable of causing death has come to be recognized. Health agencies around the world have been organized to protect the public from hazardous products being allowed to circulate in society.

N_2O is found naturally in the atmosphere in minute quantities. It is quickly reversible in action, but is it totally harmless?

Little was known of the possible effects of inhalation of minute amounts of anesthetic vapors until the late 1960s. Until that time little was done to eliminate anesthetic vapors being delivered into the ambient air from anesthesia machines. In 1967 Vaisman[1] published the results of a survey of Russian anesthesiologists in which it was demonstrated that they suffered a higher incidence of irritability, headache, fatigue, nausea, pruritus, spontaneous abortion, and fetal malformation than non–operating room personnel. This was the first report that inhalation gases may exert a negative influence on human physiology. Subsequent retrospective studies followed that seemed to confirm Vaisman's result.[2-4] It must be emphasized that in these studies, N_2O was but one of many gases under investigation. Because it is the most commonly used inhalation anesthetic, N_2O is found in all samples of air taken from operating rooms. It is used in conjunction with O_2 and other more potent inhalation anesthetics such as halothane, enflurane, sevoflurane, and isoflurane. Therefore it has been impossible to separate the effects of any one of these gases from the others. In other words, the findings presented here are potentially produced by any one of the drugs found in the operating room. Because of the special nature of dental practice, in which virtually the only inhalation anesthetic used is N_2O, the findings of these operating room studies were not applicable to the dental profession.

In the United States, Cohen et al.[5,6] published articles in the 1970s dealing with anesthetic health hazards in the dental setting. One article contained a study that surveyed more than 50,000 dentists and dental assistants who were exposed to trace anesthetics. The results suggested that long-time exposure to anesthetic gases could be associated with an increase in general health problems and with disease of the reproductive system in particular. This study was of course retrospective in nature, and it only fueled the concern regarding the safety of N_2O in the dental office. Unfortunately, this "study" did not contain any measured data on these trace gases that were involved in any of the environs reported.

In 1974, Bruce, Bach, and Arbit[7] "investigated the possibility of N_2O affecting perceptual cognition and psychomotor skills of personnel exposed to varying concentrations of the gas." They reported that just hours of exposure to as little as 50 ppm could result in audiovisual impairment. Despite multiple attempts to duplicate their results, all efforts failed. The National Institute of Occupational Safety and Health (NIOSH) and the Occupational Safety Health Administration (OSHA) became interested in these studies and established 50 ppm to be the maximum exposure limit for personnel in the dental setting. It was determined that 25 ppm was achievable in the operating room, and therefore this became the standard for that setting. Multiple attempts to reproduce the research results of Bruce, Bach, and Arbit[8] have failed; interestingly, these researchers have retracted their conclusions, indicating that the results were not based on biologic factors.[9]

The results of this "research," as one would expect, caused a concern and subsequent decline in the use of N_2O-O_2. Indeed, there was alarm in the manufacturing and equipment industry for N_2O-O_2 that bordered on a crisis. In 1995 I conducted a worldwide literature search on the topic of biohazards associated with N_2O-O_2 use. I retrieved 850 citations, of which 23 met the predetermined criteria for scientific merit.[10] The conclusion drawn from this literature review was that there was no scientific basis for the previously established threshold levels for the hospital operating room or the dental setting. This research became the impetus for a meeting of interested parties representing dentistry, government, and manufacturing. A result of the September 1995 meeting, sponsored by the American Dental Association's Council of Scientific Affairs and Council of Dental Practice, was the formal position statement that a maximum N_2O exposure limit in parts per million has not been determined.[11]

The specific biologic issue is the inactivation of methionine synthase. This enzyme is linked to vitamin B_{12} metabolism. Vitamin B_{12} is necessary for DNA production and subsequent cellular reproduction. The fact is that N_2O does affect methionine synthase and does, in high concentration and long exposure (24 hours or greater), have an effect on reproduction.[12] However, to date there is no evidence that a direct causal relationship exists between reproductive health and scavenged low levels of N_2O.[13,14] Sweeney et al.[15] were the first to link reproductive problems in humans with long-term N_2O exposure. They used a sensitive test—the deoxyuridine suppression test—to accurately determine the first signs of this biologic effect in humans. Sweeney et al. found that long-term exposure levels of 1800 ppm of N_2O did not exert any detectable biologic effect in humans. They suggest that a level of 400 ppm is a reasonable exposure level that is both attainable and significantly below the biologic threshold.

An additional specific biologic issue surrounding N_2O includes the fact that N_2O in very high nontherapeutic doses can cause leukopenia and reduction in megaloblastic erythropoiesis resembling pernicious anemia. Neurologic disorders associated with long-term N_2O exposure appear as myeloneuropathy.[16-20] Symptoms such as sensory and proprioception impairment may be permanent but are usually temporary with a slow recovery.

Scavenging

Today, it is below the standard of care to not have a scavenging nasal hood[10] (Figure 17-1). They are cheap,

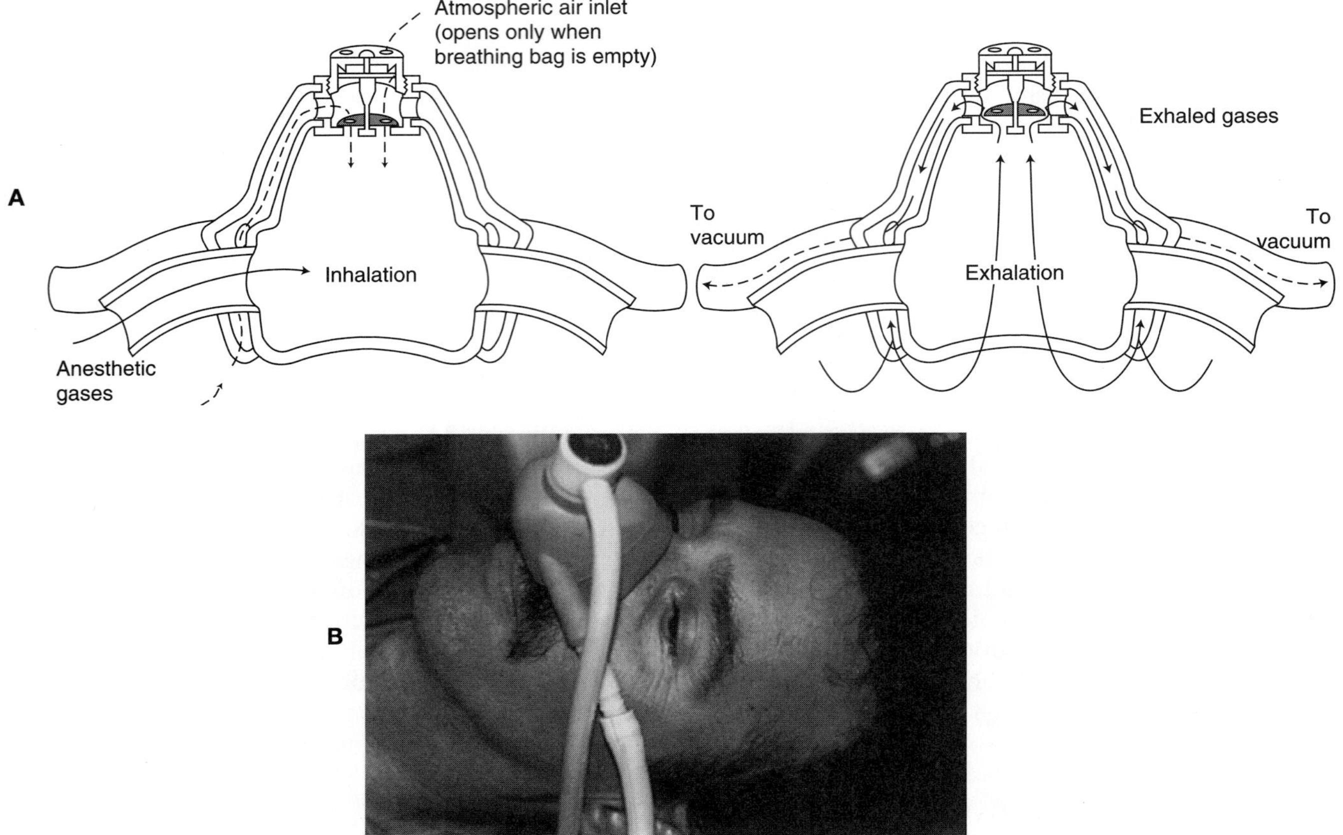

Figure 17-1 **A,** Scavenging nasal hood. **B,** Scavenging mask in use.

disposable, and readily available. The scavenging nasal hood is a double mask—an inner mask contained within a slightly larger outer mask. Each mask has two tubes entering into it so that the entire apparatus has four tubes, two on either side of the nasal hood. The inner mask receives a fresh supply of N_2O-O_2 from the inhalation sedation unit and delivers gas to the nose of the patient through two tubes that are slightly larger in diameter than the other two tubes. The outer, slightly larger, mask connects to the two slightly smaller tubes that connect with the vacuum system. Thus a small vacuum is present in the space between the inner and outer masks. On exhalation through the nose, all exhaled gases are vented into the outer nasal hood and then, via the vacuum, are carried away from the patient and the treatment area (Figure 17-2).

An additional benefit of the scavenging nasal hood is that peripheral leakage of gases resulting from improper fit of the mask is prevented because the outer nasal hood is attached to the vacuum system and will remove any such gases before they reach the ambient air.[21] The optimal and recommended vacuum flow rate is 45 L/min. At this rate leakage of N_2O-O_2 into the room is prevented even when the mask is removed from the patient and a gas flow of 4 L of each nitrous oxide and oxygen is delivered through the nasal hood.[22] It is important to remember that the vacuum should not be so strong as to prevent adequate ventilation of the lungs with N_2O-O_2 to achieve sedation. Allowing the patient to adjust the mask will invariably create a snugger fit and seal of the nasal hood periphery than the administrator would be able to achieve alone.

The ventilation system in the operatory can be extremely effective as a scavenging tool. A strategically placed, well-designed venting system can not only minimize trace N_2O levels in one operatory but can expedite separation of gas from one area of a building to another. This tremendous source of scavenging is often overlooked and underused. It can also be achieved relatively inexpensively.

Air sweeps are just oscillating fans that can be placed in such a way as to "sweep" the trace N_2O from a specific area. The problem that arises is that if it is not taken completely to the outside, the predictability of actual trace gas does not exist. The air sweep is probably most useful in interrupting the transfer of gas from

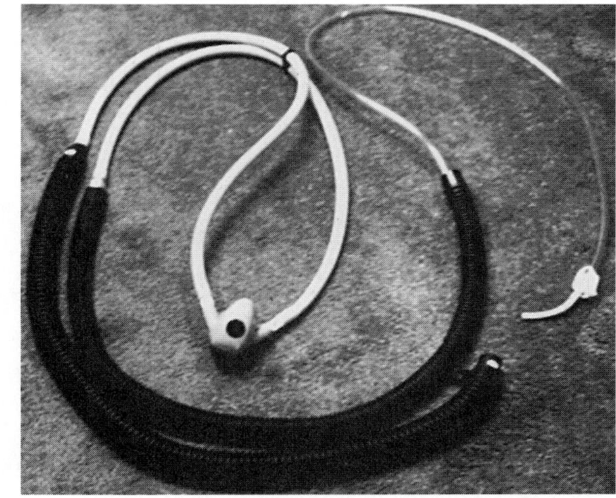

A

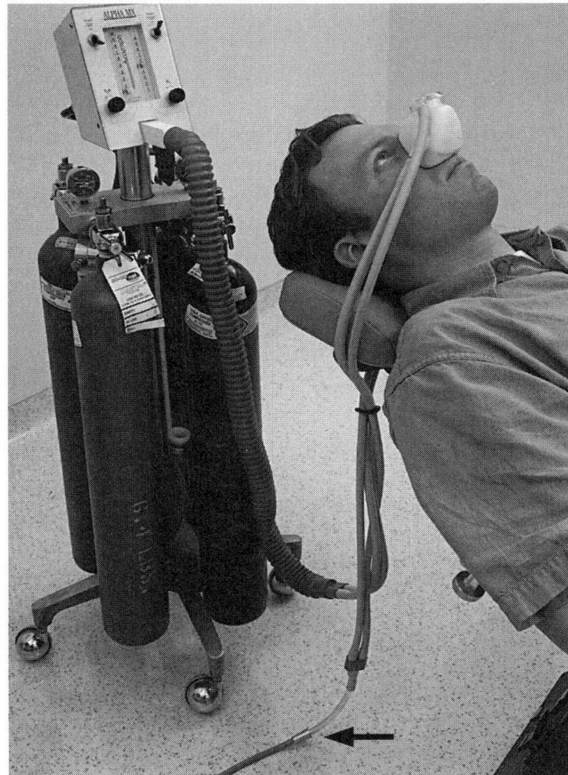

B

Figure 17-2 **A,** Bain-Littell breathing system. **B,** Through insertion of one-way valves in tubing, gases are carried from sedation unit to patient and then evacuated into the vacuum system *(arrow)*.

patient to operator. This 12-inch area, sometimes called the *breathing zone*, of possibly high concentrations of gas may be directed toward the venting system (Table 17-1).

The number one cause of N_2O contamination in the office is from the patient talking (Box 17-1). The clinician should recognize this and attempt to modify the situation to make the interaction with the patient as brief and concise as possible. This is best done by simple explanation to the patient that N_2O-O_2 works best with the lips sealed. The use of a rubber dam is highly effective to decrease trace N_2O exposure. Remember that all vocal discourse, laughing, and so forth creates a direct source of N_2O into the treatment area.[23]

Monitoring of Trace Nitrous Oxide

The most accurate and effective method of determining N_2O levels in ambient air is through an

BOX 17-1 Potential Sources of Nitrous Oxide

1. Normal gas flow
   - Exhaling valve
   - Around perimeter of nasal hood
2. Patient
   - During the procedure—mouth breathing, talking, laughing
   - After the procedure—30 L N_2O exhaled within 3-5 minutes
3. Inhalation sedation unit
   - High-pressure system
     - Worn wall connectors
     - Loose high-pressure hose connections
     - Deformed compression fittings
   - Low-pressure system
     - Loose, defective, or missing gaskets and seals
     - Worn or defective bags and breathing tubes
     - Loosely assembled slip joints and threaded connections
     - Loose flowmeters
4. Air conditioning

TABLE 17-1 Levels of N_2O (ppm) in Breathing Zones When Using Conventional Nasal Hood with Expiratory Valve

Categories	Dentist	Assistant	Room Average
General dentist's office	775 ± 63	440 ± 52	310 ± 37
Pediatric dentist's office	940 ± 92	112 ± 23	280 ± 52
Oral surgeon's office	1000 ± 130	1600 ± 250	310 ± 47

infrared (IR) N_2O analyzer.[24] Infrared light is absorbed at different wavelengths by different gases. The advantage of infrared spectrophotometry is the ability to detect minute levels of gases, such as N_2O, in ambient air at levels of as low as 1 ppm. The IR analyzer takes surrounding air samples into a nozzlelike opening and transfers them to a sampling cell. Differences in N_2O concentrations in the sampled air result in proportional change in the quantity of IR energy that is transmitted through the sampling cell, sensed by the detector, and then amplified and displayed on the monitor. This can be almost instantaneous. The IR can be used to detect many different gases in addition to N_2O, and can detect gases from the previously mentioned 1 ppm to an upper limit of 2000 ppm. The machine is extremely accurate to within a half of a percentage point. These devices are very expensive but can be rented from a gas service company. The supplier of your gases will have the resource for contacts to allow you to rent an infrared spectrophotometer for N_2O analysis.

Time-weighted monitoring devices are commonly used in medical/dental offices.[25] The devices detect the amount of N_2O absorption over a given period. The dosimeter badge is worn by anyone (usually staff) who desires to know the amount of N_2O he or she has been exposed to in a particular setting. The dosimeters are sent back to the company laboratory with the history of exposure time to N_2O. The laboratory returns a time-weighted value of exposure to N_2O. Although they are not nearly as accurate as IR, they serve a useful purpose (Figure 17-3).

The American Dental Association published in its March 1997 Journal recommendations for responsible maintenance and monitoring of N_2O and its equipment (Box 17-2).[11]

In conclusion, we hope always to challenge ourselves to deliver the very best to our patients. We are

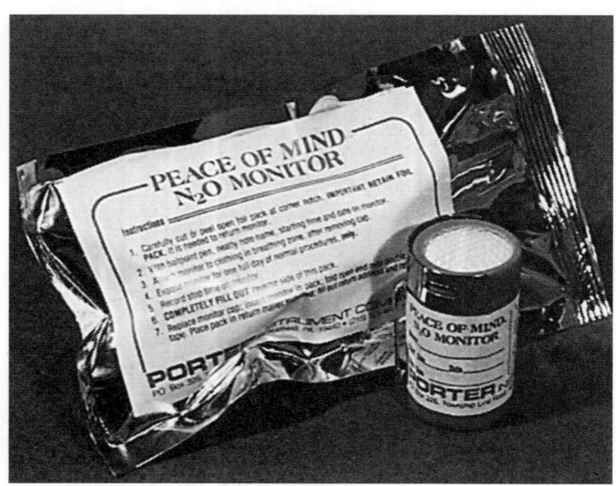

Figure 17-3 N_2O monitoring device is worn by doctors or auxiliary personnel.

guided by our conscience and our knowledge. To date, no direct evidence of any causal relationship between long-term low-level exposure to N_2O and potential biologic effects exist.

RECREATIONAL ABUSE OF NITROUS OXIDE

N_2O causes euphoria and therefore, as Sir Humphrey Davy discovered in 1798, has a potential for abuse.[26,27] It is usually not as addictive as some drugs but nonetheless can be a "steppingstone" to other drugs and can cause incapacitation of the affected person. Dr. Gardner Colton traveled the world displaying the "exhilarating" effect of N_2O. These same pleasant effects are used to abate fear in our practices. N_2O should be given the same respect that is given to all drugs.[28,29] When chronically abused, N_2O can have serious health consequences.[30] Agents that can produce euphoria when inhaled are readily available. This includes such products as solvents, model glue, nail polish remover, or typewriter correction fluid, to name a few. These products are sold commercially to everyone. It is particularly unfortunate that children and adolescents have a higher incidence of abuse than even older adolescents and young adults. It also appears that these inhalation products are attractive because they are cheap and easily attained. N_2O is legally available in small cylinders called *whippets*. These are used in the manufacturing of whipping cream, N_2O being the propellant gas in whipped cream cylinders (Figure 17-5). When these cylinders are used properly, whipping cream fluffed up by N_2O emerges; if they are held improperly, 100% N_2O escapes. A quick glance at a can of whipping cream on the grocer's shelf will reveal N_2O as an ingredient. Often, these whippets can be purchased at music concerts or areas of repute for good times such as Bourbon Street in New Orleans, Louisiana. The pharmacokinetics of N_2O does not allow for screening detection as with other drugs. This does not imply that there is no physiologic affect on the user.

Typical abusers of N_2O are usually older and probably from middle- to upper-class society. If they have an inhalation sedation unit available, it has probably been altered in an attempt to deliver a higher concentration of gas. A dentist living very close to my home in Colorado placed a blanket over his head to increase the concentration as well. He became asphyxiated because of this and his alteration of the machine and could not be revived. Chronic inhalation (abuse) of N_2O may lead to various neuropathies. This is particularly disconcerting if the loss of tactile sensation is associated with interference with their occupation

BOX 17-2 Recommendations for Responsible Maintenance and Monitoring of Nitrous Oxide and Equipment

1. The dental office should have a properly installed nitrous oxide delivery system. This includes appropriate scavenging equipment with a readily visible and accurate flowmeter (or equivalent measuring device), a vacuum pump with the capacity for up to 45 L of air per minute per workstation, and a variety of sizes of masks to ensure proper fit for individual patients.
2. The vacuum exhaust and ventilation exhaust should be vented to the outside (e.g., through the vacuum system) and not close to fresh-air intake vents.
3. The general ventilation should provide good room air mixing.
4. Each time the nitrous oxide machine is first turned on and every time a gas cylinder is changed, the pressure connections should be tested for leaks. High-pressure-line connections should be tested for leaks on a quarterly basis. A soap solution may be used to test for leaks. Alternatively, a portable infrared spectrophotometer can be use to diagnose an insidious leak.
5. Before their first daily use, all nitrous oxide equipment (reservoir bag, tubings, mask, connectors) should be inspected for worn parts, cracks, holes, or tears (Figure 17-4). Replace as necessary.
6. The mask may then be connected to the tubing and the vacuum pump turned on. All appropriate flow rates (i.e., up to 45 L/min or per manufacturer's recommendations) should be verified.
7. A properly sized mask should be selected and placed on the patient. A good, comfortable fit should be ensured. The reservoir (breathing) bag should not be overinflated or underinflated while the patient is breathing oxygen (before administering nitrous oxide).
8. The patient should be encouraged to minimize talking and mouth breathing while the mask is in place.
9. During administration, the reservoir bag should be periodically inspected for changes in tidal volume and the vacuum flow rate verified.
10. On completion of administration, 100% oxygen should be delivered to the patient for 5 minutes before the mask is removed. In this way, both the patient and the system will be purged of residual nitrous oxide. Do not use an oxygen flush.
11. Periodic (semiannual interval is suggested) personal sampling of dental personnel, with emphasis on chairside personnel exposed to nitrous oxide, should be conducted (e.g., use of diffusive sampler [dosimeters] or infrared spectrophotometer).

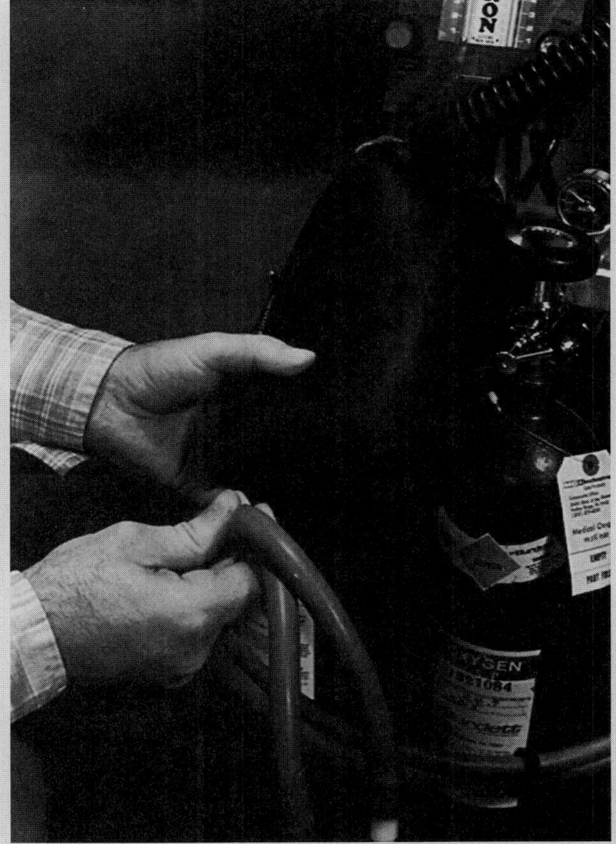

Figure 17-4 The reservoir bag is checked for leaks by overinflating the bag, occluding conducting tubes, and squeezing the bag. If the bag deflates, a leak is present in the system.

Modified from ADA Council on Scientific Affairs, ADA Council on Dental Practice: *J Am Dent Assoc* 128:364, 1997.

(e.g., dentist). The neuropathy is generally reversible but can be permanent.

N_2O is used for mood alteration, sedation, and analgesia. It is the weakest of all general anesthetic agents. In the right circumstances it has the potential to cause unconsciousness. Today, there are programs in most states that are part of the licensing board to help practitioners to effectively treat addictive and self-abusive drug issues. All drug addiction requires just "a little bit more" to maintain or reach that desired "high." It is the principle of addiction and always, if not aborted, leads to death.[31,32] The stakes are high when a decision is made by anyone to abuse a substance. Finally, as we should have learned from Horace Wells, whose life

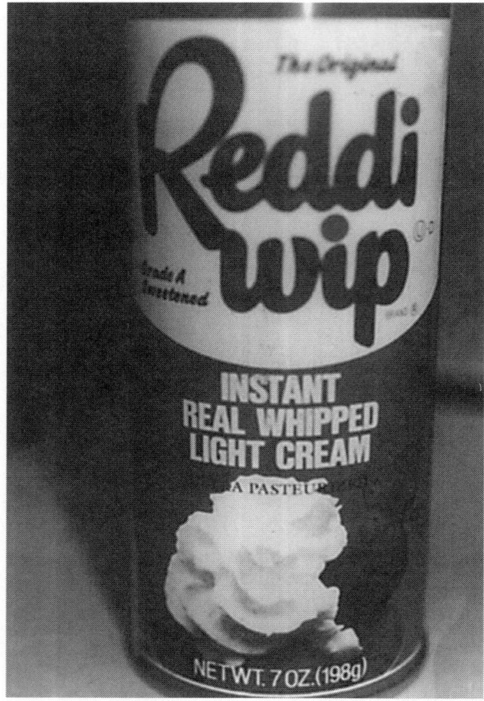

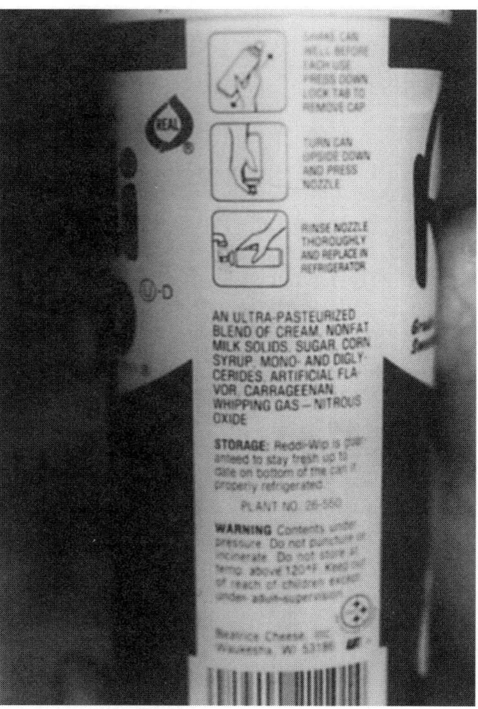

Figure 17-5 Whipped cream container utilizes nitrous oxide as its whipping gas *(right).*

took a tragic turn because of abuse, "Let's make original mistakes."

SEXUAL AWARENESS REGARDING NITROUS OXIDE

There have been reports of sexual abuse against patients while they are under the influence of a variety of anesthetics.[33-35] As expected, N_2O has also been associated with scattered reports of impropriety between male practitioners and female patients. N_2O does cause euphoria and, in high concentrations, dreaming hallucinations and, as described by Sir Humphrey Davy in 1798, "voluptuous sensations." The cases of record that I have personally reviewed always involve three elements that place the practitioner at risk: (1) treatment of a patient alone without the benefit of an assistant in the operatory, (2) high concentrations of N_2O, or (3) failure to titrate the patient to avoid the extension beyond his or her range of therapeutic sedation (Figure 17-6).

N_2O requires hosing that can drape around the shoulders for retention of the mask. It is important to allow the patient to adjust the mask on his or her face and to let the patient understand that it is connected to the hosing. The hosing in a euphoric patient can be misconstrued to be an inappropriate contact. Also allow the patient to fully recover. It may take longer than 3 to 5 minutes for this to occur. Jastak and Malamed have reported a series of cases (1980) that one may review.[33] Malamed reports in an unpublished survey that a percentage of dental hygiene students reported increased feelings of sexuality and/or arousal while under the effects of N_2O.[36,37] They also reported some instances of orgasm. N_2O should be administered with confidence. Employing simple guidelines will ensure that the administrator of N_2O has no difficulties with any sexual issues.

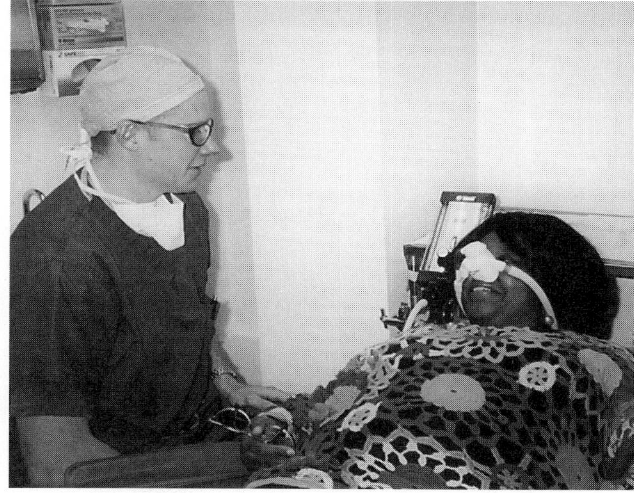

Figure 17-6 In all instances of allegations of sexual misconduct, the male dentist was alone in the treatment room with the female patient.

REFERENCES

1. Vaisman A: Work in surgical theatres and its influence on the health of anesthesiologists, *Eksp Khir Anestheziol* 3:44, 1967.
2. Askrog V, Harvald B: Teratogen effect of inhalation anesthetics, *Nord Med* 83:498, 1970.
3. Lencz L, Nemes C: Morbidity of Hungarian anesthesiologists in relation to occupational hazard. In Corbett TH, ed: Anesthetics as a cause of abortion, *Fertil Steril* 23:866, 1972.
4. Bruce D, Eide KA, Linde HM et al: Causes of death among anesthesiologists: a 20 year survey, *Anesthesiology* 35:348, 1971.
5. Cohen EN, Brown BW Jr, Bruce DL et al: A survey of anesthetic health hazards among dentists, *J Am Dent Assoc* 90:1291, 1975.
6. Cohen EN, Brown BW Jr, Wu ML et al: Occupational disease in dentistry and chronic exposure to trace anesthetic gases, *J Am Dent Assoc* 101:21, 1980.
7. Bruce DL, Bach MJ, Arbit J: Trace anesthetic effects on perceptual, cognitive, and motor skills, *Anesthesiology* 40:453, 1974.
8. Cohen EN, Belville JW, Brown BW: Anesthesia, pregnancy and miscarriage: a study of operating room nurses and anesthetists, *Anesthesiology* 35:343, 1971.
9. Yagiela JA: Health hazards and nitrous oxide: a time for reappraisal, *Anesth Prog* 38:1, 1991.
10. Clark M, Brunick A: *Handbook of nitrous oxide and oxygen sedation*, St Louis, 1999, Mosby.
11. ADA Council on Scientific Affairs, ADA Council on Dental Practice: Nitrous oxide in the dental office, *J Am Dent Assoc* 128:364, 1997.
12. Fujinagra M, Baden JM, Mazze RI: Susceptible period of nitrous oxide teratogenicity in Sprague-Dawley rats, *Teratology* 40:439, 1989.
13. Rowland AS, Baird DD, Weinberg CR et al: Reduced fertility among women employed as dental assistants exposed to high levels of nitrous oxide, *N Engl J Med* 327:993, 1992.
14. Eger EI II: Fetal injury and abortion associated with occupational exposure to inhaled anesthetics, *AANA J* 59:309, 1991.
15. Sweeney B, Bingham RM, Amos RJ et al: Toxicity of bone marrow in dentists exposed to nitrous oxide, *BMJ* 291:567, 1985.
16. Layzer RB, Fishman RA, Schafer JA: Neuropathy following abuse of nitrous oxide, *Neurology* 28:504, 1978.
17. Lassen HC, Henriksen E, Neukirch R et al: Treatment of tetanus, severe bone marrow depression after prolonged nitrous oxide anesthesia, *Lancet* 1:527, 1956.
18. Stacy CB, DiRocci A, Gould RJ: Methionine in the treatment of nitrous oxide-induced neuropathy and myeloneuropathy, *J Neurol* 239:401, 1992.
19. Sahenk Z, Mendell JR, Couri D et al: Polyneuropathy from inhalation of N_2O cartridges through a whipped cream dispenser, *Neurology* 28:485, 1978.
20. Heyer EJ, Simpson DM, Bodis-Wollner I et al: Nitrous oxide: clinical and electrophysiologic investigation of neurologic complications, *Neurology* 36:1618, 1986.
21. Whitcher CE, Zimmerman DC, Tonn EM et al: Control of occupational exposure to nitrous oxide in the dental operatory, *J Am Dent Assoc* 95:763, 1977.
22. Borganelli GN, Primosch RE, Henry RJ: Operatory ventilation and scavenger evacuation rate influence on ambient nitrous oxide levels, *J Dent Res* 72:1275, 1993.
23. Allen WA: Nitrous oxide in the surgery; pollution and scavenging, *Br Dent J* 159:222, 1985.
24. Lane GA: Measurement of anesthetic pollution in oral surgery offices, *J Oral Surg* 36:444, 1978.
25. Landauer RS Jr & Co, Division of Tech Ops Inc, Products and Sevices Division, Landauer, Inc. Glenwood Science Park, Glenwood, Ill 40425.
26. Gillman MA: Nitrous oxide abuse in perspective, *Clin Neuropharmacol* 15:297, 1992.
27. Malamed SF, Orr DL II, Hershfield S et al: The recreational abuse of nitrous oxide by health professionals, *J Calif Dent Assoc* 8:38, 1980.
28. Gillman MA: Nitrous oxide: an opioid addictive agent, *Am J Med* 81:97, 1986.
29. Aston R: Drug abuse: its relationship to dental practice, *Dent Clin North Am* 28:595, 1984.
30. Layzer RB, Fishman RA, Schafer JA: Neuropathy following abuse of nitrous oxide, *Neurology* 28:504, 1978.
31. Wagner SA, Clark MA, Wesche DL et al: Asphyxial deaths from recreational use of nitrous oxide, *J Forensic Sci* 37:1008, 1992.
32. Suruda AJ, McGlothlin JD: Fatal abuse of nitrous oxide in the workplace, *J Occup Med* 32:682, 1990.
33. Jastak JT, Malamed SF: Nitrous oxide and sexual phenomena, *J Am Dent Assoc* 101:38, 1980.
34. Lambert C: Sexual phenomena, hypnosis, and nitrous oxide sedation, *J Am Dent Assoc* 105:990, 1982.
35. Gillman MA: Assessment of the effects of analgesic concentrations of nitrous oxide on human sexual response, *Int J Neurosci* 43:27, 1988.
36. Malamed SF, Serxner K, Wiedenfeld AM: The incidence of sexual phenomena in females receiving nitrous oxide and oxygen inhalation sedation, *J Am Analg Soc* 22:9, 1988.
37. Malamed SF: Results of N_2O survey, 1983, unpublished manuscript.

CHAPTER 18

Practical Considerations

CHAPTER OUTLINE

In previous chapters of this section, the technique of administration, complications, and current concerns associated with inhalation sedation have been discussed. In this chapter a number of additional factors are discussed in an attempt to reflect on and evaluate other factors that are important in the completeness of the overall training of the administrator of nitrous oxide–oxygen (N_2O-O_2). Many of these questions do not usually arise until the doctor has been using inhalation sedation for a while. It should be remembered that realistically, complications of N_2O-O_2 sedation are indeed rare, and N_2O is a very safe agent for use in the health sciences.

DETERMINATION OF PROPER TITRATION AT SUBSEQUENT VISITS

One of the most important factors to consider when using inhalation sedation is that the gases have a very rapid onset of action. Because of this rapid onset, it becomes possible for patients to be titrated to a precise level of sedation. The ability to titrate with inhalation sedation is of considerable importance because it is quite possible that a patient may require different concentrations of N_2O-O_2 to achieve the same level of sedation at subsequent visits. The absence of titration leads to increased patient reports of negative reactions to N_2O-O_2, and their doctors begin to shy away from its use. Titration is the only means for the administrator to satisfactorily determine the appropriate level. Factors that may influence the concentration of N_2O-O_2 necessary for adequate sedation include the patient's dental anxiety level, nondental stresses, the time of day, and the patient's level of restfulness.

Dental Anxiety

As the patient's dental anxiety decreases, the percentage of N_2O necessary to achieve a given level of sedation will correspondingly decrease, with all other variables remaining equal. With proper patient management by both the doctor and the office staff, a fearful patient should become less apprehensive about the prospect of dental treatment with each succeeding visit. If the patient is titrated carefully to his or her "ideal sedation level," it will likely be observed that the patient requires somewhat lower N_2O concentrations as he or she becomes progressively less phobic over time.

Although this is true for most patients and for most forms of dental treatment, it is also possible that a patient who has been responding quite well at 30% N_2O will have an inadequate clinical effect from that concentration when a different type of dental treatment is undertaken. For example, this patient may respond well at 30% N_2O for restorative treatment; however, when undergoing periodontal surgery, the patient may require 45% N_2O. This is explained by the increased level of anxiety produced in this patient by the prospect of a surgical procedure in contrast to the more benign (in this patient's mind) restorative treatment.

Nondental Stresses

A significant influence on the level of N_2O required for sedation is nondental stress. The patient's state of mind has a significant bearing on the manner in which central nervous system (CNS) depressant drugs act. A patient may arrive at the dental office on a day when things have just not gone well. If this patient has any degree of dental anxiety, it becomes obvious that our sedation technique has a formidable task facing it. Contrast this with the same patient who arrives at the dental office having had a simply wonderful day. The concentration of N_2O required to sedate this patient will probably be lower than that required in the first situation.

It is impossible, and indeed foolhardy, to discount the influence of outside stresses on the dental patient. All practicing dentists, dental hygienists, physicians, and podiatrists have encountered remarkably different behavior patterns from the same patient at different visits. The process of titrating N_2O will help compensate for the effects of these outside influences.

Time of Day

The time of day at which a patient is treated may have considerable bearing on the concentration of N_2O required for sedation. Although this situation occurs most often in pediatric dentistry, many adult patients will exhibit these same tendencies.

As discussed in Chapter 4, it is recommended that the phobic patient, as well as the medically compromised patient, be scheduled for dental treatment earlier in the day. At this time, presumably following a period of restful sleep, the medically compromised patient is rested and better able to tolerate any additional stresses imposed by dental treatment. The fearful patient ought to be treated early in the day for the simple reason that the patient will want to get "it" over with as soon as possible. The dental appointment might well be the most unpleasant part of this patient's day. An appointment scheduled late in the day allows the patient more time to worry and for a level of anxiety to increase. Scheduled later in the day, this patient might require significantly greater levels of N_2O to achieve sedation than would have been necessary if he or she had been treated earlier in the morning.

Level of Restfulness

The level of restfulness has an effect on the patient's pain reaction threshold and therefore on the response to inhalation sedation. Patients who are tired and unable to sleep the night before the appointment because of fear of dentistry overreact to most stimuli. With their "nerves on edge," they interpret usually nonpainful stimuli as being painful. N_2O-O_2 inhalation sedation may still prove to be effective; however, the patient may require considerably greater concentrations of N_2O.

When a patient appears to be apprehensive about an upcoming treatment, it is prudent for the doctor to address this fact and consider prescribing a sedative-hypnotic for the patient 1 hour before bedtime the evening before the scheduled treatment. A well-rested patient may require lower concentrations of N_2O to achieve comparable levels of sedation than the overtired patient.

When the four factors mentioned are considered, it becomes obvious that the same person may respond to N_2O-O_2 in an entirely different manner at subsequent appointments. When titration is not used, it is entirely possible that the level of N_2O used at prior visits will produce either the same level of sedation, decreased levels of sedation, or overly deep sedation of the same patient. The use of titration at each and every dental appointment minimizes the significance of these factors.

POOR PATIENT EVALUATION

Patient evaluation relates to the administrator observing the many signs and symptoms that the patient will be exhibiting during the procedure. One of the most important safety features of all pharmacosedative techniques is that the patient remains conscious and is able to respond to verbal and physical stimuli. To ignore a patient's input during the important induction phase of sedation is foolhardy. The sedation should be to a level at which the patient feels comfortable. Information imparted by the patient is quite important in the overall assessment of his or her well-being. The patient should be used as a vital component of the overall monitoring of conscious sedation.

PATIENT UNATTENDED DURING SEDATION

Occasions may develop during the treatment of a particular patient when the doctor will be called away for a few moments to attend to some other business. When a patient is undergoing treatment without the concurrent use of sedative medications, leaving him or her unattended is usually acceptable. However, in any situation in which a patient has received, or is receiving, any CNS depressant drug (e.g., N_2O), the patient must never be left unattended.

This is quite important during inhalation sedation. When N_2O-O_2 is administered, a constant flow of gases is delivered to the patient. Dental treatment serves as a stimulus to the patient to lighten the level of sedation. When dental treatment stops but the N_2O level is left constant, the depth of sedation will become increasingly deep. The lack of treatment stimulation is the primary reason for this occurrence. This normally does not result in any serious difficulty when someone is present in the treatment room and monitoring the patient. In the absence of a trained person to monitor the patient and to promptly recognize and manage the situation, significant morbidity or mortality may result.

Should it become essential for the doctor to have to leave a patient receiving N_2O-O_2 for even a few short minutes, a well-trained assistant should be available to remain with the patient in the treatment area. In addition, because of the lack of treatment-induced stimulation of this patient, the level of N_2O should be decreased by approximately 10% whenever there is a pause in treatment for more than a few minutes. In the absence of a second person to monitor the patient, the doctor must terminate the flow of N_2O, reestablish a flow of 100% O_2, and return the patient to the presedative state before leaving the treatment area. Although this second option is more cumbersome, it should be followed whenever there is no other person available to monitor the patient.

As mentioned in Chapter 17, there is yet another, more important, reason for the doctor to have a second person available during sedative procedures—that of minimizing the possibility of being accused (perhaps falsely) of sexual improprieties. It is my recommendation that a second person be present in the treatment area whenever a patient receives any pharmacosedative technique.

IMPROPER RECOVERY PROCEDURES

Too many doctors will terminate the flow of N_2O and simply remove the nasal hood, permitting the patient to breathe atmospheric air rather than 100% O_2. As is noted in the following situation, such practice leads to an increased incidence of postinhalation sedation complications. I have also become aware of the fact that many doctors who do administer 100% O_2 to their patients following N_2O-O_2 sedation do so for a fixed period of time (e.g., 2 minutes), regardless of the length of the inhalation sedation that preceded it. As was discussed in earlier chapters on pharmacology and technique of administration, a minimum period of from 3 to 5 minutes of 100% O_2 is required for the majority of the N_2O to be eliminated from the patient's body. A period of 3 to 5 minutes is considered a minimum. After 3 to 5 minutes, the degree of recovery is assessed and, if necessary, the patient continues to receive 100% O_2 for an additional period of time.

Means of assessing recovery ought to be employed routinely whenever inhalation sedation is used if the patient is to be permitted to leave the office alone to drive a vehicle or return to work. If it is the doctor's habit to require an escort to take the patient home after inhalation sedation, the requirement of complete recovery is not as critical.

Two means of assessment of recovery from sedation are recommended: (1) monitoring of vital signs and (2) the Trieger test. These have been discussed earlier in this section. Vital signs, especially blood pressure, heart rate and rhythm, and respiratory rate, are monitored at a patient's first visit to the dental office to establish baseline vital signs. The postoperative recordings are compared with both the preoperative and baseline values; if they are reasonably close to these readings, it may be assumed that the drugs administered to the patient are no longer exerting a depressant action on the cardiorespiratory systems. Proper oxygenation at the end of inhalation sedation and proper assessment of recovery before discharge will prevent virtually all of the uncomfortable side effects and potential problems associated with inhalation sedation.

POSTSEDATION NAUSEA, HEADACHE, AND LETHARGY

After inhalation sedation, the patient, feeling symptom free and having completed appropriate recovery tests, may be discharged from the office. In most instances the patient will continue to feel normal, with no evidence of any side effects from the N_2O. A few patients will experience a postsedation feeling of being hung over; this effect may deter these few patients from future inhalation sedation appointments. Among the signs and symptoms of this postsedation hangover effect are nausea, headache, and lethargy.

In most cases this effect does not develop within the first few minutes after the termination of the sedative procedure. In fact, most patients will have returned to their home or business when the symptoms develop. Management is symptomatic. In most cases tincture of time is the recommended treatment.

It is also possible for a patient to have received O_2 for the recommended 3 to 5 minutes or even longer and still encounter these same effects postoperatively. The normal distribution curve provides evidence that there are some persons who still respond to the very low levels of N_2O found in their blood after at least 3 to 5 minutes (or longer) of 100% O_2. It is usually not possible for the doctor to prevent this occurrence the first time that the patient receives inhalation sedation, but on subsequent visits the patient, having informed the doctor of this unpleasant experience, will be administered 100% O_2 for a longer period. Although this increased period of oxygenation may prove adequate to prevent a recurrence of the signs and symptoms, it is entirely possible that even careful attention to the patient's recovery will fail to produce the desired result in extremely sensitive patients.

The term *diffusion hypoxia* is often mentioned in regard to this situation.[1] As discussed in Chapter 15, N_2O is rapidly removed from a patient's blood after the cessation of the N_2O gas flow. If the patient breathes atmospheric air rather than 100% O_2 at this time, the alveoli become filled with a mixture of N_2, O_2, carbon dioxide (CO_2), water vapor, and N_2O. Some N_2O will be reabsorbed into the circulatory system of the patient, and the O_2 present in the alveoli will be diluted to approximately 10% during the first few minutes following termination of the N_2O flow. These factors produce the signs and symptoms described. It appears that this effect is more commonly noted in cigarette smokers.[2]

One of these symptoms, specifically lethargy, may not be caused completely by the mechanisms just described. A feeling of "not quite being back to normal" does occur in some patients who have received N_2O-O_2. When asked to describe this feeling, the patient usually describes a feeling similar to that experienced when first arising from a pleasant sleep. The patient, although not tired, is not quite fully awake, feeling perhaps 90% normal. After a few moments of activity, the patient is fully functional. This type of postsedation response is not uncommon and will develop immediately after treatment. If this occurs, the patient should be permitted to move about for a few moments. If this added movement does not return the patient to the presedative state, he or she should be placed back into the chair and given 100% O_2 for several minutes.

WHO ADMINISTERS NITROUS OXIDE?

The following points are mentioned because of the legalities of inhalation sedation administration within the dental or medical office. It is not at all uncommon within the practice of dentistry for the dental assistant to be the person to administer N_2O-O_2 to the patient. In some states it is permissible for a dental assistant, under the direct supervision of the dentist (the doctor is physically present in the room at all times), to adjust the flow of gases being delivered to the patient. In this situation the doctor would tell the dental assistant to "raise the N_2O 1 L/min" or "decrease the O_2 by one half a liter per minute." The doctor controls the sedative process, the assistant being but an extension of the doctor in this case.

However, in other dental offices it is common practice for the dental assistant to administer the N_2O-O_2 without the doctor being physically present in the treatment area. In this situation it is considered by the parties involved to be acceptable because the dental assistant remains with the patient. In other cases the doctor is the one to place the nasal hood on the patient; however, the doctor will then leave the room, permitting the assistant to complete the sedative procedure alone with the patient.

Because of the legalities involved in the delegation of expanded functions to auxiliaries, such liberties as described cannot be condoned unless (1) such delegation of duty is specifically permitted under the specific state or provincial dental practice act and (2) the auxiliary being permitted to administer the inhalation sedation has received thorough training in all aspects of inhalation sedation, including the recognition and management of side effects and complications. For this reason, dentists using N_2O-O_2 sedation must be aware of their state's dental practice act and its provisions in this area.

A similar situation involves the use of N_2O-O_2 inhalation sedation by the dental hygienist. Although a number of states permit a certified registered dental hygienist to administer N_2O-O_2 to patients, in all cases the dental practice act specifies that a dentist must be physically present in the dental office. The certified registered dental hygienist is not permitted to administer inhalation sedation to patients when the dentist is not present within the office. Unfortunately, such desirable practices do not always develop, and in many instances N_2O-O_2 is in fact administered to the patient without the presence of the doctor in the office.

From a purely medicolegal perspective, it must be stated that this practice cannot be condoned. It is, at this time, the doctor's ultimate responsibility should anything undesirable result from the administration of inhalation sedation. Although the well-trained dental hygienist is fully capable of recognizing and managing such situations, the doctor should always be immediately available to direct the patient's management and to render such additional assistance as is deemed necessary under the specific circumstances of the situation.

The doctor should always be present in the office when inhalation sedation is being administered by the certified registered dental hygienist, and the doctor must always be physically present in the treatment area, directing the administration of N_2O-O_2 by the dental assistant if this is permitted in the state or province. As dental practice acts continue to be revised, it is recommended that the doctor, hygienist, and assistant regularly keep abreast of such changes as might affect their practices.

EQUIPMENT

It is important that you and your staff feel knowledgeable and comfortable around the N_2O-O_2 sedation unit. This is essential for patient comfort and reassurance. Old and outdated equipment should be replaced with more modern equipment. Updated and safe equipment will allow the practitioner to maximize skills and take full advantage of one of the most time-tested positive adjuncts in our armamentarium for the reduction of patient anxiety.

REFERENCES

1. Papageorge MB, Noonan LW Jr, Rosenberg M: Diffusion hypoxia: another view, *Anesth Pain Control Dent* 2:143, 1993.
2. Burrows B, Knudson RL, Cline MG et al: Quantitative relationships between cigarette smoking and ventilatory function, *Am Rev Respir Dis* 115:195, 1977.

CHAPTER 19

Teaching Inhalation Sedation: History and Present Guidelines

CHAPTER OUTLINE

The history of inhalation sedation and its use are well documented. Inhalation sedation with nitrous oxide (N_2O) and oxygen (O_2) has withstood the test of time as the safest of all sedation techniques used in the history of medicine and dentistry. The story of N_2O began with its discovery by Sir Joseph Priestley and the experimentation and subsequent documentation of some of the effects by Sir Humphrey Davy. The involvement of Gardner Colton and even Samuel Colt, inventor of the popular revolver, as entrepreneur showmen added color, entertainment, and most importantly clinical experience to the use of N_2O. Horace Wells, a dentist and acknowledged discoverer of anesthesia, ushered into the medical field the tremendous possibility for pain control. However, this initial discovery did not burst onto the scene; in fact, it was almost overlooked but ended up changing human history forever.

Reading the history of N_2O can give one a special appreciation for Gardner Quincy Colton. His unselfishness in teaching Horace Wells how to manufacture N_2O led to its discovery. His documentation of more than 170,000 cases of N_2O administration without mortality gave testimony to his clinical skill and dedication to the advancement of pain control.

As has been mentioned throughout this section, inhalation sedation with N_2O and O_2 is the safest of all sedation techniques currently available. Factors responsible for this include the nature of the gases being used, the manner in which they are administered (with not less than 30% O_2), the addition of failsafe devices to inhalation sedation units, and the upgrading of education in the use of inhalation sedation. This last factor is discussed in this chapter, for although great strides have been taken in improving the educational process in teaching inhalation sedation, there remain many persons who seek an easy way out, looking for shortcuts to make the technique even simpler to learn. To maintain the safety of inhalation sedation, high standards for education must be ensured and gradually increased as our knowledge of the technique continues to grow.

As mentioned in Chapter 11, one reason for the failure of inhalation sedation to maintain its popularity among the dental profession in the 1930s and 1940s was the absence of educational programs. Dental schools did not include the use of N_2O-O_2 in their curricula, and continuing education programs were essentially nonexistent at that time. Drs. Harry Langa and Harry M. Seldin were instrumental in providing education with some uniformity and baseline criteria for didactic and clinical training of dental students.

In an effort to provide a uniform level of education in the teaching of different techniques of anesthesia and sedation within the dental school curriculum, three groups—the American Dental Society of Anesthesiology (ADSA), the American Dental Association (ADA), and the American Association of Dental Schools (AADS; now American Dental Education Association [ADEA])—sponsored four workshops on pain control in 1964, 1965, 1971, and 1977. From these conferences emerged the *Guidelines for Teaching the Comprehensive Control of Pain and Anxiety in Dentistry.*[1,2] The guidelines provide outlines for a curriculum in pain control at three levels: (1) the undergraduate dental student (doctoral student), (2) graduate dental student (postdoctoral student), and (3) in a continuing education program. These guidelines were approved by the ADA's Council on Dental Education in May 1971.[2] In 1977 part III of the guidelines, relating to continuing education programs, was revised. The revised guidelines were approved by the House of Delegates of the ADA in 1978.[3] Part I of the guidelines underwent revision in 1979,[4] with the entire document revised again in 1992.[5] Sections of the most recent revision of the guidelines (as adopted by the ADA House of Delegates in 2000) relating to conscious sedation and then more specifically inhalation sedation in continuing education programs are discussed here.[5]

GENERAL PRINCIPLES OF CONSCIOUS SEDATION

Course Level

Continuing education courses in conscious sedation techniques may be offered at three different levels: intensive, supplemental, and incidental. The course descriptions follow:

1. *Intensive courses* in conscious sedation are programs designed to meet the needs of dentists who wish to become knowledgeable and proficient in the safe and effective use of N_2O-O_2 inhalation sedation. . . . They should consist of lectures, demonstrations, and sufficient clinical participation to ensure the faculty that the dentist understands the procedure[s] and can safely and effectively apply them. Faculty must be prepared to assess the individual's competency on successful completion of such training.
2. *Supplemental (or refresher) courses* are designed for persons with previous training in conscious sedation techniques. They are intended to provide a review of the subject and an introduction to recent advances in the field. They should be designed didactically and clinically to meet the specific needs of the participants. Participants must be able to document previous training (equivalent, at a minimum, to the intensive continuing education course described in this document) and current experience in conscious sedation to be eligible for enrollment in a supplemental or refresher course. This does not preclude allied health personnel from attending such courses with the dentist to enhance skills needed for assisting the dentist in the administration of conscious sedation.
3. *Incidental courses* are overview or survey programs designed to provide general information about subjects related to pain and anxiety control. Such courses should be didactic and not clinical in nature because they are not intended to develop clinical competency. Practitioners seeking to develop clinical competency in any given conscious sedation technique are expected to complete successfully an intensive continuing education course teaching that technique.

Objectives

On completion of an intensive continuing education course in conscious sedation techniques, the dentist should be able to complete the following:

1. Describe the anatomy and physiology of the respiratory, cardiovascular, and central nervous systems (CNS) as they relate to the techniques of conscious sedation.
2. Describe the pharmacologic effects of drugs used for conscious sedation.
3. Describe the methods of obtaining a medical history and conduct an appropriate physical evaluation of a dental patient.
4. Apply these methods clinically to obtain an accurate evaluation of the dental patient.
5. Use this information clinically for ASA classification and risk assessment.
6. Choose the most appropriate technique of conscious sedation for the individual dental patient.
7. Use appropriate physiologic monitoring equipment.

INHALATION SEDATION (NITROUS OXIDE–OXYGEN)

Course Objectives

On completion of a course in N_2O-O_2 inhalation sedation techniques, the dentist should be able to complete the following:

1. Describe the basic components of inhalation sedation equipment.
2. Discuss the function of each of these components.
3. List and discuss the advantages and disadvantages of inhalation sedation with N_2O-O_2.
4. List and discuss the indications and contraindications for the use of N_2O-O_2 inhalation sedation.
5. List the complications associated with N_2O-O_2 inhalation sedation.
6. Discuss the prevention, recognition, and management of these complications.
7. Administer N_2O-O_2 inhalation sedation to patients in a clinical setting in a safe and effective manner.
8. Discuss the abuse potential, occupational hazards, and other untoward effects of inhalation agents.

Course Content

The following course content is generally applicable to both inhalation and parenteral sedation programs:

1. Historical, philosophical, and psychological aspects of pain and anxiety control
2. Patient evaluation and selection through review of medical history, physical diagnosis, and psychological profiling
3. Definitions and descriptions of physiologic and psychological aspects of pain and anxiety
4. Description of the stages of drug-induced CNS depression through all levels of consciousness and unconsciousness, with special emphasis on the distinction between the conscious and the unconscious state
5. Review of respiratory and circulatory physiology and related anatomy
6. Pharmacology of agents used in inhalation sedation, including drug interaction and incompatibilities
7. Indications and contraindications for use of inhalation sedation
8. Review of dental procedures possible under inhalation sedation
9. Patient monitoring using observation and monitoring equipment, with particular attention to vital signs and reflexes related to consciousness
10. Importance of maintaining proper records with accurate chart entries recording medical history, physical examination, vital signs, drugs administered, and patient response
11. Prevention, recognition, and management of complications and life-threatening situations
12. Administration of local anesthesia in conjunction with inhalation sedation techniques
13. Description and use of inhalation sedation equipment
14. Introduction to potential health hazards of trace anesthetics and proposed techniques for limiting occupational exposure
15. Discussion of abuse potential
16. Discussion of hallucinatory effects

Course Duration

Although length of a course is only one of the many factors to be considered in determining the quality of an educational program, the course should include a minimum of 14 hours, including a clinical component during which competency in inhalation sedation technique is demonstrated.

Participant Evaluation and Documentation of Inhalation Sedation Instruction

Intensive courses in inhalation sedation techniques must afford participants sufficient clinical experience to enable them to achieve competency. This experience must be provided under the supervision of qualified faculty and must be evaluated. The course director must certify the competency of participants on satisfactory completion of training in each conscious sedation technique, including instruction, clinical experience, and airway management.

Records of the didactic instruction and clinical experience (including the number of patients managed by each participant in each pain and anxiety control modality) must be maintained and available for review by appropriate credentialing agencies. Such documentation must not be, or resemble, a certificate or diploma.

Faculty

For all facets of training, the course should be directed by a dentist or physician qualified by training. This individual should have had at least 3 years of experience, including the individual's formal training in anxiety and pain control. Dental faculty with broad clinical experience in the particular aspect of the subject under consideration should participate. In addition, the participation of highly qualified individuals in related fields, such as anesthesiologists, pharmacologists, internists, cardiologists, and psychologists, should be encouraged.

A participant/teacher ratio of not more than 10:1 when inhalation sedation is being used allows for adequate supervision during the clinical phase of instruction; a 1:1 ratio is recommended during the early stage of participation. The faculty should provide a mechanism whereby the participant can evaluate the performance of those individuals who will be presenting the course material.

Facilities

Intensive courses should be presented only in a dental or medical school, hospital, dental society–sponsored educational institution, or other institution where adequate facilities are available for proper patient care, including drugs and equipment for the management of emergencies.

The guidelines are intended to educate, elevate, and provide our patients with a comfortable and safe experience. The best years for N_2O-O_2 sedation are ahead.

REFERENCES

1. Guidelines for postgraduate and continuing education in pain and anxiety control, *Anesth Prog* 20:167, 1973.
2. American Dental Association, Council on Dental Education: Guidelines for teaching the comprehensive control of pain and anxiety in dentistry, *J Dent Educ* 36:62, 1972.
3. American Dental Society of Anesthesiology: Guidelines for the teaching of pain and anxiety control and management of related complications in a continuing education program, part III, *Anesth Prog* 26:51, 1979.
4. American Association of Dental Schools: Curricular guidelines for comprehensive control of pain and anxiety in dentistry, Special Report, *J Dent Educ* 44:279, 1980.
5. American Dental Association, Council on Dental Education: *Guidelines for teaching the comprehensive control of pain and anxiety in dentistry,* Chicago, 1992, The Association.

SECTION V

INTRAVENOUS SEDATION

The intravenous (IV) route of sedation is the subject of Section V. Drugs administered directly into the cardiovascular system produce clinical actions significantly more rapidly than drugs administered via other routes (e.g., oral or intramuscular). Rapid onset of action is both beneficial and of potential danger. It is beneficial because it permits the doctor to effectively titrate the drug to a desired clinical effect; it is potentially dangerous because the effects of intravenously administered drugs develop more rapidly and because their actions are more pronounced than those of drugs administered via other routes with slower onsets and less complete absorption. It is therefore of the utmost importance that every person using the IV route of drug administration or contemplating its use receive thorough training in the procedures involved in its safe and effective use.

The chapters that follow provide the basic didactic material for an intensive course in IV conscious sedation and consist of two parts: The first, a discussion of venipuncture, includes the anatomy for venipuncture, the armamentarium for the continuous IV infusion, and the technique of venipuncture. The second portion of an IV sedation program is the discussion of drugs and specific techniques of IV sedation, including the clinical pharmacology of intravenously administered drugs, the techniques of administering these agents, and the complications associated with the use of this route of drug administration.

Chapter 29 may prove to be the most important chapter in this section. This chapter is titled Guidelines for Teaching, and it outlines the fundamentals of training required for this very valuable, yet potentially dangerous technique. It is my belief that IV sedation is an important part of the dentist's armamentarium in the management of pain, fear, and anxiety; however, because of the nature of this technique (e.g., its rapid onset of action, more profound effects of drugs), the doctor using it must undergo a degree of training that is beyond that required for employment of many of the techniques already discussed in Sections III and IV.

All 50 states in the United States and 6 provinces in Canada have passed legislation requiring a dentist to possess a special permit in order to use the IV route for sedation.[1] Minimum educational requirements have been established by these states and by various organizations (the American Dental Society of Anesthesiology). These requirements are presented in Chapter 29. It is strongly recommended that all doctors either currently using or contemplating the use of the IV route for conscious sedation read this section carefully. Courses not meeting the requirements presented in this chapter are not considered adequate to properly prepare the doctor and the office staff to use IV conscious sedation.

Like Section IV on inhalation sedation, this section is presented in chapters that are shorter than those in other parts. Its purpose is to better enable the reader to locate the specific material that is of importance to him or her.

The IV route of drug administration is extremely valuable. It is only through proper education of those doctors wishing to use the technique that IV sedation can remain a relatively safe procedure. The reader must always keep in mind that this section was designed to be used in conjunction with an intensive course in IV conscious sedation, a course containing both didactic and clinical components. Use of IV conscious sedation after having simply read this part should never even be considered.

REFERENCE

1. American Dental Association, Department of State Government Affairs: Unpublished data, Chicago, 2002.

CHAPTER 20

Intravenous Sedation: Historical Perspective

CHAPTER OUTLINE

The historical development of intravenous (IV) anesthesia and sedation is reviewed in this chapter. Although the impact made by the development of the IV route of drug administration was not quite as dramatic as was that of inhalation anesthesia (see Chapter 11), the ability to administer medications directly into the cardiovascular system has proved to be a boon to the medical and dental professions.

THE EARLY DAYS

As was true with inhalation anesthetics, it seems as though some of the techniques and drugs had been available for a good many years before the thought occurred to put them to any therapeutic use. Indeed, with the IV route, it was not until well after the development of inhalation anesthesia that the administration of drugs directly into the cardiovascular system of a human being occurred.

William Harvey[1] (1578-1657) (Figure 20-1) provided much of the groundwork for the future of IV medication with the publication of the results of experiments on the circulation of blood. Harvey stated that there was a continuous circulation of blood within a closed system. Before Harvey's findings, a multitude of theories relating to the flow of blood in the human body abounded. Most of these suggested that blood flowed to tissues within the body in an open system. Harvey was born in England and received his medical training at Oxford University. Following graduation he went to Padua, Italy, then the major medical center in the world, where he began to formalize his theories on the circulation of blood. Andrea Cesalpino (1519-1603) was an important predecessor of Harvey's. Cesalpino was the first person to use the word *circulation* in reference to blood and its travels throughout the body.[2] Cesalpino was also first to propose that capillaries connect arteries and veins, meaning that there is no free flow of blood into the tissues of the body, as had been assumed for many years. The one major drawback to Cesalpino's theory was that he also proposed that there were direct connections between major arteries and veins.

On returning to England in 1602, Harvey entered into private medical practice and prospered. He became the court physician for King James I and for King Charles I. Despite his busy practice, Harvey continued to experiment; most of his research involved the circulation of blood. As early as 1615, Harvey spoke of the circulation of blood within a closed system; however, it was not until 1628 that he published one of the most important textbooks in the history of medicine and biology: *Exercitatio Anatomica de Motu*

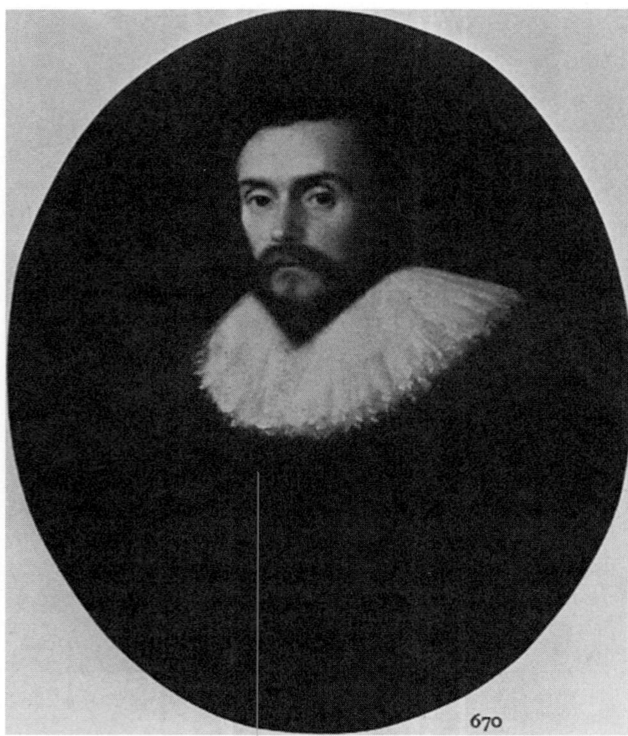

Figure 20-1 William Harvey (1579-1657).

Cordis et Sanguinis in Animalibus (On the Movement of the Heart and Blood in Animals).[1]

Harvey demonstrated for the first time that because of the presence of valves within the heart and veins, blood flow within the circulatory system was unidirectional. In addition, he discussed capillaries—microscopic vessels that connect smaller arteries and smaller veins, thus providing a closed circulatory system. Despite his description of capillaries, Harvey was never able to see them, for it was not until after his death that Marcello Malpighi (1628-1694) first saw capillaries through the microscope.

Harvey's book produced great controversy, for it attempted to disprove theories relating to blood flow that had been held for many years. In fact, controversy over Harvey's book raged for approximately 20 years after its publication. Today, Harvey's work is considered the seventeenth century's most significant achievement in physiology and in medicine.

As a logical extension of Harvey's work, the first IV administration of a drug occurred in the same century (1657). Sir Christopher Wren and Robert Boyle administered tincture of opium intravenously into a dog by using a sharpened quill to which a bladder had been attached.[3] Eight years later, Richard Lower successfully transfused blood from one animal to another.

THE 1800s

The late 1700s and early 1800s saw the development of anesthesiology, with the advent of ether, chloroform, and nitrous oxide–oxygen (N_2O-O_2). This history is chronicled in Chapter 11.

In 1839 in New York, Isaac E. Taylor and James Augustus Washington administered a solution of morphine in an Anel syringe.[4] The Anel syringe had originally been designed for entry into the lacrimal duct and had a finely elongated tapering nozzle instead of a sharp point. Taylor and Washington had to make a skin incision with a knife in order to deposit the morphine under the skin of the patient. This was not an IV injection but more than likely was subcutaneous. By 1842 modifications in syringes had occurred that eliminated the necessity to make a separate skin incision. The Jayne syringe was similar to the earlier Anel syringe; however, a sharp point had replaced the tapered nozzle, permitting a direct puncture of the skin. Charles Gabriel Pravaz (of Lyons, France) was the first to design a syringe with a separate needle. His syringe, manufactured from glass, was introduced in 1853. The Anel, Jayne, and Pravaz syringes were used primarily to deposit morphine along or near the path of a nerve in cases of neuralgia.

Professor W. W. Green,[5] from the University of Maine School of Medicine, published in 1868, in the *American Journal of Dental Sciences*, a paper entitled "The Hypodermic Use of Morphia during Anesthesia."[5] Green advocated the subcutaneous administration of 0.5 to 1 grain of morphine while the patient was receiving ether anesthesia. Green's reasons for his recommendation included the probability of pain, prevention of shock, a shortening of the anesthetic's influence, and the prevention of delirium and nausea.

Pierre-Cyprien Oré of Bordeaux, France, was the first person to administer a drug intravenously when he administered chloral hydrate to animals to achieve general anesthesia in 1872.[6] Two years later he administered chloral hydrate general anesthesia to a human being.

THE 1900s

Further development of the IV route was somewhat slow. The major developments in anesthesia during the late 1800s occurred in local anesthesia and in the refinement of the techniques of inhalation anesthesia. However, in 1903, Emil Fisher and J. von Mering synthesized the first barbiturate, barbitone (Veronal).[7] For his part in the development of this important drug, Fisher received the Nobel Prize in Medicine in 1903.

In 1929 sodium amobarbital (Amytal) was administered intravenously by L. G. Zerfas.[8] This represented the first IV administration of a rapidly acting barbiturate. However, amobarbital was not administered by Zerfas for the purpose of producing anesthesia. Rather, amobarbital was used primarily as an anticonvulsant. Its function as an anesthetic was limited to those patients in whom inhalation anesthetics could not be administered. A year later, in 1930, pentobarbital (Nembutal) was synthesized.

In 1935 John S. Lundy[9] at the Mayo Clinic in Rochester, Minnesota, introduced sodium thiopental (Pentothal).[9] This rapid-acting, short-duration IV anesthetic eventually became the most popular drug (in the United States) for the induction of general anesthesia via the IV route.

At approximately the same time in England, Stanley L. Drummond-Jackson[10] pioneered the use of IV barbiturate anesthesia for both oral surgery and conservative dental procedures.[10] The agent employed by Drummond-Jackson was methohexital, marketed as Brevital in the United States and Brietal in Europe.

Studying at the Mayo Clinic with Lundy was Adrian Hubbell. Hubbell, along with two others, B. S. Wyckoff and O. K. Bullard, was a pioneer in the administration of IV general anesthesia for ambulatory oral surgical patients.[11] In addition, Hubbell was the first person in North America to use IV general anesthesia without premedication as a sole agent for ambulatory patients having oral operations in a dental office. In 1933 Victor Goldman[12] published the first English-language article dealing with the subject of IV anesthesia for dental surgery.

Thus far we have discussed the evolution of IV general anesthesia. As also occurred with the use of N_2O general anesthesia in the early to mid-1900s, an evolutionary process was taking place. With the advent of better, more effective local anesthetics for pain control, the requirement of anesthesia and analgesia from IV medications was diminishing.

In 1945 Niels Bjorn Jorgensen became probably the first person to use the IV route to provide what Jorgensen himself termed *intravenous premedication*.[13] Jorgensen refined the technique of administering IV barbiturates and combined pentobarbital administration with an opioid (meperidine) and scopolamine. This technique was first used in 1945 at the Loma Linda University School of Medicine. In 1955 this technique for producing IV sedation was first taught to the junior (third-year) dental students at the Loma Linda School of Dentistry, where it has been taught to all succeeding classes. This technique gradually became known as the "Loma Linda technique" and is now known as the "Jorgensen technique," after Niels Bjorn Jorgensen, its founder and the father of IV sedation in dentistry.[14]

In 1965 A. Davidau[15] in Paris, France, first used diazepam (Valium) as a sedative agent in dentistry. Shortly thereafter, D. M. G. Main[16] reported on his first case of diazepam sedation in dentistry. Main used diazepam as an adjunctive agent in the Jorgensen technique.

R. O'Neil and P. J. Verrill[17,18] used diazepam as the sole sedative agent for patients undergoing oral surgical procedures. The Verrill sign, considered by some an indicator of the proper level of sedation, came from these studies. Diazepam became the most commonly employed IV sedative agent within dentistry. Interestingly, the Jorgensen technique, the original IV sedative technique, is still used, primarily for longer procedures. In 1986 midazolam, a water-soluble benzodiazepine, was introduced into clinical practice in the United States following its earlier introduction elsewhere in the world. Although similar in many respects to diazepam, midazolam has a number of distinct advantages and has become very popular as an IV conscious sedative in both medicine and dentistry, rivaling the popularity of diazepam.[19]

Another major change in IV sedation has been the increased attention placed on patient monitoring during sedation and general anesthesia. Noninvasive forms of monitoring have become available that help increase patient safety during IV conscious sedation and general anesthesia.[20,21] Examples of these devices include automatic vital sign monitors, pulse oximeters, and end-tidal carbon dioxide monitors.

REFERENCES

1. Harvey W: *Exercitatio anatomica de motu cordis et sanguinis in animalibus*, 1628, (Leake CD transl), Springfield, Ill, 1931, Charles C Thomas.
2. Lee JA, Atkinson RS: *A synopsis of anesthesia*, ed 5, Baltimore, 1964, Williams & Wilkins.
3. Bankoff G: *The conquest of pain: the story of anesthesia*, London, 1946, MacDonald.
4. Archer WH: *A manual of dental anesthesia*, Philadelphia, 1952, WB Saunders.
5. Green WW: Hypodermic use of morphia during anaesthesia, *Am J Dent Sci* (3rd ser) 2:207, 1868 (extracts).
6. Sykes WS: *Essays on the first hundred years of anaesthesia*, Edinburgh, 1960, E & S Livingstone.
7. Driscoll EJ: Dental anesthesiology: its history and continuing evolution, *Anesth Prog* 25:143, 1978.
8. Zerfas LG: Induction of anesthesia in man by intravenous injection of sodium iso-amyl-ethyl barbiturate, *Proc Soc Exp Biol Med* 26:399, 1929.
9. Lundy JS: Intravenous anesthesia: preliminary report of use of two new thiobarbiturates, *Proc Staff Meetings Mayo Clin* 10:536, 1935.
10. Drummond-Jackson SL: Epival anesthesia in dentistry, *Dental Cosmos* 77:130, 1935.

11. Hubbell AO, Adams RC: Intravenous anesthesia for dental surgery with sodium ethyl (1-methylbutyl) thiobarbituric acid, *J Am Dent Assoc* 27:1186, 1940.
12. Goldman V: "Evipan" in dentistry, *Dent Mag Oral Top* 50:1153, 1953.
13. Jorgensen NB, Leffingwell FE: Premedication in dentistry, *J South Calif Dent Assoc* 21:1, 1953.
14. Jorgensen NB, Hayden J Jr: *Sedation, local and general anesthesia in dentistry*, ed 2, Philadelphia, 1972, Lea & Febiger.
15. Davidau A: New methods in anaesthesiology and their use in dentistry: treatment of difficult patients and execution of complex procedures, *Rev Assoc Med Israelites (France)* 16:663, 1967.
16. Brown PRH, Main DMG, Lawson JM: Diazepam in dentistry, report on 108 cases, *Br Dent J* 125:498, 1968.
17. O'Neil R, Verrill PJ: Intravenous diazepam in minor oral surgery, *Br J Oral Surg* 7:12, 1969.
18. O'Neil R, Verrill PJ, Aellig WH et al: Intravenous diazepam in minor oral surgery, *Br Dent J* 128:15, 1970.
19. Trieger N: Intravenous sedation in dentistry and oral surgery, *Int Anesth Clin* 27:83, 1989.
20. Eichhorn JH, Cooper JB, Cullen DJ et al: Standards for patient monitoring during anesthesia at Harvard Medical School, *JAMA* 256:1017, 1986.
21. Holzman RS, Cullen DJ, Eichhorn JH et al: Guidelines for sedation by nonanesthesiologists during diagnostic and therapeutic procedures. The Risk Management Committee of the Department of Anaesthesia of Harvard Medical School, *J Clin Anesth* 6:265, 1994.

CHAPTER 21

Intravenous Conscious Sedation: Rationale

CHAPTER OUTLINE

Intravenous (IV) conscious sedation is a relatively new technique in dentistry. IV general anesthesia has a long history in dentistry, but only in the past 25 to 35 years has IV conscious sedation gained a foothold. Until the late 1960s the IV route was used almost exclusively by oral and maxillofacial surgeons, primarily because their postdoctoral training placed great emphasis on the IV route of drug administration. Until recently, most dental schools in the United States did not include training in IV drug administration in their curricula, and today woefully few courses are available wherein the postgraduate doctor can receive such training. The past 15 years, however, has seen the implementation of predoctoral courses in IV conscious sedation by a small, but still growing, number of U.S. dental schools. Because of this and the present availability of a handful of excellent postgraduate programs in IV conscious sedation, as well as the continuing, although diminished, availability of 2-year residencies in general anesthesia for dentists, the number of dentists using IV conscious sedation has slowly continued to grow. It is impossible to even guess at the number of dentists employing the IV route today; however, for the patient who requires this form of treatment, it has become somewhat easier to locate a doctor who administers IV conscious sedation for nonsurgical procedures.

A factor that deterred many doctors from the use of IV conscious sedation was the high cost of professional liability insurance. The 1980s saw a dramatic increase in the cost of liability insurance in many areas of life in the United States, not only in the health professions. However, the fact was that the cost of liability insurance for a dentist using IV conscious sedation was, in many states, extremely high. This became a major consideration in a doctor's decision of whether to use this valuable technique of patient management. As the mid-1990s arrived, the cost of liability insurance leveled off and in certain circumstances, for example, for the periodontist using IV conscious sedation (in the state of California), actually decreased. As more complete risk assessment surveys were completed, the cost of liability insurance for dentists using IV conscious sedation continued along this promising pathway.

ADVANTAGES

1. The onset of action of intravenously administered drugs is the most rapid of all techniques discussed

in this book. The arm-brain circulation time is approximately 20 to 25 seconds. Although there may be some individual variation in this and in the onset of action for different drugs, overall, the IV route of drug administration permits the most rapid onset of action.

2. Because of the rapid onset of action of most intravenously administered drugs, drug dosage may be tailored to meet the specific needs of the patient. Guesswork involved in determining proper dosage of a drug administered orally, rectally, or intramuscularly is eliminated when the IV route is used. This concept of individualizing drug dosages is termed *titration* and represents one of the most important safety factors associated with IV drug administration.
3. Because of the rapid onset of action of most IV drugs, the doctor is able to provide the patient with a suitable level of sedation. The level of sedation must never, of course, exceed that level to which the doctor has been trained. Light, moderate, and deep levels of "conscious" sedation can easily be achieved via the IV route, and the doctor must always remain cognizant of his or her limitations, as based on prior experience and training.
4. The recovery period for most intravenously administered drugs is significantly shorter than that seen for the same drug administered via the oral, rectal, intranasal (IN), or intramuscular (IM) route. Recovery from intravenously administered drugs will, however, be considerably longer and less complete than that following nitrous oxide–oxygen (N_2O-O_2) inhalation sedation.
5. In the continuous IV infusion technique recommended in this book, a patent vein is maintained throughout the procedure. This facilitates the reinjection of any additional drug (although this is rarely necessary). However, the major significance of the patent vein is that through it a portal exists for the administration of emergency drugs that may be required in the unlikely event of an emergency arising during IV therapy.
6. The side effects of nausea and vomiting are extremely uncommon when drugs are administered intravenously, as recommended.
7. Control of salivary secretions is possible through the IV administration of anticholinergics. This will be of benefit to the doctor during various types of dental therapy.
8. The gag reflex is diminished. Patients receiving IV conscious sedation rarely experience difficulty with gagging. This action is similar to that occurring with N_2O-O_2 inhalation sedation. If the only requirement in a patient is to minimize the gag reflex, inhalation sedation is preferred over IV conscious sedation. Only in the event that inhalation sedation fails to diminish the overactive gag reflex should IV conscious sedation be employed solely for this purpose.
9. Many of the medications employed intravenously for sedation effectively diminish motor disturbances (e.g., seizure activity and cerebral palsy), making this route advantageous for seizure-prone patients.
10. The ability to readily gain IV access (venipuncture) may prove to be important in any emergency situation. Although antidotal drug therapy is not recommended as the initial step in the effective management of all emergency situations, the ability to establish an IV line provides immediate access to the cardiovascular system should it become necessary to administer drugs to the victim. Through the use of IV conscious sedation on a regular basis, the doctor is better able to maintain proficiency in the technique of venipuncture.

DISADVANTAGES

1. Venipuncture is necessary. Although most adult patients tolerate venipuncture with little or no difficulty, some patients are psychologically unable to accept needles anywhere in their body. Children may be particularly difficult to manage via this route because veins are proportionally smaller in smaller patients, making venipuncture itself more difficult. Younger children requiring IV conscious sedation will usually pose severe management problems (the "precooperative" patient) or be physically unable to control themselves. Not all patients, even adults, have veins that are easy to visualize and gain access to with a needle. Probably the most significant hurdle facing the doctor learning to use IV conscious sedation is to develop a degree of proficiency at venipuncture. Venipuncture is a learned skill, one that becomes easier to perform as experience is gained.
2. Complications may arise at the site of the venipuncture. As discussed in Chapter 27, a variety of minor and some major complications might develop at the venipuncture site. These include hematoma, phlebitis, and intraarterial injection of a drug.
3. Monitoring of the patient receiving IV conscious sedation must be more intensive than that required in most other conscious sedation techniques. Because intravenously administered drugs act rapidly, the entire dental team must be trained to assess the physical and mental status of the patient throughout the procedure. The greater the depth of sedation is, the greater is the need for increased patient monitoring.

4. Recovery from intravenously administered drugs is not complete at the end of the dental treatment. All patients receiving any intravenously administered central nervous system (CNS) depressant must be escorted from the dental office by a responsible adult companion.
5. Although the depth of sedation provided by intravenously administered drugs can be increased rapidly (by administration of additional drug), the converse is not true. Many intravenously administered drugs cannot be reversed by specific antagonist drugs. Although antagonists do exist for several drug groups, specifically opioids, benzodiazepines, and anticholinergics, they are not recommended for routine administration.[1,2] Should a patient become overly sedated, the most effective management in all situations is the maintenance of basic life support: Assess the patient's airway, assist or support ventilation, and provide for the effective circulation of oxygenated blood. Following these steps (P-A-B-C: basic life support) consideration may be given to antidotal drug therapy.

Box 21-1 summarizes the advantages and disadvantages of the intravenous route of drug administration.

CONTRAINDICATIONS

1. Unless a doctor has received specific training in the administration of CNS depressant drugs to patients younger than 6 years and older than 65 years, IV conscious sedation is relatively contraindicated in these groups. The major reason for this recommendation is that in both of these groups there is a greater than usual incidence of overreaction to usual therapeutic dosages of CNS depressants. In other words, many of these patients require smaller dosages of a drug to achieve a desired clinical level of sedation. This ought not to be a problem because the doctor administering the drug should always titrate slowly; however, extreme caution must be exercised whenever the younger or older patient receives CNS depressants via any route. Because of the rapid onset of action of intravenously administered drugs, this route should be reserved for use by the individual specifically trained or experienced in managing these patients (e.g., pediatric dentist).
2. Pregnancy represents a relative contraindication to the administration of IV conscious sedation because most CNS depressants cross the placenta into the fetus. With some drugs, there is an increased risk of birth defects in the developing fetus. The subject of sedation in pregnancy is more fully discussed in Chapter 4.
3. A history of significant hepatic disease contraindicates the use of IV conscious sedation. Most intravenously administered drugs are biotransformed in the liver into pharmacologically inactive products. The presence of significant liver dysfunction (American Society of Anesthesiologists [ASA] III or IV) may alter the rate at which these drugs are metabolized. This may lead to both a prolongation of the clinical actions of the drug and a more profound effect from the same dose. Most patients with serious liver dysfunction (e.g., cirrhosis, hepatitis) are not ambulatory; however, when presented with a history of liver disease, the doctor should pursue an in-depth dialogue history and consider medical consultation should any doubt remain as to the patient's physical status.
4. Thyroid dysfunction is a relative contraindication to the use of IV conscious sedation. Patients who are clinically hypothyroid are particularly sensitive to CNS depressants such as sedative-hypnotics, antianxiety agents, and opioid analgesics. Patients exhibiting clinical signs of hypothyroidism should

BOX 21-1 Advantages and Disadvantages of Intravenous Sedation

Advantages

1. Rapid onset of action
2. Titration is possible
3. Highly effective
4. Recovery shorter than other techniques (intramuscular, oral)
5. Patent vein is safety factor
6. Nausea and vomiting are uncommon
7. Control of salivary secretions possible
8. Gag reflex diminished
9. Motor disturbances (epilepsy, cerebral palsy) diminished
10. Ability to perform IV is benefit in serious emergency situations

Disadvantages

1. Venipuncture is necessary
2. Venipuncture complications may occur
3. More intensive monitoring required
4. Recovery not complete—escort needed
5. Most IV agents cannot be reversed

not be administered IV conscious sedation. Box 21-2 lists clinical signs and symptoms of hypothyroidism. This represents a relative (not an absolute) contraindication, for in the event that other sedative techniques (e.g., inhalation sedation) prove inadequate, lighter levels of IV conscious sedation may be provided. Titration ought to be carried out even more slowly than is usually recommended. Patients who are hypothyroid but are currently being treated with thyroid medications (e.g., levothyroxine [Synthroid]) can safely receive IV conscious sedation. Patients who are clinically hyperthyroid are likely to prove extremely difficult to sedate. In addition, drugs such as the anticholinergics atropine and scopolamine ought not be administered to the clinically hyperthyroid patient. Both drugs possess vagolytic properties, increasing the heart rate. Because hyperthyroid individuals have a significant elevation in their heart rate already, additional increases might well prove deleterious to the patient by increasing the workload of the heart and the risk of possible myocardial ischemia and decreasing cardiac output. Patients with a hyperthyroid history but who, through surgery, radiation, or drug therapy, are presently euthyroid (normal thyroid function) may receive IV conscious sedation with minimal increase in risk.

5. Adrenal insufficiency represents a relative contraindication to the use of IV conscious sedation. Patients receiving chronic corticosteroid therapy or patients with Addison's disease may be less able physiologically to handle the stresses associated with dental care than are patients with normal adrenal cortices. Although these patients require careful management (see stress-reduction protocol, Chapter 4), deeper levels of sedation are not recommended. IV conscious sedation may be used; however, only light to moderate sedation levels are suggested.
6. Patients receiving either monoamine oxidase inhibitors (MAOIs) or tricyclic antidepressants (TCAs) should be evaluated carefully before the administration of any CNS depressant. These drugs are used in the management of depression. Before administration of any other drug that is able to alter mental function (e.g., CNS depressants), medical consultation with the patient's psychiatrist or physician is recommended. Opioid agonists and barbiturates are synergistic with these two groups of drugs.
7. IV conscious sedation is not contraindicated in patients with a history of psychiatric disorders; however, it is strongly recommended that medical consultation be obtained before CNS depressant drugs are given.
8. Patients who are extremely obese present with a variety of potential problems. Because of the excessive amounts of skin and superficial fat, venipuncture might prove to be extremely difficult. Of greater importance is the fact that, in markedly obese persons, there is usually a concomitant decrease in cardiovascular and pulmonary reserve. Other forms of sedation, especially inhalation sedation, should be considered first, with IV conscious sedation considered only when other techniques prove ineffectual.
9. One of the most significant contraindications to the use of IV conscious sedation in the dental office is a dearth of visible superficial veins. All IV procedures in a dental office environment will be of an elective nature. It seems patently unfair for an already phobic patient to have to endure multiple unsuccessful venipuncture attempts so that we can give them a drug to help them to relax. As is discussed in Chapter 24, the preliminary IV visit is used to determine whether the patient is an acceptable candidate for the proposed IV procedure. One of the objectives of this visit is to look for the presence of superficial veins.
10. When using IV conscious sedation, the doctor must specifically question the patient regarding any history with each of the drugs being considered for the procedure. Allergic responses and "hyperresponders" may be discovered before the offending drug is administered. In addition, each drug has specific contraindications to its use. The drug package insert or Chapter 25 of this book should be reviewed for this important information. These contraindications include opioids (specifically meperidine)—asthma; barbiturates—asthma, porphyria; anticholinergics—glaucoma, prostatic hypertrophy.

BOX 21-2 Signs and Symptoms of Hypothyroidism and Hyperthyroidism

Hypothyroidism	*Hyperthyroidism*
Weakness	Nervousness
Dry skin	Increased sweating
Lethargy	Hypersensitivity to heat
Slow speech	Palpitation
Sensation of cold	Fatigue
Gain in weight	Eye signs (exophthalmos)
Cold skin	Increased appetite
Thick tongue	Tachycardia
Edema of face	Goiter
Pallor of skin	Tremor
Memory impairment	Weight loss
Decreased sweating	Weakness
Loss of hair	

INDICATIONS

The major indications for the use of IV conscious sedation are essentially those of other sedative techniques. However, there are a number of indications for IV conscious sedation that are unique to this technique. These include the control of salivary secretions and the production of amnesia.

IV conscious sedation is not a technique that should be used as readily as is inhalation sedation. Before employing IV techniques the doctor should carefully consider other procedures, especially inhalation sedation. IV conscious sedation should be considered for use only in situations in which there exists a specific indication for it.

Anxiety

As with inhalation sedation and the other sedation techniques discussed in this book, the primary indication for use of sedation is the presence of fear and anxiety. Unlike inhalation sedation, however, the use of the IV route should be reserved for those patients in whom other techniques have proved inadequate or for patients in whom prior history or the doctor's experience indicates that the IV route is the only method that might be effective.

In most instances the IV route should be reserved for patients exhibiting pronounced levels of apprehension and fear of the dental situation. Inhalation sedation can often effectively manage the patient with a lesser degree of fear and anxiety. However, there will be occasions when IV conscious sedation is required even for these patients.

Amnesia

An advantage of IV drug administration is the ability to provide a degree of amnesia (or a lack of recall). Whether amnesia develops or does not develop after IV drug administration depends on several items. Some drugs are much more likely to provide amnesia than others. Diazepam, midazolam, lorazepam, and scopolamine are examples of drugs that have a greater degree of amnesia associated with their administration; meperidine and pentobarbital are less likely to provide an amnestic effect.

The depth of CNS depression (sedation) has an effect on whether amnesia develops and on the duration of the amnestic period. In general, given the same patient and the same drug (e.g., diazepam), more profound levels of sedation will provide greater degrees of amnesia. This factor is the reason for my considering amnesia to be "the icing on the cake" during a sedation procedure. The major goal of sedation is to relax the patient. In most cases this result can be obtained with the patient only lightly sedated. The patient may tolerate the procedure quite well but at its conclusion may not be amnesic. In this situation the sedation procedure must be considered a success. The primary goal, that of managing the difficult patient more easily and effectively, was accomplished. Should there also be a lack of recall of events that occurred during the procedure, so much the better. It is safer to provide a patient comfortable dental treatment with total recall (no amnesia) at a lighter level of sedation than it is to provide comfortable dental treatment with total lack of recall at deeper levels of sedation. With the loss of consciousness, lack of recall (amnesia) is virtually 100%, yet risk to the patient is greater.

As with all other factors relating to drug response, there is a significant degree of individual variation in the occurrence of amnesia. Some patients will be amnesic following seemingly very light levels of sedation, whereas others may demonstrate no apparent amnesia with deeper levels of sedation. Such response is consistent with normal variation in response to drug administration.

Medically Compromised Patients

The IV route of sedation is indicated in the management of persons who are medically compromised and unable to tolerate stress in a normal manner. Although inhalation sedation is the preferred technique in most of these patients, light levels of IV conscious sedation may also be used in many of these situations.

ASA II or III Cardiovascular-Risk Patients. Examples of cardiovascular situations in which the IV route may be considered include angina pectoris, previous myocardial infarction, certain dysrhythmias, congestive heart failure, and high blood pressure. The preferred route of sedation for all of these disorders is inhalation sedation with N_2O and O_2. In each of these cardiovascular disorders, the clinical status of the patient will deteriorate should the level of O_2 in the myocardium or in the blood become inadequate to meet the demands of the heart. With N_2O-O_2 sedation the occurrence of such situations is minimized. Whenever IV conscious sedation is used in the management of the ASA III patient, there are two recommendations:

1. Employ light levels of sedation only.
2. Administer 3 L/min of O_2 via nasal cannula, or 6 L/min via nasal hood, throughout the sedative procedure.

Previous Cerebrovascular Accident. The patient who has suffered a cerebrovascular accident (CVA, stroke) falls into the ASA II, III, or IV category.

The ASA status of the patient is determined by the duration of time since the CVA and by the presence or absence of residual signs and symptoms of CNS dysfunction.

As with the cardiovascular-risk patient, the CVA patient may require sedation during dental treatment. Although N_2O-O_2 is the preferred technique because of the increased percentage of O_2 being administered, IV conscious sedation can be used if these same recommendations (as listed for cardiovascular-risk patients) concerning depth of sedation (light only) and the administration of O_2 are followed.

Epilepsy. Epileptic patients are acceptable candidates for IV conscious sedation. In most cases the seizure activity of the patient is controlled through daily administration of anticonvulsant drugs (many of which, coincidentally, are used intravenously as sedatives). Such patients will be able to tolerate almost any technique of sedation with little or no difficulty. It is in the patient whose seizure activity has not been controlled effectively that the IV route may prove particularly beneficial. Stress is a factor that acts to precipitate acute seizure activity; therefore utilization of the stress-reduction protocol is recommended. Although inhalation sedation may prove to be effective, the use of intravenously administered benzodiazepines, particularly diazepam and midazolam, is recommended. The Jorgensen technique, which includes pentobarbital, is also indicated in epileptic patients. These drugs are effective anticonvulsants and can be administered intravenously when a protracted seizure develops. Their use as IV sedatives will greatly diminish (although not entirely eliminate) the likelihood of a seizure developing during treatment. Consultation with the patient's physician is recommended before use of IV conscious sedation in these patients. The use of O_2 via nasal cannula or nasal hood is strongly recommended in epileptic patients because any degree of hypoxia may precipitate a seizure. Light to moderate levels of sedation may be safely employed in these patients.

Other Medically Compromised Patients. The IV route can also be used for many other medically compromised patients. ASA IV patients should not receive IV conscious sedation within the dental office, such treatment being relegated to the operating room or the hospital dental clinic, where medical consultation and a more controlled treatment environment can be provided. ASA II and III patients are usually acceptable candidates for sedation. Whether or not the IV route is appropriate can be determined through consultation with the patient's physician. The administration of supplemental O_2 throughout the IV procedure is recommended for all ASA II, III, and IV patients.

Control of Secretions

Occasions arise during dental treatment when it is beneficial to decrease the volume of salivary secretions. The major indication for this will be impression taking following the preparation of teeth for full coverage. A dry mouth may also prove to be beneficial during restorative dentistry and surgical procedures. Anticholinergics can be administered orally, intramuscularly, and intravenously, but the IV route provides the most effective and reliable results. Agents such as atropine, scopolamine, and glycopyrrolate may be administered intravenously either alone or in conjunction with other CNS depressants.

Analgesia

Although far from being the ideal method of pain control in dentistry, intravenously administered opioid analgesics assist in obtaining clinically adequate pain control. Local anesthetics remain the ideal drug for eliminating pain during dental treatment; however, occasions do arise where these drugs do not provide entirely adequate relief of discomfort. In such situations the administration of CNS depressants, such as N_2O-O_2 or opioid analgesics, elevates the pain reaction threshold of the patient, thereby decreasing or at least modifying the patient's response to noxious stimulation.

The use of intravenously administered drugs as the sole means of achieving pain control is ineffective in the absence of general anesthesia. General anesthesia should not be considered unless the doctor has completed a residency in anesthesiology (see Section VI).

Diminished Gagging

Some dental patients have a significant problem with gagging whenever instruments or fingers are placed in the posterior part of their oral cavity. Whatever the underlying reason for this response, it becomes difficult, if not impossible, for the doctor to treat these patients successfully. Several sedation techniques possess the added benefit of diminishing the gag reflex. Most notable among these is IV conscious sedation, followed closely by inhalation sedation with N_2O-O_2.

In most instances, the use of inhalation sedation is recommended to control a hyperactive gag reflex. To obtain a few intraoral radiographs or an impression takes but a few minutes, and because IV sedative techniques are too long acting for these procedures, inhalation sedation is recommended. If a patient has difficulty whenever anything is placed in his or her mouth (e.g., handpiece, explorer) and treatment is to last for an hour or more, the use of IV conscious sedation becomes more reasonable.

Indications for the use of intravenously administered drugs are quite numerous. Although the obvious indication is fear and apprehension, the doctor should be aware that many other indications for the use of IV conscious sedation do exist.

REFERENCES

1. Brogden RN, Goa ZL: Flumazenil. A reappraisal of its pharmacological properties and therapeutic efficacy as a benzodiazepine antagonist, *Drugs* 42:1061, 1991.
2. The Flumazenil in Intravenous Conscious Sedation with Diazepam Multicenter Study Group II: Reversal of central benzodiazepine effects by flumazenil after intravenous conscious sedation with diazepam and opioids: report of a double-blind multicenter study, *Clin Ther* 14:910, 1992.

CHAPTER 22

Armamentarium

CHAPTER OUTLINE

INTRAVENOUS DRUG ADMINISTRATION

The equipment required for venipuncture and for intravenous (IV) drug administration is discussed in this chapter. IV drugs can be administered in a number of ways, including the following:

1. Direct IV drug administration; vein not kept patent
2. Needle maintained in the vein without a continuous infusion; patency maintained by periodic flushing
3. Continuous IV infusion; patency maintained by a continuous infusion of solution

Direct Intravenous Administration

In direct IV administration a tourniquet is placed on the patient's arm, the veins become engorged, the injection site is prepared, and the needle of the syringe containing the drug(s) is placed into the lumen of the vein. After ensuring that the needle is within the vein (aspiration of blood back into the syringe), the doctor or assistant removes the tourniquet and the drug is slowly deposited into the vein. After drug administration the needle is removed from the vein, pressure is applied to the site to stop bleeding, and the treatment is begun. No access to the vein is maintained during the procedure (Figure 22-1).

Needle Maintained in the Vein without Continuous Infusion

When the needle is maintained in the vein without an infusion being used, the tourniquet is placed, the veins are engorged, and the tissues are prepared in the usual manner. A winged infusion set or a hollow metal needle is used for venipuncture. Following successful venipuncture, the tourniquet is removed and the syringe (without a needle attached) is connected to the needle that has been left in the vein and taped into place. After the drug is titrated to effect, the syringe is detached from the needle, and a second syringe containing a solution

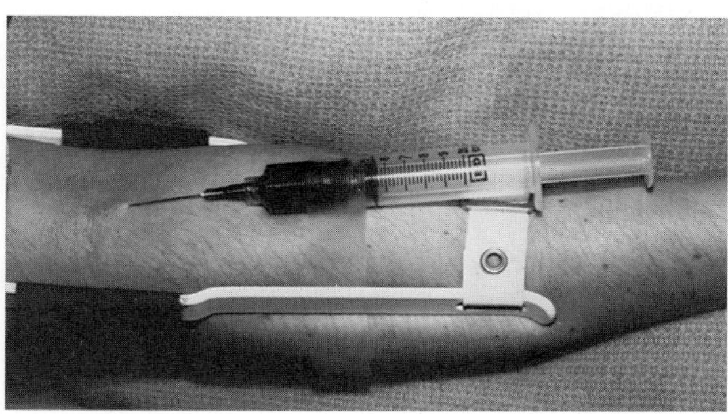

Figure 22-1 Direct IV drug administration. Blood is aspirated into syringe before injection to determine that needle is still within lumen of vein.

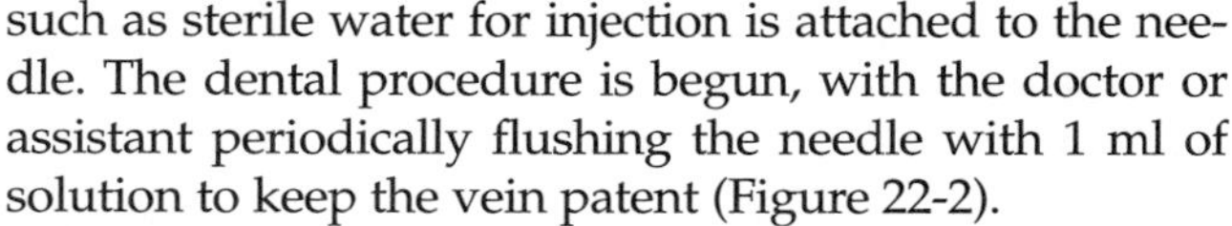

such as sterile water for injection is attached to the needle. The dental procedure is begun, with the doctor or assistant periodically flushing the needle with 1 ml of solution to keep the vein patent (Figure 22-2).

Continuous Intravenous Infusion

In a continuous IV infusion an indwelling needle or catheter is attached to a length of tubing that in turn is connected to a bag of infusate. The same venipuncture procedure is carried out that was described for the first two techniques. Following removal of the tourniquet, the flow of IV solution is started and the needle or catheter is securely taped. The IV drugs are administered through an injection site located on the tubing, and the syringe is then removed. The rate of the IV infusion is adjusted to maintain a slow flow that will prevent needle occlusion during the dental procedure, which is then begun (Figure 22-3).

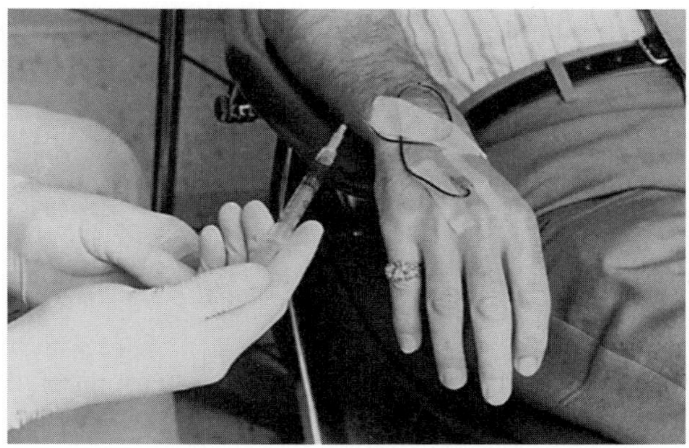

Figure 22-2 Needle maintained in the vein without continuous infusion.

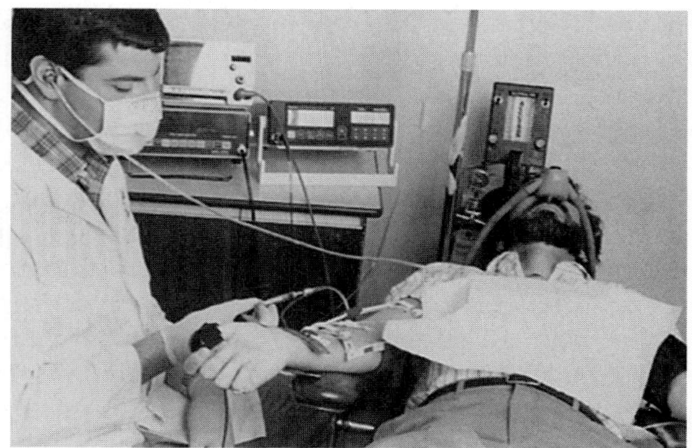

Figure 22-3 Continuous IV infusion.

ADVANTAGES AND DISADVANTAGES OF VARIOUS METHODS

The first technique, direct IV administration, in which the syringe is removed from the vein after drug administration, cannot be recommended for routine use in IV sedation. In fact, the only reasons for considering use of this technique, in my opinion, follow:

1. Emergency situations in which IV drug administration is required and time or the lack of equipment does not permit establishment of an IV infusion
2. Situations in which the needle needs to be maintained in the vein for only a very brief period of time (as in drawing of blood for laboratory analysis)

Why do I believe this technique should not be used? As is evident in later chapters and during training in IV conscious sedation, the most difficult part of learning to use IV conscious sedation is becoming technically proficient in venipuncture. Although not a hard technique to master, venipuncture can be difficult on some occasions in even the most experienced of hands. Why, therefore, if placing a needle into the vein is the most difficult task in IV conscious sedation, should the needle be removed from the patient's vein after a successful venipuncture? Adherents of the needle removal technique claim that the patient is bothered by the needle remaining in the vein and that the presence of the needle in the vein throughout the procedure reminds the patient of a hospital. However, once the needle is placed into a vein, the patient has little, if any, awareness of its being there, be it in for 1 minute or several days. In response to the belief about the hospital setting, I can only state that the presence of a needle within the vein throughout the procedure is routine in hospital practice simply because it adds to the safety of the procedure. Patients will accept as normal most practices within the dental office. A valid argument in favor of the needle removal technique is that removal of the needle from the vein makes it difficult for additional drugs to be administered following the initial titration, minimizing the chance of a drug overdose.

Removal of the needle from the vein is illogical because, on occasion, additional IV sedative drugs may be required later in the procedure or an emergency situation may develop in which antidotal therapy will be needed. Drugs such as flumazenil, naloxone, or physostigmine may be required during or at the end of the IV conscious sedation procedure. In both of these situations a venipuncture will have to be reestablished. Because the venipuncture is the only part of the IV conscious sedation procedure that might be considered difficult, is it not logical to leave the needle in situ during the entire procedure? In addition, should the patient's blood pressure decrease significantly, superficial veins will become difficult to visualize and to cannulate.

The second technique, in which the needle is left in the vein throughout the procedure, its patency maintained by periodic flushing with some solution, is an improvement on the previous technique. The only drawback to this technique is that periodic flushing of the needle is necessary to prevent clotting of the lumen from occurring. During a busy dental procedure it is not uncommon for the doctor and the assistant to become deeply engrossed in the oral cavity and to neglect to flush the needle, in which case the lumen of the needle becomes clotted with blood and a vein must be recannulated.

Continuous IV infusion is the most highly recommended technique in all situations in which a patent vein is to be maintained for a period of time exceeding but a few minutes. In this technique, patency of the needle and vein are maintained by the constant infusion of IV solution from the bag into the needle and the patient's vein. The only drawback to this procedure is the possibility of (1) the infusate being contaminated (a highly unlikely occurrence) and (2) the drip rate being too rapid, causing the bag of solution to be emptied during the procedure.

Readministration of sedative or emergency IV drugs is easily carried out by simply inserting the syringe needle into the injection site on the IV tubing. The ease of maintaining a patent vein and the increased safety afforded the patient by the continuous IV infusion are the primary reasons for considering this technique as the ideal for IV drug administration. The equipment and techniques discussed in this section relate to continuous IV infusion.

Armamentarium for Venipuncture and Intravenous Infusion

Basic Equipment

IV infusion solution*
IV administration set*
Needle*
IV stand
Tourniquet
Adhesive tape*
Sterile gauze pad, 2 × 2 inch*
Alcohol wipe*
Armboard
Bandage*

Additional Items

Sphygmomanometer
Stethoscope
Monitoring devices
O_2 delivery system
Emergency kit
Antidotal drugs

IV, Intravenous.
*Single-use, disposable item.

INTRAVENOUS INFUSION SOLUTION

Choice of Solution

A variety of fluids are available for IV therapy. Although the type of solution chosen is of some significance in the hospitalized patient during prolonged IV therapy, for a short-duration IV procedure (less than 1 hour to several hours' duration) on a relatively healthy patient, the choice of infusate becomes academic. Solutions available for IV administration include the following:

Solution	Abbreviation
Lactated Ringer's	LR
Sterile water for injection	SW
5% dextrose in water	D_5W
Sodium chloride injection	¼NS

Although other infusion solutions are available, these represent the most commonly used solutions.

In the ambulatory American Society of Anesthesiologists (ASA) I, II, or III patient being considered as a candidate for IV conscious sedation on an outpatient basis, there will be no contraindication to the use of any of these solutions. The question of whether a patient with insulin-dependent diabetes mellitus (type 1, or IDDM) should receive 5% dextrose in water often arises—won't this solution elevate the patient's blood sugar level?

The answer is that a 5% dextrose and water solution is not contraindicated in the diabetic patient. First, the concentration of dextrose (5%) is not great enough to produce any significant change in the blood sugar level of this patient.[1] Second, as stressed in Chapter 26, the patient receiving IV conscious sedation will be requested to fast (be NPO) for approximately 4 hours before the planned procedure. The patient will arrive at the dental office with a decreased blood sugar level, perhaps not quite hypoglycemic but definitely not hyperglycemic. The addition of 100 to 200 ml of 5% dextrose and water will produce a slight elevation in blood sugar level, a desirable effect at this time. It must be remembered that when a person with diabetes becomes clinically hypoglycemic, treatment of choice is the administration of 50% dextrose, a solution 10 times that which is being infused during IV conscious sedation. The most commonly used IV infusate is 5% dextrose and water (Figure 22-4).

Volume of Solution

All IV infusion solutions are packaged in plastic bags (see Figure 22-4). Obvious advantages of plastic bags include their unbreakability and the ease of packaging and shipping as compared with the older glass bottles.

IV solutions are available in a variety of sizes. The most commonly used sizes include 1000, 500, and 250 ml.

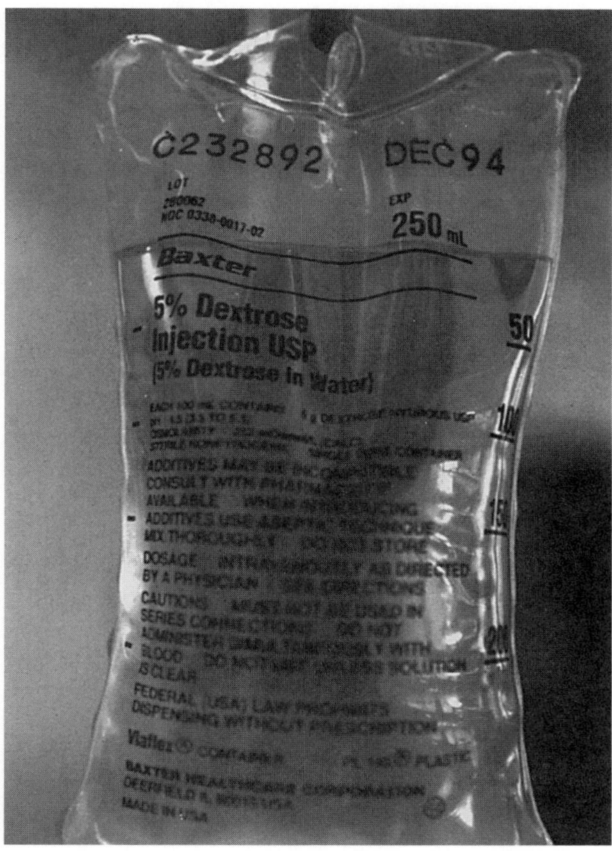

Figure 22-4 IV infusion solution of 5% dextrose in water (D_5W).

The 1000-ml (1-L) size is commonly used in the hospital setting when a patient is receiving long-term IV therapy. The patient usually receives 3 L of IV solution daily. During general anesthesia, during which the patient must be kept hydrated throughout surgery, 1-L bags are also commonly used. Use of the 1-L bag for dental outpatient procedures is not the most highly recommended, although there is no significant reason why it should not be used. However, for the typical IV procedure in the dental office, the 1-L bag is simply too large. For example, during a 1-hour procedure a patient may receive 125 to 200 ml of infusion solution. At the conclusion of the procedure the infusion bag represents one of the three items in the IV armamentarium that must be discarded. It is a single-use item and must never be reused despite the fact that, in this example, approximately 800 ml of infusate remains unused. I have seen situations in which well-meaning doctors have reused the bag of IV solution on from two to five patients, rather than discard it, on the theory that it is extremely unlikely that blood or microorganisms can travel uphill against gravity the 72 inches from the patient's vein to the IV bag. Using a 500-ml bag decreases the likelihood of the same type of situation arising.

The 250-ml bag of IV fluid represents the most nearly ideal size for the typical 1- to 4-hour dental IV conscious sedation procedure. With proper management of the flow rate (as discussed in Chapter 26), the 250-ml bag can be made to last for 3 to 4 hours. Discarding the small volume of solution remaining is quite easy, and doctors are less likely to be tempted to reuse this size bag.

The solution found within the IV bag is sterile. However, problems with contaminated solutions have developed in the past.[2] Care must be exercised by the user of such solutions to try to ensure the sterility of this solution. Administration of contaminated solutions directly into the cardiovascular system of the patient can produce bacteremia or septicemia and has led to deaths and to significant morbidity.[3]

The following should be checked before using a bag of solution:

1. *All IV infusion solutions are clear.* A solution that has any coloration to it or has any particulate matter floating within it should never be used.
2. In addition to the name of the solution, the bag will have an expiration date. *IV infusion solution should never be used after its expiration date has passed* (see Figure 22-4).
3. *Once the seal on the bag of infusate has been opened, the solution cannot be stored for any length of time without the possibility of contamination.* If a bag of solution is prepared for an IV procedure and the appointment is canceled, the bag could still be used if another procedure is scheduled for that same day. However, the bag should be discarded

if it would not be used for a day or more. Bags of IV solution do not contain preservatives or bacteriostatic agents; therefore they represent excellent culture media for bacterial growth.

4. *If there is ever any doubt as to the sterility of the IV infusion solution, it should not be used.* However, the bag should not be thrown away. On the contrary, the bag should be returned to the manufacturer so that the solution may be assayed. The manufacturer will be very concerned about the possibility of a contaminated IV solution being used clinically.
5. In the extremely rare case in which a glass bottle of IV solution is being used, there is an additional concern: When the rubber seal on the glass bottle (Figure 22-5) is punctured, the vacuum within the bottle is dissipated as air is forced into the bottle. The person preparing the IV drip will normally notice air bubbles entering into the glass bottle as the IV tubing is forced into it. Absence of these bubbles or a glass bottle with no seal over the rubber stopper should give the doctor reason to think that perhaps the seal had been broken and the solution is not sterile.

The following checklist summarizes precautions for IV infusion solution:

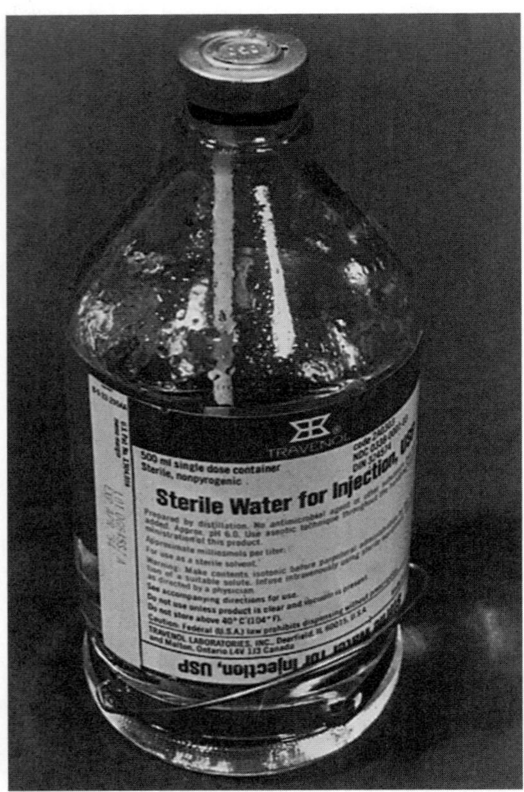

Figure 22-5 Sterile water for injection in glass bottle.

1. Is the IV solution clear?
2. Has the expiration date of the IV solution passed?
3. If an opened IV bag, has it been stored for more than a few hours?
4. Is there any doubt regarding its sterility? (Never use a bag of IV solution when any doubt exists as to its sterility.)

INTRAVENOUS ADMINISTRATION SET

Delivery of the IV infusion solution from the bag to the patient requires tubing. Infusion sets, as they are known, have several components in common (Figure 22-6).

The *piercing pin* is that part of the IV tubing that is inserted into the bag of IV solution. It is a solid plastic piece that should be kept sterile before its insertion into the bag of solution.

Located immediately below the piercing pin is the *drip chamber*. The drip chamber is an enlarged clear plastic chamber into which solution from the bag will drip. The drip chamber has two functions: to prevent air from entering into the IV tubing and to permit regulation of the solution's flow rate.

The drip chamber should be filled with IV solution approximately halfway to prevent air bubbles from being trapped in the IV tubing. Although isolated air bubbles within the tubing are of little consequence (see Chapter 27), the unknowing patient may be quite disturbed to see any bubble of air enter into his or her body. An unfilled drip chamber or one just barely filled with solution will continually permit air bubbles to enter the tubing as each drop of solution falls from the bag into the drip chamber.

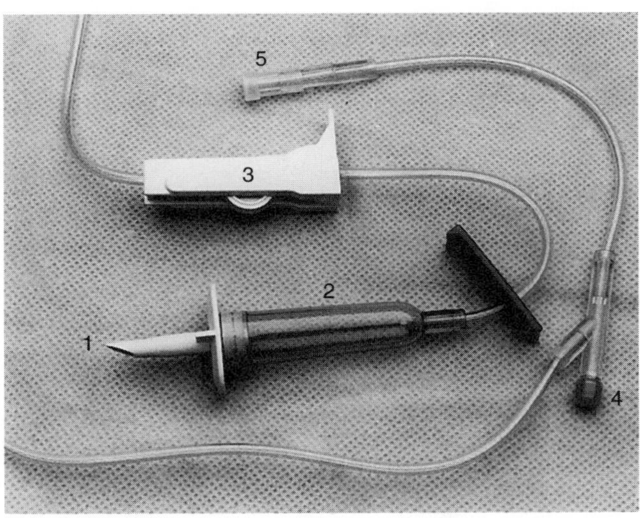

Figure 22-6 IV administration set: *1,* piercing pin; *2,* drip chamber; *3,* rate adjustment knob; *4,* injection site; and *5,* needle adapter.

Conversely, overfilling the drip chamber prevents the doctor from assessing the flow rate of the IV solution. Although this factor is not as critical in the ambulatory dental or surgical patient as it is in the hospitalized patient, the flow rate does require adjustment at various times during the procedure (see Chapter 26). In addition, in two groups of patients—the smaller child and the patient with serious congestive heart failure (ASA III or IV)—overhydration is a complication to be avoided. The ability to determine the precise rate of flow is of importance in these situations.

When the usual adult IV infusion set is used, 10 drops equals 1 ml of solution. Therefore, for a 250-ml bag of IV solution to last for 2 hours (120 minutes), we can adjust the flow rate to 20 drops per minute (2 ml/min × 120 min = 240 ml).

Pediatric infusion sets provide a finer adjustment such that 60 drops equals 1 ml of solution. Use of the pediatric infusion is recommended in the smaller child and in the adult with serious congestive heart failure (ASA III) (Figure 22-7).

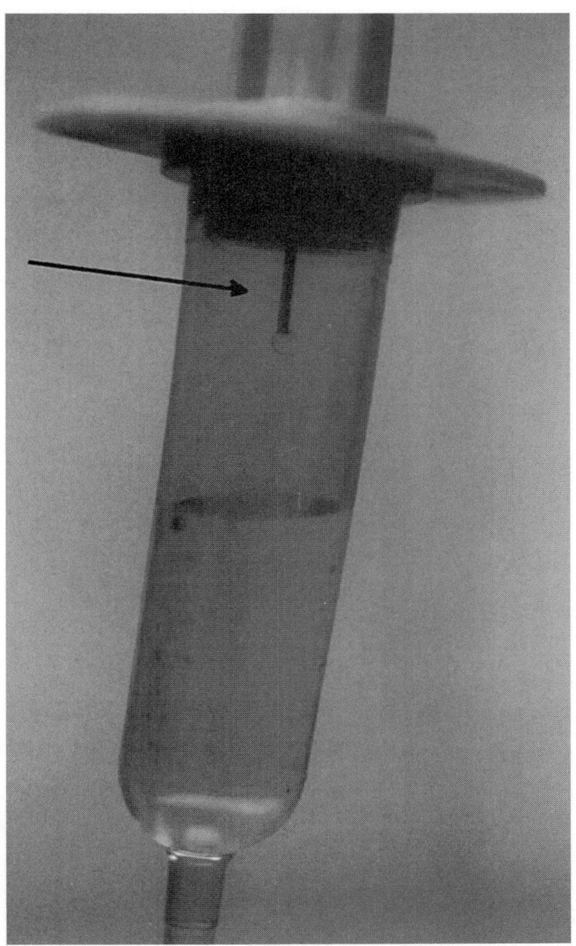

Figure 22-7 Pediatric IV drip. Note small pin within drip chamber *(arrow)*.

Extending from the drip chamber is a variable length of plastic tubing, usually 72 inches long, that attaches to the IV needle. Along the length of this tubing are found several items (see Figure 22-6):

- Rate adjustment knob
- Injection port or syringe port
- Rubber bulb
- Adapter for needle or syringe

The *rate adjustment knob* permits the rate of flow of solution into the drip chamber to be regulated.

The *injection port* is usually a rubber diaphragm that fits over a hard plastic spur off of the main IV tubing. The needle of the syringe containing the drug to be injected is placed into this port, and the drug is injected into the flowing infusion. The rubber diaphragm should not be removed from the plastic before injection.

Because of the potential danger of needlestick injury, infusion sets have been developed in which the syringe connects to the injection port through a Luer-Lok connection.

On some IV sets, near the distal end of the IV tubing, just above where the needle adapter is found, is a rubber bulb. This bulb is larger than the plastic tubing and serves as a means of checking if a needle or catheter tip lies within the lumen of a vein. The bulb need only be squeezed and released. If the needle or catheter tip lies within the lumen of a vein, a flash of blood appears in the tubing just above the entry point of the needle into the patient's skin. A second possible use of the rubber bulb is to serve as an alternative site for injection of a drug. The syringe needle is inserted into the bulb (with care not to perforate the other side of the tubing), and the drug is injected into the infusion. Multiple punctures of the rubber bulb, however, lead to leakage of infusate. When present, the injection port is the recommended site for drug administration on the IV tubing.

At the very end of the IV tubing is the *needle adapter*. A variety of shapes and sizes of needles may be used for venipuncture. In addition, there are a multitude of manufacturers of each needle. To ensure that needles and tubing from different manufacturers can be used interchangeably, a standard female Luer connector is used. Any needle in the following discussion easily attaches onto standard IV tubing.

Under no circumstances should the reuse of the IV infusion tubing ever be considered, for the tubing is always contaminated at its distal end with the patient's blood. This blood may be quite visible as it surges back into the tubing as the needle tip enters the lumen of the vein during venipuncture, or it may be quite dilute and perhaps not visible to the eye. Reuse of the IV tubing runs an unacceptably high risk of transmission of potentially very serious diseases. Do not do it!

NEEDLES

To deposit a drug underneath the skin, as in the case of intramuscular or subcutaneous injection, or directly into a blood vessel, as in the case of IV administration, a needle must be used. Needles are usually referred to by gauge and type.

Gauge

Gauge usually refers to the outside diameter of the needle. However, in discussions of the hypodermic needle, standard gauge numbers have come to be associated with the size of the lumen. Therefore the gauge number of a needle may refer to the internal diameter (ID) or the outside diameter (OD) of the needle lumen. Needles used for venipuncture generally range from 14 gauge to approximately 23 gauge. The lower (smaller) the gauge number, the larger the size of the lumen. Therefore a 16-gauge needle has a larger lumen than a 23-gauge needle.

The term *gauge* is often quite confusing. The term derives from the number of pieces of wire (in this case needles) that can be placed into a 1-mm circle. Therefore only 16 needles of 16 gauge will fit into the same space occupied by 23 needles of 23 gauge. Table 22-1 lists commonly used needle gauges and their major functions.

Types

Several types of needle are available for venipuncture; all have their adherents, their advantages, and disadvantages. The following are the three most commonly employed needles (Figure 22-8):

1. Hollow metal needle
2. Winged needle (scalp vein needle)
3. Indwelling catheter

The *hollow metal needle* is the prototypical needle, that is, the traditional IV needle. This needle represents the basic design from which other needles in the following discussions have been modified. Figure 22-9 illustrates the components of the hollow metal needle.

The needle is inserted directly into the vein and then attached via its hub to the IV tubing or directly to the syringe containing the drug to be administered. Since the development of the scalp vein needle and the indwelling catheter, use of the hollow metal needle for venipuncture has been limited to emergency situations in which other needles are not readily available or situations in which blood is to be drawn from a patient for laboratory analysis.

The hollow metal needle may be used to review the anatomy of the IV needle. At one end of the needle is a sharp tip. A triple bevel slopes backward from this tip and ends at the heel of the shaft. The shaft runs from this point to the hub. The length of the shaft

TABLE 22-1 Needle Gauge and Function

Gauge	Function
14	Phlebotomy Administration of blood
16	Phlebotomy Surgical procedures in which blood is likely to be required
18	Common during general anesthesia in which blood administration is unlikely
20, 21	Intramuscular drug administration Occasionally IV during short procedure on ASA I or II patients IV sedation in dentistry
23	IV sedation in dentistry
25, 27	Intraoral local anesthetic administration
30	Intraoral local anesthetic administration Acupuncture

ASA, American Society of Anesthesiologists; *IV*, intravenous.

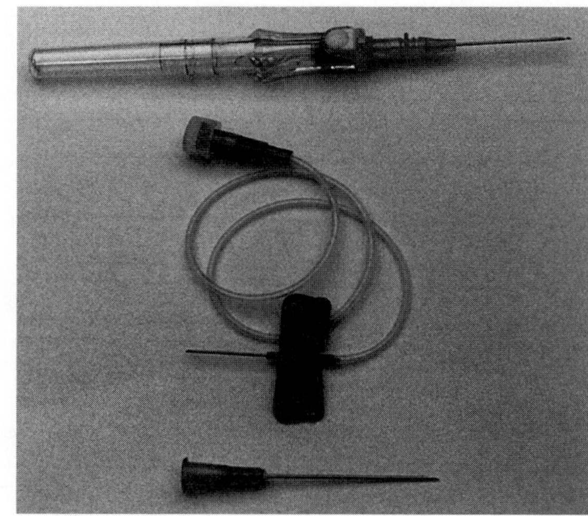

Figure 22-8 Indwelling catheter *(top)*, winged needle *(middle)*, and hollow metal needle *(bottom)* are available for IV drug administration.

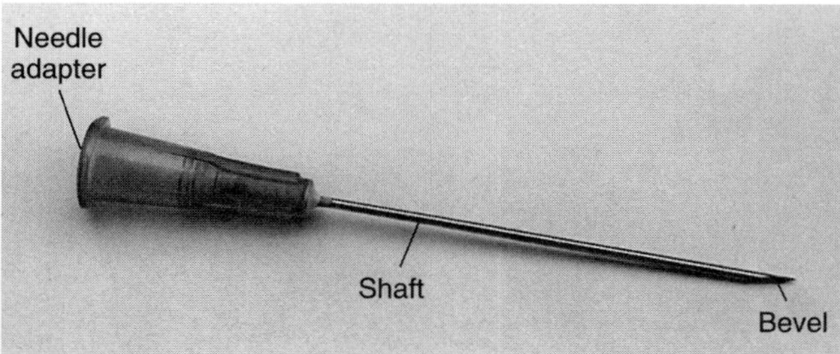

Figure 22-9 Components of the hollow metal needle.

varies but is commonly between 5/8 inch and 1.2 inches in length. The hub is an enlarged metal or plastic portion that permits the needle to be attached to the intravenous tubing or a syringe.

The *winged needle* is a popular needle for IV conscious sedation procedures in the ambulatory patient within both dentistry and medicine. Some regard the winged needle as the device of choice for venipuncture of superficial veins in patients of all ages. The primary advantage over other types of needles is its ease of manipulation.

The winged needle (Figure 22-10) consists of a sharp stainless steel needle, one or two flexible winglike projections mounted to the shaft of the needle, a variable length of flexible tubing, and a female Luer adapter that connects with any standard IV administration set.

The wings allow the user to hold onto the needle more firmly, permitting greater ability to manipulate the needle and to gain greater "feel" during the procedure. In addition, following successful venipuncture the wings may be taped down to better secure the needle within the vein. The winged needle has several synonyms: *winged infusion set, Butterfly needle*, and *scalp vein needle*.

Butterfly is a proprietary name for the winged infusion set. However, like other proprietary names, such as Ping Pong and Linoleum, common usage has turned the proprietary name into the most commonly used name of the device. The term *butterfly needle* is very commonly used and is acceptable, although technically not correct.

The winged infusion set evolved from what was termed the *scalp vein needle*. Superficial veins in most neonates and infants are quite small and frequently inaccessible. Often, the physician had to surgically expose a vein (called a *venous cutdown*) to manually insert a catheter. The scalp vein needle evolved because among the most prominent veins found in the neonate or infant are those on their scalp. The scalp vein needle contains a shorter needle, thereby minimizing the problem of needle perforation of the back wall of the vein, which can lead to either an infiltration or a hematoma.

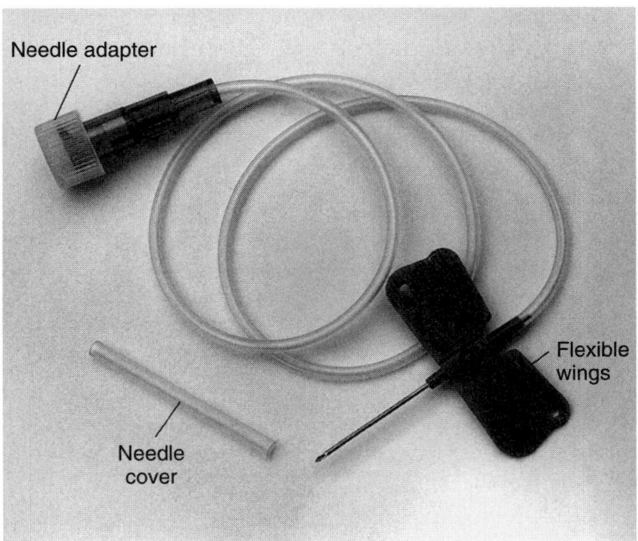

Figure 22-10 Components of the winged needle.

Although they are available in a variety of different gauges, the 21- and 23-gauge winged infusion sets are most commonly used in dentistry, with the 21-gauge needle preferred because it will permit a greater volume of solution to flow through it per minute than the 23-gauge needle (13 to 3 ml/min).[4]

A potential problem with both the hollow metal needle and the winged infusion set is that they are rigid. Should they be placed into a vein in a mobile area, such as the wrist or the antecubital fossa, special precautions must be observed to prevent the patient from moving that area, or the needle, lying in the lumen of the vein, will perforate the posterior wall, requiring reentry into the vein. Common terminology says that "we have lost the vein."

To minimize this risk, the flexible *indwelling catheter* was devised. Several types of indwelling catheter are available, among them the catheter-over-needle unit and the catheter-inside-needle unit. Within dentistry only the catheter-over-needle is recommended for use. Recently "safety catheters" have been developed that minimize risk of needlestick injury. Following successful venipuncture the metal needle retracts into a protective plastic sheath, preventing inadvertent needlestick injury. Materials used for the plastic catheter include polyvinyl chloride (PVC), Silastic, and Teflon. Modern catheters are radiopaque so that they may easily be visualized on x-ray examination.

The indwelling catheter, called the *catheter-over-needle*, when first designed consisted of a metal hub to which was attached a plastic catheter. The catheter was physically connected to the separate metal hub by means of a piece of plastic. The safety of this design was questioned because the link between the catheter and the hub may not be secure and the catheter could come loose and migrate through the patient's veins. In fact, such occurrences did occur, leading to the development of the modern indwelling catheter in which the catheter is of one-piece design (Figure 22-11).[5] The catheter migration problem is virtually nonexistent with the catheter-over-needle unit.

Regardless of the particular design of the indwelling catheter, the basic format is the same. A metal needle (called the *introducer* because it introduces the catheter into the vein), ranging in gauge from 14 to 23, has a very tight-fitting plastic catheter placed over it. The catheter is just slightly shorter than the needle so that several millimeters of the metal needle protrude beyond the catheter.

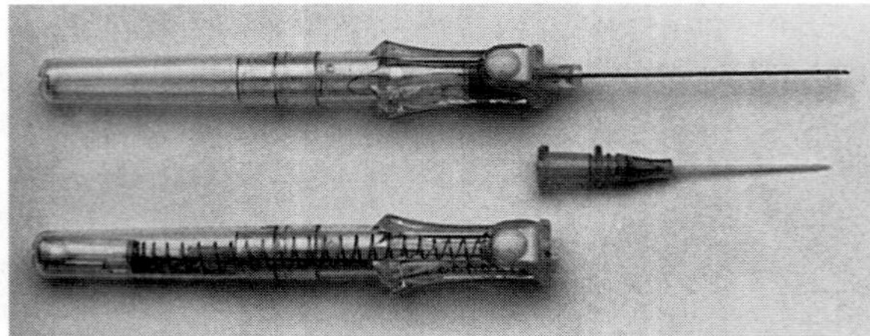

Figure 22-11 Components of the indwelling catheter. Intact unit *(top)* and catheter with "safe" needle retracted *(middle, bottom)*.

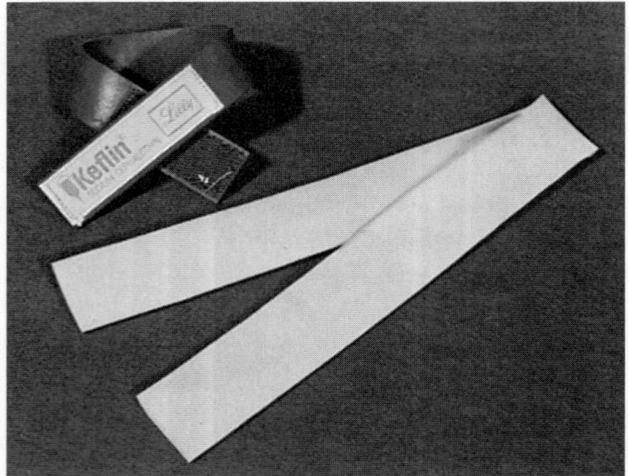

Figure 22-12 Tourniquets: Velcro tourniquet *(top)* and rubber tubing *(bottom)*.

Following successful venipuncture with the metal needle, the catheter is advanced into the vein, the metal needle removed, the appropriate infusion set attached, and the catheter secured with tape. The actual technique of venipuncture using the indwelling catheter is presented in Chapter 24.

The indwelling catheter is recommended for use within the operating room or in most general anesthetic procedures. It has also become a favorite needle in IV conscious sedation. In situations in which maintenance of a patent vein is essential, indwelling catheters are recommended. The reason indwelling catheters are not taught as the primary venipuncture needle for most ambulatory procedures is that the winged infusion set is somewhat easier for a beginner to master. After some experience has been gained with the winged infusion set, the student will have little or no difficulty moving to the indwelling catheter. *The IV infusion, the administration set, and the needle are all single-use, disposable items.*

OTHER ITEMS

A number of additional items are of importance during venipuncture. An *IV stand* is used to elevate the bag of

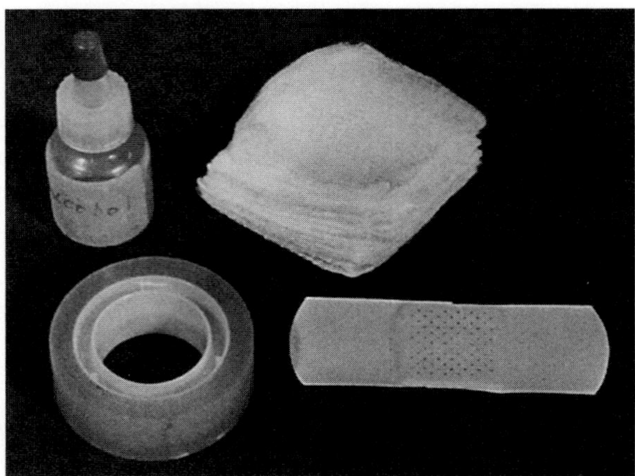

Figure 22-13 Additional items for venipuncture: alcohol, sterile gauze, transparent tape, and bandages.

IV solution. As is discussed in Chapter 24, the height of the bag of IV solution above the patient's heart will, in part, determine the rate of flow of the solution.

IV poles mounted on a portable stand are commonly used within the operating room. Such devices are usually too cumbersome for use within the dental environment; there simply not being enough room for the doctor, an assistant, and the IV pole. In addition, portable IV stands are somewhat expensive, whereas the following device is inexpensive but functional.

To conserve precious floor space, the bag of IV fluids may be hung from the ceiling. A bolt and hook, as used for hanging plants, with several links of chain placed on the ceiling to the side of the patient's head, functions quite well as an IV stand.

A *tourniquet* is used to prevent the return of venous blood from the periphery to the heart while allowing for the unimpeded flow of arterial blood into the limb. A variety of items may be used as tourniquets (Figure 22-12):

1. Thin rubber tubing (e.g., Penrose drain)
2. Velcro tourniquet
3. Blood pressure cuff (sphygmomanometer)

Adhesive tape is needed to secure the needle to the patient's arm (Figure 22-13). An inexpensive tape such as transparent adhesive tape is usually adequate. Traditional white surgical adhesive tape may be used but is not highly recommended because it is not as easy to work with as are other tapes. Some patients are allergic to the adhesive used on tape and will require the use of a hypoallergenic tape. Always ask this question of the patient before the start of the IV procedure.

A simple, inexpensive tape such as transparent tape is recommended because it is easy to manipulate, adheres quite well to skin, and, being clear, can be

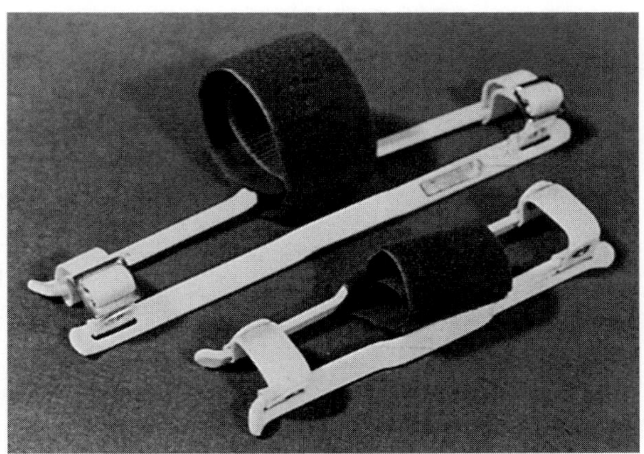

Figure 22-14 Elbow immobilizers: adult and pediatric.

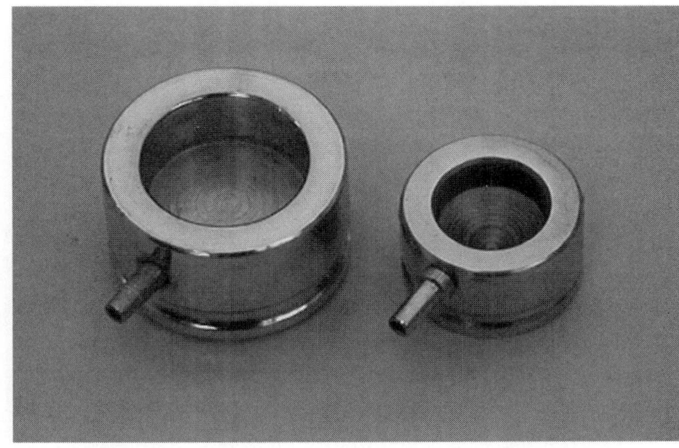

Figure 22-15 Weighted metal stethoscope head for pretracheal/precordial stethoscope. Adult and pediatric are shown.

placed in areas where a nontransparent tape should not be placed (e.g., directly over the point of entry of the needle into the skin).

To cleanse the skin before venipuncture and to dry the tissue, a number of *sterile 2-×-2-inch gauze wipes* are needed. These gauze squares can also be used as pressure dressings or to protect the hairs on the hand from adhesive tape.

Prepackaged *alcohol wipes*, or simply a 2-×-2-inch gauze pad moistened with isopropyl alcohol, will be needed to cleanse the skin before venipuncture. Alcohol can also be used to cleanse the rubber covering of the injection site on the IV tubing and the rubber stopper on multiple-dose vials of drugs.

An *armboard* is important when IV conscious sedation is contemplated. The armboard is used to immobilize a portion of the arm, preventing it from being flexed by the patient with the metal needle becoming dislodged from the vein. Armboards are commonly used for the wrist and the antecubital fossa whenever rigid metal needles are used. They are not necessary where flexible catheters have been inserted.

A number of devices are available for use as armboards. A rigid piece of cardboard with a disposable paper sleeve is relatively inexpensive and may be used multiple times, simply replacing the sleeve between uses. It is available in a short length, for use as a wrist immobilizer, and in a longer length for use in the antecubital fossa. Another device is known as an *elbow immobilizer* (Figure 22-14). It consists of two rigid metal pieces connected at either end by two adjustable plastic straps. In the center is a Velcro strap that is used to fasten the immobilizer in position. The elbow immobilizer is available in both adult and pediatric sizes, is easy to work with, does an excellent job of immobilizing the antecubital fossa, and is not very expensive. This device does not effectively immobilize the wrist.

Adhesive bandages are used at the end of the procedure to protect the site of venipuncture.

The items described previously are the essentials for venipuncture and IV conscious sedation. Several other items should always be available not only for IV conscious sedation but also in every dental office.

A *sphygmomanometer* and *stethoscope* are required for monitoring of the patient's blood pressure before, during, and after the sedative procedure. In addition, the stethoscope may be used to auscultate both the heart and lungs at any time before or during the procedure. A *pretracheal stethoscope* head taped to the patient either in the precordial region or on the neck above the trachea functions as a device for continuous listening to the patient's breath and heart sounds (Figures 22-15 and 22-16).

The blood pressure cuff (sphygmomanometer) can be used as a tourniquet by simply inflating it to a reading above the patient's diastolic pressure but below their systolic pressure.

Patients must be monitored throughout the IV sedation procedure. A variety of *monitoring devices* have become available, ranging from the inexpensive (pretracheal stethoscope) to the more costly (end-tidal carbon dioxide [CO_2] monitor). The use of these monitors and recommendations for monitoring during various forms of sedation are discussed in Chapters 5 and 26.

Oxygen (O_2) should be available in all dental offices whether or not IV conscious sedation is being used. Although its primary use is in the management of

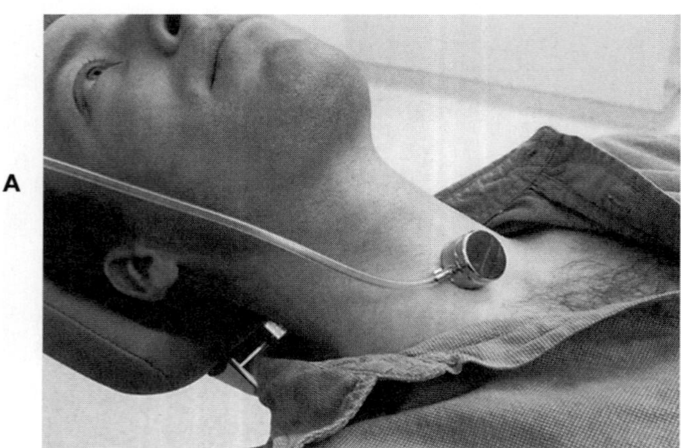

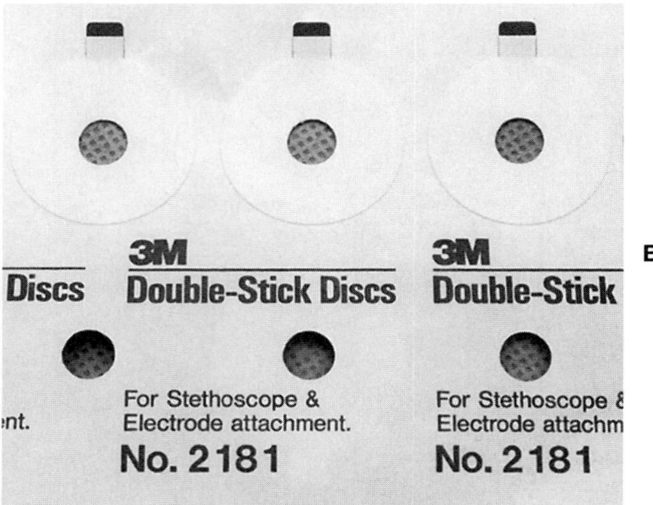

Figure 22-16 A, Pretracheal stethoscope on patient's neck. B, Double-sided tape for pretracheal stethoscope.

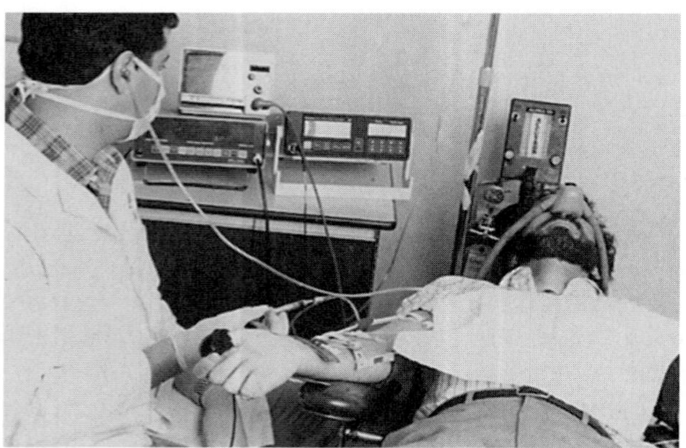

Figure 22-17 Patient receives oxygen during intravenous sedation.

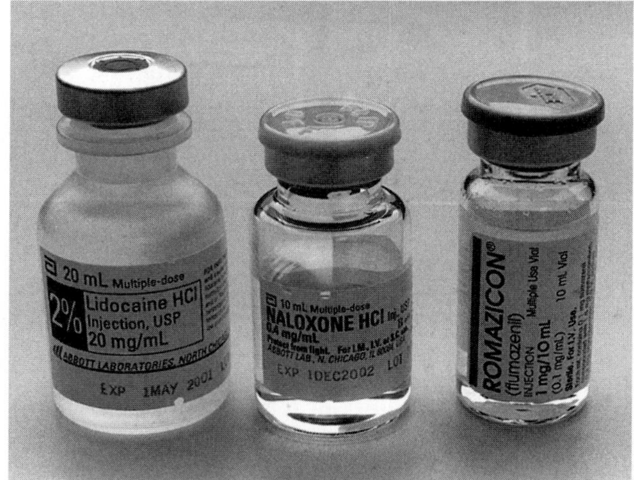

Figure 22-18 Vasodilator: lidocaine *(left)*; opioid antagonist: naloxone *(center)*; and benzodiazepine antagonist: flumazenil *(right)*.

emergency situations, the routine administration of O_2 through a nasal cannula or nasal hood (Figure 22-17) to patients receiving IV conscious sedation is recommended (see Chapter 26).

An *emergency drug kit* and *emergency equipment* must also be available in all dental offices. The emergency kit in the dental office in which IV conscious sedation is used will contain several drugs that are not considered necessary in the typical emergency drug kit (Figure 22-18):

1. Opioid antagonist: naloxone or nalbuphine
2. Benzodiazepine antagonist: flumazenil
3. Antiemergence delirium: physostigmine
4. Vasodilator: procaine 1% or 2%

These important items and their uses are discussed in detail in Chapter 27, and the emergency kit and equipment are reviewed in Chapter 33.

REFERENCES

1. Milaskiewicz RM, Hall GM: Diabetes and anaesthesia: the past decade. *Br J Anaesth* 68:198, 1992.
2. Fleer A, Senders RC, Visser MR et al: Septicemia due to coagulase-negative staphylococci in a neonatal intensive care unit: clinical and bacteriological features and contaminated parenteral fluids as a source of sepsis, *Pediatr Infect Dis* 2:426, 1983.
3. Matsaniotis NS, Syriopoulou VP, Theodoridou MC et al: *Enterobacter* sepsis in infants and children due to contaminated intravenous fluids, *Infect Control* 5:471, 1994.
4. Trieger NT: *Pain control*, ed 2, St Louis, 1994, Mosby.
5. Galdun JP, Paris PM, Weiss LD et al: Central embolization of needle fragments: a complication of intravenous drug abuse, *Am J Emerg Med* 5:379, 1987.

CHAPTER 23

Anatomy for Venipuncture

CHAPTER OUTLINE

Venipuncture is a technique that is separate and distinct from intravenous (IV) conscious sedation. All health-care professionals should become proficient with this route of drug administration whether IV conscious sedation is practiced or not, for the ability to start an IV line may prove to be important in emergency situations.

Venipuncture is not a difficult technique to learn. Indeed, Malamed[1] has demonstrated that an initial attempt at venipuncture by untrained dental students has a greater than 90% success rate. However, to become proficient requires practice. Once learned, knowledge of the technique remains with the doctor forever, yet because it is an acquired skill, if it is not used regularly, the level of the doctor's ability will diminish.

In theory, venipuncture may be attempted in any superficial vein of a size sufficient to accommodate the needle. Figure 23-1 illustrates the major superficial veins in the human body. In practice, however, elective venipuncture is usually confined to one of the patient's extremities. Either an arm or leg may be used. Usual preference is the arm, with the leg being used when arm veins are inadequate or in emergency situations in which the arm may be unavailable or unsuitable for use.

IV conscious sedation in the dental setting in an ambulatory patient will almost always be an elective procedure. The selection of a venipuncture site will therefore usually be limited to one of the arms. Use of the leg for venipuncture is usually reserved for the infant or child, in whom arm veins are smaller and less superficial than in the adult, and the adult with a disability, in whom a venipuncture site in the foot may be more easily secured than one on the arm.

In this chapter the anatomy of the circulation to the arm is described in detail. Both the venous circulation and the arterial circulation are discussed, for it is essential to be aware of those sites where anatomically important structures, such as arteries and nerves, lie in close proximity to veins. Knowing

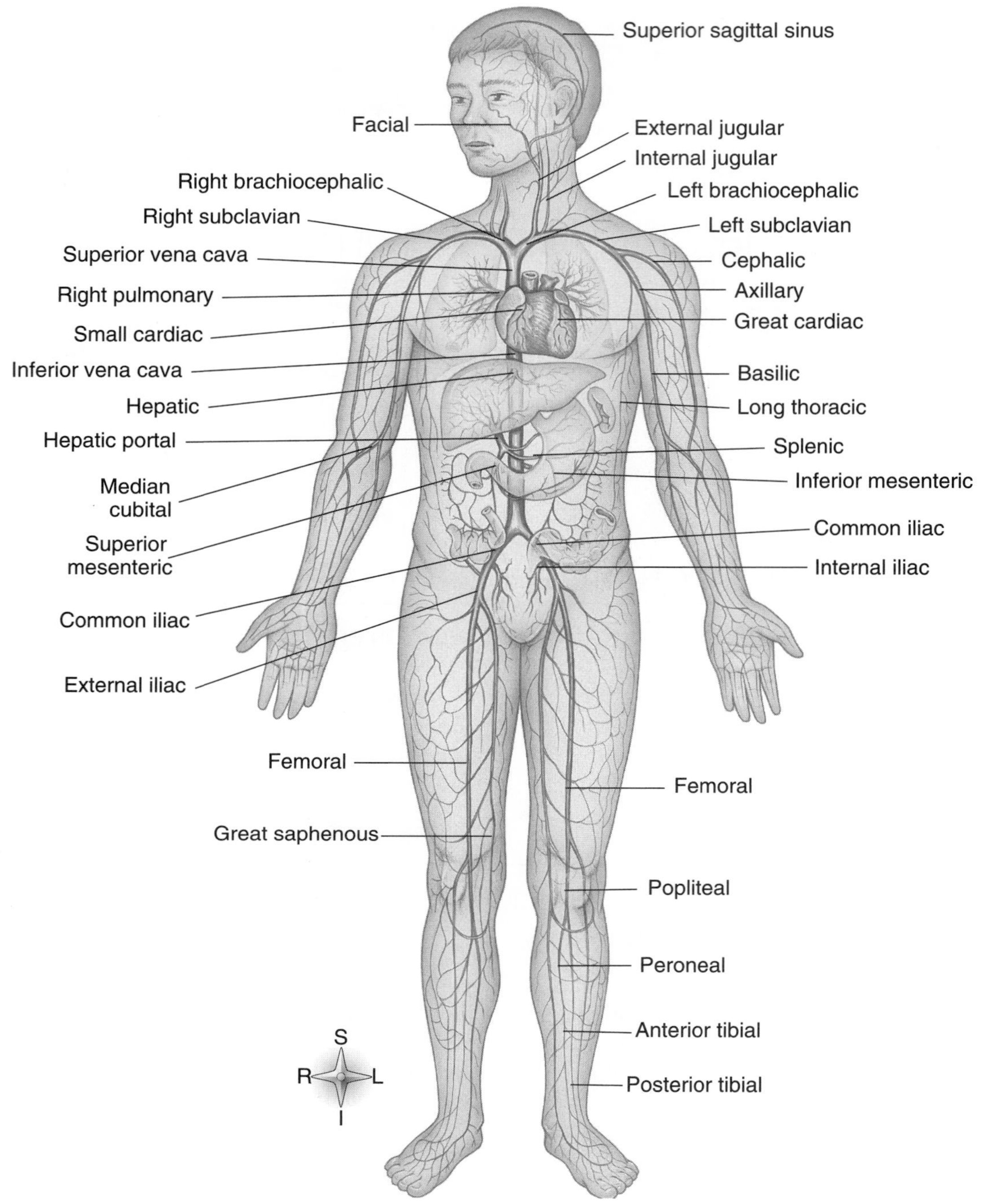

Figure 23-1 Principal veins of the human body. (From Thibodeau GA, Patton KT: *The human body in health & disease,* ed 3, St Louis, 2002, Mosby.)

where not to attempt a venipuncture is valuable knowledge.

ARTERIES OF THE UPPER LIMB

Blood to the right upper limb leaves the aortic arch through the short, wide brachiocephalic (innominate) trunk, which divides into the right common carotid and right subclavian arteries, the latter delivering arterial blood to the upper limb. On the left side the subclavian artery is a direct branch of the arch of the aorta. From this point onward the arteries of the two sides are symmetric.[2]

At the outer border of the first rib the *subclavian artery* turns laterally to enter into the axilla. At this point it is termed the *axillary artery.* The axillary artery leaves the axilla at the lower border of the

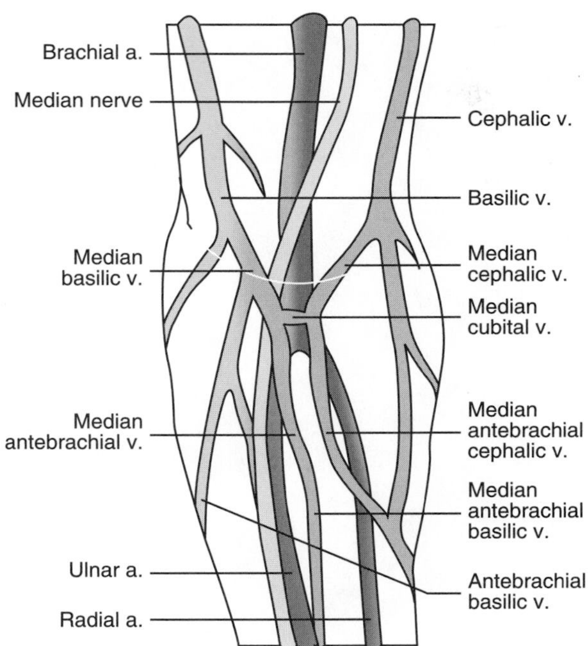

Figure 23-2 Relative location of major arteries in upper arm.

teres major muscle to enter the arm or brachium as the *brachial artery.* Approximately 1 inch below the antecubital fossa the brachial artery bifurcates into the *radial* and *ulnar arteries* (Figure 23-2), which travel distally in the forearm and terminate in the palm as an *arterial arch.* The ulnar artery forms the *superficial palmar arch,* which travels to the level of the web of the thumb, where it is completed by a small branch arising from the radial artery, the superficial palmar branch. The radial artery crosses the bottom of the so-called snuffbox (the hollow at the base of the thumb), reaching the dorsum of the hand and then entering the palm. There it forms the *deep palmar arch,* which is completed by a small branch from the ulnar artery, the deep palmar branch.

The location of these arteries has great clinical significance. Within the antecubital fossa, the brachial artery is commonly found beneath the median basilic vein, usually the most prominent vein in the antecubital fossa. The brachial artery is located just medial of the midline in the antecubital fossa and is the primary reason that the medial aspect of the antecubital fossa is low on my list of preferred venipuncture sites for the neophyte phlebotomist.

Approximately 1 inch below the antecubital fossa, the radial and ulnar arteries arise from the brachial artery. The radial artery lies on the lateral aspect of the ventral surface of the forearm, the ulnar on the medial aspect. Although it is not superficial at its origin, approximately 5% of the population does possess a recurrent radial artery, which is located on the lateral side of the antecubital fossa and is relatively superficial.

The radial artery continues down the ventral aspect of the forearm, not lying near the surface until it reaches the lateral aspect of the wrist, at the base of the snuffbox. At this point, on the ventral surface of the wrist, the radial artery is quite superficial. It is at this point that the radial pulse and arterial blood for blood gas analysis may be obtained. Care must be exercised whenever venipuncture is contemplated in this region. Fortunately, venous anatomy does not readily lend itself to venipuncture at this site.

The ulnar artery descends through the forearm lying more deeply within the tissues than does the radial. It lies on the medial aspect of the forearm, but at no point does it become superficial enough to be palpable.

VEINS OF THE UPPER LIMB

The primary venous return from the arm is through the *axillary vein,* which continues centrally as the *subclavian* and *brachiocephalic (innominate) veins* before emptying into the *superior vena cava.*

The veins of the arm may be divided into two groups: deep veins and superficial veins. The deep veins, for the most part, accompany arteries within the fascial sleeve, whereas the superficial veins lie for most of their course outside the fascial sleeve.

Deep veins, except for the axillary veins, are arranged in pairs, one on either side of the various arteries. The axillary vein, which is a direct continuation of the basilic vein, crosses the axilla and becomes the subclavian vein at the outer border of the first rib. Its branches correspond to those of the axillary artery, except for the thoracoacromial, which joins the cephalic vein. The axillary vein receives the brachial veins in the lower portion of the axilla and the cephalic vein in the upper portion of the axilla. The deep veins will not be of significance in venipuncture.

The superficial veins of the upper limb are the veins that will be selected for most elective venipuncture. Their anatomy is discussed in the following sections (see Figure 23-1).

Blood to the digits is drained through an anastomosis of *palmar* and *dorsal digital veins.* From the palmar aspect of the hand most blood flows to the dorsum of the hand, especially through the *intercapitular veins* that lie between the heads of the metacarpal bones and around the margins of these heads. Blood from the digits and palm therefore drains primarily into the *dorsal venous network* on the back of the hand. Two major veins arise from this dorsal venous network. The *cephalic vein* arises from the radial aspect of this network, and the *basilic vein* rises from the ulnar side. These veins ascend the forearm, the cephalic on the lateral aspect, the basilic medially. Within the forearm the *median vein of the forearm* arises and ascends the forearm on its medial aspect.

At the antecubital fossa a number of veins are usually visible. From lateral to medial are the *cephalic vein,* the *median cephalic,* the *median vein,* the *median basilic,* and the *basilic.* The cephalic vein continues upward through the clavipectoral fascia to drain into the *axillary vein,* and the *basilic vein* runs to the axilla, where it continues directly as the axillary vein.

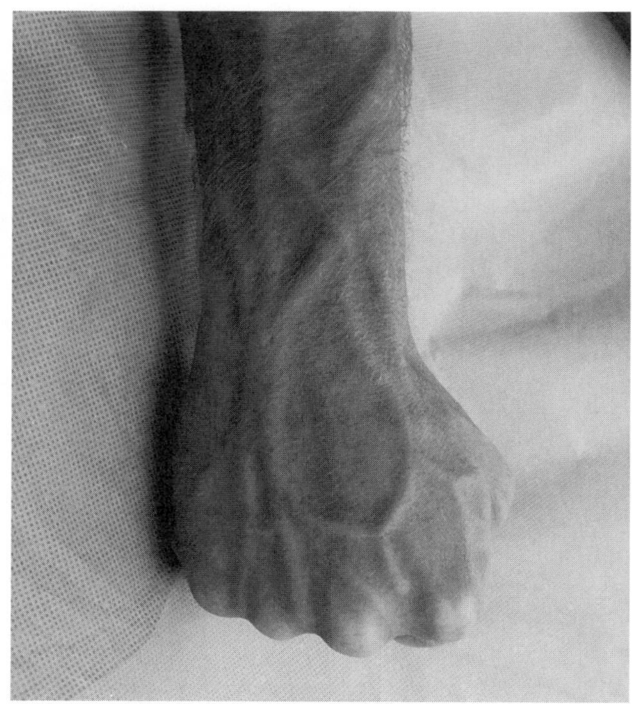

Figure 23-3 Superficial veins of dorsum of hand and wrist.

ANATOMY

Clinically, the arm provides the phlebotomist with four distinct areas for venipuncture. Starting at the upper part of the arm are found the antecubital fossa, which is discussed as two separate areas: (1) the medial aspect of the antecubital fossa and (2) the lateral aspect of the antecubital fossa. In our descent down the arm the ventral aspect of the forearm is next, followed by the dorsum of the wrist and of the hand. Each of these potential venipuncture sites presents its own advantages and disadvantages.

Dorsum of the Hand

The dorsum of the hand is the preferred site for venipuncture among anesthesiologists (Figure 23-3). It has several distinct advantages over other sites and has few disadvantages. It is one of my two preferred sites.

Anatomically, it is extremely rare to find arteries on the dorsal aspect of the hand, most arteries being located on its palmar aspect. In addition, most blood returning to the heart is routed into the veins that form the dorsal venous network, a group of superficial veins. The location of most veins on the dorsum of the hand and of most arteries in the palm obviates the obstructive pressures that occur on the dorsum when a fist is formed, thereby maintaining intact the arterial blood supply to the hand during a "fight or flight" situation. This pattern is similar to the dorsal venous arch of the foot, which is distant from the pressure applied to the sole when a person stands.

The veins within the dorsal venous network have the obvious advantage of being quite superficial. Ease of accessibility is important when elective venipuncture is being considered. A second advantage of the dorsum of the hand is the anatomic safety of the region. Rarely (but not never) will an artery be found on the dorsal aspect of the hand.

There are two disadvantages to these dorsal veins on the hand. First, the veins are smaller than veins found more proximally. Second, because these veins are superficial, they tend to be mobile.

As to the first disadvantage, it is common practice within anesthesia to start an IV infusion on the dorsum of the hand using a needle not smaller than 18 gauge. Quite frequently, a 16-gauge needle is used in this area. In virtually all children and adults the dorsum of the hand can readily accommodate these large-gauge needles. In dentistry a 21- or, rarely, a 23-gauge needle will be used for venipuncture, needles easily accommodated by the lumens of these smaller veins.

The mobility of veins on the dorsum of the hand can in some cases make venipuncture more difficult to accomplish. Fortunately, several techniques are available for immobilizing these veins during venipuncture:

1. Holding the hand in a fist during venipuncture
2. Pulling the skin of the dorsum toward the knuckles during venipuncture
3. Use of the inverted Y configuration, if present

These immobilization techniques are discussed more fully in Chapter 24.

It is sometimes said that venipuncture on the dorsum of the hand is more painful for the patient than at other sites. I personally have found that venipuncture in the dorsum is neither more comfortable nor uncomfortable than at any other site on the arm. The most important factor determining comfort or discomfort is the technical prowess of the person attempting the venipuncture. With experience usually comes increasing technical ability and greater comfort for the patient.

Wrist

The dorsal venous network continues proximally, draining subcutaneously along the margins of the hand and wrist into two major veins (see Figure 23-3). In most persons the veins of the wrist are not so uniform that they can be assigned names. However, on the lateral (radial) aspect of the wrist, in the snuffbox, is found the so-called intern's or resident's vein. This vein becomes the cephalic vein as it ascends the forearm. Although usually visible, this vein has the disadvantage of being quite mobile and of being located in an area that is very difficult to immobilize.

Another vein, which ultimately becomes the basilic vein, is commonly found on the ulnar aspect of the dorsum of the wrist. It too is located in an area where mobility is great and immobilization difficult. Another vein may be found toward the middle of the dorsal aspect of the wrist. Of the three veins, this last represents the most logical choice for venipuncture in this region. It is both superficial and mobile, but immobilization may usually be achieved through the techniques discussed previously.

The ventral aspect of the wrist is not a desirable area for elective venipuncture. Although several veins are usually visible, they possess several undesirable characteristics: They are not as large as those on the dorsum of the wrist; the anatomy of the region leaves much to be desired—relatively superficial arteries, nerves, and tendons make the region both more sensitive and more risky for attempted venipuncture; and the wrist must be immobilized if a metal needle is to be used. The ventral aspect of the wrist is more difficult to immobilize than the dorsum.

In summary, the dorsum of the wrist is greatly preferred to its ventral aspect. However, significant disadvantages to use of the wrist for venipuncture exist, including vein mobility and the need to immobilize the wrist during the entire IV procedure if a rigid metal needle is used.

Forearm

The forearm represents one of the two preferred sites for venipuncture on the upper limb (Figure 23-4). The basilic and cephalic veins are the major veins of the forearm, the basilic coursing up the medial (ulnar) aspect of the arm, the cephalic on the lateral or radial aspect. The basilic and cephalic veins are not as superficial as the veins found in the dorsum of the hand and the wrist; however, they are usually visible and often palpable, especially after application of a tourniquet.

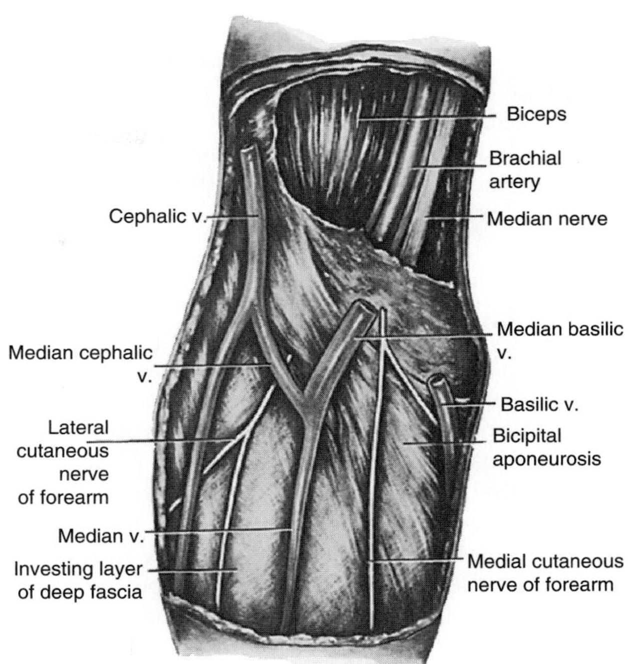

Figure 23-4 Veins of the ventral forearm and antecubital fossa. (From Drummond-Jackson SL, ed: *Intravenous anesthesia,* ed 5, London, 1971, Society for the Advancement of Anaesthesia in Dentistry.)

A third vein, the median vein of the forearm, runs subcutaneously along the midline of the ventral surface. It lies somewhat deep at the distal end of the forearm, becoming more superficial just below the antecubital fossa.

The dorsal aspect of the forearm may also be considered for venipuncture. However, because of a lack of obvious veins and the presence of hair, this site is not of primary importance.

Advantages of the veins of the forearm include the following:

1. The veins are larger than those found in the wrist and dorsum of the hand.
2. Veins, because they are not superficial, do not roll during venipuncture attempts.
3. There is no need to immobilize either the wrist or the antecubital fossa when the forearm is used for venipuncture with a rigid metal needle. (This increases patient comfort during the IV procedure.)

4. Anatomically, the superficial ventral (and dorsal) aspects of the forearm are devoid of any major arteries or nerves that might lie close to the usual venipuncture sites.

A disadvantage of the ventral aspect of the forearm is the lack of superficiality of the veins, making the venipuncture more difficult to perform in some patients.

Antecubital Fossa

The antecubital fossa, or elbow joint, has for many years been one of the most popular sites for venipuncture. The usual pattern of veins in this region is illustrated in Figures 23-1 and 23-2.

The cephalic and basilic veins traverse the lateral and medial aspects of the antecubital fossa. They represent relatively large targets for venipuncture. However, in some persons they may be located so far laterally or medially that venipuncture is technically difficult to carry out successfully, and in patients in whom venipuncture is successful, stabilization of the needle or catheter is difficult.

The median vein of the forearm usually becomes somewhat more superficial as it approaches the antecubital fossa. It lies almost directly in the midline of the forearm. Just below the border of the antecubital fossa the median vein bifurcates.

In most persons the median vein divides into two major branches: the median cephalic and the median basilic veins. The median cephalic, as its name implies, runs laterally to join with the cephalic vein, and the median basilic runs medially, joining with the basilic vein.

In this, the most common pattern, the largest of the veins in the antecubital fossa is the median basilic vein. This is so because a deep vein connects with the median basilic vein in this area. Indeed, the median basilic vein is the first choice of phlebotomists. The median cephalic vein is also large, though not as large as the median basilic vein. The cephalic and basilic veins are also large but, because of their location (lateral and medial, respectively), are more difficult to enter and to stabilize the needle in.

Although many of the veins of the antecubital fossa appear large and therefore present as inviting targets for venipuncture, there is a potential problem when venipuncture is carried out on the medial aspect of the antecubital fossa (by the neophyte). The problem lies in the anatomy of this region.

As is evident in a cross-sectional diagram of the antecubital fossa (Figure 23-5), important structures are located directly below the medial aspect of the fossa. Centrally, the biceps tendon passes deeply down to the upper end of the radius. Medial to

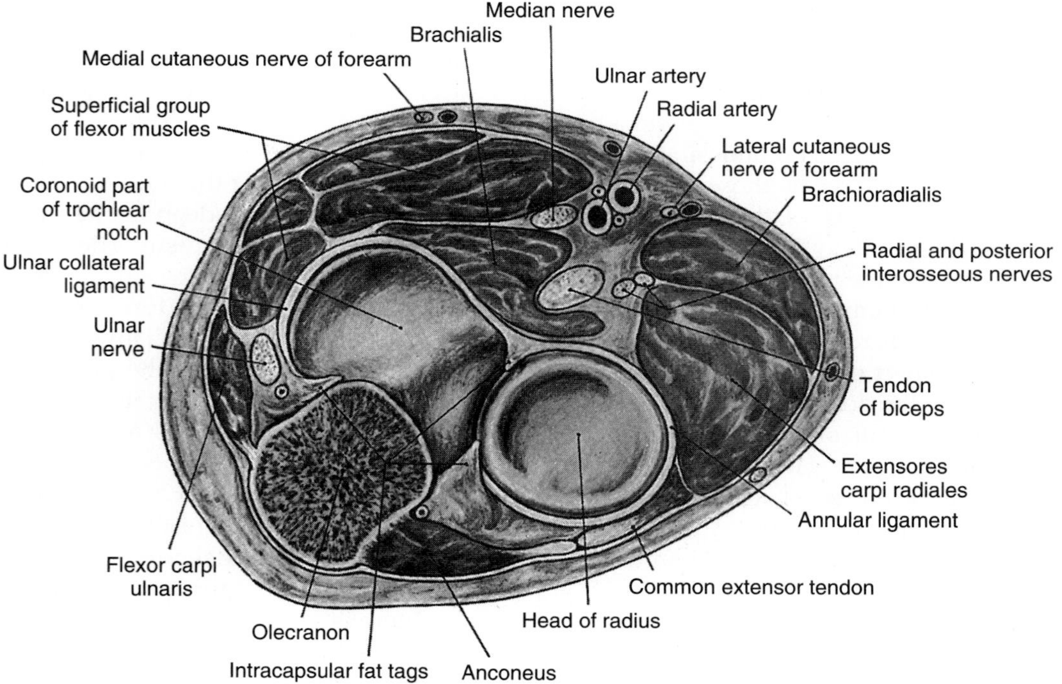

Figure 23-5 Cross section of antecubital fossa (ventral area on top). (From Williams PL: *Gray's anatomy,* ed 38, New York, 1995, Churchill Livingstone.)

this lies the bicipital aponeurosis. On the aponeurosis lies the large median basilic vein with the median cutaneous nerve of the forearm on its medial side. This vein is somewhat mobile (although not as mobile as the dorsal wrist veins) and may slip away from the needle tip during venipuncture if it is not immobilized adequately. Should the vessel be nicked, a large hematoma will develop. During immobilization the vein may be flattened, making venipuncture more difficult.

Of far greater importance, however, is the fact that immediately below the bicipital aponeurosis and the median basilic vein lie the median nerve and the brachial artery. It is not impossible for a novice to miss the median basilic vein and to enter into the brachial artery or to injure the median nerve.

No such potential problem exists on the lateral aspect of the antecubital fossa. The median cephalic vein, although smaller in size than the median basilic, is relatively immobile and can readily accommodate a 21-gauge needle. The lateral cutaneous nerve of the forearm lies nearby, but no important structures lie deep to the fascia. The radial nerve is lateral to the biceps tendon, but it lies in an intramuscular groove deep on the bone, well out of harm's way.

Advantages of the antecubital fossa as a venipuncture site include the following:

1. Veins are larger than other sites on the arm.
2. Veins are not mobile or as mobile as those on the wrist and dorsum of the hand.
3. The lateral aspect of the antecubital fossa is anatomically safe.

Disadvantages of the use of the antecubital fossa for venipuncture are as follows:

1. Veins are not as superficial as in other sites, making venipuncture more difficult in some patients.
2. Anatomically, the medial aspect of the fossa has important anatomy that should be avoided.
3. The antecubital fossa must be immobilized throughout the procedure when a rigid metal needle is used for venipuncture.

It is strongly recommended that the lateral aspect of the antecubital fossa be used preferentially, especially by the more inexperienced phlebotomist. As technical prowess increases, the medial aspect may also be used.

Foot

On a few occasions it may be impractical or impossible to use the arm for venipuncture. Within the dental setting in an elective procedure on an American Society of Anesthesiologists (ASA) I or II patient, it might be advisable to forgo the IV route in lieu of another technique of sedation. However, in pediatric dentistry, where superficial veins of the arm may be small and difficult to locate and cannulate, the foot may be considered as an IV route as more of a necessity than as an elective procedure. In addition, many younger children are not willing to sit quietly in the chair while venipuncture is performed on the arm. This is especially so in pediatric patients who require IV conscious sedation for their management. A child can relatively easily move the arm or grab at it with the opposite hand, dislodging the needle. In this situation the foot may prove a more appropriate site for venipuncture.

The superficial veins of the foot are illustrated in Figure 23-6. Anatomically, the dorsum of the foot

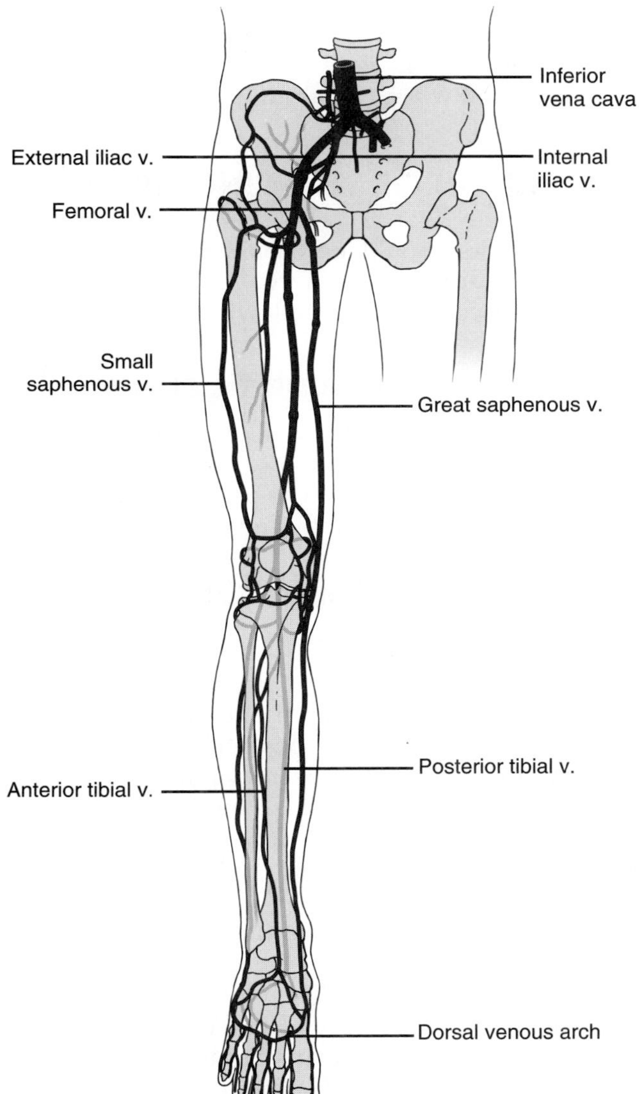

Figure 23-6 Venous drainage of lower limb. (From Liebgott B: *The anatomical basis of dentistry*, ed 2, St. Louis, 2001, Mosby.)

and the medial and lateral aspects of the ankle offer safe sites for venipuncture. In addition, the dorsal veins of the foot are usually quite superficial.

The dorsum of the foot contains a dorsal venous network similar to that found on the dorsum of the hand. As these veins progress toward the ankle, they drain into two major superficial vessels. Located immediately above the medial malleolus is the great saphenous vein, the largest superficial vein in the ankle or foot. On the opposite side, just below the lateral malleolus is found the small saphenous vein.

Advantages of the foot or ankle for venipuncture include the following:

1. Superficial vessels
2. Relatively large vessels
3. Anatomically safe
4. No need to immobilize venipuncture site

Disadvantages of the foot and ankle as a venipuncture site include the following:

1. Accessibility is more limited than upper limb.
2. Veins roll when contacted by needle.

SELECTION OF VENIPUNCTURE SITE

Several factors should be considered when determining the ideal site for a venipuncture attempt.[3] These are discussed in the following sections.

Condition of the Superficial Veins

Veins may appear tortuous, straight, hardened by age, scarred from previous use, sore, or inflamed from recent venipuncture. The preferred vein is one that is unused, easily visible, and relatively straight.

Relation of the Vein to Other Anatomic Structures

Potential venipuncture sites in which other anatomic structures of importance might be damaged should be avoided if possible. In the arm the primary area where this is of significance is the medial aspect of the antecubital fossa.

Duration of the Venipuncture

During prolonged IV infusion (more than 2 hours), a site that permits the patient the greatest freedom of movement is important. Thus a vein traversing a joint, such as the antecubital fossa or wrist, is not ideal for prolonged IV therapy because the joint will require immobilization if a rigid metal needle is used. Venipuncture on the dorsum of the hand or the ventral forearm will be better tolerated in this situation. Patients have complained bitterly, during 2- to 4-hour IV conscious sedation, that their elbow has become quite stiff or sore because of the necessity for immobilization. For shorter durations (less than 2 hours), venipuncture may be established at any site on the limb.

Clinical Status of the Patient

Injury or disease involving one of the limbs may preclude the use of that area for venipuncture. Recent venipuncture in the selected site should lead the doctor to search for another potential site.

A history of phlebitis in the patient should forewarn the doctor to either reconsider the use of IV conscious sedation or to search for the largest vein possible in the selected limb. Patients who have undergone major surgical reconstruction in the upper limb may have deficits in venous drainage from that arm.

Age (Size) of the Patient

In neonates, who are unlikely to be patients in a dental office, scalp veins are preferred because of their accessibility and to simplify the problem of restraint of the infant. In seriously ill newborn infants the umbilical vein may be used during the first 24 to 48 hours of life.

Smaller children may have superficial veins of the upper limb that are very difficult to visualize. The foot may prove a more acceptable site for venipuncture.

In very obese adult patients, veins may prove difficult or impossible to locate. Careful search of both arms and if necessary the feet will usually be fruitful in locating one or more veins. If the planned dental procedure is elective, the absence of superficial veins should be considered a contraindication to the use of IV conscious sedation. Should it be essential to establish an IV line, hospitalization of the patient, with subsequent surgical cutdown to cannulate a vein, may be the most prudent course of action.

Type of Intravenous Procedure

The chemical nature of the drugs being administered, the size of the vein to be cannulated, and the size of the needle are important, for they all may produce irritation of the inner wall of the vein, a situation leading to an increased risk of phlebitis.

In general, the larger the vein is in relation to the size of the needle or catheter, the less likelihood there is that irritation and phlebitis will develop. This is because the drugs and infusion solution will undergo more rapid dilution in the blood where the caliber of the vein exceeds the outside diameter of the needle or cannula. Mechanical irritation by the needle or cannula against the endothelial wall of the vein is another cause of phlebitis. Cannulation of larger veins is a means of decreasing risk of venous irritation and subsequent phlebitis.

Two drugs discussed in this section are capable of producing significant venous irritation. These drugs, diazepam and pentobarbital, are also commonly used IV sedatives in dentistry and medicine. Methods of minimizing the risk of phlebitis when these drugs are administered are discussed in Chapter 26. These drugs should be administered slowly into a rapidly running IV infusion. The use of larger veins will minimize but not eliminate the risk of developing venous irritation.

RECOMMENDED SITES FOR VENIPUNCTURE

Five potential sites for venipuncture in the upper limb have been reviewed in this chapter. They are, in my order of preference (Figure 23-7), as follows:

1. Dorsum of hand
2. Ventral forearm
3. Lateral antecubital fossa
4. Dorsal wrist
5. Medial antecubital fossa

The *dorsum of the hand* is the most preferred site because the veins are superficial and because of the anatomic safety of the site. However, the dorsum is not always an appropriate site for drugs that may produce venous irritation. A close second on the list is the *ventral forearm.* This site is preferred for longer-duration procedures and when the dorsum of the hand is not available. The absence of a need for immobilization of a joint, anatomic safety, and larger veins make this site suitable for most venipuncture procedures.

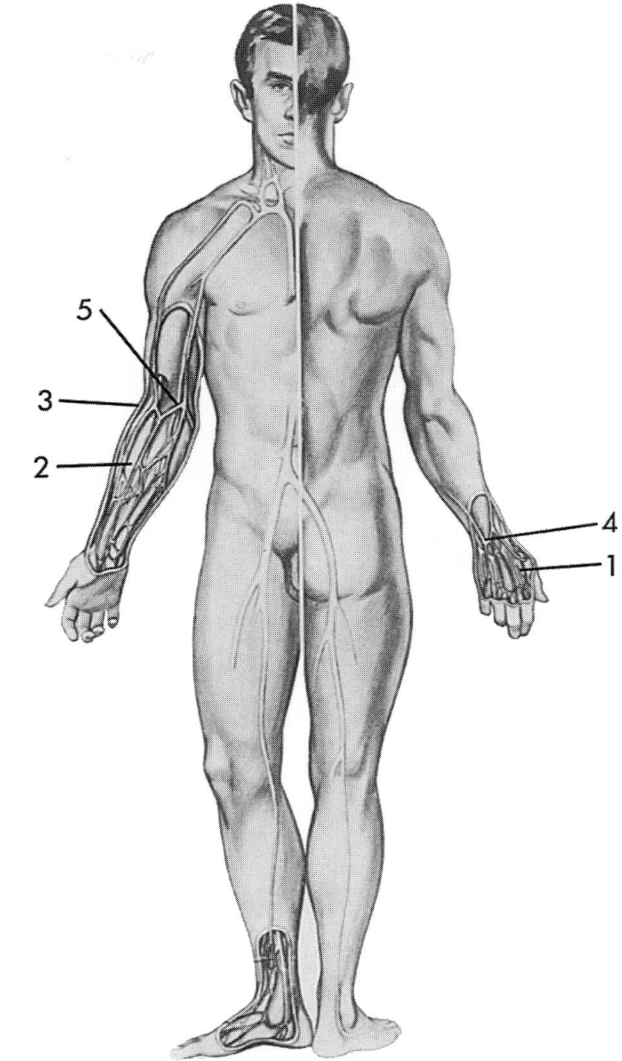

Figure 23-7 Sites of venipuncture in order of preference: *1,* dorsum of hand; *2,* ventral forearm; *3,* lateral antecubital fossa; *4,* dorsal wrist; and *5,* medial antecubital fossa. (From Abbott Laboratories: *Venipuncture and venous circulation,* Chicago, 1971, Abbott Laboratories.)

TABLE 23-1 Comparison of Venipuncture Sites

Order of Preference	Site	Proximity to Important Anatomy	Significant "Roll" or Movement of Vein	Joint Immobilization (Metal Needle Only)
1	Dorsum of hand	No	Yes	No
2	Ventral forearm	No	No	No
3	Lateral antecubital fossa	No	No	Yes
4	Dorsal wrist	No	Yes	Yes
5	Medial antecubital fossa	Yes	No	Yes

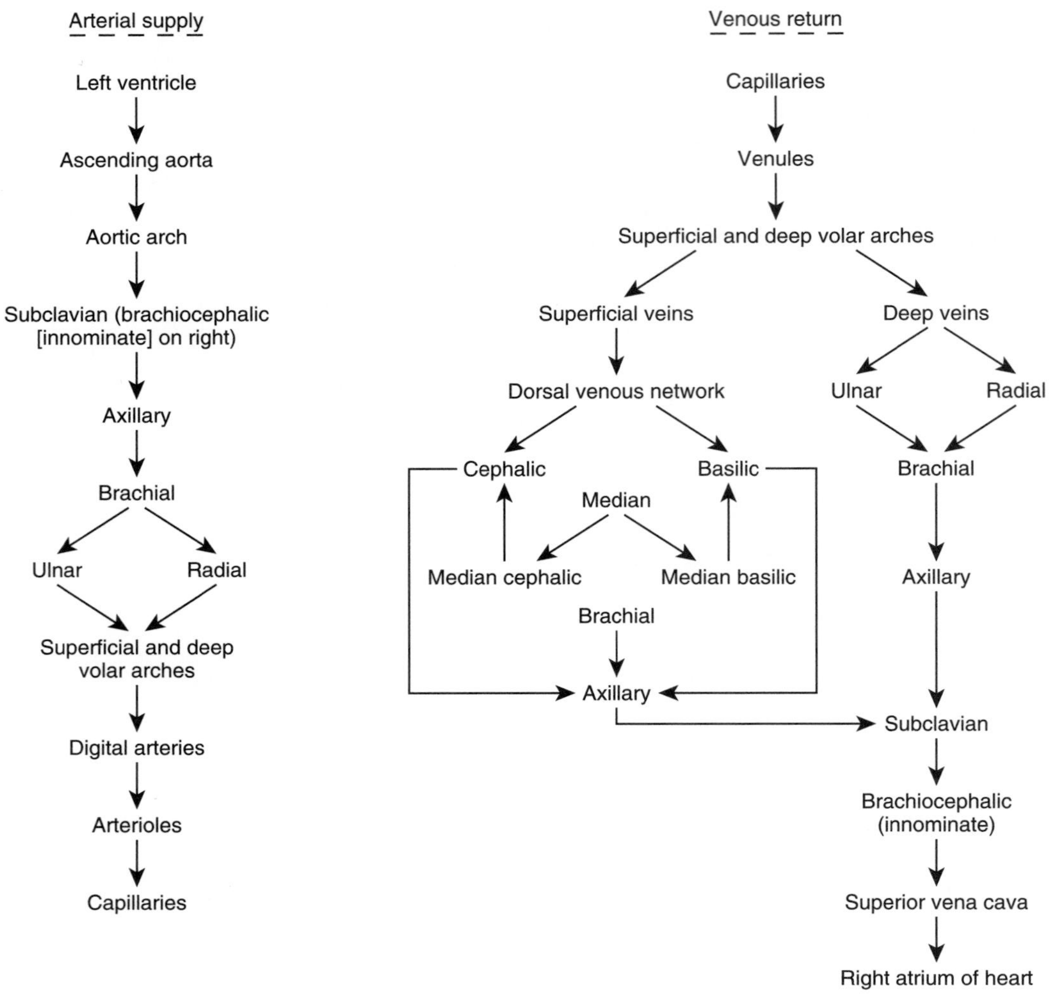

Figure 23-8 Blood circulation in the upper extremity. Blood leaves the left ventricle; traverses arteries, arterioles, capillaries, venules, and veins; and returns to the right atrium via the superior vena cava.

Running far behind the first two sites are the *lateral antecubital fossa,* chosen for its larger veins and anatomic safety; the *dorsal wrist,* with its superficial veins; and last, the *medial antecubital fossa,* with its larger veins but with its significant anatomy just below the surface. All three of these sites will also require immobilization of a joint if rigid metal needles are used.

Table 23-1 summarizes some of the important features of the five venipuncture sites on the upper limb. Figure 23-8 summarizes blood flow through the arm.

REFERENCES

1. Malamed SF: Unpublished data, 1993.
2. Grant JCB: *An atlas of anatomy,* Baltimore, 1962, Williams & Wilkins.
3. Abbott Laboratories: *Venipuncture and venous cannulation,* Chicago, 1971, Abbott Laboratories.

CHAPTER 24

Venipuncture Technique

CHAPTER OUTLINE

The preparation of the equipment for a continuous intravenous (IV) infusion and venipuncture technique is described in this chapter.

PREPARATION OF EQUIPMENT

1. The armamentarium discussed in Chapter 22 is laid out and removed from its packaging.
2. The flow-regulating clamp or screw on the IV infusion set is turned to the closed position so that no fluid will run through the tubing when it is inserted into the bag of IV solution (Figure 24-1).
3. If a winged infusion set is used, it is removed from its box and attached to the end of the IV tubing. The protective sheath covering the needle is left on (Figure 24-2). If an indwelling catheter is to be used, it is not attached to the IV tubing.
4. The cap or cover is removed from the entry ports on the bag of IV infusion solution (Figure 24-3).
5. The protective covering over the piercing pin on the IV tubing is removed carefully so as not to contaminate the pin.
6. The IV infusion bag is held securely in one hand while the piercing pin is firmly pushed through the entry port into the IV solution (Figure 24-4).
7. The bag of IV solution is inverted and suspended from the IV pole.
8. The drip chamber on the IV tubing should be filled approximately halfway with IV solution. If it is not, the chamber can be squeezed and released to draw additional fluid into it (Figure 24-5). If the chamber is overfilled to the extent that it is impossible to visualize individual drops of solution as they exit the IV bag, the bag and drip chamber are inverted and the drip chamber squeezed to force the solution back into the IV bag (Figure 24-6). Care must be taken to avoid the entry of air bubbles into the IV tubing at this time.
9. The flow-regulating clamp or screw is slowly opened, allowing fluid to run through the entire length of the IV tubing and the attached needle, removing all the air bubbles, if possible, from the tubing. On occasion, it will be impossible to remove every bubble from the tubing. Although there is little significance to a few air bubbles entering the

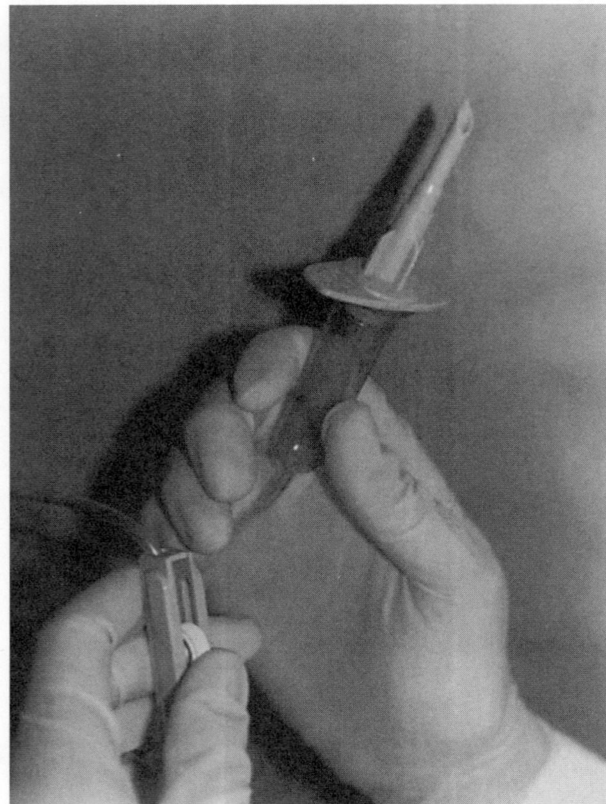

Figure 24-1 The flow-regulating clamp is placed in the closed position.

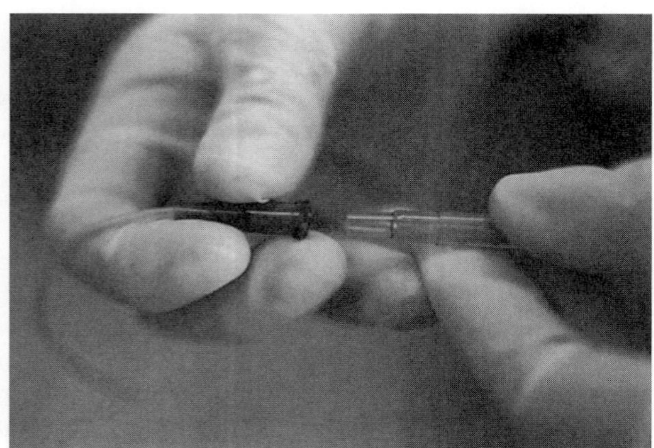

Figure 24-2 The needle is attached to the infusion set.

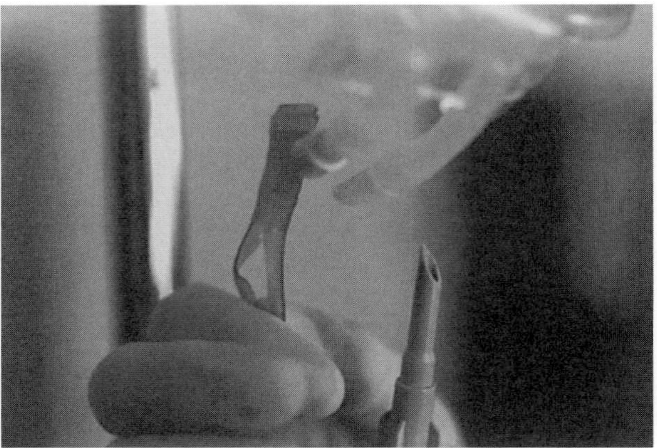

Figure 24-3 Protective caps are removed from the infusion solution and the piercing pin.

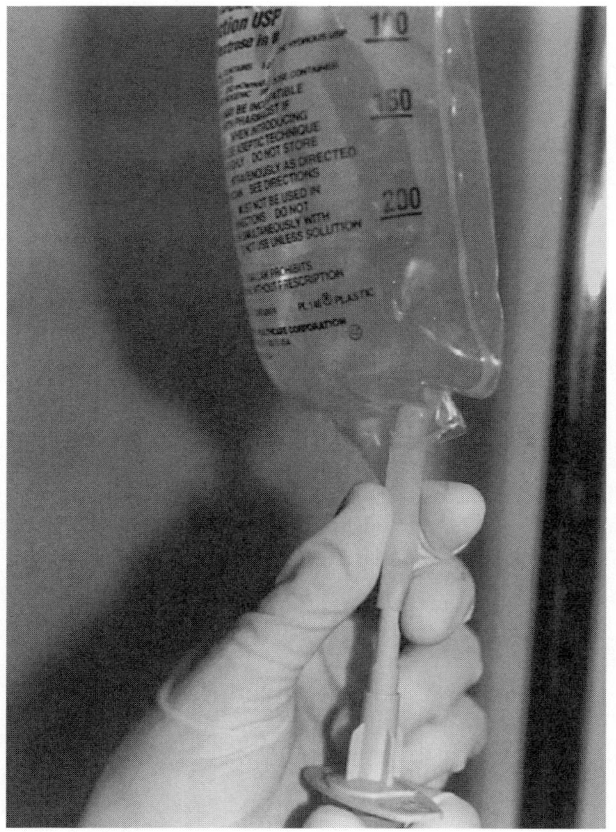

Figure 24-4 The piercing pin is inserted into the entry port on the IV solution container.

patient's cardiovascular system, it is best to attempt to eliminate them. The highly unlikely problem of air embolism is discussed in Chapter 27.

10. The flow-regulating screw is closed to stop the flow of solution. The IV infusion is now ready for use.

Additional equipment required for venipuncture includes the following:

- Tourniquet
- Three to five 3- to 6-inch strips of tape
- Alcohol wipe
- Dry 2-×-2-inch gauze squares
- Armboard: wrist or elbow immobilizer
- Bandage
- Sphygmomanometer
- Stethoscope

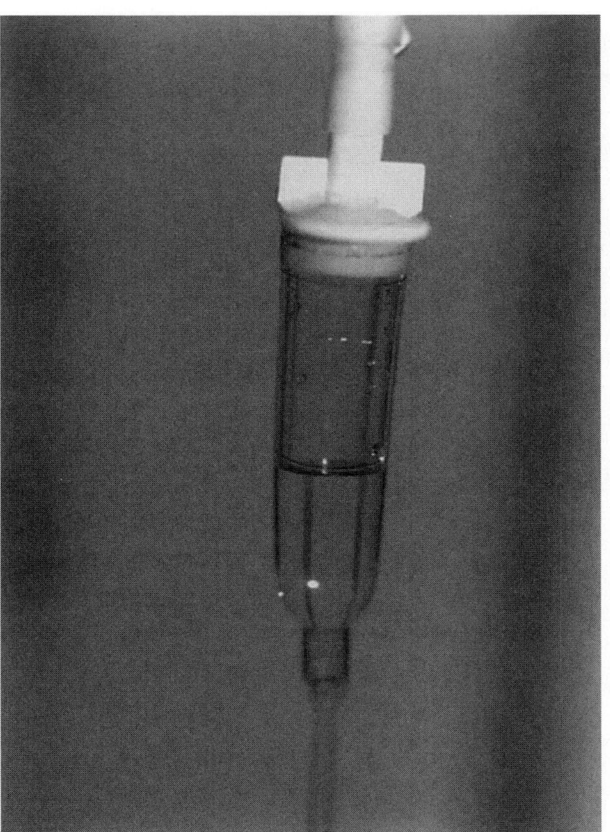

Figure 24-5 The drip chamber should be approximately half filled with solution.

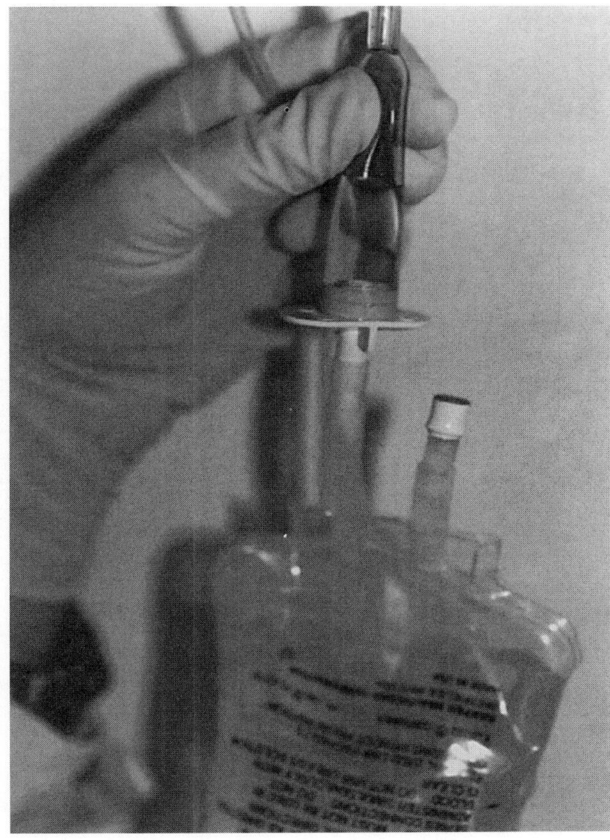

Figure 24-6 If the drip chamber is overfilled, the bag is inverted, and the chamber is squeezed to remove solution.

- Monitoring devices
- Oxygen (O_2) and emergency kit

PREPARATION FOR VENIPUNCTURE

The patient is asked to visit the restroom, if necessary, before the start of the venipuncture. Once the IV has been started with central nervous system (CNS) depressant drugs administered, it will be more difficult for the patient, with the help of the office staff, to accomplish a visit to the restroom.

The patient is seated comfortably in the dental chair. A semireclined to supine position is recommended as being physiologically superior to the upright position for maintenance of blood pressure and adequate respiration.

Preoperative vital signs are recorded on the patient's sedation record sheet (Figure 24-7). Included should be the blood pressure, heart rate and rhythm, respiratory rate, and O_2 saturation. The patient's baseline vital signs have been recorded at a prior visit to the dental office.

The blood pressure cuff (sphygmomanometer) is placed on the left arm and permitted to remain in place throughout the IV procedure. The right arm should be used if the doctor is left-handed.

The patient's arms (without the tourniquet in place) are scanned for obvious veins. Often, veins will be made readily visible if the arm is permitted to hang down below the level of the patient's heart for a few minutes, as this augments venous distention (Figure 24-8). One of the functions of the preoperative visit was to determine whether the patient has suitable veins for the IV procedure.

On occasion, a patient who had very visible, superficial veins at the preoperative visit will appear in the office on treatment day with no obvious veins. This is explained by the presence of a greater degree of anxiety and higher levels of circulating catecholamines. When veins are not readily apparent, the patient should be asked at what site on the arm he has previously had blood drawn successfully. Sometimes a patient will boast that "they had to try four times before they found a vein" or that "three people had to try before they succeeded." This should alert the doctor that a difficult venipuncture might be in the offing. However, such a statement by the patient may also be used to the doctor's advantage. If, by using "special care," the doctor is able to successfully

Patient's Name: S.S. #: Age: DATE ____/____/____

Medical Hx: CVS
Respiratory System
CNS
Liver
Kidneys
Other

Current Medications:

Allergy:

IV started at ________ a.m./p.m.
Venipuncture Site________
Type of Needle ________
IV d/c'd at ________ a.m./p.m.
IV solution & Volume________ML

DRUGS ADMINISTERED
– SUMMARY –

Base Line Vital Signs:
Date of V.S.:
B.P.: P.R.:
R.: T.:
Ht.: Wt.:
Age:

ASA: I, II, III, IV

Reason for Sedation:

Evaluator:

Name of Driver:

PREOPERATIVE time	INTRAOPERATIVE time	time	time	time	time	POST-OP time	DISCHARGE time
Blood Pressure							
Heart Rate							
Respirations							
O_2 LPM							
N_2O LPM							
(mg)							
(mg)							
(mg)							
(mg)							
(mg)							
(mg)							
(mg)							

List all drugs and route of administration (IV, IM)

DRUGS DISCARDED
– SUMMARY –

DENTISTRY TREATMENT

Start ____ Finish ____
Name of person discharged to: ________
Post-Op Medicarions (if any) ________

Additional Monitoring: precordial stethoscope ________ pulse oximeter ________
(check as appropriate) ECG ________ automatic blood pressure ________

COMMENTS

Student Doctor: ________ AMED Faculty: ________ ☐ Informed Consent
IV Student: ________ Assistants: ________ ☐ Post-Operative Instructions

SAM/USC/SOD
02/85

Figure 24-7 Sample of a sedation record for IV sedation procedure.

complete the venipuncture on the first or second attempt, the patient will feel more confident in that doctor's overall ability. Several methods of distending veins are available and are discussed later.

If the Trieger test for evaluation of recovery is to be used (see Chapter 5), the baseline Trieger test is now completed by the patient. Any other monitoring devices, such as the pulse oximeter, pretracheal stethoscope, or electrocardioscope, are now placed on the patient.

Because of the possibility of accidental inoculation of health professionals with viral and other organisms found in some patients' blood, universal precautions are essential in situations involving potential contact with blood. All persons working with the venipuncture should wear masks, glasses, and gloves. Gloves must be worn throughout the procedure, from the point of preparation until the IV is removed, the bleeding stops, and a bandage is in place. For doctors and personnel who have performed venipuncture for many years without using gloves, this may present a little difficulty at first. However, with perseverance, the wearing of gloves will no longer seem an added burden, only an additional safety measure.

> **Caution**
> Latex gloves should *always* be worn by all personnel while preparing for and performing venipuncture.

A tourniquet is next applied to the limb (arm or leg) selected for venipuncture. On the arm the tourniquet is applied superior to the antecubital fossa. The commonly used soft rubber tubing is applied in a slipknot (Figure 24-9). The tourniquet should be sufficiently tight to prevent venous drainage from the arm without obstructing arterial flow into the arm. A radial pulse should still be present with the tourniquet in place.

When a blood pressure cuff is used as a tourniquet, the pressure in the cuff is raised and locked at a point between the patient's systolic and diastolic pressures (e.g., 120 mm Hg if the blood pressure is 140/90 mm

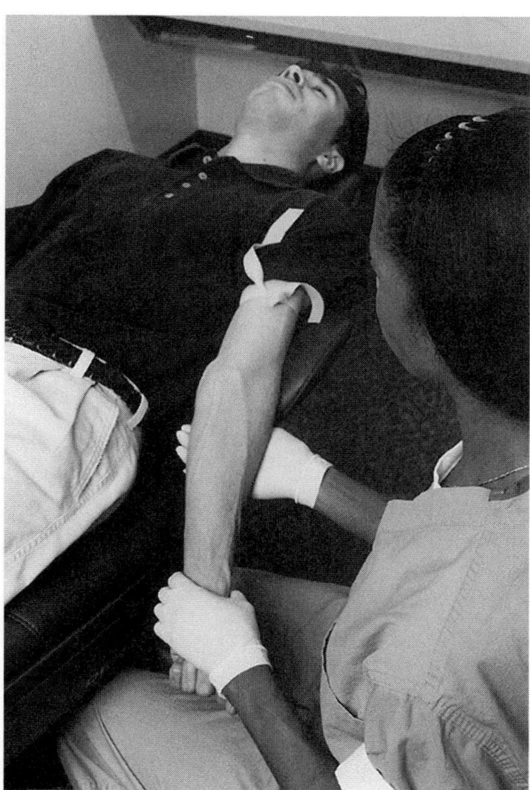

Figure 24-8 Distention of veins may be augmented by permitting the arm to hang below heart level.

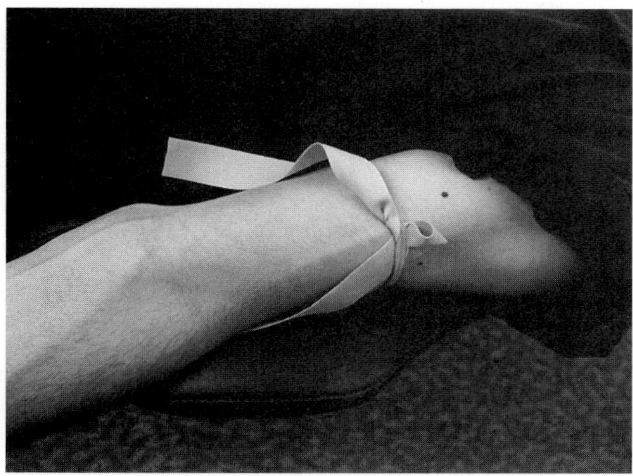

Figure 24-9 A tourniquet is applied, using a slipknot, above the antecubital fossa. Opening and closing of the hand further aids venous distention.

Hg). This produces venous distention in the same manner as the tourniquet.

The patient is then asked to repeatedly open and close her or his hand into a fist. Muscular activity forces more blood into the veins, allowing additional arterial blood to enter into the limb and further distend the veins. Once the veins have been distended, the patient is asked to keep the fist clenched until the venipuncture has been successfully completed.

At this point, most persons will have one or more readily visible veins; however, some others will as yet have no visible or even palpable veins. Several methods are available to increase venous distention.

1. *Light slapping* or *rubbing of the skin* over the vessel will aid in venodilation.
2. Anything that produces heat aids in dilating a blood vessel. The direct application of heat to the area is also a great aid.
   a. A *warm, moist towel* may be applied for several minutes to the entire region proximal and distal to the proposed venipuncture site.
   b. It has been suggested that an *electric hairdryer* can be used as a quick method to produce vasodilation at almost any site.
3. Another means of producing vasodilation is to use nitrous oxide–oxygen (N_2O-O_2) sedation, which produces the following beneficial effects during venipuncture:
   a. Peripheral vasodilation
   b. A degree of analgesia, making the venipuncture less traumatic

When N_2O-O_2 is used as an aid during venipuncture, the patient should be sedated as in Chapter 15 (titrated) and returned to a nonsedated state before the administration of any IV medications.

Once the vein chosen for cannulation has been adequately distended, the site must be prepared. Physical restraints are seldom required in adults because most patients rarely object strenuously to venipuncture (although they may not "like it"). When a vein in the antecubital fossa is selected, an elbow immobilizer should be placed before the start of the venipuncture (Figure 24-10). When the wrist is selected, the wrist immobilizer is applied after the venipuncture.

Some experts recommend that any solution used to cleanse the injection site be warmed to body temperature. Because the arm is warm, it is more sensitive to cold, so that the blood vessel may contract (i.e., disappear or "collapse") almost immediately on exposure to a cold or rapidly evaporating solution such as alcohol.

When needles larger than 20 gauge (18, 16, or 14 gauge) are used, venipuncture can be rendered virtually painless by simply raising a wheal in the skin over the vein by injecting 0.2 to 0.3 ml of a 1% lidocaine hydrochloride solution (Figure 24-11). A 25-gauge needle should be used. However, use of needles of 20 gauge or smaller is not associated with excessive discomfort, so the preceding technique is not necessary. Indeed, the injection of lidocaine itself produces a stinging sensation.

For truly needle-phobic patients, the use of EMLA should be considered. EMLA, eutectic mixture of local anesthetics, is a local anesthetic ointment consisting of

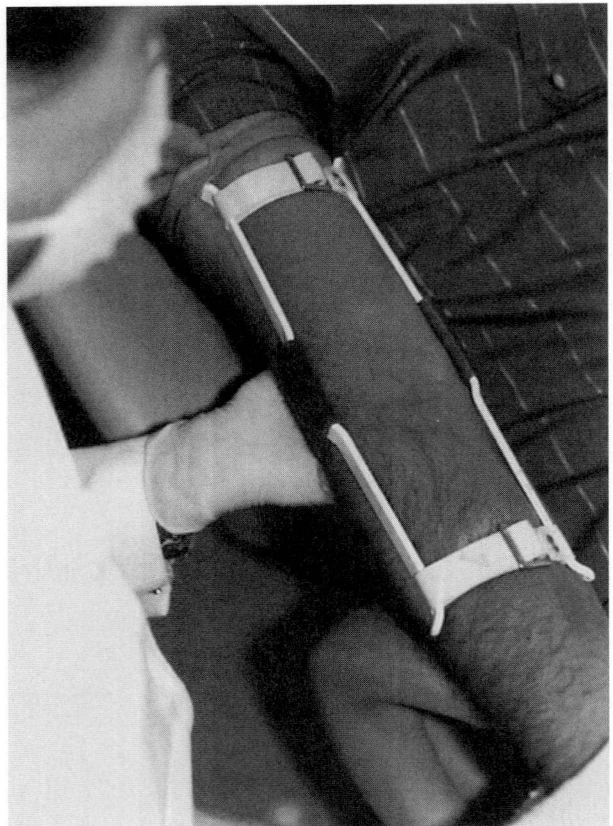

Figure 24-10 Elbow immobilizer is placed before venipuncture.

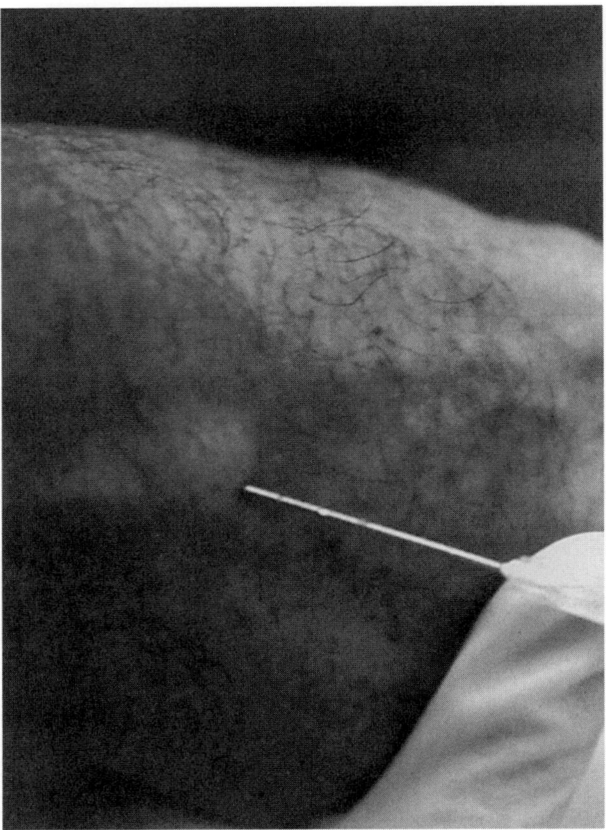

Figure 24-11 One percent lidocaine wheal is raised at site of venipuncture.

base forms of prilocaine and lidocaine.[1] It is applied to the proposed venipuncture site 1 hour before the procedure and covered with an occlusive bandage. In most instances it is recommended that two sites, one on either arm, be treated with EMLA.

Patients who are fearful about both the dental and the IV procedure should have received preoperative oral sedative drugs approximately 1 hour before the planned start of the procedure. Sedation with N_2O-O_2 should also be considered at this time.

The venipuncture site must now be cleansed. In many large hospitals it is common to prepare the venipuncture site using both a defatting agent and an antibacterial agent. Commonly available preparations are benzalkonium chloride tincture and 70% alcohol solution and 99% isopropyl alcohol and Betadine (povidone-iodine). Povidone-iodine solution is preferred to tincture of iodine because it is considerably less irritating and equally effective; on the other hand, tincture of iodine is more rapidly acting. In most short-term IV situations, the traditional isopropyl alcohol wipe is still used and is considered the minimal preparation recommended at the IV site. The site is thoroughly cleansed with the alcohol wipe and permitted to air-dry, or a sterile, dry 2-×-2-inch gauze wipe may be used to dry the area before venipuncture.

WINGED INFUSION SET

Dorsum of Hand

The wings of the needle are held by the thumb and middle fingers, with the index finger placed between the wings (Figure 24-12).[2] This permits the operator the greatest control over the needle. Holding the needle as illustrated in Figure 24-13 with the finger beneath the needle interferes with the venipuncture. The sheath over the needle is removed, and care must be taken from this point on not to contaminate the needle by touching it to any object. Should this occur, the needle is immediately replaced with a new, sterile one. Air in the tubing of the new needle must be removed by running the IV infusion solution through the needle.

The patient's hand is kept in a clenched fist until the venipuncture is completed. The patient's fist is supported in the doctor's left hand, with the thumb of the doctor's left hand placed below the patient's knuckles

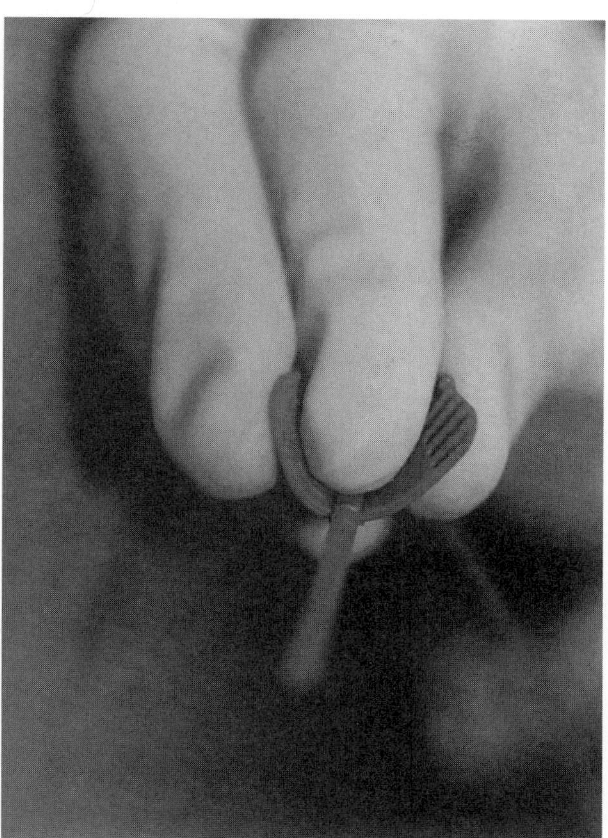

Figure 24-12 The index finger is placed between the wings of the needle, and the wings are folded over by thumb and middle fingers. This provides the doctor with increased tactile sensation during venipuncture.

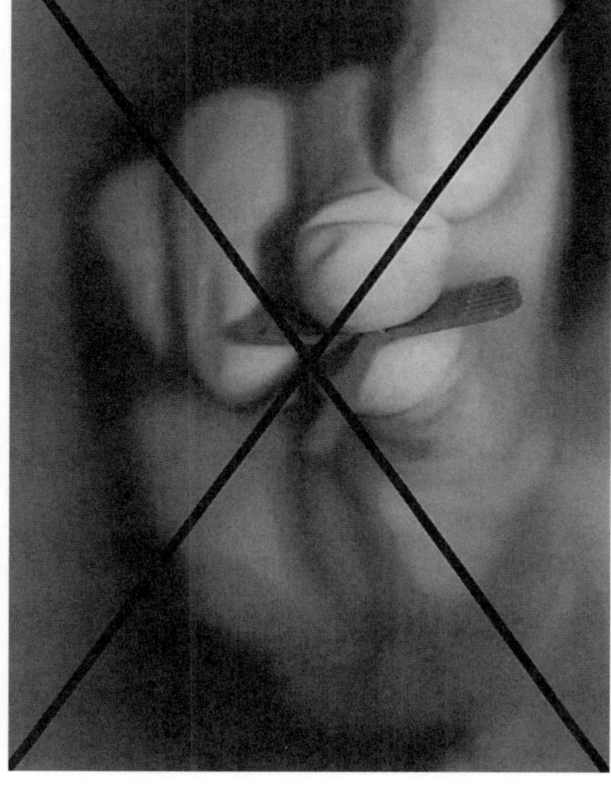

Figure 24-13 The thumb and index finger are placed on either side of the wings of the needle. This technique makes it more difficult to successfully complete venipuncture.

and the skin of the dorsum of the hand pulled toward the doctor (Figure 24-14).

These two techniques minimize mobility of the vein during venipuncture. Should this be ineffective, the patient should bend the fist down. This further immobilizes the vein. Care is taken in these techniques because in some patients the vein may actually collapse when attempts are made to immobilize it.

When the dorsum of the hand is used for venipuncture, the site of needle entry into the skin is lateral to the vein and approximately ¼ inch below the desired point of entry of the needle into the vein (Figure 24-15). This takes into account the mobility of these veins. Should the needle be placed directly atop the vein, as pressure is applied on the needle, the vein will invariably roll out from under the needle.

The optimal angle of entry of the needle through the skin is 30 degrees (Figure 24-16). Angles greater than this increase the risk of the needle traveling through the entire vein, and angles less than 30 degrees are associated with increased discomfort during passage of the needle through the skin. *The bevel of the needle will always be facing up.* The point of the needle is placed gently against the skin at the site of entry with the needle directed parallel to the course of the vein. With the skin of the dorsum still pulled over the knuckles, the point of the needle penetrates the skin lateral to the vein. Resistance will be noted as the needle passes through the skin. Once through the skin, resistance markedly decreases. At this point, the angle of the needle is decreased so that the needle shaft is held parallel to the skin (Figure 24-17). The veins of the dorsum are quite superficial, and if the needle is directed deeper, the vein may be missed entirely. The direction of the needle is also altered at this time. The needle should be angled toward the spot on the vein where the needle tip is about to enter the lumen of the vessel. Angulation should be gentle so that the needle meets with the vein about 10 mm above the point of entry into the skin.

The needle is gently advanced toward the vein. There should be little resistance and no discomfort to the patient at this time. As the needle tip comes into contact with the vein wall on the dorsum of the hand, the doctor may observe the vein move as the needle tip pushes it. This is a common occurrence and is easily

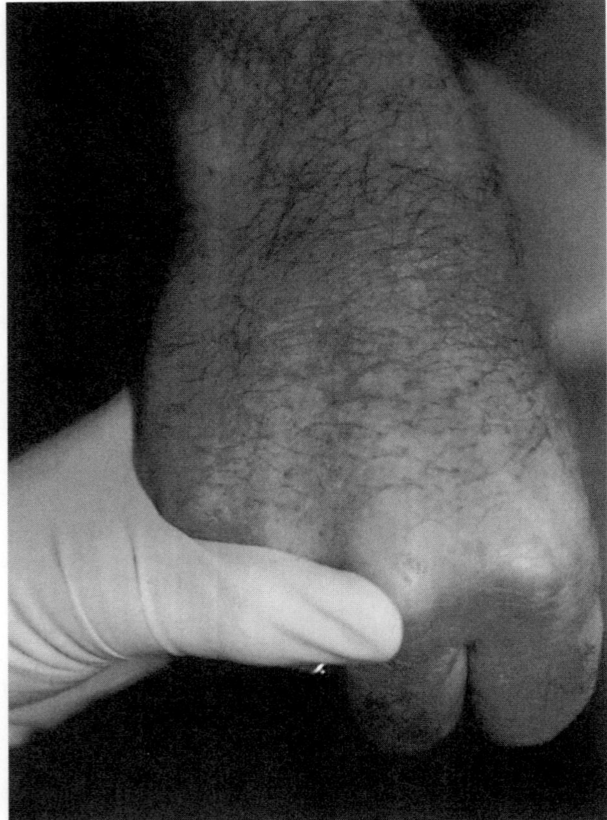

Figure 24-14 The doctor supports the patient's hand and pulls the skin of the hand over the knuckle.

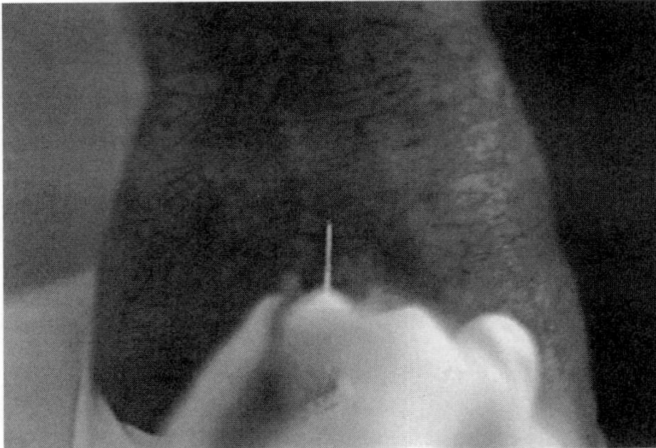

Figure 24-15 Entry point of the needle is just lateral to the vein

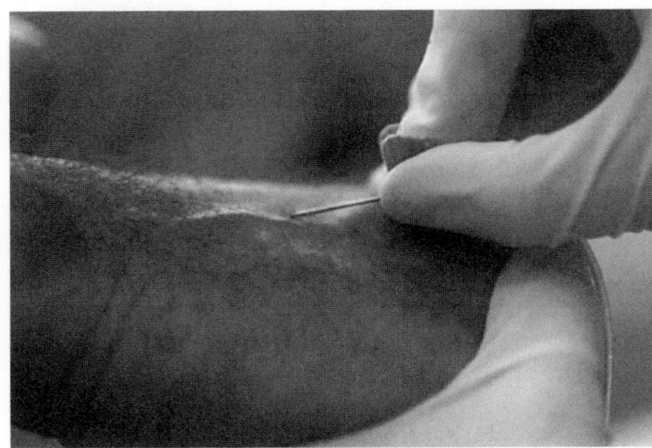

Figure 24-16 Optimum angle of needle entry is 30 degrees.

managed. The needle tip has yet to enter the lumen of the vein, but the tip has contacted the vein wall. As the needle continues to move in the same direction, the vein may continue to be pushed along with the needle. Because the vein cannot move indefinitely within the confines of the skin, it will soon appear to "pop" and to move back to its original position on the hand. (This is similar to increasing pressure being applied to the outside of an inflated balloon until the balloon finally pops.) This occurs as the needle enters into the lumen and resistance is lost. On some occasions, the patient may also be aware of this "popping" feeling.

A backflow of blood into the tubing is the one sure sign of successful venipuncture (Figure 24-18). The needle is redirected so that it lies parallel to the direction of the vein, and it is advanced very gently several more millimeters into the lumen of the vessel. This minimizes the risk of a needle that is tenuously placed within a vein, becoming dislodged as it is being secured or if the patient accidentally moves his or her hand.

Care must be taken during this procedure so that the sharp tip of this rigid needle does not puncture or perforate the inferior wall of the vessel. To prevent this, the needle tip is angled so that it is held upward within the lumen of the vein as the needle is being advanced. The shaft of the needle need be placed only a few millimeters into the lumen of the vein. Attempts to advance the entire needle shaft into the vessel often result in loss of the vein through puncture of the wall ("blowing the vein") and in the formation of a hematoma.

Once the needle is inside the vein, the plastic wings of the needle are placed against the patient's skin and held in position by the doctor while the assistant performs several important tasks. The doctor's primary job at this time is to maintain the needle within the vein.

The assistant releases the tourniquet on the patient's arm, resulting in a significant drop in venous blood pressure. The blood leaves the IV tubing, reentering the blood vessel. The tourniquet is removed and the IV infusion started. The assistant opens the flow screw or knob on the tubing and drops of solution should form in the drip chamber. This is done immediately to prevent clotting of blood within the needle or tubing. The next task is to secure the needle within the vein by taping the needle into position.

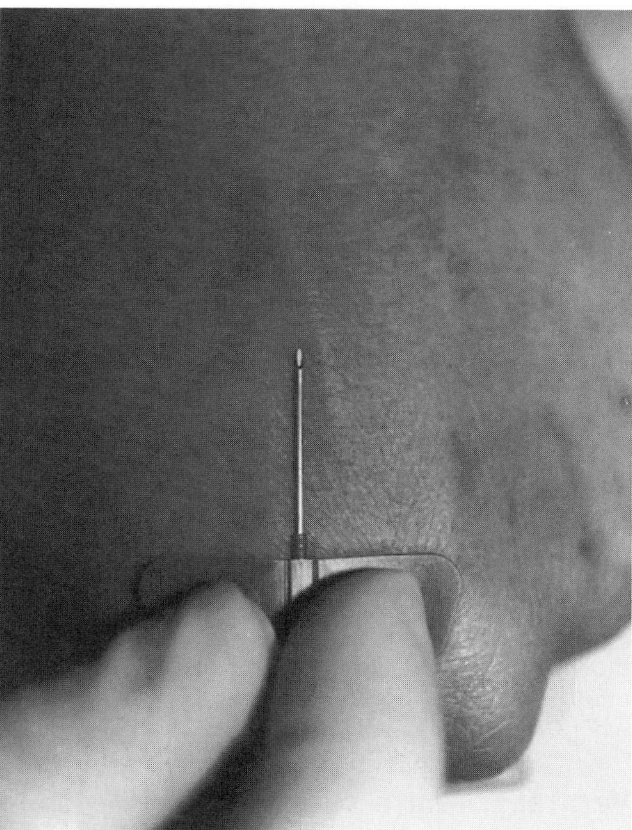

Figure 24-17 The angle of the needle is decreased, and the needle tip is directed toward the vein.

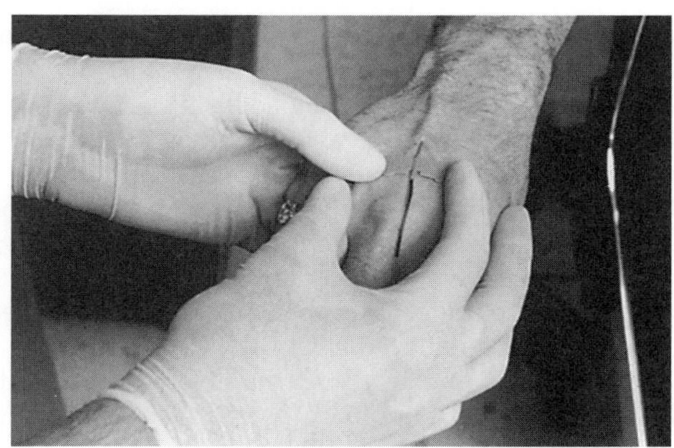

Figure 24-18 Return of blood into IV tubing signifies successful venipuncture. The doctor holds the wing securely until the needle is secured.

Many variations on taping exist, but only one is offered here. The goal in taping, of course, is to secure the needle in position for the duration of the planned procedure. With the doctor holding the needle gently against the patient's skin, a 3-inch piece of tape is placed across one of the wings, parallel to the direction in which the needle is pointing. A second piece of tape is placed on the other wing in the same exact manner.

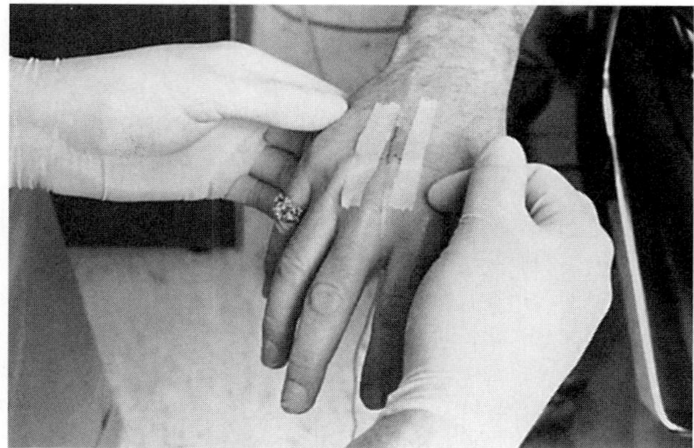

Figure 24-19 Tape is placed across each wing and secured from below needle proximally.

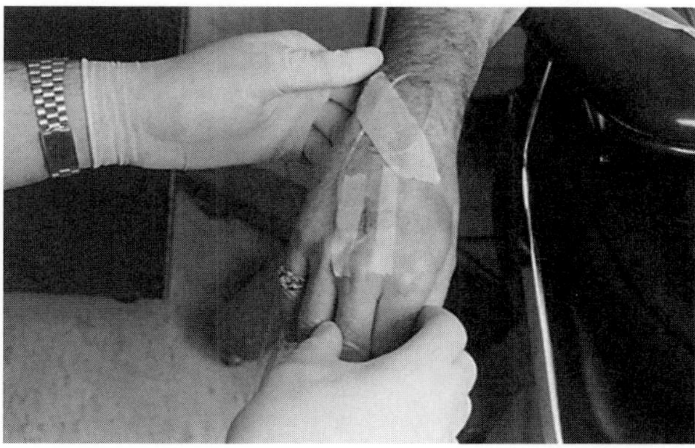

Figure 24-20 Loop of tubing is secured with the third piece of tape, and the fourth piece is placed at the site of needle penetration of the skin.

It is strongly recommended that as the tape is being secured against the skin, it be applied from the site away from the needle entry point into the skin toward the needle tip (Figure 24-19). Although this may seem a trivial point, I have observed many doctors accidentally dislodge the needle from the vein as they sought to secure it with tape and applied pressure from the needle tip toward the wings.

A 5- to 6-inch length of tape is next placed across a loop made in the IV tubing. This loop serves as a shock absorber in the event that the IV tubing is accidentally pulled. The loop of tubing serves to prevent the needle from being easily dislodged from the vein.

A fourth piece of tape, about 3 inches long, is placed over the site at which the needle enters the skin to keep the site clean. This is done only if the tape is transparent. The site of needle entry into the skin should remain visible during the procedure in the event of swelling or discomfort at the site (Figure 24-20). The patient is now ready for the administration of IV drugs.

The most pressing problem in establishing an IV infusion on the dorsum of the hand is the mobility of the veins; any method of immobilization is appreciated. Three means of so doing have been described (clenched fist, bending hand, and thumb pulling skin over knuckles). A fourth, a naturally occurring anatomic configuration of veins, may also be used to advantage. This configuration involves the formation of an inverted Y from the merging of two smaller veins to form a larger one. Often, this configuration is located just above the knuckles as two digital veins converge (Figure 24-21). Basic venipuncture technique is identical to that just described, the primary difference being that entry of the needle into the vein occurs at the point of confluence of these three vessels. If the needle is inserted between the two digital veins and aimed for the point at which they meet, the veins are prevented from rolling away from the needle.

The needle enters into the skin about ¼ inch to ½ inch below the convergence of the veins and is directed toward that spot. Pressure is exerted on the needle, which then enters the lumen of the vein; the needle is advanced and then secured as previously described. The inverted Y is a highly recommended site for venipuncture on the dorsum of the hand.

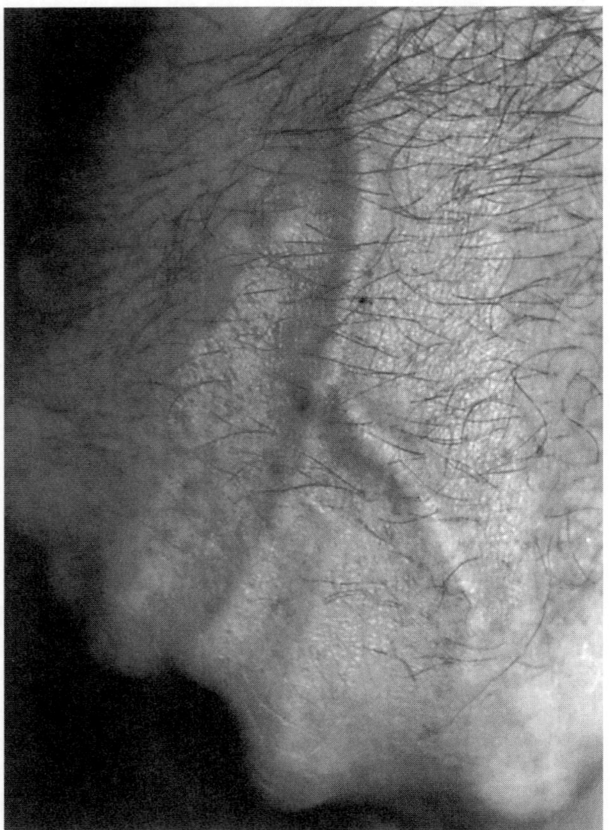

Figure 24-21 Y formed by merging of two veins is ideal configuration for venipuncture. Needle is placed approximately 1/4 to 1/2 inch below convergence of veins.

Following successful venipuncture on the dorsum of the hand, immobilizing the wrist should be considered if the needle tip is located in its proximity. Needles placed further away from the wrist do not require the use of an arm immobilizer (Figure 24-22).

The patient holds the armboard securely while tape is placed around the fingers and the armboard. The proximal end of the armboard is then taped to the patient's forearm. A piece of gauze placed between the patient's skin and the tape will prevent hair from sticking to the tape and minimize patient discomfort when the tape is removed.

Dorsum of Wrist

The technique of venipuncture on the dorsum of the wrist with the winged infusion set is identical to that just described for the dorsum of the hand. It is extremely rare to find the inverted Y configuration on the wrist; however, where it is present, its use is recommended. The use of an armboard is necessary whenever a rigid needle tip is located in the wrist.

Ventral Forearm

The ventral aspect of the forearm is a recommended site for venipuncture. Because veins at this site are less superficial than those of the dorsum of the hand and wrist, they tend to be less mobile. Because of this decreased mobility, there is a slight variation in the venipuncture technique on the ventral forearm.

On the ventral forearm, the needle is placed directly atop the vein to be entered rather than on its side. Held in the same 30-degree angle, the needle is directed into the skin and then directly into the vein. Once blood returns into the tubing, signifying successful entry into the vein, the angle of the needle is decreased so that it is held almost parallel to the skin and slowly advanced several millimeters into the vein.

During venipuncture, the thumb of the opposite hand of the doctor should be placed on the skin several inches below (distal to) the planned entry site, pulling skin at the site in a direction opposite to that of the needle (Figure 24-23). This facilitates entry of the needle through the skin. All other components of venipuncture at this site are identical to the basic procedure described above. Immobilization of the wrist or antecubital fossa is not required when the forearm is used for venipuncture with a rigid needle.

Antecubital Fossa

The technique of venipuncture at either the medial or lateral antecubital fossa is identical to that of the ventral forearm, with the important exception that the elbow *must* be immobilized. It is suggested that immobilization of the joint occur before venipuncture rather than after, when any accidental movement by the patient might dislodge the needle (Figure 24-24).

Occasionally, veins in the antecubital fossa will be superficial. In this case it is possible that the vein will roll out from under the needle as venipuncture progresses. Should this occur, the attempt is continued using the technique described for the dorsum of the hand, with the needle entering from the side of the vein.

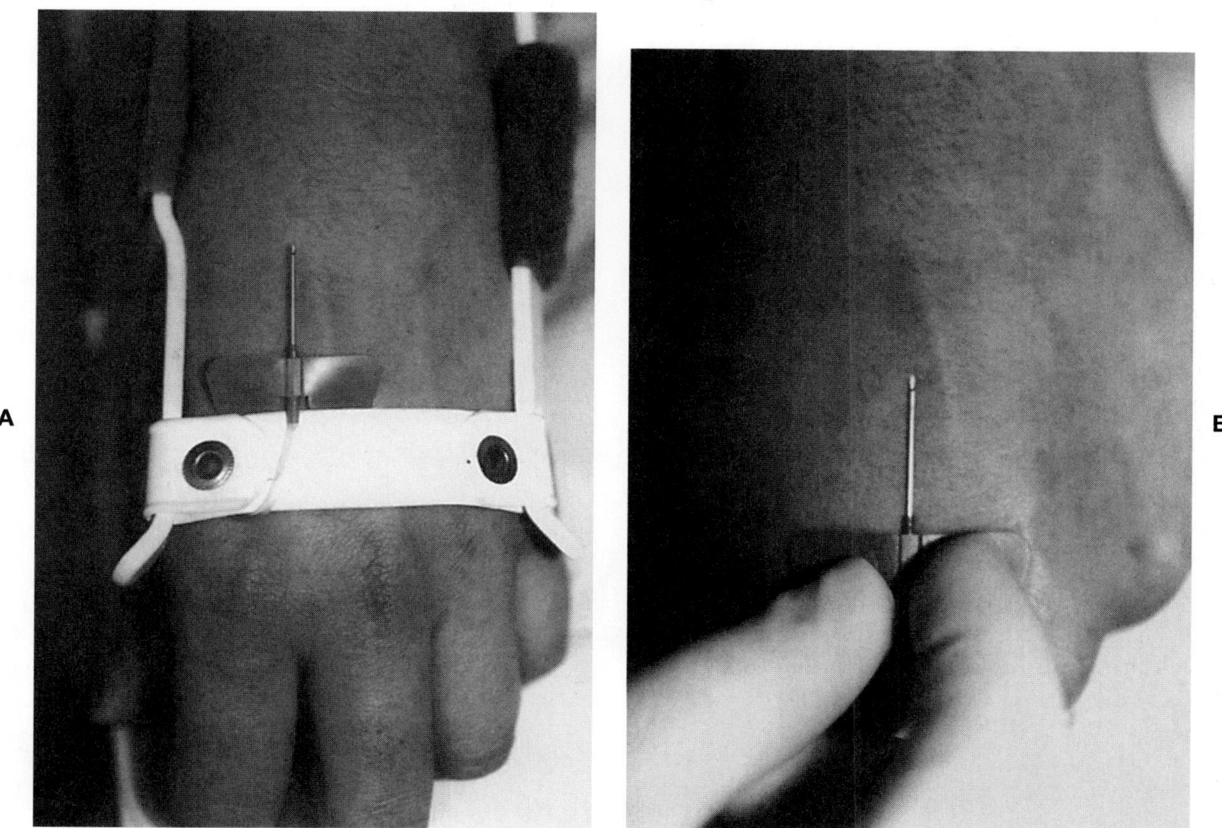

Figure 24-22 The needle placed in dorsum of wrist requires wrist to be immobilized **(A)**, whereas needle placed in dorsum of hand does not **(B)**.

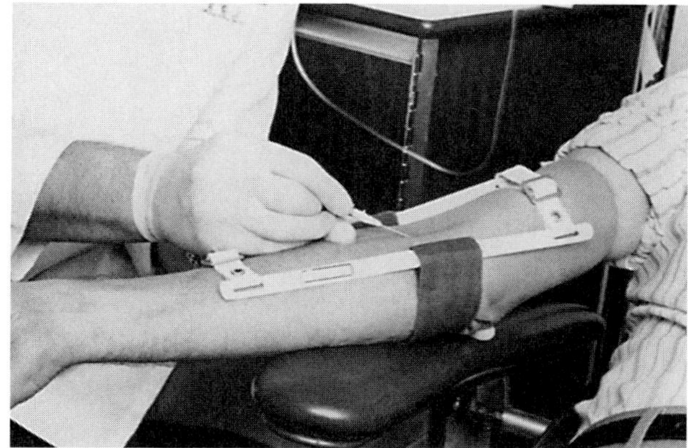

Figure 24-23 Angle of penetration of skin is 30 degrees. Skin is retracted by the fingers of the other hand.

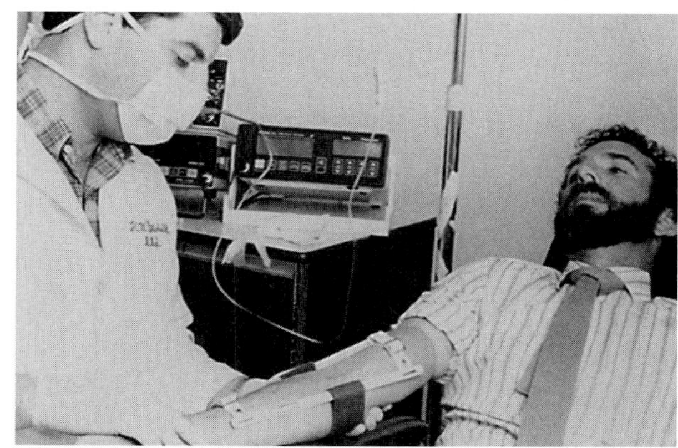

Figure 24-24 The antecubital fossa is immobilized before venipuncture.

INDWELLING CATHETER: ALL INJECTION SITES

The indwelling catheter requires a somewhat different venipuncture technique from that just described for the winged infusion set, a device that is somewhat more manageable by the beginner. The IV infusion is prepared for use as described previously, with the exception that the catheter is not attached to the IV tubing.

The vein is selected, distended, and prepared for venipuncture in the usual manner. The indwelling catheter is held at a 30-degree angle to the skin, either lateral to the vein or directly atop it, depending on the site of venipuncture.[3,4] The skin is pulled in the direction opposite to which the needle is being advanced to facilitate passage through the skin. Resistance is lost once skin is penetrated, the angle of the needle is decreased, and the needle is directed toward the vein. On entry of the needle into the vein, blood is noted in the needle (Figure 24-25). The needle is angled parallel to the course of the vein and advanced a few more millimeters into the vessel. It is at this point that the technique of venipuncture with the indwelling catheter differs from the technique with the winged infusion set.

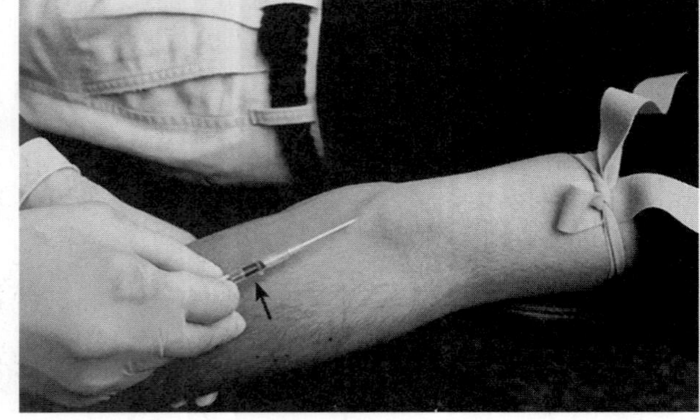

Figure 24-25 The needle is inserted into vein at 30-degree angle *(arrow)* **(A)** until blood return is observed in plastic window *(arrow)* **(B)**.

The hub of the metal needle is held securely in one hand while the other hand is placed on the catheter hub. The entire length of the plastic catheter is slowly and gently advanced into the vein (Figure 24-26). It is important that *the catheter not be forced if any resistance is encountered.* It is also important that only the catheter *be advanced into* the vein and that the metal introducer (the metal needle) *not be withdrawn* from the catheter.

The tourniquet is removed to decrease venous pressure. The assistant holds the needle adapter end of the IV tubing while the doctor removes the metal introducer needle from the indwelling catheter. The needle adapter is expeditiously connected to the catheter hub, and the IV flow is begun (Figure 24-27). The needle adapter and catheter must not be released at this time because they have yet to be secured. Once the introducer needle is removed from the catheter, blood will flow

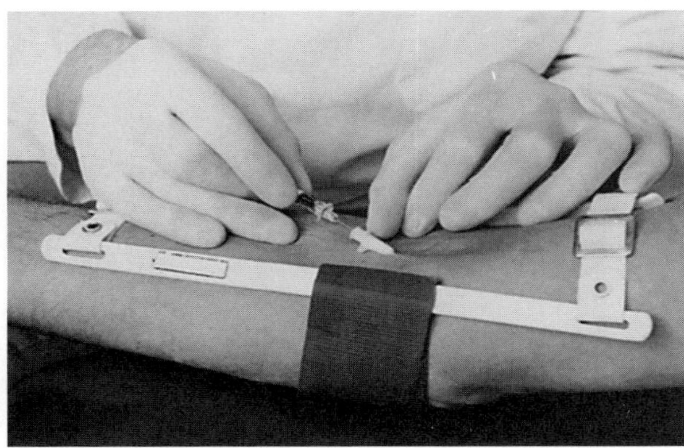

Figure 24-26 Once the vein is entered, decrease the needle angle, advance the needle several millimeters into vein, and advance the catheter to its hub.

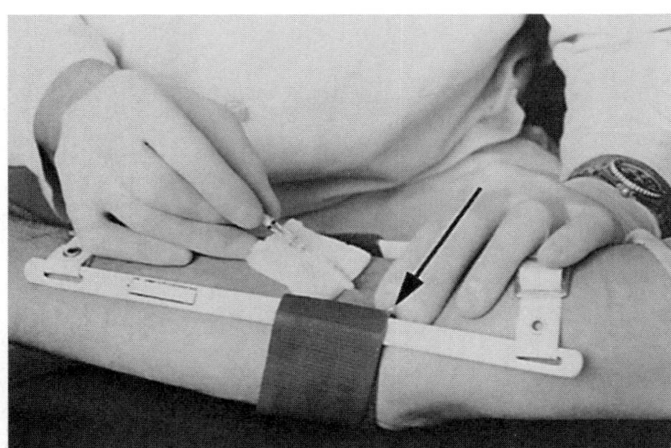

Figure 24-27 The catheter is inserted slowly into the vein, and the metal needle is removed. Note the placement of the doctor's finger over the tip of the catheter *(arrow)*. This prevents any bleeding when the metal needle is removed.

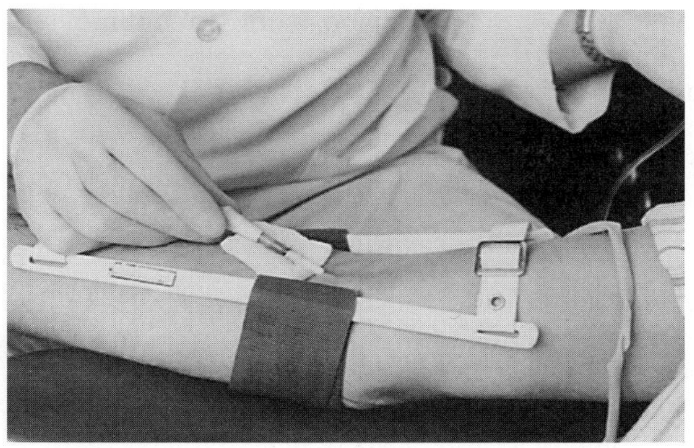

Figure 24-28 IV tubing is attached to the catheter, the drip is started, and the flash bulb is squeezed to check adequacy of venipuncture.

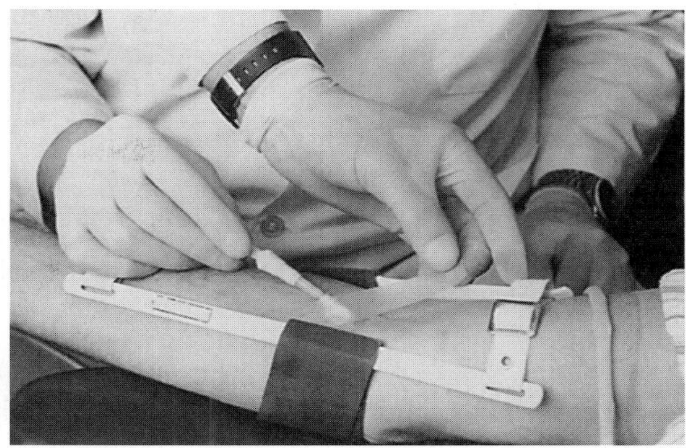

Figure 24-29 Adhesive is placed beneath the catheter and then brought forward onto the skin.

back into the catheter and onto the patient if the catheter is not attached to the IV tubing. The importance of removing the tourniquet before this step is obvious, for what amounts to a mere oozing of blood out of the catheter without the tourniquet would be a river of blood if the tourniquet were left in place. Even for experienced hands, this step can become untidy. To minimize this possibility the following is suggested:

1. Release the tourniquet.
2. Place a dry 2-×-2-inch gauze wipe beneath the end of the catheter (see Figure 24-27). This will absorb the small volume of blood that might be lost.
3. Press your fingertip onto the skin directly above the tip of the plastic catheter within the vein. This occludes the catheter, preventing any blood loss.
4. Connect the needle adapter and the catheter (Figure 24-28).

If step 3 is done properly, this entire process can be completed at a leisurely pace, without the loss of any blood.

The IV drip is now started and the catheter secured with tape. Although several taping techniques are available, just one is presented here. A 5- or 6-inch piece of narrow tape is used for taping the catheter. (This tape is prepared by tearing a full piece of tape in half lengthwise.) Standard-size Scotch-brand tape (uncut) is of suitable width (not more than 1 inch wide). The center of the tape is placed beneath the catheter just below the needle adapter with the adhesive side of the tape facing upward (away from the skin). One end of the tape is then crossed over the top of the catheter and secured against the skin (Figure 24-29). The same process occurs for the other end of the tape, crossing the catheter and the first piece of tape. This technique results in the catheter being securely placed within the lumen of the vein, with little possibility of its being accidentally removed.

The connection between the needle adapter and the catheter is checked to ensure that it is secure. A 5- to 6-inch piece of tape is then placed over the connection (Figure 24-30).

A loop is made with the IV tubing and taped against the skin. Whenever tape is used to secure a venipuncture, it should be secured to the patient's skin, not to another piece of tape. If one piece of tape becomes loose, any tape that is attached to it will also become loose, jeopardizing the venipuncture.

Because the flexible catheter lies within the vein, neither armboards nor elbow immobilizers are

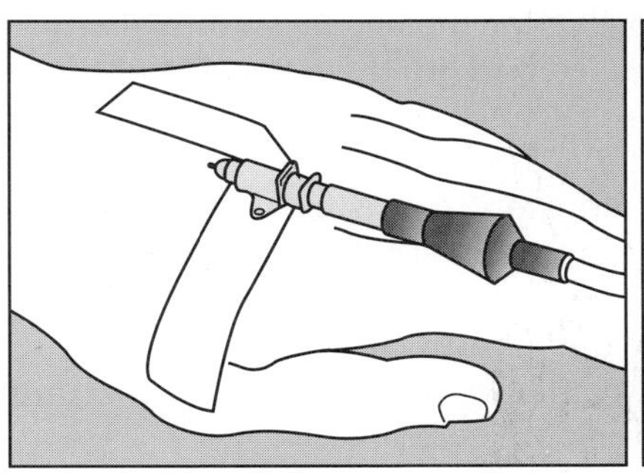

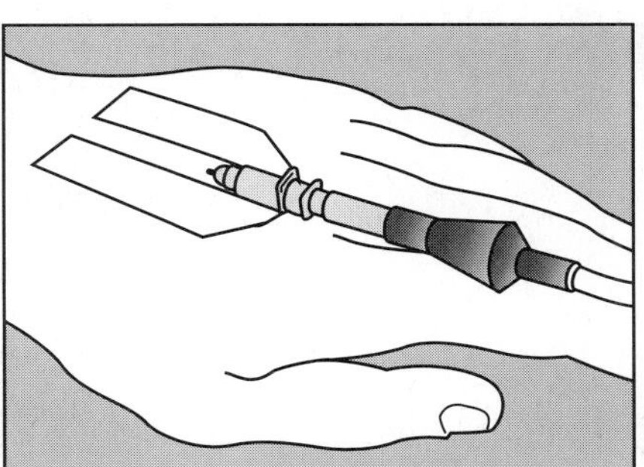

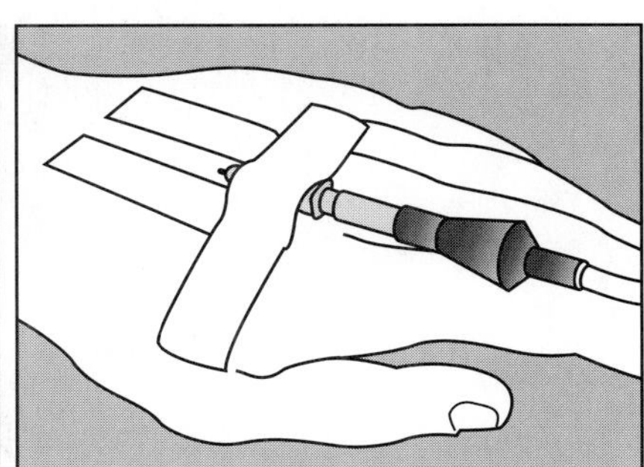

Figure 24-30 A second piece of tape is placed over the catheter hub.

necessary. The patient is now ready for the administration of the IV medications.

HOLLOW METAL NEEDLE

Dorsum of Hand and Ventral Forearm

Although not recommended for use in routine IV sedation, the hollow metal needle may be used for venipuncture in emergency situations or in procedures, such as the drawing of blood samples for laboratory analysis, when only short-term cannulation is required. The hollow metal needle will almost always be attached to a syringe, which contains a drug to be injected or into which blood is to be drawn.

The basic technique of venipuncture is the same as that described earlier for the winged infusion set. However, once the metal needle enters the vein, great care must be taken as the needle is advanced because it is often difficult to obtain the correct needle angulation within the vein with a syringe attached (syringes are available that have an eccentrically placed needle, making venipuncture somewhat easier). The tourniquet is removed and the syringe held securely in place.

Before the administration of the drug, an aspiration test must be performed to confirm that the needle tip remains within the vessel's lumen. With one hand holding the syringe in position, the other hand gently pulls the plunger of the syringe until a backflow of blood is observed. This technique (drawing of blood into syringe) is called *barbitage* (Figure 24-31). The drug is then administered.

Dorsal Wrist and Antecubital Fossa

Venipuncture with the hollow metal needle on the dorsum of the wrist or the antecubital fossa differs from the technique described above only in that movement of the joint must be prevented. An elbow immobilizer or armboard may be used.

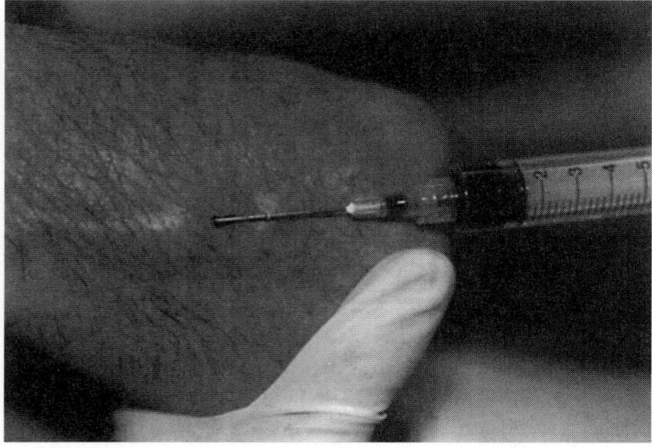

Figure 24-31 Barbitage. Blood pulled into syringe to dilute drug.

Before a discussion of the termination of an intravenous infusion, a few comments are warranted concerning the technique of venipuncture.

1. Experienced phlebotomists often devote more time to locating a suitable vein than actually performing the venipuncture. Time spent in distending veins is time well spent because the likelihood of successfully entering a larger diameter vein is greater than that of entering a small vein.
2. If the tourniquet is placed on the leg or arm for an extended time, the skin will become mottled, then purple, and will feel cool. The patient will probably complain of discomfort as a period of hyperesthesia develops. Should this occur, the tourniquet should be removed and circulation in the tissue permitted to be restored. After 2 to 3 minutes, the tourniquet may be reapplied and the procedure restarted. Venipuncture should not take long to accomplish. Each of the steps described is performed sequentially. As experience and technical ability are acquired, the speed with which venipuncture is completed will increase.
3. If the needle gets "lost" within the tissues during venipuncture (e.g., the needle should be in the vein, but it is not), do *not* use the needle as a probe in an attempt to locate the vein. Using the needle as a probe simply traumatizes the tissues, increasing patient discomfort and greatly increasing the risk of accidentally puncturing the vein and producing a hematoma. The following sequence is recommended in this situation:
   a. Locate the tip of the needle by lifting the needle tip up and looking for the imprint it makes under the skin.
   b. If the tip is located under and beyond the vein, withdraw the needle slightly so that the tip is pulled back on the other side of the vein. Elevate the tip of the needle and readvance it toward the vein.
   c. If the needle tip has advanced over and beyond the vein, withdraw the needle slightly so that the tip is pulled back to the original side of the vein. Readvance the needle with the tip pointed more parallel to the vein than in the previous attempt.

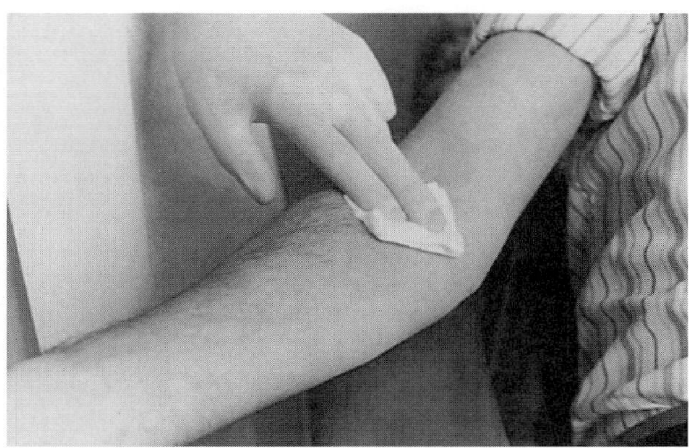

Figure 24-32 Firm, direct finger pressure over the site of venipuncture prevents postoperative hematoma.

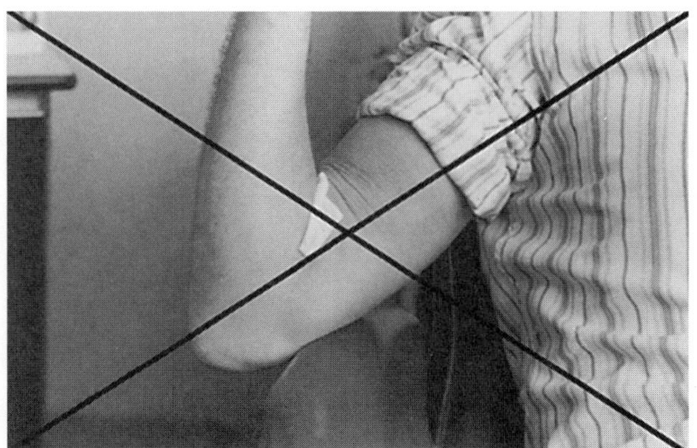

Figure 24-33 Placing gauze over the injection site and bending the elbow does *not* provide adequate pressure and often results in hematoma formation.

TERMINATING THE INTRAVENOUS INFUSION

At the conclusion of the IV procedure, the needle or catheter must be removed before the patient can be discharged from the office. Criteria for terminating the IV infusion are discussed in Chapter 26. It is assumed here that all criteria have been satisfactorily met by the patient.

1. If an IV infusion is being used, the drip is stopped by tightening the rate-control screw or knob.
2. The needle or catheter is held gently in position while all tape is carefully removed from the skin.
3. A sterile 2-×-2-inch gauze square is placed over the site of needle entry into the skin. No pressure is exerted because pressure on the skin while a rigid metal needle is still within the vein will be uncomfortable for the patient and might injure the vein as the needle is withdrawn. This does not occur with a catheter.
4. The needle or catheter is carefully withdrawn from the vein. The assistant should cap or discard the needle immediately so that no one will be accidentally stuck with a contaminated needle.
5. As soon as the needle is withdrawn from the skin, firm, direct finger pressure is applied onto the gauze square over the site of penetration of the skin (Figure 24-32). Pressure is maintained for at least 3 to 5 minutes. Failure to do so may result in the formation of a hematoma.
6. When the antecubital fossa is used for venipuncture, a common mistake is to place a gauze square on the site and have the patient bend his or her elbow (Figure 24-33), assuming that this will provide pressure adequate to stop the bleeding. *Bending of the elbow does not provide adequate pressure and will result in a hematoma!* Regardless of the location of the venipuncture, it is important that firm, direct pressure with a gloved hand be applied for at least 3 to 5 minutes.
7. A bandage is placed over the puncture site.
8. The needle is destroyed (Figure 24-34), and the IV needle, tubing, and bag are discarded.

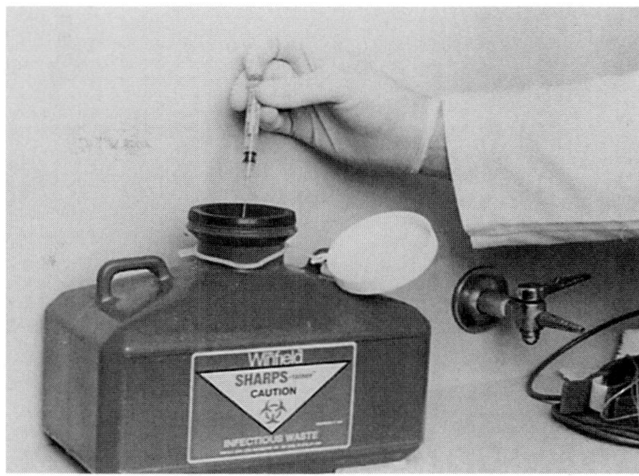

Figure 24-34 An appropriate disposal should be available for used needles.

REFERENCES

1. Fetzer SJ: Reducing the pain of venipuncture, *J Perianesth Nurs* 14:95, 1999.
2. Abbott Laboratories: *I.V. tips #6: how to use the butterfly infusion set*, Chicago, 1972, Abbott Laboratories.
3. Travenol Laboratories: *Quik-Cath, product information sheet*, Deerfield, Ill, 1978, Travenol Laboratories.
4. Abbott Laboratories: *Venipuncture and venous cannulation*, Chicago, 1971, Abbott Laboratories.

CHAPTER 25

Pharmacology

CHAPTER OUTLINE

A variety of drugs are available for intravenous (IV) conscious sedation. These include a number of categories, primarily sedative-hypnotics, opioids, and anticholinergics. The drugs most commonly used in IV conscious sedation are listed in Box 25-1. Also listed in Box 25-1 are several drugs (indicated by ‡) that are not recommended for IV use by doctors who have not completed a 2-year residency in anesthesiology. These drugs are discussed briefly in this chapter so that the doctor may more fully understand the rationale for their not being recommended.

BOX 25-1 Drugs Available for Intravenous Conscious Sedation

Sedative-Hypnotics and Antianxiety Drugs

Benzodiazepines
Diazepam
Midazolam
Lorazepam*
Flunitrazepam†
Chlordiazepoxide

Barbiturates
Pentobarbital
Secobarbital
Methohexital‡
Thiopental‡
Thiamylal‡

Histamine Blockers
Promethazine
Hydroxyzine*

Opioid Agonists
Meperidine
Morphine
Fentanyl
Sufentanil
Alfentanil
Remifentanil*

Opioid Antagonist
Naloxone

Anticholinergics
Atropine
Scopolamine
Glycopyrrolate

Antidotal Drugs
Flumazenil
Naloxone
Nalbuphine
Physostigmine
Procaine

Others
Innovar (droperidol + fentanyl)‡
Ketamine‡
Propofol‡

*Not recommended for use in intravenous conscious sedation.
†Not available for clinical use in the United States (as of July 2002).
‡Not recommended for use in intravenous conscious sedation without anesthesiology training.

BENZODIAZEPINES

The benzodiazepines have become the most commonly used IV sedative drugs in both dentistry and medicine. Five benzodiazepines are discussed here (Table 25-1); four of them are presently available in the United States, and one (flunitrazepam) is available outside the United States.

Diazepam

Diazepam was synthesized in 1959 by Sternbach and Reeder. The drug became available as Valium (Hoffmann-LaRoche) in 1963 and shortly thereafter became the most prescribed oral drug in the Western world.[1] Diazepam is also available in a parenteral preparation for intramuscular (IM) and IV use (see Chapter 10).

IV administration of diazepam appears to have begun with the work of Davidau[2] in Paris in 1965. This was followed shortly thereafter by a report by Main[3] in 1967, who used diazepam as an adjunct to the Jorgensen technique. In 1968 Brown reported on 40 cases in which diazepam was used alone, the drug being administered until the patient felt sleepy.[4]

In 1969 O'Neill and Verrill[5] reported on the use of IV diazepam for sedation in minor oral surgical procedures, with good to excellent results in 51 of 52 patients treated. In 1970 O'Neill et al. reported on 55 patients undergoing dental surgical procedures lasting between 20 and 45 minutes. IV diazepam provided successful sedation and cooperation in 49 patients; four others moved and spoke occasionally but were able to be treated, and two patients required additional IV medications (methohexital) for treatment to be completed successfully.[6]

The dosage used in these patients was that required to produce marked ptosis (drooping of the upper eyelid; Figure 25-1). Halfway ptosis of the upper eyelid is now recognized as the Verrill sign.[7] The practice of

TABLE 25-1 Benzodiazepines for Intravenous Conscious Sedation

Generic Name	Proprietary Name	Usual Concentration (mg/ml)	Duration of Action (min)	Average Sedation Dose (mg)
Diazepam	Valium	5	45	10-12
Lorazepam	Ativan	2.4	6-8 hours	2-4
Midazolam	Versed, Dormicum, Hypnovel	1.5	45	2.5-7.5

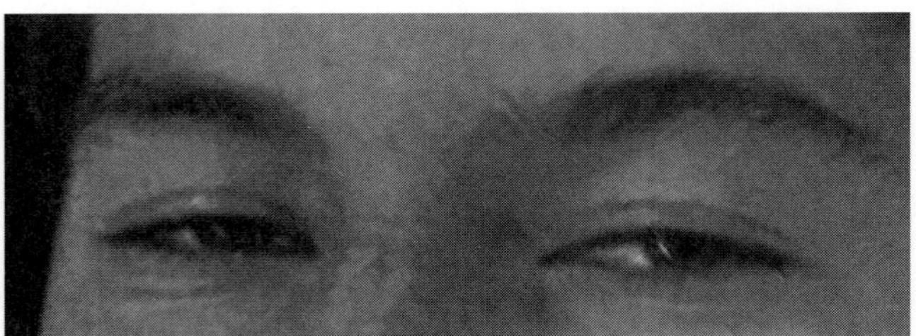

Figure 25-1 Verrill sign: eyelids at "half-staff."

administering diazepam until the appearance of the Verrill sign produces a level of sedation (central nervous system [CNS] depression) that is considered by some to be more profound than is usually necessary and is therefore not recommended for routine use.[8]

Peter Foreman,[9] in New Zealand, used diazepam in combination with atropine and incremental doses of methohexital. Although successful, he stated that the addition of even small amounts of methohexital greatly increased the risk of overdosage. In a subsequent study, Foreman used diazepam alone for a variety of dental therapies, finding that although the degree of amnesia produced by diazepam varied significantly from patient to patient, virtually all patients agreed that dental treatment had been at least tolerable rather than an ordeal. He found that IV diazepam had made it possible to treat those patients who may not have received proper treatment in the past because of fear. Foreman stated, "Diazepam has become the drug of choice for the trained general dental practitioner, as well as for the introduction of dental students to intravenous sedation."[10]

With the introduction of midazolam into clinical practice, the use of IV conscious sedation with diazepam has decreased somewhat. However, as discussed in Chapter 26, there are still significant reasons to consider diazepam as a first-line agent for IV conscious sedation.

Chemistry. Diazepam is a member of the 1,4-benzodiazepine group of compounds. The chemical formula for diazepam is 7-chloro-1,3-dihydro-1-methyl-5-phenyl-2H-1,4-benzodiazepin-2-one. It is a pale yellow-white crystalline powder with virtually no odor. It is considerably soluble in chloroform and acetone, moderately soluble in ethanol and ether, and poorly soluble in water.[11]

General Pharmacology. It is believed that emotions are largely controlled by the limbic system, that is, the portion of the brain comprised of the amygdala, hippocampus, and septal areas.[12] The midbrain reticular formation, hypothalamus, and thalamus are also involved with the experience or transmission of emotions.

In very small doses, diazepam appears to act on the hippocampus, whereas other areas of the brain remain unaffected and the patient remains alert.[13] Following oral administration of diazepam, this action of the drug would be appropriate; however, when diazepam is administered intravenously, a greater effect is normally desirable. Administered to the point at which sedation and ataxia (loss of muscular coordination) occur, a more generalized depression of the CNS is observed.

Research suggests that the anxiolytic properties of benzodiazepines are mediated by increased inhibitory nerve transmission.[14] γ-Aminobutyric acid (GABA) is an important inhibitory neurotransmitter in the brain. Glycine (aminoacetic acid), the simplest nonessential amino acid, may be the major inhibitory transmitter of the spinal cord. The anticonvulsant and sedative properties of benzodiazepines may result from a direct agonist effect on stereospecific benzodiazepine receptors, which in turn facilitate the inhibitory action of GABA on its own postsynaptic receptors.

Fate of Intravenous Diazepam. Following IV administration, diazepam reaches a peak blood level in approximately 1 to 2 minutes. The onset of clinical activity is therefore quite rapid.[15] Blood levels of approximately 1.0 μg/ml may be achieved after an IV dose of 10 to 20 mg of diazepam.[16] Clinically, this would equate with a deeper level of conscious sedation and a period of anterograde amnesia.

As mentioned in Chapters 7 and 10, diazepam has a plasma half-life of approximately 30+ hours.[17]

A commonly held misconception is that a drug with a long half-life will possess a long duration of action, whereas one with a shorter half-life will have a shorter duration of action. This is not true, and diazepam is an excellent example of this. The β-half-life is an indicator of the rate at which a drug undergoes biotransformation (in the liver for diazepam), whereas the factor most responsible for a drug's duration of action is its degree of receptor-site (protein) binding.

Over a period of approximately 45 minutes after the titration of an appropriate dose of diazepam, the patient will remain sedated and free of anxiety. In many patients the following distinct phases of this sedation can be observed, each lasting approximately 15 minutes.

Phase 1: 0 to 15 Minutes. During phase 1 of IV conscious sedation with diazepam, the cerebral blood level of diazepam is at its peak and the patient is sedated to the maximum degree. The patient remains responsive to verbal and physical stimulation, but response time is increased, speech is slurred, and the patient may have difficulty enunciating words. The patient may not appear to be aware of the presence of the doctor or the assistant during this phase. Anterograde amnesia, if it is to occur, usually involves procedures occurring at this time.

Phase 2: 16 to 30 Minutes. The level of sedation is somewhat lessened (the patient becomes more aware of the surroundings than in phase 1; however, he or she is definitely still sedated, because the cerebral blood level of diazepam begins to decrease as the drug undergoes redistribution: [α-half-life] to those organs and parts of the body that are less vessel rich than the brain). Patient response to stimulation (verbal and physical) is more rapid, the slowing of responses in phase 1 having diminished or disappeared. Patients can usually recall events occurring during this phase, although in isolated cases amnesia may occur in this phase too.

Phase 3: 31 to 45 Minutes. During this period the typical patient will state that he or she feels "normal" again; in other words, the feeling of sedation has dissipated. It may be tempting to administer additional diazepam to the patient; however, this is normally not necessary. Although no longer feeling sedated, the patient is also no longer apprehensive. The now decreasing cerebral blood level of diazepam is no longer adequate to maintain the earlier depth of sedation, but it is sufficient to provide an anxiolytic state (similar to the desired actions of oral diazepam). With treatment nearing completion and the patient free of pain (as a result of the administration of local anesthetics), there is usually no need for the readministration of diazepam at this time.

Phase 4: 46 to 60 Minutes. At this time after receiving diazepam, virtually all patients will feel, and in fact look, recovered. This is not a result of the β-half-life of the drug (30+ hours) but because of redistribution: α-half-life. The blood level of diazepam at 60 minutes after IV administration of 20 mg is 0.25 μg/ml.[16] The patient is not recovered at this time. Under no circumstances should the doctor ever believe that this patient is capable of operating a car or leaving the dental or surgical office unescorted.

As redistribution of diazepam continues during this first hour after IV administration, the level of the drug increases in several storage sites: the fat, the walls of the intestines, and the gallbladder. Diazepam stored in fat will usually remain there because diazepam is quite lipid soluble and the blood supply of fat is relatively poor.

A clinically significant phenomenon can arise at this point, a result of the diazepam stored in the gallbladder and intestinal walls. Known as the *rebound effect* or *second-peak effect*, it involves a recurrence of symptoms of sedation and drowsiness approximately 1 hour after the first meal taken after the patient leaves the treatment site.[18] In most cases this will be about 4 to 6 hours following the start of the procedure. After a meal, particularly one rich in lipids, the gallbladder constricts, releasing its contents of bile and unmetabolized diazepam into the small intestine, where over the next hour or so diazepam is reabsorbed back into the cardiovascular system. In some patients the diazepam blood level may reach a level at which clinical signs and symptoms of sedation recur: The patient feels quite tired and will want to lie down for a few minutes. It becomes absolutely essential, therefore, that the patient receiving diazepam, as well as his or her escort, be advised of this possibility before their discharge from the dental office. The rebound effect is less likely to be observed in a patient whose gallbladder has been removed.

Because diazepam is extremely lipophilic, it cannot be excreted through the kidneys and therefore must undergo biotransformation in the liver.

Biotransformation. Diazepam is biotransformed by one of two pathways. In the first the diazepam molecule undergoes demethylation to desmethyldiazepam, which possesses anxiolytic, but not sedative, effects. Desmethyldiazepam is too lipophilic to permit its excretion by the kidney. Desmethyldiazepam has a half-life of 96 hours and eventually undergoes hydroxylation to oxazepam.[19]

The second pathway involves the hydroxylation of the diazepam molecule to 3-hydroxydiazepam, another pharmacologically active metabolite also known as *temazepam*. Temazepam undergoes demethylation into oxazepam.

Oxazepam is yet another water-insoluble anxiolytic benzodiazepine. It is used as an anxiolytic agent by the oral route of administration. The pharmacology of oxazepam (Serax) is discussed in Chapter 7. The half-life of oxazepam is short, ranging between 3 and 21 hours. It is rapidly biotransformed into its major metabolite, oxazepam glucuronide.

Effects of Age and Disease. It is often stated that drug dosages should be decreased in very young and the elderly patients as well as in patients with significant liver disease. The pharmacokinetics of diazepam have been well studied in these groups of patents.[20-23] The following is presented as a summation of that research:

In patients 2 years and older, diazepam is handled as in the adult. The only significant clinical advice is to adjust the dose of the drug appropriately. With titration via the IV route, clinical results are usually achieved at smaller doses than in adults (assuming a cooperative patient—not a very likely situation).

In elderly patients the dose of diazepam by the IV (or any other) route should be decreased for several reasons. The rate at which the diazepam undergoes biotransformation is decreased in older patients. In addition, when administered orally, the drug is absorbed in the gastrointestinal tract somewhat more slowly. However, the most important reason for the apparent increased sensitivity of older patients to diazepam (and other drugs) is related primarily to protein binding. Older patients exhibit decreased protein binding of drugs.[20] This means that there will be more of the free, unbound drug available within the blood to cross the blood-brain barrier and produce CNS depression. Diazepam is offered as an example: In the younger patient, diazepam is approximately 98.5% protein bound.[21] Therefore the clinical effects of diazepam are produced by but 1.5% of the dosage administered: the non–protein-bound diazepam. In the older patient, in whom protein binding has decreased, diazepam may be 97% protein bound, still a significant figure, but one permitting 3% (or twice as much) non–protein-bound diazepam to be available to produce CNS depression. It becomes obvious that when administered the same dose of the drug, the clinical actions on the older patient will be exaggerated. The dosages of diazepam by the oral and IM routes must be decreased in older patients. With IV administration, titration will provide effective sedation at what will probably be a smaller dose of the drug than is usually given.

Skeletal Muscle Relaxation. Diazepam and other benzodiazepines produce skeletal muscle relaxation. Research has demonstrated that the muscle-relaxant properties of benzodiazepines are caused by central rather than peripheral effects.[24] Monosynaptic reflexes such as the knee jerk are essentially unaffected by even large doses of diazepam, whereas polysynaptic reflexes are depressed by rather small doses.

Anticonvulsant Activity. Benzodiazepines have important anticonvulsant properties. Diazepam, midazolam, chlordiazepoxide, and nitrazepam (as well as other benzodiazepines) have the ability to antagonize the convulsive effects of local anesthetic overdose produced by lidocaine, mepivacaine, bupivacaine, cocaine, and procaine.

In one study the seizure threshold for lidocaine-induced tonic-clonic seizure activity was 8.5 mg/kg.[25] When IM diazepam was administered 60 minutes before treatment in a dose of 0.25 to 0.5 mg/kg, the seizure threshold was elevated to 16.8 mg/kg of lidocaine. Although barbiturates also provide protection (e.g., pentobarbital 10 mg/kg), they also produce profound behavioral, cardiovascular, and respiratory depression compared with the minimal effects produced by the benzodiazepines.[26]

In the management of generalized tonic-clonic seizures the benzodiazepines have not supplanted phenytoin and phenobarbital as oral maintenance anticonvulsants. IV diazepam is the drug of choice, however, in the management of status epilepticus and acute seizure activity.[27] Once the seizure has been controlled, maintenance therapy with other anticonvulsants is initiated.

Cardiovascular System. Hemodynamic studies show that diazepam produces little effect on the cardiovascular system of healthy human subjects.[28] IV diazepam, in a dose of 0.3 mg/kg, produces no clinically significant changes in either blood pressure or cardiac output.

Diazepam has been compared with thiopental as a preanesthetic induction agent in the cardiovascularly compromised patient (American Society of Anesthesiologists [ASA] III and IV).[29] Administered intravenously in a dose of 0.2 mg/kg, less than 1% of the patients studied experienced a reduction of cardiac output of more than 15%, and none had a mean blood pressure reduction of more than 15%. In contrast, on receiving 2 mg/kg of thiopental, 85% of the patients exhibited more than a 15% reduction in cardiac output, whereas 68% demonstrated more than a 15% reduction in blood pressure. Adverse hemodynamic effects attributable to the benzodiazepines are rare in humans, even in patients with significant cardiac or pulmonary disease.[30]

Respiratory System. All sedative-hypnotics, including the benzodiazepines, are potential respiratory depressants. When these drugs are studied in patients without pulmonary disease, respiratory depression produced by intravenously administered benzodiazepines is barely detectable.[31] In addition, and quite significantly, the benzodiazepines do not potentiate the respiratory depressant actions of opioids.[32]

Hepatic Disease. Agitation and combativeness are occasionally encountered in patients with liver disease. Murray-Lyon et al.,[33] in a study of patients with severe parenchymal liver disease, administered diazepam intravenously.[33] Adequate sedation was achieved in all patients with no deterioration of their clinical status. Diazepam, administered with care, is an appropriate sedative for patients with impaired liver function.

Pain. In general, studies have failed to demonstrate specific analgesic properties of the benzodiazepines; however, large doses of these agents will impair motor response to painful stimulation.[34] These studies show that benzodiazepines are much more capable of attenuating the emotional response to pain than of altering the actual sensation of pain.

More recent studies have demonstrated that diazepam may possess some slight analgesic properties.[35] These findings do not, however, alter the fact that in clinical situations in which pain control is a factor during dental treatment, local anesthetics must still be administered in the usual manner.

Amnesia. Intravenously administered diazepam produces *anterograde amnesia,* that is, a lack of recall occurring from the time of injection onward.[36] Retrograde amnesia, a lack of recall of events occurring before drug administration, is quite rare. Amnesia after diazepam IM administration is uncommon and is essentially nonexistent after oral administration.

After IV diazepam administration, the duration of the amnesic period is approximately 10 minutes; however, considerable variation is noted. During this time, patients respond normally to stimulation, but at a later time (immediately postoperatively or 24 hours later), they will be unable to recall the event.

In my experience with IV diazepam sedation, amnesia developed in approximately 75% of patients in whom diazepam had been titrated to a clinically adequate level of conscious sedation. The length of amnesia has varied, but it has been limited in most persons to the first 10 to 15 minutes after diazepam administration. In fewer patients the amnesic effect has lasted through the entire appointment.

The importance of the amnesic phase is that traumatic procedures may be completed, with the patient responding normally to them; however, at the end of the procedure, the patient will have no recall of the procedure. The most commonly used procedure during this period is the administration of local anesthetic. It is common for the patient to respond to the initial administration of the local anesthetic (although administration of the local anesthetic should be performed as atraumatically as possible). At the end of the dental or surgical procedure, patients often question the doctor to find out either how their lips or tongue became numb without a "shot" or how the drug that was injected into their arm (the diazepam) kept them from feeling the procedure. Unfortunately, the amnesic period does not encompass the time period preceding the administration of the diazepam (retrograde amnesia); therefore patients almost always remember the venipuncture attempt or attempts.

Although amnesia is usually a welcome benefit of IV conscious sedation, the absence of amnesia does not imply that the procedure was a failure. The primary goal of sedation is relaxation of the patient so that the treatment can be completed in a more ideal manner. The presence or absence of amnesia does not alter this fact. Lack of recall should be considered to be the "icing on the cake."

Contraindications. Injectable diazepam is contraindicated in patients with the following: known allergy to diazepam or other benzodiazepines and acute narrow-angle glaucoma and open-angle glaucoma, unless the patient is receiving appropriate therapy. Other contraindications include alcohol intoxication, CNS depression, and age less than 6 months.

Cautions include psychosis, impaired pulmonary function, impaired renal function, impaired liver function, and advanced patient age.

Warnings. Probably the most significant side effect of intravenously administered diazepam is the occurrence of venous thrombosis, phlebitis, local irritation, or swelling. Although these complications are rare with the administration of IV diazepam as recommended in Chapter 26, one of the manufacturers of diazepam, Roche Laboratories, Inc., recommends the following as a means to minimize this possibility[37]:

1. The solution should be injected slowly, taking at least 1 minute for each milliliter (5 mg).
2. Small veins, such as those on the dorsum of the hand or wrist, should not be used.
3. Extreme care should be taken to avoid intraarterial administration or extravasation.
4. Diazepam should not be mixed or diluted with other solutions or drugs in a syringe or infusion flask.
5. If it is not feasible to administer diazepam directly intravenously, it may be injected slowly through the infusion tubing as close as possible to the vein insertion.

Other warnings include the following:

1. Extreme care must be exercised when diazepam is administered to elderly or debilitated patients and to those with limited pulmonary reserve because of the possibility of apnea or cardiac arrest or both.
2. Concomitant use of barbiturates, alcohol, or other CNS depressants increases depression with increased risk of apnea.
3. When diazepam is administered with an opioid analgesic, the dosage of the opioid should be reduced by at least one third and should be administered in small increments.

The administration of IV diazepam as recommended in Chapter 26 takes into account these warnings. Titration will prevent accidental overdose in the preceding situations.

Use in Pregnancy. Any drug that crosses the blood-brain barrier also crosses the placenta into the fetus. An increased risk of congenital malformation associated with the administration of benzodiazepines during the first trimester of pregnancy has been suggested in several studies.[38] Because the administration of these drugs in dentistry is rarely a matter of urgency, their use at this time cannot be recommended. The possibility that a woman of childbearing potential may be pregnant at the time diazepam is used should always be considered.

Pediatric Use. Children 2 years and older handle diazepam as adults do. The major consideration is the dosage. If diazepam is administered intravenously, titration will provide the proper safeguard to prevent overdosage.

The administration of IV diazepam alone to younger children in the dental setting has not always provided ideal sedation. Difficulties exist in establishing venipuncture in any of these patients. Even more significant, however, is the child's response to the feeling of being lightly sedated (IV conscious sedation). Whereas the adult will become more relaxed and cooperative as the effect of the diazepam increases, many younger children will appear to "fight" the effect, becoming increasingly agitated and uncomfortable. Some may call this a "paradoxical reaction" to the drug. It is my belief that the child is simply responding to the altered sensations he or she is experiencing (in his or her head). Being unaccustomed to this feeling, the child moves around so as to "get away" from it. IV diazepam, when used as a sole agent in younger children, does not provide a consistently adequate level of sedation.

Precautions. When diazepam is combined with other psychotropic agents, careful consideration must be given to possible potentiation of drug effect.[37] Categories such as the phenothiazines, opioids, barbiturates, monoamine oxidase inhibitors (MAOIs), and other antidepressants are included.

Because metabolites of diazepam are excreted in the kidneys, the administration of diazepam in patients with compromised renal function should be undertaken with care. Lower dosages may be required for elderly or debilitated patients.

Patients receiving diazepam intravenously must be cautioned against engaging in hazardous occupations requiring complete mental alertness, such as operating machinery or driving a motor vehicle. Patients should also be advised against the use of alcoholic beverages after the administration of IV diazepam. In general, it is my policy to recommend that patients neither drive their car nor consume alcohol for the remainder of the treatment day at least, and not the next day if recovery at that time is not complete.

Adverse Reactions. The most frequently reported adverse reaction to intravenously administered diazepam is phlebitis at the site of injection. This is discussed in Chapter 27. Other less frequently occurring adverse reactions include the following:

- Hyperactivity
- Confusion
- Nausea (extremely rare)
- Changes in libido
- Hiccoughs (not uncommon; more annoying than anything)
- Decreased salivation (a benefit in dental treatment)

Paradoxical reactions such as acute hyperexcited states, anxiety, hallucinations, increased muscle spasticity, rage, and stimulation are also seen. The general term for this phenomenon is *emergence delirium.* It is seen more frequently with scopolamine administration and is discussed thoroughly in Chapter 27.

Dosage. The following directions regarding recommended dosage are taken from the diazepam package insert[37]:

> Dosage should be individualized for maximal beneficial effect. The usual recommended dose in older children and adults ranges from 2 to 20 mg IV, depending on the indication and its severity. Lower doses, usually 2 to 5 mg . . . should be used for elderly or debilitated patients.

The dose of intravenously administered diazepam will always be determined by titrating the drug slowly into a rapidly running IV infusion. In this manner each patient will receive only the dose appropriate for sedation, and overdosage should not occur.

Availability. Valium (Roche): 5 mg/ml in 2-ml ampules, 10-ml multiple-dose vials, and 2-ml preloaded syringe. Injectable diazepam consists of the following ingredients[37]:

- 40% propylene glycol
- 10% ethyl alcohol
- 5% sodium benzoate and benzoic acid as buffers
- 1.5% benzyl alcohol as preservative

Diazepam is classified as a DEA Schedule IV drug. Propylene glycol and ethyl alcohol are included because diazepam is lipid soluble and relatively water insoluble; therefore it requires a nonaqueous solvent system. Many of the complications and side effects attributed to diazepam, especially phlebitis, are in fact produced by the propylene glycol, which is also a major component of antifreeze.[39]

The IV administration of diazepam can produce a sensation of burning in some patients. This is caused not by the diazepam but rather by the propylene glycol vehicle. It is recommended that the patient be advised of this possibility as the drug is administered. The doctor will tell the patient, "There may be a feeling of warmth as the drug is administered. This is entirely normal and will pass within a few minutes." As the drug is carried in venous blood away from the injection site, this sensation fades. Its occurrence may be minimized by opening the IV infusion to a rapid rate before injecting the diazepam. Some persons recommend the administration of 1 ml of 1% lidocaine or procaine into the IV line immediately before the administration of diazepam. The analgesic properties of lidocaine and procaine prevent the burning sensation from occurring. In my experience with diazepam, slow injection of diazepam into a rapidly running infusion prevents this sensation from arising. IV lidocaine administration is not necessary.

Dizac (Ohmeda Pharmaceutical) is diazepam in an emulsion form that does not produce the same burning sensation as is often noted with the diazepam formulation described above. It is available as 2.5, 5, and 10 mg/ml injectable solutions.[40]

The search for a water-soluble benzodiazepine with clinical properties similar to diazepam but without its potential for venous irritation led to the development of midazolam. Diazepam is presently the most commonly used IV sedative within dentistry. When used as recommended, it is safe and extremely effective in the management of severe apprehension and fear of the dental or surgical situation. IV diazepam is recognized as one of the two "basic" IV conscious sedation techniques in dentistry.

Diazepam
The medical history of patients receiving diazepam should be checked for the following:
- Allergy or hypersensitivity to benzodiazepines
- Glaucoma (untreated)
- Phlebitis, thrombophlebitis

Diazepam
Proprietary name: Valium
Classification: benzodiazepine
Availability: 5 mg/ml
Average sedative dose (IV): 10-12 mg
Maximal single dose: 20 mg
Maximal total dose: 30 mg

Diazepam	
Pregnancy category	D
Lactation	NS
Metabolism	Liver
Excretion	Urine
DEA schedule	IV

Midazolam

Midazolam is a 1,4-benzodiazepine compound that is similar in most pharmacologic aspects to diazepam. It possesses several attributes, however, that make it somewhat more attractive than diazepam in certain clinical situations.

Midazolam was synthesized in 1975 by Walser and Fryer at Hoffmann-LaRoche, Inc. Midazolam was available in many parts of the world in the early 1980s and was released for use in the United States in 1986. The chemical formula is 8-chloro-5(2′-fluorophenyl)-1-methyl-4H-imidazo (1,5-a)(1,4) benzodiazepine maleate. It is a colorless crystal in an aqueous solution. Each milliliter contains either 1 or 5 mg midazolam maleate buffered to a pH of 3.3.[41] The acidic pH maintains the benzodiazepine ring in an open configuration, which is required for its water solubility (the diazepam ring is closed, and it is insoluble in water). Once in the body, the physiologic pH (7.4) acts to close the ring, providing the chemical structure of the drug that is required for its clinical efficacy.

Its water solubility differentiates midazolam from other parenteral benzodiazepines—diazepam, lorazepam, and chlordiazepoxide. The need for potentially irritating solvents, such as propylene glycol, is eliminated with midazolam. The water solubility of midazolam is produced by the substitution of imidazole at the 1,2 position of the 1,4-benzodiazepine ring structure and is aided because midazolam is the salt of an acid. This water solubility is responsible for the positive findings of a lack of burning sensation on injection and the absence of phlebitic sequelae at the injection site.

Pharmacokinetics and Biotransformation. Midazolam undergoes metabolism in the liver by hydroxylation into three major metabolites.[42] Whereas the major metabolites of diazepam are pharmacologically active anxiolytics, the major metabolites of midazolam have no pharmacologic activity. In addition, because of its lack of active metabolites and shorter half-life, a rebound effect is not evidenced with midazolam.

The α-half-life (distribution and redistribution) of midazolam has been recorded as 4 to 18 minutes. The β-half-life (metabolism and excretion) is 1.7 to 2.4 hours. By contrast, diazepam's β-half-life is 31.3 hours.[43] The shorter half-lives of midazolam make the drug more suitable for ambulatory sedation procedures: a relatively short duration of action combined with a relatively rapidly inactivated and excreted drug.

Midazolam is 94% protein bound, the binding occurring primarily in serum albumin. Midazolam possesses a relatively rapid onset of action, the induction of general anesthesia having ranged from 55 to 143 seconds.[44]

Amnesia. Midazolam, like the other parenteral benzodiazepines, has the ability to produce anterograde amnesia. Conner et al.[45] demonstrated the incidence of amnesia in patients receiving IV midazolam (Table 25-2).[45]

The results shown in Table 25-2 indicate that midazolam is superior to other benzodiazepines or IV drug combinations in providing anterograde amnesia. In one study 71% of the patients did not recall being in the recovery room.[45] Other studies have not demonstrated these same remarkable results, but in all cases the degree of anterograde amnesia provided by midazolam was at least equal to that produced by diazepam.[46] Retrograde amnesia is not produced by midazolam.

Since the introduction of midazolam to clinical use in the United States, I have seen the dramatic effects of midazolam-induced amnesia; most are beneficial, but some are potentially dangerous. For the typical 1-hour IV conscious sedation procedure in dental or outpatient surgical practice, most patients have little recall of most or all of the procedure, and for most patients this is quite acceptable and positive. One case, however, must be mentioned as a caution:

> A young, healthy (ASA I) woman received IV midazolam and local anesthesia for the removal of three third molars. Following the 20-minute procedure, the patient appeared alert and was quite responsive to questions. Gauze packs had been placed at the sites of extraction, and the patient had been told to bite down hard on the gauze and not to swallow. She responded verbally that she would do as directed. Within 2 minutes the patient was complaining of a lump in her throat. Observation of the mouth indicated that all gauze packs had disappeared—the patient had swallowed them. Fortunately, they were located in the esophagus and were of no great consequence. However, when questioned, the patient had absolutely no recall either of receiving the instructions given her by the doctor or of swallowing the gauze pads.[47]

It becomes imperative, therefore, for the patient to be observed much more carefully during the in-office recovery period, that special precautions be taken to prevent such events from recurring, and that postoperative instructions (verbal and written) be given to both the patient and his or her escort. The benzodiazepine antagonist flumazenil has been shown to decrease the duration of midazolam's amnesic period.[48]

Duration of Clinical Activity. Because of its short α-half-life, the duration of clinical sedation noted with midazolam is somewhat shorter than that of diazepam. Its duration of action is therefore quite compatible with the typical 1-hour dental or surgical procedure.

Midazolam differs in another manner from diazepam. It appears that midazolam is much more effective than diazepam when amnesia is a desired result of the drug's administration. However, when sedation is of higher priority, diazepam is a more effective agent. These are personal observations (anecdotes) that have not received the careful scientific study (evidenced-based medicine) required to make a categorical statement.

Cardiorespiratory Activity. Midazolam, as a typical member of the benzodiazepines, has minimal effect on the cardiovascular and respiratory dynamics of the ASA I or II patient in usual doses. IV doses of 0.15 mg/kg of midazolam in healthy persons have produced statistically significant, but clinically insignificant, decreases in arterial blood pressure and increases in heart rate.[49] However, other researchers noted no untoward cardiovascular response with similar doses.[50] In fact, Gath et al.[51] recommend midazolam as an induction agent for patients with ischemic

TABLE 25-2 Incidence of Amnesia in Patients Receiving Intravenous Midazolam

Time after Injection (min)	Amnesic Patients (%)
2	96
30	87.5*
32	69
43	57

*Data from Fragen RJ, Caldwell NJ: *Anesthesiology* 153:511, 1980.

heart disease because of its rapid onset of action and minimal effects on the cardiovascular system.

Diazepam and midazolam both produce the same effects on the respiratory system. Doses of 0.3 mg/kg of diazepam and 0.15 mg/kg of midazolam produced comparable depression of respiratory response to CO_2 in healthy volunteers.[49] It was concluded that midazolam and diazepam injected intravenously in equipotent doses depress respiration significantly and similarly. The results of the study indicate that this is mediated by direct depression of central respiratory drive rather than being caused by a simultaneous depression of the muscles of respiration, although this possibility cannot be excluded. In the doses administered, equivalent to 21 mg of diazepam and 10 mg of midazolam for the typical 70-kg adult male, such a response might be expected. Since publication of this study in 1980, it has been demonstrated that equipotent doses of midazolam are approximately one fourth of the diazepam dose.

In all cases the cardiovascular and respiratory depression noted with midazolam were typical for parenteral benzodiazepines and significantly less than those observed following equipotent doses of barbiturates (thiopental, pentobarbital). No cardiac dysrhythmias were provoked by midazolam administration.

In November 1987 Roche Laboratories, Inc., the manufacturer of midazolam, sent a warning to doctors about the use of midazolam in conscious sedation.[52] It stated that the administration of midazolam had been associated with respiratory depression and respiratory arrest. Guidelines for the safe administration of this agent were offered (see Dosage and Administration). These guidelines emphasized the need for the slow titration of midazolam to all patients, especially the medically compromised.

Side Effects. The most frequently noted complaint after midazolam administration is dizziness. In the study by Conner et al.,[45] 46% of patients mentioned experiencing dizziness. Despite this, 92% stated that they enjoyed the feeling produced by midazolam, and 100% said that they would accept the drug again if they required another operation.

Dosage and Administration. When midazolam was introduced, initial reports implied that midazolam was 1.5 times as potent as diazepam. Subsequent clinical experience with midazolam has shown it to be approximately two to four times as potent as diazepam. The mean effective dose for 50% of subjects (MED_{50}) for the induction of general anesthesia is 0.2 mg/kg, although significant patient variation exists.[53] Clinically adequate IV conscious sedation with midazolam should always be achieved by slow titration. In its recent letter, Roche recommends "an initial intravenous dose for conscious sedation as little as 1 mg, but not exceeding 2.5 mg for a normal, healthy adult."[52]

> Lower doses are necessary for older (over 60 years) or debilitated patients and in patients receiving concomitant opioids or other CNS depressants. The initial dose and all subsequent doses should never be given as a bolus; administer over at least 2 minutes and allow an additional 2 or more minutes to fully evaluate the sedative effect. The use of the 1 mg/ml or dilution of the 5 mg/ml formulation is recommended to facilitate slower injection."[52]

Doses of midazolam administered to normal, healthy (ASA I) adult patients at the University of Southern California School of Dentistry have ranged from as little as 2 to 10 mg for an initial titrating dose. As with all drugs, there is significant patient variation in response to dosage.

Availability. Versed (Roche Laboratories): 1 and 5 mg/ml in 2- and 10-ml vials. (Hypnovel, Dormicum [Roche Laboratories] in the United Kingdom and other parts of the world.) Midazolam is classified as a DEA Schedule IV drug.

As with other CNS depressants, the dosage of midazolam must be decreased when other CNS depressants are being administered concomitantly. In addition, following IV conscious sedation, the patient must be escorted from the dental office in the company of a responsible adult and be advised not to have any alcohol and not to engage in any hazardous occupation requiring complete mental alertness, such as operating machinery or driving a motor vehicle, for approximately 24 hours.

Midazolam
The medical history of patients receiving midazolam should be checked for the following:
- Allergy or hypersensitivity to benzodiazepines
- Acute pulmonary insufficiency
- Respiratory depression

Midazolam
Proprietary name: Versed (USA); Hypnovel, Dormicum (UK)
Classification: benzodiazepine
Availability: 1 mg/ml, 5 mg/ml
Average sedative dose (IV): 2.5-7.5 mg
Maximal single dose: 6-8 mg
Maximal total dose: 10 mg

Midazolam	
Pregnancy category	D
Lactation	?
Metabolism	Liver
Excretion	Feces and urine
DEA schedule	IV

Lorazepam

Lorazepam is a benzodiazepine with sedative and antianxiety effects. It may be administered either intramuscularly or intravenously. Chemically, it is 7-chloro-5-(*o*-chlorophenyl)-1,3-dihydro-3-hydroxy-2H-1, 4-benzodiazepin-2-one. Lorazepam, like diazepam, is virtually insoluble in water. Although available for IV use, lorazepam is seldom used in the outpatient ambulatory patient because of the relative inability to titrate the drug and its prolonged duration of action.[54]

Lorazepam differs from most IV drugs in that its onset of clinical action is quite slow. After IV administration, lorazepam produces little or no clinical effect for about 5 minutes, with its maximal effect noted approximately 20 minutes after administration. This extremely slow onset of action prevents lorazepam from being titrated. "Average" dosages must be administered, a situation that takes away one of the most important safety features of the IV route of drug administration.

From personal experience with IV lorazepam I have found that it is rather easy to oversedate the patient. Administration of 1 or 2 mg of lorazepam usually provides adequate sedation, but because of the bell-shaped curve, some patients become overly sedated at this same dose.

The duration of clinical action of lorazepam is too long for the typical dental procedure. The usual duration of sedative effects of lorazepam is 6 to 8 hours; however, some degree of unsteadiness and sensitivity to the CNS depressant effects of other drugs (e.g., opioid analgesics prescribed for postsurgical pain control) may persist for as long as 24 hours. I vividly recall a patient who contacted me 36 hours after having received 2 mg of lorazepam intravenously and asked me when the effect of the drug would go away.

The introduction of flumazenil offers a means of reversing the sedative effects of lorazepam at the conclusion of the procedure. However, the clinical actions of flumazenil, especially after IV administration, are shorter than the clinical actions of lorazepam, leading to the possible recurrence of sedation after the patient is discharged from the office, a possibly dangerous situation. As discussed in the section on flumazenil, antidotal drugs and complications (see Chapter 27), consideration should be given for IM flumazenil administration whenever IV flumazenil is used.

The amnesic properties of lorazepam are impressive and include both anterograde and a degree of retrograde amnesia. Lack of recall is maximal approximately 15 to 20 minutes after IV administration and may include events occurring throughout the treatment day. This feeling of "losing a day" may not be very comfortable for the ambulatory patient. Lorazepam is more highly recommended for use in the hospitalized, monitored patient as a preoperative IM or IV drug than in the ambulatory outpatient.

Warnings and Precautions. Patients receiving lorazepam must be warned against operating a motor vehicle or machinery or engaging in hazardous occupations for 24 to 48 hours after its administration. Dosages of lorazepam should be decreased in patients older than 50 years to minimize the risk of oversedation.[55]

The use of scopolamine with lorazepam is not recommended as there is no beneficial effect to be gained; however, additive CNS depression, hallucination, and irrational behavior may be more likely to occur.

Patients must be advised that getting out of bed unassisted may result in falling and injury if undertaken within 8 hours of receiving parenteral lorazepam. Alcohol should not be consumed for at least 24 to 48 hours after lorazepam injection. Other warnings and precautions for lorazepam are similar to those for diazepam and other benzodiazepines.

Pediatric Use. Data are insufficient to support the use of lorazepam in patients younger than 18 years. Its administration in outpatient pediatric dentistry appears unwarranted at this time, especially in light of its prolonged clinical action.

Adverse Reactions. The most frequently noted adverse reactions to lorazepam are caused by a direct extension of its CNS depressant properties and include the following[56]:

1. *Excessive sleepiness* that interfered with regional nerve block developed in 6% of patients studied. Patients older than 50 years had a significantly greater incidence of excessive sleepiness than did younger patients.
2. Restlessness, confusion, depression, and delirium occurred in 1.3% of patients.
3. Visual and self-limiting hallucinations developed in 1% of patients.

Because of its lack of water solubility, lorazepam may produce a burning sensation at the site of IV administration similar to that of diazepam. This occurred in 1.6% of patients receiving the drug. At 24 hours after injection, 0.5% still complained of discomfort. Patients should be advised that there may be a slight warmth felt at the injection site as the drug is administered and that this is entirely normal and will pass within a few minutes. Slow injection of lorazepam into a rapidly running IV infusion minimizes this reaction.

Dosage. The following directions regarding recommended dosage are taken from the lorazepam package insert:

> For the primary purpose of sedation and relief of anxiety, usual recommended initial IV dose of lorazepam is 2 mg total, or 0.02 mg/lb (0.044 mg/kg), whichever is smaller. This dose will suffice for sedating most adults, and should not ordinarily be exceeded in patients over 50 years.[55]

Administration. Lorazepam should be diluted immediately before IV administration with an equal volume of a compatible solution. When properly diluted, lorazepam may be administered directly into a vein or into the tubing of an existing IV infusion. The rate of injection of lorazepam should not exceed 2.0 mg/min. Lorazepam may be diluted with the following:[55]

- Sterile water for injection
- Sodium chloride injection
- 5% dextrose injection

Availability. Ativan (Wyeth): 2 and 4 mg/ml in 10-ml vials and 1-ml preloaded syringes. Each milliliter of solution consists of the following:

- 2 or 4 mg lorazepam
- 0.18 ml polyethylene glycol 400 in propylene glycol
- 2% benzyl alcohol as a preservative

Lorazepam is not highly recommended for use in outpatient sedation because of its prolonged clinical action, its extreme amnesic properties, and primarily the lack of ability of the administrator to titrate the drug to clinical effect. Lorazepam is classified as a Schedule IV drug. Lorazepam is an excellent IV sedative for nonambulatory hospitalized patients for whom close posttreatment monitoring is available for extended periods.[56]

Lorazepam
The medical history of patients receiving lorazepam should be checked for the following:

- Allergy or hypersensitivity to benzodiazepines

Lorazepam
Proprietary name: Ativan
Classification: benzodiazepine
Availability: 2 and 4 mg/ml
Average sedative dose (IV): 2 mg
Maximal single dose: 2 mg
Maximal total dose: 4 mg

Lorazepam	
Pregnancy category	D
Lactation	NS
Metabolism	Liver
Excretion	Urine
DEA schedule	IV

Flunitrazepam

Flunitrazepam is a water-soluble benzodiazepine derivative that is chemically and pharmacologically related to diazepam and other drugs of this group. The chemical formula for flunitrazepam is 5-(*o*-fluorophenyl)-1,3-dihydro-1-methyl-7-nitro-2H-1,4-benzodiazepin-2-one. The sedative, antianxiety, amnesic, and muscle-relaxing properties of flunitrazepam are similar to those of diazepam except that its sedative and sleep-inducing properties are more pronounced and longer lasting than those of diazepam.[57] Foreman[58] reported flunitrazepam to be approximately 15 times as potent as diazepam and suggested that the drug be diluted before administration to ensure precise titration.

Flunitrazepam is available in a 1-ml ampule containing 2 mg. The manufacturer suggests diluting the drug with 1 ml of sterile water for injection before use, providing a solution of 1 mg/ml.[58] Foreman, however, suggests that further dilution is warranted, recommending the dilution of 2 mg (1 ml) of flunitrazepam in 9 ml of sterile water, providing a solution of 0.2 mg/ml.[58]

Following IV administration for the induction of general anesthesia, flunitrazepam produces its clinical effects within 1 to 3 minutes, and the peak effect is noted in 5 minutes. The duration of clinical action ranged from 10 to 60 minutes, with significant variation with dosage (1 to 6 mg). The α- and β-half-lives of flunitrazepam are 19 and 34 hours.

Side Effects and Complications. The side effects and complications associated with flunitrazepam administration are similar to those of other benzodiazepines. As with most benzodiazepines, flunitrazepam is remarkably free of respiratory or cardiovascular depressant effects. The most frequently reported side effects associated with flunitrazepam administration are diaphoresis, ataxia, erythema, blurred vision, hypersalivation, dry mouth, weakness, hypothermia, hypoventilation, and prolonged drowsiness.[59] The dosage of flunitrazepam should be decreased in elderly and debilitated patients. The use of alcohol and driving should be prohibited for 24 hours after the administration of flunitrazepam.

Flunitrazepam Sedation in Dentistry. Foreman reported on 10 patients who received IV flunitrazepam for conscious sedation.[58] The dosages ranged from 1.4 to 2 mg. Treatment conditions ranged from good to excellent in 8 of the 10 patients. No patient recalled receiving a local anesthetic during treatment (although they all did receive local anesthetics), nor in fact did they recall any of the dental treatment. They did remember being escorted to the recovery area and being driven home after discharge from the office.

The duration of sedation produced by flunitrazepam is somewhat longer than that produced by diazepam. This would contraindicate its use in shorter procedures (those lasting less than 1 hour) but would be an indication for its administration in longer procedures. Recovery from sedation was less complete than that seen with diazepam, even at 24 hours. In cases in which a more rapid patient recovery is important, flunitrazepam may not be the desired drug for IV conscious sedation.

Availability. Rohypnol (Roche Laboratories): 2 mg in 1-ml ampules. Flunitrazepam is not available in the United States at this time. It is available in both oral and parenteral preparations in the United Kingdom and other countries.

Chlordiazepoxide

Chlordiazepoxide is also available for injectable use; however, because of the more ready accessibility of other benzodiazepines, it is rarely used parenterally, especially intravenously.

Because of the instability of parenteral forms of chlordiazepoxide, chlordiazepoxide for IV and IM use must be prepared immediately before its administration by mixing a 5-ml dry-filled ampule containing 100 mg of chlordiazepoxide with 5 ml of either sterile physiologic saline or sterile water for injection.[60] This produces a concentration of chlordiazepoxide of 20 mg/ml, which is then injected at a rate of 1 ml/min. In view of the current availability and efficacy of diazepam and midazolam, there appears to be little reason for considering the IV administration of chlordiazepoxide.

Summary

The benzodiazepines represent the most nearly ideal agents for IV conscious sedation in the ambulatory patient. Pharmacologically, they normally demonstrate little significant effect on the cardiovascular and respiratory systems when administered in recommended doses via recommended techniques. Diazepam and midazolam are the drugs of choice for IV conscious sedation procedures with a duration of 60 minutes or less. Midazolam appears to possess several advantages over diazepam, most important of which are its amnesic qualities, lack of irritation to blood vessels, and the lack of a rebound, or second-peak, effect. Flunitrazepam is recommended for administration where procedures in excess of 1 hour are contemplated, whereas lorazepam should be reserved, in most instances, for nonambulatory well-monitored patients undergoing longer procedures.

BARBITURATES

The barbiturates have served as an important group of sedative drugs in dentistry for almost 50 years. Niels B. Jorgensen, the father of IV sedation in dentistry, used a barbiturate in his technique of IV premedication, now known worldwide as the *Jorgensen technique.*[61]

Although several barbiturates are available for IV administration (Table 25-3), only one, pentobarbital, has retained any popularity.

Secobarbital is used intravenously in the Berns technique.[62] Other barbiturates used intravenously include

TABLE 25-3 Barbiturates for Intravenous Administration

Generic Name	Proprietary Name	Usual Concentration (mg/ml)	Duration of Action	Average Sedative Dose (mg)
Pentobarbital	Nembutal	50	2-4 hr	125-175
Secobarbital	Seconal	50	2-4 hr	100-150
Methohexital	Brevital (USA) Brietal (UK)	10	5-7 min	‡
Thiopental	Pentothal	25	—	‡
Thiamylal	Surital	25	—	‡

‡Not recommended for intravenous conscious sedation without anesthesiology training.

the ultrashort-acting general anesthesia–induction agents methohexital, thiopental, and thiamylal.

Pentobarbital Sodium

Chemically, pentobarbital sodium is sodium 5-ethyl-5-(1-methylbutyl) barbiturate. The sodium salt is freely soluble in water and alcohol. Pentobarbital is classified as a short-acting barbiturate. It possesses characteristics of the entire group of barbiturates, which are now discussed.

Pharmacology. Barbiturates are frequently classified according to their duration of clinical action following oral administration (see Table 7-3). After oral and IV administration, the clinical actions of pentobarbital will be observed for approximately 2 to 4 hours.

All barbiturate sedative-hypnotics are generalized depressants, with the CNS being the most sensitive system. Barbiturates produce a characteristic pattern of CNS depression: The cerebral cortex and the reticular activating system (RAS) are most sensitive to the actions of the barbiturates; the cerebellar, vestibular, and spinal systems less so, and the medulla least sensitive of all.[63]

The RAS is important in the maintenance of a conscious alert state. Sedative doses of barbiturates act on this system to depress ascending neuronal conduction to the cerebral cortex; as a result, consciousness is diminished or lost.

Unlike true analgesic drugs, such as the opioids or nonsteroidal antiinflamatory drugs (NSAIDs), barbiturates have no effect on pain threshold except in doses affecting the level of consciousness (as in deep IV conscious sedation). In the presence of severe pain it is found that barbiturates frequently render the patient restless and more difficult to manage. This occurs because of decreased control over emotions by the cortical centers of the brain. The adult patient becomes less inhibited and more likely to respond to noxious stimulation as would a typically uninhibited child. Barbiturates should not be used as the sole agent for sedation when a painful procedure is planned. Analgesics, such as meperidine, and local anesthetics are almost always used when IV barbiturates are administered to counteract this negative effect on the pain reaction threshold.

Parenteral barbiturates are effective anticonvulsants and are administered in the management of seizures produced by tetanus, epilepsy, and local anesthetic overdose. However, with the availability of benzodiazepines, which are equally effective anticonvulsants, but with a smaller potential for respiratory depression, the use of barbiturates as anticonvulsants has declined.

Respiratory System. The barbiturates produce respiratory depression by a direct action on the medullary respiratory center. The degree of respiratory depression is dose related.[64] Respiratory arrest is the usual cause of death from barbiturate overdose. As respiratory depression develops from barbiturate administration, the rate of respiration increases while the tidal volume decreases. Respiratory reflexes, such as coughing, sneezing, hiccoughing, and laryngospasm, are only slightly depressed until the degree of CNS depression is pronounced. Laryngospasm is one of the chief respiratory complications of IV barbiturate general anesthesia (see Chapter 31).

Cardiovascular System. In comparison to the respiratory system, the cardiovascular system is relatively resistant to the depressant actions of barbiturates. Usual hypnotic doses are associated with only a slight fall in heart rate and blood pressure, similar to that seen in normal sleep. IV thiopental anesthesia will produce more significant depression of the cardiovascular system.[65] The slight drop in blood pressure observed with IV barbiturate sedation or anesthesia is a result of depression of the vasomotor center with consequent peripheral vasodilation. Larger doses of barbiturates act directly on smaller blood vessels to produce dilation and increased capillary permeability.

Absorption, Metabolism, and Excretion. Parenteral barbiturates are highly lipid soluble, a property that facilitates their rapid redistribution from the blood to other tissues within the body. When administered intravenously, the ultrashort-acting barbiturates reach peak concentration in the brain within 30 seconds. During this time, the other so-called vessel-rich tissues—heart, liver, and kidneys—also reach saturation levels. Lipid solubility and plasma protein binding of the barbiturates vary (Table 25-4) and are responsible for onset and duration of action. Drugs with greater lipid solubility (greater partition coefficient) have a more rapid onset of action, whereas protein binding relates to the relative duration of action of the agent.

Barbiturates rapidly diffuse out of the blood and are redistributed to all tissues. This leads to a rapid decrease in the blood level of the drug and a termination of clinical activity (α-half-life). The liver and muscles account for most of the volume of barbiturate that is withdrawn from the blood. Body fat, with a sparse blood supply, requires approximately 1.5 to 2 hours to become saturated. When equilibrium between the barbiturate in the tissues and the blood occurs, the decline in barbiturate blood level is slowed and becomes a measure of the rate of metabolism of the drug.

It is this rapid removal (redistribution) from the blood that accounts for the brief action of the so-called ultrashort-acting barbiturates, not their rapid metabolism. Thiopental, for example, undergoes metabolism at the

TABLE 25-4 Characteristics of Intravenous Barbiturates

Drug	Partition Coefficient	Plasma Protein Binding	Delay in Onset of Action (min)
Barbital	1	0.05	22
Phenobarbital	3	0.20	12
Pentobarbital	39	0.35	0.1
Secobarbital	52	0.44	0.1
Thiopental	580	0.65	<0.1

rate of 15% per hour. This important aspect of barbiturate pharmacology is discussed more fully in Chapter 31.

Barbiturates are eliminated in one of two methods: biotransformation in the liver and excretion through the kidneys. A few barbiturates are largely excreted, others are almost completely inactivated by the liver, and still others are partially excreted and partially metabolized (Box 25-2).

The liver is the most important organ for metabolism of barbiturates, although other organs, such as the kidneys, brain, and muscle, are also involved. Any form of liver disease or dysfunction may tend to prolong the action or intensify the depth of depression produced by the barbiturate and should be considered a relative or absolute contraindication to barbiturate administration.

The β-half-lives (the time required for biotransformation and excretion) of some of the barbiturates are listed in Table 25-5. The slow release of the barbiturates from these tissue depots may be somewhat responsible for the hangover effects so often noted after barbiturate administration.[66] The day after the administration of IV pentobarbital, some patients will still exhibit clinical signs of CNS depression.

BOX 25-2 Method of Elimination of Barbiturates

Primarily excreted by kidney
Barbital
Phenobarbital
Degraded by liver and excreted by kidney
Aprobarbital
Primarily metabolized by liver
Amobarbital
Pentobarbital
Secobarbital
Distributed to body fat, eventually dependent on liver and kidney
Thiopental
Thiamylal

Unwanted Effects. The most commonly observed unwanted effects from barbiturate administration are hangover and excitement. Hangover, or unwanted posttreatment lethargy, is produced by the slow reabsorption of the barbiturate from tissue depots (e.g., fat, muscle) into the blood and is more likely to develop with the longer-acting barbiturates.

In some patients the barbiturates produce excitation rather than depression; the patient appears to be inebriated and becomes quite talkative. This represents an idiosyncratic response and is more likely after administration of phenobarbital, although it can develop with other barbiturates.

Patients with a personal or familial history of acute intermittent porphyria represent one of the few absolute contraindications to barbiturate administration. (See Chapter 4 for a discussion of acute intermittent porphyria.)

Allergy to barbiturates, although uncommon, is more likely to develop in patients with histories of allergy, urticaria, and angioedema. Barbiturate use, especially chronic, can produce drug dependence and tolerance. In addition, drug-drug interactions with other CNS depressants must be considered whenever concomitant drug therapy is used.

Warnings. Patients receiving pentobarbital must be advised against performing any potentially hazardous tasks such as driving a vehicle or operating machinery.

TABLE 25-5 β-Half-Lives of Selected Barbiturates

Drug	β-Half-Life (hr)
Hexobarbital	4.35
Amobarbital	21.1
Pentobarbital	21.8
Secobarbital	28.9
Phenobarbital	86

It has been my clinical experience that patients who have received IV pentobarbital do not want to do anything other than return home and go to sleep in the immediate postsedation period. Patients are advised that the next day they will probably be fully capable of functioning normally; however, in a few instances, signs and symptoms may persist and the patient may be advised to continue resting.

The use of alcohol or other CNS depressants after pentobarbital administration must be cautioned against because potentially significant additive effects may develop. Prescriptions for postoperative analgesics must take this into consideration. The use of a long-acting local anesthetic, such as bupivacaine or etidocaine, as well as NSAIDs, is recommended. Chronic use of barbiturates induces liver microsomal enzyme activity and may influence the dosage of pentobarbital required for sedation. Because pentobarbital crosses the placenta, its use is contraindicated in pregnancy.

Precautions. Pentobarbital should be used with caution in patients with impaired liver function or a history of drug dependence or abuse. A history of cirrhosis or recent hepatitis represents a relative contraindication to pentobarbital administration, as does recent or chronic alcoholism. The alcoholic may respond in one of three ways to administration of the barbiturate: In most instances the response will approximate the usual response with doses within the normal range. In the second possible response the alcoholic's liver will have produced a greater volume of hepatic microsomal enzymes, which will decrease the patient's response to the usual barbiturate dosage. Significantly larger doses may be required to provide a sedative effect with pentobarbital. This response is usually noted in the "early" alcoholic, before the development of liver dysfunction—0fatty degeneration (cirrhosis)—making the patient less able to manage the usual dose of barbiturates. In this third situation the alcoholic patient will overrespond to usual dosages of pentobarbital and other barbiturates.

Patients with any respiratory disorder, especially asthma, should be administered pentobarbital with caution. Because barbiturates are potent respiratory depressants, they should be administered carefully in all patients with a suspicion of pulmonary dysfunction. The parenteral solution of pentobarbital is quite alkaline (pH 9.5). Extravascular injection of the drug may produce tissue irritation and possible damage, such as sloughing or sterile abscess formation (see Chapter 27). Hypotension may occur after rapid IV administration of pentobarbital. When the agent is administered at the recommended rate of 1 ml/min, such a response is rare.

Patients must be warned against operating a motor vehicle for the remainder of the day on which the drug is administered. As mentioned, most patients receiving pentobarbital have no desire to drive a car.

Adverse Reactions. Possible adverse reactions to pentobarbital administration include the following:[67]

- Respiratory depression
- Apnea
- Circulatory collapse
- Pain
- Skin rash
- Allergic reaction
- Residual sedation (hangover)
- Nausea and vomiting
- Paradoxical excitement

Coughing, hiccoughing, laryngospasm, and chest wall spasm have been observed after IV pentobarbital sedation. Slow administration minimizes the occurrence of these effects. With more than 1450 administrations of pentobarbital (at the University of Southern California School of Dentistry), laryngospasm and chest wall spasm have never been encountered. Bronchospasm may occur, particularly in patients with a history of asthma. This represents a relative contraindication to pentobarbital. Thrombophlebitis may also occur at the site of drug administration, although its incidence from pentobarbital is quite insignificant.

Dosage. When administered intravenously, pentobarbital must be titrated to effect. As used in the Jorgensen technique, pentobarbital will be used to provide the suitable level of sedation. The dosage range observed with pentobarbital is quite wide, with as little as 30 mg to as much as 300 mg providing the same clinical signs and symptoms in different patients. This wide range of safety with pentobarbital is one of the reasons why this drug may be recommended in IV conscious sedation procedures. Other barbiturates do not possess the same relatively flat dose-response curve and are therefore not recommended for sedative use by any doctor not trained in general anesthesia.

Although doses of pentobarbital as high as 500 mg have been used to achieve sedation in some patients, it is my recommendation that a single dose not exceed 300 mg. Repeated titration (if needed) could bring the dose up to a maximum of 500 mg for one appointment. The average dose of pentobarbital required for adequate sedation in the Jorgensen technique is 125 to 175 mg.[68]

Availability. Nembutal (Abbott): 50 mg/ml of 2-ml ampules and 20- and 50-ml multidose vials. Each milliliter of pentobarbital sodium contains the following:

- 40 mg pentobarbital sodium
- 40% propylene glycol

- 10% alcohol
- Water for injection
- pH adjusted to 9.5 with hydrochloric acid and/or sodium hydroxide
- Air in container displaced by nitrogen

Pentobarbital is classified as a DEA Schedule II drug.

Pentobarbital
The medical history of patients receiving pentobarbital should be checked for the following:
- Allergy or hypersensitivity to barbiturates
- Porphyria
- Hepatic dysfunction
- Asthma
- Respiratory depression
- Alcoholism

Pentobarbital
Proprietary name: Nembutal
Classification: barbiturate
Availability: 50 mg/ml
Average sedative dose (IV): 125-175 mg
Maximal single dose: 300 mg
Maximal total dose: 500 mg

Pentobarbital	
Pregnancy category	D
Lactation	?
Metabolism	Liver
Excretion	Urine
DEA schedule	II

Secobarbital

Secobarbital is a short-acting barbiturate similar in action to pentobarbital that is used intravenously in the Berns technique, a combination of secobarbital with an opioid and ultrashort-acting barbiturate.[62] The basic pharmacology, warnings, precautions, and side effects of secobarbital are similar to those for pentobarbital.

Dosage. In the Berns technique, when used in combination with other drugs, the maximal recommended dose of secobarbital is 50 mg.[62] When used as the sole agent for sedation, doses of 100 to 150 mg may be used, injected slowly.

Availability. Seconal (Lilly): 50 mg/ml in 1-, 2-, 10-, 20-, and 30-ml vials. Secobarbital sodium is available as a powder that is diluted with sterile water for injection. Bacteriostatic water and Ringer's lactate solutions are incompatible with secobarbital sodium. As a powder it comes in ampules containing 250 mg of the drug. It is diluted with 5 ml of diluent to produce a concentration of 5%, or 50 mg/ml. It is also available generically. Secobarbital is classified as a Schedule II drug.

Secobarbital
The medical history of patients receiving secobarbital should be checked for the following:
- Allergy or hypersensitivity to barbiturates
- Porphyria
- Hepatic dysfunction
- Asthma
- Respiratory depression
- Alcoholism

Secobarbital
Proprietary name: Seconal
Classification: barbiturate
Availability: 50 mg/ml
Average sedative dose (IV): 50-150 mg
Maximal single dose: 150 mg
Maximal total dose: 250 mg

Secobarbital	
Pregnancy category	D
Lactation	NS
Metabolism	Liver
Excretion	Urine
DEA schedule	II

Methohexital Sodium

Methohexital sodium is an ultrashort-acting barbiturate most commonly used for the rapid induction of general anesthesia (stage III) or the production of short-duration ultralight general anesthesia as frequently used for oral surgical procedures (Guedel stage II). Methohexital was synthesized by Stoelting in 1957 and popularized as an agent for outpatient dental anesthesia by Adrian Hubbell in the early 1960s.[69]

Although used primarily as a general anesthetic, methohexital sodium may be used in smaller doses as a sedative-hypnotic. Several IV conscious sedation techniques have been developed in which methohexital is used: intermittent methohexital sedation, the Berns technique (secobarbital, meperidine, and methohexital), the Shane technique (hydroxyzine, alphaprodine, and methohexital), and diazepam and methohexital sedation. These techniques are discussed in the following chapter, but the use of methohexital by any person not trained in general anesthesia cannot be recommended.

The chemical formula for methohexital sodium is sodium-a-*dl*-1-methyl-5-ally 1-5-(1-methyl-2-pentyl) barbiturate. It differs from other barbiturate anesthetics in that it does not contain any sulfur. When compared with the actions of other IV barbiturate anesthetics (e.g., thiopental, thiamylal), methohexital possesses several advantages:

- Shorter duration of action
- Faster clinical recovery
- Relative absence of local complications
- Amnesia
- Relatively stable solution

The usual duration of action of an induction dose of methohexital is 4 to 7 minutes. It is therefore suitable for short procedures requiring less than 20 minutes. Foreman[58] recommends its use as a sedative only for restorative and minor oral surgical procedures of short duration and says that if this limitation is observed, and if the patency of the airway is ensured at all times by effective mouth packing, intermittent methohexital sedation is a safe and useful technique.[9] Because of the steeper dose-response curve of methohexital, it is possible to produce overly deep sedation or light general anesthesia quite by accident. This relative lack of safety with methohexital is the basis for my recommendation against its use as a sedative by anyone without advanced training in general anesthesia. Methohexital is used as a 1% (10 mg/ml) solution. Contraindications and warnings for methohexital are similar to those for pentobarbital.

Adverse Reactions. The following are the major adverse reactions observed after the administration of methohexital sodium[70]:

- Circulatory depression: most often seen after overly rapid administration of larger doses (>10 to 20 ml)
- Thrombophlebitis: not a significant problem
- Respiratory depression, apnea: probably the most significant adverse responses to use of methohexital sodium; usually dose related; however, in sensitive individuals respiratory depression or apnea may develop at unusually small doses
- Laryngospasm: a serious complication that will develop as the patient becomes more deeply sedated if the pharynx contains fluid or foreign matter
- Bronchospasm: much more likely to develop in the patient with a history of asthma
- Hiccoughs: usually associated with rapid administration
- Skeletal muscle hyperactivity: not uncommon as the patient enters stage 2 of anesthesia; this should not develop with the small doses (10 to 20 mg) recommended for sedation
- Emergence delirium
- Nausea and vomiting
- Acute, life-threatening allergic reactions, although rare, have developed after administration of methohexital sodium

Dosage. When used as an adjunct to IV conscious sedation in dentistry, methohexital sodium must always be titrated in extremely small doses not exceeding 10 mg. On rare occasion a 20-mg dose may be used by the experienced individual, but this is never to be exceeded.

Because dental procedures in which methohexital sodium is used for sedation should not exceed 20 minutes, the maximum suggested total dose of methohexital is 100 mg. In procedures expected to require more than 20 minutes, other IV drugs should be considered for use. In both the Berns and Shane techniques, 10- to 20-mg increments of methohexital sodium are administered after the injection of other IV drugs.[62,71]

Availability. Brevital (Lilly), Brietal: 500 mg in 50-ml vials. Methohexital is prepared before use by adding 50 ml of suitable diluent to the vial to produce a 1%, or 10 mg/ml, solution. Suitable diluents include sterile water for injection, in which case the solution may be stored for up to 6 weeks, and 5% dextrose in water or isotonic (0.9%) sodium chloride solution, in which case the solution is only stable for 24 hours. Each vial of methohexital sodium contains 500 mg methohexital sodium and 30 mg anhydrous sodium carbonate. It contains no preservative. Methohexital is classified as a Schedule IV drug.

Methohexital	
Pregnancy category	B
Lactation	?
Metabolism	Liver
Excretion	Urine
DEA schedule	IV

Thiopental and Thiamylal

Two other ultrashort-acting barbiturates, thiopental and thiamylal, are available for IV administration. Thiopental (Pentothal, Abbott) and thiamylal (Surital, Parke-Davis) are used for the induction of general anesthesia (stage III) and as solo agents for general anesthesia in surgical procedures requiring 30 minutes or less. Thiopental was introduced into clinical practice by Lundy in 1934, whereas thiamylal was first described in 1935 by Volwiler and Tabern.[72] Thiopental is the most widely used ultrashort-acting barbiturate in current anesthesia practice. The duration of action of both thiopental and thiamylal is longer than that of methohexital. These drugs are rarely used in sedative procedures and cannot be recommended for use in this regard. They are discussed further in Chapter 31.

Summary

Although a number of barbiturates are available for IV administration, there are important reasons for some not being recommended for use in IV conscious sedation. The potent respiratory depressant properties of the barbiturates, combined with the steep dose-response curves of methohexital, thiopental, and thiamylal, are reason enough to recommend against their use by any doctor not extensively trained in general anesthesia and in the management of the airway of the unconscious patient. It is simply too easy to get into trouble (e.g., inadvertent loss of consciousness and airway obstruction) with these drugs. There are, however, two barbiturates—pentobarbital and secobarbital—that are recommended for use as IV sedatives. Although pharmacologically similar, pentobarbital is the more commonly used. Possessing a relatively flat dose-response curve, pentobarbital is an excellent drug for sedative procedures requiring 2 to 4 hours.

HISTAMINE BLOCKERS (ANTIHISTAMINICS)

Two drugs that are classified as histamine blockers—promethazine and hydroxyzine—are occasionally employed for IV conscious sedation. The basic pharmacology of these two drugs is discussed in Chapters 7 and 10. In this section only those aspects of their pharmacology relevant to IV administration are reviewed.

Promethazine

Promethazine is a phenothiazine derivative that is commonly used in dentistry, primarily in pediatric dentistry, as a sedative-hypnotic administered either orally or intramuscularly. Promethazine may also be administered intravenously either as a solo drug or in combination with an opioid.

The clinical duration of action of promethazine after IV administration is approximately 1 to 2 hours. Clinical recovery of the patient at this time is somewhat greater than that observed after pentobarbital administration; however, it is significantly less than that seen with diazepam or midazolam. Promethazine fills the void between the diazepam/midazolam sedative actions of approximately 1 hour and the 2- to 4-hour sedation provided by pentobarbital.

The most significant adverse reaction to the administration of promethazine is the occurrence of extrapyramidal reactions. Clinical signs and symptoms of extrapyramidal reactions and their management are discussed in Chapter 7.

Dosage. The usual dose of promethazine required for sedation after IV administration is approximately 25 to 35 mg. This drug should be administered in a concentration of 25 mg/ml. Promethazine may be administered intravenously to children. The drug should be titrated to clinical effect. In most cases the pediatric dose will not exceed that for the average adult.

Availability. Phenergan (Wyeth), Fellozine (O'Neal, Jones & Feldman), Lemprometh (Lemmon), Provigan (Reid-Provident), and Zipan (Savage): 25 mg/ml in 1-ml ampules and 10-ml vials. It is also available in a 50 mg/ml concentration that is recommended for IM use only. Promethazine is not a scheduled drug.

Promethazine	
Pregnancy category	C
Lactation	NS
Metabolism	Liver
Excretion	Feces and urine
DEA schedule	Not controlled

Hydroxyzine

Hydroxyzine is a histamine blocker that has sedative properties, although it is not as potent as promethazine. The chemical formula for hydroxyzine is 1-(*p*-chlorobenzhydryl)4-(2-[2-hydroxyethoxy]ethyl) piperazine hydrochloride. The pharmacology of hydroxyzine is discussed in Chapters 7 and 10.

Clinically important properties of hydroxyzine include its antiemetic actions and its ability to potentiate the actions of other CNS depressants, such as opioids and barbiturates. Hydroxyzine has been recommended for IV use in the Shane technique (which involves the administration of hydroxyzine, alphaprodine, and methohexital).[71] Despite the reported success of the Shane technique, there are limitations to its use, not the least of which is the fact that hydroxyzine is not recommended by its manufacturer for IV use.[73]

The drug package insert accompanying hydroxyzine lists the following as contraindications[73]:

Hydroxyzine hydrochloride intramuscular solution is intended only for intramuscular administration and should not, under any circumstances, be injected subcutaneously, intraarterially, or intravenously.

Hydroxyzine appears to be quite irritating to blood vessel walls, producing a high incidence of local complications ranging from mild phlebitis to more serious thrombosis. Because of the availability of other equally effective IV sedative-hypnotics not associated with the same degree of complications and adverse effects, the administration of hydroxyzine intravenously cannot be recommended.

Summary

Promethazine is an effective IV sedative. Its primary indication is for IV procedures requiring more than 1 but less than 2 hours to complete.

Hydroxyzine, although an effective sedative, is associated with an unacceptably high rate of localized complications and is not recommended for use intravenously.

PROPOFOL

Propofol, a 2,6-diisopropylphenol compound, is virtually insoluble in aqueous solution. After its initial introduction in a chromophore EL formulation, propofol was withdrawn from clinical use because of a high incidence of anaphylactic reactions to the chromophore solvent (1 in 1000 administrations). Propofol has subsequently been reintroduced as a 1% solution in an egg lecithin emulsion formulation consisting of 10% soya bean oil, 2.25% glycerol, and 1.2% egg phosphatide.[74] Pain on injection into small veins occurs in a high proportion of patients, but injection into larger veins or the prior administration of lidocaine or an opioid analgesic ameliorates the pain.[75] Propofol may be administered into an IV infusion of dextrose or saline but should not be mixed with other drugs or IV fluids.

Pharmacodynamics

Central Nervous System. Propofol decreases cerebral metabolism, blood flow, and intracranial pressure.[76,77] However, when larger doses are administered, marked lowering of systemic arterial pressures can significantly diminish cerebral perfusion.[78]

Respiratory System. Propofol, like most other IV CNS depressants, possesses respiratory depressant properties. Propofol depresses respiration similarly to the barbiturates in normal patients (ASA I) but to a greater degree than the benzodiazepines.[79]

Cardiovascular System. Propofol's cardiovascular depressant effects are more profound than those of thiopental.[80] Both a direct myocardial depression and decreased systemic vascular resistance have been implicated in producing profound hypotension following large bolus doses of propofol.[80,81] Age also affects cardiovascular response to propofol, and caution is mandatory when propofol is administered to elderly patients.[82]

Miscellaneous Effects

Propofol may have antiemetic effects. Studies have demonstrated an extremely low incidence of emetic sequelae after outpatient anesthesia with propofol.[83] Propofol has a distribution half-life of 2 to 4 minutes and an elimination half-life of 1 to 3 hours.[79]

Like most IV anesthetics, propofol is eliminated via hepatic metabolism followed by renal excretion of the more water-soluble metabolites. There is some evidence that an extrahepatic route of elimination, such as the lungs, contributes to the clearance of propofol.[79] Propofol is rapidly and extensively metabolized to inactive, water-soluble sulphate and glucuronic acid conjugates that are eliminated by the kidney.[84] No changes in propofol's pharmacokinetics have been reported to date in the presence of hepatic or renal disease.

Clinical Use. IV administration of propofol results in a rapid onset of action that is comparable to that of barbiturates.[85,86] Recovery from propofol's sedative-hypnotic effects is equally rapid.[87] The duration of propofol's central depressant effects increases in a dose-dependent fashion.[88] In contrast to the barbiturates, there appears to be less residual postoperative sedation, fatigue ("hangover"), and cognitive and psychomotor impairment with propofol.[89]

Propofol has received extensive interest in the area of conscious sedation and may offer advantages over other sedative-hypnotics because of its short duration of effect, rapid recovery, and minimal side effects.[90-92] A carefully titrated subhypnotic dose of propofol (0.5 to 1 mg/kg followed by 3 to 4.5 mg/kg/hr) produces excellent sedation with minimal respiratory depression and a short recovery period.[93]

Warnings. Propofol is not recommended for use in pediatric patients because safety and effectiveness have not been established.[94] Propofol administration is contraindicated in patients with a known hypersensitivity to the drug or its components.

Patients receiving propofol should be continuously monitored by persons not involved in the conduct of the surgical or diagnostic procedure; oxygen supplementation should be immediately available and provided where clinically indicated; and oxygen saturation should be monitored in all patients.[94]

Adverse Reactions. The most common adverse reactions, which occurred in more than 3% of patients receiving propofol, included hypotension, nausea, headache, and injection site pain or hotness.

Dosage and Administration. Drug dosages should always be individualized. The following are general dosage guidelines:[94]

Induction of Anesthesia. Adults: 2 to 2.5 mg/kg or approximately 40 mg every 10 seconds until induction. Elderly, debilitated patients: 1 to 1.5 mg/kg or approximately 20 mg every 10 seconds until induction. Variable-rate infusion: titrated until the desired clinical effect is obtained.

Maintenance of Anesthesia. Adults: most patients require 100 to 200 μg/kg/min, or 6 to 12 mg/kg/hr. Elderly, debilitated, and ASA III or IV patients: most require 50 to 100 μg/kg/min, or 3 to 6 mg/kg/hr. With an intermittent bolus of propofol a dose of 25 to 50 mg as needed is suggested. Variable-rate infusion: titrated to desired clinical effect.

Sedation. Dosage and rate should be individualized. A slow infusion or slow injection is preferred to rapid bolus administration. Most require an infusion of 100 to 150 μg/kg/min (6 to 9 mg/kg/hr) or a slow injection of 0.5 mg/kg over 3 to 5 minutes.

Most elderly, debilitated, and ASA III or IV patients require doses similar to healthy adults, but they must be given as a slow infusion or slow injection and not as a rapid bolus. Bolus and rate should be titrated to clinical effect. A variable-rate infusion technique is preferred over an intermittent bolus technique. Most patients require an infusion of 25 to 75 μg/kg/min (1.5 to 4.5 mg/kg/hr) or incremental bolus doses of 10 or 20 mg.

Elderly, debilitated, and ASA III or IV patients require a 20% reduction of the adult dose. A rapid (single or repeated) bolus dose should not be used.

Propofol has been shown to be compatible with the following IV fluids when administered into a running IV catheter:

- 5% dextrose injection
- Lactated Ringer's injection
- Lactated Ringer's and 5% dextrose injection
- 5% dextrose and 0.45% sodium chloride injection
- 5% dextrose and 0.2% sodium chloride injection

Strict aseptic technique must always be maintained during handling because propofol is a single-use parenteral preparation and contains no antimicrobial preservative. The vehicle is capable of supporting rapid growth of microorganisms. Failure to follow recommended handling procedures may result in microbial contamination causing fever, infection or sepsis, or other adverse consequences that could lead to life-threatening illness. Propofol should be prepared for use just before administration. Administration should be completed within 6 hours after opening of the ampules or vials.

Availability

Propofol (Diprivan; Stuart Pharmaceuticals) is available in ready-to-use 20-ml ampules and 50-ml infusion vials containing 10 mg/ml of propofol. Propofol is not a scheduled drug.

Propofol

The medical history of patients receiving propofol should be checked for the following:

- Allergy or known hypersensitivity to propofol or its components
- Nursing women

Propofol

Proprietary name: Diprivan
Classification: intravenous anesthetic/sedative-hypnotic
Availability: 10 mg/ml
Average sedative dose (IV): an infusion of 100 to 150 μg/kg/min (6 to 9 mg/kg/hr) or a slow injection of 0.5 mg/kg over 3 to 5 min
Maximal single dose: remains to be determined
Maximal total dose: remains to be determined

Propofol

Pregnancy category	B
Lactation	NS
Metabolism	Liver
Excretion	Kidney
DEA schedule	Not controlled

OPIOID ANALGESICS

Opioids are administered primarily for their analgesic properties. They are excellent drugs for the relief of moderate to severe pain.[95] Although they affect many systems throughout the body, their primary therapeutic actions derive from their effects on the CNS. Opioids are able to produce analgesia, drowsiness, changes in mood, and mental clouding. Of significance is the fact that analgesia is produced without the loss of consciousness. The use of these drugs by the oral and IM routes is discussed in Chapters 7 and 10, with relevant pharmacology reviewed in Chapter 10. In this section the use of these drugs in IV conscious sedation is discussed.

Opioid analgesics may be divided into the following categories: (1) opioid agonists, (2) opioid agonist/antagonists, and (3) opioid antagonists. *Opioid agonists* are those drugs that interact with an opioid receptor producing a physiologic change. An *opioid antagonist* is a drug that occupies a receptor site with no resultant pharmacologic effect. Opioids of the third group, *opioid agonist/antagonists,* possess properties of opioids of both of the preceding groups. With the appearance in the 1960s of drugs such as pentazocine, which had both agonist and antagonist properties, it became necessary to formulate a concept of multiple opioid receptors in the CNS.

In 1976 Martin[96] proposed a theory of multiple receptors rather than a single target for opiate agonists. Three separate opioid receptors, mu (μ), kappa (κ), and sigma (σ), were defined. A fourth, delta (δ), has since been identified. Table 10-3 lists the opioid receptors as well as agonist and antagonist drugs for each. Box 25-3 lists the various physiologic responses attributed to the various opioid receptors.[97,98]

OPIOID AGONISTS

A number of opioid agonists—meperidine, morphine, fentanyl, alfentanil, sufentanil, and remifentanil—are available for use intravenously during sedation in dentistry.

BOX 25-3 Opioid Receptor Activation and Physiologic Effects

Mu (μ) Receptor	Kappa (κ) Receptor
Euphoria	Sedation
Supraspinal analgesia	Spinal analgesia
Indifference to stimuli	Miosis
Respiratory depression	Limited respiratory depression
Catalepsy	Depressed flexor reflexes
Locomotion	
Hypothermia	
Muscular rigidity	
Dependence	

Sigma (σ) Receptor	Delta (δ) Receptor
Dysphoria	Sedation
Hallucinations	Euphoria
Catatonia	
Mydriasis	
Tachycardia	
Respiratory stimulation	
Vasomotor stimulation	

From Pallasch TJ, Gill CJ: *Oral Surg* 59:15, 1985.

Meperidine

Meperidine is the most commonly used IV opioid in dentistry. The basic pharmacology of meperidine is discussed in Chapter 10. After IV administration, meperidine exhibits clinical actions in 2 to 4 minutes. Its duration of action is approximately 30 to 45 minutes, with considerable variation noted between patients and with administration of larger doses.

Meperidine has atropine-like properties, having been synthesized in the 1930s as an anticholinergic.[99] Patients receiving meperidine may demonstrate decreased salivary secretions and an increased heart rate because of its vagolytic properties. In the doses recommended here, these responses are normally minimal.

Meperidine may also produce localized histamine release, resulting in the phenomenon of "tracking" at the site of meperidine administration. The skin overlying the vein into which meperidine is injected will appear red, and the patient may mention that itching is present. As meperidine is carried by veins up the patient's arm toward the heart, the reddening may continue to follow the path of the vein. It is important to remember that this is a normal response to meperidine administration, not an allergic reaction. Meperidine-induced histamine release will be localized to the path of the vein, whereas an allergic response will be more generalized over the entire region. Management of meperidine-induced histamine release is simply to allow it to dissipate spontaneously, which occurs over the next 10 to 15 minutes.

Dosage. When meperidine is administered intravenously during conscious sedation in most dental situations, the recommended maximal dose is 50 mg. When this dose is administered, the usual patient response is an increase in the pain reaction threshold (analgesia) without any significant change in the depth of sedation. Opioids are usually administered *after* administration of a sedative-hypnotic (the primary drugs used to produce sedation). At a maximal dose of 50 mg, meperidine produces virtually no cardiovascular or respiratory depression in the typical patient.[100] Meperidine should be administered in a concentration not exceeding 10 mg/ml. When the 50-mg/ml concentration is used, 1 ml of meperidine is placed into a 5-ml syringe and 4 ml of diluent (e.g., 5% dextrose and water) is added. The resulting solution contains 50 mg of meperidine in 5 ml of fluid, or 10 mg/ml.

Availability. Demerol (Winthrop) (Pethidine in the United Kingdom): 10 mg/ml in 1-ml ampules, 25 mg/ml in 0.5- and 1-ml ampules, 50 mg/ml in 0.5- and

1-ml ampules and 30-ml vials, 75 mg/ml in 1- and 1.5-ml ampules, and 100 mg/ml in 1- and 2-ml ampules and 20- and 30-ml vials. Meperidine is classified as a Schedule II drug (DEA). Each milliliter of solution contains the following:

- *x* mg meperidine
- pH adjusted to 3.5 to 6 with sodium hydroxide or hydrochloric acid
- Multidose vials that contain 0.1% metacresol as a preservative; no preservatives are added to the ampules

It has been my clinical experience that the 50-mg/ml dosage form of meperidine is the most convenient to work with. More concentrated solutions are potentially dangerous because it is too easy for a mistake in calculation to lead to the administration of an overly large dose. The 10- and 25-mg/ml dosage forms are also appropriate; however, with the 10-mg/ml form larger volumes of solution will be used.

Single-use 1-ml ampules are recommended instead of multidose vials unless meperidine is used on a regular basis. The 20- or 30-ml vial may become contaminated if permitted to remain unused for a considerable time. Because meperidine (and other opioid analgesics) is a Schedule II drug, precise records must be kept of the drug's administration. Use of 1-ml ampules simplifies this task considerably.

Meperidine
The medical history of patients receiving meperidine should be checked for the following:

- Allergy or known hypersensitivity to opioid analgesics
- MAOIs taken within 14 days
- COPD and decreased respiratory reserve

Meperidine
Proprietary name: Demerol
Classification: opioid agonist
Availability: 10, 25, 50, 75, and 100 mg/ml
Average sedative dose (IV): 37.5-50 mg
Maximal single dose: 50 mg
Maximal total dose: 50 mg

Meperidine	
Pregnancy category	C
Lactation	?
Metabolism	Liver, mostly
Excretion	Urine
DEA schedule	II

Morphine

Morphine sulfate is the classical opioid agonist. It is useful but rarely used for IV conscious sedation in outpatient situations because of its long duration of action (1.5 to 2 hours). The pharmacology of morphine is discussed in Chapter 10.

Dosage. When it is administered for IV conscious sedation in dentistry, the maximal dose of morphine should not exceed 8 mg. The drug is diluted to a concentration of 1 mg/ml before use. Little change in the depth of sedation will normally occur at this dose level, yet the patient's pain reaction threshold will be elevated.

Availability. Morphine sulfate: 2, 4, 8, 10, and 15 mg/ml. Morphine sulfate is classified as a Schedule II drug. The use of morphine sulfate should be restricted to dental procedures requiring more than 2 hours.

Morphine
The medical history of patients receiving morphine should be checked for the following:

- Allergy or known hypersensitivity to opioid analgesics
- Asthma
- MAOIs taken within 14 days
- COPD and decreased respiratory reserve

Morphine
Proprietary name: Morphine
Classification: opioid agonist
Availability: 2, 4, 8, 10, 15 mg/ml
Average sedative dose (IV): 5-6 mg
Maximal single dose: 8 mg
Maximal total dose: 8 mg

Morphine	
Pregnancy category	C
Lactation	?
Metabolism	Liver
Excretion	Urine
DEA schedule	II

Alphaprodine

In response to a number of unfortunate incidents involving its administration, the manufacturer of alphaprodine (Roche Laboratories, Inc.) removed the agent from the U.S. market in 1986.[101] This was the second time that this action had been taken and probably represented the end of alphaprodine's clinical use in the United States. The agent is still available, and used successfully, in many other parts of the world.

Alphaprodine is a rapid-onset, short-acting opioid agonist used primarily in pediatric dentistry by the submucosal (SM) route of administration.[102] Its pharmacology is reviewed in Chapter 10. Onset of action after IV administration is 1 to 2 minutes. Duration of action of IV alphaprodine is approximately 30 minutes, which makes this a potentially very useful drug in dentistry.

Alphaprodine is no longer available in the United States. When available, it was classified as a Schedule II drug.

Fentanyl

Fentanyl is a rapid-onset, short-acting opioid agonist that is approximately 100 times more potent than morphine (0.1 mg of fentanyl is equianalgesic to 10 mg of morphine).[103] It was originally synthesized and introduced as one of the components of the drug combination known as Innovar.

After IV administration the onset of analgesia and sedation occurs almost immediately (less than 1 minute), although the maximal analgesic and respiratory depressant effects of fentanyl do not develop for several minutes. Average duration of clinical action is 30 to 60 minutes, which makes fentanyl an almost ideal drug for outpatient procedures requiring approximately 1 hour to complete.[104]

Respiratory depression is a side effect of all opioid agonists, with the respiratory depressant effect of fentanyl lasting longer than its analgesic properties. This potential must always be considered before discharge of an apparently "recovered" patient from the office in the custody of a person who is not trained to recognize respiratory depression and to manage it.

As with other opioid agonists, fentanyl slows the respiratory rate. This action of fentanyl is rarely observed for more than 30 minutes after the drug's administration. After IV administration of a single dose of fentanyl, peak respiratory depression is noted 5 to 15 minutes later.[105] Depression of breathing (decreased sensitivity to CO_2 stimulation) has been demonstrated for up to 4 hours in healthy volunteers.

Indications. Fentanyl is indicated for use as the following:

- As an analgesic in short anesthetic procedures and in the recovery room
- As an analgesic to supplement general or regional anesthesia
- In combination with a neuroleptic as a premedication for the induction of anesthesia and as an adjunct in the maintenance of general and regional anesthesia

Contraindications. Fentanyl is contraindicated for use in patients with known allergy or intolerance to it.

Warnings. Fentanyl may cause muscular rigidity, especially involving the muscles of respiration (thoracic and abdominal).[106] This action appears to be related to rate of injection, occurring more frequently when the drug is administered rapidly. This can usually be prevented by the slow IV administration of the drug.

Should muscular rigidity develop, management consists of assisted or controlled ventilation or, if necessary, the administration of a neuromuscular blocking agent such as succinylcholine. This latter step must never be considered unless the doctor has been trained to administer skeletal muscle relaxants and is intimate with the technique of controlled ventilation. Patients who have received MAOIs within the past 14 days should not receive fentanyl or any other opioid agonist because of the potential for severe and unpredictable potentiation of the opioid effect.[107]

The safety of fentanyl in patients younger than 2 years has not been established; therefore it cannot be recommended for use in dental outpatient sedation in this population. Fentanyl should not be administered to pregnant patients unless the benefits of its administration clearly outweigh the potential hazards of opioid administration.[108]

Precautions. Fentanyl should be administered with caution to patients with chronic obstructive pulmonary disease (COPD) and to patients with decreased respiratory reserve (ASA III through V). In these patients opioids may decrease respiratory drive to an even greater degree than usual. Significant liver and renal dysfunction also represent relative contraindications to fentanyl administration.

Adverse Reactions. The most frequently noted adverse reactions to fentanyl administration include respiratory depression, apnea, muscular rigidity, and bradycardia. If untreated, these may progress to respiratory arrest, circulatory depression, or cardiac arrest. Other adverse reactions include hypotension, dizziness, blurred vision, nausea and vomiting, laryngospasm, and diaphoresis.[108]

Dosage. Fentanyl is administered in conjunction with other antianxiety or sedative-hypnotic medications for sedation. The recommended dose of fentanyl is therefore predicated on the fact that the patient has already received one or more other CNS depressants.

The maximal dose of fentanyl recommended for use in outpatient sedative procedures is 0.05 to 0.06 mg (1.0 to 1.2 ml). This dose is equivalent to approximately 8 mg morphine and about 50 mg of meperidine. Fentanyl should always be diluted from its initial concentration of 0.05 mg/ml by adding 4 ml of diluent (e.g., 5% dextrose and sterile water) to produce a final concentration of 0.01 mg/ml.

Availability. Sublimaze (Janssen, McNEILAB): 0.05 mg/ml in 2-, 5-, 10-, and 20-ml ampules. Each milliliter of solution contains 0.05 mg fentanyl citrate and sodium hydroxide for adjustment of pH to 4.0 to 7.5.

Fentanyl (Abbott, Elkins-Sinn): 0.05 mg/ml in same forms as Sublimaze. Fentanyl is classified as a Schedule II drug.

Fentanyl

The medical history of patients receiving fentanyl should be checked for the following:

- Allergy or known hypersensitivity to opioid analgesics
- MAOIs taken within 14 days
- COPD and decreased respiratory reserve

Fentanyl

Proprietary name: Sublimaze
Classification: opioid agonist
Availability: 0.05 mg/ml
Average sedative dose (IV): 0.05-0.06 mg
Maximal single dose: 0.08 mg
Maximal total dose: 0.08 mg

Fentanyl

Pregnancy category	C
Lactation	NS
Metabolism	Liver
Excretion	Urine
DEA schedule	II

Alfentanil, Sufentanil, and Remifentanil

Three analogs of fentanyl—alfentanil, sufentanil, and remifentanil—are in clinical use in the United States. Clinical actions of these drugs are similar to those of fentanyl, but there are significant differences. Although the onset of clinical action of alfentanil is very rapid, occurring within 1 minute after injection, its duration is very short (11 minutes at twice its MED_{50}).[109] The elimination half-life of alfentanil is 97 ± 22 minutes in adults, whereas in geriatric patients and persons with liver dysfunction, clearance rates are slower.[110-112] Alfentanil is a tetrazole derivative of fentanyl with many pharmacologic actions similar to those of fentanyl and sufentanil; however, alfentanil has a quicker onset of action than fentanyl and a shorter duration of action than either fentanyl or sufentanil.[113] In addition, alfentanil has a shorter half-life and may produce less respiratory depression than either fentanyl or sufentanil.

The use of alfentanil and sufentanil in general anesthesia has been evaluated in depth,[114,115] they are quite well accepted, especially for short surgical procedures. Alfentanil has received considerable attention in dentistry and other outpatient surgical procedures.[116-118] Alfentanil is frequently administered in conjunction with propofol.[119] Both alfentanil and sufentanil are opioid agonists and as such should be managed with the same care as other members of this group.

Remifentanil, an ultrashort-acting opioid agonist, is the most recent addition to the fentanyl family.[120-123] It is used as a supplement in the maintenance of balanced general anesthesia. Because of its short duration of action, its use as a sole agent for induction of anesthesia is not recommended; remifentanil should be used in combination with other induction agents. An infusion pump is the recommended means of remifentanil administration. Onset of action is 1 minute, with a duration of action of between 5 and 10 minutes. Bolus doses are not recommended for sedation cases and in the treatment of postoperative pain because of the risk of respiratory depression and muscle rigidity. Because of remifentanil's extremely short duration of action, when postoperative pain is anticipated, a postoperative analgesic (e.g., morphine or meperidine) should be administered before discontinuation of the remifentanil infusion.

Availability. Alfenta (Janssen): 500 μg (alfentanil as hydrochloride) per milliliter in 2-, 5-, 10-, and 20-ml ampules. Sufenta (Janssen): 50 μg (sufentanil as citrate) per milliliter in 1-, 2-, and 5-ml ampules. Ultiva (Glaxo Wellcome): (remifentanil) 1 mg/3 ml vial; 2 mg/5 ml vial; 5 mg/10 ml vial. Alfentanil, sufentanil and remifentanil are classified as Schedule II drugs.

OPIOID AGONIST/ANTAGONISTS

Because of the potentially significant side effects associated with administration of opioid agonists, considerable research was conducted to find a potent analgesic that possesses the efficacy of morphine but lacks its respiratory depressant actions, its drug dependence, and abuse liability.

In the 1960s success was attained with the introduction of pentazocine, the first drug with both opioid agonist and opioid antagonist properties to be marketed (1967).[124] In succeeding years some of the initial fervor for pentazocine waned as significant side effects were reported.[125-126] Two other drugs in this same category—nalbuphine and butorphanol—have been developed and are used in IV conscious sedation in both dental and medical outpatient procedures.[127-128] The three drugs classified as opioid agonist/antagonists are pentazocine, nalbuphine, and butorphanol.

Pentazocine

The chemical formula for pentazocine is 1,2,3,4,5,6-hexahydro-6,11-dimethyl-3-(3-methyl-2-butenyl)-2,6-methano-3-benzazocin-8-ol lactate. Pentazocine was introduced in 1967 as a nonnarcotic opioid in both oral and parenteral formulations.[124]

A dose of 30 mg of pentazocine is equivalent to approximately 10 mg of morphine or 75 mg of meperidine. Administered intravenously, pentazocine's onset of action is 1 to 2 minutes, with a duration of approximately 1 hour, although the patient may still exhibit alterations in consciousness for a number of hours after discharge from the office.

Pentazocine has opioid antagonist effects as well as sedative properties. Administered to patients receiving morphine-type opioids, pentazocine weakly antagonizes the analgesic, cardiovascular, respiratory, and CNS depressant effects produced by these agents.[129] The sedative effect of a 30-mg IV dose of pentazocine is equivalent to that of approximately 10 mg of IV diazepam.[130] Pentazocine does not provide the same degree of amnesia as does diazepam.

Pentazocine is indicated for use in the management of moderate to severe pain (usually administered orally or intramuscularly) and is also used as a preoperative or preanesthetic medication (usually administered intramuscularly) and as a supplement during general anesthesia (administered intravenously). Pentazocine initially gained some popularity within dentistry as an alternative to the opioid agonists.[131] However, with the introduction of butorphanol and nalbuphine, the dental use of pentazocine decreased substantially.

Contraindications. Pentazocine is contraindicated for use in patients with documented allergy to it.

Warnings. Despite early claims to the contrary, experience with pentazocine has demonstrated that both psychological and physical dependence can develop.[132] Abrupt discontinuance of pentazocine has produced a clinical syndrome consisting of abdominal cramps, elevated temperature, rhinorrhea, restlessness, anxiety, and lacrimation.[133] Pentazocine is a drug with significant abuse potential, being combined (orally) with the histamine blocker pyribenzamine in a combination called "Ts and blues."[134]

In the 1980s the manufacturers of oral pentazocine (Talwin) reformulated its compound, taking into account this abuse potential. Its new formulation, Talwin Nx, combines pentazocine (50 mg) with the opioid antagonist naloxone (0.5 mg). The intent of this combination is obvious, but its effectiveness is not yet known.[135]

Pentazocine should be administered to the pregnant patient only in situations in which the benefits of administration clearly outweigh its potential hazards. For routine outpatient sedation in a typical dental setting, there is little indication for pentazocine administration in pregnant patients.

Another significant untoward effect of pentazocine is the occurrence of acute neuropsychiatric manifestations, such as visual hallucinations, disorientation, confusion, mental depression, disturbing dreams, and dysphoria.[136] These responses usually resolve spontaneously within a few hours. The responsible mechanism is as yet unknown. Administration of naloxone may end in recovery. Management of reactions that do occur is symptomatic, with vital signs being monitored and recorded regularly during the reaction, although stimulation of the sigma receptor will produce these same responses. Readministration of pentazocine to this same patient at future dates should be avoided if possible to minimize the possibility of recurrence.

The administration of pentazocine to patients younger than 12 years is not recommended because of a lack of clinical data. The drug package insert for pentazocine recommends that ambulatory patients receiving parenteral pentazocine be cautioned not to operate machinery, drive cars, or unnecessarily expose themselves to hazards.[137]

Precautions. Patients with asthma, COPD, or other conditions associated with decreased respiratory reserve should be given pentazocine with caution, if at all. Patients with extensive liver disease appear to exhibit a greater number of adverse side effects from the usual clinical dose, a response indicating a decreased rate of metabolism of the drug by the liver. The plasma half-life of pentazocine is approximately 2 hours.

Pentazocine should be administered with caution to patients with seizure disorders. Seizures have developed after administration of pentazocine, although a direct cause-and-effect relationship has never been established.[138]

Adverse Reactions. Pentazocine exhibits the same adverse reactions as the opioid agonists discussed, including nausea and vomiting, xerostomia, diarrhea, constipation, blurred vision, euphoria, dysphoria, respiratory and cardiovascular depression, and allergic reactions. In addition, pentazocine produces the neuropsychiatric reactions noted.

Dosage. Pentazocine is commonly administered in conjunction with an antianxiety or sedative-hypnotic agent for conscious sedation. It is therefore usually administered after the patient has received one or more drugs. The maximal recommended dose of pentazocine in IV conscious sedation is 30 mg. When titrated slowly, the usual dose required (in combination with other drugs) for sedation is approximately 20 mg.

Availability. Talwin (Winthrop): 30 mg/ml in 1-ml, 1.5-ml, and 2-ml ampules and in 10-ml vials. Each milliliter of solution in the ampule contains the following:

- 30 mg pentazocine lactate
- 1 mg acetone sodium bisulfite
- 2.2 mg sodium chloride
- Water for injection

Each milliliter of solution in the vial contains the following:

- 30 mg pentazocine lactate
- 2 mg acetone sodium bisulfite
- 1.5 mg sodium chloride
- 1 mg methylparaben as preservative
- Water for injection

The pH of both solutions is adjusted to 4 to 5 with lactic acid or sodium hydroxide. Air in both the ampules and vials has been displaced with nitrogen. Pentazocine is classified as a Schedule IV drug.

Nalbuphine

Nalbuphine, 17-(cyclobutylmethyl)-4,5a-epoxymorphinan-3,6a,14-triol hydrochloride, was synthesized in 1965. The chemical incorporates the molecular features of the opioid agonist oxymorphone hydrochloride (Numorphan) with that of the opioid antagonist naloxone hydrochloride (Narcan).[139]

Pharmacology. Nalbuphine is a potent analgesic with an analgesic potency approximately 0.8 to 0.9 times that of morphine. In clinical practice nalbuphine is considered equianalgesic to morphine when administered in equal doses (e.g., 10 mg of nalbuphine is equal to 10 mg of morphine).[140]

After IV administration, nalbuphine's onset of action is 2 to 3 minutes. Its duration of action is slightly longer than that of morphine (approximately 3 to 6 hours). A 10-mg dose of nalbuphine is equivalent to approximately 50 to 75 mg of meperidine.[141]

Studies of the effectiveness of nalbuphine as a preoperative sedative agent are lacking, and there are few studies evaluating IV nalbuphine in dental procedures.[142-144] Over the past 10 years I have used nalbuphine several hundred times in IV conscious sedation on dental outpatients, usually with acceptable results.

Nalbuphine possesses opioid antagonist effects at the μ-opioid receptor. Nalbuphine is 10 times as effective as pentazocine as an opioid antagonist and one fourth as potent as nalorphine in morphine-dependent subjects. Quite interesting, and potentially very significant, is the fact that nalbuphine may be used as an opioid antagonist in place of naloxone. Magruder et al.[145] substituted nalbuphine (0.1 mg/kg) for naloxone to reverse respiratory depression produced by oxymorphone or hydromorphone. They noted a dramatic reversal of respiratory depression and a restoration of normal ventilation within 5 minutes. Of greater importance is the fact that nalbuphine provided substantial analgesia *after* reversal of the opioid-induced respiratory depression, which extended well into the postoperative period. These differential μ-opioid (opioid antagonism) and μ-opioid (agonist analgesia) receptor actions of nalbuphine may be of value in avoidance of the adverse cardiovascular stimulation observed in some patients suffering from surgical pain when naloxone is administered to reverse opioid-induced CNS depression; unfortunately, however, naloxone also acts to reverse the analgesia produced by the opioid.[146]

Pharmacokinetics. After IV administration the analgesic effects of nalbuphine appear in 2 to 3 minutes. The analgesic effects of the drug persist for approximately 3 to 6 hours. The plasma half-life of nalbuphine is 5 hours. The drug undergoes metabolism in the liver; oral doses of nalbuphine undergo a significant hepatic first-pass effect, with only 20% of an orally administered dose being biologically available.[147]

Nalbuphine is physically compatible with most aqueous drugs and can thus be combined in the same syringe. Nalbuphine cannot, however, be combined with either diazepam or pentobarbital because a milky white precipitate forms.

Adverse Effects. When nalbuphine is used solely as an analgesic, the most frequently noted adverse effect is sedation, which is reported in 36% of patients.[148] This "side effect" is used to advantage in IV conscious sedation procedures. Other common adverse responses (occurring in more than 3% of patients) include the following:

Sweaty, clammy feeling	9%
Nausea and vomiting	6%
Dizziness, vertigo	5%
Dry mouth	4%
Headache	3%

Psychotomimetic effects occurred only rarely and included depression, confusion, dysphoria, euphoria, feelings of unreality, feelings of hostility, and hallucinations. The incidence of these is significantly less than that seen with pentazocine.[148]

Possibly the most potentially serious adverse effect associated with nalbuphine administration is respiratory depression. When the classic opioid agonists (morphine, meperidine, and fentanyl) are administered, both the rate and depth of respiration are depressed in a dose-related manner until apnea occurs. For outpatient ambulatory procedures, the potential for respiratory depression is the factor most significantly limiting the use of opioid agonists. Nalbuphine possesses ceiling effects for respiratory depression, whereas its analgesic effects may become more pronounced with increasing doses. Gal et al.[149] demonstrated a plateau effect for both respiratory depression and analgesia for nalbuphine in doses up to 0.6 mg/kg. In other studies it was demonstrated that the normal dose of nalbuphine (7 to 10 mg/70 kg) produced the same degree of respiratory depression as an equivalent dose of morphine; however, nalbuphine-induced respiratory depression peaked at 30 mg/70 kg (equivalent to 20 mg/70 kg morphine) and remained the same even at nalbuphine doses of 3 mg/kg (210 mg/70 kg), whereas morphine-induced depression continued in a dose-related manner.[150,151] Larger doses of nalbuphine do not extend the duration of respiratory depression beyond the usual 3 hours. Nalbuphine therefore possesses a ceiling effect to both the degree and the duration of respiratory depression. This is in contrast to butorphanol, which has a ceiling effect only for the degree of respiratory depression, not its duration.[152]

In the area of administration to medically compromised patients, especially the cardiovascular-risk patient, nalbuphine produces a slight decrease in the cardiac workload, a potentially beneficial effect. Romagnoli and Keats[153] considered nalbuphine an ideal drug for patients with heart disease because it was devoid of hemodynamic effects except those associated with the relief of pain and anxiety. Lefevre et al. compared clinically equivalent doses of fentanyl with nalbuphine for "IV analgesia" in medically compromised patients (ASA III or IV).[154] Respiratory rates and SpO_2 were significantly lower ($p < .05$) for the patients receiving fentanyl.

One of the potential benefits of the opioid agonist/antagonist analgesics is a limited or absent drug dependence and abuse liability (e.g., psychic dependence, physical dependence, tolerance) as a result of their opioid antagonist actions when compared with complete μ-receptor agonists such as morphine.[155]

Overdose. Overdose of nalbuphine is exceptionally rare but possible. Signs and symptoms of overdose include CNS depression and respiratory depression, both of which are managed with basic life support and completely reversed with the IV administration of naloxone.

Contraindications. Nalbuphine is contraindicated for use in patients who are allergic or hypersensitive to it.

Warnings. Because nalbuphine produces CNS depression, patients receiving this drug must be cautioned against the performance of potentially dangerous tasks such as driving a car and operating machinery.[139] Nalbuphine is not recommended for administration to patients younger than 18 years because of a lack of clinical experience in patients in this age group. Pregnant patients should not receive nalbuphine unless the advantages of its administration clearly outweigh its potential disadvantages.

Nalbuphine may exhibit additive effects with other CNS depressants administered concurrently. The dosage of one or both of the drugs should be reduced. This should not be a significant problem with IV administration if the drugs are titrated to effect.

Precautions. Nalbuphine should be administered with caution, at reduced dosages, to patients with impaired respiratory drive, including asthma and COPD (ASA III, IV, and V). Because nalbuphine is metabolized in the liver and excreted through the kidneys, it is possible that patients with impaired hepatic or renal function may overrespond to usual dosages. Dosages should be reduced in these patents. Titration minimizes this risk.

Dosage. When administered intravenously, nalbuphine should be titrated to clinical effect. The maximal dose of nalbuphine recommended for IV conscious sedation is 10 mg. This represents both the maximal single and total doses. Onset of action after IV administration is 2 to 3 minutes, with a duration of analgesic effect of 3 to 6 hours. The average IV dose of nalbuphine is approximately 7 to 8 mg.

When nalbuphine is administered after diazepam or midazolam, the depth of sedation is rarely increased. However, recovery from sedation is somewhat less complete than that observed when diazepam or midazolam is administered alone.

Because of the doses recommended here, the beneficial effects of nalbuphine's ceiling level for respiratory depression will not be observed. It is only at dosages considerably greater than these that the ceiling effect on respiratory depression will be noted. In doses up to 10 mg of nalbuphine, the degree of respiratory depression should not be profound but will be equivalent to that induced by 10 mg of morphine or 50 to 75 mg of meperidine.

Availability. Nubain (Endo): 10 mg/ml in 1- and 2-ml ampules and 10-ml vials. Each milliliter of solution contains the following:

- 10 mg nalbuphine hydrochloride
- 0.1% sodium chloride
- 0.94% sodium citrate
- 1.26% citric acid anhydrous
- 0.1% sodium metabisulfite
- 0.2% 9:1 mixture of methylparaben and propylparaben as a preservative
- Hydrochloric acid to adjust pH

Nalbuphine is not a scheduled drug.

Nalbuphine
The medical history of patients receiving nalbuphine should be checked for the following:

- Allergy or known hypersensitivity to nalbuphine
- Known or suspected opioid dependence
- Pregnancy or childbearing potential
- Asthma, COPD, or other types of decreased respiratory drive

Nalbuphine
Proprietary name: Nubain
Classification: opioid agonist/antagonist
Availability: 10 mg/ml
Average sedative dose (IV): 7-8 mg
Maximal single dose: 10 mg
Maximal total dose: 10 mg

Nalbuphine	
Pregnancy category	B
Lactation	S?
Metabolism	Liver
Excretion	Feces and urine
DEA schedule	Not controlled

Butorphanol

Butorphanol was synthesized in 1971 by Monkovic and introduced in the United States in 1978. Butorphanol is a synthetic agonist/antagonist analgesic similar in pharmacology to nalbuphine. The chemical formula of butorphanol is *levo-N*-cyclobutylmethyl-6,10a, b-dihydroxy-1,2,3,9,10,10a-hexahydro-(4H)-10, 4a-iminoethanophenanthrene tartrate.

Pharmacology. When butorphanol is compared with morphine for analgesia, 2 mg of butorphanol (administered intramuscularly) is approximately as effective as 10 mg of morphine, 80 mg of meperidine, and 40 mg of pentazocine. Data indicate that butorphanol is approximately 3.5 to 7 times as potent as morphine, 15 to 20 times more potent than pentazocine, and 30 to 40 times more potent than meperidine on a weight basis.[156]

Pharmacokinetics. After IV administration, butorphanol's analgesic actions are noted within minutes. Maximal blood levels occur in 5 minutes and thereafter decline in a biphasic manner. The α-half-life of rapid elimination (distribution) is approximately 0.1 hour, and the β-half-life (metabolism and excretion) is 2.15 to 3.5 hours. Duration of analgesic properties is 3 to 4 hours.[157]

Butorphanol undergoes extensive metabolism in the liver before excretion through the kidneys. Less than 5% of a dose is excreted unchanged in the urine. The major route of elimination of butorphanol and its metabolites is through the kidney (75%), with biliary excretion accounting for 15% of the dose. It is 80% bound to human serum protein and distributed extensively to tissues. Butorphanol is highly lipid soluble and concentrates in adipose tissue and excretory organs. Accumulation may occur with repeated doses of the drug.[158]

Effect on Respiration. Butorphanol has properties similar to those of pentazocine and nalbuphine with respect to respiratory depression and opioid antagonist properties.[159] As an antagonist, butorphanol is 30 times as potent as pentazocine but only one fortieth as potent as naloxone. In a study by Nagashima et al., 2- and 4-mg IV doses of butorphanol were compared with 10- and 20-mg doses of morphine.[160] Respiratory depression produced by 4 mg of butorphanol was found to be statistically and clinically equivalent to that produced by 2 mg of butorphanol or 10 mg of morphine. This and other studies have demonstrated that butorphanol does not produce a dose-related effect on respiration in contrast to that observed with opioid agonists such as morphine and meperidine.

Increasing doses of butorphanol did, however, produce a longer duration of respiratory depression, although the degree of depression did not increase.[161] Butorphanol possesses a ceiling effect only for the degree of respiratory depression but not for its duration, whereas nalbuphine possesses a ceiling effect for both the depth and duration of respiratory depression. As with other opioid agonists and opioid agonist/antagonists, these respiratory depressant properties of butorphanol are reversible with naloxone.

Cardiovascular Effects. Unlike nalbuphine, butorphanol does possess cardiovascular effects similar to, but less intense than, those of pentazocine.

These include increased pulmonary artery pressure, increased pulmonary wedge pressure, increased left ventricular end-diastolic pressure, increased systemic arterial pressure, and increased pulmonary vascular resistance. Both the cardiac index and cardiac workload are increased with butorphanol.[162]

Butorphanol and pentazocine administration should be restricted in patients with acute myocardial infarction, coronary insufficiency or ventricular dysfunction, and high blood pressure (ASA IV and V). Butorphanol, like nalbuphine, is an agonist/antagonist analgesic with a low physical-dependence liability, which distinguishes it from traditional potent opioid agonists.

When butorphanol is administered in large doses, the incidence of unpleasant psychotomimetic effects is increased. This factor may serve to limit the abuse potential of butorphanol.

Side Effects. Side effects reported after butorphanol administration are similar to those for other parenteral analgesics. The most frequently reported side effect was sedation (37%), a side effect that is used to advantage during IV conscious sedation. Other common side effects were as follows:

Floating, pleasant feelings	7%
Nausea	7%
Clamminess, sweating	5%
Headache	2%
Vertigo	2%
Dizziness	2%
Lethargy	2%

Overdosage. Overdose of butorphanol is extremely unlikely; however, it is a clinical possibility. Signs and symptoms relate to exaggerated CNS and respiratory depression. Management consists of basic life support, with consideration for airway patency and ventilation, followed by the administration of naloxone or other opioid antagonists.

Warnings. Because of its opioid antagonist properties, the use of butorphanol is not recommended in patients known to be physically dependent on opioids. Administration in such patients may induce an acute abstinence syndrome (withdrawal).[163] Because of the increased workload of the heart occurring with butorphanol administration, this drug is not recommended in patients with ventricular dysfunction or coronary insufficiency.

Precautions. Because butorphanol produces some respiratory depression, it should be administered with caution to patients with preexisting respiratory depression, such as patients receiving other CNS depressants; patients with asthma, COPD, or other types of decreased respiratory reserve; or patients with high blood pressure (ASA III, IV, or V).

Patients with hepatic or renal dysfunction may overrespond to usual doses of butorphanol. If it is administered to these patients, the dosage should be adjusted to account for this response. With IV administration, slow titration will minimize this possibility.

Use of butorphanol in patients younger than 18 years or in pregnant patients is not recommended because of a lack of clinical experience to indicate its safety in these groups. Ambulatory patients receiving butorphanol must, of course, be cautioned against possible hazardous situations such as driving a car or operating machinery.

Dosage. My experience with butorphanol administered for IV conscious sedation has been limited to approximately 112 cases at this time (July 2002). However, it has been my impression that butorphanol may effectively be substituted for the traditional opioid agonists with no decrease in effectiveness and with the possible addition of decreased risk of respiratory depression. The doses recommended for IV use should preclude significant respiratory depression regardless of the pharmacologic properties of butorphanol.

After IV administration of 1 to 2 mg, onset of analgesic and sedative actions is quite rapid (1 to 2 minutes). Administered after diazepam, titrated butorphanol usually will not deepen the sedative level of the patient; therefore the maximal recommended dose (2 mg) is usually given. Recovery from diazepam-butorphanol sedation is not as complete clinically as from diazepam sedation alone.

Availability. Stadol (Bristol): 1 mg/ml in 1-mg single-dose vial and 2 mg/ml in 1-, 2-, and 10-ml vials. Each milliliter of solution contains sodium chloride, sodium citrate, and citric acid as buffers.

The 10-ml multidose vial also contains the preservative benzethonium chloride. Butorphanol is a DEA Schedule IV drug.

Butorphanol
The medical history of patients receiving butorphanol should be checked for the following:
- Allergy or known hypersensitivity to butorphanol
- Known or suspected opioid dependence
- Asthma, COPD, or other types of decreased respiratory drive
- High blood pressure
- Cardiovascular disease

Butorphanol
Proprietary name: Stadol
Classification: opioid agonist/antagonist
Availability: 1 and 2 mg/ml
Average sedative dose (IV): 1.5 mg
Maximal single dose: 2 mg
Maximal total dose: 2 mg

Butorphanol	
Pregnancy category	C
Lactation	S
Metabolism	Liver, extensively
Excretion	Urine
DEA schedule	IV

Summary

The opioid agonist/antagonists offer several advantages over traditional opioid agonists such as meperidine, fentanyl, and morphine. When respiratory depression was a significant consideration in opioid agonist administration, this risk has been reduced (although not eliminated). Problems may still develop with administration of these newer agents, but they appear to be less common.

Pentazocine has been available for more than 30 years. It is rarely used intravenously in conscious sedation because of the significant incidence of negative psychotomimetic effects. In addition, it is known today that physical dependence to pentazocine does occur.

Butorphanol, a more recent addition to the armamentarium, appears to have fewer significant adverse effects than pentazocine. However, it produces an increase in cardiovascular workload, which mitigates against its use in cardiovascular-risk patients.

Nalbuphine appears to have all the advantages of butorphanol, with the additional advantages of not increasing cardiovascular workload and of being an excellent opioid antagonist. One additional benefit of butorphanol and nalbuphine is that they are nonscheduled drugs, requiring no special forms or paperwork for their purchase or administration. Pentazocine is a Schedule IV drug, whereas the opioid agonists are Schedule II drugs.

Note: Throughout this discussion of the opioid agonists and opioid agonist/antagonists, it has been mentioned in the Warnings and Precautions sections that the use of these agents in patients with significant liver or renal dysfunction, or both, and in patients with significant pulmonary disease (COPD) is contraindicated. Please bear in mind that the use of IV conscious sedation was earlier recommended for patients who have been categorized as ASA physical status classifications I and II, with only a selected few ASA III patients being considered acceptable. The patients mentioned in the "Warnings" and "Precautions" sections are considered at best ASA III and are usually ASA IV. Adherence to basic tenets of patient selection for IV conscious sedation will minimize the number of problems that may develop in these patients.

OPIOID ANTAGONISTS

The only drug presently available that possesses pure opioid-antagonist properties is naloxone. The pharmacology and clinical importance of this drug are reviewed in the section on antidotal drugs (p. 366).

ANTICHOLINERGICS

The anticholinergics, also known as *belladonna alkaloids* and *cholinergic blocking agents,* are important to the practice of anesthesia and are valuable adjuncts to intravenously administered sedatives. Indications for the use of anticholinergics in the practice of anesthesia and IV conscious sedation include the following: (1) as preoperative medication to reduce salivary secretions, (2) to correct vagally induced bradycardia, and (3) to reverse curarization (in general anesthesia) when administered with neostigmine. Three anticholinergics—atropine, scopolamine, and glycopyrrolate—are discussed here. These drugs are very popular during IV conscious sedation in dentistry, administered primarily for their antisalivary actions.

Pharmacology

The belladonna alkaloids are widely distributed in nature. Atropine, chemically a racemic mixture of *levo-* and *dextro*-hyoscyamine (only the *levo* form is pharmacologically active), is found in the following botanicals:

- *Atropa belladonna,* known as the *deadly nightshade*
- *Datura stramonium,* Jamestown weed, jimson weed, stinkweed, thorn-apple, and devil's apple

Scopolamine, chemically *levo*-hyoscine, is found in the following:

- *Hyoscyamus niger,* black henbane
- *Scopolia carniolica*

Glycopyrrolate, a synthetic anticholinergic, was introduced in 1961. It is a quaternary ammonium compound with the chemical name 1-methyl-3-pyrrolidyl-phenyl-cyclopentane-glycolate methobromide.

Mechanism of Action

The anticholinergics act as competitive antagonists to acetylcholine at the postganglionic receptor located at the neuroeffector junction of the parasympathetic nervous system. Although the actions of these drugs are essentially similar, the degree to which the individual drug possesses a certain property may differ. For example, scopolamine has a greater effect on salivary glands than does atropine, but atropine has a greater effect on the heart and bronchial musculature. In clinical doses, atropine does not produce CNS depression; however, scopolamine does and is therefore commonly used for preoperative medication.

Central Nervous System

Atropine produces a stimulation of the medulla and higher cerebral centers. In clinical doses of 0.5 to 1.0 mg, this effect is noted as a mild vagal stimulation in which both the rate and depth of breathing are increased.[164] This effect is a result of bronchiolar dilation and increased physiologic dead space. Atropine is not effective in reversing significant respiratory depression.

Scopolamine in therapeutic doses produces a degree of CNS depression, clinically noted as drowsiness, euphoria, amnesia, fatigue, and dreamless sleep. Unfortunately, in some patients the same clinical dose may produce excitement, restlessness, hallucinations, and delirium and is more likely to occur in the presence of pain.

Glycopyrrolate, a quaternary ammonium compound, does not cross the blood-brain barrier. It also does not produce the CNS actions noted for atropine and scopolamine.

In cases in which sedation is a desirable effect, the administration of scopolamine is preferred to either atropine or glycopyrrolate. Scopolamine provides 5 to 15 times the sedative effects of the other two drugs.[165]

Amnesia may be a desirable action of an anticholinergic drug. Of the three, only scopolamine produces this effect. Although amnesia may occur after scopolamine administration, it is not as consistent a finding as it is with diazepam or midazolam. When present, however, amnesia tends to be prolonged, often persisting for 2 to 4 hours. Although anterograde amnesia—lack of recall of events occurring after administration of scopolamine—is most common, retrograde amnesia—the lack of recall of events occurring before administration of the drug—may also occur.[166]

Eye

Anticholinergics block the responses of the sphincter muscle of the iris and the ciliary muscle of the lens to cholinergic stimulation. They therefore produce mydriasis (dilation of the pupil) and cycloplegia (paralysis of accommodation). Administered in therapeutic doses, atropine (0.4 to 0.6 mg) produces little ocular effect. However, scopolamine in therapeutic doses produces significant mydriasis and cycloplegia.

Administered parenterally, the anticholinergics have little effect on intraocular pressure, except in patients with acute narrow-angle glaucoma, in whom dangerously high intraocular pressures may develop. This occurs when the iris, which is crowded back into the angle of the anterior chamber of the eye, interferes with drainage of the aqueous humor.[167] In the more commonly seen wide-angle glaucoma, such an increase in intraocular pressure seldom occurs, and the anticholinergics may be used with little increase in risk to the patient. The administration of anticholinergics is contraindicated for patients who wear contact lenses.

Respiratory Tract

The anticholinergic drugs decrease secretions of the nose, mouth, pharynx, and bronchi, thereby drying the mucous membranes of the respiratory tract. This of course represents one of the indications for administration of these drugs as preanesthetic medications. Clinically, the antisialagoric actions of 0.4 mg of atropine are equal to those of a dose of 0.2 mg of glycopyrrolate.

Bronchial smooth muscle is also dilated after administration of anticholinergic drugs, atropine being considerably more potent in this regard than either scopolamine or glycopyrrolate. Atropine, scopolamine, and glycopyrrolate decrease the incidence of laryngospasm during general anesthesia. This is because of the decrease in respiratory tract secretions that might precipitate reflex laryngospasm, which is produced by contraction of laryngeal skeletal muscle.

Cardiovascular Actions

The principal effect of the anticholinergics on the heart is an alteration in rate. Clinical doses of 0.4 to 0.6 mg of atropine produce a decrease in heart rate of 4 to 8 beats/min. This effect is not seen if the drug is administered rapidly intravenously. Larger doses produce a tachycardia by blocking the effects of the vagus nerve at the sinoatrial (SA) pacemaker. The rate may rise as much as 35 to 40 beats above the resting rate (in a study with young men receiving 2 mg of atropine intramuscularly).[168] This action of the anticholinergics is most notable in young healthy adults in whom vagal tone is great. In very young patients and geriatric patients, atropine may fail to accelerate the heart rate.

Scopolamine in small doses (0.1 to 0.2 mg) produces even more profound cardiac slowing than atropine. With larger doses, the resultant tachycardia is equal to that of atropine but shorter lived. The heart rate will return to baseline or perhaps result in bradycardia.

Glycopyrrolate produces less tachycardia than either atropine or scopolamine and thus is indicated for use in patients in whom atropine- or scopolamine-induced tachycardia is not desirable. Conversely, in situations in which significant bradycardia has developed, the administration of glycopyrrolate will not provide the desired increase in heart rate. Atropine or scopolamine is necessary at this time.

Gastrointestinal Tract

Therapeutic doses of anticholinergics do not greatly affect gastric secretion. Doses in excess of 1 mg (atropine) must be administered to alter gastric secretion significantly. The anticholinergics have little effect on the secretion of pancreatic juice, bile, or succus entericus.

On the other hand, anticholinergics have profound actions on gastrointestinal motility. In both healthy patients and in those with gastrointestinal disease, therapeutic doses inhibit the motor activity of much of the small and large intestine. Motility is reduced along with muscle tone, as well as the amplitude and frequency of peristaltic activity. This is termed the *antispasmodic effect of the anticholinergics.*[169]

Secretory Glands

The actions of the anticholinergics on respiratory and digestive tract secretions have been discussed. Even small doses inhibit the activity of sweat glands. The skin becomes hot and dry. If sweating is depressed, body temperature may rise, a finding usually noted only after toxic doses. The lacrimal glands are also inhibited by the anticholinergics, but to a smaller extent than other secretory glands. The secretion of milk is not significantly affected.

Biotransformation

The anticholinergics are rapidly removed from the blood and are distributed throughout the body. Atropine is approximately 50% protein bound in the blood. The metabolism of the anticholinergics is not very well understood. Approximately 13% to 50% of a dose of atropine is found unchanged in the urine. The liver is the primary organ of biotransformation. A small amount of the drug is found in the feces, and an even smaller amount is found in expired air.[170] Less than 1% of a dose of scopolamine is recovered unchanged in the urine.

Atropine

In clinical doses (0.5 to 1 mg), atropine produces stimulation of the medulla and higher cerebral centers, resulting in a mild central vagal stimulation and moderate respiratory stimulation. Its primary IV use is for the reduction of salivary and bronchial secretions.[171]

Contraindications to the administration of atropine include glaucoma, adhesions (synechiae) between the iris and the lens of the eye, and asthma.[172] The effects of atropine on the developing fetus are not known with any degree of certainty; therefore the use of atropine during pregnancy should be reserved for those cases in which its effects are truly important. This will rule out its use in most dental situations.

Adverse Reactions. Although systemic tolerance to drug effects varies greatly, Table 25-6 lists the "normal" response to increasing doses of atropine.

Intoxication to atropine has been described as follows: "Dry as a bone, red as a beet, and mad as a hatter." Fortunately, atropine intoxication is rarely fatal if rapidly diagnosed and antidotal therapy instituted. Physostigmine, 1 to 5 ml of a dilution of 1 mg of

TABLE 25-6 Normal Response to Increasing Doses of Atropine

Dose (mg)	Effect
0.5	Slight dryness of nose and mouth Bradycardia
1.0	Greater dryness of nose and mouth, with thirst Slowing, then acceleration, of the heart Mydriasis
2.0	Very dry mouth Tachycardia with palpitation Mydriasis Slight blurring of near vision Flushed, dry skin
5.0	Increase in the preceding symptoms plus the following: Disturbance of speech Difficulty in swallowing Headache Hot, dry skin Restlessness with asthenia (lack of energy)
10.0	The preceding symptoms to an extreme degree plus the following: Ataxia Excitement Disorientation Hallucinations Delirium Coma

physostigmine in 5 ml (0.2 mg/ml) administered intravenously, is the drug of choice in the management of this reaction. The dose may be repeated every 5 minutes if necessary for a total dose of 2 mg in children and 6 mg in adults.[173]

Dosage. The usual adult dose of atropine is 0.4 to 0.6 mg. Table 25-7 shows the recommended doses for children.

Availability. Atropine sulfate: 0.3, 0.4, 0.5, 0.6, 1, and 1.3 mg/ml. Each milliliter of atropine sulfate solution contains 0.4 mg atropine sulfate and 0.5% chlorobutanol as a preservative. Atropine is not a scheduled drug.

TABLE 25-7 Atropine Doses for Children

Weight kg	Weight lb	Dose (mg)
3-7	7-16	0.1
8-11	17-24	0.15
12-18	25-40	0.2
19-29	41-65	0.3
30-41	66-90	0.4
>41	>90	0.4-0.6

Atropine Sulfate
The medical history of patients receiving atropine sulfate should be checked for the following:
- Glaucoma
- Prostate disease
- Asthma
- Adhesions between iris and lens of eye
- Myasthenia gravis
- Contact lenses

Atropine Sulfate
Classification: anticholinergic
Availability: 0.3-1.3 mg/ml
Average therapeutic dose: 0.4-0.6 mg
Maximal single dose: 0.4-0.6 mg
Maximal total dose: 0.4-0.6 mg

Atropine Sulfate

Pregnancy category	C
Lactation	S
Metabolism	Other
Excretion	Urine
DEA schedule	Not controlled

Scopolamine Hydrobromide

Scopolamine hydrobromide differs in several significant ways from atropine. It can produce a degree of CNS depression, whereas atropine does not. Scopolamine is a commonly used constituent of preanesthetic medication. In this regard, scopolamine provides the following beneficial effects:
- Decreases in salivary and bronchial secretions
- Some sedative effect (minor)
- Anterograde amnesia

The latter two effects are unique to scopolamine and form the basis for its widespread use in anesthesia practice.[174] Unfortunately, scopolamine is also more apt to produce the phenomenon known as *emergence delirium* than either atropine or glycopyrrolate. Because this reaction, which involves vivid dreaming, nightmares, and hallucinations, develops most often in very young and elderly patients, the use of scopolamine in patients younger than 6 years and older than 65 years is discouraged.[175]

Dosage. The usual adult therapeutic dose is 0.32 to 0.65 mg. Table 25-8 shows the recommended doses for children.[176]

Availability. Scopolamine hydrobromide: 0.3 mg/ml, 0.4 mg/ml in 0.5- and 1.0-ml ampules, and 0.6 mg/ml. Each milliliter of scopolamine hydrobromide solution contains the following:
- 0.3 mg scopolamine hydrobromide
- 1% alcohol
- 10% mannitol
- Water for injection

Scopolamine is not a scheduled drug.

TABLE 25-8 Scopolamine Hydrobromide Doses for Children

Age	Dose (mg)
6 mo to 3 yr	0.1-0.15
3-6 yr	0.15-0.2
6-12 yr	0.2-0.3

Scopolamine Hydrobromide
The medical history of patients receiving scopolamine hydrobromide should be checked for the following:
- Glaucoma
- Adhesions between iris and lens
- Asthma
- Prostatic disease
- Myasthenia gravis
- Contact lenses

Scopolamine Hydrobromide
Classification: anticholinergic
Availability: 0.3-0.6 mg/ml
Average therapeutic dose: 0.3 mg
Maximal single dose: 0.3 mg
Maximal total dose: 0.3 mg

Scopolamine Hydrobromide	
Pregnancy category	C
Lactation	S
Metabolism	Liver
Excretion	Urine
DEA schedule	Not controlled

Glycopyrrolate

Glycopyrrolate is a quaternary ammonium compound. As such it does not cross lipid membranes, such as the blood-brain barrier; this is in contrast to both atropine and scopolamine. Glycopyrrolate is less likely to produce unwanted CNS depression or delirium-type reactions.

After IV administration, the onset of clinical action develops within 1 minute. Glycopyrrolate has a duration of action of vagal blocking effects for 2 to 3 hours and antisialagogue effects for up to 7 hours.[177] This latter effect may be undesirable in the ambulatory patient.

Warnings. Ambulatory patients receiving glycopyrrolate must be advised not to perform hazardous work, operate machinery, or drive a motor vehicle because the drug may produce drowsiness or blurred vision.[178] In the presence of a high environmental temperature, heat prostration (heat stroke and fever caused by decreased sweating) can occur with the use of glycopyrrolate.

Precautions. Glycopyrrolate should be used with caution in patients with tachycardia because the drug may cause a further increase in the heart rate.[178] In addition, patients with ischemic heart disease, coronary artery disease, heart failure, dysrhythmias, hypertension, or hyperthyroidism should be evaluated carefully before administration of glycopyrrolate.

Although glycopyrrolate has been shown to be nonteratogenic in animal studies, its effect on the human fetus is unknown; therefore the use of glycopyrrolate in pregnancy is not recommended and should be reserved for those cases in whom it is truly required.

Dosage. The usual therapeutic dose of glycopyrrolate in adults is 0.1 mg (0.5 ml) as needed and may be repeated every 2 to 3 minutes. In children the IV dose of glycopyrrolate is 0.02 mg (0.1 ml) per pound of body weight, not to exceed a dose of 0.1 mg (0.5 ml) in a single dose. As with the adult, this dose may be repeated every 2 to 3 minutes as needed.

Availability. Robinul (Robins): 0.2 mg/ml in 1-, 2-, 5-, and 20-ml ampules and vials. Each milliliter of glycopyrrolate contains the following:
- 0.2 mg glycopyrrolate
- Water for injection
- 0.5 to 0.9% benzyl alcohol as preservative
- pH adjusted to 2 to 3 with sodium hydroxide or hydrochloric acid

Glycopyrrolate is not a scheduled drug.

Glycopyrrolate
The medical history of patients receiving glycopyrrolate should be checked for the following:
- Allergy to glycopyrrolate
- Glaucoma
- Prostatic disease
- Asthma
- Myasthenia gravis
- Ischemic heart disease
- Contact lenses

Glycopyrrolate
Proprietary name: Robinul
Classification: anticholinergic
Availability: 0.2 mg/ml
Average therapeutic dose: 0.1 mg
Maximal single dose: 0.1 mg
Maximal total dose: 0.2 mg

Glycopyrrolate	
Pregnancy category	B
Lactation	NS
Metabolism	Unknown
Excretion	Feces, primarily
DEA schedule	Not controlled

Summary

The anticholinergics serve primarily as adjunctive drugs during IV conscious sedation in outpatients. The selection of the appropriate anticholinergic will be based on the indication for its use; for example:

- Longer procedures (more than 2 to 3 hours): glycopyrrolate
- Amnesia: scopolamine
- Sedation: scopolamine
- Decreased cardiovascular action: glycopyrrolate
- Short procedure, no amnesia, no sedation: atropine

Anticholinergics may be administered in combination with any of the drugs discussed in this section, with the notable exception of lorazepam (Ativan). The use of scopolamine is not recommended in conjunction with lorazepam because of the intense amnesic effect and the increased possibility of emergence delirium produced by this combination.[179]

INNOVAR

Innovar is the proprietary name of a combination of two drugs: (1) the long-acting, potent, nonphenothiazine tranquilizer of the butyrophenone type, droperidol, and (2) the potent, short-acting opioid agonist fentanyl. When administered intravenously, this combination of drugs produces a state termed *neuroleptanesthesia* or *neuroleptanalgesia,* depending on the dosage of drugs administered.[180]

The term *neuroleptic* is defined as a state of consciousness in which the patient has the following characteristics:

- Is sleepy but not unconscious
- Is psychologically detached from the environment
- Retains the ability to obey commands
- Has diminished motor activity

The concept of neuroleptanesthesia, introduced in 1959, proposed combining the neuroleptic state with analgesia and amnesia to provide ideal circumstances for surgery.[181] The combination of droperidol and fentanyl provides neuroleptanalgesia, a state in which the patient retains consciousness, yet is detached from the environment. The addition of nitrous oxide (N_2O) and oxygen (O_2) renders the patient unconscious in a state called *neuroleptanesthesia.*

Within the operating room, neuroleptanesthesia is a popular technique of general anesthesia, especially in medically compromised patients (ASA III and IV). In the hospital environment in which the patient is nonambulatory, the use of Innovar is rational. In typical ambulatory outpatient dental situations or in short-stay surgery centers, however, the use of Innovar makes less sense. The pharmacology of the component drugs will demonstrate this point.

Droperidol

Droperidol was synthesized in 1962 by Janssen Pharmaceutica in Belgium.

Pharmacology. Droperidol produces marked tranquilization and sedation. Other pharmacologic actions of droperidol include the following[182]:

- Antiemetic actions
- Potentiation of CNS depressant drugs
- Mild α-adrenergic blockade (producing peripheral vasodilation) and a decrease in the pressor effects of epinephrine (Droperidol can produce hypotension and a decrease in peripheral vascular resistance; however, this effect is not usually observed in therapeutic doses.)
- Reduced incidence of epinephrine-induced cardiac dysrhythmias by the α-adrenergic properties of droperidol—however, no effect on the incidence of other types of dysrhythmias

After IV administration the clinical actions of droperidol are noted within 3 to 10 minutes; however, the full effect may not be observed for as long as 30 minutes. This is a negative factor in the use of droperidol for ambulatory outpatient procedures, which are usually short. Even more significant than the relatively slow onset is the fact that although the duration of clinically evident sedation and tranquilization produced by droperidol usually lasts for 2 to 4 hours, alterations in the patient's state of consciousness may persist for up to 12 hours. This is the primary reason for not recommending this drug for use in outpatient procedures.

Indications. The following three indications are listed in the drug package insert for droperidol[183]:

1. To provide tranquilization and reduce the incidence of nausea and vomiting in surgical procedures
2. For premedication, induction, and as an adjunct in the maintenance of general and regional anesthesia
3. In neuroleptanalgesia, in which droperidol is administered concurrently with fentanyl to aid in tranquilization and decrease pain and anxiety

Warnings. Fluids and other countermeasures must be readily available to counteract hypotension if it should develop after administration of droperidol. Droperidol potentiates the CNS depressant properties of other drugs, including opioid agonists such as fentanyl. The initial dose of opioid should be decreased to about one fourth or one third of the usually recommended dose.

Droperidol may be used safely in children older than 2 years. However, there are insufficient data to recommend its use in younger patients.

The safety of droperidol in pregnancy has not been established with respect to its possible effect on the fetus. Therefore droperidol should be reserved for use in pregnant women and women of childbearing potential only when the benefits clearly outweigh the potential hazards of its use. In elective, ambulatory, outpatient procedures, the use of droperidol is rarely indicated.

Precautions. The initial dose of droperidol should be reduced appropriately in the elderly, debilitated, and other high-risk patients (ASA III and IV). Other CNS depressant drugs (e.g., opioids, phenothiazines, barbiturates) have additive or potentiating effects when administered in conjunction with droperidol. When a patient has received one of these before droperidol, the dose of droperidol should be reduced. In the same manner, the dose of the other CNS depressant is decreased when it is administered following droperidol. Patients with significant liver or kidney disease should receive droperidol with caution because it is metabolized and excreted through these organs.

Adverse Reactions. The most frequently reported adverse reactions to droperidol are hypotension and a mild tachycardia. Both of these effects usually resolve without additional drug management. The management of hypotension, if severe or prolonged, is to administer IV fluids to the patient in an effort to increase fluid volume. Other adverse reactions include the following:

- Postoperative drowsiness
- Extrapyramidal symptoms, such as dystonia, akathisia, and oculogyric crisis (Management requires IV administration of diphenhydramine.)
- Restlessness, hyperactivity, anxiety
- Dizziness
- Chills, shivering, or both
- Laryngospasm, bronchospasm
- Postoperative hallucinations

Respiratory depression, apnea, and muscular rigidity can develop when droperidol is administered with fentanyl. If permitted to remain untreated, these may lead to respiratory arrest.

The use of droperidol in the ambulatory outpatient is not recommended.

Droperidol is combined with the short-acting opioid agonist fentanyl to produce the combination marketed as Innovar. Fentanyl has previously been discussed (see p. 351).

> **Droperidol**
> The medical history of patients receiving droperidol should be checked for the following:
> - Possible hypovolemia (increases risk of hypotension with droperidol)
> - Allergy or hypersensitivity to droperidol

Effects of Innovar

The administration of Innovar alone does not normally produce loss of consciousness. It does produce the state of neuroleptanalgesia, which was described at the beginning of this section.

When Innovar is administered, both pharyngeal and laryngeal reflexes are obtunded and care must be taken to protect the patient's airway. Fentanyl possesses mild emetic properties that are effectively counterbalanced by the potent antiemetic properties of droperidol.

One of the most significant concerns when Innovar is used is the potential for the production of respiratory depression. Innovar produces depression of the medullary respiratory center, raising the threshold to arterial carbon dioxide (CO_2) tension.[184] Large doses of fentanyl may produce apnea.

The fentanyl component may also produce skeletal muscle rigidity of the thoracic and abdominal walls. Although not common, this action is most often related to the speed of administration of the drug and may be effectively prevented by the slow injection of Innovar or fentanyl. Should it develop, assisted or controlled ventilation is required, with the possible need for a neuromuscular blocking agent such as succinylcholine.

Contraindications. Contraindications to the administration of Innovar are allergy or hypersensitivity to either the droperidol or fentanyl component.

Warnings. The safety of fentanyl in patients who have received MAOIs within 14 days has not been established and is therefore not recommended.[185] The safety of Innovar in patients younger than 2 years of age has not been established and is therefore not recommended.

Pregnant patients should not be administered Innovar unless the benefits of its administration clearly outweigh the potential hazards of its use. For this reason, the use of Innovar cannot be recommended for the pregnant patient in the outpatient environment.

Adverse Reactions. Adverse reactions to Innovar are the same as those previously discussed for droperidol and fentanyl. The two most common adverse reactions are hypotension and respiratory depression.

Orthostatic hypotension, primarily caused by the droperidol, is another factor to consider in the ambulatory patient. Positional changes (from supine to upright) may produce dramatic decreases in the patient's blood pressure after droperidol administration. Droperidol's duration of activity is approximately 8 hours, requiring the patient and the escort to be made fully aware of this possibility.

Dosage. As with all intravenously administered drugs, the dose of Innovar should be individualized. Anesthesia is induced with a dose of 1 ml of Innovar per 20 to 25 pounds (1 ml/9 to 11 kg). This dose must be administered slowly (over 5 to 6 minutes) to minimize the risk of muscular rigidity. Once the patient is heavily sedated with Innovar, N_2O-O_2 is added, unconsciousness occurs, and other general anesthetic drugs may be added. In the absence of N_2O-O_2, the patient remains conscious, yet sedated.

Availability. Innovar (McNEILAB): 0.05 mg/ml fentanyl citrate (Sublimaze) and 2.5 mg/ml droperidol (Inapsine) in 2- and 5-ml ampules. Lactic acid is added to adjust the pH of the solution to 3.5 ± 0.3. Innovar is classified as a Schedule II drug.

Droperidol	
Pregnancy category	C
Lactation	S?
Metabolism	Liver
Excretion	Feces and urine
DEA schedule	Not controlled

Innovar
Proprietary name: Innovar
Classification: neuroleptic
Availability: Droperidol, 2.5 mg/ml
Fentanyl, 0.05 mg/ml
Average sedative dose: 1-2 ml
Maximal single dose: 0.5-1 ml
Maximal total dose: 0.5-1 ml

Note: Innovar is not recommended for use in outpatient procedures.

Summary

Innovar is a popular drug combination for the production of neuroleptanalgesia or neuroleptanesthesia. As used in the hospitalized patient in whom postoperative recovery can be monitored carefully, neuroleptanesthesia and neuroleptanalgesia are excellent techniques. Because the duration of action of one of its components, droperidol, is 8 hours, entirely too long for ambulatory patients, Innovar cannot be recommended for use in the typical outpatient environment.

The combination of droperidol and fentanyl appears to be illogical. Fentanyl, with its 45-minute duration of action, combined with droperidol's 8-hour duration of action, does not seem logical. In the operating room environment, a patient will receive an initial dose of the Innovar combination, after which there is no longer a need to readminister droperidol for approximately 2 to 4 hours (usual duration of its sedative actions); however, the opioid actions of fentanyl will disappear within 45 minutes. Individual doses of fentanyl are therefore readministered, as needed, during the procedure. In surgical procedures of longer duration an initial dose of Innovar or droperidol is administered and a longer-acting opioid such as morphine substituted for fentanyl.

A word of caution is needed before this discussion on Innovar is concluded. Some doctors employ nurse anesthetists to administer outpatient sedation or general anesthesia in their offices. Many of these hospital-based persons favor the use of Innovar in the dental patient. Remember that most of the procedures that these persons usually perform are on hospitalized patients in whom postoperative recovery is closely monitored for however many hours are required. Such is not the case in the typical dental patient. The use of Innovar should be discouraged in this environment. Other highly effective drugs for IV conscious sedation are available in its place.

KETAMINE

Ketamine hydrochloride is a cyclohexane derivative closely related chemically and pharmacologically to phencyclidine, a veterinary anesthetic and drug of abuse (known as *angel dust*).

Anesthesia produced by ketamine has been termed dissociative anesthesia.[186] It is a state in which the patient appears awake, has his or her eyes open, and is capable of (involuntary) muscular movement but appears to be unaware of, or dissociated from, the environment. Another term for the state induced by ketamine is *cataleptic anesthesia.* Profound analgesia and amnesia are associated with ketamine administration.

The dissociative state produced by ketamine is an excitatory state, completely dissimilar from that seen after administration of traditional general anesthetics such as halothane, thiopental, and meperidine. Blood pressure and heart rate, usually somewhat depressed during general anesthesia, are elevated after ketamine administration. Respiration is spontaneous, with the airway affected very little by the drug, the patient retaining the ability to maintain a patent airway throughout the procedure. Laryngeal and pharyngeal reflexes are intact or even hyperactive during ketamine anesthesia. When used in dental procedures, it is important to place an oropharyngeal pack to prevent contamination of the pharynx and/or larynx with debris.

In the operating room, IV ketamine is used for short procedures, such as dilatation and curettage (D&C), surgical procedures on the skin, or dental procedures such as extraction or restorative dentistry in pediatric patients. Another use of ketamine is in patients in whom numerous surgical procedures will be required, such as burn victims requiring multiple debridements and skin grafts over a brief period.

The onset of action of ketamine after IV administration is rapid (less than 1 minute), with a duration of clinical effect of approximately 10 minutes.[187] The usual IV induction dose of ketamine is 1 to 4.5 mg/kg (approximately 0.5 to 2 mg/pound) administered over 1 minute. More rapid administration results in respiratory depression and an exaggerated pressor response. The duration of anesthesia may be extended with readministration of ketamine in doses of 0.5 mg/kg. Recovery from ketamine anesthesia is prolonged when larger doses of ketamine are administered. An even more effective method of prolonging ketamine anesthesia is by administering local anesthesia for pain control and N_2O-O_2 for additional CNS depression. Administration of these drugs along with ketamine reduces the dose of ketamine required, speeds recovery, and minimizes adverse recovery room phenomena (hallucinations).

Recovery from ketamine-induced anesthesia is prolonged and often associated with vivid dreams, hallucinations, and delirium.[188] These emergence reactions are significantly more common in adults than in children and may last from minutes to hours. Flashbacks—recurrence of these experiences—have occurred months after the administration of ketamine. This is somewhat similar to flashbacks occurring after administration of LSD. Sussman reported that 24% of patients older than 16 years reported emergence reactions, whereas only 8% of those younger than 16 years had the same response.[189] Patients older than 65 years have decreased incidence of adverse emergence phenomena. The incidence of recovery phenomena may be minimized if the patient is permitted to remain undisturbed in a quiet, darkened recovery area.[190] IM administration of ketamine is associated with a decreased incidence of these reactions.

Ketamine is commonly used in the younger patient as an induction agent (via IM administration), after which an IV infusion is started and the patient maintained with IV ketamine, or other agents, as needed. Ketamine is also used as an anesthetic agent for diagnostic procedures, for minor operations of shorter duration, and for patients undergoing multiple procedures under general anesthesia.

Having considerable experience with ketamine anesthesia with both inpatients and outpatients, I believe that ketamine use should be limited to doctors who have completed a residency in anesthesiology, have experience with ketamine (because it is so different from "traditional" general anesthetics), and have adequate recovery room facilities and monitoring available in the office.

ANTIDOTAL DRUGS

In concluding this section on the pharmacology of IV conscious sedation drugs, several additional agents demand attention. These drugs are used but rarely; however, like an umbrella on a cloudy day, their presence is important. This group is called *antidotal drugs*, for their use is reserved for reversing adverse effects of drugs that have been previously administered. The following categories of drugs are included:

- Opioid antagonist
- Benzodiazepine antagonist
- Agent for reversal of emergence delirium
- Vasodilator for extravascular or intraarterial drug administration

Each of these categories should be represented in the emergency kit of doctors administering parenteral sedation by the subcutaneous (SC), IM, or IV routes or by IV general anesthesia.

Opioid Antagonists

The most significant side effect of opioid analgesics is respiratory depression. This, more than anything else, limits their use in outpatient dentistry. Less-than-adequate monitoring of respiratory efforts in the sedated patient has led to significant morbidity and death.[191] Management of respiratory depression is reviewed in Chapter 27 and includes the administration of an opioid antagonist. IV administration of an opioid antagonist rapidly reverses the respiratory depressant effects of the opioid agonist.

The first opioid antagonist, nalorphine, became available in 1951, followed a year later by levallorphan. Both of these drugs reverse the analgesic effects of opioids and their respiratory depressant properties. Administered to an opioid-dependent individual, these drugs induce acute abstinence syndrome (withdrawal). When administered in the absence of opioid-induced respiratory depression, both nalorphine and levallorphan are capable of producing respiratory depression and of enhancing respiratory depression produced by barbiturates.[192]

In the late 1960s naloxone was introduced and has replaced both levallorphan and nalorphine as the drug of choice in reversing opioid-induced respiratory depression. It is the only opioid antagonist currently available that is free of opioid agonist effects.[193]

Nalbuphine is an opioid agonist/antagonist analgesic that is used in both anesthesia and sedation. Magruder et al.[194] used nalbuphine in place of naloxone for reversal of opioid-induced respiratory depression, noting dramatic improvement within minutes without any reversal of analgesia or euphoria. Further study is necessary before nalbuphine can be recommended as the drug of choice for reversal of opioid-induced respiratory depression.

Naloxone. Naloxone is a synthetic congener of the opioid analgesic oxymorphone from which it differs by the replacement of the methyl group on the N_2 atom by an allyl group.[193] Naloxone hydrochloride is soluble in water and dilute acids and strong alkali. It is only slightly soluble in alcohol and practically insoluble in ether and chloroform.

Naloxone hydrochloride is an essentially pure opioid antagonist. It does not possess any "agonistic" or opioid-type properties. Naloxone does not produce respiratory depression, unlike levallorphan and nalorphine, nor does it produce psychotomimetic effects or miosis. When administered in the absence of opioids, naloxone exhibits essentially no pharmacologic activity. Administered to a patient who is physically dependent on opioids, naloxone induces withdrawal symptoms. Naloxone in and of itself does not produce tolerance or lead to physical or psychological dependence.

After IV administration of naloxone, improvement in respiration may be observed within 2 minutes. The duration of naloxone's effect is relatively short after IV use (about 30 minutes). The duration of respiratory depression produced by the opioid varies considerably with different opioids. It is therefore possible for naloxone to successfully reverse opioid-induced respiratory depression, only to have respiratory depression recur later after the clinical activity of naloxone has regressed. For this reason, it has become common practice to administer an IM dose of naloxone following the IV dose. The IM dose provides a longer duration of clinical action. After the administration of naloxone, the patient should not be discharged from the office for approximately 1 hour so that any recurrence of respiratory depression may be recognized and managed by readministration of naloxone, if necessary.

Naloxone is indicated for use in opioid depression, including respiratory depression, induced by any of the natural or synthetic opioids, propoxyphene, and the opioid agonist/antagonists pentazocine, nalbuphine, and butorphanol.

Contraindications. Naloxone is contraindicated for use in patients who are allergic or hypersensitive to it.

Warnings. Naloxone must be administered with extreme care to persons with known or suspected physical dependence on opioids. The abrupt and complete reversal of opioid agonist effects may precipitate an acute abstinence syndrome. After naloxone reversal of opioid-induced respiratory depression, the patient must be kept under surveillance in the event that repeated doses of naloxone might be needed. Respiratory depression produced by nonopioids (e.g., barbiturates) is not reversible by naloxone or other opioid antagonists.

Precautions. In the event of opioid-induced respiratory depression, naloxone is neither the most important nor the first step in patient management. Of greater importance is patency of the airway and adequate ventilation. All persons administering parenteral opioid analgesics must be capable of maintaining the airway of the unconscious patient and of assisting or controlling the ventilation of the patient.

Adverse Reactions. Administered to patients in the absence of opioids, naloxone is essentially free of any side effects. In the presence of opioids, abrupt reversal of opioid depression may produce the following:

- Nausea and vomiting
- Sweating
- Tachycardia
- Increased blood pressure
- Tremulousness

In the presence of pain, reversal of opioid depression by large doses (greater than 0.4 mg) of naloxone may also significantly reverse analgesia, resulting in extreme discomfort and excitement. It has been reported in cardiac-risk patients that rapid reversal of opioid-induced respiratory depression by large doses of naloxone has produced tachycardia and dramatic elevations in blood pressure, resulting in left ventricular failure and pulmonary edema.[195]

Dosage. Naloxone may be administered subcutaneously, intramuscularly, or intravenously. As mentioned, the onset of action after IV administration is within 2 minutes. After IM or subcutaneous administration, approximately 10 minutes may be required for onset of action. Duration of action is 30 minutes after IV administration and 1 to 4 hours following IM or subcutaneous administration. The potency of naloxone will be greater after IV administration.[196]

For the adult naloxone is diluted to a concentration of 0.1 mg/ml. This is accomplished by taking 1 ml of the 0.4-mg/ml concentration and adding 3 ml of diluent (e.g., 5% dextrose and water). Every 2 to 3 minutes, 0.1 to 0.2 mg should be injected slowly intravenously while the patient is observed for adequate reversal of respiratory depression: increased ventilation effort and increased alertness without significant pain or discomfort.

Additional doses of naloxone may be required in some patients, depending on the type and dose of opioid administered and the patient's response to naloxone. If repeated administration of naloxone is necessary, it is recommended that the IM route be given serious consideration because the duration of action of naloxone will be prolonged by this route of administration.

In children the initial dose of naloxone is 0.01 mg/kg of body weight administered intravenously, intramuscularly, or subcutaneously. This dose may be repeated every 2 to 3 minutes (IV) if the patient's response, or lack of response, dictates its administration.

If, for some reason, naloxone must be administered subcutaneously or intramuscularly, the adult dose is 0.4 mg and the pediatric dose is 0.01 mg/kg. The onset of action is slower; however, the duration of action will be significantly longer than noted after IV administration.

Availability. Narcan (Endo): adults and children, 0.4 mg/ml in 1-ml ampules and 10-ml vials; neonates, 0.02 mg/ml in 2-ml ampules. Each milliliter of naloxone contains the following:

- Either 0.02 or 0.4 mg/ml naloxone
- 8.6 mg sodium chloride
- 2.0 mg methylparaben and propylparaben in a ratio of 9:1 as preservatives
- pH adjusted with hydrochloric acid

Naloxone is not a scheduled drug.

Naloxone
The medical history of patients receiving naloxone should be checked for the following:
- Allergy or known hypersensitivity to naloxone
- Opioid dependence

Naloxone
Proprietary name: Narcan
Classification: opioid antagonist
Availability: 0.02 and 0.4 mg/ml
Average reversal dose (IV): 0.4 mg (adult)
Maximal single dose: 0.4 mg (adult)
Maximal total dose: 1.2 mg (adult)*

*Lack of improvement after two or three doses usually indicates that respiratory depression is not produced by opioids.

Naloxone	
Pregnancy category	B
Lactation	S?
Metabolism	Liver
Excretion	Urine
DEA schedule	Not controlled

Nalbuphine. As mentioned in the introduction to opioid antagonists, nalbuphine, an opioid agonist/antagonist, has been used to reverse opioid-induced respiratory depression. It appears to be as effective as naloxone but possesses the added benefit of not reversing analgesia when used in large doses. The dosage of nalbuphine used by Magruder et al.[194] was 0.1 mg/kg. Although nalbuphine is a very promising addition to the armamentarium of opioid antagonists, additional research is required before it can be recommended over naloxone.

Summary. The availability of drugs capable of reversing significant undesirable effects of opioids is quite important. However, it is significantly more important to remember that the occasion to use these drugs will almost never develop if IV sedatives and opioids are administered in a reasonable manner. The maximal doses of opioids recommended in this and in succeeding chapters will not produce respiratory depression in any but the most debilitated or acutely sensitive patients. However, maximal doses rarely need be administered. Adequate clinical effects are usually obtained with doses below these maximal doses. The secret to success and safety with opioids, as with all drugs, is the slow titration of the drug to the desired effect.

In 29 years of teaching IV conscious sedation on the doctoral, postdoctoral, and continuing education levels, I have never treated a patient who required an opioid antagonist for reversal of opioid-induced respiratory depression. Having the drug readily available is absolutely essential if opioids of any type are administered by any route. Routine opioid reversal, recommended by some, is unnecessary and may in some cases increase patient risk (as in cases in which postoperative pain is present, overstressing the cardiovascular system).

Benzodiazepine Antagonist

Although the benzodiazepines have been described as the most nearly ideal drugs for anxiety control and sedation, there are still adverse reactions associated with their administration. Emergence delirium, excessive duration of sedation, and possible respiratory depression are but a few of these. Although rare, their occurrence can wreak havoc on a procedure. Flumazenil, a specific benzodiazepine antagonist, was introduced into clinical practice in the late 1980s and in the United States in 1992.

Flumazenil, administered intravenously after the IV administration of diazepam or midazolam, produces a rapid reversal of sedation and improved ability to comprehend and obey commands.[197] Flumazenil also reduces the duration of anterograde amnesia produced with midazolam: 91 minutes (with flumazenil) compared with 121 minutes (no flumazenil).[198,199] When administered in a geriatric population (72 ± 9 years) following midazolam sedation, patients required less recovery time from sedation and demonstrated increased alertness and a decreased amnesic effect. Two patients became somewhat anxious following flumazenil administration.[199]

The dose administered in trials has varied considerably, from 0.5 mg to 0.6 to 1 mg to 20 to 40 mg.[200-202] The elimination half-life of flumazenil is short, less than 1 hour, and there appear at this time to be few side effects, aside from the possibility of producing anxiety states in the patient after use of flumazenil.[202] Sage et al.[200] concluded that "in doses up to 0.5 mg [flumazenil] provided safe and effective antagonism of midazolam-induced sedation in a clinical setting."[200]

Flumazenil is used clinically as a means of terminating undesirable actions of injected benzodiazepines. However, the "routine" administration of flumazenil at the termination of every IV benzodiazepine procedure is unnecessary.

Dosage. Initial IV dose of 0.2 mg (2 ml) with subsequent doses administered every minute as needed, to a maximum dosage of 1.0 mg.

Availability. Romazicon (Roche) is supplied in 5-ml multiple-use vials containing 0.1 mg/ml flumazenil.

Flumazenil

The medical history of patients receiving flumazenil should be checked for the following:

- Allergy or known hypersensitivity to flumazenil or benzodiazepines
- Patients who have been given benzodiazepines for control of a life-threatening condition such as status epilepticus or control of intracranial pressure

Flumazenil

Proprietary name: Romazicon
Classification: benzodiazepine antagonist
Availability: 0.1 mg/ml
Average reversal dose (IV): 0.2 mg
Maximal single dose: 0.2 mg every 60 seconds
Maximal total dose: 1.0 mg

Flumazenil	
Pregnancy category	C
Lactation	S?
Metabolism	Liver
Excretion	Feces and urine
DEA schedule	Not controlled

Agents for Reversal of Emergence Delirium

Several of the drugs previously discussed in this chapter have the disturbing ability to produce what is known as *emergence delirium*.[203] During recovery from clinical sedation with a benzodiazepine or scopolamine (the drugs most likely to produce emergence delirium), the patient appears to lose contact with reality. There may be increased muscular activity, and the patient may be speaking, but the sounds are unintelligible. A variety of clinical responses may be noted; however, in all of them it is apparent that the patient is not returning to his or her "normal" state of consciousness. Until the mid-1970s management of emergence delirium consisted of monitoring the patient and symptomatic treatment. Antidotal therapy was not available.

Physostigmine. Physostigmine is a reversible anticholinesterase similar in action to neostigmine, with the important difference that neostigmine, a quaternary compound, does not cross the blood-brain barrier, whereas physostigmine, a tertiary ammonium compound, readily crosses it.

Actions. Physostigmine is extracted from the seeds of *Physostigma venenosum* (Calabar bean). It is a reversible anticholinesterase that increases the concentration of acetylcholine (ACh) at cholinergic transmission sites. The action of ACh is normally quite transient because of its rapid hydrolysis by the enzyme anticholinesterase. Physostigmine inhibits this action of anticholinesterase and thereby prolongs and intensifies the actions of ACh.[204]

Being a tertiary ammonium compound, physostigmine crosses the blood-brain barrier to reverse the central toxic effects of anticholinergia and emergence delirium: anxiety, delirium, disorientation, hallucinations, hyperactivity, and seizures. Physostigmine is rapidly metabolized (60 to 120 minutes).

Contraindications. Physostigmine should not be administered to patients with asthma, diabetes, cardiovascular disease, or mechanical obstruction of the gastrointestinal or genitourinary tracts.[205]

Warnings. Physostigmine may produce excessive salivation, emesis, urination, and defecation. These are unlikely to develop if the drug is administered intravenously at a rate of 1 mg/min. More rapid administration can produce the preceding signs and symptoms and bradycardia; hypersalivation, leading to respiration difficulties; and possibly convulsions.

Precautions. Atropine sulfate should always be available whenever physostigmine is administered because it is an antagonist and antidote for physostigmine.

Dosage. The usual adult dose of physostigmine for reversal of emergence delirium is 0.5 to 2 mg. The drug is administered slowly through the IV infusion at a rate of not more than 1 mg/min. Maximal dose should not exceed 4 mg.

Availability. Antilirium (O'Neal, Jones & Feldman): 1.0 mg/ml in 2-ml ampules. Each milliliter of solution contains the following:

- 1.0 mg physostigmine salicylate
- 0.1% sodium bisulfite
- 2.0% benzyl alcohol
- Water for injection

Physostigmine is not a scheduled drug.

Physostigmine

The medical history of patients receiving physostigmine should be checked for the following:

- Asthma
- Diabetes mellitus
- Cardiovascular disease
- Mechanical obstruction of gastrointestinal or genitourinary tract

Physostigmine

Proprietary name: Antilirium
Classification: reversible anticholinesterase
Availability: 1 mg/ml
Average therapeutic dose (IV): 0.5 to 2.0 mg
Maximal single dose: 2 mg
Maximal total dose: 4 mg

Physostigmine

Pregnancy category	C
Lactation	?
Metabolism	Other or unknown
Excretion	Other or unknown
DEA schedule	Not controlled

Summary. Although emergence delirium is an uncommon complication of sedative procedures, it can occur. It is most often seen after the administration of scopolamine to a patient who is younger than 6 years old or older than 65 years old. Management of emergence delirium is based primarily on symptomatic treatment. Physostigmine administration hastens the reversal of signs and symptoms.

It is important to note that agitation and excessive movement during or after sedation may also be a sign of hypoxia. The patency of the patient's airway and oxygenation of the lungs must always be considered before administration of a drug for what is presumed to be emergence delirium.

Vasodilator for Extravascular or Intraarterial Drug Administration

Procaine. Procaine, the last of the antidotal drugs recommended for the emergency kit of the doctor administering parenteral sedation or general anesthesia, is a local anesthetic with significant vasodilating properties. The following are indications for use of this drug:

- Extravascular administration of an irritating chemical
- Intraarterial administration of a drug

In both cases the major problem is that of compromised circulation to either a localized area of tissue (extravascular injection) or a limb (intraarterial). Proper management requires the restoration of blood flow.

A property of all injectable local anesthetics (with the notable exception of cocaine) is vasodilation. Of the available injectable local anesthetics, procaine (Novocain) possesses the most vasodilating effects. This property makes procaine less effective as a local anesthetic (without the addition of a vasopressor) but makes it eminently suitable for the reversal of blood vessel spasm.

Procaine should be used in a 1% concentration without vasopressor. More detailed discussion of management of these problems is found in Chapter 27.

Dosage. For management of extravascular drug administration, 1 to 5 ml of 1% procaine is administered as described in Chapter 27. For intraarterial administration, 1 to 2 ml of 1% procaine is usually sufficient.

Availability. Novocain (Breon): 1% procaine in 2-ml and 6-ml ampules and 30-ml vials. Each milliliter of solution of 1% procaine contains the following:

- 10 mg procaine
- Less than 1 mg acetone sodium bisulfite as preservative

- Less than 2.5 mg chlorobutanol (in vial form only) as preservative

Procaine
The medical history of patients receiving procaine should be checked for the following:
- Allergy or known hypersensitivity to ester-type local anesthetics
- Familial history of atypical plasma cholinesterase

Procaine
Proprietary name: Novocain
Classification: local anesthetic
Availability: 1% (10 mg/ml)
Average reversal dose (IV): 1-5 ml
Maximal single dose: 1-5 ml
Maximal total dose: 5 ml

Procaine

Pregnancy category	C
Lactation	S
Metabolism	Plasma cholinesterase
Excretion	Urine
DEA schedule	Not controlled

REFERENCES

1. Giovannitti JA, Trapp LD: Adult sedation: oral, rectal, IM, IV. In Dionne RA, Phero JC, eds: *Management of pain and anxiety in dental practice,* New York, 1991, Elsevier.
2. Davidau A: New methods in anaesthesiology and their use in dentistry: treatment of difficult patients and execution of complex procedures, *Rev Assoc Med Israelites (France)* 16:663, 1967.
3. Main DMG: The use of diazepam in dental anaesthesia. In Knight PF, Burgess CG, eds: *Diazepam in anaesthesia,* Bristol, 1968, John Wright.
4. Brown PRH, Main DMG, Wood N: Intravenous sedation in dentistry: a study of 55 cases using pentazocine and diazepam, *Br Dent J* 139:59, 1975.
5. O'Neill R, Verrill P: Intravenous diazepam in minor surgery, *Br J Oral Surg* 7:12, 1969.
6. O'Neill R, Verrill PF, Aellig WH et al: Intravenous diazepam in minor oral surgery, *Br Dent J* 128:15, 1970.
7. Trieger N: Intravenous sedation in dentistry and oral surgery, *Int Anesthesiol Clin* 27:83, 1989.
8. Trieger N: *Pain control,* Chicago, 1974, Quintessence.
9. Foreman PA: Diazepam in dentistry: clinical observations based on the treatment of 167 patients in general dental practice, *Anesth Prog* 15:253, 1968.
10. Foreman PA: Intravenous diazepam in general dental practice, *NZ Dent J* 65:243, 1969.
11. Danneberg P, Weber KH: Chemical structure and biological activity of the diazepines, *Br J Clin Pharmacol* 16(suppl 2):231S, 1983.
12. Joseph R: The limbic system: emotion, laterality and unconscious mind, *Psychoanal Rev* 79:405, 1991.
13. Medina JH, Novas ML, DeRoberts E: Chronic RO 15-1788 treatment increases the number of benzodiazepine receptors in rat cerebral cortex and hippocampus, *Eur J Pharmacol* 90:125, 1983.
14. Haefely W: The biological basis of benzodiazepine actions, *J Psychoactive Drugs* 15:19, 1983.
15. Jack ML, Colburn WA, Spirt NM et al: A pharmacokinetic/pharmacodynamic/receptor binding model to predict the onset and duration of pharmacological activity of the benzodiazepines, *Prog Neuro-Psychopharmacol Biol Psychiatr* 7:629, 1983.
16. Ghoneim MM, Mewaldt SP, Hinrichs JV: Behavioral effects of oral versus intravenous administration of diazepam, *Pharmacol Biochem Behav* 21:231, 1984.
17. Colburn WA, Gibson M: Composite pharmacokinetic profiling, *J Pharm Sci* 73:1667, 1984.
18. Baird ES, Hailey DM: Delayed recovery from a sedative: correlation of the plasma levels of diazepam with clinical effects after oral and intravenous administration, *Br J Anaesth* 144:803, 1972.
19. Vree TB, Hekster CA, vander Kleijn E: Significance of apparent half-lives of a metabolite with a higher elimination rate than its parent drug, *Drug Intell Clin Pharm* 16:126, 1982.
20. Salzman C, Shader RI, Greenblatt DJ et al: Long v. short half-life benzodiazepines in the elderly. Kinetics and clinical effects of diazepam and oxazepam, *Arch Gen Psychiatr* 40:293, 1983.
21. Greenblatt DJ, Divoll M, Abernethy DR et al: Benzodiazepine kinetics: implications for therapeutics and pharmacogeriatrics, *Drug Metab Rev* 14:251, 1983.
22. Pacifici GM, Cuoci L, Placidi GF et al: Elimination of kinetics of desmethydiazepam in two young and two elderly subjects, *Eur J Drug Metab Pharmacokinet* 7:69, 1982.
23. Pomara N, Stanley B, Block R et al: Adverse effects of single therapeutic doses of diazepam on performance in normal geriatric subjects: relationship to plasma concentrations, *Psychopharmacology* 84:342, 1984.
24. Zbinden G, Randall LO: Pharmacology of benzodiazepines: laboratory and clinical correlations, *Adv Pharmacol* 5:213, 1967.
25. Ausinch B, Malagodi MH, Munson ES: Diazepam in the prophylaxis of lignocaine seizures, *Br J Anaesth* 48:309, 1976.
26. de Jong RH: Clinical physiology of local anesthetic action. In Cousins MJ, Bridenbaugh PO, eds: *Neural blockade,* ed 2, Philadelphia, 1988, Lippincott.
27. Ramsay RE: Treatment of status epilepticus, *Epilepsia* 34(suppl 1):S71, 1993.
28. Darmansjah I, Muchtar A: Dose-response variation among different populations, *Clin Pharmacol Ther* 52:449, 1992.
29. Luo A, Huang Y, Liu Y et al: Midazolam as a main anesthesia induction agent: a comparison with thiopental and diazepam, *Chin Med Sci J* 6:172, 1991.

30. Jacka MJ, Johnson GD, Milne B: Diazepam's effect on systemic vascular resistance during cardiopulmonary bypass is not caused by its vehicle (alcohol-propylene glycol), *J Cardiothorac Vasc Anesth* 7:28, 1993.
31. Taburet AM, Tollier C, Richard C: The effect of respiratory disorders on clinical pharmacokinetic variables, *Clin Pharmacokinet* 19:462, 1990.
32. Paakkari P, Paakkari I, Landes P et al: Respiratory μ-opioid and benzodiazepine interactions in the unrestrained rat, *Neuropharmacology* 32:323, 1993.
33. Murray-Lyon IM, Young J, Parkes JD et al: Clinical and electroencephalographic assessment of diazepam in liver disease, *Br Med J* 4:265, 1971.
34. DeFeudis FV: GABA-ergic analgesia: a naloxone-insensitive system, *Pharmacol Res Commun* 14:383, 1982.
35. Sawynok J: GABAergic mechanisms of analgesia: an update, *Pharmacol Biochem Behav* 26:463, 1987.
36. Unrug-Neervoort A, van-Luijtelaar G, Coenen A: Cognition and vigilance: differential effects of diazepam and buspirone on memory and psychomotor performance, *Neuropsychobiology* 26:146, 1992.
37. Roche Laboratories: Valium. Drug package insert, Nutley, NJ, 1990, Roche Laboratories.
38. Bergman U, Rosa FW, Baum C et al: Effects of exposure to benzodiazepines during fetal life, *Lancet* 340:694, 1992.
39. Doenicke A, Lorenz W, Hoernecke R et al: Histamine release after injection of benzodiazepines and of etomidate. A problem associated with the solvent propylene glycol, *Ann Fr Anesth Reanim* 12:166, 1993.
40. van Vlymen JM, Sa Rego MM, White PF: Benzodiazepine premedication: can it improve outcome in patients undergoing breast biopsy procedures? *Anesthesiology* 90:740, 1999.
41. Amrein R, Hetzel W: Pharmacology of drugs frequently used in ICU's: midazolam and flumazenil, *Intens Care Med* 17:S1, 1991.
42. Fraser AD, Bryan W, Isner AF: Urinary screening for midazolam and its major metabolites with the Abbott ADx and TDx analyzers and the EMIT d.a.u. benzodiazepine assay with confirmation by GC/MS, *J Anal Toxicol* 15:8, 1991.
43. Jones RD, Chan K, Rouolson CJ et al: Pharmacokinetics of flumazenil and midazolam, *Br J Anaesth* 70:286, 1993.
44. Ouellette RG: Midazolam: an induction agent for general anesthesia, *Nurse Anesth* 2:134, 1991.
45. Conner JT, Katz RL, Pagano RR et al: RO 21-3981 for intravenous surgical premedication and induction of anesthesia, *Anesth Analg* 57:1, 1978.
46. Hennessy MJ, Kirkby KC, Montgomery IM: Comparison of the amnesic effects of midazolam and diazepam, *Psychopharmacology* 103:545, 1991.
47. Malamed SF, Nikchevich D Jr, Block J: Anterograde amnesia as a possible postoperative complication of midazolam as an agent for intravenous conscious sedation, *Anesth Prog* 35:160, 1988.
48. Longmire AW, Seger DL: Topics in clinical pharmacology: flumazenil, a benzodiazepine antagonist, *Am J Med Sci* 306:49, 1993.
49. Forster A, Gardaz JP, Suter PM et al: Respiratory depression by midazolam and diazepam, *Anesthesiology* 53:494, 1980.
50. Brown CR, Sarnquist FH, Canup CA et al: Clinical, electroencephalographic, and pharmacokinetic studies of a water-soluble benzodiazepine, midazolam maleate, *Anesthesiology* 50:467, 1979.
51. Gath I, Weidenfeld J, Collins GI et al: Electrophysiological aspects of benzodiazepine antagonists, Ro 15-1788 and Ro 15-3505, *Br J Clin Pharmacol* 18:541, 1984.
52. Roche Laboratories: Important new information on the administration of Versed (midazolam hydrochloride/Roche) injection for conscious sedation, Letter, November 1987.
53. Jones RD, Lawson AD, Andrew LJ et al: Antagonism of the hypnotic effect of midazolam in children: a randomized, double-blind study of placebo and flumazenil administered after midazolam-induced anaesthesia, *Br J Anaesth* 66:660, 1991.
54. Saano V, Hansen PP, Paronen P: Interactions and comparative effects of zopiclone, diazepam and lorazepam on psychomotor performance and on elimination pharmacokinetics in healthy volunteers, *Pharmacol Toxicol* 70:135, 1992.
55. Wyeth-Ayerst Laboratories: Ativan. Drug package insert, Philadelphia, 1992, Wyeth-Ayerst Laboratories.
56. Eldor J: High dose flunitrazepam anesthesia, *Med Hypotheses* 38:352, 1992.
57. Young C, Knudsen N, Hilton A, Reves JG: Sedation in the intensive care unit, *Crit Care Med* 28:854, 2000.
58. Foreman PA: Flunitrazepam in outpatient dentistry, *Anesth Prog* 29:50, 1982.
59. Dixon RA, Bennett NR, Harrison MJ et al: I.V. flunitrazepam in conservative dentistry: a cross-over trial, *Br J Anaesth* 52:517, 1980.
60. Steen SN, Martinez LR: Some pharmacologic effects of intravenous chlordiazepoxide, *Clin Pharmacol Ther* 5:44, 1964.
61. Jorgensen NB: Local anesthesia and intravenous premedication, *Anesth Prog* 13:168, 1966.
62. Berns J: Twilight sedation: a substitute for lengthy office intravenous anesthesia, *J Conn State Dent Assoc* 37:4, 1963.
63. Andrews PR, Mark LC: Structural specificity of barbiturates and related drugs, *Anesthesiology* 57:314, 1982.
64. Harvey SC: Hypnotics and sedatives: the barbiturates. In Goodman LS, Gilman A, eds: *Pharmacological basis of therapeutics,* ed 8, Elmsford, NY, 1990, Pergamon.
65. Lebowitz P, Cote W, Daniels AL et al: Comparative cardiovascular effects of midazolam and thiopental in healthy patients, *Anesth Analg* 61:771, 1983.
66. Burch PG, Stansk DR: The role of metabolism and protein binding in thiopental anesthesia, *Anesthesiology* 58:146, 1983.
67. Abbott Laboratories: Nembutal. Drug package insert, Chicago, 1992, Abbott Laboratories.
68. Everett GB, Allen GD: Simultaneous evaluation of cardiorespiratory and analgesic effects of intravenous analgesia using pentobarbital, meperidine, and scopolamine with local anesthesia, *J Am Dent Assoc* 83:155, 1971.
69. Breimer DD: Pharmacokinetics of methohexitone following intravenous infusion in humans, *Br J Anaesth* 48:643, 1976.
70. Lilly Laboratories: Brevital. Drug package insert, Indianapolis, 1989, Eli Lilly Laboratories.

71. Shane SM: Intravenous amnesia for total dentistry in one sitting, *Oral Surg* 24:1, 1966.
72. Van Hemelrijck J, Gonzales JM, White PF: Pharmacology of intravenous anesthetic agents. In Rogers MC, Tinker JH, Covino BG et al, eds: *Principles and practice of anesthesiology,* St Louis, 1993, Mosby.
73. Roerig Laboratories: Vistaril. Drug package insert, New York, 1992, Roerig Laboratories.
74. Briggs LP, White M: The effects of premedication on anaesthesia with propofol (Diprivan), *Postgrad Med J* 61:35, 1985.
75. Briggs LP, Clarke RS, Dundee JW et al: Use of diisopropylphenol as main agent for short procedures, *Br J Anaesth* 53:1197, 1981.
76. Vandesteene A, Trempont V, Engelman E et al: Effect of propofol on cerebral blood flow and metabolism in man, *Anaesthesia* 43:37, 1988.
77. Van Hemelrijck J, Fitch W, Mattheussen M et al: Effect of propofol on the cerebral circulation and autoregulation in the baboon, *Anesth Analg* 71:49, 1990.
78. Van Hemelrijck J, Van Aken H, Plets C et al: The effects of propofol on ICP and cerebral perfusion pressure in patients with brain tumors, *Anesthesiol Rev* 15:67, 1989.
79. Hemelrijck JV, Gonzales JM, White PF: Pharmacology of intravenous anesthetic agents. In Rogers MC, Tinker JH, Covino BG et al, eds: *Principles and practice of anesthesiology,* St Louis, 1993, Mosby.
80. Grounds RM, Twigley AJ, Carli F et al: The haemodynamic effects of intravenous induction, comparison of the effects of thiopentone and propofol, *Anaesthesia* 40:735, 1985.
81. Patrick MR, Blair IJ, Feneck PO et al: A comparison of the hemodynamic effects of propofol (Diprivan) and thiopentone in patients with coronary artery disease, *Postgrad Med J* 61:23, 1985.
82. Dundee JW, Robinson FP, McCollum JS et al: Sensitivity to propofol in the elderly, *Anaesthesia* 41:482, 1986.
83. McCollum JSC, Milligan KR, Dundee JW: The antiemetic action of propofol, *Anaesthesia* 43:239, 1988.
84. White PF: Propofol, pharmacokinetics and pharmacodynamics, *Semin Anesth* 7:4, 1988.
85. Rogers KM, Dewar KM, McCubbin TD et al: Preliminary experience with ICI 35868 as an IV induction agent: comparison with althesin, *Br J Anaesth* 52:807, 1980.
86. Rutter DV, Morgan M, Lumley J et al: ICI 35868 (Diprivan): a new intravenous induction agent, *Anaesthesia* 35:1188, 1980.
87. Weightman WM, Zacharias M: Comparison of propofol and thiopentone anaesthesia (with special reference to recovery characteristics), *Anaesth Intens Care* 15:389, 1987.
88. Kay B, Stephenson DF: Dose-response relationship for disoprofol (IC 135868; Diprivan), *Anaesthesia* 36:863, 1981.
89. MacKenzie N, Grant IS: Comparison of the new emulsion formulation of propofol with methohexitone and thiopentone for induction of anaesthesia in day cases, *Br J Anaesth* 57:725, 1985.
90. MacKenzie N, Grant S: Comparison of propofol with methohexitone in the provision of anesthesia for surgery under regional blockade, *Br J Anaesth* 57:1167, 1985.
91. MacKenzie N, Grant IS: Propofol for intravenous sedation, *Anaesthesia* 42:3, 1987.
92. MacKenzie N, Grant IS: Propofol infusion for sedation in the intensive care unit, *Br Med J* 294: 774, 1987.
93. White PF, Negus JB: Sedative infusions during local or intravenous regional anesthesia: a comparison of propofol and midazolam, *J Clin Anesth* 3:32, 1991.
94. Stuart Pharmaceuticals: Diprivan. Drug package insert, Wilmington, Del, 1992, Stuart Pharmaceuticals.
95. Stanley TH: Opiate anaesthesia, *Anaesth Intensive Care* 15:38, 1987.
96. Martin WR: Naloxone, *Ann Intern Med* 85:765, 1976.
97. Phillips WJ: Central nervous system pain receptors. In Faust RJ, ed: *Anesthesiology review,* New York, 1991, Churchill Livingstone.
98. Shields SE: Pharmacokinetics of epidural narcotics. In Faust RJ, ed: *Anesthesiology review.* New York, 1991, Churchill Livingstone.
99. Pallasch TJ: *Clinical drug therapy in dental practice,* Philadelphia, 1973, Lea & Febiger.
100. Rosow C: Pharmacology of opioid analgetic agents. In Rogers MC, Tinker JH, Covino BG et al, eds: *Principles and practice of anesthesiology,* St. Louis, 1993, Mosby.
101. Lambert LA, Nazif MM, Moore PA et al: Nonlinear dose-response characteristics of alphaprodine sedation in preschool children, *Pediatr Dent* 10:30, 1988.
102. Lunt RC, Howard HE: A descriptive study of 201 uncombined alphaprodine HC1 conscious sedations in pediatric dental patients (1982-1985), *Pediatr Dent* 10:121, 1988.
103. Wedell D, Hersh EV: A review of the opioid analgesics fentanyl, alfentanil, and sufentanil, *Compendium* 12:184, 1991.
104. Gracely, RH, Dubner R, McGrath PA: Fentanyl reduces the intensity of painful tooth pulp sensations: controlling for detection of active drugs, *Anesth Analg* 61:751, 1982.
105. Shook JE, Watkins WD, Camporesi EM: Differential roles of opioid receptors in respiration, respiratory disease, and opiate-induced respiratory depression, *Am Rev Respir Dis* 142:895, 1990.
106. Rosenberg M: Muscle rigidity with fentanyl: a case report, *Anesth Prog* 24:50, 1977.
107. Mackenzie JE, Frank LW: Influence of pretreatment with a monoamine oxidase inhibitor (phenelzine) on the effects of buprenorphine and pethidine in the conscious rabbit, *Br J Anaesth* 60:216, 1988.
108. Elkins-Sinn: Fentanyl citrate injection. Drug package insert, Cherry Hill, NJ, 1992, Elkins-Sinn.
109. Janssens F, Torremans J, Janssen PA: Synthetic 1,4-disubstituted-1,4-dihydro-5H-tetrazol-5-one derivatives of fentanyl: alfentanil (R 39209), a potent, extremely short-acting narcotic analgesic, *J Med Chem* 29:2290, 1986.
110. Meistelman C, Saint-Maurice C, Lepaul M et al: A comparison of alfentanil pharmacokinetics in children and adults, *Anesthesiology* 66:13, 1987.
111. Helmers JH, Noordiun H, van-Leeuwen L: Alfentanil used in the aged: a clinical comparison with its use in young patients, *Eur J Anaesthesiol* 2:347, 1985.
112. Shafer A, Sung ML, White PF: Pharmacokinetics and pharmacodynamics of alfentanil infusions during general anesthesia, *Anesth Analg* 65:1021, 1986.
113. Reitz JA: Alfentanil in anesthesia and analgesia, *Drug Intell Clin Pharm* 20:336, 1986.

114. Fone KC, Wilson H: The effects of alfentanil and selected narcotic analgesics on the rate of action potential discharge of medullary respiratory neurones in anesthetized rats, *Br J Pharmacol* 89:67, 1986.
115. Bagshaw ON, Singh P, Aitkenhead AR: Alfentanil in daycase anaesthesia. Assessment of a single dose on the quality of anaesthesia and recovery, *Anaesthesia* 48:476, 1993.
116. Phitayakorn P, Melnick BM, Vuicinie AF: Comparison of continuous sufentanil and fentanyl infusions for outpatient anaesthesia, *Can J Anaesth* 34:242, 1987.
117. Davis PJ, Chopyk JB, Nazif M et al: Continuous alfentanil infusion in pediatric patients undergoing general anesthesia for complete oral restoration, *J Clin Anesth* 3:125, 1991.
118. Edgin WA, Ford ML, Mansfield MJ: Alfentanil for general anesthesia in oral and maxillofacial surgery, *Oral Maxillofac Surg* 47:1039, 1989.
119. Bostek CC, Fiducia DA, Klotz RW et al: Total intravenous anesthesia with a continuous propofol-alfentanil infusion, *CRNA* 3:124, 1992.
120. Donnelly AJ, Cunningham FE, Baughman VL: *Anesthesiology & critical care drug handbook, 1999-2000,* ed, 2, Cleveland, 1999, Lexi-Comp.
121. Burkle H, Dunbar S, Van Aken H: Remifentanil: a novel, short-acting, μ-opioid, *Anesth Analg* 83:646, 1996.
122. Glass PS: Remifentanil: a new opioid, *J Clin Anesth* 7:558, 1995.
123. Kapila A, Glass PS, Jacobs JR et al: Measured context-sensitive half-times of remifentanil and alfentanil, *Anesthesiology* 83:968, 1995.
124. Goldstein G: Pentazocine, *Drug Alcohol Depend* 14:313, 1985.
125. Burstein AH, Fullerton T: Oculogyric crisis possibly related to pentazocine, *Ann Pharmacother* 27:874, 1993.
126. Wilkinson DJ: Opioid agonist/antagonists in general anaesthesia, *Br J Hosp Med* 38:130, 1987.
127. Pallasch TJ, Gill CJ: Butorphanol and nalbuphine: a pharmacologic comparison, *Oral Surg* 59:15, 1985.
128. Zallen RD, Cobetto GA, Bohmfalk C et al: Butorphanol/diazepam compared to meperidine/diazepam for sedation in oral and maxillofacial surgery: a double-blind evaluation, *Oral Surg* 64:395, 1987.
129. Woolverton WL, Schuster CR: Behavioral and pharmacological aspects of opioid dependence: mixed agonist/antagonists, *Pharmacol Rev* 35:33, 1983.
130. Donadoni R, Rolly G, Devulder J et al: Double-blind comparison between nalbuphine and pentazocine in the control of postoperative pain after orthopedic surgery, *Acta Anaesthesiol Belg* 39:251, 1988.
131. Davidson-Lamb R: Nalbuphine hydrochloride (Nubain) versus pentazocine for analgesia during dental operations. A double blind, randomized trial, *SAAD Dig* 6:76, 1985.
132. Baum C, Hus JP, Nelson RC: The impact of the addition of naloxone on the use and abuse of pentazocine, *Public Health Rep* 102:426, 1987.
133. Kewitz H: Rare but serious risks associated with non-narcotic analgesics: clinical experience, *Med Toxicol* 1 (suppl 1):86, 1986.
134. Schnoll SH, Chasnoff IJ, Glassroth J: Pentazocine and tripelennamine abuse: T's and blues, *Psychiatr Med* 3:219, 1985.
135. Challoner KR, McCarron MM, Newton EJ: Pentazocine (Talwin) intoxication: report of 57 cases, *J Emerg Med* 8:67, 1990.
136. Jago RH, Restall J, Stonham J: The effect of naloxone on pentazocine induced hallucinations, *J Roy Army Med Corps* 130:64, 1984.
137. Winthrop Laboratories: Talwin. Drug package insert, New York, 1992, Winthrop Laboratories.
138. Roytblat L, Bear R, Gesztes T: Seizures after pentazocine overdose, *Isr J Med Sci* 22:385, 1986.
139. Facts and Comparisons: *Nalbuphine,* St Louis, 2000, Facts and Comparisons.
140. Miller RR: Evaluation of nalbuphine hydrochloride, *Am J Hosp Pharm* 37:942, 1980.
141. Lefevre B, Freysz M, Lepine J et al: Comparison of nalbuphine and fentanyl as intravenous analgesics for medically compromised patients undergoing oral surgery, *Anesth Prog* 39:13, 1993.
142. Hunter PL: Use of nalbuphine for analgesia in combination with methohexital sodium, *Anesth Prog* 36:150, 1989.
143. Dolan EA, Murray WJ, Ruddy MP: Double-blind comparison of nalbuphine and meperidine in combination with diazepam for intravenous conscious sedation in oral surgery outpatients, *Oral Surg* 66:536, 1988.
144. Maupome G, Cannon J: Intravenous sedation in pediatric dentistry using midazolam, nalbuphine and droperidol. *Pediatr Dent* 22:113, 2000.
145. Magruder MR, Delaney RD, DiFazio CA: Reversal of narcotic-induced respiratory depression with nalbuphine hydrochloride, *Anesth Rev* 9:34, 1982.
146. Pallasch TJ, Gill CJ: Naloxone-associated morbidity and mortality, *Oral Surg* 52:602, 1981.
147. Schmidt WK, Tam SW, Shotzberger GS et al: Nalbuphine, *Drug Alcohol Depend* 14:339, 1985.
148. Hameroff SR: Opiate receptor pharmacology: mixed agonist/antagonist narcotics, *Contemp Anesth Pract* 7:27, 1983.
149. Gal TJ, DiFazio CA, Moscicki J: Analgesic and respiratory depressant activity of nalbuphine: a comparison with morphine, *Anesthesiology* 57:367, 1982.
150. Errick JK, Heel RC: Nalbuphine: a preliminary review of its pharmacological properties and therapeutic efficacy, *Drugs* 26:191, 1983.
151. Crul JF, Smets MJ, van Egmond J: The efficacy and safety of nalbuphine (Nubain) in balanced anesthesia. A double blind comparison with fentanyl in gynecological and urological surgery, *Acta Anaesthesiol Belg* 41:261, 1990.
152. Bowdle TA: Clinical pharmacology of antagonists of narcotic-induced respiratory depression. A brief review, *Acute Care* 12(suppl 1):70, 1988.
153. Romagnoli A, Keats AS: Ceiling effect for respiratory depression by nalbuphine, *Clin Pharmacol Ther* 27:478, 1980.
154. Lefevre B, Freysz M, Lepine J et al: Comparison of nalbuphine and fentanyl as intravenous analgesics for medically compromised patients undergoing oral surgery. *Anesth Prog* 39:13, 1993.

155. Preston KL, Jasinski DR: Abuse liability studies of opioid agonist-antagonists in humans, *Drug Alcohol Depend* 28:49, 1991.
156. Bowdle TA: Clinical pharmacology of antagonists of narcotic-induced respiratory depression. *Acute Care* 12 Suppl 1:70, 1988.
157. Vogelsang J, Hayes SR: Butorphanol tartrate (Stadol): a review, *J Post Anesth Nurs* 6:129, 1991.
158. Vandam LD: Butorphanol, *N Engl J Med* 302:381, 1980.
159. Vogelsang J, Hayes SR: Butorphanol tartrate (Stadol): a review, *J Post Anesth Nurs* 6:129, 1991.
160. Nagashima H, Karamanian A, MaLovany R et al: Respiratory and circulatory effects of intravenous butorphanol and morphine, *Clin Pharmacol Ther* 19:738, 1976.
161. Roscow CE: Butorphanol in perspective, *Acute Care* 12 (suppl 1):2, 1988.
162. O'Hair KC, Dodd KT, Phillips YY et al: Cardiopulmonary effects of nalbuphine hydrochloride and butorphanol tartrate in sheep, *Lab Anim Sci* 38:58, 1988.
163. Facts and Comparisons: *Butorphanol* (package insert), St Louis, 1982, Facts and Comparisons.
164. From RP: Substance dependence and abuse by anesthesia care providers. In Rogers MC, Tinker JH, Covino CG et al, eds: *Principles and practice of anesthesiology,* St Louis, 1993, Mosby.
165. Finder RL, Bennett CR: Use of scopolamine for dental anesthesia and analgesia techniques, *J Oral Maxillofac Surg* 42:802, 1984.
166. Izquierdo I: Mechanism of action of scopolamine as an amnestic, *Trends Pharmacol Sci* 10:175, 1988.
167. Fassi A, Rosenberg M: Atropine, scopolamine and glycopyrrolate, *Anesth Prog* 26:155, 1979.
168. Das G: Therapeutic review: cardiac effects of atropine in man: an update, *Int J Clin Pharmacol Ther Toxicol* 27:473, 1989.
169. Noronha-Blob L, Lowe VC, Peterson JS et al: The anticholinergic activity of agents indicated for urinary incontinence is an important property for effective control of bladder dysfunction, *J Pharmacol Exp Ther* 251:586, 1989.
170. Kanto J, Klotz U: Pharmacokinetic implications for the clinical use of atropine, scopolamine and glycopyrrolate, *Acta Anaesth Scand* 32:69, 1988.
171. Bryant DH: Anti-cholinergic drugs and their use in asthma, *Prog Clin Biol Res* 263:379, 1988.
172. Astra Pharmaceuticals: Atropine. Drug package insert, Westboro, Mass, 1996, Astra Pharmaceuticals.
173. Repreht J: The central muscarinic transmission during anaesthesia and recovery: the central anticholinergic syndrome, *Anaesth Reanim* 16:250, 1991.
174. Nuotto E: Psychomotor, physiological and cognitive effects of scopolamine and ephedrine in healthy man, *Eur J Clin Pharmacol* 24:603, 1983.
175. Schneck HJ, Rupreht J: Central anticholinergic syndrome (CAS) in anesthesia and intensive care, *Acta Anaesthesiol Belg* 40:219, 1989.
176. Helfaer MA, Rock P: Formulary: guide to physiologic assessment and pharmacologic dosing in common anesthetic practice. In Rogers MC, Tinker JH, Covino CG et al, eds: *Principles and practice of anesthesiology,* St Louis, 1993, Mosby.
177. el-Hakim M: Cardiac dysrhythmias during dental surgery, comparison of hyoscine, glycopyrrolate and placebo medication, *Anaesth Reanim* 16:393, 1991.
178. AH Robins: Robinul Injectable. Drug package insert, Richmond, Va, 1996, AH Robins.
179. Preston GC, Broks P, Traub M et al: Effects of lorazepam on memory, attention and sedation in man, *Psychopharmacology* 95:208, 1988.
180. Henschel WF: 30 years of neuroleptanalgesia: the current status, *Anaesth Reanim* 15:267, 1990.
181. Greenfield W: Neuroleptanalgesia and dissociative drugs, *Dent Clin North Am* 17:263, 1973.
182. Mehrotra RG, Gupta NR: Neuroleptanalgesia with fentanyl-droperidol: an appreciation based on 100 anesthetics for dental surgery on ambulatory patients, *J Indian Dent Assoc* 54:95, 1982.
183. Janssen: Inapsine injection. Drug package insert, Piscataway, NJ, 1997, Janssen.
184. Dangers of Innovar, *Med Lett Drugs Ther* 16:42, 1974.
185. Janssen: Innovar. Drug package insert, Piscataway, NJ, 1996, Janssen.
186. Reich DL, Silvay G: Ketamine: an update on the first twenty-five years of clinical experience, *Can J Anaesth* 36:186, 1989.
187. Haas DA, Harper DG: Ketamine: a review of its pharmacologic properties and use in ambulatory anesthesia, *Anesth Prog* 39:61, 1992.
188. Becsey L, Malamed SF, Radnay P et al: Reduction of the psychotomimetic and circulatory side effects of ketamine by droperidol, *Anesthesiology* 37:536, 1972.
189. Sussman DR: A comparative evaluation of ketamine anesthesia in children and adults, *Anesthesiology* 40:459, 1974.
190. White PF, Way, WL, Trevor AJ: Ketamine: its pharmacology and therapeutic uses, *Anesthesiology* 56:119, 1982.
191. Goodson JM, Moore P: Life-threatening reactions following pedodontic sedation: an assessment of narcotic, local anesthetic and antiemetic drug interaction, *J Am Dent Assoc* 107:239, 1983.
192. Lasagna L, Beecher HK: The analgesic effectiveness of nalorphine and nalorphine-morphine combinations in man, *J Pharmacol Exp Ther* 112:356, 1954.
193. Sharts-Engel NC: Naloxone review and pediatric dosage update, *Am J Maternal Child Nurs* 16:182, 1991.
194. Magruder MR, Delaney RD, DiFazio CA: Reversal of narcotic-induced respiratory depression with nalbuphine hydrochloride, *Anesth Rev* 9:34, 1982.
195. Wride SR, Smith RE, Courtney PG: A fatal case of pulmonary edema in a healthy young male following naloxone administration, *Anaesth Intens Care* 17:374, 1989.
196. DuPont: Narcan. Drug package insert, Wilmington, Del, 1993, DuPont Multi-Source Products.
197. Rodrigo MR, Rosenquist JB: The effect of Ro 15-1788 (Anexate) on conscious sedation produced with midazolam, *Anaesth Intens Care* 15:185, 1987.
198. Wolff J, Carl P, Clausen TG et al: Ro 15-1778 for postoperative recovery: a randomized clinical trial in patients undergoing minor surgical procedures under midazolam anaesthesia, *Anaesthesia* 41:1001, 1986.
199. Ricou B, Forster A, Bruckner A et al: Clinical evaluation of a specific benzodiazepine antagonist (Ro 15-1788):

studies in elderly patients after regional anaesthesia under benzodiazepine sedation, *Br J Anaesth* 58:1, 1986.

200. Sage DJ, Close A, Boas RA: Reversal of midazolam sedation with Anexate, *Br J Anaesth* 59:459, 1987.
201. Kirkegaard L, Knudsen L, Jensen S et al: Benzodiazepine antagonist Ro 15-1788: antagonism of diazepam sedation in outpatients undergoing gastroscopy, *Anaesthesia* 41:1184, 1986.
202. Roncari G, Ziegler WH, Guentert TW: Pharmacokinetics of the new benzodiazepine antagonist Ro 15-1788 in man following intravenous and oral administration, *Br J Clin Pharm* 22:421, 1986.
203. Olympio MA: Postanesthetic emergence delirium: historical perspective, *J Clin Anesth* 3:60, 1991.
204. Lauven PM, Stoeckel H: Flumazenil (Ro 15-1788) and physostigmine, *Resuscitation* 16(suppl):S41, 1988.
205. Forest Pharmaceuticals: Antilirium. Drug package insert, St Louis, 1992, Forest Pharmaceuticals.

CHAPTER 26

Intravenous Sedation: Techniques of Administration

CHAPTER OUTLINE

In this chapter techniques of intravenous (IV) conscious sedation are discussed. These techniques employ many of the drugs discussed in Chapter 25 and are grouped into four levels, based on the degree of complexity, the level of training required by the doctor before he or she should consider use of the technique, and the requirement for patient monitoring during the procedure. These four categories are (1) basic techniques, (2) modifications of basic techniques, (3) advanced techniques, and (4) other techniques (Box 26-1).

MONITORING INTRAVENOUS SEDATION

Whenever drugs are administered parenterally, it is of paramount importance that the patient be monitored more closely than after oral or inhalation sedation. Guidelines for monitoring during conscious sedation have been developed.[1-5] I recommend the following regimen for monitoring during IV conscious sedation:

1. Baseline vital signs are recorded at preliminary appointment.
   a. Blood pressure
   b. Heart rate and rhythm
   c. Respiratory rate
   d. Height/weight (optional)
   e. Temperature (optional)
2. Vital signs are recorded preoperatively on the day of treatment.
3. Immediately after IV drug administration, vital signs are recorded.
4. Every 10 to 15 minutes, vital signs should be recorded.
5. Postoperatively, vital signs are recorded.
6. Following recovery and immediately before patient discharge from the office, a final set of vital signs is recorded.

BOX 26-1 **Intravenous Conscious Sedation Techniques**

Basic Techniques
Benzodiazepine
Jorgensen technique
Promethazine

Modifications of Basic Techniques
Benzodiazepine with anticholinergic

Advanced Techniques
Benzodiazepine with opioid plus anticholinergic
Promethazine with opioid
Jorgensen technique plus benzodiazepine
Opioid with group A drug

Others
Diazepam with methohexital (Foreman technique)
Berns technique
Shane technique

In addition, the protocol for IV conscious sedation at the University of Southern California (USC) requires the use of two continuous monitors during IV conscious sedation procedures.[6] The following methods are available (see discussion in Chapter 5):

1. Precordial/pretracheal stethoscope
2. Pulse meter
3. Pulse oximeter
4. End-tidal carbon dioxide (CO_2) monitor (capnography)
5. Electrocardiograph (ECG)
6. Vital signs monitor

A pretracheal stethoscope should be used in all IV conscious sedation procedures. It is very effective and inexpensive. The pulse oximeter has become a standard monitoring device for IV conscious sedation. Functioning as a continuous monitor of arterial oxygen saturation as well as heart rate, use of a pulse oximeter is considered the standard of care in parenteral sedation. As an aside, recent graduates from U.S. dental schools who use IV conscious sedation would never consider starting an IV case in the absence of an oximeter.[7] End-tidal CO_2 monitors are rapidly gaining entry into the monitoring armamentarium of doctors using general anesthesia or IV deep sedation and somewhat more gradually for IV conscious sedation. The pulse meter and ECG are less essential during parenteral sedation procedures than are techniques for monitoring the respiratory system. The ECG, although desirable, should be considered an optional monitor for IV conscious sedation.

The most important monitor used during IV conscious sedation is that of the central nervous system through direct verbal contact with and response from the patient. Patients should be able to respond appropriately to verbal or physical stimulation throughout parenteral conscious sedation procedures.

Classification of Intravenous Drugs

Group A (Antianxiety/Sedative-Hypnotic Drugs)
Diazepam
Midazolam
Pentobarbital
Promethazine

Group B (Opioid-Type Analgesics)
Meperidine
Morphine
Fentanyl
Alfentanil
Sufentanil
Remifentanil
Pentazocine
Nalbuphine
Butorphanol

Group C (Anticholinergics)
Atropine
Scopolamine
Glycopyrrolate

BASIC INTRAVENOUS TECHNIQUES

The first group of sedation techniques are those that form the backbone of IV conscious sedation. With these techniques available, the trained doctor will be able to meet the needs of a dental or surgical procedure of any duration and achieve satisfactory sedation in virtually all patients requiring IV conscious sedation.

The *Jorgensen technique* is arguably the original IV conscious sedation technique.[8] Despite attempts at improving it, the original Jorgensen technique is still taught today, providing excellent sedation with few reports of any significant complications. The primary indication for the Jorgensen technique is a procedure requiring 2 hours or more to complete.

IV conscious sedation using a benzodiazepine has become the most popular technique in dentistry.[9] IV benzodiazepine sedation meets the needs of contemporary dental practice, that is, sedation for approximately 1 hour. In the years since its introduction (1986), midazolam has challenged diazepam for supremacy in the area of 1-hour IV conscious sedation.

With the availability of these two techniques, virtually all patients who require IV conscious sedation will be treated successfully. However, with the major effect of diazepam or midazolam lasting less than 1 hour and the Jorgensen technique effective for more than 2 hours, a procedure providing effective sedation of from 1 to 2 hours may be needed. This need is effectively met by promethazine.

These three basic techniques are described next. The benzodiazepine and Jorgensen techniques are described in detail. These provide the basic format for the techniques to follow, which are described in somewhat less detail.

Intravenous Benzodiazepine (Diazepam or Midazolam)

Preliminary Appointment. When either diazepam or midazolam is being considered for IV use, specific questions must be asked of the patient concerning any prior experience with the drugs to be used and, if "yes," the response to it, any adverse responses, and any specific contraindications to their use. For diazepam and midazolam, these include the following:

1. Allergy or hypersensitivity to benzodiazepines
2. Glaucoma (untreated)
3. History of phlebitis, thrombophlebitis (contraindication to diazepam)
4. Acute pulmonary insufficiency (contraindication to midazolam)
5. Preexisting respiratory depression

Patients classified as American Society of Anesthesiologists (ASA) I and II are candidates for IV conscious sedation. Only selected ASA III patients should be considered, and then only on a case-by-case basis.

Before the day of treatment, the following items concerning the patient's suitability for IV conscious sedation are evaluated by the doctor and staff:

1. Degree of Apprehension. Which route of sedation (oral, intramuscular [IM], inhalation, IV) is most appropriate for this patient? If the IV route is selected, which of the techniques is most appropriate for this patient?

2. Informed Consent. If the IV route is selected, informed consent must be provided to the patient, describing the IV procedure, its alternatives (e.g., IM, general anesthesia), and the most likely complications associated with its use. The patient is asked to sign the consent form, which is then added to the patient's dental record.

3. Medical History. The medical history questionnaire, dialogue history, and vital signs are reviewed to determine the presence of contraindications, either relative or absolute, to the use of the drugs being considered.

4. Nature and Length of Dental Procedure Being Contemplated. The degree of trauma associated with the planned procedure must be considered in evaluating a potential sedative technique. In addition, the length of the procedure is also a consideration. Selection of appropriate IV drugs can tailor the length of sedation to almost any duration.

5. Presence of Superficial Veins. The presence of suitable superficial veins is a primary requisite for elective IV sedative procedures. Lack of suitably visible veins is an acceptable reason for avoiding the IV route and selecting an alternative route of drug administration.

6. Recording of Vital Signs. Baseline vital signs are obtained at this visit if they have not yet been recorded.

7. Preoperative Instructions. Following is an example of preoperative instructions for IV conscious sedation:

1. Arrangements must be made for a responsible adult to drive the patient home after the IV conscious sedation appointment. The patient will be unable to leave the office alone.

COMMENT: When the patient arrives for treatment, the name, address, and telephone number of the escort should be obtained immediately. If treatment is planned to last up to 1 hour, the escort is requested to accompany the patient to the office and remain during the procedure. For procedures lasting more than 2 hours, the escort is still requested to accompany the patient to the office. However, the doctor may elect to permit the escort to leave the office for the duration of the procedure and to return before the procedure is scheduled to end. In either case it is extremely important to have seen or at least spoken to the patient's escort before the start of the procedure. It is my policy to cancel the planned procedure whenever a suitable escort is not available at the start of treatment.

When oral sedation is prescribed preoperatively, an escort *must* accompany the patient to the office.

2. The patient should have had nothing to eat for approximately 4 hours before the procedure.

COMMENT: The attempt here is to provide an empty stomach and gastric fluids with a higher pH in the unlikely event that the patient should become nauseous or vomit during or following the IV procedure. There is less likelihood of aspiration if food is not present in the stomach. Patients may be permitted to ingest clear liquids such as water or apple juice along with any medications they may be required to take (e.g., antihypertensives). If the scheduled appointment is before noon, the patient is told not to eat anything that morning. For an afternoon IV conscious sedation case, the patient is advised to avoid anything by mouth after 8 AM. A light, carbohydrate-rich breakfast consisting of dry cereal and juice may be taken before 8 AM that morning. Medications may be taken, normally, with water.

3. The patient is advised to wear loose-fitting garments.

COMMENT: This will prevent any possibly excessive respiratory depression caused by mechanical means. The upper garment worn by the patient should be of short-sleeved length or have no sleeves so that access may readily be gained to both arms.

Many doctors using IV conscious sedation or general anesthesia have the patient change into a surgical shirt (or "scrubs"). Loose fitting and sleeveless, this permits the anesthesia team immediate and unimpeded access to the patient's chest and upper body throughout the procedure.

4. The patient should plan to arrive at the office approximately 15 minutes before the scheduled appointment.

5. Should the patient develop a cold, flu, sore throat, or any other illness, the appointment will be canceled and rescheduled at a time when the patient is more physically fit. The patient should call if any of these symptoms develop.

COMMENT: Research has demonstrated that morbidity and mortality following anesthesia in patients with upper respiratory infections (URI) are actually greater in the time following the patient's apparent "recovery" from the URI.[10] Most of this morbidity is related to respiratory disease.

6. The medications to be taken before arrival in the office for treatment are prescribed, and the names of drugs, dosages, and instructions are given.

7. The time, date, and place of appointment are given to the patient.

8. Day of Treatment. The day of the scheduled IV conscious sedation and dental treatment arrives, and the patient is in the waiting room. Knowing that the patient is fearful of the upcoming procedures, the doctor will not wish to prolong his or her wait any longer than necessary because the patient's anxiety and fears will increase during this time.

An exception to this will be the patient receiving oral sedation in addition to IV conscious sedation. If the oral drug is not taken at home, the patient should be scheduled to arrive in the office approximately 45 minutes before the scheduled start of the IV conscious sedation, the oral drug administered, and the patient asked to remain in the waiting room.

During this time the assistant prepares the IV infusion and drugs for use (see Chapter 24). Once all is ready, the assistant asks the patient to go to the restroom and void, if necessary, following which the patient is taken to the treatment chair and seated in a semiupright (comfortable) position. The availability of the patient's escort should be determined at this time. Preoperative vital signs are monitored and recorded on the anesthesia record sheet for the patient (Figure 26-1).

Once these procedures are completed, monitors are placed. The blood pressure cuff is placed on the arm opposite the working side of the doctor and left in place throughout the procedure. The pretracheal stethoscope, ECG electrodes (if used), and pulse oximeter and/or end-tidal CO_2 monitor or pulse monitor are also placed at this time. A nasal canula or nasal hood is positioned, and a 3- to 6-L/min flow of oxygen is administered throughout the IV procedure. This is standard IV protocol at USC.

Because of an increased incidence of phlebitis when diazepam is administered, it is suggested that, when possible, smaller veins such as those on the dorsum of the hand or wrist be avoided when venipuncture is performed.[11,12] This is not the case with water-soluble midazolam. Venipuncture is completed, and the IV infusion is established and secured (see Chapter 24).

Diazepam. Diazepam may now be administered to the patient. The diazepam has previously been readied for use by the dental assistant. This is now reviewed.

Diazepam is available in a 10-ml vial at a concentration of 5 mg/ml. The assistant takes a sterile, disposable 3- or 5-ml syringe and, after wiping the rubber diaphragm of the vial with isopropyl alcohol (and waiting 1 minute for the alcohol to dry), injects 3 ml of air into the vial of diazepam and withdraws an equal volume of the yellowish diazepam solution. The syringe is recapped, labeled "diazepam 5 mg/ml," and put aside for later use. Syringes containing drugs must always be labeled, even when only one drug is being used.

Drug Administration. The patient is placed in a supine position before drug administration. It is good practice to open up the IV infusion so that the rate of flow is rapid during the administration of any drug. This further dilutes the drug, minimizing any local irritation that might develop as the drug comes into contact with the vein wall.

Immediately before beginning drug administration, the assistant or doctor should make one final check to confirm that the IV infusion is still patent. Squeezing the flash bulb of the tubing (Figure 26-2) or holding the bag of IV solution below the patient's heart level should disclose blood in the tubing, a sign of a patent IV line (Figure 26-3).

Diazepam, an oily viscous liquid, has a propensity to cause a burning sensation in some patients as the drug is administered, the sensation lasting until the diazepam is flushed from the injection site. A rapidly running IV drip minimizes this effect. In addition, it is advisable to tell the patient that he or she may experience a brief period of warmth when the drug is injected and that this is normal and will subside quickly.

A test dose of 0.2 ml (each small delineation on the 5-ml [5-cc] syringe is 0.2 ml) is administered to deter-

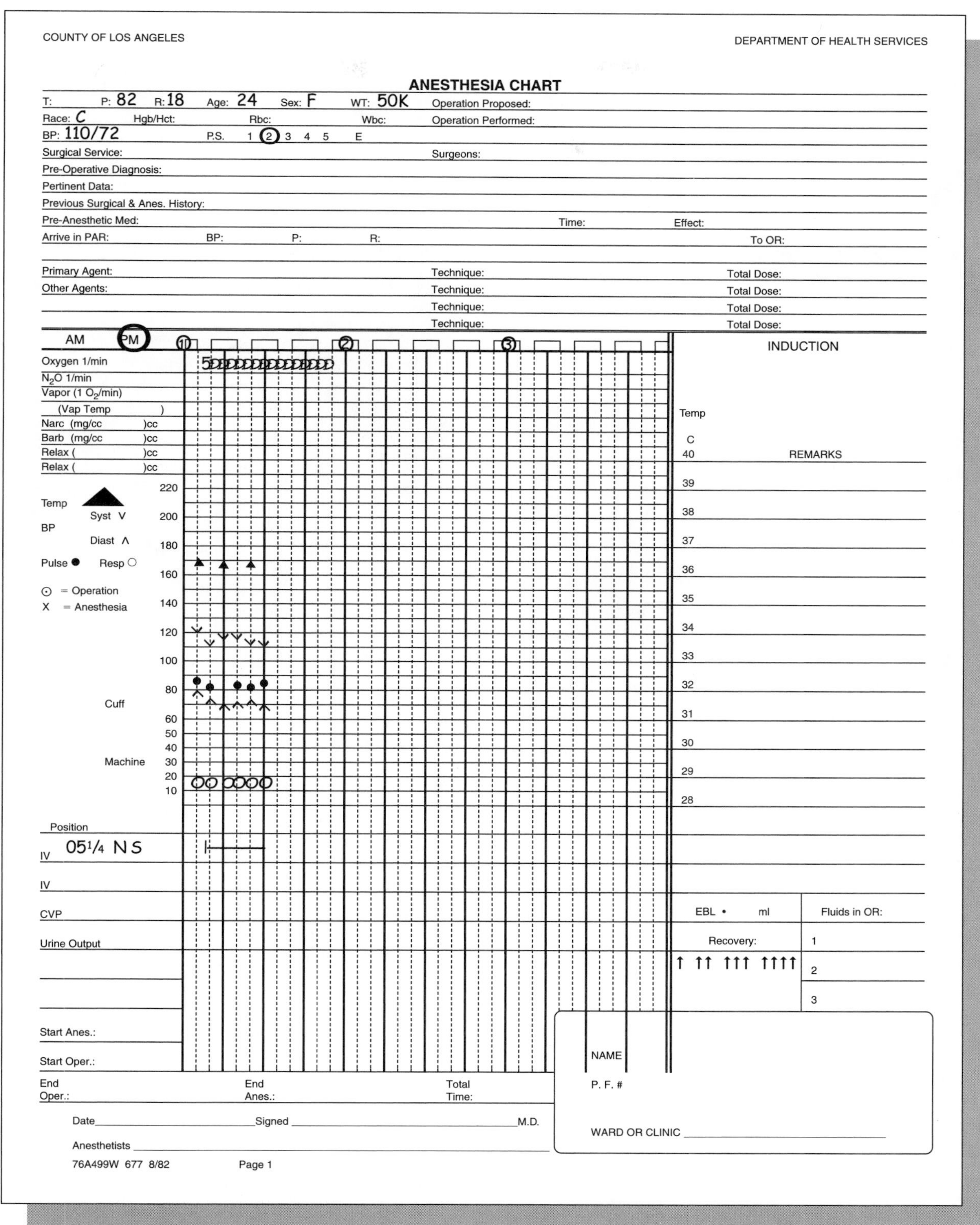
COUNTY OF LOS ANGELES

DEPARTMENT OF HEALTH SERVICES

ANESTHESIA CHART

T: P: 82 R: 18 Age: 24 Sex: F WT: 50K Operation Proposed:

Race: C Hgb/Hct: Rbc: Wbc: Operation Performed:

BP: 110/72 P.S. 1 (2) 3 4 5 E

Surgical Service: Surgeons:

Pre-Operative Diagnosis:

Pertinent Data:

Previous Surgical & Anes. History:

Pre-Anesthetic Med: Time: Effect:

Arrive in PAR: BP: P: R: To OR:

Primary Agent: Technique: Total Dose:

Other Agents: Technique: Total Dose:

Technique: Total Dose:

Technique: Total Dose:

AM (PM) (1) (2) (3)

INDUCTION

Oxygen 1/min 5

N_2O 1/min

Vapor (1 O_2/min)

(Vap Temp)

Narc (mg/cc)cc

Barb (mg/cc)cc

Relax ( )cc

Relax ( )cc

Temp ▲

BP Syst V Diast Λ

Pulse ● Resp ○

⊙ = Operation

X = Anesthesia

Cuff

Machine

220 200 180 160 140 120 100 80 60 50 40 30 20 10

Temp C 40 39 38 37 36 35 34 33 32 31 30 29 28

REMARKS

Position

IV 05¹/₄ N S

IV

CVP

Urine Output

EBL • ml

Fluids in OR: 1 2 3

Recovery: ↑ ↑↑ ↑↑↑ ↑↑↑↑

Start Anes.:

Start Oper.:

NAME

P. F. #

WARD OR CLINIC

End Oper.: End Anes.: Total Time:

Date Signed M.D.

Anesthetists

76A499W 677 8/82 Page 1

Figure 26-1 Preoperative vital signs are recorded and entered onto the patient's chart.

mine whether any unusual response (e.g., hypersensitivity, allergy) is to develop (Figure 26-4).

After waiting about 20 seconds, the titration of diazepam starts. The recommended rate of injection of diazepam is 1 ml/min, equivalent to 5 mg of diazepam per minute.

The doctor should start by administering 0.5 ml slowly and continuously over 30 seconds. Because of

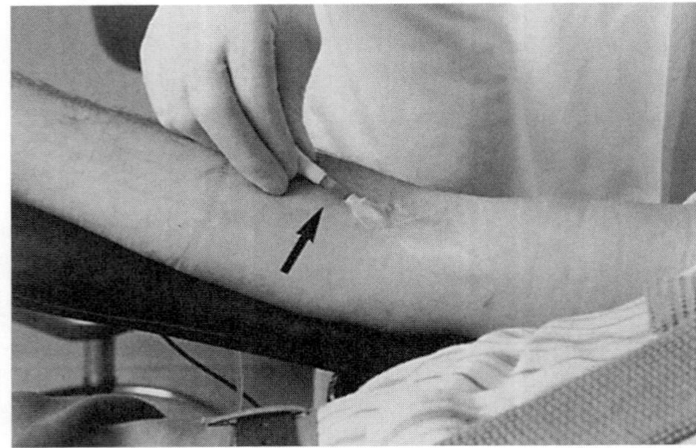

Figure 26-2 Squeezing and releasing flash bulb should elicit return of blood *(arrow)* as final check of patency of vein.

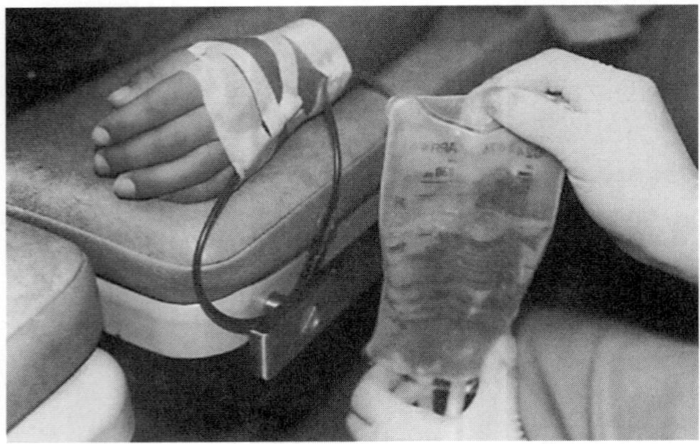

Figure 26-3 Holding bag of IV solution below level of vein should produce a return of blood into the tubing, a sign of a patent IV.

the great individual variation in drug response, the doctor must always titrate carefully to each patient's precise level of sedation. Diazepam should continue to be titrated at a rate of 1 ml/min until this ideal level of sedation is achieved.

When a doctor is first learning to use IV conscious sedation, his or her natural tendency will be to cease titration of diazepam at the very first sign of a change in the patient's level of consciousness. Because of the uncertainty of the doctor, many patients may, in fact, be undersedated. As clinical experience is gained, the doctor will develop a "feel" for the proper level of sedation.

The following are clinical signs and symptoms associated with the desired level of sedation:

- The patient will appear to become more relaxed in the dental chair in contrast to his or her earlier, tenser demeanor. The patient may stretch out, uncross the legs, and relax his or her grip on the arm of the chair.
- The patient's response to questions will be somewhat slower than it was before the sedation, and the patient may appear to have some difficulty in putting thoughts together into words.

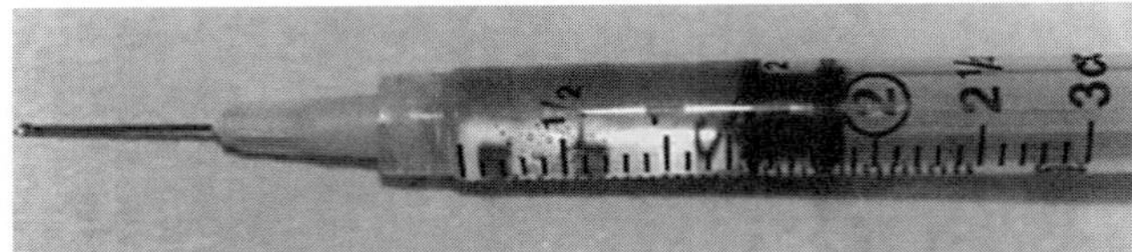

Figure 26-4 A test dose of 0.2 ml (each small delineation on the syringe is 0.1 ml) is administered to determine if any unusual response (e.g., hypersensitivity, allergy) develops.

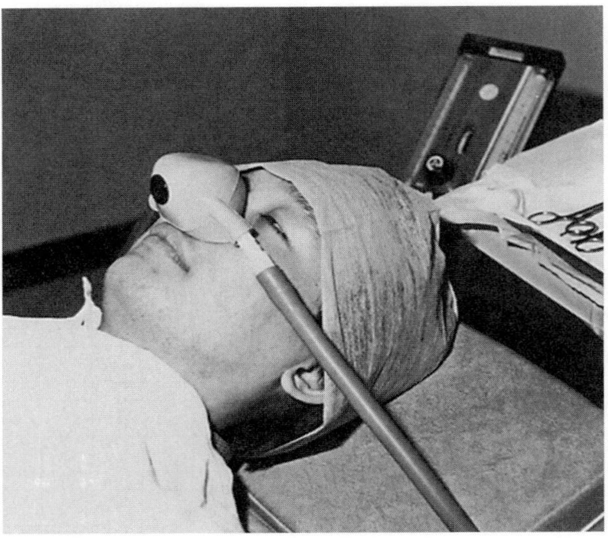

Figure 26-5 Halfway ptosis of the upper eyelid is often seen when diazepam is employed as an IV sedative. (The patient is receiving 100% O_2 via nasal hood.)

- The patient's eyelids may appear to be drooping. This is *not* to be considered the primary criterion for proper sedation. Halfway ptosis of the upper eyelid, the Verrill sign (Figure 26-5), usually occurs when the patient is somewhat too heavily sedated.[12,13]

When diazepam is administered at the recommended rate, the typical patient (middle of the "bell-shaped" curve), who requires approximately 10 to 12 mg of diazepam, will be sedated within 2 to 3 minutes of the start of drug administration. Once the desired level of sedation is reached, the rate of the IV infusion is slowed. Whenever a drug is not being administered, the infusion rate is adjusted to approximately 1 drop every 5 to 10 seconds. The purpose is to prevent a blood clot from forming in the needle during the procedure. This slow drip rate is commonly abbreviated as *t.k.o.* (to keep open).

Immediately after the administration of diazepam, vital signs and the drug dose (in milligrams) are recorded on the anesthesia record. Vital signs should be recorded immediately after any subsequent IV drug administration and at 5- to 10-minute intervals throughout the procedure. All drugs administered during IV conscious sedation, including local anesthetics, must be recorded on the anesthesia record.

Dosage. The average dose of diazepam required for clinically adequate IV conscious sedation is between 10 and 12 mg (based on an average of more than 3200 cases). The range of these doses is of far greater importance, for it illustrates the tremendous individual variability in response to diazepam (and all drugs). In my experience with diazepam as a sole agent for sedation, clinically adequate sedation has been achieved with as little as 2.5 mg (0.5 ml) in some patients, whereas others have received in excess of 30 mg and have not even approached the desired level of sedation.

The following is suggested as a means of determining the maximum dose of diazepam for a given patient. Diazepam is titrated at a rate of 5 mg (1 ml) per minute until ideal sedation is achieved. The average dose of diazepam required to produce this clinical effect is 10 to 12 mg. Once this effect is achieved, titration ceases, the IV infusion is slowed to t.k.o., and the operative phase of treatment is begun (see later discussion).

However, if a diazepam dose of 20 mg has been administered and the patient demonstrates some clinical sedation, although not quite at the desired level, additional diazepam may be titrated up to a total of 25 mg. On the other hand, if the patient has received 20 mg of diazepam but exhibits virtually *no signs or symptoms* of sedation, it is prudent to cease the administration of diazepam. Experience with diazepam has demonstrated that when no evidence of sedation occurs with a 20-mg dose, the addition of another 10 or 20 mg probably will not prove beneficial to the patient but may, in fact, increase the risk of occurrence of several dose-related complications. My recommendation to the neophyte at IV conscious sedation is that when a dose of 20 mg diazepam fails to produce any signs or symptoms of clinical sedation, the administration of diazepam be terminated, and the planned dental/surgical procedure attempted without the administration of any additional IV drugs.

The doctor experienced in IV conscious sedation and/or general anesthesia has several additional options available at this time, but in the hands of the doctor without anesthesiology training, the most prudent course of action at this time is to cease IV drug administration and begin the planned procedure. I am continually surprised by the number of patients who, without any obvious signs or symptoms of sedation, do extremely well and have a significant degree of amnesia at the end of the procedure. Should this attempt to treat fail, the patient should be dismissed (following recovery) and rescheduled for a different IV conscious sedation technique at a later date.

Diazepam	
Average sedative dose	10-12 mg
Sedative dose range	2.5 to >30 mg
Maximum dose, no sedation	20 mg
Maximum dose, some sedation	25 mg

Intraoperative Period. Local anesthetic is administered to the patient exactly as it would be if the patient were not sedated. This includes the use of topical anesthetic and all of the other steps involved in the atraumatic administration of local anesthesia.[14] The patient may react to any pain associated with the local anesthetic injection, but this usually is nothing more than a slight moan, grimace, or minor movement. Adequate time should be allowed for the local anesthetic to take effect (3 to 5 minutes) before the start of the planned procedure.

During the first 3 to 5 minutes following IV diazepam titration, the level of sedation is greatest. Although overresponse to the drug can occur, the patient who has overresponded to diazepam will be somewhat sluggish in response to verbal commands, such as "open your mouth." For this reason, the use of a mouth prop should be considered, at least at the outset of the IV diazepam procedure. Within 5 to 10 minutes the depth of sedation has usually lessened so that the patient's mouth can be voluntarily kept open. A rubber bite block with a piece of string (dental floss) tied around it or a ratchet-type (Molt) mouth prop may be used at this time (Figure 26-6).

Lack of response to verbal command or, more significantly, a lack of response to a painful stimulus (i.e., local anesthetic injection) may indicate that the patient is overly sedated. Lack of response to sensory stimulation is always an indication for the doctor to stop treatment and reevaluate the patient's level of consciousness and airway and ventilatory status.

Following local anesthetic administration, a rubber dam should be applied, if feasible, for the planned procedure. The rubber dam serves two important functions during IV conscious sedation:

1. It aids in maintaining the mouth in an open position (it may be used in place of the mouth prop).
2. It prevents extraneous material from falling into the posterior part of the mouth, throat, and pharynx.

Dental treatment begins at this time. Because of the 45-minute duration of sedation provided by IV diazepam, treatment should be planned to fit into this time period.[15] Also, diazepam produces a period of anterograde amnesia in approximately 75% of patients, lasting approximately 10 minutes.[16] It is recommended that potentially painful or traumatic procedures be completed at the start of the treatment, if possible, to take advantage of this amnesic period.

In this manner, as the sedative effect begins to wane (about 30 minutes after drug administration), relatively innocuous procedures will be performed, such

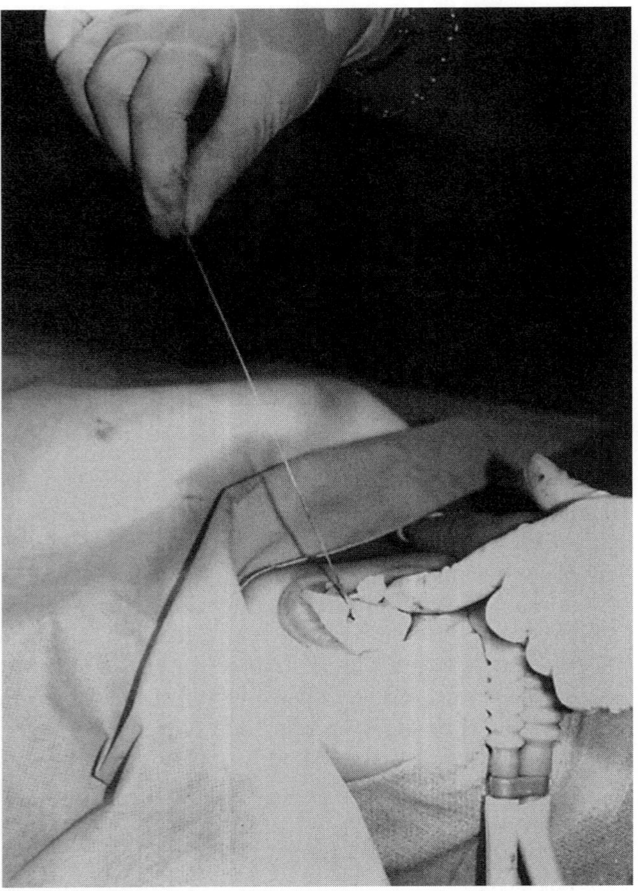

Figure 26-6 Rubber bite block with string (dental floss) tied to it placed into mouth of sedated patient.

as completing restorations, suturing, or adjusting occlusion. In addition, having received local anesthesia earlier, the patient will be pain free at this time and able to tolerate these procedures without complaint. In most patients actual treatment time, with one initial titrating dose of diazepam, can usually be extended well beyond 1 hour because of the lack of pain and the relative innocuousness of the procedures being carried out at the end of the treatment period.

It is rare for a patient to require a second dose of diazepam if the duration of the planned procedure was appropriate (about 1 hour). As discussed in Chapter 25, diazepam sedation may be divided into three phases: stage I: decreased awareness, good sedation, amnesia; stage II: increasing awareness, good sedation, no amnesia; stage III: alert, aware. With entry into the third phase the patient may opine that he or she feels "normal" once again, and the doctor might be tempted to readminister additional diazepam. However, by this time treatment should be nearing completion, the procedure being performed is usually atraumatic, the patient has effective local anesthesia, and although the patient feels normal, he or she is still anxiety free, if not visibly sedated. Thus it is clear that readministration of diazepam is rarely necessary in the typical 1-hour IV conscious sedation procedure.

Occasionally, readministration of diazepam might become necessary to permit successful completion of the procedure. For example, a patient is scheduled for restorative procedures with IV diazepam. All goes well, but one of the teeth requires endodontic treatment. The patient begins to become increasingly aware of the surroundings approximately 40 minutes into the procedure and has become somewhat apprehensive again. The treating doctor has two options: first, to temporarily fill the canal, dismiss the patient, and reschedule for another IV visit; or second, to retitrate additional diazepam and continue with endodontic care at the same visit.

Should the decision be made to retitrate and continue treatment, the assistant increases the rate of the IV drip and additional diazepam is titrated slowly until the patient becomes sedated once again or until a total dose (including the initial titration) of 30 mg diazepam is administered. Following retitration, the IV drip rate is again slowed to t.k.o. and treatment continued.

Retitration with diazepam almost always requires a smaller dose than that required initially. For example, if 12 mg was required at first, a dose of 3 or 8 mg might produce the same clinical level of sedation on retitration. For reasons that are explained in Chapter 27, the total, combined dose of diazepam administered at one appointment should, if possible, be kept to less than 30 mg. When diazepam is readministered, the vital signs are recorded on the anesthesia record sheet.

Posttreatment Period. Following completion of the planned treatment, the IV infusion is discontinued if, in the opinion of the doctor, there is no further need for it. The patient should be responding normally at this time, with no adverse or bizarre signs or symptoms noted (e.g., emergence delirium). The technique for termination of the IV infusion is discussed in Chapter 24. Nasal oxygen (O_2) can also be terminated at this time.

Recovery Criteria. The patient is never to be discharged alone from the office after IV conscious sedation, regardless of the patient's apparent state of recovery or the degree to which the patient protests. Criteria for discharge from the office include the vital signs and the reaction of the patient.

Vital signs should be approximately at baseline level (taken at the preliminary visit). If blood pressure appears significantly depressed (more than 30 mm Hg below baseline) and clinical signs and symptoms of sedation are present, the patient should be permitted to recover for a few more minutes while receiving O_2.

The most important criterion for discharge is the patient's response. Under no circumstances should a patient ever be permitted to leave the office feeling poorly or unable to walk without assistance. In a few cases the patient may feel dizzy, mildly nauseous, or weak. In such cases the patient should be permitted to rest until he or she feels better (thus the importance of a recovery area in the office supervised by a trained assistant). A sedated patient should never be left unattended in any room for any length of time; the doctor or a trained member of the staff should be physically present at all times.

When it is thought that the patient has recovered sufficiently to be discharged, all monitoring devices are removed and the patient permitted to stand. A member of the dental team, the doctor or assistant, should position himself or herself in front of the patient so that if the patient's legs are a little weak, that person can support the patient, preventing injury and possible litigation.

The position of the chair is adjusted from the semisupine to an almost 90-degree position. This is done slowly, preferably in several steps, to allow the patient's cardiovascular system to readapt to the increasing effect of gravity, thereby preventing postural hypotension, possible dizziness, and syncope.

The patient then sits with his or her legs touching the floor and then stands. If the patient is able to accomplish this without difficulty (following diazepam or midazolam IV conscious sedation, there is rarely difficulty in standing after 45 minutes), the patient is requested to take a few steps toward the doctor or assistant. If all is well, the patient is reseated in the dental chair and the patient's escort brought in.

The foremost criterion in permitting patients to be discharged from the office is their ability to take care of themselves should they, for any reason, be left alone during the remainder of the day. They should be able to walk without assistance. If such is not the case, the patient is permitted additional time to recover.

When diazepam or midazolam is used for IV conscious sedation, clinical recovery usually appears to be quite complete at 45 to 60 minutes. However, with other drugs (e.g., pentobarbital, promethazine), recovery may not appear nearly as complete.

Once recovery is deemed adequate for discharge, the patient is returned to the dental chair and the escort called in. In the presence of both persons postoperative instructions are presented verbally and in writing. It is potentially possible, although highly unlikely with diazepam, that the patient may still be amnesic at this time in the procedure, thus the necessity of the escort and written instructions. Instructions given to the patient should be recorded on the anesthesia record and/or included in the patient's dental chart.

Usual postsedation instructions are presented in Box 26-2. Additional instructions should be included if mandated by the dental treatment. This might include restrictions on diet or the need for ice or heat applications. Once again, these are presented verbally to both the patient and escort, given to the patient in writing, and recorded on the patient's chart.

The companion accompanies the patient from the office. A member of the office staff should remain with the patient until the patient is safely in the car with the seat belt secured (in the passenger seat, *not* the driver seat!).

The anesthesia record sheet and the patient's treatment chart are completed, disposable IV equipment (needle, tubing, syringes, and infusion solution) discarded, and any unused drug discarded. A note in the chart and anesthesia record sheet is made: "*x* mg diazepam discarded." Recording of the disposition of all drugs, especially the Schedule II barbiturates and opioid agonists, is a very important part of the IV procedure.

Figure 26-7 illustrates a typical anesthesia record at the conclusion of the IV conscious sedation procedure. The following entry is made in the patient's dental chart when the anesthesia record sheet is included in the chart:

> Date. Patient received intravenous conscious sedation. Anesthesia record enclosed. Dental treatment: extraction 27, 30, 31; MOD 15, etc., signature or initials of doctor.

BOX 26-2 **Postsedation Instructions**

1. Go home and rest for the remainder of the day.
2. Do not perform any strenuous activity. You should remain in the company of a responsible adult until you are fully alert.
3. Do not attempt to eat a heavy meal immediately. If you are hungry, a light diet (liquids and toast) will be more than adequate.
4. A feeling of nausea may occasionally develop after conscious sedation. The following may help you feel better: (a) lying down for a while; (b) a glass of cola beverage.
5. Do not drive a motor vehicle or perform any hazardous tasks for the remainder of the day.
6. Do not take any alcoholic beverages or any medications for the remainder of the day unless you have contacted me first.
7. The following medication(s) have been ordered for you by the doctor. Take them only as directed.
8. If you have any unusual problems you may call (office telephone number).

Patient Name: *John Smith* Date: *2-14-03*

IV infusion was started at *915* a.m./p.m with a *21* gauge Butterfly needle in *(2) AC FOSSA*.

Height/weight: *6' 182 LBS*

TIME (1 box = 15 minutes)

	pre-op																				
	9:10	925		940		1025	1030														
B.P.	116/74	120/86		110/70		112/70	114/77														
Pulse	62	70		64		66	66														
Resp	18	21		16		16	18														
N_2O_2%																					
2% Lidocaine 1/100			1.8ml																		
2% Lidocaine 1/50																					
2% Carbocaine 1/20																					
4% Citanest 1/200																					
mg. Valium (5 mg/ml)		11																			
mg. Scopolamine																					
mg. Demerol (50 mg/ml)																					
mg. Nembutal (50 mg/ml)																					
mg.																					
mg.																					
mg.																					
mg.																					

The procedure lasted *1* hrs. *05* minutes and the patient received *180* ml of D5W. The patient tolerated the procedure well and was discharged at *10:30* a.m./p.m. in good condition to the custody of *MARY SMITH*. Postoperative instructions were given verbally to the patient and the companion.

AMED Faculty Signature: *HM* Student: ______

Figure 26-7 Completed sedation record for an IV diazepam procedure.

When an anesthesia record is not available (every effort should be taken to avoid this), the following chart entry is suggested:

> IV started with a 21-gauge indwelling catheter in the left ventral forearm. The patient received 13 mg diazepam in one dose. Duration of IV procedure = 45 minutes, the patient receiving 5 L/min 100% O_2 via nasal hood throughout the procedure. A total of 180 ml of 5% dextrose and water was administered. Monitoring included continuous pulse oximetry and BP q15min. The patient tolerated the procedure well and was discharged from the office in the custody of Mary Smith at 12:05 PM. Postoperative instructions were given verbally and in writing to both the patient and companion.

Although this may appear to be voluminous and perhaps excessive, especially considering the nature of the usual entry in dental records, this type of recordkeeping is absolutely essential whenever sedative procedures are employed. There should be no doubt at a later date as to exactly what transpired during the sedative procedure.

One more important task remains on the day of the IV conscious sedation: Each and every patient who receives IV (or IM) sedation should be contacted by telephone, by the doctor in the late afternoon if the IV was in the morning or early that evening if the IV was in the afternoon. This is one of the most important actions a professional can perform for his or her patient. It demonstrates to the patient the doctor's sincerity and concern and is a means of circumventing potential problems (e.g., the development of pain or bleeding) before they become significant. This conversation is recorded in the patient's chart.

Midazolam. The technique of IV conscious sedation with midazolam is similar to that described for diazepam, with the following exceptions. Midazolam

	Baseline	*Preoperative*	*Post-IV Drug Administration*	*Postoperative*
Blood pressure (mm Hg)	124/68	132/74	128/70	124/72
Heart rate (beats/min)	66	78	74	74
Respiratory rate (breaths/min)	16	18	14	16
O_2 saturation (%)	97	97	98	98

Doctor's signature: ______

should be administered intravenously in a concentration of 1 mg/ml. A letter from the drug's manufacturer, Roche Laboratories, Inc., recommends use of the 1 mg/ml concentration.[17] When the 5 mg/ml formulation of midazolam is used, 1 ml of the drug is placed in a 5-ml syringe and 4 ml of D_5W or 0.9% sodium chloride added. This provides a final concentration of 1 mg/ml midazolam.

Because midazolam is water soluble and phlebitis is rarely noted, the IV infusion may be started at any available site, including the dorsum of the hand and wrist. After increasing the rate of the IV drip, midazolam is administered slowly. The manufacturer recommends a rate of 1 ml every 2 minutes, followed by an additional 2 minutes or more to fully evaluate the sedative effect. The range of midazolam required for "ideal" sedation varies from 1 to 10 mg or more. It is suggested that titration be terminated if sedation is not evident at a dose of 6 to 8 mg. Clinical experience suggests that midazolam is anywhere from two to four times as potent as diazepam.[18] If additional doses of midazolam are required, it is suggested that the total midazolam dose not exceed 10 mg for the entire appointment, if possible.

Patients who are receiving benzodiazepines orally for prolonged periods may exhibit a tolerance to the IV administration of diazepam or midazolam. Robb and Hargrave[19] reported three cases of patients who required doses of 47 and 50 mg midazolam, 26 mg midazolam, and 30 and 34 mg midazolam for IV sedation. Discontinuance of the oral benzodiazepine produces a return to more normal response.

The duration of midazolam-induced sedation is slightly shorter than that of diazepam. Clinical experience has demonstrated that recovery is as complete as with diazepam. Some patients may exhibit a degree of residual sedation up to 60 minutes after drug administration, although this is rare. It also appears, subjectively, that the depth of sedation provided by midazolam is not as intense as that noted with diazepam; however, the degree and length of midazolam-induced anterograde amnesia is far greater than that produced by diazepam.

The decision as to which benzodiazepine to use must take into account several factors, including the following:

1. Possibility of phlebitis (venous inflammation)
2. Requirement for sedation
3. Requirement for amnesia

Posttreatment instructions—verbal and written—must always be given to both the patient and the adult escort. This is especially important with midazolam because of the greater likelihood of amnesia persisting into the recovery period. The administration of flumazenil, a benzodiazepine antagonist, may be indicated at this time if continued amnesia is not desirable. Early studies indicated that flumazenil decreased the length of midazolam-induced amnesia.[20]

Midazolam	
Average sedative dose	6-8 mg
Sedative dose range	2.5-7.5 mg
Maximum dose, no sedation	6-8 mg
Maximum dose, some sedation	10 mg

The administration of a single titrating dose of either midazolam or diazepam for sedation provides the doctor with approximately 45 to 60 minutes of sedation. When combined with adequate local anesthesia treatment, time easily exceeds 1 hour. There are occasions, however, when treatment requires in excess of 2 hours to complete. For these procedures, use of the Jorgensen technique is indicated.

The Jorgensen Technique

The Jorgensen technique is a combination of three drugs administered intravenously to provide more than 2 hours of conscious sedation. Niels Bjorn Jorgensen first used this technique, which he called *intravenous premedication*, in 1945 at the Loma Linda University School of Medicine.[21] Jorgensen introduced the technique because of his dissatisfaction with the vagaries of oral and intramuscular routes of sedation. IV drug administration permitted a more precise and reliable level of sedation than was possible with any of the other techniques then available.

The Jorgensen technique has been used successfully at the Loma Linda University School of Dentistry in excess of 15,000 times since 1965. Originally designed for use during oral surgical procedures, its appropriateness in all branches of dentistry has been reaffirmed many times. The technique became known as the *Loma Linda technique* because of Jorgensen's affiliation with that school and is now known as the *Jorgensen technique,* after the man considered by many to be the father of IV sedation in dentistry.

Three drugs are administered in the Jorgensen technique:

1. Pentobarbital, a barbiturate
2. Meperidine, an opioid agonist
3. Scopolamine, an anticholinergic

As is discussed later in this chapter, polypharmacy (the use of multiple drugs to achieve a therapeutic goal) should, if possible, be avoided. The incidence of drug-drug interactions greatly increases as additional drugs are administered to a patient. The Jorgensen technique is a positive example of polypharmacy, but unlike many drug combinations in which there appears to be no relevance for the drugs being administered, each of the drugs in the Jorgensen technique serves an important function.

Everett and Allen[22] discussed the physiologic effects of the Jorgensen technique and demonstrated that there is minimal physiologic alteration produced, although three of their subjects did develop nausea. This latter effect was most likely caused by the opioid. In my experience with the Jorgensen technique, nausea and vomiting are extremely rare and are rarely significant complications.

Function of the Individual Drugs. Detailed pharmacology of the drugs used in the Jorgensen technique is found in Chapter 25.

Pentobarbital. Pentobarbital is the drug used to produce the desired level of sedation in the Jorgensen technique. Pentobarbital is also the drug that provides the 2- to 4-hour duration of action associated with the Jorgensen technique. Pentobarbital, a generalized central nervous system (CNS) depressant, has the disquieting effect of making patients more likely to overreact to stimulation. This is a negative action of the drug and is one reason for inclusion of the opioid in the technique.

Meperidine. Meperidine is an opioid agonist and as such has a number of potentially adverse side effects, including respiratory depression, postural hypotension, nausea, and vomiting. Its functions in the Jorgensen technique are threefold:

1. To provide some additional sedation
2. To provide some analgesia, counterbalancing the negative actions of the barbiturate
3. To provide some euphoria

In the dosage of meperidine used in the Jorgensen technique (not greater than 25 mg), the major effect of meperidine is its analgesic action. Patients who have received pentobarbital alone usually overreact to painful or traumatic stimulation; however, with the addition of up to 25 mg of meperidine this response is moderated, most patients responding to stimulation "normally."

Scopolamine. Scopolamine is an anticholinergic with several functions in the Jorgensen technique:

1. Scopolamine provides anterograde amnesia in some patients
2. It inhibits salivary secretions, thus providing a drier operating field
3. It produces a degree of CNS depression, although this is rarely of any significance

Scopolamine may also produce emergence delirium, which is why it is contraindicated in patients younger than 6 years and those older than 65 years.

Preliminary Appointment. At the visit prior to actual treatment, the patient is evaluated as discussed in the diazepam technique section. The Jorgensen technique is described to the patient in general terms, mentioning that the drugs are to be administered intravenously and that the patient will feel quite relaxed, perhaps somewhat sleepy. It is important to mention to the patient that he or she will not be unconscious, for this is not general anesthesia, but a safer, equally effective technique called conscious sedation.

The patient's previous responses (if any) to the drugs included in the technique must also be determined. Whether the patient has ever received Nembutal, Demerol, or scopolamine is determined, and if so, the patient's reaction is noted. In addition, the patient is questioned about the presence of possible contraindications to the use of one or more of these drugs. These include the following.

Contraindications to the Jorgensen Technique

1. Allergy or hypersensitivity to any of the three drugs
2. Porphyria (contraindication to barbiturate)
3. Liver disease (contraindication to barbiturate, opioid)
4. Asthma (contraindication to barbiturate, opioid, scopolamine)
5. Respiratory depression (contraindication to barbiturate, opioid)
6. Alcoholism (contraindication to barbiturate, opioid)
7. Monoamine oxidase inhibitors (MAOIs) within 14 days (contraindication to opioid)
8. Glaucoma (contraindication to scopolamine)
9. Adhesions between iris and lens (contraindication to scopolamine)
10. Prostate disease (contraindication to scopolamine)
11. Myasthenia gravis (contraindication to scopolamine)
12. Contact lenses (contraindication to scopolamine)

Baseline vital signs are recorded, the presence of superficial veins determined, preoperative instructions given to the patient, and the sedation appointment scheduled.

Day of Treatment. On treatment day, the patient is prepared for the IV procedure as previously described for the benzodiazepines. Because of the inherent length of the Jorgensen technique, the importance of asking the patient to void before the start of the procedure is stressed. Venipuncture may be started at any site where suitable veins are located, there being no prohibitions concerning selection of an IV site with any of the three drugs.

Preparation of Drugs. Two 5-ml syringes are required when preparing drugs for use in the Jorgensen technique. The drugs are available as follows:

- Pentobarbital: 50 mg/ml in 2-ml ampules and multidose vials
- Meperidine: 50 mg/ml in 0.5- and 1-ml ampules
- Scopolamine: 0.3 mg in 1.0-ml ampules

Into the first syringe is placed 3 ml (if using the multidose vial) or 4 ml (two 2-ml ampules) of pentobarbital. The syringe is labeled "pentobarbital 50 mg/ml."

To remove a drug from an ampule, the doctor or assistant holds the ampule in his or her fingers as illustrated in Figure 26-8. A gauze square is used to prevent injury from sharp pieces of glass. Making certain that all of the drug is in the bottom of the ampule, the doctor or assistant cracks the glass at its prescored neck. A micropore filter needle (optional) is placed onto the syringe and the drug drawn up. The micropore filter is designed to stop any small fragments of glass that may have fallen into the solution from entering the syringe and being injected into the patient. After the syringe is filled with solution, the micropore filter needle is replaced with the original needle. The filter needle can be used in only one direction—either to withdraw solutions into the syringe or to inject them out of the syringe—and it must be replaced with the original needle for the other function.

When a drug is removed from a multidose vial, the rubber stopper is cleansed with an alcohol wipe and permitted to dry. Placing the needle of the syringe into the bottle at an angle to prevent coring (the placing of small pieces of rubber into the solution), a volume of air is injected into the vial equal to the volume of solution to be withdrawn. This makes it much easier for the drug to be withdrawn from the vial.

Into the second syringe will be placed meperidine (25 mg), scopolamine (0.3 mg), and a volume of diluent that may be withdrawn from the IV infusion bag. Assuming in this instance that the meperidine ampule contains 50 mg in 1.0 ml (or 25 mg in 0.5 ml) and the scopolamine contains 0.3 mg in 1.0 ml, the doctor or assistant first inserts the empty syringe into the injection site on the IV infusion bag or the injection site on the IV tubing and withdraws 3.5 ml of solution. Each of the ampules is carefully opened and its contents withdrawn into the syringe. A total of 5 ml of solution should now be in the syringe (3.5 ml of IV solution, 0.5 ml meperidine, and 1 ml scopolamine), containing 25 mg meperidine and 0.3 mg scopolamine. The syringe is labeled "meperidine 5 mg/ml, scopolamine 0.06 mg/ml."

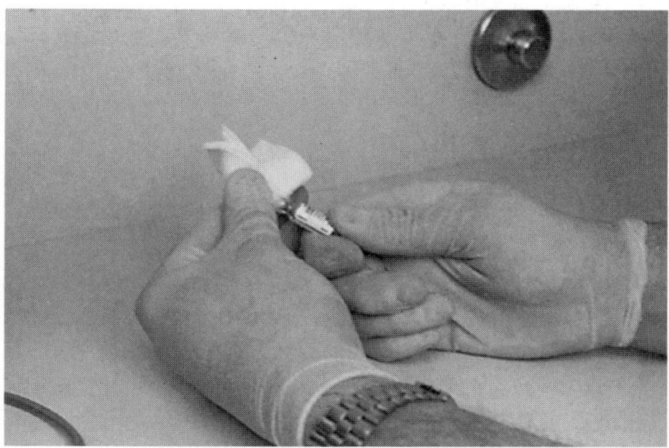

Figure 26-8 Ampule is held in gauze and cracked at its prescored neck.

> Always read the label of the drug being prepared for use to confirm its mg/ml formulation

The patient is placed in a semisupine position, monitoring devices attached, preoperative vital signs recorded, and the venipuncture established. There are no prohibitions on venipuncture site for any of the drugs in the Jorgensen technique. Nasal O_2 through either a cannula or nasal hood at a rate of 3 to 5 L/min is initiated at this time.

The rate of the IV infusion is increased, and patency of the IV infusion is rechecked as described for the benzodiazepines. The pentobarbital syringe is placed into the injection site on the IV tubing, and a test dose of 0.2 ml of solution (one small delineation on the syringe) is administered to rule out any allergic reaction or hypersensitivity response. After 30 seconds the doctor or assistant begins the administration of pentobarbital at a rate of 10 mg every 30 seconds (0.2 ml or one small delineation) while continuously conversing with the patient.

The pentobarbital is injected until the patient mentions the presence of the first symptoms of cortical depression. These usually are the following:

- Slight dizziness
- A feeling of being tired
- Decreased apprehension
- Difficulty in focusing on distant objects

Clinical signs that may be noted at this time are the following:

- Relaxation in patients who were initially agitated
- Slight slurring of speech
- Slower response to commands
- Heaviness of the eyelids

It is suggested that a mouth prop be placed in the patient's mouth at this time so that should responses become even more sluggish, the patient will have no difficulty in maintaining an open mouth. It is important to administer the pentobarbital slowly, for the lag time between injection and the onset of clinical signs and symptoms is somewhat slower than that noted with either diazepam and midazolam, approximately 2 to 4 minutes. In other words, the clinical effect seen at any moment in time was produced by the pentobarbital administered up to 4 minutes earlier.

Jorgensen[23] termed the point of appearance of the first signs of cortical sedation *baseline.* The average dose of pentobarbital required to reach baseline is between 125 and 175 mg. The range, however, is quite broad, baseline sedation having been achieved with pentobarbital doses from 30 to 300 mg.

In Jorgensen and Leffingwell's[21] original description of the technique, they stated that at this point an additional volume of pentobarbital is injected equal to 10% to 15% of the baseline dosage. Thus, if 100 mg was required to reach baseline, an additional 10 to 15 mg will be injected and the syringe removed. Having used this technique for 25 years, I have found that this additional 10% to 15% need not always be administered, for in many patients additional pentobarbital leads to a greater depth of sedation than is desired. Additional pentobarbital can always be administered if necessary, but once the drug has been injected, there is no way of removing it or of reversing its actions.

Once baseline sedation has been achieved, the second syringe, containing meperidine (5 mg/mL) and scopolamine, is placed into the injection site. The dose administered is based on the meperidine: It is suggested that it be injected at a rate of 10 mg/min or, in this instance, 1 ml every 30 seconds.

The maximum dose of meperidine is based on the dose of pentobarbital required to reach baseline sedation. The ratio of pentobarbital to meperidine will be 4:1 mg/mg up to a maximal dose of 25 mg meperidine (Table 26-1). Thus a patient who received 100 mg pentobarbital may receive up to 25 mg meperidine. If 60 mg pentobarbital was required, a maximal dose of 15 mg meperidine may be administered. If the patient required 180, 200, or 300 mg pentobarbital to reach baseline, the maximal meperidine dose is still 25 mg. No more than 25 mg meperidine is administered.

As the meperidine-scopolamine combination is administered, the patient must be observed carefully for signs of increasing sedation. In most instances no noticeable change in depth of sedation occurs and the maximal calculated dose of meperidine-scopolamine is administered.

In some instances, however, the patient is noted to become more deeply sedated as meperidine is administered. Further administration of meperidine-scopolamine should be halted before the patient reaches an overly deep level of sedation. In this situation the maximal calculated dose of meperidine might not be reached.

The rate of the IV infusion is now slowed to a rate just fast enough to keep the needle from occluding (t.k.o.). Vital signs are recorded on the anesthesia record sheet following the completion of IV drug administration.

The combination of pentobarbital (for its sedation), meperidine (for its analgesia, euphoria, and some additional sedation), and scopolamine (for its amnesic and antisialagogue actions) usually results in a cooperative, relaxed, and sedated patient who willingly accepts 2 hours or more of concentrated restorative or surgical procedures under local anesthesia yet remains conscious and able to assist the doctor when necessary.

TABLE 26-1 Ratio of Barbiturate to Meperidine in Jorgensen Technique

Barbituate Dose (mg) (Syringe 1)	Maximum Meperidine Dose (Syringe 2) mg	ml
30	7.5	1.5
50	12.5	2.5
60	15	3
80	20	4
100	25	5
200	25	5
300	25	5

Perioperative Period. Local anesthesia is administered and treatment begun. Although virtually all patients will be well sedated and cooperative at this point, it is possible that some will overreact when treatment is started. This may be an indication for the administration of either additional pentobarbital or of local anesthetic to the patient. If it appears that the patient's movements are related only to painful dental procedures (e.g., excavating cavities, manipulating tissue), pain control may be incomplete, requiring the administration of additional local anesthetic. However, if the patient's movements are more generalized, occurring in response to nontraumatic procedures, the patient is asked how he or she is feeling. If the patient responds that he or she is still fearful of the procedure ("Doctor, I'm too awake!"), the IV infusion rate is increased and additional pentobarbital titrated until relaxation occurs. Pentobarbital is responsible for the proper level of sedation in the Jorgensen technique. Once an appropriate sedation level is achieved, the pentobarbital syringe is removed and the IV infusion rate slowed (t.k.o.). No additional meperidine-scopolamine is administered at this time.

In the event that there is a sluggish or absent response, additional drug is not administered. Airway patency is checked immediately. Restlessness is often a sign of hypoxia and/or hypercarbia. Ventilation is assessed and controlled if necessary until the patient recovers (sedation lightens) sufficiently to permit resumption of the dental procedure.

The duration of the depth of ideal sedation during the Jorgensen technique is considerably longer than that seen with diazepam or midazolam. Recovery is correspondingly slower: The patient appears sedated even after 3 or 4 hours.

The following are several points to bear in mind during treatment of the sedated patient:

1. *Work efficiently and quietly.* Remember that your patient is awake and able to hear you. Be careful in what you do and say while treating the sedated patient, who may not hear every word that you utter and may misinterpret those they do hear. Be especially careful where you place your hands and instruments. The patient may consider a perfectly innocent gesture as an assault on his or her body (see Chapter 17).
2. *When the patient is female (or male if the operator is female), it is important (medicolegally) for another person of the patient's gender to be present in the room at all times during the procedure.*
3. *Some patients may complain about the dryness that accompanies the administration of scopolamine.* It may be necessary for the doctor or assistant to moisten the soft tissues of the patient's mouth and throat with small squirts of water from the air-water syringe.
4. *When a scalp vein or straight metal needle is used in the antecubital fossa for the Jorgensen technique, immobilization is required.* Some patients complain during the procedure that their elbow is sore. They are unable to flex the joint because of the mandatory presence of an elbow immobilizer whenever a rigid needle is used for venipuncture. It is therefore suggested that the operator use either an indwelling catheter for venipuncture at any site (including the antecubital fossa) or a scalp vein or straight metal needle in either the ventral aspect of the forearm or dorsum of the hand where joint immobilization is not necessary.

Postoperative Period. Recovery from the Jorgensen technique is considerably less complete than that seen after benzodiazepine sedation. This is perversely beneficial because the patient is unlikely to want to drive a car or do other potentially hazardous chores after sedation with the Jorgensen technique. The typical patient simply wants to go home and go to bed and sleep. Fitness for discharge is based on the patient's ability to walk without assistance and on a comparison of the vital signs obtained before, during, and after the procedure, as described in the discussion on benzodiazepine sedation. Recordkeeping in the patient's chart includes the anesthesia record sheet or a written statement similar to that recommended for the benzodiazepines placed in the patient's treatment record.

Postoperative instructions are given verbally and in writing to both the patient and his or her companion. Postoperative analgesics administered during the first 6 to 8 hours should be nonopioid (if possible) to minimize any additive effects of opioids with those administered intravenously. If pain is expected to be a significant problem postoperatively, administration of a long-acting local anesthetic such as bupivacaine immediately before discharge of the patient is suggested.

The patient is escorted out of the office by his escort and a staff member and safely secured in the passenger seat of the car. A telephone call is made later that day to see how the recovery is progressing and to review postoperative instructions.

There is a greater possibility that the patient will not be fully recovered from the effects of the pentobarbital the next day, especially if the sedation procedure occurred during the afternoon. It is therefore preferable for sedation with the Jorgensen technique to be carried out during the morning hours.

Intravenous Promethazine

The third of the basic techniques of IV conscious sedation is the administration of promethazine, a phenothiazine derivative with significant sedative and histamine-blocking properties. Because promethazine does possess histamine-blocking and anticholinergic properties, the addition of an anticholinergic, such as atropine or scopolamine, is usually unnecessary.

The primary indication for promethazine is a dental or surgical procedure expected to require between 1 and 2 hours to complete. Procedures of less than 1 hour are well managed with diazepam or midazolam, whereas with procedures taking more than 2 hours, the Jorgensen technique is suggested. The following relative and absolute contraindications to promethazine must be sought at the preoperative visit:

1. Allergy or hypersensitivity to promethazine
2. Glaucoma
3. Prostatic hypertrophy
4. Stenosing peptic ulcer
5. Bladder neck obstruction

If any of these are present, alternative IV techniques should be sought. Diazepam or midazolam is recommended in place of promethazine in most of these patients. The Jorgensen technique is not as suitable, primarily because these same contraindications are present for the anticholinergics used in that technique.

Promethazine is prepared for injection by placing 3 ml of 5% dextrose and water into a 5-ml syringe and then adding 2 ml of promethazine (25 mg/ml). This produces a concentration of 10 mg/ml, the recommended concentration for injection of promethazine. The IV infusion may be established at any convenient site when promethazine is used.

The drug is titrated at a rate of 1 ml/min to clinical effect. The average dose of promethazine required for sedation is 32.5 mg, the range between 25 and 35 mg.

If adequate sedation is not present by 50 mg, drug administration is terminated and the planned treatment begun if possible, or the patient rescheduled for another appointment, at which time a different IV technique will be used.

Although readministration of promethazine is usually not required once the initial titrating dose has been given, readministration may be necessary on occasion. In this situation the suggested absolute maximal dose of promethazine is 75 mg.

Promethazine	
Average sedative dose	32.5 mg
Sedative dose range	25-35 mg
Maximum dose, no sedation	50 mg
Maximum dose, some sedation	75 mg

Recovery from promethazine sedation is not as clinically complete as that for diazepam or midazolam. Rather the patient still retains some degree of CNS depression on departing from the office.

Summary

Three basic techniques of IV conscious sedation have been presented. It is my belief that these techniques form the backbone of the doctor's IV sedative armamentarium. When these techniques are used as described, serious complications will not arise. Retrospective studies on the Jorgensen technique and IV diazepam have demonstrated beyond doubt that these procedures are sound, safe, and effective.[24,25]

Availability of these three procedures enables the doctor to pick an appropriate IV technique based on the time allotted for treatment:

- Up to 1 hour: diazepam or midazolam
- From 1 to 2 hours: promethazine or midazolam or diazepam (retitrated)
- More than 2 hours: Jorgensen technique

In addition, the following applies to IV drug administration:

- Titrate the drugs slowly.
- Remain within the dosage limits recommended for each technique.
- Failures (the inability to provide adequate sedation within the dosage recommended), although rare, will occur. When this happens, no other drug should be administered to the patient (this includes nitrous oxide–oxygen [N_2O-O_2] for the relatively inexperienced operator). An attempt is made to treat the patient as best as is possible. If this proves to be futile, the procedure is terminated and rescheduled for another time, at which a different technique of sedation will be used. The administration of additional drug or of a different drug to the patient increases the risk of problems (e.g., unconsciousness, airway obstruction), especially in the hands of the less experienced doctor. Finding out the hard way that this is true is not recommended.

MODIFICATION OF BASIC TECHNIQUES

In this section a modification of basic technique is described: the addition of an anticholinergic to diazepam or midazolam. The Jorgensen technique already includes an anticholinergic, and promethazine possesses anticholinergic properties, so addition of anticholinergics is unnecessary.

Selection of a suitable anticholinergic is based on the needs of the patient and the desired duration of its action. Where a slight degree of sedation and amnesia is desired, scopolamine (0.3 mg) is recommended. Its use is appropriate in a procedure of any duration. If the patient is younger than 6 years or older than 65 years, scopolamine is not recommended because of an increased risk of emergence delirium.

Atropine (0.4 mg) is used when a drying effect is desired without amnesia or additional sedation and the

TABLE 26-2 Indications for Anticholinergics

	Salivary Secretions	Amnesia	Sedation	Duration (hr)
Atropine	+	–	–	<2
Glycopyrrolate	+	–	–	>2
Scopolamine	+	+	+	<2

duration of the procedure is less than 2 hours. Glycopyrrolate (0.2 mg) is recommended for procedures in excess of 2 hours when a drying effect is required. Table 26-2 summarizes the properties of anticholinergics.

Technique

When anticholinergics, which are aqueous solutions, are administered with diazepam, which is lipid soluble, they must be administered in a separate syringe. The patient receives diazepam as discussed previously, and the anticholinergic is then administered. The anticholinergic drug is slowly injected over 1 minute.

The use of diazepam and scopolamine (0.3 mg) will provide a greater degree of amnesia in most patients than will either drug alone. Rather than the amnesic period being approximately 10 minutes in duration, it may extend over greater lengths of time. Being water soluble, midazolam and anticholinergics may be mixed in a single syringe before administration and injected together, although in most situations it is more practical to administer the anticholinergic separately, as previously discussed.

One of the disadvantages of employing anticholinergics is that some patients will complain that the drying effect is bothersome, both during the procedure and in some cases after the procedure on returning home. Although drugs are available to reverse anticholinergics (the reversible cholinesterase inhibitors neostigmine and physostigmine), their use is not recommended because of possible undesirable side effects.

ADVANCED TECHNIQUES

In this section techniques are discussed that include the addition of an opioid to an antianxiety or sedative hypnotic drug. Box 26-1 presents a categorization of the drugs discussed in this section.

When used for a well-defined purpose, the combination of a drug from group A (antianxiety/sedative-hypnotic) and one from group B (opioid) is quite rational. As discussed in the preceding section, the addition of an anticholinergic (group C) is suggested whenever a drying effect or amnesia is desirable.

Use of techniques described in this section should be limited to doctors meeting one or both of the following requirements:

1. Doctors who have successfully completed training in general anesthesia techniques and in the management of the airway of an unconscious patient
2. Doctors with extensive experience in the basic techniques of IV conscious sedation

Because these techniques involve administration of two or more CNS depressants, there is an increased likelihood of additive drug effects being observed. Clinically, this would produce an increased depth of sedation beyond that which is desirable, requiring the doctor to terminate dental treatment momentarily and evaluate the patient's status.

When the listed drugs are administered as suggested (dosage, rate of injection, and monitoring), clinical problems are extremely unlikely to develop. Deviation from these guidelines will increase the potential for adverse side effects.

Rationale for Advanced Techniques

Why discuss the addition of a second drug to the basic IV conscious sedation technique? Two reasons are presented.

First, maximum, safe, and effective doses of each of the basic drugs have been presented. If no clinical effect has developed at that dose, further administration of the same drug is unlikely to provide acceptable sedation until extremely large doses are given. It was strongly recommended in the discussion of basic techniques that the inexperienced doctor abort the procedure and attempt a different IV technique at a subsequent appointment.

The doctor who meets one or both of the aforementioned criteria listed may, however, elect to administer a second CNS depressant to this patient. Opioids are an excellent choice, with small doses usually providing the additional sedation required for the patient to accept dental treatment and remain comfortable.

Second, a degree of analgesia is provided during painful procedures, or in some cases (barbiturates) the opioid counterbalances the negative effect of a drug on the pain reaction threshold. When used in this regard, a larger dose of opioid is desirable.

The sequence in which the antianxiety or sedative-hypnotic and opioid are administered will depend on the reason for its inclusion in the technique.

Requirement: Sedation

In the situation in which the group A drug (diazepam, midazolam, pentobarbital, or promethazine) has been administered to its maximal recommended dose yet the patient remains unsedated, the addition of an opioid will aid in providing the desired sedation. The opioid is slowly titrated, the doctor and assistant carefully observing the patient for signs of increasing sedation. Titration of the opioid ceases when the desired sedation occurs or the maximum dose of 50 mg meperidine is administered. The depth of sedation achieved in this manner should be no greater than that observed with the basic techniques.

In this first technique, in which the primary requirement is sedation, the patient will have received a larger dose of the antianxiety drug and a smaller dose of the opioid analgesic, for example, diazepam 20 mg and meperidine 10 mg or promethazine 50 mg and morphine 6 mg.

Requirement: Analgesia

When the planned dental procedure involves a significant potential for pain, such as oral surgery or endodontic or periodontal surgery, the benefits of an opioid analgesic may be desirable. The primary technique of pain control during dental treatment will always be local anesthesia. The addition of IV analgesics will help the patient during the procedure should the local anesthetic effect begin to lessen. The nature of the discomfort experienced by the patient will be altered.

When used for this reason the analgesic is administered first, titrated until one of two things occurs: (1) clinically adequate sedation develops or (2) the maximal recommended opioid dose has been administered. In most situations the slow administration of the opioid does not produce significant sedation, so the maximal recommended dose is usually administered; however, the opioid must always be titrated slowly to prevent a hyperresponding patient from overreacting. Following opioid administration, if additional sedation is desired, a drug from group A may be slowly titrated.

It is obvious that when this technique is used, the patient will receive a larger dose of the opioid analgesic and a smaller dose of the antianxiety or sedative hypnotic drug, for example, meperidine 50 mg and diazepam 7 mg or pentazocine 30 mg and promethazine 15 mg.

Some patients are quite sensitive to the CNS depressant actions of opioids and will become adequately sedated at a dose below the maximum recommended for that drug. Should this occur, titration of the opioid is ceased when the desired sedative level is reached, no other group A drug is administered, and the treatment is started. The maximal doses and the recommended dilutions of group B drugs (opioids) are presented in Table 26-3.

Techniques

Diazepam or Midazolam with Opioid. When either diazepam or midazolam is the primary drug for sedation, the most appropriate opioids to use are short-acting meperidine, fentanyl, alfentanil, and sufentanil. Duration of sedation will usually not be increased; however, it is possible that clinical recovery at 60 minutes will not be as complete as that seen when diazepam or midazolam is administered alone. Administration of longer-acting opioids (morphine) will only delay recovery.

Diazepam or Midazolam with Opioid Plus Anticholinergic. Addition of an anticholinergic is based on the criteria previously discussed. The use of glycopyrrolate is not recommended because of its prolonged duration of action compared to diazepam or midazolam. The anticholinergic may be mixed in the same syringe as the opioid (see the Jorgensen technique for procedure).

Promethazine with Opioid. Because the clinical action of promethazine is somewhat longer than that of diazepam or midazolam, longer-acting opioids may be given if indicated. Nalbuphine, butorphanol, morphine, and meperidine are recommended. Morphine should be used for procedures requiring very close to, or more than, 2 hours to complete, whereas meperidine is used for procedures approximately 1 hour in length.

Promethazine with Opioid plus Anticholinergic. There is little need for this combination because of the anticholinergic properties of promethazine.

Pentobarbital with Opioid. The administration of pentobarbital intravenously as a sole agent for sedation is rarely justified because of the negative action of the drug on the patient's pain reaction threshold. Patients receiving IV barbiturates may overreact to painful stimulation. In addition, many patients become quite

TABLE 26-3 Group B Drugs: Doses and Dilutions

	Availability (mg/ml)	Maximal Dose (mg)	Dilution for Use (mg/ml)
Meperidine	50	50	10
Morphine	10	8	1
Fentanyl	0.05 (50 μg/ml)	0.08	0.01
Pentazocine	30	30	10
Nalbuphine	10	10	2
Butorphanol	2	2	0.4

talkative and demonstrate increased movement in the dental chair following pentobarbital administration.

The administration of an opioid analgesic therefore is almost a requirement whenever pentobarbital is used, unless, of course, the doctor does not wish to increase the sedative level of the patient any further. Pentobarbital will normally be used for procedures requiring 2 hours or more to complete. Therefore our choice of opioid is limited to the longer-acting ones.

Meperidine	If duration is just 2 hr
Morphine	2-4 hr
Butorphanol	2-3 hr
Nalbuphine	2-3 hr

Jorgensen Technique Plus Benzodiazepine. As the dental or surgical procedure extends beyond the second hour, some patients may require additional sedation for their treatment to be completed. Because of its long duration of action (2 to 4 hours), the readministration of pentobarbital is not recommended at this time. For this reason, in those few cases in which patients do require additional sedation, a benzodiazepine may be administered. Either diazepam (at 5 mg/min) or midazolam (at 1 mg/min) is titrated slowly to clinical effect. This provides the additional sedation necessary in the doctor's judgment while not unnecessarily prolonging the duration of the entire sedative procedure.

Opioid with a Group A Drug. In reversing the order of drug administration we seek a greater analgesic effect from our drugs. Anxiety reduction is not the primary reason for the IV procedure.

Selection of the opioid and antianxiety or sedative-hypnotic should be based on the anticipated duration of the procedure, as discussed. Anticholinergics (group C) may be added to the opioid syringe if desired. Table 26-4 illustrates the different doses of group A and B drugs required when administered alone or in combination. These results are taken from more than 25 years of IV conscious sedation continuing education courses.

When any of these advanced IV techniques are used, the drugs must always be titrated slowly (1 ml/min) unless otherwise recommended. The patient is observed for signs of increasing sedation so that oversedation does not occur.

Never combine the opioid in the same syringe as the group A antianxiety or sedative-hypnotic. The administrator loses control over drug action when this is done.

OTHER TECHNIQUES

Other IV conscious sedation techniques are available. It is my belief, however, that the techniques discussed in this section *cannot* be recommended unless the doctor has completed a residency program in anesthesiology and is conversant with and able to maintain the airway of an unconscious patient. The depth of sedation provided with these techniques is considered "deep sedation" as compared with the conscious sedation techniques described in the previous sections of this chapter. The point at which deep sedation ends and general anesthesia (the loss of consciousness) starts is a gray area to be avoided by all but the most well-trained individuals. Indeed, many state dental boards and legislative bodies have determined that deep sedation, for all intents and purposes, *is* general anesthesia and must be treated in the same manner.

These techniques are mentioned for historical accuracy and to make our discussion more inclusive. Doctors Sylvan Shane, Joel Berns, and Peter Foreman were pioneers in the administration of IV drugs in dentistry.

TABLE 26-4 Average Drug Doses from 2153 Cases

Drug 1	Dose (mg)	Drug 2	Dose (mg)
Diazepam	12.5	—	—
Diazepam	19.1	Meperidine	35.1
Meperidine	48.2	Diazepam	8.4
Midazolam	4.8	—	—
Midazolam	7.5	Meperidine	38.0
Meperidine	46.7	Midazolam	3.6
Promethazine	41.2	—	—
Promethazine	48.6	Meperidine	31.1
Meperidine	45.2	Promethazine	21.4

Diazepam with Methohexital (Foreman Technique)

The combination of diazepam with methohexital, an ultrashort-acting barbiturate, has been used with success by many persons, foremost among whom is Peter Foreman of New Zealand.[26-29] After initially titrating diazepam to baseline sedation (see diazepam technique discussion), a dose of 5 to 10 mg of methohexital is administered in anticipation of unpleasant procedures. This includes the administration of local anesthetics or surgery on osseous structures. The 5- to 10-mg increments of methohexital provide a deepening of sedation (into deep sedation) that lasts for from 5 to 7 minutes.

Foreman has found this technique to be valuable in dental procedures requiring 30 to 90 minutes for completion. In his experience the usual dose of drugs administered in a procedure lasting more than 1 hour is diazepam 10 to 20 mg and methohexital 50 to 100 mg (in 5- to 10-mg increments). Amnesia is greatly enhanced by addition of the methohexital.

Care must be taken to administer only small increments of methohexital with this technique because larger doses will produce deep sedation bordering on loss of consciousness, with attendant depression of protective reflexes, skeletal muscle relaxation, difficulty in maintaining a patent airway, and possible laryngospasm.

The Berns Technique

Joel Berns[30] describes a technique involving the administration of three drugs: the barbiturate (group A) secobarbital, the opioid (group B) meperidine, and the barbiturate (group A) methohexital. Secobarbital is administered first and slowly titrated to baseline sedation (the dose range being from 25 to 75 mg), followed by 25 to 50 mg meperidine. Local anesthesia is administered and the procedure started. Methohexital in increments of 10 to 20 mg is administered just before any traumatic procedure, which may include administration of local anesthesia or extractions.

This technique is similar to the Foreman technique previously described, with the barbiturate secobarbital replacing diazepam. The same benefits and potential problems exist in this procedure. An additional consideration is the absence of any pharmacologic antagonist for the barbiturates, whereas flumazenil is available to reverse any unwanted actions of the benzodiazepines.

The Shane Technique

Sylvan Shane,[31,32] from Maryland, developed a technique, first described in 1966, that he calls *intravenous amnesia.* The technique consists of two components: (1) a verbal component that precedes drug administration and (2) a drug component that involves the IV administration of alphaprodine, hydroxyzine, atropine, and methohexital and local anesthesia for pain control.

The verbal component is extremely important in the Shane technique. Before drug administration, the patient is told the following:

1. You will be asleep during the procedure.
2. Before falling asleep you will feel the calming effects of the medications.
3. "Pentothal" is being administered.
4. No pain will be felt during the procedure.
5. When the procedure is complete, you will express disbelief and insist that you were never asleep. (This must be said to the patient before the patient says it to the dentist.)
6. You will know when the procedure is over, for your lips, tongue, and teeth will feel numb. When you feel the numbness, you will know that "something must have happened," and this numbness confirms the fact that the procedure is over.
7. (The patient is then exposed to the sound of the drill, air blower, and amalgam condenser.) You will hear these sounds, and they also mean that the procedure is over. These instruments are used to polish, carve, and smooth the fillings, and this is done during the hour required for you to awaken sufficiently to get up out of the chair.
8. (Gauze is placed over the patient's eyes [taped in place].) The gauze will be over your eyes when you awaken to keep the polishing dust out of your eyes.
9. (The patient's later response to all of the above is anticipated.) You will swear that you were never asleep, yet the treatment will be completed and you will feel as though only a minute has passed.

The drugs are then administered as listed in Table 26-5. Shane recommends combining alphaprodine, hydroxyzine, and atropine in one syringe, the methohexital in a second syringe.

Following the administration of the drugs in the first syringe to clinical effect, 1 to 2 ml (10 to 20 mg) of methohexital is administered. Local anesthesia of the entire oral cavity (as needed) is obtained. On completion of local anesthetic administration, the patient is told to close his or her mouth and nothing is said or done for the next 2 minutes.

The dentist then tells the patient that the treatment is completed, all the fillings are done, and the patient may now go home. Of course, the doctor has not even started treatment yet. Patients normally respond to this by saying, "You're fooling me" or "You're kidding."

The doctor counters this by reminding the patient that the mouth is numb and that he or she was told

TABLE 26-5 Shane Technique Drug Schedule

	Dose (mg)*		
Drug	Age 2 to 6 yr	Age 7 to 18 yr	Adult
Alphaprodine	6	7-18 (same as age in years)	18-24
Hydroxyzine	25	25-50	50
Atropine	0.3	0.4	0.6

*Normal saline is added to dilute the mixture as needed to a total of 5 ml in the syringe.

previously that when awakened, he or she would be numb. The patient will then lie back in the chair and begin sleeping.

At this point the doctor states, "I am going to be polishing your fillings or trimming your bony spicules from the extraction sites." The actual dental procedure starts.

Shane et al.[33,34] term the verbal component of the procedure the *therapeutic lie.* They have reported on at least 15,000 sedations without fatality.

The level of CNS depression noted during the Shane technique is deep sedation. The doctor using this technique must be well trained (and in most states in the United States have a general anesthesia "permit") in the management of patients at this level of CNS depression. Factors that severely limit use of the Shane technique are the recommendation by the manufacturer of hydroxyzine that the drug not be administered intravenously and the removal of alphaprodine from clinical use in the United States.

Propofol

Propofol has been used for IV sedation in a number of medical specialties, including ophthalmology,[35] radiology,[36] gynecology,[37,38] gastroenterology,[39] neurosurgery,[40] intensive care medicine,[41,42] and pediatric surgery,[43] as well as dentistry.[44-46] Among propofol's advantages is a very rapid onset of action and an extremely rapid recovery following termination of administration. Following propofol sedation patients are ready for discharge in a considerably shorter period than following the IV benzodiazepines, diazepam and midazolam, or barbiturates (methohexital).[47]

Disadvantages attendant with the administration of propofol include the possibility of a burning sensation on IV administration and the expense of the drug and infusion pumps. The infusion pump costs approximately $3000 (as of July 2002). Not the least of the disadvantages of propofol administration is its potential to produce levels of sedation and respiratory depression that may be beyond the training of the IV conscious sedation dentist.

When propofol is administered intravenously, many patients mention a "burning sensation" at the site of injection.[48] This may be prevented or minimized by the initial administration (IV) of 1 ml of lidocaine (1%) or any other IV drug (midazolam, diazepam, or meperidine).

Because of the short duration of action of propofol, microcomputer-based syringe pumps have been developed that enable a continuous controlled dose of drug to be administered. This enables the doctor to maintain a therapeutic blood level of propofol for prolonged periods. Drugs administered via infusion pumps are administered on a dose/weight/time basis (e.g., microgram/kilogram/minute).

Oei-Lim et al.[46] found that a syringe-infusion pump set at an initial rate of 3 mg/kg/hr induced *conscious sedation* in approximately 11.6 minutes in severely apprehensive patients and/or those with mental or physical disabilities. The infusion rate was then adjusted to accommodate for variations in the level of sedation during the dental procedure (average duration of treatment = 55 minutes). The mean infusion rate was 3.6 mg/kg/hr. Sedation was successful in 17 of 19 patients. Cohen et al.[49] used an initial bolus of dose of 0.5 mg/kg, followed by an infusion of 4 mg/kg/hr to provide deep sedation for ambulatory oral surgery.

Propofol may also be administered as a bolus by syringe without an infusion pump. Propofol must be administered frequently by this method to maintain the patient in a sedated state. It is my recommendation that propofol *not* be used by doctors trained solely in IV conscious sedation.

SUMMARY

A number of techniques of IV conscious sedation are presented in this chapter. As a rule, there is no

TABLE 26-6 Summary of Intravenous Drug Doses, Duration, Amnesia

Drug	Concentration Used (mg/ml)	Average Dose (mg)	Minimal Dose (mg)*	Maximal Dose (mg)†	Duration	Amnesia‡ Induced
Group A						
Diazepam	5	10-12	20	30	45 min	Yes
Midazolam	2	2.5-7.5	6-8	10	45 min	Yes
Pentobarbital	50	125-175	300	500	2-4 hr	Somewhat
Promethazine	10	25-35	50	75	1-2 hr	Somewhat
Group B						
Meperidine	10	37.5	50	50	<1 hr	No
Morphine	1	5-6	8	8	1.5-2.5 hr	No
Fentanyl	0.01	0.05-0.06	0.08	0.08	30-45 min	No
Pentazocine	10	20	30	30	1 hr	No
Nalbuphine	2	7-8	2	2	1.5-2 hr	No
Butorphanol	0.4	1.5	2	2	1.5-2 hr	No
Group C						
Atropine	0.4	0.4-0.6	0.4-0.6	0.4-0.6	3-4 hr	No
Scopolamine	0.3	0.3	0.3	0.3	3-4 hr	Yes
Glycopyrrolate	0.1	0.1	0.1	0.2	7 hr	No

*Maximal dose at one titration.
†Maximal total dose at appointment.
‡Amnesic effect when used in maximal dose recommended.

necessity for any one doctor to have all of these techniques available for use in his or her dental practice.

The most rational way of employing these techniques is to start out by initially working with the basic techniques. To learn them well will require at least 50 to 100 cases with each technique.

The only means of obtaining the knowledge and training in the safe and effective use of IV conscious sedation techniques is through dental school undergraduate, postgraduate, and continuing education courses. The safe administration of IV conscious sedation cannot be learned by reading a textbook.

Strict adherence to the recommendations presented for each of the drugs and techniques, without exception, no matter how tempting alterations might appear, is essential. If these simple rules are followed, problems do not often occur. A summary of recommended drugs, dosages, and durations is presented in Table 26-6.

REFERENCES

1. Rosenberg MB, Campbell RL: Guidelines for intraoperative monitoring of dental patients undergoing conscious sedation, deep sedation, and general anesthesia, *Oral Surg* 71:2, 1991.
2. Council on Dental Education, American Dental Association: *Guidelines for teaching the comprehensive control of pain and anxiety in dentistry,* Chicago, 1992, The Association.
3. American Academy of Periodontology, Subcommittee on Anxiety and Pain Control of the Pharmacotherapeutics Committee: *Guidelines for the use of conscious sedation in periodontics,* Chicago, 1990, The Academy.
4. American Association of Oral and Maxillofacial Surgeons, Committee on Anesthesia: *Office Anesthesia Evaluation Manual,* ed 4, Rosemont, Ill, 1991, The Association.
5. American Academy of Pediatric Dentistry: Guidelines for the elective use of conscious sedation, deep sedation, and general anesthesia in pediatric patients. Revised May 1998. *Pediatr Dent* 21:58, 1999.
6. University of Southern California School of Dentistry: *Guidelines for parenteral sedation,* Los Angeles, 1991, University of Southern California.
7. Malamed SF: Survey of doctors using IV conscious sedation, unpublished data, 1993.
8. Jorgensen NB, Hayden J Jr: *Premedication, local and general anesthesia in dentistry,* Philadelphia, 1967, Lea & Febiger.
9. Coughlin MW, Panuska HJ: Direct comparison of midazolam and diazepam for conscious sedation in outpatient oral surgery, *Anesth Prog* 36:160, 1989.

10. Tait AR, Knight PR: The effects of general anesthesia on upper respiratory tract infection in children, *Anesthesiology* 67:930, 1987.
11. Valium, drug package insert, Nutley, NJ, 1990, Roche Laboratories.
12. O'Neill R, Verrill PJ, Aellig WH et al: Intravenous diazepam in minor oral surgery, *Br Dent J* 128:15, 1970.
13. Trieger N: *Pain control.* Chicago, 1974, Quintessence.
14. Malamed SF, Sykes P, Kubota Y et al: Local anesthesia: a review, *J Anesth Pain Contr Dent* 1:11, 1992.
15. O'Boyle CA, Barry H, Fox E et al: Controlled comparison of a new sublingual lormetazepam formulation and I.V. diazepam in outpatient minor oral surgery, *Br J Anaesth* 60:419, 1988.
16. O'Boyle CA: Benzodiazepine-induced amnesia and anaesthetic practice: a review, *Psychopharmacol Series* 6:146, 1988.
17. Roche Laboratories: Dosing and titration of midazolam (Versed), Letters to doctors, Nutley, NJ, 1987.
18. Nuotto EJ, Kortilla KT, Lichtor JL et al: Sedation and recovery of psychomotor function after intravenous administration of various doses of midazolam and diazepam, *Anesth Analg* 74:265, 1992.
19. Robb ND, Hargrave SA: Tolerance to intravenous midazolam as a result of oral benzodiazepine therapy: a potential problem for the provision of conscious sedation in dentistry, *J Anesth Pain Contr Dent* 2:94, 1993.
20. The Flumazenil in General Anesthesia in Outpatients Study Group I: Reversal of the central effects of midazolam by intravenous flumazenil after general anesthesia in outpatients: a multicenter double-blind clinical study, *Clin Ther* 14:966, 1992.
21. Jorgensen NB, Leffingwell FE: Premedication in dentistry, *J South Calif State Dent Assoc* 21:25, 1953.
22. Everett GB, Allen GD: Simultaneous evaluation of cardiorespiratory and analgesic effects of intravenous analgesia using pentobarbital, meperidine, and scopolamine with local analgesia, *J Am Dent Assoc* 83:155, 1971.
23. Jorgensen NB, Hayden J Jr: *Sedation, local and general anesthesia in dentistry,* ed 2, Philadelphia, 1972, Lea & Febiger.
24. Shepherd SR, Sims TN, Johnson BW et al: Assessment of stress during periodontal surgery with intravenous sedation and with local anesthesia only, *J Periodontol* 59:147, 1988.
25. Daniel SR, Fry HR, Savard EG: Intravenous "conscious" sedation in periodontal surgery: a selective review and report of 1,708 cases, *J West Soc Periodontol/Periodont Abstr* 32:133, 1984.
26. Foreman PA: Pharmacosedation: intravenous route. In McCarthy EM, ed: *Emergencies in dental practice,* ed 3, Philadelphia, 1979, WB Saunders.
27. Foreman PA: Control of the anxiety/pain complex in dentistry: intravenous psychosedation with techniques using diazepam, *Oral Surg* 37:337, 1974.
28. Foreman PA: Intravenous diazepam in general dental practice, *NZ Dent J* 65:243, 1969.
29. Foreman PA, Neels R, Willetts PW: Diazepam in dentistry, *Anesth Prog* 15:253, 1968.
30. Berns JM: "Twilight sedation": a substitute for lengthy office intravenous anesthesia, *J Conn Dent Assoc* 37:4, 1963.
31. Shane SM: Intravenous amnesia to obliterate fear, anxiety and pain in ambulatory dental patients, *J Md Dent Assoc* 9:94, 1966.
32. Shane SM: Intravenous amnesia for total dentistry in one sitting, *J Oral Surg* 24:27, 1966.
33. Shane SM, Carrel R, Vandenberge J: Intravenous amnesia: an appraisal after seven years and 10,500 administrations, *Anesth Prog* 21:36, 1974.
34. Shane SM: Intravenous amnesia for total dentistry in one sitting: an appraisal after 15,000 administrations. Fifth annual Continuing Education Seminar in Practical Considerations in IV and IM Dental Sedation, Miami Beach, 1979.
35. Kost M, Emerson D: Propofol-fentanyl versus midazolam-fentanyl: a comparative study of local sedation techniques for cataract surgery, *CRNA* 3:7, 1992.
36. Bloomfield EL, Masaryk TJ, Caplin A et al: Intravenous sedation for MR imaging of the brain and spine in children: pentobarbital versus propofol, *Radiology* 186:93, 1993.
37. Sherry E: Admixture of propofol and alfentanil: use for intravenous sedation and analgesia during transvaginal oocyte retrieval, *Anaesthesia* 47:477, 1992.
38. Silverman DG: New anesthetic approaches to gynecologic surgery, *Curr Opin Obstet Gynecol* 3:375, 1991.
39. Chin NM, Tai HY, Chin MK: Intravenous sedation for upper gastrointestinal endoscopy: midazolam versus propofol, *Singapore Med J* 33:478, 1992.
40. Silbergeld DL, Mueller WM, Colley PS et al: Use of propofol (Diprivan) for awake craniotomies: technical note, *Surg Neurol* 38:271, 1992.
41. Niccolai I, Barontini L, Paolini P et al: Long-term sedation with propofol in ICU: hemocoagulation problems, *Minerva Anestesiol* 58:375, 1992.
42. Ewart MC, Yau KW, Morgan M: 2% propofol for sedation in the intensive care unit: a feasibility study, *Anaesthesia* 47:146, 1992.
43. Bifarini G, Spaccatini A, Ciammitti B et al: Sedation with continuously infused propofol in caudal block for elective pediatric surgery, *Minerva Anestesiol* 58:181, 1992.
44. Oei-Lim VL, Kalkman CJ, Bouvy-Berends EC et al: A comparison of the effects of propofol and nitrous oxide on the electroencephalogram in epileptic patients during conscious sedation for dental procedures, *Anesth Analg* 75:708, 1992.
45. Rudkin GE, Osborne GA, Curtis NJ: Intra-operative patient-controlled sedation, *Anaesthesia* 46:90, 1991.
46. Oei-Lim LB, Vermeulen-Cranch DM, Bouvy-Berends EC: Conscious sedation with propofol in dentistry, *Br Dent J* 170:340, 1991.
47. Dembo JB, Kirkwood CA, Marsh RA: A comparison of propofol (Diprivan) and methohexital for outpatient oral surgery. Proceedings of the 40th annual meeting of the American Society of Anesthesiology, Toronto, Ontario, 1993.
48. Cillo JE Jr: Propofol anesthesia for outpatient oral and maxillofacial surgery, *Oral Surg Oral Med Oral Pathol Oral Radiol Endo* 87:530, 1999.
49. Cohen M, Eisig S, Kraut RA: Infusion pump for deep conscious sedation with propofol and methohexital. Proceedings of the 40th annual meeting of the American Society of Anesthesiology, Toronto, Ontario, 1993.

CHAPTER 27

Intravenous Sedation: Complications

CHAPTER OUTLINE

A number of complications are possible when the intravenous (IV) route of drug administration is used. Fortunately, most are relatively benign and easily managed. Some, however, are more significant and can lead to serious morbidity and to death.

The complications associated with IV drug administration are divided into four groups: (1) those associated with venipuncture, (2) localized complications related to drug administration, (3) general drug-related problems, and (4) drug-specific complications. These are outlined in Box 27-1.

VENIPUNCTURE COMPLICATIONS

Nonrunning Intravenous Infusion

One of the most common complications of venipuncture and IV sedation is a nonrunning or very slowly running IV infusion. Once venipuncture has been successfully completed, the tourniquet is removed and the IV drip started. During drug administration the drip rate should be increased; at other times the rate should be slowed. The causes of a nonrunning or

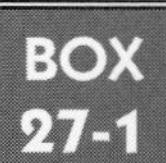

BOX 27-1 **Complications Associated with IV Drug Administration**

Venipuncture Complications
- Nonrunning IV infusion
- Venospasm
- Hematoma
- Infiltration
- Local venous complications
- Air embolism
- Overhydration

Local Complications of Drug Administration
- Extravascular drug administration
- Intraarterial injection
- Local venous complications

General Drug-Related Complications
- Nausea and vomiting
- Localized allergy
- Respiratory depression
- Emergence delirium
- Laryngospasm

Specific Drug Complications

Benzodiazepines
- Local venous complications
- Emergence delirium
- Recurrence of amnesia
- Oversedation

Pentobarbital
- Oversedation
- Respiratory depression

Promethazine
- Oversedation
- Extrapyramidal reactions

Opioids
- Nausea and vomiting
- Respiratory depression
- Rigid chest

Scopolamine
- Emergence delirium

slowly running IV infusion are listed in the following sections.

IV Infusion Bag Too Close to the Heart Level. Gravity forces the IV infusate from the bag down into the patient. The greater the difference in height between the bag and the patient's heart is, the more rapid the flow of solution will be. A simple experiment demonstrates this: The IV bag is held high above the patient's heart level, and the rate of flow is checked. With the rate-adjusting knob opened fully, the drip should be rapid. When the bag is gradually lowered toward the level of the patient's heart, the rate of flow of the drip decreases until, when held at the patient's heart level, the flow ceases entirely. As the bag is lowered below the level of the patient's heart, blood returns into the tubing (Figure 27-1).

This is a situation that might arise when the dental chair is placed low to the floor at the start of a procedure and is elevated at a later time. Increasing the distance between the bag of IV infusion solution and the patient's heart will correct the situation.

Bevel of Needle against Wall of Vein. It was recommended that the bevel of the needle be facing upward during venipuncture to make entry into the skin as atraumatic as possible. Following entry into the skin, the needle is advanced into the vein. At this point the tourniquet is removed and the infusion started. If the IV drip rate is rapid until the scalp vein or metal needle is taped into position and then slows considerably, it is quite possible that in taping the needle into position, the bevel was lifted and now lies against the wall of the vein. This would prevent or restrict the flow of fluid from the IV drip into the patient.

To determine whether this is the cause of the slow or nonrunning drip, the needle is carefully untaped and the wings of the butterfly needle gently lifted. This lowers the bevel of the needle off the wall of the vein. If this increases the drip rate, then the protective cap from the scalp vein needle (Figure 27-2) or a 2-×-2-inch gauze square is carefully placed under the wings of the needle and the needle retaped.

This is unlikely to occur when an indwelling catheter is used for venipuncture because there is no bevel on the catheter. However, when the catheter is positioned in either the dorsum of the hand or the antecubital fossa, it is possible for the tip of the catheter to lie in a bend in the vein, creating a slow flow of IV solution. Determine this by straightening the patient's wrist or elbow and looking for an increase in the rate of flow of the IV drip. Minimize this by preventing the patient from bending the joint through the use of an elbow immobilizer or wrist board.

Tourniquet Left on Arm. An embarrassing but not uncommon cause of a nonrunning IV drip following successful venipuncture may simply be that the tourniquet is covered by a sleeve that inched down. Following the return of blood into the IV tubing, the doctor or assistant opens up the control knob to start the IV drip. It is noted that the drip is not flowing and that blood does not leave the IV tubing as normally occurs. It is usually noted that more blood appears to be entering the IV tubing (as it is forced from the vein into the tubing). Once excessive blood is noticed in the tubing, simply removing the tourniquet will alleviate the problem.

Infiltration. Following successful entry into the vein the needle becomes dislodged during the securing (taping) of the needle. The doctor and assistant, unaware of this, open the rate knob, but little or no solution flows. If no solution is flowing, the three causes of nonrunning IVs discussed should be checked. If the drip rate is extremely slow and cannot be increased, one should look at the site where the needle tip is located beneath the patient's skin. If the needle has left the vein and fluid is still flowing, a small colorless swelling will develop at this site. This is termed an *infiltration*.

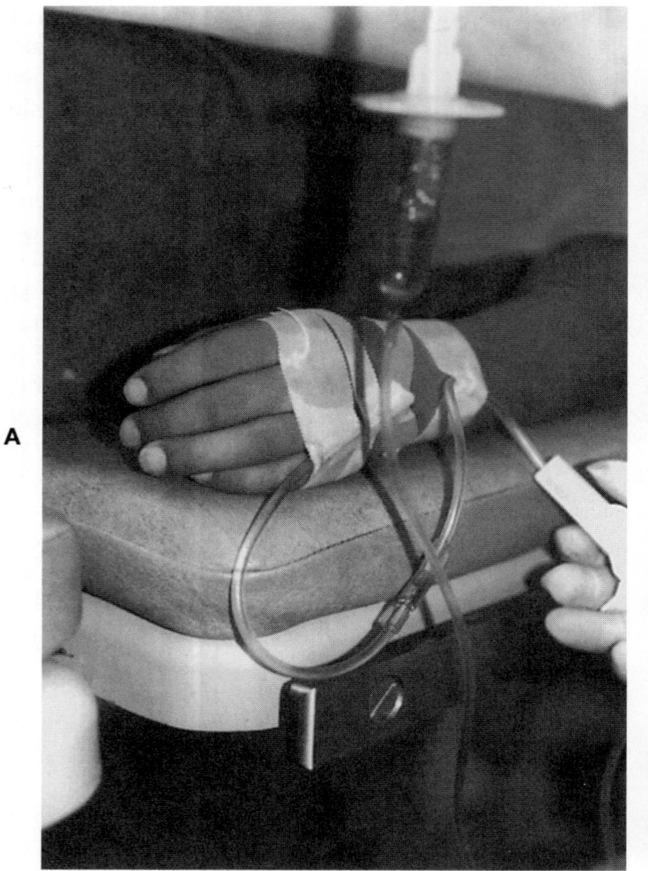
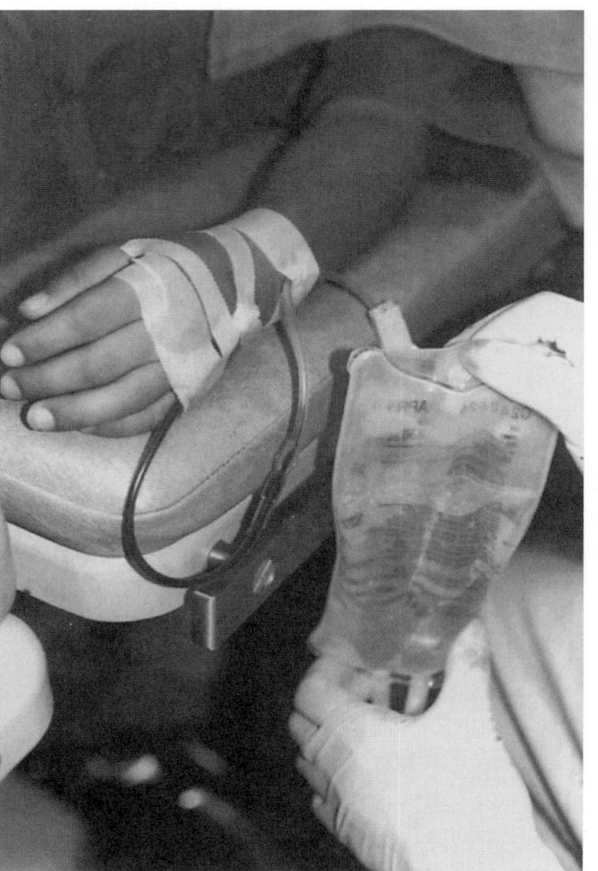

Figure 27-1 **A,** Bag of IV solution held *above* level of patient's heart (vein) allows fluid to run *into* patient. **B,** Lowering bag of IV solution *below* level of patient's heart (vein) allows blood to *return into tubing* from patient.

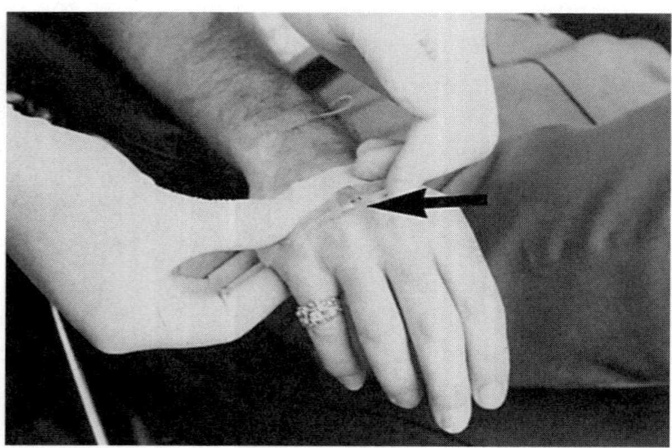

Figure 27-2 Placing the protective sheath of the needle (or gauze) beneath the wings of the needle *(arrow)* increases the rate of IV infusion if the bevel is pressing against the vein wall.

In all cases in which an IV drip that was previously running well has either slowed or stopped running entirely, the needle should not be removed from the vein until it has been determined definitely that the needle is no longer within the vein. The following procedure should be followed to determine the cause of the slow or nonrunning IV drip:

1. Open the drip rate knob.
2. Elevate the IV bag. Does flow rate increase?
3. Place the IV bag below heart level. Does blood return?
4. Check the IV site. Is tissue swelling present? Does the skin at the needle site feel cooler than surrounding tissues? (See Infiltration, p. 404.)
5. Elevate wings of needle or straighten patient's arm or wrist, as appropriate. Does flow improve?

Venospasm

Venospasm is a protective mechanism in which the vein wall responds to stimulation from the needle by going into spasm. As the needle approaches the vein, the vein appears to disappear or "collapse." Venospasm is occasionally accompanied by a burning sensation in the immediate area. This burning sensation resolves without treatment. Venospasm may occur before or after entry of the needle into the vein, securing of the needle, or starting of the IV drip.

Prevention. Venospasm cannot be prevented.

Recognition. Venospasm is identified by the disappearance of a previously visible vein during attempted venipuncture. A burning sensation may or may not accompany venospasm.

Management. The needle should not be removed from the site, for the vein has not yet been entered or damaged. The needle is pulled back slightly (1 to 2 mm), and heat is applied to the site in an effort to dilate the vessel. If and when the vein reappears, the venipuncture may be reattempted.

A sensation of burning is associated with several other complications and with one noncomplication. The IV administration of diazepam occasionally is associated with a sensation of warmth or burning; however, this sensation travels up the patient's arm as the drug passes through the veins. Intraarterial (IA) injection of a drug produces a burning sensation or pain traveling down the arm toward the fingers. Extravascular injection of a drug produces a burning sensation at the site of injection that remains at the site of administration. The injection of meperidine may cause the release of histamine and a burning or itching sensation along the path of the vein. Venospasm occurs more frequently in apprehensive patients, presumably as a result of their higher levels of circulating catecholamines (predisposing them to peripheral vasoconstriction).

Hematoma

Hematoma is the most common complication associated with venipuncture. It is the extravasation of blood into interstitial spaces surrounding a blood vessel. The presence of blood in this space leads to localized swelling and discoloration.

When venipuncture is successful, the needle itself acts as an obturator, sealing the hole within the vein made during entry of the needle. In some patients, particularly older patients in whom vein walls are less elastic, leakage of blood around the needle may occur during the IV procedure although the needle is still within the vein.

Hematoma may occur at two times during the IV procedure. First, it may develop during the venipuncture attempt if the vessel is damaged. This is not always preventable. The second cause of hematoma is usually preventable. In this situation the IV procedure has been completed and the needle removed from the vein. Improper application of pressure or inadequate duration of pressure at the venipuncture site can lead to a hematoma.

Prevention. It is not always possible to prevent a hematoma during venipuncture, although careful adherence to recommended technique minimizes its occurrence. Hematoma developing after the procedure can be prevented with the application of firm pressure for a minimum of 5 to 6 minutes. The commonly used technique of placing gauze over the venipuncture site in the antecubital fossa and having the patient flex his or her arm (illustrated in Figure 27-3) does *not* provide pressure adequate to prevent hematoma.

Recognition. Hematoma is a painless, bluish discoloration noted under the skin at the site of the needle puncture. It develops during the venipuncture attempt or at the conclusion of the IV procedure.

Management. *When hematoma develops during attempted venipuncture,* swelling increases rapidly because the tourniquet is still on the patient's arm (increasing blood pressure in the vein). Immediate management consists of the following:

1. Remove the tourniquet to decrease venous blood pressure.
2. Remove the needle from the skin.
3. Apply firm pressure with sterile gauze for 5 to 6 minutes.
4. If the site is tender, ice may be applied in the first few postoperative hours. Ice acts as a vasoconstrictor and as an analgesic.

When *hematoma develops following removal of the IV needle,* immediate management consists solely of direct pressure with gauze and ice. Subsequent management of either form of hematoma can best be described as "tincture of time." It will require approximately 7 to 10 days for the subcutaneous blood to be resorbed by the body. Nothing can be done to speed up this process. Should the patient complain of discomfort or soreness (more likely if the hematoma is located in a joint), he or

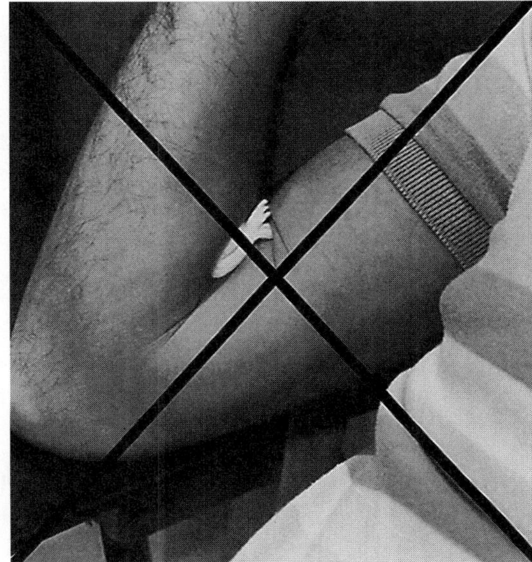

Figure 27-3 Placing gauze over the injection site and bending the elbow does *not* provide adequate pressure and often results in hematoma formation.

she can be advised to use moist heat on the area for 20 minutes every hour. Heat should not be used within the first 4 hours after the onset of the hematoma because it acts as a vasodilator and might induce further bleeding.

Infiltration

Infiltration is similar to a hematoma in that a fluid is being deposited into the tissues surrounding a blood vessel. In fact, a hematoma is the infiltration of blood outside of a blood vessel. Extravascular injection of a drug is an infiltration of drug outside of a blood vessel. Infiltration may be defined as a painless, colorless swelling developing at the site of the needle (canula) tip when the IV infusion is started.

In this situation we are discussing the deposition of the IV infusate into the tissues surrounding the blood vessel. The infiltration discussed here differs from hematoma in that the swelling that develops will not occur until the IV drip is turned on, whereas the hematoma occurs as soon as the vein is punctured.

In a continuous IV infusion technique, when infiltration does occur, it will only be a solution such as 5% dextrose and water or normal saline, which does not produce any tissue irritation or damage. In contrast, in IV sedation techniques in which a drug is injected directly into a blood vessel, it is much more likely that the drug will produce tissue damage and/or a delayed onset of sedation if deposited outside the blood vessel.

Prevention. Infiltration can be prevented by careful venipuncture technique and by not starting the IV drip or injecting drugs until it is confirmed that the needle tip lies within the lumen of the vein. Checking for this is quite easy. The rubber flash bulb on the IV tubing may be squeezed with blood returning into the tubing when the pressure is released, or the IV bag may be held below the level of the patient's heart (Figure 27-4).

Cause. Movement of the metal needle either while it is being secured or through movement of the patient's arm during the sedation procedure may cause the rigid metal needle to perforate the vein wall and produce an infiltration. The most common causes of a needle becoming dislodged are (1) attempting to thread (insert) a rigid metal needle too far into the vein and (2) being careless during taping of the needle. Infiltration is much less likely to occur when catheters are used for venipuncture.

Recognition. Infiltration is a painless, colorless swelling that occurs around the tip of the needle when the IV drip is started. The tissue around the needle tip is raised, and the skin at this site feels cooler than skin at a distance away from this site. This is because the infusate is at room temperature (72° F), not body temperature.

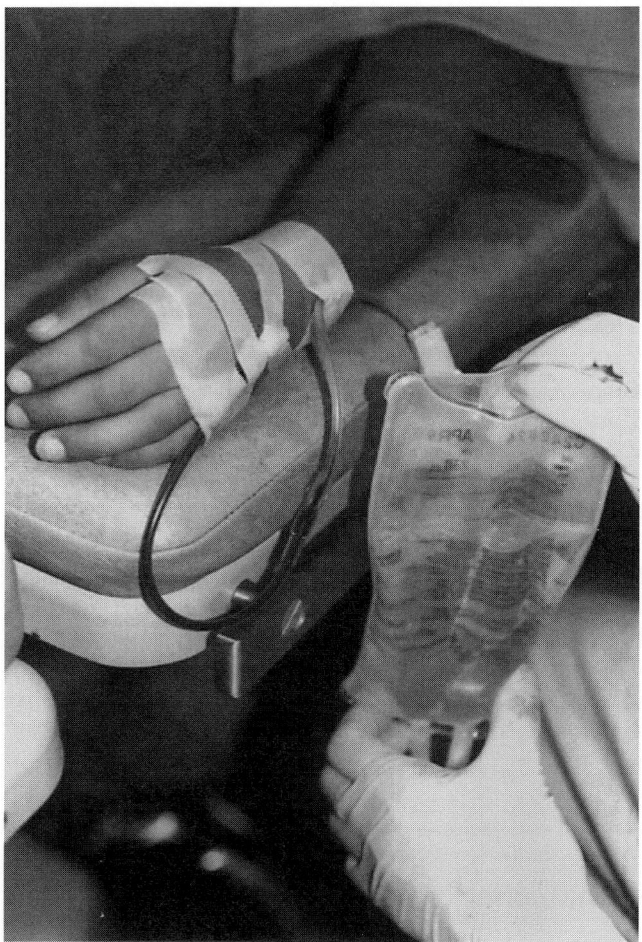

Figure 27-4 Lowering bag of IV solution below level of patient's heart (vein) allows blood to return into tubing from patient.

Management. The IV infusion must be stopped immediately and the needle removed. A piece of 2-×-2-inch gauze is placed at the site, and pressure is applied for 5 to 6 minutes. Pressure will stop any bleeding and also spread out any fluid within the tissue. The fluid will be resorbed into the cardiovascular system. Little or no residual soreness will be noted.

Localized Venous Complications

Localized venous complications can develop after IV sedation procedures. Many factors are responsible for their development, and indeed, there are a number of different clinical expressions that venous complications take. Trauma to the vein wall produced by the needle or cannula is a possible cause of this problem. In the dental outpatient environment the most likely cause of venous complications is chemical irritation of the vein wall produced by the drug being administered, usually diazepam or pentobarbital. Localized venous complications are discussed further later in this chapter (see Local Complications of Drug Administration).

Air Embolism

Air embolism is a possible, although extremely unlikely, complication of IV sedation. It is best prevented by using a technique that is free of air: eliminating air bubbles from syringes and from the IV tubing before the procedure and periodically observing the IV infusion bag to prevent its becoming emptied.

In the highly likely event that one or more small bubbles of air enter into the venous circulation, they will be absorbed quite rapidly by the blood with no clinical problem developing. It is not always possible for all air bubbles to be removed from the IV tubing or syringes, and it is quite probable that they will enter into the venous circulation of the patient. The patient, sighting an air bubble moving slowly down the IV tubing toward his or her arm, may become quite agitated, thinking that as little as one bubble of air is lethal. Fortunately, this is not so. A rule of thumb in a hospital environment is that a patient can tolerate up to 1 ml/kg of body weight of air in the peripheral venous circulation without adverse effect.[1]

The average IV administration set will hold approximately 13 ml of air.[2] Because 10 drops of solution (or air) equals 1 ml (adult infusion set), the chances of introducing large volumes of air into the patient's circulation are quite low. A 50-kg (110-lb) patient can tolerate 50 ml of air. This is equivalent to 500 to 750 drops of air from an adult IV administration set (10 or 15 drops per ml).

In small children air embolism is a more significant problem because their bodies cannot tolerate large volumes of air. A 30-lb (13-kg) child is at greater risk of this complication than is a larger patient.

Management. Should air embolism occur, management is based on the attempt to prevent this air from entering into the cerebral and pulmonary circulations. This is accomplished by positioning the patient in the dental chair lying on his or her left side (preventing entry into the pulmonary circulation) and in a head-down position (preventing entry into the cerebral circulation).

Overhydration

Overhydration of the patient is not a very common problem during IV sedative procedures in the dental office. The two most likely candidates for overhydration, however, are the patient with congestive heart failure and the child. Signs of overhydration include pulmonary edema, respiratory distress, and an increase in the heart rate and blood pressure. These are also the signs and symptoms occasionally noted in a patient with acute pulmonary edema.

A rule of thumb for replacement of fluid in a patient is that the initial dose of IV solution administered is equal to 1.5 times the number of hours a patient has gone without food times the patient's weight in kilograms.[3] This is the volume of fluid in milliliters required to replace the fluid deficit created by the patient's taking nothing by mouth (NPO) before the procedure. If a patient has been NPO for 6 hours before coming to the office, the initial volume of IV solution administered is nine times the patient's body weight in kilograms. The maintenance dose of IV solution is 3 ml/kg. The problem of underhydration is not significant in the usual outpatient environment.

When IV drugs are given to pediatric patients, it is recommended that a pediatric infusion set be used. This set, which permits 60 drops per milliliter instead of the usual 10 or 15, allows for a more careful administration of fluids to the younger, smaller patient or to the adult with serious congestive heart failure. In most instances these two classes of patients are not candidates for elective IV conscious sedation procedures in the outpatient setting.

LOCAL COMPLICATIONS OF DRUG ADMINISTRATION

Extravascular Drug Administration

When a drug is injected into subcutaneous tissues instead of a blood vessel, three problems may develop:

1. Pain
2. Delayed absorption of the drug
3. Tissue damage

Pain associated with extravascular drug administration occurs at the site of the needle tip under the skin and tends to remain localized to that area. This distinguishes extravascular injection from IA and IV injections, where a burning sensation radiates either peripherally or centrally. The patient will complain of discomfort as the drug is being injected in all three situations.

A potentially greater problem is delayed absorption of the drug into the cardiovascular system, especially if larger volumes have been deposited into the tissues. In essence the drug has been administered subcutaneously instead of intravenously. Uptake of the drug is slow, with an onset of clinical activity occurring anywhere from about 10 to 30 minutes later.

A third problem that might arise is damage to the tissues into which the drug has been deposited. Some drugs used intravenously are potentially irritating to tissues. This is especially true for diazepam and pentobarbital. The initial reaction in the tissues is for arteriolar and capillary constriction, which decreases the blood supply to the area. If vascular constriction is prolonged or if the chemical is irritating enough, necrosis and sloughing of tissue may occur.

Causes. There are two causes of extravascular drug administration. The first is the needle or cannula slipping out of the vein. This usually leads to an immediate formation of a hematoma that is quickly recognized. No drug is usually injected at this time. The second cause is the needle entering the vein and then being pushed through the other side as the doctor attempts to advance it farther into the vein. Blood will have returned into the tubing as the needle entered the vein originally, thereby giving the (false) impression that the needle tip is still in the vein. However, with removal of the tourniquet, it is unlikely that the blood will leave the tubing, as normally occurs, because the tip of the needle no longer lies in the vein but in subcutaneous tissue. On rare occasion the blood will reenter the patient and the IV infusion will be running even though the needle tip is no longer in the vein. This will occur when the bag of IV solution is quite high above the patient's heart or if the patient's skin and underlying soft tissues are not "firm," allowing gravity to force the solution into the tissues.

The continuous IV drip technique really minimizes the possibility of extravascular injection of a drug because an infiltration of infusate produces a swelling immediately. Second, before administration of any drug it is recommended that patency of the vein be reconfirmed by squeezing the flash bulb or holding the IV bag below the level of the patient's heart. Despite these precautions, a subtle movement of a patient's wrist or elbow just after this check but just before drug administration can produce this complication if rigid metal needles are used. The administration of a 0.2-ml test dose of a drug is a means of detecting this complication before a larger, potentially more damaging bolus of drug is deposited.

Recognition. As the irritating drug, especially diazepam or pentobarbital, is injected extravascularly, the patient will complain of a more intense pain that occurs at the site of the needle tip but does not migrate up or down the arm. In addition, as a volume of the drug is injected, the tissue at the site of the needle tip is raised as the solution is forced into the subcutaneous tissues. If the chemical is irritating, the skin overlying the raised tissue will become ischemic as blood vessels in the area constrict in response to the irritation. A second possible reaction is for the tissues to become erythematous as a result of inflammation.

Management. The two major problems to be managed are possible delayed absorption of the drug and its effect on the patient and potential damage to the tissues at the site of injection. Management initially consists of removing the needle and applying pressure at the site of injection to (1) stop the bleeding and (2) disperse the solution deposited under the skin. If less than 1 or 2 ml of drug has been deposited extravascularly, these steps are all that are required for effective management.

In the highly unlikely situation that larger volumes of drug have been deposited extravascularly and the overlying tissue is raised and ischemic, two problems must be addressed: (1) tissue damage and (2) delayed-onset sedation. Pressure alone may not be adequate to spread the solution, and additional drug management may be required. The drug of choice is 1% procaine, a local anesthetic with profound vasodilating properties. Several milliliters of procaine can be infiltrated into the affected tissues, using a single puncture point and a "fan-type" injection. This increases the rate of drug absorption and eliminates any discomfort that may be present.

The possible delayed onset of sedation produced by the slow absorption of the drug must be managed symptomatically, with basic life support procedures—maintaining the airway, ventilation, and circulation—implemented as needed.

In the conscious patient receiving drugs via an IV infusion, it is unlikely that a large volume of drug will be administered extravascularly. If the drug is titrated at the recommended rate of 1 ml/min, it will become obvious well within a minute that the needle is not in the vein. Further administration of the drug is immediately stopped and the IV patency rechecked.

Intraarterial Injection

The most significant of the localized complications of IV conscious sedation is IA injection of a drug. There are numerous reasons why this serious complication occurs only infrequently. However, when it does occur, immediate and vigorous therapy is indicated to prevent tissue damage, gangrene, and possible loss of the limb.[4-8] Drugs injected into an artery produce irritation of the artery wall as the drug is carried peripherally. As the diameter of the artery decreases, the drug is increasingly in contact with the artery wall. The immediate response of the artery to this chemical insult is spasm. Arterial spasm, especially if it occurs in one of the larger arteries of the upper limb, as is likely in this situation, will compromise the circulation to all, or a large portion, of the tissue distal to the injection site.

Prevention. Prevention is the most important feature in this discussion of IA injections. Fortunately, it is rather difficult to accidentally enter into an artery and even more difficult to accidentally administer a drug intraarterially. Many signs and symptoms develop that alert the doctor and assistant to the fact that the needle is not within a vein.

1. The vessel should be palpated before venipuncture. *Arteries conduct a pulse that can be palpated before the tourniquet is placed on the patient's arm.* Once a tourniquet is in place, the artery may not pulsate and the vessel may be mistaken for a vein. This is especially likely to happen on the

medial aspect of the antecubital fossa, where the brachial artery is somewhat superficial.

2. As the needle approaches the arterial wall, the vessel will begin to spasm. Arterial spasm is much more intense than venospasm and is associated with a more intense burning sensation. For this reason alone it is usually very difficult to accidentally (and on many occasions even purposefully) enter into an artery.
3. If the needle enters the artery (or any vessel, for that matter), blood will return into the IV tubing. With the tourniquet in place the return of blood will be similar to that seen in venipuncture; however, the color of the blood differs: Arterial blood is a brighter cherry red, whereas venous blood is a darker maroon.
4. On removal of the tourniquet a significant difference is noted. Venous blood leaves the IV tubing when the tourniquet is released, lowering the venous blood pressure to 4 to 6 mm Hg in the arm, and the IV drip is started. Following removal of the tourniquet, arterial blood, with a much higher blood pressure (e.g., 120/80 mm Hg), remains in the IV tubing and demonstrates a pulsatile flow with every contraction of the heart.

To this point, nothing damaging has been done to the patient or the artery. If the IA puncture is noted at this time, the needle is carefully removed and firm pressure exerted over the site for at least 10 minutes. If, however, a drug is injected into the artery, problems may develop rapidly.

Recognition. A number of signs and symptoms are associated with IA injection of a drug:

1. The patient complains of a severe pain that radiates peripherally from the site of injection of the drug toward the hand and fingers.
2. The radial pulse should be checked. Absence of the radial pulse indicates that the arterial spasm is quite severe and that immediate management is essential. Presence of the radial pulse, even though it may be quite weak, indicates that at least some arterial blood is entering the hand and fingers. A serious problem may exist, but it is not as acute.
3. The skin color of the affected hand should be compared with that of the opposite hand. Lack of blood flow into the affected limb produces a loss of normal skin color. A paler color or a mottled appearance may be noted initially.
4. Both limbs should be felt to determine temperature. The flow of blood into the hand provides warmth. When blood flow to the limb is compromised, that limb becomes cooler than the opposite limb with normal blood flow.

The major cause of injury from IA injection is chemical endarteritis that results in thrombosis and ischemia. Crystals of the drug precipitate as a result of the change in pH, leading to further occlusion of vessels. Results of this range from small areas of gangrene to the loss of fingers or a limb (Figure 27-5).

Management. Management of IA injection is best achieved by the following steps:

1. *Leave the needle in place.* Do not remove the IA needle that has been accidentally placed. It provides an avenue for the administration of the drug used in management of this situation.
2. *Administer procaine.* Slowly inject 1% procaine, to a volume of between 2 and 10 ml, into the artery. Procaine serves four functions at this time: (1) anesthetic, to decrease pain; (2) vasodilator, to break the arterial spasm and initiate return of blood flow; (3) pH about 5, counterbalance for drugs with alkaline pH (pentobarbital); and (4) diluent, decreasing the concentration of the

A

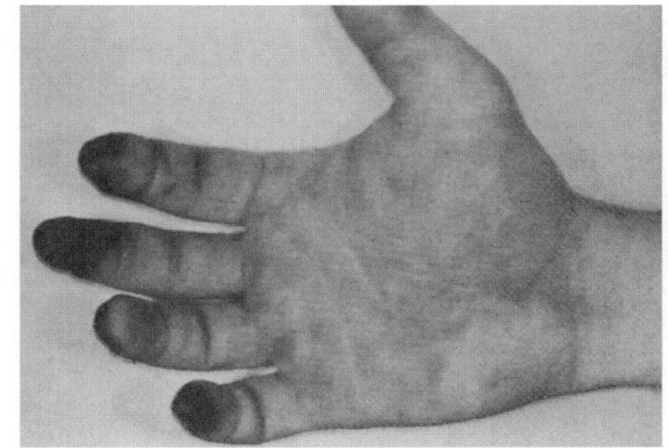

B

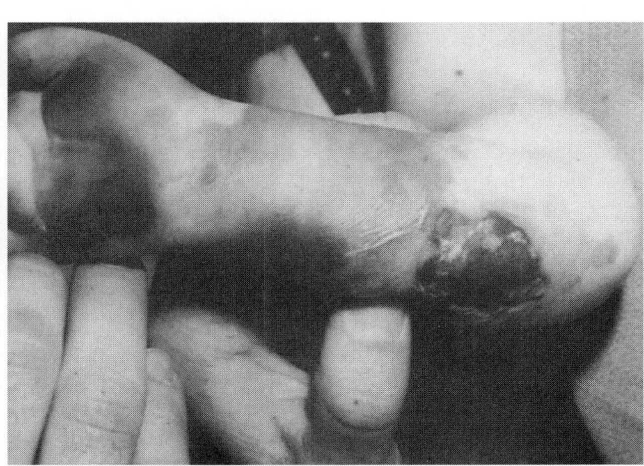

Figure 27-5 **A,** Gangrenous fingers secondary to intraarterial drug administration. **B,** Gangrene of forearm, hand, and fingers.

previously administered IA drug. Procaine frequently breaks the arterial spasm, which is noted by a return of color and warmth to the limb, as well as a return of a pulse wave equal in strength to that of the opposite limb.

3. *Hospitalize the patient.* All patients having had accidental IA drug administration should be seen in the emergency room of a hospital where a vascular surgeon or anesthesiologist will be consulted. The doctor should accompany the patient to the hospital so that the physicians can be advised of the drug(s) administered intraarterially and the treatment rendered. Additional treatment may also be deemed necessary. Such treatment may consist of a sympathetic nerve block, such as stellate ganglion block or brachial plexus block. When indicated, general anesthesia or surgical endarterectomy may be required. Heparinization may be used, if needed, to prevent further thrombosis. If treatment fails to reestablish effective blood flow to the limb, amputation of gangrenous parts may be required. Hyperbaric oxygen is often used to force oxygen into the tissues when IA spasm is not readily broken by the aforementioned procedures.[9]

The IA injection of a drug is a serious complication that should not occur if basic concepts of venipuncture and IV drug administration, recommended in earlier chapters of this section, are followed. In the unlikely situation that IA drug administration does occur, management as described is recommended, followed by accurate recordkeeping and contacting the doctor's insurance carrier immediately.

IA Drug Injection

Prevention

Palpate vessel before placement of tourniquet.
Avoid anatomically risky sites (e.g., median antecubital fossa), if possible.

Recognition

Intense pain during venipuncture attempt
Bright cherry red blood
Pulsating flow of blood in IV tubing when tourniquet is released
Intense pain radiating *down* arm toward fingers as drug is injected
Loss of color in limb
Loss of warmth in limb
Weakening or loss of radial pulse in limb

Local Venous Complications

Following a successful IV conscious sedation procedure, the patient is discharged home. The patient may feel fine through the next day only to find, 2 days after the procedure, that the hand in which the needle and drug were placed is swollen, red, hot, and painful.

The general category of local venous complications is being used here because of the multiple names given to the situation being discussed.

Phlebitis is the inflammation of a vein.

Thrombophlebitis is a condition in which inflammation of the vein wall has preceded the formation of a thrombus (blood clot).

Phlebothrombosis is the presence of a clot within a vein, unassociated with inflammation of the wall of the vein.

Gelfman and Driscoll[10,11] have reported on several prospective and retrospective studies of the problem of local venous complications. Criteria that they established for identification of these entities were the following:

- Thrombophlebitis: pain, induration, and a delay in onset of these symptoms
- Phlebothrombosis: a condition of venous thrombosis without inflammation; occurs much more immediately, and pain is not a prominent feature

It appears that the primary problem developing after IV conscious sedation is thrombophlebitis. Clinical features of thrombophlebitis include the following:

- Edema
- Inflammation
- Tenderness
- Delayed onset: 24 to 48 hours but may develop up to a week after venous insult

Causes of thrombophlebitis include anything that produces either mechanical or chemical irritation of a vein. Among the factors involved in the development of thrombophlebitis are those listed in Box 27-2.

IV solutions, be they infusions or drugs, that have pH values at either end of the spectrum are associated with

BOX 27-2 Factors Involved in the Development of Thrombophlebitis

pH of the infusion liquid
Components of the infusate
pH of the drug(s)
Duration of the IV infusion
Mechanical factors:

- Bevel and dullness of needle
- Technique of venipuncture
- Improper fixation of needle
- Size of needle in relation to vein lumen
- Type of needle (metal vs. plastic catheter)
- Presence of infection or disease
- Age and sex of the patient
- Site of venipuncture

a greater incidence of venous complications. Some drugs injected intravenously have vehicles, such as propylene glycol and alcohol, that are irritating to vein walls. Diazepam is an example of a drug containing such a vehicle (propylene glycol). It was mentioned earlier in this section that some patients experience pain on IV administration of diazepam. Gelfman and Driscoll[11] reported that in patients experiencing such discomfort on injection, the incidence of phlebothrombosis, but not thrombophlebitis, was increased.

The duration of the IV infusion is not as great a concern in outpatient sedation as it is within the hospital, where an IV infusion may be maintained for days at a time. It is common practice within hospitals for an IV team to change the site of the infusion every few days, thereby minimizing the development of local venous complications.

Improper technique, use of dull needles (highly unlikely with disposable needles), and improper fixation of the needle are mechanical causes of irritation. A needle that is not well secured will continually irritate the walls of the vein.

Placement of a very large needle within the lumen of a smaller vein will potentially produce greater irritation and an increased risk of thrombophlebitis. As recommended in this section, the 21-gauge needle will not impinge on the walls of any vein within the upper limb.

The site of venipuncture is also a factor. Venipuncture of the femoral or saphenous vein of the leg is associated with a higher incidence of thrombophlebitis and thromboembolism. There are significantly fewer complications with superficial veins of the arm and the dorsum of the hand. Within the upper limb, there are differences in the incidence of thrombophlebitis. Nordell et al.[12] reported five cases of thrombophlebitis in 52 patients. Table 27-1 is a summary of sites of venipuncture and incidence of thrombophlebitis.

Other studies have demonstrated similar statistics. Chambiras found a twofold greater incidence of venous complications in the hand than in the antecubital fossa.[13]

Prevention. It is not always possible to prevent local venous irritation when one of the factors responsible for its development is mechanical irritation produced by the venipuncture or the needle being used. Fortunately, the superficial veins of the upper limb are less likely to suffer serious postinjection complications than are the veins of the leg. Prevention is based on the following:

- Using sharp, sterile needles
- Following atraumatic, sterile venipuncture technique
- Securing the needle firmly in position
- Injecting IV drugs slowly into a rapid infusion
- Diluting IV drugs when possible

When dilution is not possible (e.g., with diazepam or propofol), use of larger veins (antecubital fossa and forearm) is recommended.

Recognition. The patient is usually asymptomatic for 1 day or more after the IV procedure. The inflammatory process requires approximately 24 to 48 hours to fully develop, at which time the patient usually contacts the office complaining of soreness, (possibly) swelling, redness of the area, and (possibly) warmth.

Management. Management of any localized venous complication requires that the patient return to the office for evaluation. The doctor should examine the patient to determine the nature and the extent of the situation. All findings are recorded in the patient's chart, and the patient is examined regularly until the situation resolves. The key to successful management is patient cooperation and satisfaction.

Management of thrombophlebitis includes the following:

1. Activity in the limb must be limited through the use, if possible, of a sling.
2. The affected limb must be elevated when possible.
3. Moist heat must be applied for 20 minutes three to four times a day.
4. Should thrombophlebitis occur in a joint (elbow or wrist), immobilization is more difficult but should still be attempted. Constant movement of the affected area leads, in some patients, to increased discomfort. Management of pain consists of the administration of nonsteroidal antiinflammatory analgesics (NSAIDs) such as aspirin every 4 to 6 hours as needed for pain.

TABLE 27-1 Site of Venipuncture and Incidence of Thrombophlebitis

Site	No. of Venipunctures	No. of Cases of Thrombophlebitis	Incidence of Thrombophlebitis (%)
Hand, wrist	26	3	11.5
Forearm	15	2	13.33
Antecubital fossa	11	0	0

5. Anticoagulants and antibiotics are *not* part of the usual therapy and will not be required unless the situation deteriorates. By this time, however, the patient will have been referred to a physician (vascular surgeon) for definitive management.

In the usual course of events, the acute phase of thrombophlebitis, involving tenderness, swelling, and discomfort, resolves within a few days, gradually leading to a chronic phase in which the discomfort is gone but the vein remains hard and knotty. This may occur at the site of the venipuncture or anywhere along the path of this vein and its tributaries. The extent of these lumps and bumps subsides over time. Treatment of choice during this phase is tincture of time.

The patient is seen in the office on a less and less frequent basis as the situation resolves. Records are maintained of the findings at each visit. In most cases full resolution is noted within 3 to 4 weeks, although cases have been reported in which patients have suffered lingering tenderness for over 3 years (wrist vein).

In the unlikely event that fever or malaise develops, consultation with a vascular surgeon (the person most likely to be familiar with the management of this complication) is recommended. In any situation in which a patient is being referred for medical (or dental) consultation, it is recommended that the referring doctor speak with the physician (discussing management of the case) before the patient is seen. Another clinical indication for referral to a physician is patient dissatisfaction. If the patient expresses doubt over the doctor's handling of the problem (after all, this is no longer a dental problem), immediate consultation with an appropriate physician is recommended.

Management of phlebothrombosis, which is a small painless nodule located at the site of venipuncture, is essentially the same as that described for thrombophlebitis:

1. Immobilization of the affected limb
2. Moist heat applied to area
3. Tincture of time

Virtually all cases of local venous complications resolve within a short period without residual effects.

GENERAL DRUG-RELATED COMPLICATIONS

In this section systemic reactions brought about through the administration of IV drugs are discussed.

Nausea and Vomiting

The incidence of nausea and vomiting associated with IV conscious sedation is quite low. However, the potential does exist for some of the drugs being administered to produce this problem. Among the drugs recommended for use via the IV route, the opioids are most likely to induce nausea and vomiting. Promethazine and scopolamine, which possess antiemetic properties, are among those drugs least likely to produce nausea and vomiting.

Causes of Nausea and Vomiting

1. Opioid administration
2. Hypoxia
3. Swallowing blood

The potential problem is not in the development of nausea but in the act of vomiting, especially in the patient with central nervous system (CNS) depression (i.e., the sedated patient). The patient who vomits while lying supine in a dental chair faces the possibility of aspirating vomitus into the trachea and suffocating on the vomitus. The fact that a patient has received a CNS depressant drug only increases this risk because protective reflexes may be depressed.

As mentioned, it is the general category of opioids in which the incidence of vomiting is greatest. The production of nausea and vomiting related to opioid use is a dose-related response. The greater the dose of opioid is, the higher the incidence of nausea and vomiting is. In the dosages recommended in Chapters 25 and 26, the incidence of vomiting has proved to be virtually zero. When I first began the clinical use of nalbuphine, it was used in doses greater than those currently recommended. Of the first 10 patients receiving nalbuphine, 5 either became nauseous or vomited later that same day. Decreasing the dosage of the drug has eliminated this as a problem.

The incidence of vomiting following opioid administration is greater in ambulatory patients than in hospitalized, nonambulatory patients.[14] Patients receiving very large doses of opioids during general anesthesia do not have as high an incidence of postoperative vomiting, whereas patients undergoing ambulatory surgery and receiving significantly lower doses of opioids have a greater incidence of vomiting. This increased rate of vomiting is related to the more frequent changes of body position that occur in the ambulatory patient. Unfortunately, this is a fact of life with which we must live. Happily, however, when opioid dosages are kept within the limits recommended herein, the incidence of this complication is extremely low.

Management of Nausea. Should nausea develop while the patient is still in the dental office, he or she can be placed back in the dental chair and oxygen (O_2) administered. This alone usually leads to recovery. Hypoxia is a common cause of nausea. Since recommending that nasal O_2 be administered routinely during IV conscious sedation, we have seen a virtual disappearance of nausea in our patient population in the dental office. If nausea develops after discharge of the patient from the office, postoperative instructions suggest that the patient lie down for a while and drink a cola beverage, if it is available, because this may settle the stomach.

Management of Vomiting. Should nausea progress to vomiting when the patient is at home, the most important thing for the patient to remember is that he or she should not be lying supine because the possibility of aspiration of vomitus is greater in this position. This is one of the reasons for strict adherence to the discharge criteria recommendation that the patient be able to manage himself or herself at home before being discharged from the office.

If vomiting occurs during dental treatment (a situation that has occurred only once in more than 3500 cases at the University of South California), the airway must immediately be cleared of all dental equipment. The patient's head should be turned to the side (away from the operator) so that the vomitus pools on one side of the mouth, leaving a patent airway. Suction is then applied so that the remaining vomitus may be removed.

Localized Allergy

It is not uncommon for a patient receiving IV drugs to mention that the skin at the site of injection itches. There may be a localized or diffuse reddening of the tissues. Several possibilities exist as to the cause of this reaction.

The opioid agonist meperidine induces the localized release of histamine. As the drug enters and travels up the vein toward the heart, a red line tracing the course of the vein may be noted (Figure 27-6). The patient may mention that his or her arm itches. *Histamine release is a normal pharmacologic property of meperidine and does not represent allergy.* Within 5 to 10 minutes, this response resolves by itself. Treatment is usually not required. If the itching is intense, IV administration of a histamine blocker such as diphenhydramine or chlorpheniramine should be considered.

Less frequently, it will be observed that the skin around the site of the needle is diffusely erythematous with raised areas noted. The word *blotchy* may appropriately be used to describe its appearance. The site may burn or be quite itchy. The reaction is localized to the immediate area but is not as localized to the path of the blood vessels as is the meperidine-induced histamine reaction. The most frequently observed cause of this type of localized allergic response is the adhesive on the tape used to secure the needle. Many persons are allergic to the adhesives used on tape. The erythematous reaction will appear to be located around the tape. Management of this situation dictates the IV administration of a histamine blocker, either diphenhydramine or chlorpheniramine. The use of hypoallergenic tape should prevent recurrence of this reaction.

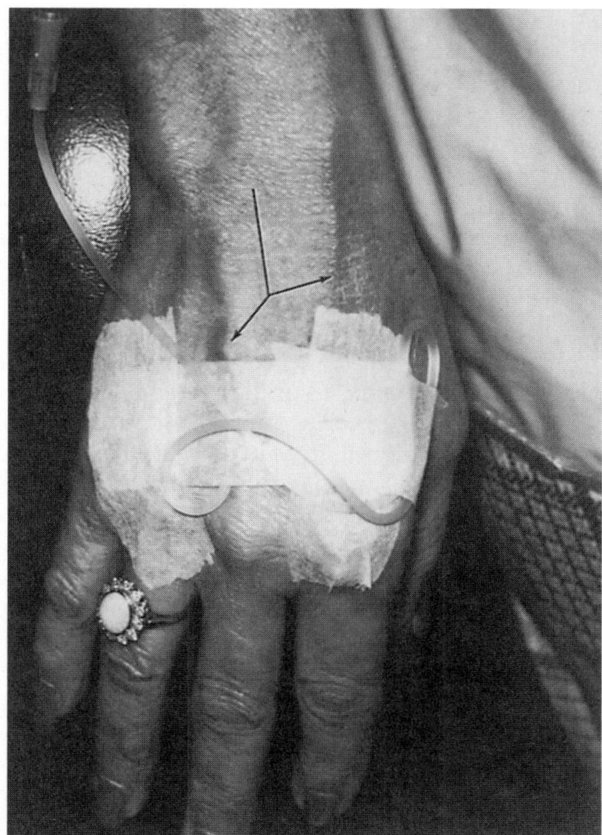

Figure 27-6 Meperidine-induced localized histamine release along path of vein *(dark lines on wrist).*

If the allergic response appears to be more directly related to drug administration, treatment need be more vigorous and more immediate. The chemical mediators of allergy that are released from mast cells into the venous circulation in response to antigenic challenge will be traveling toward the heart and may soon involve the skin and respiratory and cardiovascular systems. Management of this potentially life-threatening reaction involves placing a tourniquet high on the patient's arm as soon as the reaction is noted. This may prevent or at least slow the development of a generalized reaction. If the reaction is still limited to the limb, parenteral administration of a histamine blocker is recommended; however, once the reaction becomes more generalized, 3 to 5 ml of a 1:10,000 epinephrine solution is administered intravenously, followed by administration of a histamine blocker.

Prevention of allergic reactions is greatly preferred to their management. Prevention is based on a careful pretreatment discussion of the patient's prior allergic history and response to the drugs being administered.

The patient should be questioned about any previous reactions to adhesive tape. In addition, the 0.2-ml test dose recommended for all drugs will aid in determining whether allergy is present. Although the administration of a dose as small as 0.2 ml of an allergen can, in some cases, induce anaphylactic or anaphylactoid reactions, in most circumstances the observed reaction will be less severe and management can proceed as previously described.

Respiratory Depression

Morbidity and mortality associated with IV conscious sedation has usually been related to the presence of respiratory depression that went undetected, leading to respiratory arrest, cardiac dysrhythmias, and cardiac arrest. *All* of the sedative drugs discussed in this book are respiratory depressants (although to varying degrees at therapeutic doses). All are capable, in some doses and in some patients, of producing respiratory arrest. Respiratory depression is a more significant problem with certain drug groups, such as opioid agonists and barbiturates.

Respiratory depression occurring after drug administration is a dose-related response. Smaller doses of the drug produce little or no respiratory depression in the "average patient" (middle of the bell-shaped curve); however, increasing the drug dosage increases its CNS depressant effects and leads ultimately to respiratory depression.

Respiratory depression may occur following extremely low dosages of any drug if the patient lies on the hyperresponding slope of the bell-shaped curve. Unfortunately, there is little that can be done before drug administration to determine this fact. The patient can be questioned about his or her usual response to drugs such as analgesics and tranquilizers (e.g., oral diazepam). A response from a patient who mentions falling asleep after one 2-mg diazepam (Valium) tablet should alert the doctor to the possibility of hyperresponsiveness to benzodiazepines. The 0.2-ml test dose, followed by a wait of 30 seconds before administering any additional drug, is another means of discovering a patient's hypersensitivity to a drug. One other means of accounting for variations in patient response to drugs is titration. Drugs should *always* be titrated to clinical effect, whenever titration is possible. When this is done, oversedation and respiratory depression following IV drug administration should not occur or will do so only infrequently. The drug doses recommended in Chapters 25 and 26 will provide effective sedation with little or no respiratory depression in the typical patient.

The two drug categories most likely to produce respiratory depression are opioid analgesics and barbiturates. Opioid-induced respiratory depression is characterized by a decrease in the rate of breathing. The adult respiratory rate, normally between 14 to 18 breaths/min, may decrease to 5 or 6 deeper breaths/min. Barbiturate-induced respiratory depression is characterized by a more rapid but shallower respiratory effort than that seen with opioids.

Management. The initial steps in management of respiratory depression are universal, regardless of the cause of the problem. Following are the steps of basic life support:

- *Position:* If not already in the supine position, the patient is immediately positioned supine. The patient's feet are elevated slightly (10 to 15 degrees) to aid the return of venous blood to the heart.
- *Airway:* Probably the most important step in basic life support is maintenance of a patent airway. This is accomplished through the head-tilt/chin-lift maneuver (Figure 27-7). Proper performance of this step elevates the tongue from the hypopharynx, providing a patent airway in most circumstances.
- *Breathing:* The doctor or assistant performing the previous step places his or her ear 1 inch from the patient's mouth and nose, looking at the patient's chest while listening and feeling for air exiting the patient's mouth and nose and watching the patient's chest for signs of spontaneous ventilatory efforts (Figure 27-8). In the likely event that the patient is breathing spontaneously but the rate and depth are depressed, the rescuer must assist or control the patient's breathing. Using a positive-pressure O_2 device (Robertshaw or Elder valve) (Figure 27-9) or a self-inflating bag-valve-mask device (Ambu bag) (Figure 27-10), the rescuer inflates the patient's lungs every time a spontaneous respiration is attempted. If the patient's respiratory rate is less than 8 breaths/min, the rescuer will increase the rate of

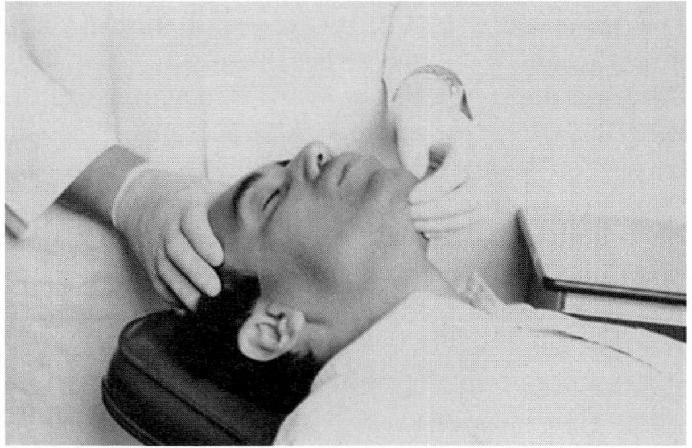

Figure 27-7 Airway maintenance employing head-tilt/chin-lift maneuver.

breathing by interposing a controlled ventilation between each of the spontaneous attempts by the patient. The self-inflating bag-valve-mask device is not recommended for use in larger adults unless a reservoir bag is added. It is, however, recommended for use in children.

- *Circulation:* The carotid pulse is checked to determine the functional status of the cardiovascular system. If respiratory depression is recognized early, the carotid pulse will still be strong and regular.
- *Definitive care:* If respiratory depression occurs after opioid administration (either as a sole drug or as one of a combination), an opioid antagonist should be administered.

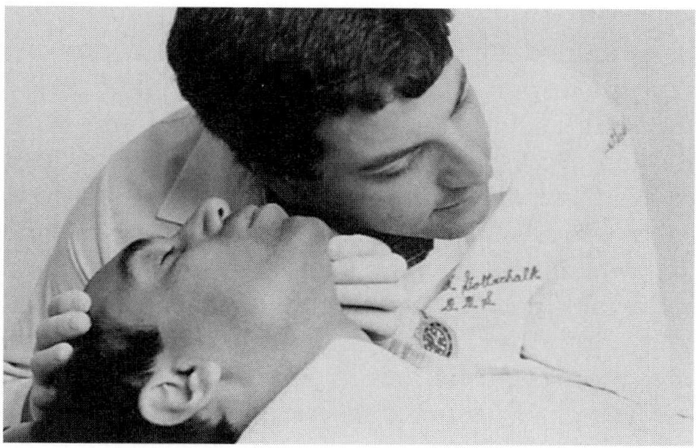

Figure 27-8 Look, listen, and feel while checking for respiration and airway patency.

Naloxone is the drug of choice for reversing opioid-induced respiratory depression. Nalbuphine has been used with great success; however, more study of this drug is required before it can be recommended for this function.[15] Naloxone should be diluted from its original 0.4 mg/ml concentration by adding 3 ml of diluent (5% dextrose and water, normal saline), producing a 0.1 mg/ml concentration for injection. The patient is continually observed for signs of increased respiration while 0.1 mg (1 ml) is slowly administered every minute. In most cases less than 0.4 mg naloxone will be required to reverse opioid-induced respiratory depression. In the not too distant past, naloxone was administered in 0.4-mg increments. It was found, however, that larger doses of naloxone also antagonize the analgesic properties of the opioid. If the patient had undergone a painful procedure (e.g., abdominal surgery), the reversal, by naloxone, of the analgesic actions of the opioid led to an acute onset of pain, which is a

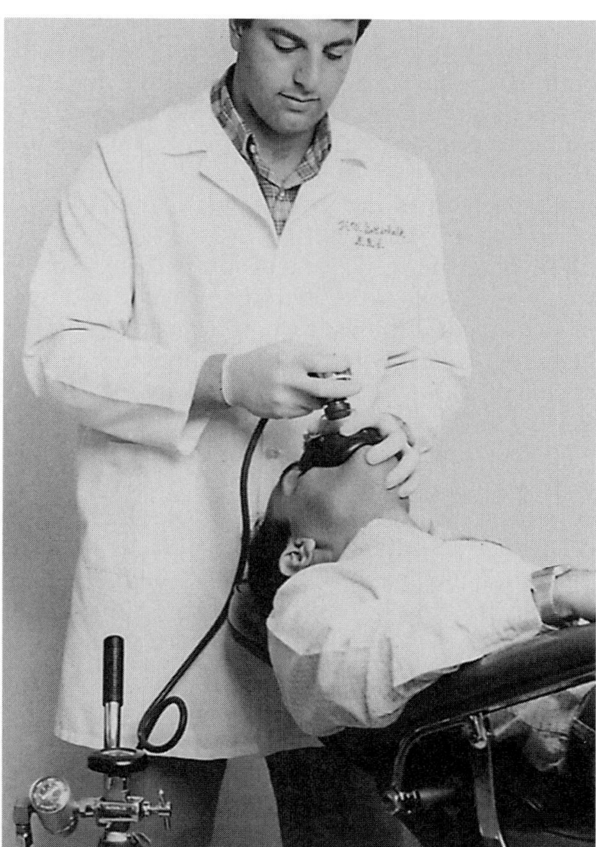

Figure 27-9 Assisted or controlled ventilation using a positive-pressure demand device.

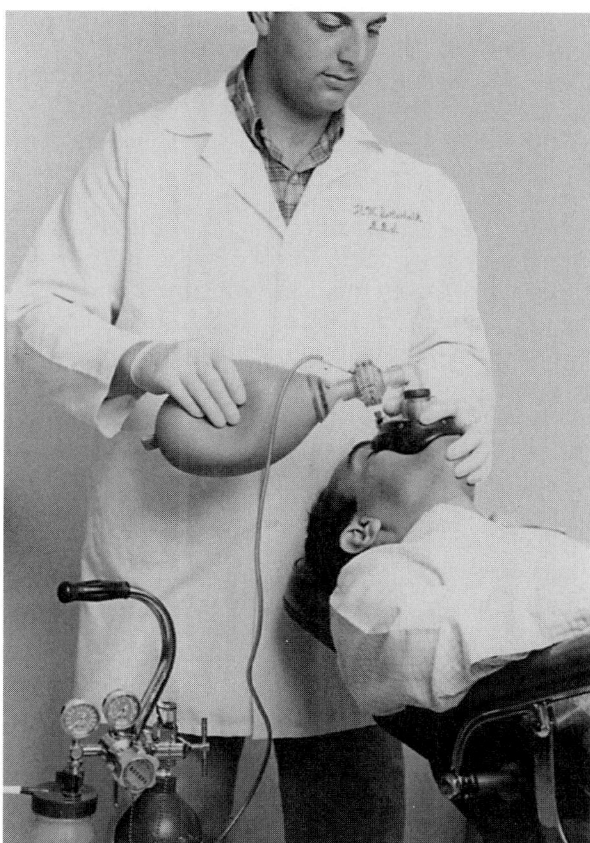

Figure 27-10 Assisted or controlled ventilation using a self-inflating bag-valve-mask device.

significant stimulus to the heart and cardiovascular system. This led to life-threatening emergencies in patients with prior histories of cardiovascular disease.[16] Slow titration of 0.1 mg per minute minimizes this reaction. During the time between the administration of naloxone and its onset of action, the steps of basic life support must be continued.

With the return of more rapid and deeper respiration, the patient begins to look and feel considerably better. The patient may be unaware of what has transpired because he or she has been deeply sedated during this time. Dental treatment may be halted, but the patient should not be discharged from the office at this time. Naloxone is a rapid-acting respiratory depressant; however, its duration of action after IV administration is fairly short. It is therefore possible, although unlikely, for respiratory depression to recur approximately 30 minutes after the initial dose of naloxone was given. With the use of the shorter-acting opioids, fentanyl, alfentanil, sufentanil, and remifentanil, this is less likely to occur. When meperidine, morphine, and butorphanol are administered, the likelihood increases. The patient should remain in the office, in a monitored recovery area with O_2 available, for at least 1 hour after the administration of naloxone.

Following the initial IV dose of naloxone and recovery of the patient, it is suggested by many persons that 0.4 mg naloxone be administered intramuscularly. The duration of clinical action of intramuscular (IM) naloxone is considerably longer than that of an IV dose, thereby minimizing the risk of recurrence of respiratory depression.

Non–opioid-induced respiratory depression is not reversible with naloxone. The barbiturates are the other drug group most likely to produce respiratory depression. Management of non–opioid-induced respiratory depression is based on the steps of basic life support—airway, breathing, and circulation—until the cerebral blood level of the offending drug has been lowered, through redistribution, to the point at which breathing is no longer depressed. There are no effective antidotal drugs for barbiturates.

Respiratory depression produced by benzodiazepines is much more uncommon within the dosage ranges presented previously. That respiratory depression can occur with these agents was brought to the attention of doctors in the United States by a letter from the manufacturer of midazolam that reemphasized this possibility and recommended appropriate measures to minimize or prevent its development.[17] Management is based on the basic life support techniques described. The IV administration of the benzodiazepine antagonist flumazenil, in an initial dose of 0.2 mg (2 ml) with subsequent doses administered every minute as needed (to a maximum dose of 1.0 mg), will reverse the respiratory depression (and other clinical actions of benzodiazepines) more rapidly.

Emergence Delirium

A complication known as *emergence delirium* has been reported after the administration of many CNS depressants, as well as with some adjunctive drugs commonly given intravenously in sedative procedures. The patient's response is one of transient delirium, hallucination, anxiety, or rage that develops at some time during or immediately after the sedative procedure. Very often, the response is associated with recall of an upsetting event in the patient's life. Minichetti and Milles[18] reported a case of a 27-year-old patient receiving 7.5 mg IV diazepam in addition to meperidine, atropine, nitrous oxide–oxygen (N_2O-O_2), and local anesthesia for extraction of several teeth. The patient felt quite comfortable and sedated. Following the administration of an additional 2.5 mg diazepam later in the procedure, the patient became progressively more excited. His eyes closed, he began crying, and he would not respond to verbal commands. Attempts made to communicate with the patient were ineffective. He became hyperexcitable and began thrashing about in the dental chair. Removal of the N_2O and administration of 100% O_2 did not resolve the situation, nor did administration of 0.4 mg naloxone. He continued to hallucinate for about 20 minutes, exhibiting rage and anxiety. He recovered gradually, calmed down, stopped crying, and began responding to his name. When questioned later about the incident he said that he thought he had merely been dreaming about an unpleasant experience he had had in Vietnam.

The drugs most likely to produce emergence delirium are scopolamine, diazepam, and midazolam. Other benzodiazepines, such as lorazepam, have also been reported to produce emergence delirium. Scopolamine, however, is far and away the drug most likely to produce emergence delirium.[19]

The reactions associated with emergence delirium are thought to be manifestations of the central anticholinergic syndrome (CAS).[20,21] CAS includes such paradoxical reactions as acute hyperactivity, anxiety, delirium, hallucinations, and recent memory impairment. In its most severe form CAS produces apnea, medullary paralysis, coma, and death, although these reactions are extremely rare. The dose of scopolamine or benzodiazepine required to produce CAS is extremely small; it is not a dose-related phenomenon. Therefore the doctor administering IV anticholinergics or benzodiazepines must be aware of the CAS, its prevention, and its management.

Prevention. The incidence of CAS and emergence delirium is considerably lower in patients between the ages of 6 and 65 years. For this reason, the use of scopolamine is not recommended in patients younger than 6 or older than 65 years. Other anticholinergics, such as atropine and glycopyrrolate, which are less likely to produce CAS, are recommended in these patients. Fortunately, the indication for IV conscious sedation in these two groups of patients is not great. Slow injection of drugs and use of minimal doses may aid in minimizing these reactions.

Management. Management of the usual form of emergence delirium, in which the patient may exhibit dreaming and appears uncomfortable but does not respond to verbal questioning, takes two forms.

Symptomatic Management. Positioning, monitoring of the patient, assurance of a patent airway and adequate blood supply to the brain (PABC) and prevention of injury to the patient are the goals of treatment. Given an appropriate time span (variable), the reaction will terminate and the patient will open his or her eyes and be able to respond to commands and questions normally. In one case of emergence delirium that I witnessed (before the availability of physostigmine and flumazenil), the patient had received scopolamine as a part of the Jorgensen technique and for almost 5 hours continued to dream and make uncoordinated movements in the chair. She was unresponsive to questioning but had a very adequate airway with her vital signs but slightly elevated over baseline. Approximately 5 hours after the administration of the scopolamine, the patient opened her eyes and was able to respond to commands.

Physostigmine Administration. The second means of managing emergence delirium is the administration of physostigmine, a reversible anticholinesterase. IV administration of physostigmine rapidly reverses emergence delirium and the CAS.

The dose of physostigmine for reversal of emergence delirium is 1.0 mg for the 70-kg adult and 0.5 mg for the child, administered intravenously. One milligram of physostigmine may be administered per minute until the reaction is terminated or a maximum dose of 4 mg is reached. Because physostigmine is metabolized within 30 minutes, the patient must be monitored closely to be certain that signs and symptoms do not recur. Rapid administration of physostigmine is associated with the possible development of bradycardia, hypersalivation, emesis, and defecation.[22]

Laryngospasm

Laryngospasm is a protective reflex of the body. In the fully conscious patient (i.e., no CNS depression), foreign objects are prevented from entry into the airway (trachea) by the swallowing reflex, the epiglottis, and the cough reflex. As a patient becomes more and more CNS depressed through the administration of drugs, these protective reflexes become progressively more depressed. In conscious sedation, as observed with N_2O-O_2, IV diazepam, midazolam, the Jorgensen technique, and IV promethazine, there is but little impairment of these reflexes. Foreign material, such as water and scraps of dental material, will be easily removed by the patient as he or she spits or swallows. Aspiration is not a common occurrence with these techniques of conscious sedation. However, as the level of CNS depression increases with increased doses or the addition of other drugs, protective reflexes are depressed to a greater degree.[23]

In stage II, ultralight general anesthesia, foreign material present in the area of the larynx provokes a protective reflex in which the vocal cords adduct in an attempt to seal off the trachea from entry of foreign material. Although truly a protective reflex, it also prevents the passage of air into and out of the trachea and lungs (Figure 27-11). Laryngospasm will not occur in stage I of anesthesia, which we have called sedation or analgesia, because the other protective reflexes are still intact. It is only when the patient enters stage II that laryngospasm will occur.

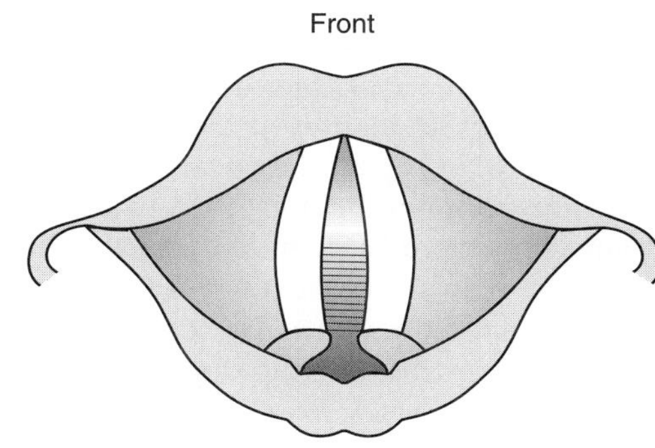

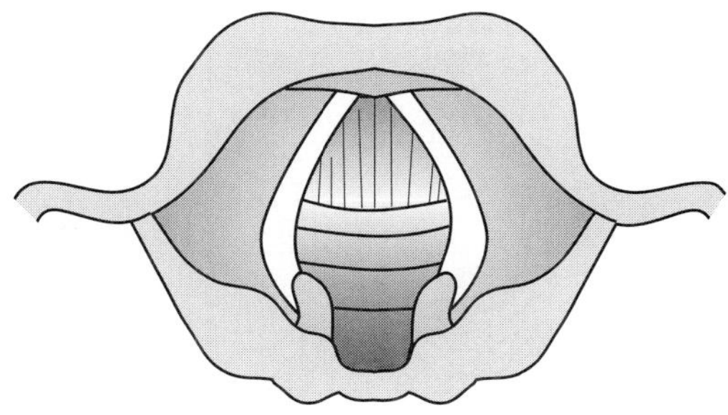

Figure 27-11 View of vocal cords. **Top,** Cords are adducted (closed), thus preventing foreign material and air from entering trachea. **Bottom,** Cords abducted (open). (From Scanlan CL, Wilkins RL, Stoller JK: *Egan's fundamentals of respiratory care,* ed 7, St Louis, 1999, Mosby.)

Recognition. Recognition of laryngospasm is based on the presence or absence of sounds. A partial laryngospasm is identified by the presence of stridor, an abnormal high-pitched, musical respiratory sound produced as air is forced out through partially adducted vocal folds. Total (complete) laryngospasm is identified by the absence of sound in the presence of respiratory efforts, an ominous "sound" indeed.

The patient attempts to breathe against this partially or completely closed airway. Respiratory efforts are exaggerated: Expansion of the chest is greater than usual, and accessory muscles of respiration are used. Substernal, supraclavicular, and intercostal soft tissue retraction may be observed (Figure 27-12). This is the sucking in of the soft tissues overlying the intercostal spaces between the ribs and sternum as the chest expands and intrathoracic pressure becomes more negative. Soft tissue retraction is a sign of a partially or totally obstructed airway.

Management

1. The first step in management of laryngospasm is the removal of any offending material from the patient's airway. A large-diameter suction tip or tonsil suction is placed into the pharynx to remove any material it finds. This step alone will break laryngospasm in many cases.
2. Following suctioning of the airway, positive-pressure O_2 is administered, either via the self-inflating bag-valve-mask device or positive-pressure demand valve. Often, it is possible to break the spasm by forcing O_2 past the vocal cords.
3. The administration of drugs to terminate laryngospasm is never recommended unless the doctor is well trained in anesthesiology and in management of the apneic patient. The drug of choice is succinylcholine, a short-acting depolarizing muscle relaxant. Administered in a concentration of 20 mg/ml, an IV dose of 20 to 40 mg is usually adequate to break laryngospasm by paralyzing the muscles of respiration. At this point, however, the patient is no longer breathing, and the doctor becomes responsible for instituting controlled ventilation for 3 to 4 minutes until the typical patient resumes spontaneous ventilation.[24]
4. If no drugs are administered during laryngospasm, the level of carbon dioxide (CO_2) in the patient's blood would increase, the level of consciousness would decrease, and laryngospasm would break spontaneously. Although this technique of managing laryngospasm is acceptable, it is not recommended for the untrained doctor.

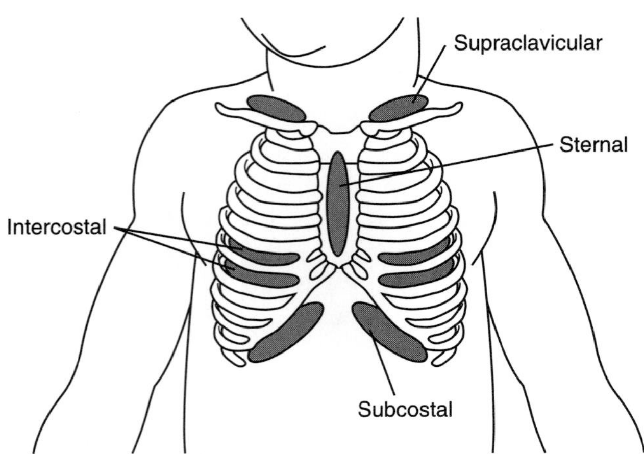

Figure 27-12 Retractions associated with respiratory distress: intercostal, supraclavicular, subcostal, and sternal.

Laryngospasm should not develop when lighter levels of sedation are maintained and the airway is kept free of debris, water, blood, and saliva.

SPECIFIC DRUG COMPLICATIONS

Benzodiazepines

The most commonly seen complications associated with diazepam and midazolam administration are as follows:

1. Local venous complications (diazepam only)
2. Emergence delirium
3. Recurrences of amnesia
4. Oversedation

Local venous complications and emergence delirium have been discussed previously. The recurrence of amnesia following diazepam administration has occurred only twice over 30 years in my experience; however, it was this phenomenon that caused me to decrease the recommended dose of diazepam used for sedation.

Two patients received diazepam, one a dose of 45 mg and the other a dose of 38 mg, and achieved clinically ideal sedation lasting for the usual 45 minutes. Recovery was normal, the patients appearing unsedated after 1 hour. It was later reported that for the first 24 hours after they left the clinic (these cases were done at different times and on different days) their recovery was normal. However, in both cases, approximately 24 hours later, the patients experienced a relapse of amnesia. One patient had driven to work, parked his car, and entered his office building when suddenly he did not remember where he was, how he had gotten there, or what day it was. Within a few minutes the patient's memory returned. No further relapses occurred. The same type of response occurred in the second patient. I am unaware of similar responses developing in patients who have received less than 30 mg of diazepam at a single treatment, thus the recommendation that this dose not be exceeded as a total for one treatment session.

Oversedation is unlikely to develop with diazepam or midazolam if the drug is titrated at the recommended rate of 1 ml/min. However, if a patient does become oversedated, management is to ensure a patent airway and ventilation (PAB). Within a few minutes redistribution of the drug leads to a lessening of the level of sedation and increased responsiveness. The administration of flumazenil will speed recovery (D).[25,26]

Pentobarbital

The most common problems associated with pentobarbital administration are oversedation and respiratory depression. Management of both situations requires implementation, as needed, of basic life support: position, airway, breathing, and circulation (PABC). No antidotal drugs are available to reverse barbiturate-induced oversedation or respiratory depression. Unfortunately, because of the prolonged duration of action of pentobarbital, it may take 30 minutes to an hour for the patient to become considerably more responsive.

Promethazine

Promethazine-related complications include oversedation and extrapyramidal reactions. Oversedation is managed through basic life support (PAB). There is no effective antidote for promethazine-induced oversedation or respiratory depression. Extrapyramidal reactions, although quite rare, do develop after promethazine administration. Four types of reaction are identified: akathisia (motor restlessness), acute dystonias, parkinsonism, and tardive dyskinesias. These are described in Chapter 7. Management requires administration of IV diphenhydramine, 50 mg for the adult and 25 mg for the child.

Opioids

The major side effects of opioid administration are nausea and vomiting, respiratory depression, and rigid chest. The first two complications are discussed earlier in this chapter.

Rigid chest is an uncommon phenomenon that has been observed primarily after administration of fentanyl but can develop with any opioid.[27-30] It is most commonly seen when N_2O-O_2 has been administered concomitantly.[31] In this situation the skeletal muscles of the thorax appear to be paralyzed and inflation of the chest is impossible. The cause of rigid chest is unknown. The patient will be unable to breathe. Efforts to force air into the patient will prove futile as the chest does not expand. The chest has a firm board-like feel during this reaction. Management of rigid chest involves the following:

1. The airway is supported, and an attempt is made to force O_2 into the lungs.
2. IV succinylcholine, 20 to 40 mg, is administered (only recommended for those trained in anesthesiology).
3. Following the release of the rigid chest (caused by the actions of succinylcholine), the patient will be apneic for approximately 3 to 5 minutes, during which time controlled ventilation is absolutely necessary.

TABLE 27-2 Percentage of Doctors Who Have Witnessed IV Complications*

	Malamed (n = 114)		*Trieger (n = 117)*	
	no.	%	no.	%
Hematoma	39	34.2	32	27.0
Infiltration	38	33.3	41	35.0
Pain on injection	29	25.4	50	42.0
Hyperexcitement	29	25.4	11	9.0
Thrombophlebitis	28	24.5	24	20.0
Prolonged sedation	19	16.6	12	10.0
Vomiting	16	14.0	8	6.0
Hypotension	12	10.5	11	9.0
Apnea	1	0.8	0	0.0
Arterial injection	0	0.0	3	2.5

From Malamed SF: *Anesth Prog* 28:158, 1981.

*The statistics illustrate the *number of doctors* who have seen the complication listed, not the *number of times* they have seen it occur. Therefore a doctor may have seen one case of vomiting in 5000 IV procedures, but because 16 of the 114 reporting doctors reported at least one case of vomiting, it is listed as a 14% incidence.

Rigid chest has been observed in conjunction with the fentanyl and N_2O combination. Use of this combination is therefore not recommended for routine use in outpatient sedation procedures. The use of combinations of techniques is discussed in Chapter 28.

Scopolamine

The major problem associated with scopolamine administration is emergence delirium, which was discussed earlier.

SUMMARY

Complications do occur during IV conscious sedation. Trieger[31] and Malamed[32] conducted independent surveys of doctors having completed basic IV conscious sedation programs to determine which complications did in fact develop most often. Table 27-2 presents their findings.

REFERENCES

1. Woodring JH, Fried AM: Nonfatal venous air embolism after contrast-enhanced CT, *Radiology* 167:405, 1988.
2. Trieger NT: *Pain control*, ed 2, St Louis, 1994, Mosby.
3. Philip JH: Intravenous access and delivery principles. In Rogers MC, Tinker JH, Covino BG et al, eds: *Principles and practice of anesthesiology*, St Louis, 1993, Mosby.
4. Shukla PC: Acute ischemia of the hand following intra-arterial oxymetazoline injection. *J Emerg Med* 13:65-70, 1995.
5. Ozel A, Yavuz H, Erkul I: Gangrene after penicillin injection (a case report), *Turk J Pediatr* 37:67, 1995.
6. Goldsmith D, Trieger N: Accidental intra-arterial injection: a medical emergency, *Anesth Prog* 22:180, 1975.
7. Lynes RFA, Bisset WIK: Intra-arterial thiopentone: inadvertent injection through a cannula on the back of the hand, *Anaesthesia* 24:257, 1969.
8. Topazian RG: Accidental intra-arterial injection: a hazard of intravenous medication, *J Am Dent Assoc* 81:410, 1970.
9. Myers RA, Schnitzer BM: Hyperbaric oxygen use, update 1984, *Postgrad Med* 76:83, 1984.
10. Gelfman SS, Dionne RA, Driscoll EJ: Prospective study of venous complications following intravenous diazepam and in dental outpatients, *Anesth Prog* 28:126, 1981.
11. Gelfman SS, Driscoll EJ: Thrombophlebitis following intravenous anesthesia and sedation: an annotated literature review, *Anesth Prog* 24:194, 1977.
12. Nordell K, Mogensen L, Nyquist O et al: Thrombophlebitis following intravenous lidocaine infusion, *Acta Med Scand* 192:263, 1972.
13. Chambiras PG: Sedation in dentistry, intravenous diazepam, *Aust Dent J* 17:17, 1972.
14. Watcha MF, White PF: Postoperative nausea and vomiting: its etiology, treatment, and prevention, *Anesthesiology* 77:162, 1992.
15. Blaise GA, Nugent M, McMichan JC et al: Side effects of nalbuphine while reversing opioid-induced respiratory depression: report of four cases, *Can J Anaesth* 37:794, 1990.
16. Pallasch TJ, Gill CJ: Naloxone-associated morbidity and mortality, *Oral Surg* 52:602, 1981.
17. Dosing and titration of midazolam (Versed), Letter to doctors, Nutley, NJ, 1987, Roche Laboratories.
18. Minichette J, Milles M: Hallucination and delirium reaction to intravenous diazepam administration: case report, *Anesth Prog* 29:144, 1982.
19. Olympio MA: Postanesthetic emergence delirium: historical perspective, *J Clin Anesth* 3:60, 1991.
20. Schneck HJ, Rupreht J: Central anticholinergic syndrome (CAS) in anesthesia and intensive care, *Acta Anaesth Belg* 40:219, 1989.
21. Rupreht J: The central muscarinic transmission during anaesthesia and recovery: the central anticholinergic syndrome, *Anaesth Reanim* 16:250, 1991.
22. Physostigmine: drug package insert, Forest Pharmaceuticals, 1998.
23. Odom JL: Airway emergencies in the post anesthesia care unit, *Nurs Clin North Am* 28:483, 1993.
24. Roy WL, Lerman J: Laryngospasm in paediatric anaesthesia, *Can J Anaesth* 35:93, 1988.
25. Longmire AW, Seger DL: Topics in clinical pharmacology: flumazenil, a benzodiazepine antagonist, *Am J Med Sci* 306:49, 1993.
26. Kulka PJ, Lauven PM: Benzodiazepine antagonists: an update of their role in the emergency care of overdose patients, *Drug Safety* 7:381, 1992.
27. Klausner JM, Caspi J, Lelcuk S et al: Delayed muscular rigidity and respiratory depression following fentanyl anesthesia, *Arch Surg* 123:66, 1988.
28. Vacanti CA, Silbert BS, Vacanti FX: The effects of thiopental on fentanyl-induced muscle rigidity in a human model, *J Clin Anesth* 3:395, 1991.
29. Ackerman WE, Phero JC, Theodore GT: Ineffective ventilation during conscious sedation due to chest wall rigidity after intravenous midazolam and fentanyl, *Anesth Prog* 37:46, 1990.
30. Neidhart P, Burgener MC, Schwieger I et al: Chest wall rigidity during fentanyl and midazolam-fentanyl induction: ventilatory and haemodynamic effects, *Acta Anaesthesiol Scand* 33:1, 1989.
31. Trieger NT: Teaching intravenous sedation: follow-up of 200 dentists, *Anesth Prog* 25:154, 1978.
32. Malamed SF: Continuing education in intravenous sedation. Part 2: complications and non-use, *Anesth Prog* 28:158, 1981.

CHAPTER 28

Practical Considerations

The following are frequently asked questions that relate to intravenous (IV) conscious sedation.

Who can start the IV line and administer IV drugs?

Many doctors wish to delegate the duties of venipuncture and drug administration to auxiliary personnel (i.e., dental assistant, registered dental assistant, dental hygienist, or registered nurse). Although the Dental Practice Act in each state must be consulted for specific regulations, it is law in most states that only the doctor (DDS or equivalent, MD) or certified registered nurse anesthetist (CRNA) may start a venipuncture and administer IV drugs. In some states, registered nurses (RNs) may perform venipuncture. As mentioned in Chapter 24, an auxiliary may perform virtually all of the duties relating to the IV conscious sedation procedure except for venipuncture and the administration of drugs.

What if the patient doesn't respond to the maximal dose of the drug?

The manner in which patients respond to drugs differs greatly, as evidenced by the normal distribution curve. The fact that titration is possible for essentially all intravenously administered drugs (lorazepam being a notable exception) permits us to determine exactly where the patient fits into this curve. Some patients are *hyporesponders,* in whom the clinically observed effect of a drug at its maximal recommended dose is less than ideal or, in fact, may be nonexistent. The most reasonable approach to take, when the maximal recommended dose of a drug has failed to produce adequate sedation, is to cease further administration of the drug and attempt the planned dental treatment. As mentioned earlier, I have been pleasantly surprised on numerous occasions with the ease with which treatment proceeds on an apparently nonsedated patient. If sedation is truly inadequate to permit the planned procedure to continue, the patient should be allowed to recover (despite the apparent lack of symptoms), discharged, and rescheduled at a later date for a different drug technique. For patients in whom diazepam has failed to produce adequate sedation, midazolam or the Jorgensen technique has almost always been successful at subsequent visits and vice versa.

Doses of drugs beyond those recommended should not be administered unless the doctor has completed training in anesthesiology. In many cases persons with this training will not administer additional drugs because the administration of other drugs can only prolong and complicate recovery in the ambulatory outpatient setting.

The drug doses and techniques recommended in this section have withstood the test of time. When they are used as recommended, the success rate of IV conscious sedation approaches 100%. The occasional failure will occur and must be accepted by the doctor. Inability to accept failure requires the doctor to inject larger and larger doses of more and more drugs, a situation potentially fraught with disaster.

Who should escort the patient from the dental office?

On occasion, usually once in a doctor's career, a patient's escort (ride home) will disappear or never show up. If the IV conscious sedation procedure has yet to begin I strongly urge that the procedure be canceled unless another suitable escort can be arranged *before the start of the procedure.* It is tempting and natural for the doctor to want go ahead with the IV procedure because of the time that has been allotted in the day's schedule. The doctor must resist such temptation.

Patients receiving diazepam or midazolam will appear quite recovered 1 hour after drug administration. In the absence of an escort, the patient may insist that he or she is recovered enough to be allowed to leave the office unescorted. *This must never be permitted to happen.* Explain to the patient that although he or she feels recovered this is not the case. The feeling is similar to that which occurs when one has had some alcohol and feels normal but cannot function at a normal capacity.

Alternative patient escorts that may occur to the patient or to doctor are taking a taxicab, a bus, or train; walking home; or being accompanied by a member of the office staff. None of these alternatives is acceptable. The only person who should be permitted to escort the patient home is a relative or close friend of the patient, a person who can remain with the patient until he or she has recovered. The dangers involved in these other alternatives are unacceptable. It is good practice for a member of the office staff to contact the patient the day before the scheduled IV procedure to review preoperative instructions, stressing the need for an escort.

What do you recommend when I first introduce IV conscious sedation into my office?

First, members of the office staff, especially chairside assistants, should attend the IV conscious sedation course so that they can learn the techniques firsthand. Very often, remarks made in a lecture are misconstrued, and an important concept may be improperly understood. Having several office personnel attending the course will decrease the chance of this occurring.

Second, the introduction of IV conscious sedation into a dental office does disrupt the normal routine of the office, at least temporarily. It is a new technique and must be used many times before it becomes a regular part of the practice routine. One must anticipate the extra time required during the first 50 or so cases. This can best be accomplished by scheduling IV cases immediately before lunchtime or as the last appointment of the day so that if they should become delayed, the doctor will not have to worry about a reception room filled with waiting patients. As the technique becomes more accepted by the office staff, IV patients can be scheduled earlier in the day when most apprehensive patients are more ideally treated.

I have more trouble with venipuncture than anything else. How can I become more proficient?

The hardest part of learning to do IV conscious sedation is to become adept at venipuncture. Administering drugs intravenously is easy (if basic rules are followed). However, without a needle placed within a vein, drug administration is impossible.

Practice makes perfect (almost). Unfortunately, most doctors do not wish to practice venipuncture on their patients. There are several possible places where one might improve his or her technique of venipuncture. A local hospital or blood bank might welcome volunteers to help draw blood. Volunteering 1 hour a week will greatly improve venipuncture technique.

What about the use of combinations of techniques?

Unless the doctor is experienced in general anesthesia or has extensive experience with IV conscious sedation, the use of some combinations of techniques is contraindicated. These include the combination of intramuscular (IM) and IV conscious sedation (absolute contraindication) and the combination of inhalation and IV conscious sedation (relative contraindication).

When nitrous oxide–oxygen (N_2O-O_2) is added to IV conscious sedation, the degree of patient monitoring must increase significantly because the patient may drift in and out of deeper levels of sedation as the stimulation of the treatment changes. Without the training suggested, I do not believe that this combination of techniques should be used.

There are but few indications for the use of IM and IV conscious sedation together. One is the use of an IM injection for the induction of sedation in a disruptive child or disruptive adult patient who has a disability, after which an IV line is established and used for the administration of any additional drugs (see Chapters 35 and 38).

Oral sedation can be used effectively with IV conscious sedation provided that the level of sedation achieved by the oral route remains light (see Chapter 7). Oral drugs are administered the night before the appointment and/or immediately (60 minutes) before treatment in order to take the edge off the last few minutes. Oral drugs should not be used for deep sedation. When the IV line is established, as long as the IV drug is titrated, there should be no problem associated with this combination of techniques. Failure to titrate (i.e., administration of a fixed dose of drug) increases the risk of oversedation and respiratory depression or arrest.

Do I have to titrate IV drugs?

Only if you do not want problems. Fixed drug combinations are frequently mentioned in legal depositions where morbidity or mortality has occurred. A statement frequently heard is, "But I gave this same dose of drugs to 10,000 other patients without ever having a problem." Unfortunately, patient number 10,001 was on the hyperresponding side of the bell-shaped curve, and this "usual" dose was too much for this patient. Titration is a safety feature that must always be used.

Is IV sedation safe?

This is a very interesting and provocative question. Newspapers publish lurid accounts of deaths occurring in dental offices.[1-3] Often, these patients have received IV drugs; whether they received IV conscious sedation or general anesthesia is not often stated. If we were to listen solely to the newspaper account, we would have to say that intravenously administered drugs are dangerous. The fact of the matter is quite the opposite. When IV conscious sedation is implemented *as taught,* it is the safest of all techniques of parenteral drug administration, with the exception of inhalation sedation with N_2O-O_2. The degree of control maintained by the administrator over intravenously administered drugs is second only to that available with inhalation sedation.

If the techniques described in this book are followed and the doctor does not experiment with increased dosages or administer drugs with which he or she is unfamiliar or unprepared to use, then serious problems will not occur. In a review of deaths in dental offices related to anesthesia (a general term implying the use of drugs of any type), The Dentists Insurance Company of California (TDIC) stated that three factors were present in most instances where death or serious morbidity occurred[4]:

1. Inadequate preoperative evaluation of the patient
2. Lack of knowledge of the pharmacology of the drugs being administered
3. Inadequate monitoring during the procedure

Education of the doctor and staff can eliminate these sources of problems. Although no long-term studies have been published regarding morbidity and mortality associated with IV conscious sedation, several papers have been published from which numbers can be extrapolated. Although scientifically not valid, these numbers do illustrate the safety of the basic techniques discussed in this section. More than 3000 IV diazepam, midazolam, and Jorgensen techniques have been completed without any significant complication during the 17 years of the Basic Intravenous Sedation Course at the University of Southern California School of Dentistry. In a survey of 188 doctors who completed this course, it was found that they had completed more than 53,664 cases in private practice without any serious complications.[5] After 6 years of presenting a similar course at the University of Oregon, Foreman et al.[6] reported that no complications of a serious nature had been encountered during any of their courses. Extrapolation from the data presented by Foreman et al. suggests that IV conscious sedation has been successfully used more than 37,960 times by doctors completing their course.

In a 1975 study published in *The Journal of the American Dental Association,* Jastak and Paravecchio[7] analyzed 1331 cases of sedation and reported that "the safety of IV conscious sedation was also good although not quite as complication free as N_2O-O_2. However, as with N_2O-O_2 sedation, there were no incidents of hypoxia, aspiration, laryngospasm, or other serious sequelae." In their conclusion they stated, "The safety and efficacy of intravenous, oral, combination, and especially inhalation sedation given by individuals not formally trained in general anesthesia appears to have been confirmed."

At the Loma Linda School of Dentistry, where IV conscious sedation in dentistry got its start, more than 15,000 Jorgensen techniques have been successfully performed since 1965 without any serious complications.[8]

REFERENCES

1. Maxwell E: Third patient of dentist being probed dies, *Los Angeles Times*, February 20, 1983, p 1.
2. Newcomer K: Dentist waited outside while patient died, Denver, *Rocky Mountain News,* August 4, 1992.
3. Marks P: Boy lapses into coma after dental surgery, *New York Times* May 14, 1993, p B5(L).
4. DeJulien LF: Causes of severe morbidity/mortality cases, *Can Dent Assoc J* 11:45, 1983.
5. Malamed SF: Continuing education in intravenous sedation: part 2, complications and non-use, *Anesth Prog* 28:158, 1981.
6. Foreman PA, Donaldson D, Jastak JT et al: Continuing education in intravenous sedation, *Anesth Prog* 29:163, 1982.
7. Jastak JT, Paravecchio R: An analysis of 1331 sedations using inhalation, intravenous, or other techniques, *J Am Dent Assoc* 91:1242, 1975.
8. Anderson D: Personal communication, May 1988.

CHAPTER 29

Guidelines for Teaching

Education and experience are the critical elements that make intravenous (IV) conscious sedation safe. New drugs, equipment, and monitoring devices become available almost every year, and it is only through continuing education that it is possible for the doctor to evaluate these items properly, some of which are initially touted by their developers as panaceas.

In 1977 the American Dental Association (ADA), American Dental Society of Anesthesiology (ADSA), and the American Association of Dental Schools (AADS) convened a conference at which *Guidelines for Teaching the Comprehensive Control of Pain and Anxiety in Dentistry,* Part III, were developed for a continuing education program.[1,2] These guidelines have undergone periodic revision, most recently in July 1993.[3] Sections of Part III of the guidelines ("Teaching the Comprehensive Control of Pain and Anxiety in a Continuing Education Program") relating to inhalation sedation were presented in Chapter 19. Material pertaining to continuing education in intravenous (IV) sedation is presented here.

In the section on *objectives* of an intensive course in conscious sedation techniques it is stated:

Upon completion of a course in parenteral techniques of conscious sedation, the dentist should be able to:

a. Describe and demonstrate the technique of venipuncture or any other parenteral technique chosen for the patient.
b. Discuss the pharmacology of the drug(s) selected for administration.
c. Discuss the precautions, contraindications, and adverse reactions associated with the drug(s) selected.
d. Administer the selected drug(s) parenterally to dental patients in a clinical setting in a safe and effective manner.
e. List the complications associated with parenteral techniques of sedation.
f. Discuss the prevention, recognition, and management of these complications.
g. Describe a protocol for management of emergencies in the dental office.
h. List the emergency drugs and equipment required for management of life-threatening situations.
i. Discuss the use of these emergency drugs and equipment in specific life-threatening situations.
j. Discuss principles of advanced cardiac life support (ACLS). Certification in ACLS should be encouraged.
k. Demonstrate the ability to manage life-threatening emergency situations, including cardiopulmonary resuscitation.

The following information related to IV conscious sedation programs was presented later in the document in a discussion of *course content:*

Additional course content for parenteral conscious sedation programs should include:

a. Venipuncture: anatomy, armamentarium, and technique.
b. Sterile techniques in intravenous therapy.
c. Prevention, recognition, and management of local complications of venipuncture.
d. Description and rationale for the technique to be employed.
e. Prevention, recognition, and management of systemic complications of intravenous sedation, with particular attention to airway maintenance and support of the respiratory and cardiovascular systems.
f. Abuse potential of parenteral agents.

The *Guidelines* also address the length of the training programs in parenteral conscious sedation:

Parenteral conscious sedation instruction: A minimum of 60 hours of instruction, plus management of at least 20 patients per participant, is required to achieve competency in parenteral conscious sedation techniques. Clinical experience in managing a compromised airway is critical to the prevention of life-threatening emergencies. Participants should be provided supervised opportunities for clinical experience to demonstrate competence in management of the airway. Typically, clinical experience will be provided in managing healthy adult patients. Additional supervised experience is necessary to prepare participants to manage children and medically compromised adults. The faculty should schedule participants to return for additional experience if competency has not been achieved in the time allotted.

In recent years several specialty groups within dentistry have developed guidelines for their members that propose standards for the use of sedation. These groups include oral and maxillofacial surgery,[4,5] pediatric dentistry,[6,7] and periodontology.[8]

Until the early 1980s I presented a continuing education program in basic IV conscious sedation that was 5 days in length (35 hours). The success of this course was apparent, as more than 75% of doctors participating in the program still used IV conscious sedation in their practices 1 year after the program.[9,10] In a survey of these doctors it was determined that in no instance did any doctor encounter a serious emergency situation related to the administration of IV medications.[9]

However, because of a number of well-publicized unfortunate occurrences (usually involving doctors who had received little or, more commonly, no formal training in parenteral sedation or general anesthesia), it became more and more obvious that the length and depth of training in these valuable techniques had to be increased so as to enhance patient safety. As of May 29, 2001, all 50 states had adopted legislation or regulations that govern the administration of parenteral sedation.[11] In addition, at least six provinces in Canada have enacted similar regulations (Canadian Dental Association, *personal communication,* 2002).

In some extreme instances a doctor must complete a 1-year residency in anesthesiology to be eligible to administer IV conscious sedation. Other states and provinces have established less restrictive requirements based on the educational and clinical background of the doctor.

The 1- to 2-day short course in IV conscious sedation is a thing of the past. They served only to scare the doctor away from this technique or to create a potentially very dangerous person: *a doctor who thought he or she knew how to properly administer IV drugs.* Training programs, at all levels of education—doctoral (dental school), postdoctoral (residency programs), and continuing education—have been expanded to meet the growing needs of the dental profession and the dental patient.[3]

Training in IV conscious sedation, at all three levels, at the University of Southern California School of Dentistry has been expanded to a program involving approximately 174 hours. The program includes four modules that must be completed sequentially:

Module 1 consists of four prerequisite courses that must be completed before acceptance into module 2. These are courses in physical evaluation (7 hours), emergency medicine (7 hours), monitoring and the use of emergency equipment (7 hours), and basic life support (healthcare provider; 7 hours).

Module 2 is a 35-hour program in basic IV conscious sedation in which venipuncture and basic techniques of IV conscious sedation are presented. Clinical patient management is included in this module.

Module 3 (IV conscious sedation study club) provides additional experience with clinical management of patients receiving IV drugs in a supervised clinical environment. At the conclusion of modules 2 and 3 it is expected that the doctor will have completed a minimum of 20 cases of IV conscious sedation under direct supervision.

Module 4 permits the doctor to receive clinical experience in airway management of the unconscious patient (80 hours). Doctors use the operating room or outpatient general anesthesia facilities to gain hands-on experience in these invaluable and lifesaving procedures.

Following completion of the four modules it is anticipated that the doctor will begin to use IV conscious sedation in the practice of dentistry. A voluntary "certification" program has been established, which a doctor may take advantage of at this time. To receive certification in IV conscious sedation from the University of Southern California School of Dentistry, the doctor must document 50 cases of IV conscious sedation (including those performed under supervision), successfully complete both a written and oral examination in subjects relating to anesthesia (e.g., physical evaluation, emergency medicine, monitoring, pharmacology, technique), and successfully undergo an in-office evaluation in which both the doctor and staff will be observed in their management of IV conscious sedation and of staged emergency situations. It has been our experience that doctors successfully completing this intensive course of study are well trained in all aspects of the safe and effective administration of drugs via the IV and intramuscular routes and have no difficulty in receiving certification from the state or province in which they practice dentistry.

REFERENCES

1. American Dental Association, Council on Dental Education: Guidelines for teaching the comprehensive control of pain and anxiety in dentistry, *J Dent Educ* 36:62, 1972.
2. American Dental Society of Anesthesiology: Guidelines for the teaching of pain and anxiety control and management of related complications in a continuing education program, part III, *Anesth Prog* 26:51, 1979.
3. American Dental Association, Council on Dental Education: *Guidelines for teaching the comprehensive control of pain and anxiety in dentistry,* Chicago, 1993, The Association.
4. American Association of Oral and Maxillofacial Surgeons, Committee on Anesthesia: *Office anesthesia evaluation manual,* ed 4, Rosemont, Ill, 1991, The Association.
5. American Association of Oral and Maxillofacial Surgeons: Parameters of care for oral and maxillofacial surgery: a guide for practice, monitoring and evaluation (AAOMS parameters of care–92), *J Oral Maxillofac Surg* 50(suppl 2):1, 1992.
6. Committee on Drugs: Guidelines for monitoring and management of pediatric patients during and after sedation for diagnostic and therapeutic procedures, *Pediatrics* 89:1110, 1992.
7. American Academy of Pediatric Dentistry: Guidelines for the elective use of conscious sedation, deep sedation, and general anesthesia in pediatric patients, revised May 1998. *Pediatr Dent* 21:58, 1999.
8. American Academy of Periodontology, Research, Science, and Therapy Committee: *Guidelines for the use of conscious sedation in periodontics,* Chicago, 1992, The Academy.
9. Malamed SF: Continuing education in intravenous sedation: part 2, complications and non-use, *Anesth Prog* 28:158, 1981.
10. Malamed SF: Continuing education in intravenous sedation: survey of 188 dentists, *Anesth Prog* 28:33, 1981.
11. American Dental Association, Department of State Government Affairs, Chicago, 2000, The Association.

SECTION VI

GENERAL ANESTHESIA

General anesthesia has been an important part of dentistry ever since 1844, when Horace Wells first used nitrous oxide (N_2O) to induce the loss of consciousness. General anesthesia was for many years an integral part of the pain-control armamentarium of dentists, primarily because other techniques of pain control were less well developed. With the introduction of local anesthetics (cocaine) in the 1870s and their steady improvement in the 1900s with the introduction of procaine, and later of the amides in the 1940s, the need for general anesthesia as a primary means of achieving pain control during dental treatment has diminished. A second need for general anesthesia was in the management of dental fears and anxieties. For well over 100 years general anesthesia was the primary technique used for this purpose. With the introduction of newer drugs capable of relieving anxiety without inducing the loss of consciousness, our ability to manage dental fears through conscious sedation techniques increased dramatically, further diminishing the role of general anesthesia in the practice of dentistry.

Despite the decreased reliance placed on general anesthesia in contemporary dentistry, several significant indications for its use remain. These are discussed in Chapter 30. The dental profession has been a leader in the development of general anesthesia from the early days of Horace Wells and William Morton to the more recent advances in the field of outpatient general anesthesia.

I have taken the liberty of categorizing general anesthesia in the following three groups:

1. Outpatient general anesthesia using intravenous (IV) agents
2. Outpatient general anesthesia using conventional general anesthetic agents
3. Inpatient general anesthesia

As becomes clear later in this section, the techniques of general anesthesia are not amenable to teaching in a short course. Extensive training must be obtained by the doctor who contemplates using general anesthesia. The ability to render patients unconscious, safely maintain them in that state during dental treatment, and then to return them to a normal state of functioning requires at least 2 years of full-time training in an anesthesiology residency or its equivalent during an oral and maxillofacial surgery residency program. In addition to the 2 years of training, it is becoming increasingly commonplace for individual state boards of dental examiners to require the doctor to obtain a special license or permit before being allowed to use general anesthesia. As of July 2001, all 50 states required such licensure.[1]

Many excellent textbooks are available on the subject of general anesthesia. These books should be consulted by the doctor who is interested in this technique. In the two chapters comprising this section the indications for general anesthesia in dentistry as well as some of the drugs and techniques used are presented. General anesthesia does indeed form a very valuable technique for the spectrum of pain and anxiety control in both dentistry and medicine.

REFERENCE

1. American Dental Association, Department of State Government Affairs, Chicago, 2001.

CHAPTER 30

Fundamentals of General Anesthesia

CHAPTER OUTLINE

General anesthesia has been defined as a reversible state of unconsciousness produced by anesthetic agents with loss of the sensation of pain over the entire body.[1] Pallasch[2] described general anesthesia as "hypnosis (sleep or loss of consciousness) accompanied by the loss of protective laryngeal reflexes (cough). Ideally, general anesthesia represents the simultaneous presence of analgesia (loss of pain), amnesia (loss of memory) and hypnosis along with reflex inhibition and loss of skeletal muscle tone which allows for safe surgical procedures." When the central nervous system (CNS) is depressed to the extent that consciousness is lost, changes occur in the physiology of the patient that would be life threatening in the absence of a "guardian" trained in the management of the unconscious patient. These changes include partial or complete airway obstruction, hypoxia, hypercapnia, loss of the ability to clear the tracheobronchial tree, respiratory depression, blood gas and pH changes, cardiovascular depression, and depressed or absent protective reflexes.

Since the introduction of the techniques of conscious and deep sedation into clinical practice, the requirement for general anesthesia has diminished. Conscious sedation possesses a number of advantages, not the least of which is the retention of consciousness as well as the ability of the patient to maintain his or her airway and protective reflexes. One of the inherent dangers of general anesthesia is that these three factors are lost, making it the obligation of the anesthesiologist to provide a patent airway and to protect the patient during the period of unconsciousness.

Several types of general anesthesia are recognized. The most frequent use of general anesthesia in dentistry is within the specialty of oral and maxillofacial surgery. The oral and maxillofacial surgeon has been responsible, in large part, for the development of outpatient or ambulatory general anesthesia using intravenous (IV) drugs, originally barbiturates (termed *ultralight general anesthesia,* where the patient is maintained in Guedel stage II of anesthesia) or conventional general anesthetic agents (with the patient maintained in Guedel stage III of anesthesia). As hospital costs continue to rise, ambulatory general anesthesia has gained popularity within the medical profession. The dentist anesthesiologist, a dentist trained in anesthesiology (minimum of 2 years), has made ambulatory general anesthesia available to patients requiring non–oral-surgical dental care, such as periodontics, endodontics, implants, and restorative procedures.

A third type of general anesthesia available to the dental patient is traditional inpatient general anesthesia. Be the anesthesiologist a dentist or a physician, the patient is admitted into the hospital and brought to the operating theater, where general anesthesia is induced and the dental procedure completed. The dentist doing the dentistry need not be trained in general anesthesia for this type of anesthesia to be used because the anesthesiologist assumes responsibility for inducing and maintaining the appropriate depth of anesthesia. Each of these types of general anesthesia is described in Chapter 31.

ADVANTAGES

1. *Patient cooperation is not absolutely essential for the success of general anesthesia.* One of the disadvantages of all sedative techniques is that some degree of patient cooperation is required in order for the administered drugs to produce the desired clinical effect (the inhalation route), to administer the drugs (IV), or to proceed with dental treatment. In situations in which loss of consciousness is the goal (general anesthesia), patient cooperation, although desirable, is not essential. The patient may, if necessary, be premedicated with intramuscular (IM) drugs with general anesthesia induced with inhalation anesthetics. Once the patient is unconscious, IV access is established and the anesthetic procedure continued in the usual manner.
2. *The patient is unconscious.* The loss of consciousness will be considered as both an advantage and a disadvantage (see following discussion). The fearful patient, the patient with a management problem, and the patient with a mental or physical disability can receive quality dental care in a well-controlled environment, be it a dental office or the operating theater of a hospital or an outpatient surgical facility (e.g., surgi-center). Dental care may be impossible to undertake or the quality of care significantly compromised with this patient still conscious.
3. *The patient does not respond to pain.* Although many general anesthetics possess either no or only minimal analgesic properties, the level of depression of the patient's CNS in general anesthesia prevents response by the patient to the nociceptive stimuli reaching the brain. There will be variation in this response depending on the level of CNS depression. Technically, therefore, there is no need for the administration of local anesthetics during some surgical procedures, including dentistry, performed under general anesthesia. However, it is strongly recommended that local anesthetics be administered during general anesthesia to prevent painful stimuli from ever reaching the brain. In this way the concentrations or volumes of general anesthetic drugs required to maintain a smooth, even level of general anesthesia will be decreased.

   During ultralight general anesthesia with IV barbiturates (e.g., methohexital or thiopental) or propofol, the use of local anesthesia is more critical to success. In this technique the level of unconsciousness (e.g., the depth of CNS depression) is kept minimal to hasten the patient's postoperative recovery. However, when this happens, the patient may respond to noxious stimulation during the dental or surgical procedure.

   To prevent this response two things may be done: The level of anesthesia may be deepened, or local anesthesia may be administered. Deepening the level of general anesthesia through administration of additional drugs prolongs the recovery period, which in outpatient settings is undesirable. Through the administration of local anesthesia, response to painful procedures is prevented both during the operative procedure and, equally important, in the postoperative period.
4. *Amnesia is present.* With loss of consciousness amnesia occurs. For extremely fearful patients, a lack of recall of events occurring during treatment represents the major indication for the use of general anesthesia or other techniques (e.g., IV) that provide amnesia. In cases in which amnesia is the primary requirement in a procedure, general anesthesia can usually be avoided. The use of IV conscious sedation with midazolam or diazepam is recommended in place of general anesthesia.
5. *General anesthesia may be the only technique that will prove successful for certain patients,* such as the precooperative child, extremely fearful adult, and certain patients with either physical or mental disabilities such as multiple sclerosis, cerebral palsy, Down syndrome, or autism.
6. *The onset of action of general anesthesia is usually quite rapid.* In general anesthesia, drugs are administered by the IV or inhalation routes, two routes with the most rapid onset of action. In most situations loss of consciousness will occur within 1 minute.
7. *Titration is possible,* with the patient receiving the smallest volume of drug required to produce the desired effect.

DISADVANTAGES

1. *The patient is unconscious.* Previously discussed as an advantage of general anesthesia, the loss of consciousness must also be considered a disadvantage because of the many changes occurring in the patient's physiology with the loss of consciousness. These changes are deleterious to the patient's well-being. As Trieger has stated, "Such care requires extensive education and training on the part of the doctor. The management of an individual who has lost his protective reflexes depends upon his anesthetist's ability to ensure his safety and survival."[3]
2. *Protective reflexes are depressed.* Loss of consciousness is accompanied by a progressive depression of the CNS and of protective reflexes. Because the dentist is operating in the oral cavity, the potential for debris, water, saliva, or blood entering the airway and producing airway obstruction or laryngospasm is greater in dental cases than with most other surgical procedures. One of the most important tasks of the anesthesiologist is to ensure the integrity of the patient's airway.
3. *Vital signs are depressed.* With the administration of general anesthesia, it is normal to see depression of the cardiovascular and respiratory systems. The administration of ambulatory general anesthesia for elective dental procedures to high-risk, medically compromised patients (American Society of Anesthesiologists [ASA] IV and some ASA III) is contraindicated, in part because of this property of general anesthetic drugs.
4. *Advanced training is required.* In no other technique discussed in this book is the requirement for postgraduate training as important (or as difficult to obtain) as it is for general anesthesia. The doctor (physician or dentist) who wishes to administer general anesthesia must have completed a minimum of 2 years of full-time training in anesthesiology.[4] All staff members participating in the administration of general anesthesia must also have received thorough training, although it need not be as extensive as that of the doctor. Lack of proper training or education on the part of personnel represents an absolute contraindication to the administration of general anesthesia.
5. *An "anesthesia team" is required.* For the administration of general anesthesia in a dental office, there should be an anesthesia team, consisting minimally of the anesthesiologist, an anesthesia assistant, and a circulating nurse. The doctor administering the general anesthetic must not also be responsible for performing the dental therapy. Division of labor by one person in anesthesiology can only lead to an increased risk of serious complications. Lack of enough, or inadequate training of, personnel represents an absolute contraindication to the administration of general anesthesia.
6. *Special equipment is required wherever general anesthesia is administered.* Monitoring of the unconscious anesthetized patient is of greater importance than it is for those who are sedated because in the absence of the ability to communicate with the patient (CNS depression), the only means of determining a patient's status is the level of functioning of various other systems of the body, such as the cardiovascular and respiratory systems.

   In addition to monitoring equipment, other equipment is required for the administration of general anesthesia, including a laryngoscope, endotracheal tubes, and oropharyngeal or nasopharyngeal airways. The absence of adequate equipment either for monitoring or the administration of general anesthesia represents an absolute contraindication to the use of this technique.
7. *A recovery area must be available for the patient.* Following general anesthesia of any duration or depth, an area must be available in which the patient may remain until he or she has recovered sufficiently to be discharged. This area must have equipment, including oxygen and a suction apparatus, and must be monitored continually while the patient is present. Lack of adequate recovery facilities represents an absolute contraindication to the administration of general anesthesia.
8. *Intraoperative complications are more likely to occur during general anesthesia than during conscious sedation.* The patient's physiology has been altered by the administration of CNS depressant drugs to a greater degree during general anesthesia than during conscious sedation. Complications relating to the cardiovascular and respiratory systems, such as hypotension, tachycardia, bradycardia, dysrhythmias, and respiratory depression, are more frequently encountered in general anesthesia.
9. *Postanesthetic complications are more common following general anesthesia than after conscious sedation.* Postanesthetic problems can include any of those mentioned in the preceding paragraph.
10. *The patient receiving general anesthesia must receive nothing by mouth for 6 hours before the procedure.* This is usually easily provided for when the patient is hospitalized but is less of a certainty in the outpatient environment. The presence of food or liquid in the stomach can lead to the

extremely dangerous occurrence of vomiting during anesthetic induction or regurgitation during the procedure, with the possibility of airway obstruction or tracheal burning or infection of the lung. This risk is negligible during sedative procedures.

11. *Patients receiving general anesthesia must be evaluated more extensively preoperatively than patients receiving conscious sedation.* Laboratory tests are frequently required before general anesthesia is administered. Urinalysis, complete blood count (CBC), and hematocrit and/or hemoglobin determinations may be obtained. In patients older than 35 years, a chest x-ray film and electrocardiogram (ECG) are usually required. Such extensive evaluation is not required (nor is it needed) for patients receiving conscious sedation.

CONTRAINDICATIONS

The following are contraindications to the administration of general anesthesia either in a hospital environment or in an outpatient facility such as a dental office or day-surgery center for elective dental care:

1. Lack of adequate training by the doctor
2. Lack of adequately trained personnel
3. Lack of adequate equipment
4. Lack of adequate facilities
5. ASA IV and certain ASA III medically compromised patients

The first four contraindications have been mentioned in the preceding paragraphs on the disadvantages of general anesthesia; however, they are of such great importance that they must be mentioned again. Under absolutely no circumstances should general anesthesia be administered in the absence of any one of these four vital ingredients. Specifics of each of these items are discussed later in this chapter and in Chapter 31.

With the fifth contraindication (ASA IV and certain ASA III medically compromised patients), some variance will be noted between the outpatient and inpatient forms of general anesthesia. Outpatient general anesthesia, regardless of the type, is generally contraindicated in all but ASA I, II and some ASA III patients. Other ASA III and all ASA IV patients should be admitted to the hospital with their dental needs cared for in the controlled environment of the operating theater.

The severely medically compromised patient will benefit from a more thorough preoperative evaluation when hospitalized before the start of treatment and from the more immediate availability of medical consultation and emergency care should the occasion(s) arise. Medically compromised patients are readily identified during the routine medical history and physical examination performed in the dental office. Other patients who may not be candidates for outpatient general anesthesia include the following:

1. Patients with a history of poliomyelitis in whom the chest muscles have been involved
2. Patients with a history of myasthenia gravis
3. Patients with significantly decreased cardiac and/or pulmonary reserve
4. Obese patients, especially those with short, thick necks, which will provide difficulty with airway maintenance
5. Patients with a history of malignant hyperthermia (hyperpyrexia)

INDICATIONS

1. *Extreme anxiety and fear:* Conscious sedation will prove to be effective in approximately 97% of fearful adult dental patients. In these patients there is little indication for general anesthesia. However, general anesthesia will be the only technique available for dental treatment for the remaining 3%. The type of general anesthesia will vary according to the nature of the planned dental treatment: ultralight general anesthesia for surgical procedures of short duration or outpatient general anesthesia using conventional general anesthetics for longer procedures involving other types of dental treatment. In some cases it may be prudent to hospitalize the patient and utilize the services of the anesthesiologist and operating theater in managing this patient.
2. *Adults or children who have mental or physical disabilities, senile patients, or disoriented patients:* The use of conscious sedation techniques in these patients may or may not be effective. When it is ineffective, general anesthesia is indicated. These patients commonly require many forms of dental care such as periodontics, endodontics, oral surgery, and restorative procedures, procedures that generally take longer to complete. It is suggested, therefore, that when conscious sedation techniques are unavailable or have proved to be ineffective, these patients be admitted to a hospital or an ambulatory surgical facility where they can undergo a more in-depth preoperative evaluation in addition to receiving the usual high standard of care during and after the anesthetic procedure. Many of these dental procedures can be completed on an outpatient basis, but the availability of inpatient facilities is recommended in case the patient should require an extended period of recovery. Management of these patients is discussed in Chapter 38.
3. *Age—infants and children:* The techniques of conscious sedation previously discussed may be of lit-

tle utility in the very young patient, primarily because of the patient's inability to cooperate. Oral, inhalation, and IV conscious sedation may be ineffective in these patients, whereas intramuscularly administered drugs will be somewhat more effective. In Chapter 35 the use of IM/IV midazolam is presented. This technique has been quite successful in managing this patient population.

When the patient is very young, general anesthesia will be of benefit to both the patient and the dental staff. The trauma involved in dental care is minimized with a properly performed general anesthetic. Dental care may be carried out in a more calm and controlled environment, with the patient's safety being ensured by the anesthesiologist.

Smith et al.[5] have estimated that between 2% and 5% of pediatric dental patients will require general anesthesia in order for their dental treatment to be completed successfully. Trapp[6] lists the two indications for pediatric general anesthesia as (1) the healthy patient who is unable to cooperate for office procedures after the standard management armamentarium has been exhausted and (2) the patient who is medically compromised (e.g., cerebral palsy, severe mental retardation) and unable to tolerate routine dental procedures.

4. *Short, traumatic procedures:* Procedures of short duration (less than 30 minutes) that are of a traumatic nature, such as the removal of four bony impacted third molars, may be an indication for the administration of ultralight general anesthesia utilizing IV barbiturates or propofol.
5. *Prolonged, traumatic procedures:* Whereas most adult dental patients are able to tolerate procedures requiring 1 or 2 hours to complete, some patients may be unable to tolerate these same, or much longer, procedures. Although there are alternatives to the use of general anesthesia in this situation (e.g., multiple shorter appointments), in some cases general anesthesia may be a viable option. Procedures of 4 hours or longer may be performed under general anesthesia in an outpatient setting.

Within the area of general anesthesia the following are indications for the administration of outpatient, versus inpatient, general anesthesia:

1. *Economics:* The use of outpatient general anesthesia has grown in the United States since the 1980s for several reasons. One of these is the decreased cost of outpatient procedures compared with identical inpatient procedures. Schmidt has stated that the cost of outpatient procedures is between 30% and 70% less than that of identical inpatient procedures.[7]
2. *Psychological benefits:* The major psychological benefit derived from outpatient general anesthesia is in the area of pediatrics, in which the trauma associated with separation of the child from his or her parents, as well as the strange environment of the hospital, may be minimized.
3. *Reduced exposure to nosocomial infections:* Steward has stated that outpatient general anesthesia in pediatrics results in a decreased incidence of infection because the patient has a reduced exposure to health professionals, hospital wards, and their associated pathogens.[8]
4. *Parental preference:* In surveys of the parents of pediatric patients, the overwhelming majority indicate their preference for outpatient general anesthetic procedures over inpatient procedures.[7]

TYPES OF GENERAL ANESTHESIA

The following variations of general anesthesia are used in dentistry:

1. Outpatient general anesthesia
   a. IV barbiturates or propofol (less than 30 minutes)
   b. Conventional operating theater–type general anesthesia (more than 30 minutes and less than 4 hours)
2. Inpatient general anesthesia

Outpatient General Anesthesia

Intravenous Barbiturates or Propofol. The administration of IV barbiturates or propofol to induce and to maintain unconsciousness has become an accepted and relatively common technique of general anesthesia. In dentistry it is used primarily in oral and maxillofacial surgery for relatively short procedures (usually less than 30 minutes), such as the removal of impacted third molars.[9] In what is known as *ultralight general anesthesia* (Figure 30-1), the most frequently

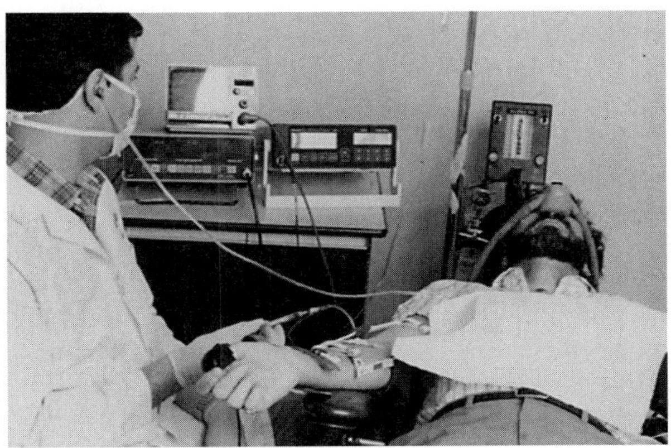

Figure 30-1 Ultralight general anesthesia employing an IV barbiturate, initial titration.

administered drugs are methohexital (Brevital, Brietal), thiopental (Pentothal), and thiamylal (Surital). Methohexital is by far the most commonly used IV barbiturate in this technique of general anesthesia. Propofol, a rapid-acting short-duration nonbarbiturate, has come to rival methohexital in popularity. Patient recovery from propofol is rapid and more complete than with barbiturates.

Patients receiving ultralight general anesthesia may, in addition, receive other drugs, including nitrous oxide–oxygen (N_2O-O_2), a benzodiazepine, opioids, and local anesthetics that assist in maintenance of a smooth level of general anesthesia. The benzodiazepine and N_2O-O_2 act to prolong the duration of the anesthesia and to potentiate the effect of the IV barbiturate or propofol, permitting a smaller dose to be used. In addition, the administration of O_2 minimizes the risk of hypoxia. Studies using pulse oximeters and end-tidal carbon dioxide (CO_2) monitors have demonstrated that some degree of hypoxia and hypercarbia is not uncommon during this form of general anesthesia unless supplemental O_2 is provided.[10] Local anesthesia is important, preventing noxious stimuli from reaching the brain, thereby minimizing the dosage of barbiturate (and other CNS depressant drugs) required, shortening recovery, and speeding the discharge of the patient. Postoperative pain control is also aided by local anesthetic administration, especially the longer-acting drug bupivacaine, in addition to either oral or parenteral nonsteroidal antiinflammatory drugs (NSAIDs).[11] The typical patient will remain pain free (from the local anesthetic) for from 6 to 12 hours after completion of the surgical procedure. The requirement for administration of opioid analgesics postoperatively is therefore minimized.

Lytle[12] and Driscoll, Herbert, and Batting[13] have reported on mortality rates from outpatient general anesthesia with IV barbiturates. The rates presented in these studies are approximately 1 death in 400,000 general anesthetic administrations, a figure that compares quite favorably with figures reported from hospital centers (see later). A more recent study provided similar statistics from Great Britain: a mortality rate of 1:338,536 for outpatient general anesthesia.[14]

The statistics from Great Britain appear to be more reliable than the others primarily because the numbers in the first two studies were extrapolations of data provided voluntarily by dentists, whereas the British numbers were based on reports from the Office of Population Censuses and Surveys, which is responsible for recording basic population data, including deaths, for England and Wales. Regardless of the source of information, it appears that outpatient general anesthesia in ASA I, ASA II, and selected ASA III patients administered by persons with adequate training possesses a remarkable safety record.

Conventional Operating Room–Type General Anesthesia. The second variety of outpatient general anesthesia is utilized for procedures ranging from 30 minutes to 4 hours or less. The patient undergoes the same general anesthetic preparation and procedure as does the inpatient. Facilities for anesthetic administration may vary from the dental office to an outpatient day-surgery facility to a hospital operating theater.

Because of the length of the dental or surgical procedure to be completed, this form of general anesthesia is usually limited to the ASA I, ASA II, and selected ASA III patients. ASA IV patients requiring general anesthesia for their dental care will be hospitalized before the procedure and remain hospitalized after the procedure.

The person administering the anesthetic must have completed training in anesthesiology (a minimum of 2 full years). This person may be a physician anesthesiologist, a dentist anesthesiologist, or a certified registered nurse anesthetist (CRNA). A dentist will be responsible for the dental care. In no circumstance may the same person administer the general anesthetic and perform the dental treatment.

Residency programs in anesthesiology for dentists are available, although the number is limited. Educational aspects of anesthesiology training are discussed in the following paragraph. The drugs and techniques used in general anesthesia are discussed in the following paragraphs and in Chapter 31.

The mortality rate associated with operating room–type general anesthesia in ASA I and II outpatients, administered by qualified persons, is equal to that for hospital inpatients.[7] Coplans and Curson[14] reported a mortality rate of 1 per 593,000 for hospital outpatient general anesthesia in which the general anesthetic was judged to be solely responsible for the death of an ASA I patient, and 1 per 148,000 in which both the anesthetic and the underlying disease (ASA II, III, and IV patients) were implicated. The incidence of hospital admissions as a complication of outpatient general anesthesia is less than 5%.[8,15] This complications rate is associated directly with the duration of the general anesthetic.[16,17] Because of the relationship between duration of anesthesia and the incidence of complications, it is recommended that the duration of an outpatient general anesthetic not exceed 4 hours.[8]

Inpatient General Anesthesia

The third form of general anesthesia is inpatient general anesthesia. The patient is admitted to the hospital before the planned procedure, is worked up to determine the potential risk of the surgery and anesthesia, undergoes the procedure, and then remains in the hospital at least 1 day postoperatively to recover and for her or his physical condition to stabilize.

In this situation the dentist need not be trained in anesthesiology. The anesthesiologist is responsible for the administration of the anesthetic for the planned procedure. The treating dentist should contact the anesthesiologist before the scheduled procedure to discuss any special needs or requirements. In many cases in which prolonged dental treatment is planned, the doctor will request that the patient be intubated through the nose (nasoendotracheal) rather than through the mouth (oroendotracheal) so that there is less danger of the dental procedure interfering with the patient's airway and vice versa.

Although it may appear at first glance that dental treatment is often a very "minor" procedure to be done under general anesthesia, especially compared with cardiac surgery, neurosurgery, or other forms of surgery, the truth is that the administration of general anesthesia for dental procedures is actually more difficult in many ways. This is because the oral cavity is always being used by the dental surgeon; therefore the potential for airway complications is increased. Many hospitals maintain a dentist anesthesiologist or a physician anesthesiologist who will administer anesthesia for all dental cases requiring general anesthesia. Familiarity with the peculiar requirements of this combination of surgery and anesthesia serves to increase patient safety.

Patients of any ASA classification may be admitted to the hospital for general anesthesia as inpatients; however, it seems prudent to limit this form of general anesthesia to ASA IV and selected ASA III patients and to any other patient for whom outpatient procedures are contraindicated or are not available.

Mortality rates for hospital inpatient anesthesia are somewhat higher than those for outpatient procedures primarily because of the difference in patient risk factor. Most ASA I and II patients are treated as outpatients when anesthesia is administered, whereas ASA III and IV patients are usually hospitalized. In the United States the anesthesia mortality rate in large teaching institutions is 1 per 1500, whereas in smaller nonteaching hospitals it is 1 per 9000. The surgical procedure most similar to a simple dental procedure is the removal of tonsils and adenoids (T and A). The mortality rate for this procedure in hospitals in the United States is approximately 1 per 40,000. The British study reported a general anesthesia mortality rate of 1 per 63,000 for hospital inpatients in cases in which the general anesthetic was solely responsible for the death of a healthy, ASA I patient and a mortality rate of 1 per 26,000 in cases in which the underlying disease and the general anesthetic was judged to be responsible.[14]

EDUCATION IN GENERAL ANESTHESIA

In no other area of patient management is thorough educational and clinical experience as important as in the administration of general anesthesia. Unlike most techniques of conscious sedation, it is impossible to teach general anesthesia in short courses. Education in general anesthesia requires not less than 2 years of full-time training of the dentist in an accredited anesthesiology residency or its equivalent during oral and maxillofacial surgery residencies.[4]

A number of dental anesthesiology residency programs are available, several of which have a long history of dental residents and tailor their training program to meet the specific requirements of the dental anesthesiology resident. A list of programs available as of July 2001 is presented at the end of this chapter in Table 30-1.

Guidelines Relative to the Establishment of a Dental Residency in Anesthesiology

In 1979 the American Dental Society of Anesthesiology (ADSA) established and approved the following guidelines[18]:

1. Trainee title: Dental Resident in Anesthesiology
2. Suggested qualifications of resident: Although this is not mandatory, it would be desirable for the resident to have satisfactorily completed a minimum of 1 year of previous hospital training, such as a general practice residency or an equivalent program in which training in hospital procedures and inpatient management is emphasized.
3. The training program must be full-time and be a minimum of 1 year's duration.*
4. Didactic and clinical program must be structured and resident schedule of duties clearly delineated.
5. The program should be a joint cooperative effort between the department of anesthesiology and the department of dentistry. Accordingly, support and cooperation of the director of anesthesiology is essential to establish and conduct a meaningful joint training program.
6. Instruction of both a didactic basic science as well as a clinical nature must be incorporated into the residency program. This instruction must be given in a seminar or conference format or may include formal courses.
7. The dental resident shall serve on an equal basis with the medical residents in anesthesiol-

*More recent guidelines require a minimum of 2 calendar years.

ogy. The programs shall include participation in all the usual duties of anesthesiology residents, including preanesthetic patient evaluation, administration of anesthesia in the operating room on a daily scheduled basis, postanesthetic care and management, and emergency call.

8. The resident's training must include significant experience in anesthetic management for ambulatory outpatient procedures, as well as the use of inhalation and IV sedation techniques. An optimum learning experience for these procedures would be provided in a hospital dental clinic that is properly equipped and staffed for the administration of general anesthesia for ambulatory patients.
9. Individuals responsible for training the resident(s) must include a qualified medical anesthesiologist and at least one qualified dentist who is a fellow in general anesthesia of the ADSA. In addition, the dental director of the program must hold fellowship status in the ADSA.
10. Clinical training should include training in a broad spectrum of pain-control techniques suitable for ambulatory patients. In addition, a clear understanding of pain and pain mechanisms should be developed.
11. The program must conform to that outlined in Part Two ("Teaching of Pain Control and Management of Related Complications at the Advanced Education Level") of the Guidelines for Teaching the Comprehensive Control of Pain and Anxiety in Dentistry as approved by the ADA Council on Dental Education and the Commission on Accreditation and endorsed by the ASA Committee on Manpower.[4]
12. Dental residents should be encouraged to take the annual In-Service Training Examination in Anesthesiology.
13. The Fellowship Committee of the ADSA will act in an advisory capacity with regard to these guidelines.

The availability of accredited training programs in general anesthesia for dentists has become increasingly important because all states in the United States have adopted regulations that act to restrict the use of this technique to qualified dentists. At the time of publication of the second edition of this textbook in July 1987, 37 states required special licensing for doctors using general anesthesia. By June 1993 this number had increased to 47.[19] Today, all states mandate special licensing for the administration of general anesthesia.[20] Although general anesthesia regulations vary, many states have proposed regulations limiting the administration of general anesthesia to doctors who meet one or both of the following criteria: (1) a licensed dentist who has completed a residency program in anesthesiology of not less than 2 calendar years that is approved by the Board of Directors of the American Dental Society of Anesthesiology for eligibility for the Fellowship in General Anesthesia or has a Fellowship in General Anesthesia or (2) a licensed dentist who has completed a graduate program in oral and maxillofacial surgery that has been approved by the Commission on Accreditation of the ADA.

The Fellowship in General Anesthesia of the American Dental Society of Anesthesiology is available to dentists and physicians who have completed at least 1 full year of anesthesiology residency in an accredited program or its equivalent in an approved oral and maxillofacial surgery residency program. At this time it appears that the fellowship has become an important means of defining adequacy of training in general anesthesia in dentistry. A second group, the American Society of Dentist Anesthesiologists (ASDA), composed of dentists who have completed 2 years of training in anesthesiology, has established a diplomate status recognizing expertise in the safe and effective administration of general anesthesia.

General anesthesia must never be taken lightly. The doctor who is considering the use of this valuable, but potentially dangerous, technique should explore the means of achieving at least 2 full years of residency training in general anesthesia.

ACCREDITED ANESTHESIOLOGY RESIDENCIES IN WHICH DENTISTS CAN ENROLL

Table 30-1 is a listing of programs that provide 2 years of training in anesthesiology for qualified dentists. This list was provided by the American Dental Society of Anesthesiology (ADSA) and the American Society of Dentist Anesthesiologists (ASDA) and is current as of January 2001.[21,22] It is suggested that persons interested in pursuing training in anesthesiology write directly to the chief of the dentistry department at the hospital of their choice.

The reader is directed to the ADSA and ASDA web sites for updated program lists:

The American Dental Society of Anesthesiology: www.adsahome.org

The American Society of Dentist Anesthesiologists: www.asdahq.org

TABLE 30-1 Accredited Dental Anesthesiology Residency Programs

Institution	Contact Name and Address	Telephone/Fax	Program Length
Loma Linda University	Dr. John W. Leyman, Director Dental Anesthesiology Residency Programs Loma Linda University School of Dentistry 11234 Anderson Avenue Loma Linda, CA 92350	Phone: 909-842-4611 Fax: 909-478-4106	2 years
University of California, Los Angeles (UCLA)	Dr. John Yagiela, Program Director University of California, Los Angeles Center for Health Sciences School of Dentistry Los Angeles, CA 90095	Phone: 310-825-9300 Fax: 310-825-3125	2 years
University of Medicine & Dentistry of New Jersey	Dr. Sanford Klein, Professor & Department Chairman Department of Anesthesia Robert Wood Johnson Medical School University of Medicine & Dentistry of New Jersey Clinical Academic Building, Suite 3100 125 Paterson Street New Brunswick, NJ 08901-1977	Phone: 908-235-7827 Fax: 908-235-6131	2 years
Long Island Jewish Medical Center	Dr. Martin R. Boorin, Program Director Department of Anesthesiology Long Island Jewish Medical Center 270-05 76th Avenue New Hyde Park, NY 11042	Phone: 718-470-7111 Fax: 718-347-4118	2 years
Mount Sinai Medical Center	Dr. David V. Valauri, Director of Dental Anesthesiology Mount Sinai Medical Center One Gustave L. Levy Place New York, NY 10029-6574	Fax: 212-996-9793	2 years
The Ohio State University	Dr. Joel M. Weaver, Director of Anesthesiology The Ohio State University College of Dentistry 2131 Postle Hall 305 West 12th Avenue Columbus, OH 43210	Phone: 614-292-5144 Web site: www.dent.ohio-state.edu/anesthesiology	2 years
Case Western Reserve University	Dr. Frank Ditzig, Clinical Director of Dental Anesthesiology Case Western Reserve University MetroHealth Medical Center 2500 MetroHealth Drive Cleveland, OH 44109	Phone: 216-459-4737 Fax: 216-778-8875	1 year, with optional 2nd year
University of Toronto	Dr. Daniel A. Haas, Program Director & Head of Anaesthesia University of Toronto Faculty of Dentistry Department of Anaesthesia 124 Edward Street Toronto, Ontario, M5G 1G6 Canada	Phone: 416-979-4922	3 years leading to MSc

Continued

TABLE 30-1 Accredited Dental Anesthesiology Residency Programs—cont'd

University of Pittsburgh	Dr. C. Richard Bennett, Chair University of Pittsburgh School of Dental Medicine G-89 Salk Hall 3501 Terrace Street Pittsburgh, PA 15261	Phone: 412-648-8606 Fax: 412-648-8219 Web site: anesthesia.dental.pitt.edu	2 years
Medical College of Virginia	Dr. Robert L. Campbell, Director Department of Oral & Maxillofacial Surgery Medical College of Virginia Box 566, MCV Station Richmond, VA 23298-0566	Phone: 804-828-0602	2 years
Johns Hopkins University	Dr. Jeffrey Kirsch Director, Resident Education Johns Hopkins University School of Medicine Department of Anesthesiology and Critical Care Medicine 600 North Wolfe Street/Blalock 1412 Baltimore, MD 21287-4963		2 years

REFERENCES

1. Snow JC: Intravenous anesthesia. In *Manual of anesthesia,* Boston, 1977, Little, Brown.
2. Pallasch TJ: *Pharmacology for dental students and practitioners,* Philadelphia, 1980, Lea & Febiger.
3. Trieger NT: *Pain control,* ed 2, St Louis, 1994, Mosby.
4. American Dental Association, Council on Dental Education: *Guidelines for teaching the comprehensive control of pain and anxiety in dentistry,* Chicago, 1993, The Association.
5. Smith F, Deputy BS, Berry FA Jr: Outpatient anesthesia for children undergoing extensive dental treatment, *J Dent Child* 45:38, 1978.
6. Trapp LD: Sedation of children for dental treatment, *Pediatr Dent* 4:164, 1982.
7. Schmidt K, ed: Outpatient anesthesia, *Int Anesthesiol Clin* 14:1, 1976.
8. Steward D: Outpatient pediatric anesthesia, *Anesthesiology* 43:268, 1975.
9. Rosenberg M, Weaver J: General anesthesia, *Anesth Prog* 38:172, 1991.
10. Jastak JT, Peskin RM: Major morbidity or mortality from office anesthetic procedures: a closed-claim analysis of 13 cases, *Anesth Prog* 38:39, 1991.
11. Acute Pain Management Guidelines Panel: *Acute pain management: operative or medical procedures and trauma, clinical practice guideline, AHCPR Pub No 92-2,* Rockville, Md, 1992, Agency for Health Care Policy and Research, Public Health Service, US Department of Health and Human Services.
12. Lytle JJ: Anesthesia morbidity and mortality survey of the Southern California Society of Oral Surgeons, *J Oral Surg* 32:739, 1974.
13. Driscoll EJ, Herbert CL, Batting CG: Research in anesthesia for ambulatory patients: practical considerations, *Trans Cong Int Assoc Oral Surg* 1970, p 538.
14. Coplans MP, Curson I: Deaths associated with dentistry, *Br Dent J* 153:357, 1982.
15. Smith F, Deputy BS, Berry FA Jr: Outpatient anesthesia for children undergoing extensive dental treatment, *J Dent Child* 45:38, 1978.
16. Fahy A, Marshall M: Postanaesthetic morbidity in outpatients, *Br J Anaesth* 41:433, 1969.
17. Steward D: Experiences with an outpatient anesthesia service for children, *Anesth Analg* 52:877, 1973.
18. American Dental Society of Anesthesiology: Guidelines relative to the establishment of a dental residency in anesthesiology, *Anesth Prog* 26:177, 1979.
19. American Dental Association, Department of State Government Affairs, Chicago, 1992, The Association.
20. American Dental Association, Department of State Government Affairs, Chicago, 2001, The Association.
21. American Dental Society of Anesthesiology: *Accredited dental anesthesiology residencies,* Chicago, 2000, The Society.
22. American Society of Dentist Anesthesiologists: *Dental anesthesia residency programs,* Holmdel, NJ, 2001, ASDA.

CHAPTER 31

Armamentarium, Drugs, and Techniques

CHAPTER OUTLINE

This chapter presents an overview of the equipment, drugs, and techniques that are vitally important to the success of general anesthesia. Many of the drugs discussed have been reviewed in depth elsewhere in this book and receive only the briefest of notice here. Other drugs are mentioned for the first time; however, their pharmacology is also reviewed briefly, for it is not the purpose of this chapter to provide the reader with a feeling that he or she is able to use these drugs safely after having read about them. As discussed in Chapter 30, this section is meant as an introduction to the vast subject of general anesthesia, not as a complete text in that area.

Following a review of the armamentarium and drugs, each of the major techniques of general anesthesia—outpatient general anesthesia with intravenous (IV) barbiturates, operating room–type outpatient general anesthesia, and inpatient general anesthesia—is discussed.

ARMAMENTARIUM

The equipment required for the administration of general anesthesia may vary according to the type of anesthesia being delivered. In general, the equipment for IV barbiturate general anesthesia varies somewhat from that required for other types of anesthesia.

The armamentarium for general anesthesia may be divided into the following five groups:

1. Anesthesia machine
2. IV equipment
3. Ancillary anesthesia equipment
4. Monitoring equipment
5. Emergency equipment and drugs

Anesthesia Machine

The anesthesia machine is able to deliver oxygen (O_2) and inhalation anesthetics to the patient. The inhalation sedation unit used in dentistry to deliver nitrous oxide–oxygen (N_2O-O_2) is a modification of the anesthesia machine used in the operating room. The primary difference between the two is the number of inhalation anesthetics the operating room unit is capable of delivering. As seen in Figure 31-1, the anesthesia machine can deliver many gases: N_2O, O_2, halothane, methoxyflurane, enflurane, isoflurane, and fluroxene. Flowmeters, as well as devices called *vaporizers* that contain the various volatile anesthetics and permit their concentrations to be controlled, are integral parts of the unit.

The anesthesia machine is capable of operating with O_2 and N_2O supplied from either a central cylinder system or portable cylinders mounted on the sides of the unit. In the operating room, many of the fail-safe devices used in dental inhalation units are not present. However, most anesthesia machines have O_2 monitors that sound an alarm if the unit fails to provide a preset minimum percentage of O_2 (i.e., 25%).

During IV barbiturate general anesthesia, an inhalation sedation unit, as discussed in Chapter 14, is used to supplement the patient's ventilation with O_2 and perhaps N_2O. In the other forms of anesthesia, a unit similar to that shown in Figure 31-1 is used.

The modern anesthesia machine also contains a number of important devices for monitoring patients receiving these agents. Attached to the anesthesia machine shown in Figure 31-1 are several monitors, including a blood pressure monitor, electrocardiogram (ECG), pulse oximeter, end-tidal carbon dioxide ($ETCO_2$) monitor, electroencephologram (EEG), and a temperature monitor. Attached to the right side of the unit is a ventilator, a device used to control or assist the ventilation of a patient during anesthesia.

Intravenous Equipment

A supply of equipment for venipuncture and IV drug administration is required during general anesthesia. A *continuous IV infusion* is recommended for all general anesthetic procedures. Winged needles are rarely used during general anesthesia, except perhaps for the shortest of procedures. Even then, however, *indwelling catheters* are recommended. The gauge of the venipuncture needle or indwelling catheter should not be smaller than 21 (for short procedures), with the 18-gauge needle being most commonly used for routine general anesthetic procedures and 16-gauge needles used whenever a transfusion of blood may be

A

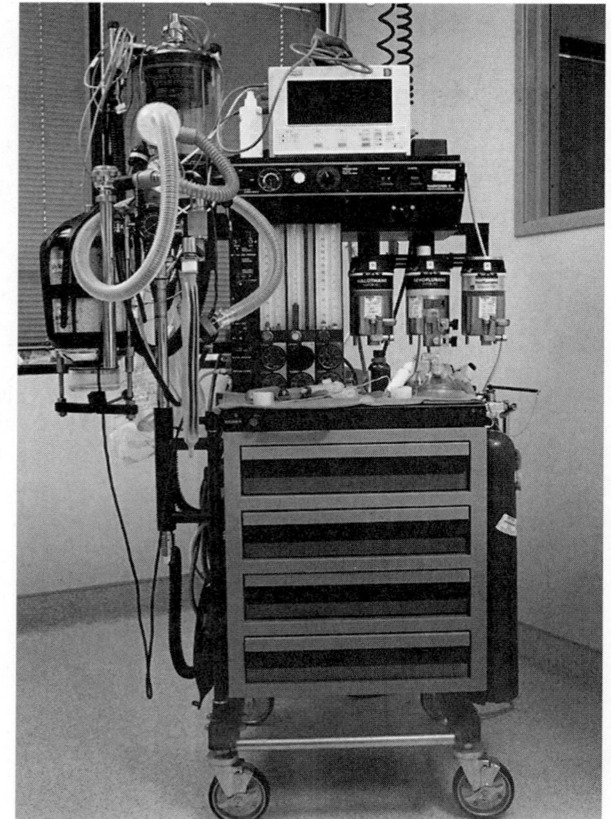

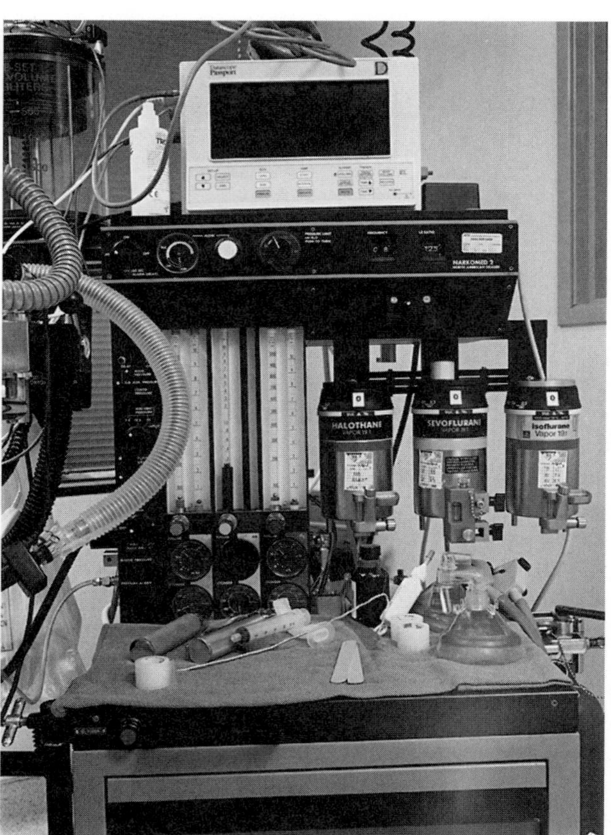

B

Figure 31-1 **A** and **B**, General anesthesia machine can deliver a variety of anesthetic gases and contains multiple monitoring devices.

required. An assortment of needles should be available.

Tubing and bags of IV solution are also required. During short procedures a 250-ml bag may be adequate; however, a 1000-ml size is usually recommended for all procedures lasting more than 30 minutes because of the possibility of the patient becoming hypovolemic as a result of a combination of having been NPO (nothing by mouth) before surgery, blood loss during surgery, and evaporation of fluids during surgery (especially where the abdominal or thoracic cavity is exposed). A variety of *disposable syringes* and *needles* should also be available as well as various *adhesive tapes* (e.g., paper, hypoallergenic).

Ancillary Anesthesia Equipment

The following items must also be available whenever general anesthesia is administered:

- Full-face masks in child and adult sizes and appropriate connectors
- Laryngoscope complete with adequate selection of blades and spare batteries and bulb
- Adequate selection of endotracheal tubes and appropriate connectors
- Adequate selection of oropharyngeal and nasopharyngeal airways
- Tonsillar suction tips
- Magill intubation forceps
- Child- and adult-size sphygmomanometers and stethoscopes

Face Masks. Face masks (Figure 31-2) are rubber or silicone masks that cover both the mouth and nose of the patient. Face masks are used to deliver O_2, N_2O-O_2, and/or other inhalation anesthetics before, during, and after the anesthetic procedure. Because of the variations in the size and shape of faces, several different sizes of full-face masks should always be available.

Face masks are frequently made of black rubber, which prevents the mouth and nose of the patient from being visualized. Much preferred is a clear plastic or rubber face mask that allows the patient's mouth and nose to be seen so that foreign material (e.g., vomitus, blood) may be observed and removed.

Metal connectors that attach the face mask to the tubing of the anesthesia machine are required. These connectors come in a variety of sizes and shapes.

Laryngoscopes. The laryngoscope (Figure 31-3) is a device designed to assist in the visualization of the trachea during intubation. It consists of two parts: a handle and battery holder, and a blade. The handle is usually made of metal (although some are made of plastic) and contains batteries that are used to operate the light bulb found in the blade.

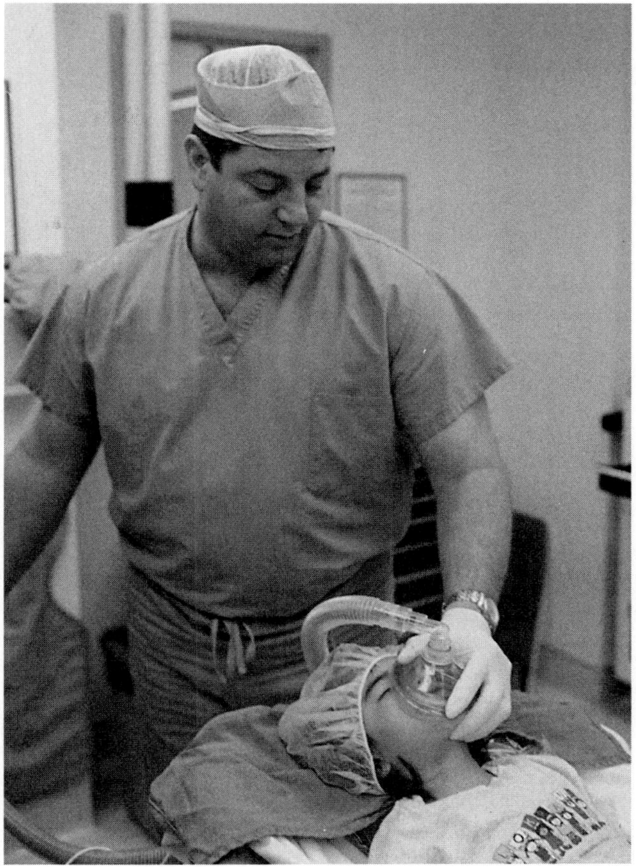

Figure 31-2 Full-face mask covers both the mouth and nose of the patient.

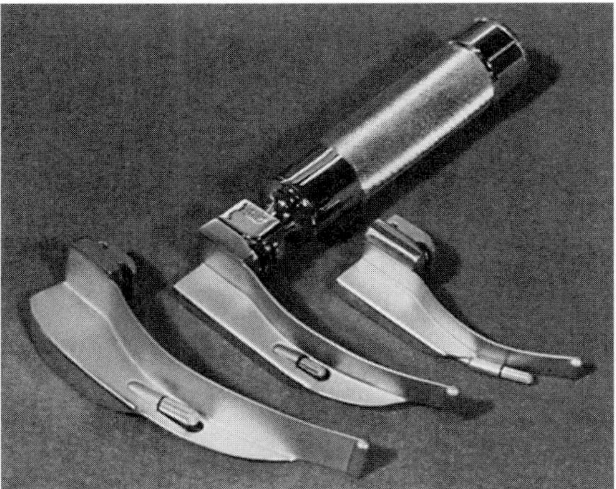

Figure 31-3 Laryngoscope handle and several sizes of curved blades.

The blade of the laryngoscope is also usually made of metal, although plastic is also used today. The laryngoscope blade is designed to be placed into the patient's mouth to aid in visualization of the larynx. A small light bulb that illuminates the laryngeal area is attached to the blade. There are two basic types of laryngoscope blade: the curved (Macintosh) and the straight (Miller) blade. Each of these blades is available in a variety of sizes. The technique for using these blades differs.

The curved blade is the more commonly used. The tip of the curved blade is inserted into the vallecula, the cul-de-sac between the base of the tongue and the epiglottis (Figure 31-4). The handle of the laryngoscope is then lifted straight up, a movement that exposes the vocal cords. When the straight blade is used, its tip is placed underneath the laryngeal surface of the epiglottis (Figure 31-5) and the larynx is exposed by an upward and forward lift of the blade.

Most laryngoscopes and blades are designed to be held in the operator's left hand, with the endotracheal tube held in the right. Special laryngoscope blades are available for left-handed operators.

Endotracheal Tubes and Connectors. Endotracheal tubes and connectors (Figure 31-6) are rubber tubes designed to be placed from the mouth (oroendotracheal) or nose (nasoendotracheal) into the patient's trachea. Reusable and disposable endotracheal tubes are available, with disposables being more popular today. Because the diameter of the laryngeal opening and of the trachea varies from patient to patient, endotracheal tubes are manufactured in a variety of diameters. Endotracheal tubes are commonly referred to by their size; for example, a no. 38 tube has an external diameter of 38 mm. For adult patients a no. 36 tube is usually appropriate for a man and a no. 34 tube for a woman. Smaller and larger tubes are available to accommodate the child or larger patient.

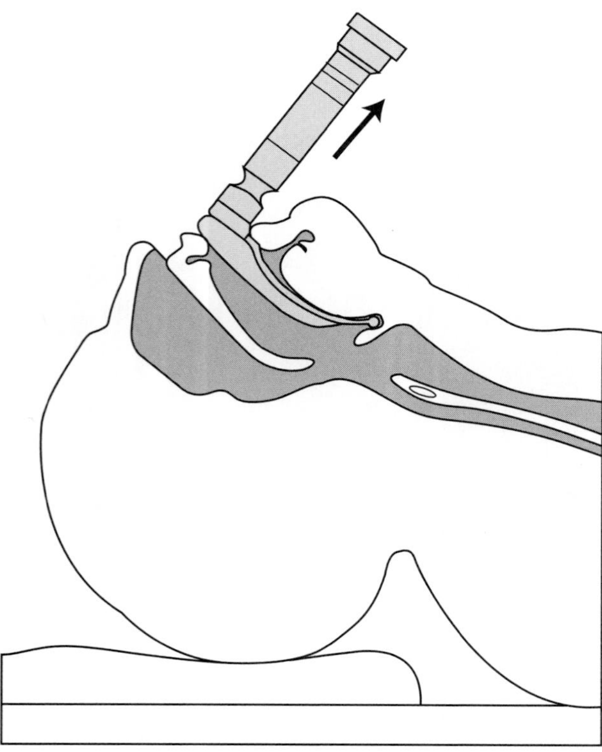

Figure 31-4 Curved blade is placed between the base of the tongue and the epiglottis. Laryngoscope is then lifted, elevating tongue and exposing larynx. (Redrawn from *Advanced cardiac life support manual*, American Heart Association.)

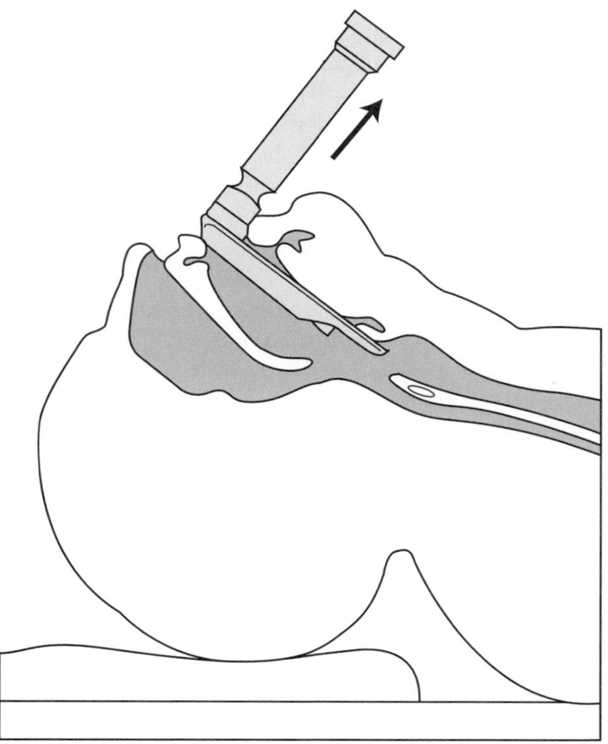

Figure 31-5 Straight laryngoscope blade is placed beneath epiglottis and lifted, thereby exposing larynx. (Redrawn from *Advanced cardiac life support manual*, American Heart Association.)

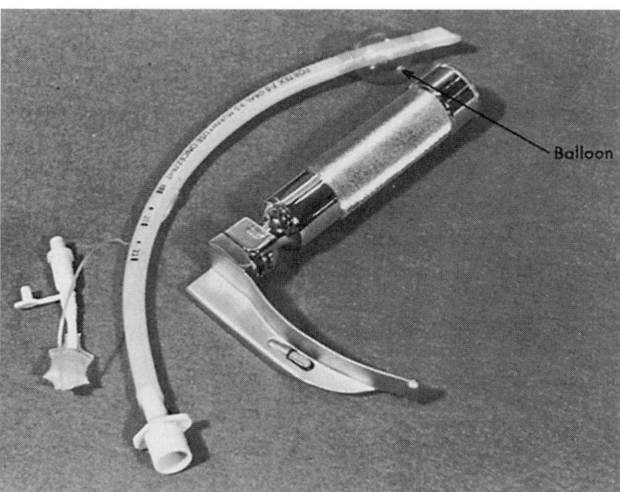

Figure 31-6 Laryngoscope and endotracheal tube. Distal end of tube has inflatable cuff *(arrow)* designed to provide an airtight seal, preventing entry of substances into the trachea.

Endotracheal tubes usually have an inflatable cuff (see Figure 31-6) located near their distal ends. When a patient is intubated, the endotracheal tube is inserted into the trachea so that the cuff disappears just beyond the level of the larynx. Air is then injected into a tube that connects with the cuff and inflates it. Enough air is injected into the cuff to seal the trachea off from the pharynx, thereby preventing foreign material, such as blood, saliva, or vomitus, from entering the trachea and bronchi.

Connectors for endotracheal tubes are the same as those used for full-face masks. They are used to connect the endotracheal tube to the anesthesia machine.

Oropharyngeal and Nasopharyngeal Airways. Oropharyngeal (Figure 31-7) and nasopharyngeal airways (Figure 31-8) are used to assist in maintaining a patent airway during and after the anesthetic procedure. Oropharyngeal airways are plastic, rubber, or metallic devices designed to fit between the base of the tongue and the posterior pharyngeal wall (Figure 31-9). The nasopharyngeal airway (also known as a nasal trumpet) is a thin, flexible rubber tube designed to be inserted through the nares and to rest between the base of the tongue and posterior pharynx (Figure 31-10). The purpose of both of these devices is to displace the tongue from the pharynx and thereby permit the patient to exchange air either around or through the airway. The nasopharyngeal airway is better tolerated by the patient, thereby minimizing the occurrence of gagging and vomiting. Nasal airways should be lubricated before their insertion to speed their placement.

Tonsillar Suction Tips. The immediate availability of suction devices is absolutely essential before general

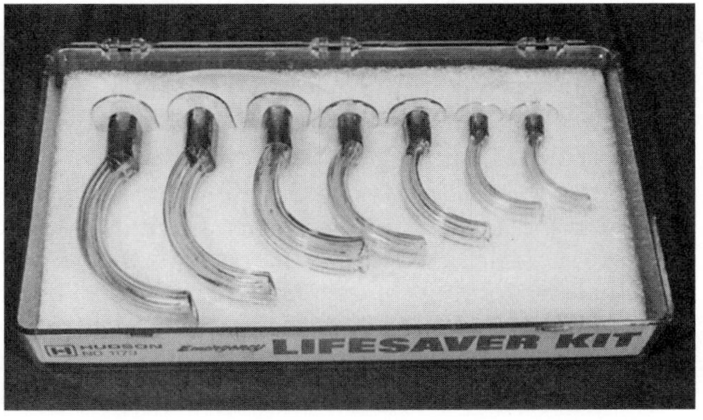

Figure 31-7 Oropharyngeal airways are available in a variety of sizes.

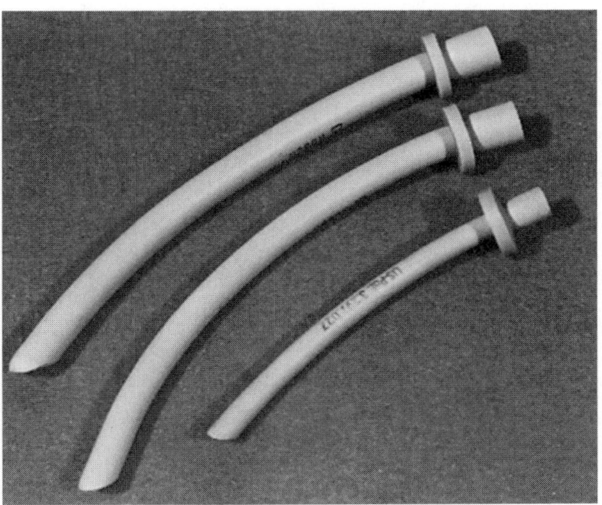

Figure 31-8 Nasopharyngeal airways.

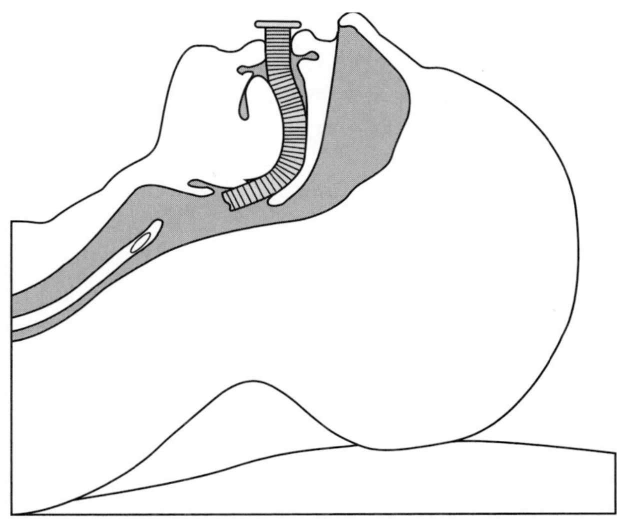

Figure 31-9 Oropharyngeal airway is designed to lift the tongue off the posterior wall of the pharynx.

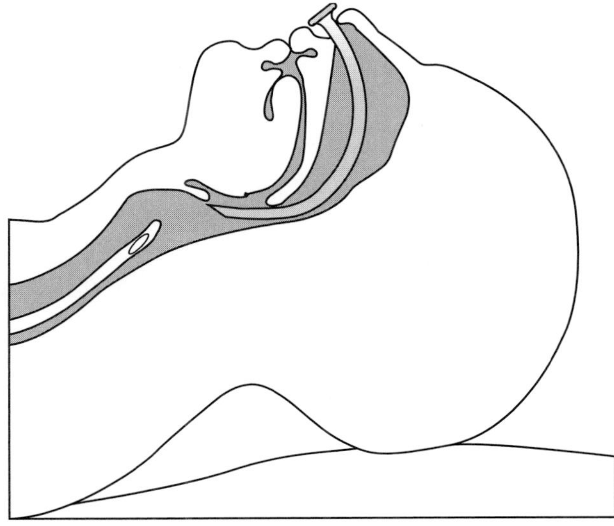

Figure 31-10 Nasopharyngeal airway is designed to rest between the base of the tongue and pharyngeal wall, thus permitting air to pass between the lungs and the nose.

anesthesia is started. Excessive salivation, bleeding in the mouth or pharynx, or vomiting can produce airway obstruction, laryngospasm, or possible infection of the trachea or bronchi. Tonsillar suction tips are recommended because they can be inserted blindly into the posterior pharynx of the patient without risk of producing bleeding. The end of the tonsillar suction tip is rounded, making this device preferable to others that have sharper tips. Several tonsillar suction tips should be available in the event that one becomes clogged.

Magill Intubation Forceps. A Magill intubation forceps (Figure 31-11) is designed to assist in placing the endotracheal tube. It is most frequently used during nasoendotracheal intubation and is therefore a very important item in the armamentarium for general anesthesia for dental procedures.

Sphygmomanometers and Stethoscopes. Sphygmomanometers and stethoscopes must also be available during general anesthetic procedures. They will be used for the monitoring of vital signs, specifically blood pressure, heart rate and rhythm, heart sounds, and breath sounds. Appropriate-size sphygmomanometers must be available if accurate blood pressure values are desired.

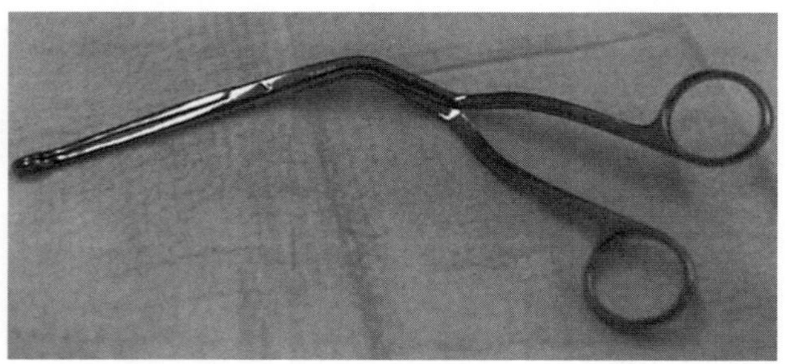

Figure 31-11 Magill intubation forceps are designed to assist in passage of an endotracheal tube, especially during nasal intubation.

Monitoring Equipment

Monitoring of the patient during sedation or general anesthesia is essential to the overall safety of the procedure. During sedative procedures monitoring of the central nervous system (CNS) via direct communication with the patient is of primary importance. Because the patient is able to respond appropriately to verbal command, other, more complex monitoring devices need not be used routinely.[1] However, once consciousness is lost (increased CNS depression), patients are unable to respond to command and other means of determining their status during anesthesia must be used. For this reason, the level of monitoring during general anesthesia is greater than that required for sedative procedures. A monitor is a device that reminds and warns. The Department of Anesthesiology at the Harvard University School of Medicine has designed monitoring guidelines for use during general anesthesia.[2] The recommendations in these guidelines have been well received and widely implemented. The following are some of the methods and devices used to monitor patients during general anesthesia:

1. The stethoscope is used with auscultation to monitor the heart rate, heart rhythm, and/or breath sounds. Taped to the chest in the precordial region, the *precordial stethoscope* (Figure 31-12) provides continuous monitoring of heart sounds, but when placed on the neck directly over the trachea, the *pretracheal stethoscope* permits

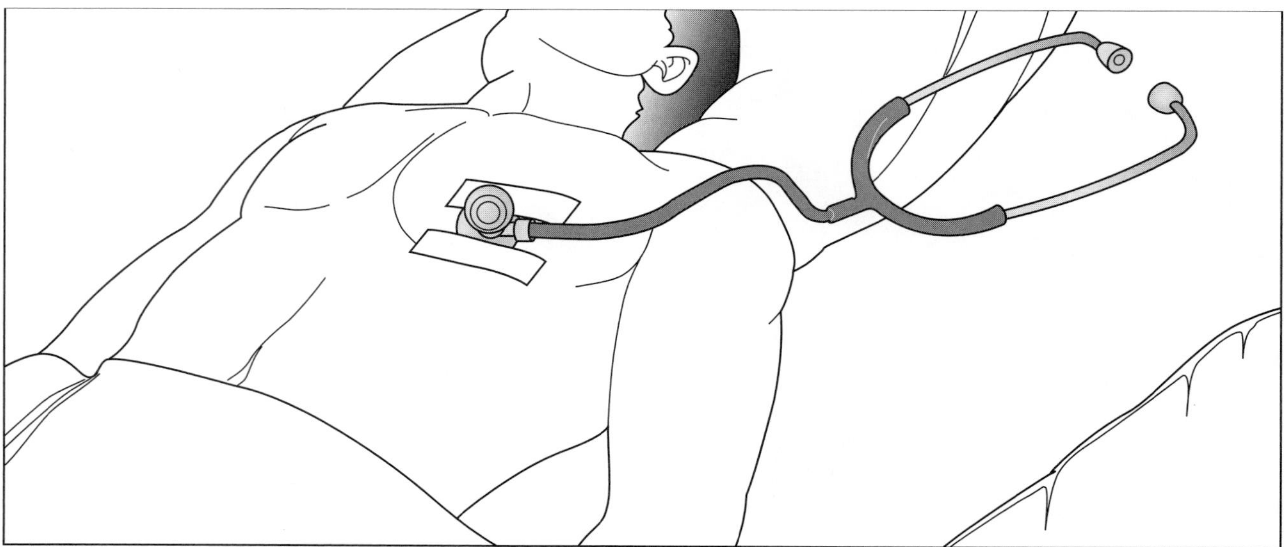

Figure 31-12 Precordial stethoscope.

monitoring of respiration. The pretracheal stethoscope is recommended for use during IV sedation procedures as well as during all forms of general anesthesia. An alternative to the precordial stethoscope during general anesthesia is the *esophageal stethoscope* (Figure 31-13), a rubber tube inserted into the patient's esophagus after intubation. This device provides continuous monitoring similar to that provided by the precordial stethoscope but is more effective because of its closer proximity to the heart and lungs. Breath and heart sounds can usually be heard more distinctly. Esophageal stethoscopes are not used during sedation procedures and brief outpatient general anesthetics.

2. The *pulse oximeter* (Figures 31-14 and 31-15) provides a noninvasive means of monitoring the degree of oxygen saturation of hemoglobin in peripheral blood vessels. Pulse oximeters provide continuous monitoring of oxygenation and of the heart rate, permitting a more rapid detection of potential airway problems (there is a time lag of about 20 seconds). The use of pulse oximetry is considered to be a standard of care during general anesthesia.
3. *$ETCO_2$ monitors* also represent standard of care in monitoring during general anesthesia. They evaluate the effectiveness of ventilation. Because the

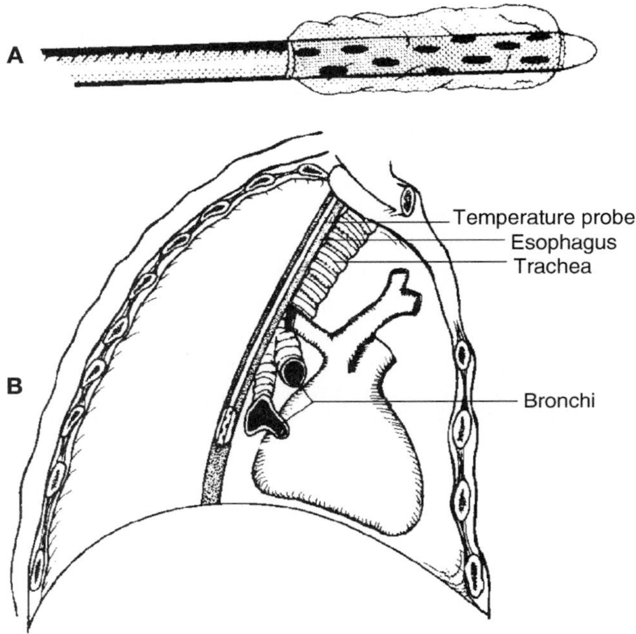

Figure 31-13 Esophageal stethoscope aids in monitoring both heart and lung sounds. **A,** Distal end of esophageal stethoscope has multiple perforations that aid in picking up sounds in thorax. **B,** Esophageal stethoscope is inserted into esophagus to the level of the heart, thereby maximizing sound amplification. (From Gravenstein JS, Paulus DA: *Monitoring practice in clinical anesthesia,* Philadelphia, 1982, Lippincott.)

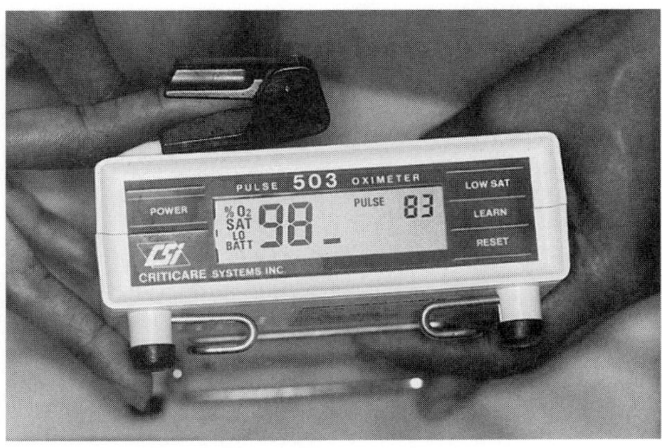

Figure 31-14 Pulse oximeter.

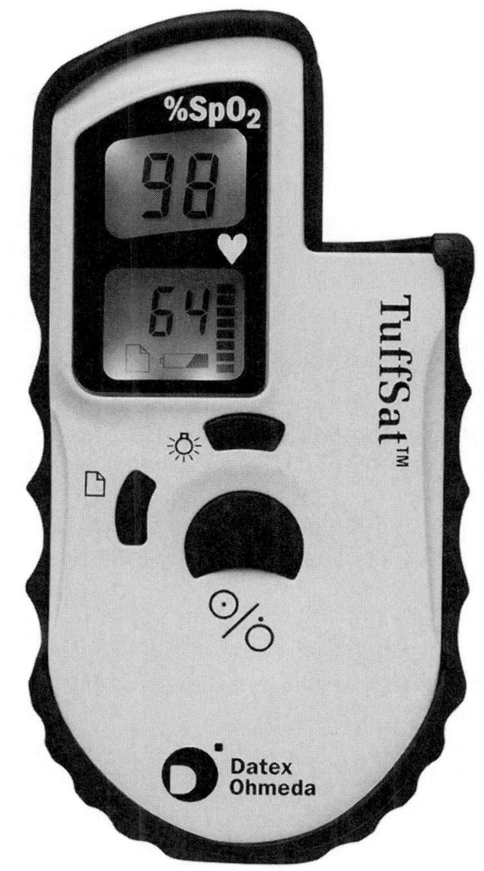

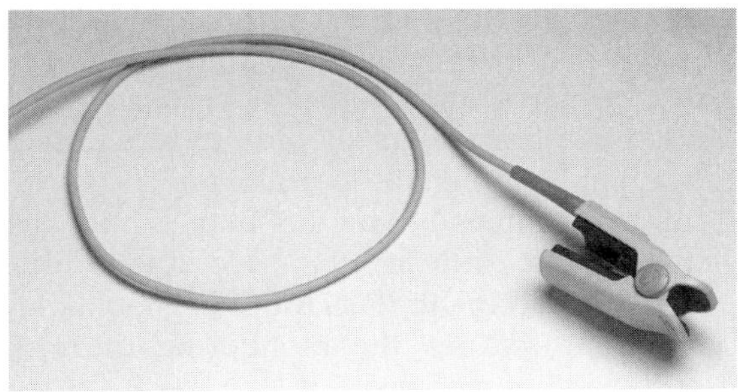

Figure 31-15 Oximeter *(top)* provides continuous monitoring of arterial O_2 saturation by a fingerprobe *(bottom)*. (Courtesy Ohmeda, Littleton, Colo.)

$ETCO_2$ monitor evaluates every breath, airway problems may be detected almost instantaneously (a lag time of several seconds exists), permitting correction before they become significant.

4. The *sphygmomanometer,* or *blood pressure cuff,* is used to monitor blood pressure by indirect determination. During general anesthesia, blood pressure, heart rate and rhythm, and respiratory rate are monitored continuously and recorded every 5 minutes. If events warrant, more frequent determinations are obtained.
5. The *electrocardiograph (ECG)* provides a means of monitoring the electrical activity and rhythm of the heart. The ECG permits continuous observation of the rate and rhythm of the heart during general anesthesia. Use of the ECG is considered a standard of care during all forms of general anesthesia.
6. *Continuous temperature monitoring* by rectal or esophageal probe has become increasingly common since the 1980s with the recognition of malignant hyperthermia. Although not used for all patients undergoing general anesthesia, temperature monitoring is considered a standard of care in children, young adults, patients with fever, and patients undergoing procedures involving induced hypothermia.[2]
7. The *EEG* reveals the electrical activity of the brain. Although not used routinely, it can easily be obtained through the use of scalp electrodes. The level of cortical depression associated with anesthesia or the effects of adverse conditions such as hypoxia or hypercapnia may be evaluated.[3]
8. Although not used routinely, *direct measurement of arterial blood pressure* is frequently of value in the critically ill patient and during cardiopulmonary bypass, major traumatic surgery, and hypotensive or hypothermic anesthesia. Its major advantage over indirect blood pressure methods is that it provides accurate values of intraarterial or intracardiac blood pressure on a continuous basis.
9. *Collection and measurement of urinary output* are easily obtained in the anesthetized patient whose bladder has been catheterized. Urinary output is a simple method of determining the degree of hydration of the body. During general anesthesia the patient should produce urine at a rate approaching the normal rate of 40 to 60 ml/hr. Volumes below this may signify dehydration and indicate the need for additional fluid replacement. For routine general anesthetic procedures the monitoring of urinary output is not required.
10. *Central venous pressure (CVP)* measures the pressure exerted by blood returning to the right side of the heart and the ability of the right heart to manage it effectively. Monitoring CVP enables the doctor to distinguish between hemorrhage and congestive heart failure. With extensive blood loss the CVP will fall, whereas in congestive heart failure or overhydration CVP is elevated.

    An invasive procedure, CVP monitoring is recommended in older patients, in patients in whom considerable blood or fluid loss is expected, during major traumatic surgery, in cases in which multiple transfusions are given, and during open heart surgery, among other indications. For the typical American Society of Anesthesiologists ASA I or II ambulatory dental patient undergoing general anesthesia, routine use of CVP is not necessary.

Emergency Equipment and Drugs

Complications occur during the administration of general anesthesia. Among the more frequently observed complications are hypotension and cardiac dysrhythmias. Monitoring of the anesthetized patient enables the entire anesthesia team to be aware of the presence of these and other potentially lethal problems and to initiate appropriate corrective treatment. The anesthesiologist will have available a supply of emergency drugs and equipment for use in these circumstances. The emergency drugs required by the Board of Dental Examiners in the state of California for doctors using general anesthesia are listed here.[4] A more thorough discussion of emergency drugs recommended for outpatient facilities is presented in Chapter 33.

Equipment	Drugs (by Category)
Portable apparatus for intermittent positive-pressure breathing (IPPB)	Vasopressor(s)
Bag-valve-mask, face masks, connectors	Corticosteroids
Portable, battery-powered light source	Bronchodilator(s)
Apparatus for emergency tracheotomy or cricothyrotomy	Succinylcholine
Electrocardiogram monitor and defibrillator	Sodium bicarbonate
	Intravenous replacement fluid
	Opioid antagonist(s)
	Histamine blocker(s)
	Anticholinergic(s)
	Antidysrhythmic(s)
	Antihypertensive(s)
	Drug for arterial dilation

Several of the drugs recommended for the emergency tray are also commonly used during the routine administration of general anesthesia. These include succinylcholine, IV replacement fluid, and opioid antagonists.

DRUGS

An array of drugs may be used during the administration of general anesthesia. Many of these drugs have been discussed in other sections of this book and are listed here with minimal discussion. Other drugs make their first appearance at this time; however, they too will receive only a brief review because it is not the goal of this textbook to provide the reader with an in-depth knowledge of general anesthesia.

The most commonly used drugs in general anesthesia may be divided into the following categories:

- IV induction agents
- Opioids (agonists and agonist/antagonists)
- Neuroleptic agents
- Dissociative agents
- Muscle relaxants
- Inhalation anesthetics

Intravenous Induction Agents

In the adult patient receiving general anesthesia, it is the desire of the anesthesiologist to achieve stage III anesthesia as rapidly as possible. In this context, IV agents are usually preferred to inhalation anesthetics because they are more rapidly acting and do not possess the unpleasant odors of some of the gases (e.g., halothane).

Barbiturates. The barbiturates remain the most commonly used IV induction agents, with methohexital, thiopental, and thiamylal most frequently administered. Other drugs used intravenously for induction of anesthesia include diazepam, midazolam, lorazepam, etomidate, ketamine, and propofol.

Methohexital is a rapid-onset, short-acting barbiturate. It is most often used as the sole agent to provide general anesthesia for short procedures (less than 30 minutes).[5] Methohexital is less frequently used as an induction agent for general anesthesia. The dosage of methohexital for induction of general anesthesia is 1 mg/kg. It is 2.5 times as potent as the thiobarbiturates (thiopental and thiamylal) and has a more rapid recovery.[6] Proprietary names of methohexital are Brevital (United States) and Brietal (Great Britain). The uses of methohexital in anesthesia are for short-duration outpatient procedures, electroconvulsive therapy,[7] and minor gynecologic or orthopedic procedures.

Thiopental (Pentothal) and *thiamylal* (Surital) are called thiobarbiturates because they possess a sulfa molecule and are quite similar pharmacologically. Following IV administration the onset of action of these drugs is rapid (within 30 to 40 seconds) and of short duration. Duration of action of thiopental and thiamylal is, however, longer than that of methohexital.[8]

The induction of general anesthesia with a thiobarbiturate is usually produced by the slow IV injection of 150 to 300 mg over a 15- to 30-second interval. Thiopental and thiamylal are used as 2.5% solutions. After induction of general anesthesia, other longer-acting anesthetics are administered for the maintenance of anesthesia.

Absolute contraindications to the administration of barbiturates include status asthmaticus and latent or manifest porphyria.

Benzodiazepines. Several benzodiazepines are also used as induction agents for general anesthesia. These include diazepam, midazolam, and lorazepam.

Diazepam and midazolam are benzodiazepines that are used on occasion to induce general anesthesia.[9] Benzodiazepines provide a slower, more gradual loss of consciousness than the barbiturates. The patient initially enters into a comfortable level of sedation, at which point additional diazepam, midazolam, or other IV (e.g., opioids) or inhalation agents (e.g., halothane) may be administered to produce the desired level of unconsciousness. Diazepam and midazolam are also used during short IV barbiturate general anesthetic procedures to potentiate the actions of the barbiturate as well as to "smooth out" the anesthesia.

Lorazepam (Ativan) is a benzodiazepine that was *not* recommended earlier for use in outpatients because of its long duration of action and the inability of the administrator to titrate the drug to clinical effect as a result of its very slow onset of action. Because the need for rapid and "complete" recovery after inpatient procedures is not as urgent, lorazepam may be used like diazepam or midazolam in these patients.

Other Agents. *Etomidate* (Amidate) was introduced in the United States in 1983 as a nonbarbiturate IV induction agent. Administered in a dose of 0.3 to 0.4 mg/kg, etomidate demonstrates a rapid onset of action combined with less respiratory depression than is seen with the barbiturates.[10] Cardiovascular stability is another positive feature of etomidate. Etomidate is highly lipid soluble, has a half-life of 60 minutes, and is short acting. Recovery of cognitive and psychomotor function is intermediate between thiopental[11] and methohexital.[12] Negative factors associated with etomidate include a burning sensation as the drug is injected in some patients, the occurrence of myoclonic jerks, the inhibition of steroid synthesis, and the occurrence of excitatory effects in approximately 30% of patients receiving it. Etomidate is used for IV induction in children where hemodynamic stability is desirable (hypovolemia) and the hypertension and tachycardia caused by ketamine are unacceptable.

Ketamine, used as either an IV or intramuscular (IM) induction agent, primarily in children, is discussed more fully in Chapter 25. Ketamine is most suitable in children who are hemodynamically unstable or hypovolemic.[13] In addition, ketamine is used in asthmatic children because of its bronchodilating properties.[14] When administered by any route, ketamine should be preceded or accompanied by the administration of atropine or glycopyrrolate to attenuate the increase in airway secretions associated with its administration.[10] In addition, concurrent benzodiazepine administration is recommended to lessen the dysphoric emergence from anesthesia that may be associated with ketamine.[15]

Propofol (diisopropylphenol) is a nonbarbiturate IV anesthetic agent that is used when rapid-onset and short-duration general anesthesia is desired.[16] Propofol is most often compared to methohexital.[17] Pecaro and Houting demonstrated that at usual dosages propofol has insignificant cardiovascular and respiratory effects.[18] Moreover, it lacks excitatory or emetic actions. The primary side effect noted with propofol administration was pain on injection (37.5% on dorsum of hand).[19]

The anesthesia induction dose of propofol is 2.5 mg/kg, which makes the drug equipotent with 4 mg/kg of thiopental.[20] McCulloch and Lees[19] suggest an induction dose of 2.25 mg/kg in "younger patients" and a dose of 1.5 mg/kg in "older patients." Pharmacokinetically, the terminal half-life of propofol is 286 ± 36 minutes, with clearance in 1803 ± 125 minutes.[21]

Cundy and Arunasalam,[22] comparing propofol with methohexital, found that propofol provided a statistically significant superior quality of anesthesia. No difference was noted in recovery time, and postoperatively methohexital patients were significantly more drowsy. Coughing and laryngospasm did not occur with propofol (0/30) as they did with methohexital (5/30). The proprietary name of propofol is Diprivan.

Opioids

The term *opioid* is used in a broad sense to include both the opioid agonists and opioid agonist/antagonists. The pharmacology of these drugs is discussed in some detail in Chapter 25.

Opioids are frequently used for the maintenance of general anesthesia in a technique involving the administration of an opioid, N_2O-O_2, and a muscle relaxant. Anesthesia is induced with one of the short-acting IV agents previously discussed and is maintained with periodic doses of an appropriate opioid. N_2O-O_2 is administered to minimize the dosage of opioid required. The most commonly used opioids in general anesthesia are morphine, meperidine, fentanyl, and its analogs sufentanil, alfentanil, and remifentanil.

Morphine is the standard opioid analgesic drug against which all others are compared. Morphine has strong analgesic and sedative properties. It is used primarily for longer-duration procedures. Morphine is usually injected as a 1-mg/ml solution.

Meperidine (Demerol) is probably the most frequently used opioid analgesic in anesthesia. It is usually used in a concentration of 10 mg/ml. Meperidine is intermediate in duration of action, between that of morphine and of fentanyl.

Fentanyl (Sublimaze) is used either as a component of Innovar (droperidol with fentanyl) to provide neuroleptanesthesia or alone during shorter surgical procedures. It is used alone in a concentration of 0.01 mg/ml.

Alfentanil (Alfenta) and *sufentanil* (Sufenta) are rapid-onset, short-duration analogs of fentanyl that have been recently introduced and have gained significant popularity.[23,24] *Remifentanil* (Ultiva) is as rapid acting as alfentanil but is even shorter acting, requiring its administration via constant infusion (infusion pump) to maintain a therapeutic blood level.[25,26]

Opioid agonist/antagonists such as *nalbuphine* and *butorphanol* are also used during general anesthesia. Their primary benefit appears to be the ceiling effect on respiratory depression that is noted with their administration.[27] This contrasts to the dose-related respiratory depression observed with opioid agonists.

The opioid antagonist *naloxone* is commonly used when opioids have been administered. At the termination of the anesthetic procedure, the anesthesiologist attempts to awaken the patient. If opioids have been used during surgery, the patient's rate of breathing may be quite slow at this time. Titration of naloxone may be necessary to reverse this opioid-induced respiratory depression. Careful monitoring of the patient following reversal with naloxone is required because several of the opioids have a longer duration of action than does naloxone and a return of respiratory depression at a later time is possible. To minimize this potential risk, the administration of an IM dose of naloxone should be considered after its IV administration.[28] The slower onset and longer duration of the IM dose of naloxone minimizes the risk of a recurrence of significant respiratory depression.

The opioid analgesics are very important anesthetic agents. Their use in a typical anesthetic procedure is as follows.

Neuroleptanesthesia

Neuroleptanesthesia and neuroleptanalgesia are discussed in Chapter 25. The neuroleptic state is produced when a neuroleptic drug (another name for a tranquilizer) and an opioid analgesic are administered together to produce a state characterized by the following[29]:

- Sleepiness without total unconsciousness
- Psychological indifference to the environment
- No voluntary movements
- Analgesia
- Satisfactory amnesia

In clinical practice neuroleptanesthesia is produced through the administration of the following drug combinations:

- Neuroleptic drug
- Opioid
- N_2O-O_2
- Muscle relaxant

Innovar, a premixed combination of droperidol (Inapsine), 2.5 mg/ml, and fentanyl (Sublimaze), 0.05 mg/ml, is the drug most frequently used to induce a neuroleptic state. The pharmacologic properties of droperidol and of fentanyl are discussed in Chapter 25. A brief review follows.

Droperidol, a tranquilizer, produces clinical actions within 5 to 10 minutes after IV administration. Long acting, its actions may be observed for 6 to 12 hours after a single injection. Additional properties of droperidol include its antiemetic and its slight α-adrenergic receptor-blocking effects. Disadvantages of droperidol include its long duration of action (a disadvantage in outpatient procedures); its peripheral vasodilating effects, which may produce hypotension; the fact that there is no pharmacologic antagonist for droperidol; and the fact that large doses produce muscle movements similar to extrapyramidal effects—dystonia, akathisia, and oculogyric crisis (see Chapter 7).

Fentanyl, a powerful opioid analgesic, acts rapidly after IV administration, with a duration of action of between 30 and 60 minutes. The analgesic potency of 0.1 mg fentanyl is equal to that of 10 mg morphine. Fentanyl does not release histamine (unlike meperidine, which does), can be reversed by opioid antagonists, produces euphoria, and has negligible effects on the cardiovascular system. Negative features of fentanyl include the fact that it is an emetic and that it produces respiratory depression, miosis, possibly bradycardia and bronchoconstriction, and, with large doses, possibly muscular rigidity (see Chapters 25 and 27).

Neuroleptanesthesia produced by droperidol, fentanyl, N_2O-O_2, and a muscle relaxant has become a very popular anesthetic technique, especially in the more severely medically compromised patient (ASA III and IV). Snow lists the following advantages of neuroleptanesthesia[30]:

- No secretions
- No venous or tissue irritation
- Stable cardiovascular system
- No sensitization of myocardial conduction system to actions of catecholamines
- No toxic effects on liver or kidney function
- Reduced cerebrospinal fluid (CSF) pressure and intraocular pressure
- Nonemetic
- Nonexplosive
- Prompt recovery
- Long periods of analgesia and amnesia
- In recovery room, longer tolerance of endotracheal tube

The following are disadvantages of neuroleptanesthesia[30]:

- Respiratory depression and apnea can be caused by fentanyl and muscle relaxants.
- Assisted or controlled ventilation is required.
- Action of muscle relaxants must be reversed.

Dissociative Anesthesia

Dissociative anesthesia and analgesia, as produced by ketamine, are described in Chapter 25. In the dissociative state, patients appear to be awake—their eyes are open, and they are capable of involuntary muscular movement—but they are unaware of, or dissociated from, the environment. After IV administration ketamine produces analgesia and unconsciousness within 30 seconds. The usual general anesthesia induction dose of ketamine is 1 to 2 mg/kg, injected at a rate of 0.5 mg/kg/min.[31]

Ketamine is used as an induction agent for general anesthesia and as the sole agent for short diagnostic and surgical procedures that do not require skeletal muscle relaxation. Ketamine is commonly used in children. It is used especially in surgical procedures in which control of the airway is difficult to maintain, especially for correction of scars and burns of the face and neck—procedures that make intubation and extension of the neck very difficult, if not impossible. The administration of dissociative anesthesia is contraindicated in intraocular surgery and in patients with a history of increased CSF pressure, cerebrovascular accident (CVA), psychiatric problems, and high blood pressure.

Ketamine is nonirritating to blood vessels and tissues. It produces profound analgesia, muscle tone is preserved, and the laryngeal and pharyngeal reflexes are not depressed; therefore a patent airway can usually be maintained without the need for intubation.

Disadvantages of ketamine include increased heart rate, blood pressure, and intraocular pressure; in addition, diplopia, eye movements, and nystagmus can occur during anesthesia—thus the recommendation that ketamine not be used in intraocular procedures. There is no antagonist for ketamine. Probably the most significant disadvantage of ketamine is its ability to produce a confused state, associated with unpleasant dreams and frightening or upsetting hallucinations, which occur most commonly in adults during the recovery period.[32,33] These appear much less frequently in children.

Muscle Relaxants (Neuromuscular Blocking Drugs)

Muscle relaxant drugs are also known as *neuromuscular blocking drugs.* They provide skeletal muscle relaxation to facilitate intubation of the trachea and controlled mechanical ventilation, and they provide optimal operating conditions. These drugs interfere with the transmission of impulses from motor nerves to muscle at the skeletal neuromuscular junction. Before the introduction of muscle relaxants into anesthesia, skeletal muscle relaxation was obtained during surgery by inducing deeper levels of anesthesia. Along with muscle relaxation, a greatly increased incidence of complications, morbidity, and mortality was seen. With the introduction of muscle relaxants, deep anesthesia can now be avoided and the concept and technique of balanced anesthesia have developed. Muscle relaxants are the most commonly used adjuvants in anesthesia practice.

During short-duration outpatient general anesthesia (e.g., with methohexital), there is little or no indication for the administration of muscle relaxants. When longer-duration outpatient procedures are performed, the patient may require intubation, a procedure that usually requires the use of the short-acting muscle relaxant *succinylcholine.* Patients undergoing inpatient dental procedures performed under general anesthesia will receive succinylcholine for intubation and may, if necessary, receive other longer-acting muscle relaxants.

There are four mechanisms in which the physiology of neuromuscular transmission may be interfered with to interrupt nerve impulses arriving at the end plate:

1. In *deficiency block* the synthesis and/or transmission of acetylcholine is interfered with. Examples of drugs that act in this manner include local anesthetics; neomycin, kanamycin, and streptomycin; *Clostridium botulinum* toxin; calcium deficiency; and magnesium excess.
2. *Nondepolarizing block* is also known as a *competitive* block. The drug attaches to cholinergic receptors, preventing acetylcholine from attaching to the receptor, a form of competitive inhibition. Most commonly used muscle relaxants act in this manner. Examples of nondepolarizing muscle relaxants include *d*-tubocurarine (Curare), pancuronium, metocurine, vecuronium, atracurium, mivacurium, and gallamine. The actions of nondepolarizing muscle relaxants may be reversed by increasing the concentration of acetylcholine, which is accomplished clinically by administering anticholinesterases such as neostigmine. Nondepolarizing muscle relaxants do not produce fasciculations (skeletal muscle contractions) when administered intravenously.
3. In *depolarizing block* (also known as *phase I* block), the drug acts in a manner similar to acetylcholine but for a prolonged time. The drug acts to produce muscle contractions, called *fasciculations* (the equivalent of acetylcholine action), followed by prolonged muscle flaccidity. Two drugs that produce this effect are succinylcholine and decamethonium.
4. *Dual block* is also called *desensitization* block. In dual block the membrane is depolarized (phase I) and is then slowly repolarized. The drug enters into the nerve fiber and acts as a nondepolarizing agent (phase II), even though the membrane potential is restored.

All neuromuscular blockers impair respiration and can produce apnea; therefore these drugs must never be administered by persons untrained in endotracheal intubation and in the administration of artificial ventilation. Nondepolarizing muscle relaxants are used more frequently during surgery than depolarizing agents because their duration is somewhat longer (20 to 45 minutes). Depolarizing agents are used for endotracheal intubation, laryngoscopy, bronchoscopy, esophagoscopy, and other short procedures.

Patients with myasthenia gravis should receive nondepolarizing muscle relaxants with great caution because they are extremely sensitive to the actions of these drugs. Such patients usually require as little as one tenth the usual dose for clinical effect.

Tubocurarine (Tubarine) is the classical nondepolarizing muscle relaxant. After IV administration the drug produces its actions within 3 minutes and with a duration of 30 to 40 minutes. The average initial dose in adults is 15 to 20 mg. Supplemental doses may be required for prolonged surgical procedures. Muscle fasciculation and postoperative muscle pain do not develop with tubocurarine. Administration of tubocurarine is contraindicated in patients with myasthenia gravis, renal disease, and bronchial asthma (because it releases histamine).

Pancuronium (Pavulon) was introduced in the United States in the early 1970s and has become a very popular nondepolarizing muscle relaxant. It is approximately five times as potent as tubocurarine and has an onset of action within 3 to 5 minutes and a duration of action of 30 to 40 minutes.

Pancuronium does not produce muscle fasciculations, nor does it produce postanesthetic muscle pain. Unlike tubocurarine, pancuronium does not release histamine. The initial IV dose range is 0.04 to 0.1 mg/kg, with supplemental doses required for prolonged procedures. Small doses of pancuronium in patients with myasthenia gravis will produce profound effects.

Recent additions to the nondepolarizing group of muscle relaxants include *metocurine, vecuronium, mivacurium, rocuronium,* and *atracurium.* The major advantage of these drugs is an elimination half-life shorter than the 2 hours possessed by pancuronium and *d*-tubocurarine. Vecuronium has an elimination half-life of 70 minutes, atracurium about 20 minutes.

Succinylcholine (Anectine) is a synthetic, short-acting depolarizing muscle relaxant. After an IV dose of 60 to 80 mg (for a 70-kg patient), relaxation develops within 1 minute. Recovery of muscle tone is rapid and complete within 5 to 15 minutes. For children the usual dose for intubation is 20 mg. Succinylcholine is used routinely for skeletal muscle relaxation before tracheal intubation. It may also be used by continuous IV drip for relaxation during abdominal operations. Succinylcholine is used during electroconvulsive therapy (ECT) and as an emergency drug during the treatment of laryngospasm (see Chapter 27). Succinylcholine is contraindicated for use in patients with penetrating injuries of the eye and patients with myotonia.

Strong skeletal muscle contractions (fasciculations) are seen after the administration of succinylcholine. Patients receiving this drug may complain of severe muscle pain for several days after its administration. Fasciculations develop first in the eyebrow and eyelids, then in the shoulder girdle and abdominal muscles, and finally in the muscles of the hands and feet. The severity of fasciculations may be diminished by slow administration of the drug or by the prior administration of tubocurarine (3 to 6 mg) or pancuronium (0.5 to 1 mg).

Succinylcholine may produce hyperkalemia (succinylcholine-induced hyperkalemia), which in certain patients may lead to cardiovascular collapse or cardiac arrest. At-risk patients include those with the following:

- Severe burns
- Massive trauma
- Tetanus
- Spinal cord injury
- Brain injury
- Uremia with increased serum potassium

Succinylcholine has been implicated as a trigger agent in malignant hyperthermia (MH). In MH-susceptible patients, succinylcholine administration is followed by exaggerated fasciculations, rigidity, and difficulty in intubation. Body temperature then increases at an alarming rate. Succinylcholine must not be administered to patients with a history of MH.

Metabolized in the serum by plasma pseudocholinesterase, succinylcholine is usually rapidly inactivated (muscle tonus returns to normal within 5 to 15 minutes). However, 1 in 3000 persons has atypical pseudocholinesterase and will exhibit a prolonged response to succinylcholine.[34] The presence of atypical pseudocholinesterase should be suspected in any patient in whom spontaneous respiration has not returned within 15 minutes after the administration of succinylcholine. Management of prolonged apnea requires continued controlled ventilation until spontaneous ventilation returns or until fresh-frozen plasma or blood is administered to restore the pseudocholinesterase level of the plasma.

Muscle relaxants are important adjuvants to general anesthesia. Their presence has permitted abdominal operations to be completed with much more ease and comfort for the patient, surgeon, and anesthesiologist alike. Their use, especially that of the longer-acting nondepolarizing muscle relaxants, is not recommended in outpatient procedures. Succinylcholine is used in outpatient procedures for intubation and in the emergency management of laryngospasm.

Inhalation Anesthetics

Inhalation anesthetics are the most frequently used means of producing general anesthesia. They are popular because of their controllability, which is based on the fact that their uptake and elimination are largely affected by pulmonary ventilation. The advantages of inhalation anesthetics are reviewed in Chapters 12 and 13.

The "ideal" inhalation anesthetic has not been found; however, volatile agents that approach the ideal are currently available. The following characteristics are desirable in an inhalation anesthetic:

1. The inhalation anesthetic should be either a gas or a liquid. If it is a gas, it should be easily liquefied at moderate pressures.
2. The blood/gas solubility coefficient (ratio) should be low (in the range of 0.3 to 2) so that a high partial pressure is obtained quickly in the alveoli. This will provide a rapid induction of anesthetic effect and an equally rapid elimination of the agent.
3. The oil/water solubility should also be low so that the drug is not stored in fat, thus avoiding prolonged recovery.

4. The inhalation anesthetic should be neither flammable nor explosive.
5. The inhalation anesthetic should be stable, not decomposing on exposure to moisture, light, or air. It should not corrode or react with rubber, plastic, metal, or carbon dioxide (CO_2) absorbers.
6. The inhalation anesthetic should have a pleasant odor, be nonirritating, and have minimal postanesthetic sequelae.
7. The inhalation anesthetic should be nontoxic to the organs and nonallergenic.
8. The inhalation anesthetic should be potent enough so that it provides good analgesia and anesthesia and so that at least 50% O_2 may be administered with it.
9. The inhalation anesthetic should be completely inert, being excreted entirely unchanged through the lungs.

The physical and chemical characteristics of major inhalation anesthetics currently used in general anesthesia are presented in Table 31-1. More commonly used inhalation anesthetics include N_2O, halothane, enflurane, isoflurane, desflurane, and sevoflurane. Other inhalation anesthetics, such as cyclopropane, chloroform, diethyl ether, divinyl ether, ethyl vinyl ether, fluroxene, methoxyflurane, and trichloroethylene, are no longer used in general anesthesia.

Among the inhalation anesthetics that are in use today, N_2O is by far the most common. In fact, N_2O is administered during almost every use of general anesthesia. The pharmacology of this very important inhalation sedative and general anesthetic is presented in Chapter 13. The primary function of N_2O administration during general anesthesia is to potentiate the actions of other, more potent drugs (IV or inhalation) being administered to produce a controlled state of unconsciousness. Its administration (along with O_2) permits a smaller dose or lesser concentration of the primary drug to be administered to produce the desired level of general anesthesia. For example, halothane administered with O_2 alone may require a 4% concentration to produce surgical-depth anesthesia; however, with the administration of 60% N_2O, halothane effectively provides the same depth of anesthesia at only a 1% concentration. With IV drug administration the same is true.

Halothane was introduced into anesthesia practice in 1956 and had profound effects on the practice of anesthesia and surgery in that it was not flammable. This permitted the use of electrocautery by the surgeon and the introduction of extensive electronic monitoring by the anesthesiologist. Unlike ether, which preceded halothane, it permitted a rapid induction and emergence from anesthesia and also allowed rapid changes of anesthetic depth during surgery. With the introduction of newer inhalation anesthetics, halothane is used less frequently in adults. Its popularity in pediatric anesthesia remains. Minimum alveolar concentration (MAC), the concentration at which 50% of patients do not respond to surgical incision, is 0.74% for halothane.

Disadvantages of halothane include inducing myocardial depression, producing cardiac dysrhythmias (at higher concentrations), resulting in sensitization of the myocardium to the actions of catecholamines, acting as a potent uterine relaxant, and possibly producing shivering or tremor during recovery in patients whose body temperature is low. Probably the most serious disadvantage of halothane is its possible

TABLE 31-1 Characteristics of Inhalation Anesthetics

	Partition Coefficient at 37° C			*Inspired Concentrations (%)*	
Agent	Fat/blood*	Blood/gas†	Minimum Alveolar Concentration (MAC)‡ (%)	Induction	Maintenance
N_2O	2.3	0.47	105.0	75	50-70
Halothane	60	2.3	0.75	1-4	0.5-2.0
Enflurane	36	1.8	1.58	2-5	1.5-3.0
Isoflurane	45	1.4	1.28	1-4	0.8-2.0
Desflurane	27	0.42	4.6-6.0	—	—
Sevoflurane	48	0.59	1.71	—	—

*Fat/blood partition coefficient—lower value, decreased lipid storage, and more rapid recovery.
†Blood/gas partition coefficient—lower value, rapid onset, and rapid recovery.
‡Minimum anesthetic concentration—gas concentration in alveoli, which, when in equilibrium with the central nervous system, causes 50% of individuals to move in response to painful cutaneous stimulation (in O_2).

hepatotoxicity. Reports also indicate that halothane may produce postanesthetic jaundice or disturbed liver function and even necrosis. The National Halothane Study concluded that if indeed halothane-induced hepatic necrosis occurs, it is rare.[35] Although most inhaled halothane is removed through the lungs, metabolites are slowly removed from the body over 2 to 3 weeks. Halothane is administered for outpatient anesthesia and on some occasions is used in lower concentrations to provide sedation.

Enflurane (Ethrane) was synthesized in 1963 and has clinical and pharmacologic properties similar to those of halothane. Enflurane, however, has the advantage of being compatible with epinephrine, up to 10 ml of a 1:100,000 concentration, with a decreased risk of dysrhythmias developing.[36]

Advantages of enflurane include the following: it has a pleasant odor, there is rapid induction and recovery, it is nonirritating (produces no secretions), it is a bronchodilator and a good muscle relaxant, it keeps the cardiovascular system fairly stable (dysrhythmias are uncommon), it is not an emetic, it is nonexplosive and nonflammable, and it is compatible with epinephrine. The MAC for enflurane is 1.68%, and anesthesia is induced at concentrations of 2% to 5% and maintained at concentrations of 1.5% to 3%.

Disadvantages of enflurane include the following: myocardial depression, progressive hypotension develops with increase in anesthetic depth, shivering may develop on emergence, the possibility of liver damage, and the production of CNS irritation at higher concentrations (especially if the patient is hypocarbic). In addition, enflurane should be avoided in patients with severely compromised renal function. Clinically, muscle twitching is noted in the jaw, neck, or extremities, and increased spike activity is noted on the EEG. Enflurane undergoes metabolism only to the extent of 2.5%, the remainder being excreted unchanged through the lungs.

Isoflurane (Forane), synthesized in 1970, is a chemical isomer of enflurane. No abnormal motor activity, such as muscle twitching or convulsions, is noted with isoflurane.

Advantages of isoflurane include that it has a pleasant odor, has a rapid induction and recovery, is nonirritating (produces no secretions), is a bronchodilator, provides excellent muscle relaxation, keeps the cardiac rhythm stable, is compatible with epinephrine, is not an emetic, and is nonexplosive and nonflammable. The MAC for isoflurane is 1.2%; anesthesia is induced at concentrations of 1% to 4% and maintained at concentrations of 0.8% to 2%.

Disadvantages of isoflurane include production of myocardial depression, depressed blood pressure as the level of anesthesia is increased, postanesthetic shivering, the possibility for hepatotoxicity, and the inadvisability of administering isoflurane to patients with severely compromised renal function.

Sevoflurane (Ultane) is noted for its low solubility and rapid induction of, and emergence from, anesthesia. It is less irritating to the airway than many other inhalation anesthetics. The MAC for sevoflurane is 2%, and the concentration at which amnesia and loss of awareness occur (MAC awake) is 0.6%.

Desflurane (Suprane) also possesses a low blood-gas partition coefficient, thereby producing a rapid onset of anesthesia and equally rapid recovery. Desflurane does not undergo biotransformation in the body. It is not recommended for the induction of anesthesia because of its unpleasant odor and airway irritant properties. Its principal advantage seems to be rapid patient emergence from anesthesia.[37] This may be a valuable property in busy surgical suites where a rapid turnover of patients is required and in surgical outpatients who would especially benefit from the rapid recovery of mental faculties.[38]

TECHNIQUES

Inpatient General Anesthesia

General anesthesia as administered to the hospitalized patient represents the fundamental technique from which the other forms of general anesthesia have developed. As a rule, this form of anesthesia is utilized in dentistry for the medically compromised patient and for patients undergoing extensive and possibly traumatic dental procedures.

The patient is usually admitted to the hospital 1 day before the scheduled procedure so that an extensive preoperative evaluation can be completed. A physical examination and laboratory tests such as hematocrit, hemoglobin, complete blood count (CBC) and differential, and urinalysis form the minimal evaluation. In adult patients scheduled for general anesthesia a chest x-ray film and ECG are required in most hospitals.

The evening before the surgical procedure the anesthesiologist will make a preanesthetic visit, the purpose of which is to evaluate the patient as to any special anesthetic risks (e.g., potential airway maintenance problems), to review the physical examination of the patient and results of the laboratory tests, to discuss the upcoming anesthetic procedure with the patient so as to allay any apprehensions, and to determine whether the patient has any special requests as to the type of anesthesia. The anesthesiologist will write preanesthetic orders for the patient. Typical orders include the patient fasting before surgery ("NPO after midnight") and preoperative medications to be administered intramuscularly either 1 hour before the scheduled procedure or "on call to the operating room" if the procedure is scheduled for later in the day. The most frequently prescribed combination of preoperative drugs includes an antianxiety drug such as diazepam or midazolam or a barbiturate such as pentobarbital, an opioid (meperidine), and an anticholinergic (scopolamine or atropine). If it is deemed necessary, the patient will also receive a sedative such as flurazepam or triazolam orally before bedtime to ensure a good night's sleep before surgery.

Before the arrival of the patient, the anesthesiologist will have prepared all of the necessary drugs and equipment. On arrival in the operating room the patient will be properly identified by the nursing staff and placed onto the operating room table. Physiologic monitors, such as a blood pressure cuff, a precordial stethoscope, ECG leads, and pulse oximeter, are attached.

An IV infusion is established, usually on the arm opposite the blood pressure cuff. An indwelling catheter, not smaller than 18 gauge, is inserted and secured. In procedures in which blood transfusion is considered likely, a 16-gauge indwelling catheter will be used for the IV infusion. A 1000-ml bag of either 5% dextrose and water or lactated Ringer's solution is used for maintenance of the infusion. Vital signs are monitored and recorded on the anesthesia record (Figure 31-16).

On arrival of the surgical team, the induction of anesthesia commences. The patient may be administered (IV) a small dose of benzodiazepine to produce a

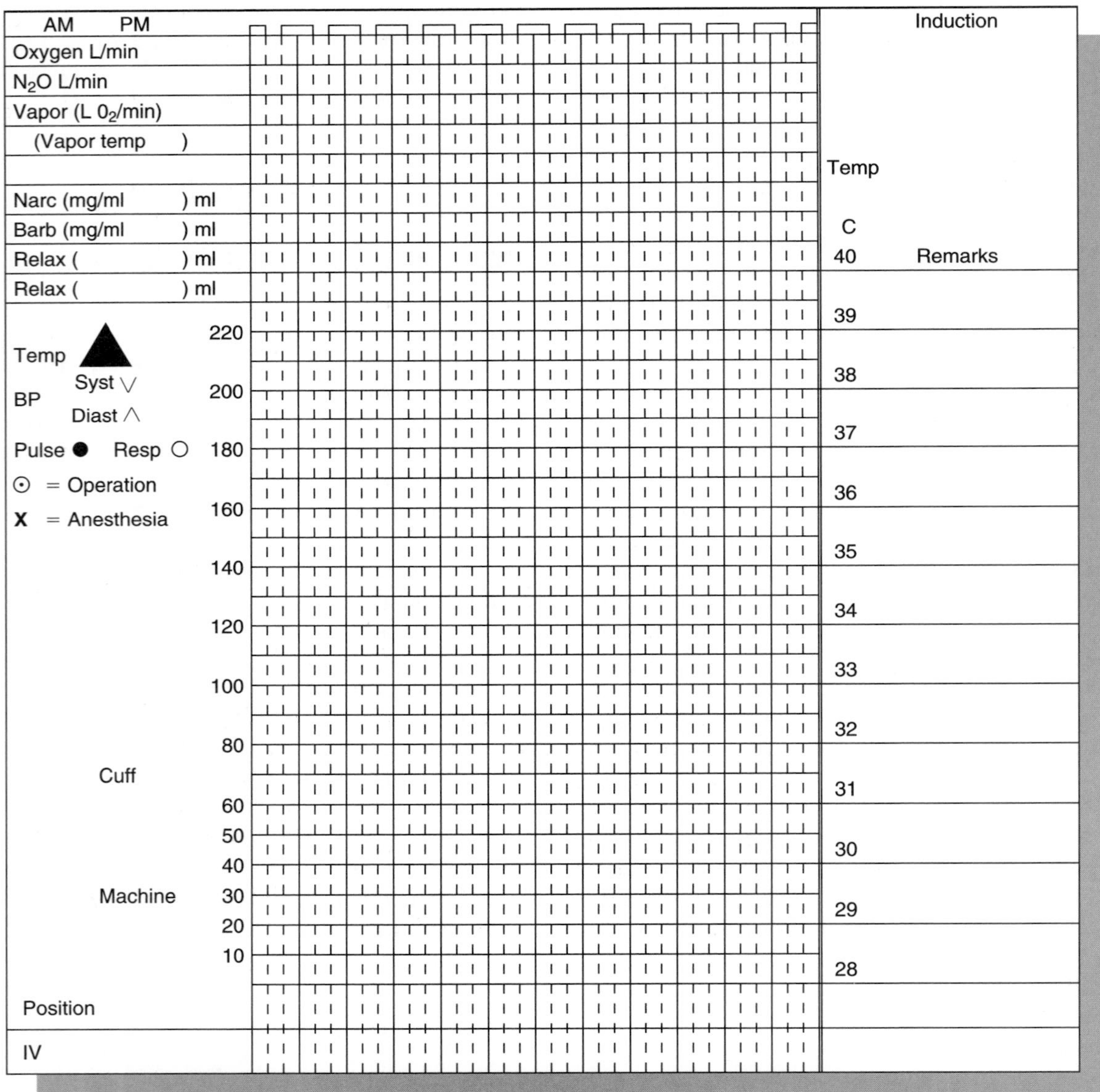

Figure 31-16 Anesthesia record: ∨, systolic blood pressure; ∧, diastolic blood pressure; ●, heart rate; ▲, temperature; O, respiration.

greater degree of sedation while awaiting the surgical team. A topical anesthetic, frequently cocaine, will be applied to each of the patient's nostrils with a cotton applicator stick to produce both analgesia and hemostasis during nasal intubation. A full-face mask is placed on the patient with a flow of approximately 5 to 7 L/min of 100% O_2.

Thiopental, thiamylal, or propofol is titrated until the patient loses consciousness. The anesthesiologist will then "bag" the patient (breathe for the patient) to confirm that a patent airway is present before the administration of a muscle relaxant. Once a patent airway is ensured, a dose of succinylcholine, a depolarizing muscle relaxant, is administered. Fasciculations occur, and then the patient ceases breathing. To prevent or minimize fasciculations, a small dose (1 to 2 ml) of a nondepolarizing muscle relaxant may be administered before the succinylcholine.

Once fasciculations occur and the patient is apneic, the lubricated nasotracheal tube is placed into a nostril and gently advanced into the nasopharynx (Figure 31-17). The anesthesiologist visualizes the larynx and the tip of the tube using the laryngoscope. With a Magill intubation forceps the endotracheal tube is gently advanced and inserted into the trachea. Once inserted, the endotracheal tube is attached to the anesthesia machine, and the patient is ventilated. The drugs to be used for maintenance of anesthesia are administered, for example, sevoflurane or an IV drug such as meperidine. The gas flow on the anesthesia machine is adjusted to 3 L/min of N_2O and 2 L/min of O_2. The endotracheal tube is secured, its cuff inflated, and the chest auscultated to determine whether breath sounds are equal on the right and left sides (the endotracheal tube may have been overinserted with its tip lying in the right mainstem bronchus). A nasogastric tube is frequently inserted through the other nostril to remove any air and gastric secretions that develop during the procedure.

The anesthetized patient is draped and prepared for surgery (Figure 31-18). During this time the anesthesiologist administers additional doses of the maintenance drug(s) and continues to monitor the patient's vital signs. For most dental procedures local anesthetics will be administered to assist in pain control and hemostasis. Following consultation with the anesthesiologist, epinephrine may be included in the local anesthetic solution. The response of the patient to stimulation as well as his or her vital signs determines the need for additional anesthetic drugs. With inhalation anesthetics the concentration of the drug will be gradually decreased to as low a level as possible (without adverse patient response). Minimal doses of injectable anesthetic drugs will be administered periodically as determined by the patient's response to surgical stimulation and his or her vital signs.

During full-mouth reconstructive dental procedures, implants, or extensive surgery, there may be a need for muscular relaxation so that the doctor can more readily gain access to the oral cavity. In most instances the degree of muscle relaxation provided by the primary anesthetic drug, especially inhalation anesthetics, is sufficient. Occasionally, however, it

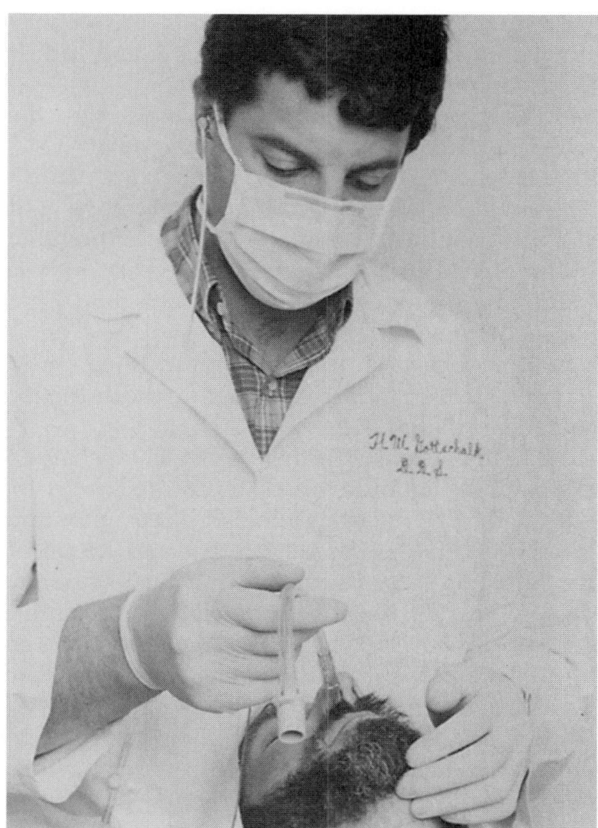

Figure 31-17 Nasoendotracheal tube is passed through nostril and into nasopharynx. Magill intubation forceps assists in its passage into trachea.

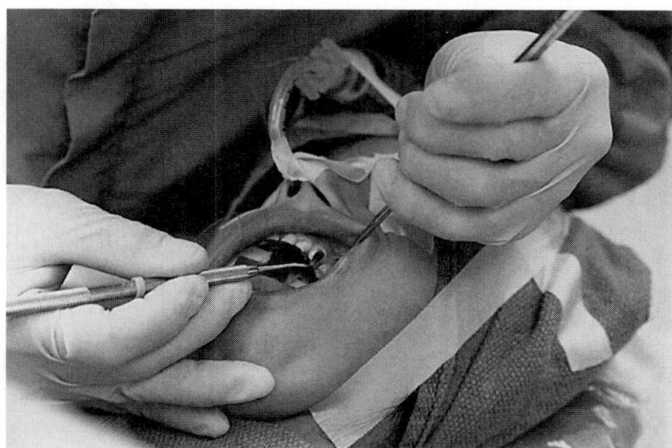

Figure 31-18 Anesthetized patient is draped and prepared for the surgical procedure.

becomes necessary to provide additional muscle relaxation through administration of a neuromuscular blocking agent such as pancuronium or atracurium.

As the surgical procedure terminates, the administration of inhalation anesthetics will be stopped and the patient permitted to breathe either 100% O_2 or a combination of N_2O-O_2 and then 100% O_2. The use of inhalation anesthetics usually provides a more rapid emergence from general anesthesia. In cases in which IV opioids, benzodiazepines, and muscle relaxants were used to provide anesthesia, it may be necessary to administer additional drugs to reverse their actions. Naloxone titrated intravenously is used to reverse opioid-induced respiratory depression, and flumazenil for residual benzodiazepine actions, whereas an anticholinesterase such as neostigmine (Prostigmin) is administered to reverse any residual muscle relaxation. Atropine will usually be administered with the neostigmine to prevent bradycardia.

After reversal of the opioid and muscle relaxant or termination of the flow of inhalation anesthetic, the patient will usually rapidly emerge from anesthesia. When the patient's respiratory movements are deemed adequate, the patient is extubated. Immediately before extubation the anesthesiologist carefully suctions the pharynx to remove any salivary secretions, fluids, or debris that may have collected in this region. The cuff of the endotracheal tube is deflated and the tube removed. A face mask is placed on the patient, and 100% O_2 is administered.

The patient is transferred to a recovery room where a trained staff of nurses and anesthesiologists look after him or her in the immediate period following recovery from anesthesia and surgery. The patient in the recovery area will receive O_2 by nasal cannula and have his or her blood pressure, pulse, respirations, and ECG monitored until the vital signs are stable (VSS) and he or she is alert and awake.

Once the patient has recovered adequately from the effects of anesthesia, he or she will be discharged from the recovery room and readmitted to the surgical ward. The patient will remain in this area until the surgeon permits him or her to be discharged from the hospital. In many inpatient dental cases the patient remains hospitalized overnight and is discharged the day after surgery. In cases of ASA IV, ASA III, and some ASA II patients, stabilization of the medical condition may require more prolonged hospitalization. For the ASA I or II patient who is to be admitted to the hospital for extensive dental treatment under general anesthesia, a minimum stay of two nights and approximately 3 days will be the norm.

Outpatient General Anesthesia

Conventional General Anesthetics. A second technique of general anesthesia is hospital-type general anesthesia on an outpatient basis. The actual anesthetic technique is quite similar to that described for the inpatient stay, with an important exception that the drugs used to produce anesthesia will be shorter acting to permit a more rapid and complete recovery on completion of the surgical procedure. For this reason, inhalation anesthetics are more often used for maintenance of anesthesia than are IV agents.

The patient, an ASA I or II (and with rare exception, an ASA III), undergoes a physical examination, including basic laboratory tests, not more than 48 hours before the scheduled procedure. The patient will have received explicit, written preoperative instructions that include being NPO for at least 6 to 8 hours before treatment.

On the morning of treatment the following must be in order:

1. The patient has been NPO for at least 6 to 8 hours.
2. Results of the basic laboratory tests have been received, have been examined, and are within normal limits.
3. The patient's medical records are complete, including the medical history and physical examination.
4. The informed consent form has been signed and witnessed.

Immediately before the start of the procedure the patient will be asked to void and to remove contact lenses and removable dental prostheses, if present.

IM premedication is not desirable before outpatient general anesthesia because most drugs used for this purpose serve to prolong the recovery period. An anticholinergic such as atropine is recommended for IM or IV administration immediately before the induction of general anesthesia.

The patient is placed either in the dental chair or on the operating table on which the procedure is to be performed. The anesthesiologist places monitoring devices—an ECG, precordial stethoscope, blood pressure cuff, and pulse oximeter—and then starts an IV infusion with an 18-gauge indwelling catheter, using either 5% dextrose and water or lactated Ringer's solution (1000 ml). The nasal mucosa is then sprayed with 4% cocaine or 0.5% phenylephrine.

Anesthesia is induced with a short-acting barbiturate, usually methohexital, propofol, or with an inhalation anesthetic. In the small child it may be difficult to start an IV infusion with the patient conscious; as a result, induction with inhalation anesthesia is more common in children.

Before the nasotracheal tube is inserted, 1 mg of pancuronium (to prevent fasciculations) and an appropriate dose of succinylcholine are administered. The technique for intubation is similar to that described on p. 453.

Once general anesthesia is induced and the patient prepared for the surgical procedure, anesthesia is maintained with a combination of N_2O, O_2, and an appropriate inhalation anesthetic (e.g., enflurane, sevoflurane). Muscle relaxation is rarely required when this procedure is used. Ventilation is spontaneous but requires assistance from the anesthesiologist. On rare occasions ventilation may be controlled.

Immediately before the start of the dental or surgical procedure, the operating dentist places a gauze pack or curtain across the posterior part of the pharynx. This will serve as a screen to collect any debris produced during the dental procedure. A rubber dam is another means of preventing the accumulation of debris in the pharynx.

The administration of local anesthesia is desirable because it decreases the requirement for additional CNS depressant administration. This hastens recovery and discharge of the patient.

At the termination of the procedure the patient receives 100% O_2, and when his or her protective reflexes are intact, he or she is extubated and taken to a recovery area that is supplied with a bed, O_2 suction, monitoring equipment, and emergency equipment and drugs and that is staffed by a trained nurse or anesthesia assistant. A minimum of 1 hour of recovery time is recommended, longer if the doctor considers it necessary. On occasion it may be necessary to admit a patient to the hospital overnight to permit more complete recovery when it appears that recovery is slow or incomplete. The possibility of hospitalization should have been discussed with the patient before the planned procedure and arrangements made with a nearby hospital for possible patient admittance. In cases in which recovery is adequate, the patient may be discharged from the facility if accompanied by a responsible adult guardian. It is recommended that the patient be contacted later that same day to determine how his or her recovery is progressing.

Intravenous General Anesthesia. Shorter procedures, usually requiring less than 30 minutes, may be facilitated with the administration of short-acting IV barbiturates or nonbarbiturates, such as propofol. Although several barbiturates are available, thiopental and methohexital have become the mainstays of ambulatory anesthesia practice in the United States and the United Kingdom. Propofol has established itself as an equally effective agent with several clinical advantages.

The patient receiving IV general anesthesia in an ambulatory care facility such as a dental office will be an ASA I, II, or rarely, III patient. Preoperative assessment will include laboratory tests (CBC, hemoglobin and/or hematocrit, and urinalysis). Patients older than about 35 years will also receive a chest x-ray film and ECG. Preoperative instructions (Box 31-1) and preoperative preparation are similar to those discussed on p. 454. Monitors include a precordial stethoscope, ECG, blood pressure cuff, and pulse oximeter.

An IV line is established using a catheter (21 gauge) and a 250-ml bag of suitable infusate. A small test dose of 1 or 2 ml of methohexital (10 mg/ml), thiopental (25 mg/ml), or propofol (10 mg/ml) is administered, and a bite block is placed between the patient's teeth to prevent their closing after the loss of consciousness. The IV anesthetic is then titrated slowly until the patient loses consciousness. The loss of the eyelid reflex is a common, although not always reliable, indicator of a light level of unconsciousness. The loss of consciousness commonly occurs approximately 30 to 40 seconds after the titration of the drugs. If a pulse oximeter or ECG is being used, a significant increase in the heart rate will be noted as methohexital begins to exert its effect.

As the patient loses consciousness, the airway must be maintained. This is accomplished by a "headholder" or "chinner," an anesthesiologist, dentist, nurse anesthetist, or anesthesia assistant who is responsible for maintenance of a patent airway during the dental procedure (Figure 31-19). The administration of additional methohexital, thiopental, or propofol may be necessary during the procedure. The response of the patient to surgical stimulation will serve as a gauge to the need for additional drug administration.

BOX 31-1 Preanesthetic Instructions

1. If the patient is an adult, he or she should have nothing to eat or drink after midnight of the night before surgery.
2. If the patient is an infant, he or she should have no solid food or milk for 6 hours before surgery. Clear fluids may be given up to 4 hours before anesthesia.
3. It must be emphasized to parents to keep a careful watch on children so that early morning snacks are not eaten.
4. No makeup is to be worn, or at least it must be kept to a minimum.
5. Children must be accompanied by parents or a legal guardian.
6. Adults must be accompanied by another adult and must not drive a motor vehicle for 24 hours after completion of anesthesia.
7. If there is any change in general health before the date of surgery, the patient is advised to contact the doctor or ambulatory care facility in which the procedure is to be performed.

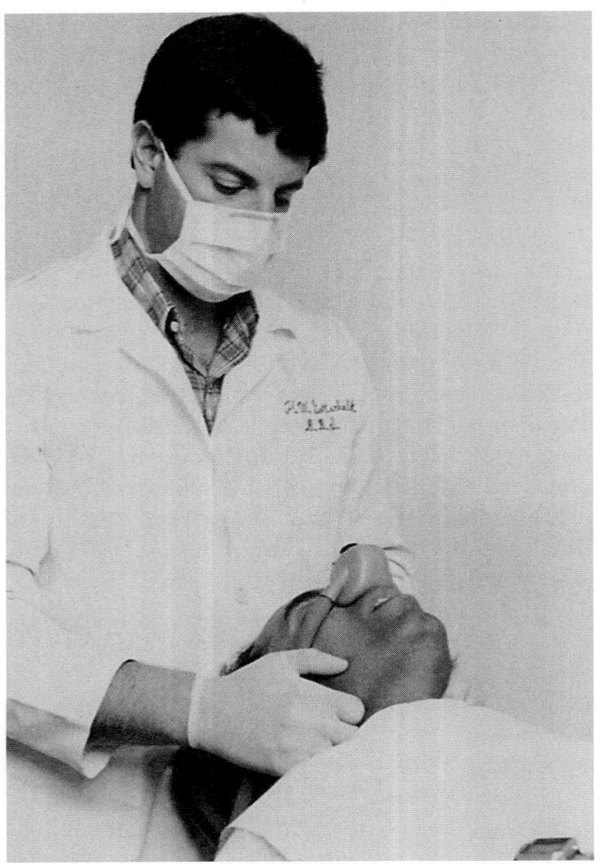

Figure 31-19 Patent airway is maintained during procedure by an anesthesiologist, nurse anesthetist, or anesthesia assistant.

Throughout the procedure a nasal hood is maintained in place, delivering either 100% O_2 or a combination of N_2O-O_2. The latter is used during longer procedures as a means of "smoothing out the anesthetic" and minimizing the dose of IV drug required. The administration of small IV doses of a benzodiazepine to smooth out the anesthetic, in addition to the O_2 or N_2O-O_2, has become increasingly popular. The IV administration of diazepam or midazolam does not increase the recovery time from this technique.

The administration of propofol, a short-acting drug, via infusion pump enables the anesthesiologist to maintain a constant level of CNS depression throughout the procedure. Recovery of consciousness is rapid and more complete than with barbiturates following cessation of the infusion.

The back of the oral cavity is screened off with a gauze curtain (a 4-×-8-inch gauze). The surgical assistant is responsible for the maintenance of a dry and relatively clean surgical field and for changing the gauze as often as is required.

Local anesthesia is recommended as a means of blocking painful stimulation, thereby decreasing the total dose of the IV anesthetic required to achieve clinically adequate anesthesia. The continued presence of local anesthesia in the immediate postoperative period enables the patient to recover from the general anesthetic without any discomfort.

After termination of the procedure the patient usually recovers consciousness quite rapidly, not from rapid metabolism of the intravenously administered drugs but, rather, from their redistribution to other organs and storage sites within the body. Be that as it may, the patient appears to recover quite rapidly and is then transferred (most frequently walking with assistance) to the fully equipped and staffed recovery area, where he or she remains until recovery is deemed adequate to permit discharge home, accompanied by a responsible adult. Contact with the patient later that day or evening is recommended.

SUMMARY

The use of general anesthesia in dentistry dates to the origins of anesthesia itself. Dentists were intimately involved in the discovery of this valuable technique of pain and anxiety control and in many of its subsequent advances. Indeed, dentistry has been in the forefront in the recent evolution of outpatient general anesthesia.

General anesthesia is a technique that requires significantly greater training on the part of the doctor and staff in order for it to be used safely. Under no circumstances should a person without a minimum of 2 years of full-time training in anesthesiology or its equivalent in an oral and maxillofacial surgery training program ever consider the administration of general anesthesia.

The indications for general anesthesia in dentistry have diminished over the years as techniques of conscious sedation have evolved. Yet, many indications for its use remain. The selection of the most appropriate type of general anesthesia for use in a given patient must be made after a thorough evaluation of the patient's physical condition, the planned dental treatment, the training and background of the doctor and staff, and the preparedness of the facility.

REFERENCES

1. Rosenberg MB, Campbell RL: Guidelines for intraoperative monitoring of dental patients undergoing conscious sedation, deep sedation, and general anesthesia, *Oral Surg* 71:2, 1991.
2. Eichhorn JH, Cooper JB, Cullen DJ et al: Anesthesia practice standards at Harvard: a review, *J Clin Anesth* 1:55, 1988.
3. Griffiths MJ, Preece AW, Green JL: Monitoring sedation levels by EEG spectral analysis, *Anesth Prog* 38:227, 1991.

4. Board of Dental Examiners: *General anesthesia statute. Extract from business and professions code, Chapter 4—Dentistry, Article 2.7—Use of general anesthesia,* Sacramento, Calif, 1993, The Board.
5. Zink BJ, Darfler K, Salluzzo RF et al: The efficacy and safety of methohexital in the emergency department, *Ann Emerg Med* 20:1293, 1991.
6. Gilman AG, Rall TW, Nies AS et al: *Goodman and Gilman's pharmacological basis of therapeutics,* ed 8, New York, 1990, McGraw-Hill.
7. Gaines GY III, Rees DI: Anesthetic considerations for electroconvulsive therapy, *South Med J* 85:469, 1992.
8. Van Hemelrijck J, Gonzales JM, White PF: Pharmacology of intravenous anesthetic agents. In Rogers MC, Tinker JH, Covino BG, eds: *Principles and practice of anesthesiology,* St Louis, 1993, Mosby.
9. Eldor J: High-dose flunitrazepam anesthesia, *Med Hypoth* 38:352, 1992.
10. Wetzel RC, Maxwell LG: Anesthesia for children. In Rogers MC, Tinker JH, Covino BG, eds: *Principles and practice of anesthesiology,* St Louis, 1993, Mosby.
11. Horrigan RW, Moyers JR, Johnson BH et al: Etomidate vs thiopental with and without fentanyl, a comparative study of awakening in man, *Anesthesiology* 52:362, 1980.
12. Miller BM, Hendry JGB, Lees NW: Etomidate and methohexital, a comparative clinical study in outpatient anesthesia, *Anaesthesia* 33:450, 1978.
13. Waxman K, Shoemaker WC, Lipmann M: Cardiovascular effects of anesthetic induction with ketamine, *Anesth Analg* 59:355, 1980.
14. Tobias JD, Martin LD, Wetzel RC: Ketamine by continuous infusion for sedation in the pediatric intensive care unit, *Crit Care Med* 18:819, 1990.
15. Reich DL, Silvay G: Ketamine: an update on the first twenty-five years of clinical experience, *Can J Anaesth* 36:186, 1989.
16. Weightman WM, Zacharias M: Comparison of propofol and thiopentone anaesthesia (with special reference to recovery characteristics), *Anaesth Intens Care* 15:389, 1987.
17. Rutter DV, Morgan M, Lumley J et al: ICI 35868 (Diprivan): a new intravenous induction agent, *Anaesthesia* 35:1188, 1980.
18. Pecaro BC, Houting T: Diprivan (ICI 35868, 2,6-di-isopropylphenol), a new intravenous anesthetic, *Oral Surg* 60:586, 1985.
19. McCulloch MJ, Lees NW: Assessment and modification of pain on induction with propofol (Diprivan), *Anaesthesia* 40:1117, 1985.
20. Grounds RM, Twigley AJ, Carli F et al: The haemodynamics of intravenous induction. Comparison of the effects of thiopentone and propofol, *Anaesthesia* 40:735, 1985.
21. Kay NH, Uppington J, Sear JW et al: Use of an emulsion of ICI 35868 (propofol) for the induction and maintenance of anaesthesia, *Br J Anaesthesiol* 57:736, 1985.
22. Cundy JM, Arunasalam K: Use of an emulsion formulation of propofol (Diprivan) in intravenous anaesthesia for termination of pregnancy. A comparison with methohexitone. *Postgrad Med J* 61(suppl 3):129, 1985.
23. Wedell D, Hersh EV: A review of the opioid analgesics fentanyl, alfentanil, and sufentanil, *Compendium* 12:184, 1991.
24. Clotz MA, Nahata MC: Clinical uses of fentanyl, sufentanil, and alfentanil, *Clin Pharm* 18:581, 1991.
25. Burkle H, Dunbar S, Van Aken H: Remifentanil: a novel, short-acting, μ-opioid, *Anesth Analg* 83:646, 1996.
26. Glass PS: Remifentanil: a new opioid, *J Clin Anesth* 7:558, 1995.
27. Lefevre B, Freysz M, Lepine J et al: Comparison of nalbuphine and fentanyl as intravenous analgesics for medically compromised patients undergoing oral surgery, *Anesth Prog* 39:13, 1993.
28. Elleby DH, Greenberg PM, Barry LD: Postoperative narcotic and nonnarcotic analgesics, *Clin Podiatr Med Surg* 9:365, 1992.
29. Bremang JA: Neuroleptic analgesia in ambulatory (nasal) endoscopies, *J Otolaryngol* 20:435, 1991.
30. Snow JC: Intravenous anesthesia. In *Manual of anesthesia,* Boston, 1977, Little, Brown.
31. Waxman K, Shoemaker WC, Lipmann M: Cardiovascular effects of anesthetic induction with ketamine, *Anesth Analg* 59:355, 1980.
32. Roelofse JA, Vander Bilj P: Adverse reactions to midazolam and ketamine premedication in children, *Anesth Prog* 38:73, 1991.
33. Klausen NO, Wilberg-Jorgensen F, Chraemmer-Jorgensen B: Psychotomimetic reactions after low-dose ketamine infusion. Comparison with neuroleptanaesthesia, *Br J Anaesth* 55:297, 1983.
34. Schweinefus R, Schick L: Succinylcholine: "good guy, bad guy," *J Post Anesth Nurs* 6:410, 1991.
35. Bunker JP and the National Research Council, Subcommittee on the National Halothane Study: *The national halothane study: a study of the possible association between halothane anesthesia and postoperative hepatic necrosis: report,* Bethesda, Md, 1969, National Institute of General Medical Science.
36. Ogawa A, Oi K: Use of N_2O/O_2 enflurane anesthesia for dental treatment of the handicapped, *J Oral Maxillofac Surg* 49:343, 1991.
37. Smiley RM, Ornstein E, Matteo RS et al: Desflurane and isoflurane in surgical patients: comparison of emergence time, *Anesthesiology* 74:425, 1991.
38. Fletcher JE, Sebel PS, Murphy MR et al: Psychomotor performance after desflurane anesthesia: a comparison with isoflurane, *Anesth Analg* 73:260, 1991.

SECTION VII

EMERGENCY PREPARATION AND MANAGEMENT

Whenever drugs are administered or prescribed, adverse reactions may occur. Fortunately, with the vast majority of drugs currently used in the management of pain and anxiety, the incidence of adverse drug reactions (ADRs) is low. Indeed, those drugs that, although therapeutically useful, have a greater incidence of ADRs are rapidly replaced in the physician's and dentist's armamentarium by newer, equally useful drugs possessing a decreased risk of ADRs.

Indiscriminate drug usage is one of the major causes of the increase in the number of serious incidents of drug-related life-threatening emergencies that are reported in the medical and dental literature.[1,2] It is hoped that whenever a drug is administered or prescribed, a rational purpose exists for its administration. Most drug-related emergency situations are classified as one aspect of iatrogenic disease, a category encompassing a spectrum of adverse effects produced unintentionally by health-care providers in the course of patient management.

The frequency of occurrence of ADRs as reported in the medical and dental literature has ranged from 3% to 20% of all hospital admissions.[1-4] Of patients hospitalized for other reasons, 5% to 40% will experience an ADR during their hospitalization. Furthermore, another 10% to 18% of those patients hospitalized because of an ADR will have yet another ADR while in the hospital, which results in the length of their hospitalization being prolonged.[4]

Because the overwhelming majority of drugs discussed in this text are CNS depressants administered to patients for the purpose of managing their treatment-related fears and anxieties, it is likely that ADRs will be noted at some time. For this reason, the doctor and the entire office staff must be able to recognize and be prepared to manage these situations rapidly and effectively.

This section is divided into three chapters. The first two chapters discuss the subject of preparation—of the office, office personnel, and the requirement for emergency drugs and equipment—and the third chapter reviews the management of systemic emergencies that might occur during conscious sedation. Localized complications have been reviewed with each of the major techniques of conscious sedation (see Chapter 10 for intramuscular sedation, Chapter 16 for inhalation sedation, and Chapter 27 for intravenous sedation).

The need for emergency preparedness exists in a dental or medical practice regardless of whether sedative techniques are used. Indeed, as discussed in Chapter 4, the medically compromised patient who is fearful or experiences unexpected pain during treatment is more likely to suffer an acute exacerbation of his or her medical problem at this time than is a more relaxed, pain-free patient with the same medical problem. In one report, 77% of systemic emergencies associated with dental care occurred either during or immediately after the administration of local anesthetic (54.9%) or during the ensuing dental treatment (22.9%), arguably the most psychologically and physiologically stressful portions of the entire dental experience.[5] The types of dental treatment most frequently being attempted at the time the systemic emergency occurred were tooth extraction and pulpal extirpation, procedures in which complete pain control may prove elusive.[5]

Occurrence of Systemic Complications	
Just before treatment	1.5%
During/after local anesthesia	54.9%
During treatment*	22.9%
After treatment	15.2%
After leaving office	5.5%

*See next box for specific treatment during emergency.

Basic preparation of the dental/medical office and office staff is the same whether or not sedative techniques are used. There are, however, some drugs and items of emergency equipment that the doctor using sedation techniques will have available that are unnecessary in the offices of doctors not using sedation. Emergency equipment is reviewed along with the components of the basic emergency kit.

Type of Dental Treatment during Occurrence of Systemic Complication	
Tooth extraction	38.9%
Pulpal extirpation	26.9%
Unknown	12.3%
Other treatment	9.0%
Preparation	7.3%
Filling	2.3%
Incision	1.7%
Apicoectomy	0.7%
Removal of fillings	0.7%
Alveolar plastics	0.3%

Most, but not all, drug-related emergencies can be prevented. The doctor administering or prescribing drugs for a patient must always keep the following three principles of toxicology in mind[6]:

1. No drug ever exerts a single action.
2. No clinically useful drug is entirely devoid of toxicity.
3. Potential toxicity of a drug rests in the hands of the user.

Ideally, the right drug in the right dose will be administered by the right route to the right patient at the right time for the right reason and will not produce any unwanted effects. Unfortunately, this clinical situation rarely, if ever, exists because no drug is so specific that it produces only desirable effects in all patients. It must also be remembered that ADRs may occur when the wrong drug is administered to the wrong patient in the wrong dose by the wrong route at the wrong time and for the wrong reason. The most important safety factors in drug administration are the knowledge and ability of the person administering the drug. Before administering any drug, the doctor should be fully prepared to manage any ADR that might develop.

REFERENCES

1. Naranjo CA, Shear NH, Lanctot KL: Advances in the diagnosis of adverse drug reactions, *J Clin Pharmacol* 32:897, 1992.
2. Waller PC: Measuring the frequency of adverse drug reactions, *Br J Clin Pharmacol* 33:249, 1992.
3. Einarson TR: Drug-related hospital admissions, *Ann Pharmacother* 27:832, 1993.
4. Bates DW, Leape LL, Petrycki S: Incidence and preventability of adverse drug events in hospitalized adults, *J Gen Intern Med* 8:289, 1993.
5. Matsuura H: Analysis of systemic complications and death during dental treatment in Japan, *Anesth Prog* 36:219, 1990.
6. Pallasch TJ: *Pharmacology for dental students and practitioners,* Philadelphia, 1980, Lea & Febiger.

CHAPTER 32

Preparation for Emergencies

CHAPTER OUTLINE

Although the prevention of life-threatening emergencies is always our primary goal, potentially catastrophic situations will develop despite our best efforts. With proper patient evaluation before the start of any treatment, appropriate treatment modification if necessary, selection of appropriate techniques and drugs for pain and anxiety control, adherence to proper technique of drug administration, and adequate monitoring throughout the procedure, it is unlikely that serious emergency situations will arise. However, in the event that an emergency does occur, it becomes extremely important for the dental office to be properly prepared and for all office personnel to be trained to recognize and to manage such situations in a prompt and effective manner. Box 32-1 summarizes the suggested preparation of the medical/dental office and staff for emergency situations.

OFFICE

With all office personnel trained to recognize and manage life-threatening situations, it is possible for each of them to maintain the life of a victim alone or as a member of a trained emergency team. Although management of most emergencies is possible with but a single rescuer, the concerted efforts of several trained persons is more efficient. Because most dental and medical offices have numerous staff persons present

BOX 32-1 Summary of Preparation

Office
Team approach to emergency management
Emergency drugs and equipment checked regularly
Emergency telephone numbers readily available:
- Emergency medical services (e.g., 9-1-1)
- Nearby oral and maxillofacial surgeon
- Nearby physician (well versed in emergency medicine)

Emergency practice drills

Office Personnel
Annual recertification in BLS (health-care provider)
Annual review program in emergency medicine

during working hours, organization of a team approach to emergency management is possible.

OFFICE PERSONNEL

An important factor in preparation of the medical/dental office for management of emergency situations will be the training of *all* office personnel, including nonchairside personnel, in their recognition and management. Training should include an annual refresher course in all aspects of emergency medicine—a course reviewing situations such as seizures, chest pain, unconsciousness, altered consciousness, drug-related emergencies, and respiratory difficulty, not simply basic life support (BLS). Such continuing education programs are available with schedules published regularly by dental organizations such as the American Dental Association.[1] In a dental office in which conscious sedation is used, refresher courses in these techniques, including their complications, are also recommended.

Basic Life Support

Of even greater importance than the overall emergency review program is the requirement for the clinical ability to perform BLS, more commonly known as *cardiopulmonary resuscitation* (CPR). It is my opinion that no other preparatory step is as important as this one because training in BLS enables a rescuer to recognize an acute life-threatening situation and to know what to do. The steps of BLS require no additional equipment, the mouth, hands, and knowledge of the rescuer being quite adequate in most cases to maintain a life. In the presence of a drug-related emergency, BLS usually proves to be the first and most important step in management.

The doctor should mandate that *all* office personnel remain proficient in BLS techniques after having received their initial course. There is a rapid decline in CPR skills following an initial BLS training program. Within 6 months of completing a provider-level training program, the average person loses approximately 60% of his or her ability to perform adequate BLS.[2] In a recent clinical experiment, only 4 of 30 postdoctoral dentists (graduate students), who had been recertified in BLS within the previous 4 months, were able to perform adequate one-person CPR on a mannequin for 1 minute.[3] Maintaining proficiency is important because even when BLS is performed perfectly (a rarely achieved goal), the delivery of oxygenated blood to the victim's brain is only 25% to 33% of normal.[4] Faulty CPR technique leads to diminished cerebral blood flow and decreased likelihood of survival.

If a doctor, an assistant, or a hygienist were present in a dental office with only one other person present and were the victim of cardiac arrest, this second person would be the only one available to provide BLS. *Making certain that* all *personnel are proficient in BLS thus becomes the single most important step in assuring that medical emergencies are managed efficiently and effectively.*

Advanced Cardiac Life Support

Advanced cardiac life support (ACLS) involves the use of adjunctive equipment and drugs to further stabilize and manage the victim of a cardiac arrest or other serious cardiac rhythm disturbance. The ACLS course includes training and evaluation in technique of venipuncture and endotracheal intubation, interpretation of electrocardiograph (ECG) rhythms, and management of cardiac dysrhythmias through drug therapy and defibrillation.[5]

Doctors using IV conscious sedation might consider becoming trained in ACLS. With the availability of the IV route for drug administration, the ACLS-trained doctor becomes better able to manage such situations. It is my contention that doctors using deep sedation or general anesthesia should become certified in advanced cardiac life support. Provider-level programs in ACLS are available in most areas to eligible persons. These include the physician, nurse, pharmacist, and dentist who have previously been certified in BLS. In some jurisdictions paramedical personnel are ACLS trained. ACLS programs are usually presented within a hospital under the auspices of the American Heart Association (AHA). Contact your local AHA affiliate for more information about these courses.

Pediatric Advanced Life Support

The doctor called on to manage the dental needs of younger children should give serious consideration to becoming trained in pediatric advanced life support (PALS). PALS training includes the following components: basic life support (infant and child); use of adjunctive equipment and special techniques to establish and maintain effective oxygenation, ventilation, and perfusion; clinical and ECG monitoring and arrhythmia detection; establishment and maintenance of vascular access; identification and treatment of reversible causes of cardiopulmonary arrest; therapies for emergency treatment of patients with cardiac and respiratory arrest; and treatment of patients with trauma, shock, respiratory failure, or other prearrest conditions.[6]

Team Approach to Emergency Management

An office emergency team consists of two or three members, each of whom has a well-defined role in the management of an emergency situation. The doctor leads the team and is responsible for directing the activities of its other members (unless it is the doctor who is the victim of the emergency). In most situations the doctor will be responsible for implementing the steps of BLS (P → A → B → C) and will administer emergency drugs to the victim, where indicated.

The second team member is responsible for the maintenance of emergency drugs and equipment. The emergency drug kit and equipment should be checked regularly to ensure that they will be available and fully stocked when needed (see Chapter 33). When an emergency does occur, this team member gathers the emergency kit and equipment and immediately brings it to the site of the emergency. Should emergency drugs be required, this team member readies the drugs for administration by the doctor. Other possible roles for this team member include administration of BLS, monitoring of vital signs, and summoning of medical assistance. In BLS this team member will be an integral part of the emergency management and will ventilate the victim and/or perform external chest compression.

A third team member may be used when available. This member reports immediately to the site of the emergency and remains available as a circulating member, assisting as required. Roles for this member include monitoring vital signs, summoning medical assistance, administering BLS, and keeping records. During BLS this member remains available to relieve the first or second member.

If the dental office is located in a large, high-rise multioffice building, a team member is directed to the lobby to ensure that an elevator is readily available for the emergency team and to expeditiously lead the emergency response team to the proper location.

It is important that all office personnel be capable of participating in the emergency team. In addition, all team members should be able to carry out any of the functions of the entire team. Practice thus becomes vitally important. Table 32-1 summarizes the role of each member of the emergency team.

TABLE 32-1 Emergency Team

Team Member	Responsibility
Member 1	Remain with victim. "Yell" for help. Administer BLS, as required.
Member 2	Retrieve emergency drug kit and oxygen. Bring items to site of emergency. Assist member 1 as needed.
Member 3	Assist members 1 and 2 as required.

EMERGENCY PRACTICE DRILLS

If life-threatening situations occurred with more frequency in medical and dental offices, there would be little need for emergency practice sessions. Team members would receive their training under actual emergency conditions. Fortunately, life-threatening situations do not occur with any degree of frequency. Because of this, team members quickly become rusty from the lack of opportunity to use their newly acquired knowledge and skill. Annual refresher courses in emergency medicine are invaluable in maintaining the level of overall knowledge of the emergency team members.

Of greater importance, however, is the team's ability to perform well in the office setting. In-office emergency drills are one means of maintaining an efficient emergency team in the absence of true emergency situations. On an irregular basis the doctor may stage a simulated life-threatening emergency. All team members should be able to respond exactly as they must under emergency conditions. Many doctors have even purchased mannequins (CPR "dummies") for practicing BLS and hold frequent practice sessions for their staff.

Oral and maxillofacial surgeons have devised a system of in-office evaluation for general anesthetic technique and emergency preparedness. A group of examiners (other doctors) assesses the preparedness of the oral surgery office by staging mock emergencies (e.g., laryngospasm, cardiac arrest, bronchospasm) and viewing the office staff's response.[7] Created by the Southern California Society of Oral and Maxillofacial Surgeons, the in-office evaluation has become a requirement for membership in the American Association of Oral and Maxillofacial Surgeons. Similar programs have been instituted by dental boards of many of the 50 states that require a dentist to obtain a permit in order to utilize general anesthesia or parenteral conscious sedation.[8] A voluntary program in office emergency preparedness, part of an IV conscious sedation certification program, has been in existence for 25 years at the University of Southern California School of Dentistry.[9]

OUTSIDE MEDICAL ASSISTANCE

Although most emergency situations are transient in nature and easily managed by the dental office emergency team, occasions arise in which outside medical assistance is required. In situations involving adverse drug reactions following the administration of CNS depressants, follow-up evaluation by well-trained medical professionals is frequently recommended. For these reasons, telephone numbers of emergency services personnel should be readily available and conspicuously posted by each telephone in the office (Figure 32-1). It is strongly suggested that the following telephone numbers be programmed into a telephone's speed-dial system:

- Local emergency medical services (EMS) (i.e., 9-1-1)
- A *well-trained* dental or medical colleague
- Emergency ambulance service with BLS- or BLS/ACLS-trained personnel
- An AHA-certified hospital emergency room

Most communities in the United States have instituted the universal emergency telephone number, 9-1-1, to expedite activation of their EMS. This number immediately connects the caller to the rescue service (usually fire, police, and medical). When emergency medical care is required in the dental office, the community EMS is usually the preferred source of immediate assistance. In the unlikely situation that 9-1-1 is unavailable in a community, the seven-digit telephone number should be conspicuously posted and programmed into the telephone.

A *well-trained* dental or medical colleague can also serve as a source of emergency medical assistance. It is important, however, to discuss this arrangement before its actual need. The doctor seeking assistance must be absolutely certain that the person called is, in fact, well versed in emergency medicine and is likely to be available during office hours.[10] In offices in which more than one well-trained doctor is usually present, such a system is easily adopted. It has been my experience that the individuals with the best training in emergency medicine are emergency medicine physicians, anesthesiologists, surgeons (physicians), and oral and maxillofacial surgeons (dentists). Unfortunately for the doctor working in a private dental practice, the first two groups are normally hospital-based and thus are not readily available to the non–hospital-based dental practitioner. A surgeon (MD) or an oral and maxillofacial surgeon may be more readily available in the nonhospital setting. Prior arrangement with these persons will avoid potential misunderstandings and increase their effectiveness in emergency situations.

Most emergency ambulance services require their personnel to be trained as emergency medical technicians (EMT) who are capable of providing BLS. This may serve as an alternative source of basic assistance should other rescuers be unavailable.

The location of a hospital close to your office that maintains a 24-hour emergency room staffed with fully trained emergency personnel should be determined in the event that a victim requires transport to that facility for evaluation or management. The AHA evaluates and certifies those emergency rooms that meet their rigid criteria.

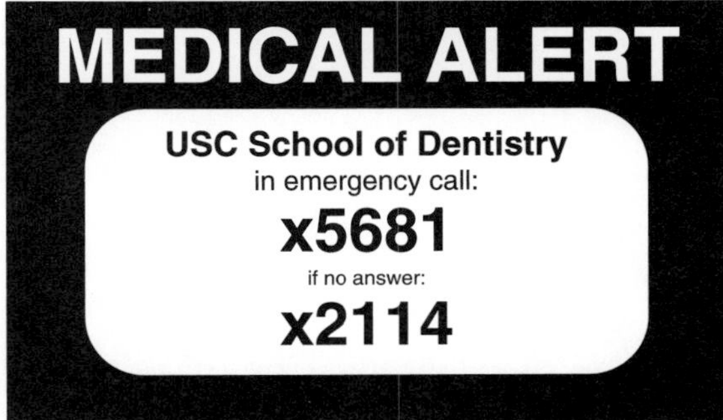

MEDICAL ALERT
USC School of Dentistry
in emergency call:
x5681
if no answer:
x2114

Figure 32-1 Emergency telephone numbers should be posted clearly at every telephone.

SUMMARY

Adequate training of all members of the office staff is absolutely essential if potentially life-threatening situations are to be adequately managed. Preparation of the staff must occur before emergencies occur. The recommended steps in preparing both the office staff and the office for such situations have been discussed. In the following chapters the components of the emergency drug kit and emergency equipment are reviewed, as is the management of specific emergency situations related to drug administration.

REFERENCES

1. Council on Dental Education: *Continuing education course list for January–June, 2001,* Chicago, 2001, ADA.
2. Bossaert LL, Putzeys T, Monsieurs KG et al: Knowledge, skills and counseling behavior of Belgian general practitioners on CPR-related issues, *Resuscitation* 24:49, 1992.
3. Malamed SF: Unpublished data. December 2000.
4. Paradis NA, Martin GB, Goetting MG et al: Simultaneous aortic, jugular bulb, and right atrial pressures during cardiopulmonary resuscitation in humans: insight into mechanisms, *Circulation* 80:361, 1989.
5. International Consensus on Science: Guidelines 2000 for cardiopulmonary resuscitation and emergency cardiovascular care. *Circulation* 102(suppl):86, 2000.
6. International Consensus on Science: Guidelines 2000 for cardiopulmonary resuscitation and emergency cardiovascular care. *Circulation* 102(suppl):291, 2000.

7. American Association of Oral and Maxillofacial Surgeons, Committee on Anesthesia: *Office anesthesia evaluation manual,* ed 4, Rosemont, Ill, 1991, The Association.
8. Department of State Government Affairs: Chicago, 2002, American Dental Association.
9. Malamed SF: Evolution of an undergraduate program in pain and anxiety control: a 15-year history, *J Dent Educ* 53:277, 1989.
10. Peter R: Sudden unconsciousness during local anesthetic, *Anesth Pain Control Dent* 2:140, 1993.

CHAPTER 33

Emergency Drugs and Equipment

CHAPTER OUTLINE

Emergency drugs and equipment must be available in every medical and dental office regardless of whether or not sedation and/or general anesthesia techniques are used. Although successful resolution of most emergency situations does not require drug administration, on occasion this may prove to be lifesaving. In the acute systemic allergic response, anaphylaxis, for example, administration of epinephrine is critical. In most other emergencies, however, drug administration is afforded a secondary role in overall management. In situations in which adverse drug reactions (ADRs) develop following administration of drugs for sedation or pain control, it may be possible, in some cases, to significantly improve the clinical picture through the administration of an antidotal drug.

The emergency drug kit is discussed at several different levels of complexity. The entry level represents the "bare bones" basic emergency kit, which I believe should be available in the offices of all practicing dentists and physicians regardless of whether sedative techniques are used. The second group of drugs is recommended for doctors who have received more advanced training in the care and handling of medical emergencies. Following this, drugs recommended for possible administration in advanced cardiac life support (ACLS) are discussed, with drugs required for the management of ADRs associated with parenteral drug administration concluding our discussion.[1]

The emergency kit need not and, indeed, should not be overly complex. As Pallasch[2] has stated, "Complexity in a time of adversity breeds chaos."

Because dentists' levels of training in emergency management can vary significantly, it is impossible to recommend any one list of emergency drugs or any one proprietary emergency drug kit that meets the needs and abilities of all dentists. For this reason, dentists should develop their own emergency drug and equipment kits based on their level of expertise in managing medical emergencies.[3]

The emergency drug kit maintained by the doctor using parenteral sedation or general anesthesia will, of necessity, include drugs and equipment not recommended for emergency kits of doctors who are not well trained in anesthesia (used in its broadest sense). The Council on Dental Therapeutics of the American Dental Association, many state dental boards, and specialty organizations have developed and published either recommendations or requirements for the inclusion of specific emergency drugs and equipment for offices in which parenteral sedation or general anesthesia is administered (Boxes 33-1 and 33-2).[4-6]

A plastic container for fishing tackle can be used to store these drugs (Figure 33-1). A more inclusive emergency kit might be developed from a mobile tool chest (Figure 33-2). Labels are applied to each container with both the generic and proprietary name of the drug and its dosage, for example, diazepam (Valium), 5 mg/ml. The emergency kit must be maintained in an area where it may be easily located. All emergency drugs and equipment should be checked weekly and reordered before their expiration dates; the oxygen (O_2) cylinder should be checked daily.

The following are guidelines for the development of an office emergency kit. Categories of drugs are listed with a suggestion for specific drug(s) within each grouping. Space precludes lengthy descriptions of the rationale for selecting each drug. Readers desiring more in-depth information are referred to appropriate textbooks.[1,3]

Each of the drug categories presented next should be considered for inclusion in the emergency kit; however, the doctor should select only those drugs with which he or she is familiar. The doctor must carefully evaluate everything that goes into the emergency kit. All drugs come with a "package insert." The insert should be saved and read and important information concerning the drug noted, such as usual dose, contraindications, adverse reactions, and expiration date. Two categories of drugs, injectables and noninjectables, are included in

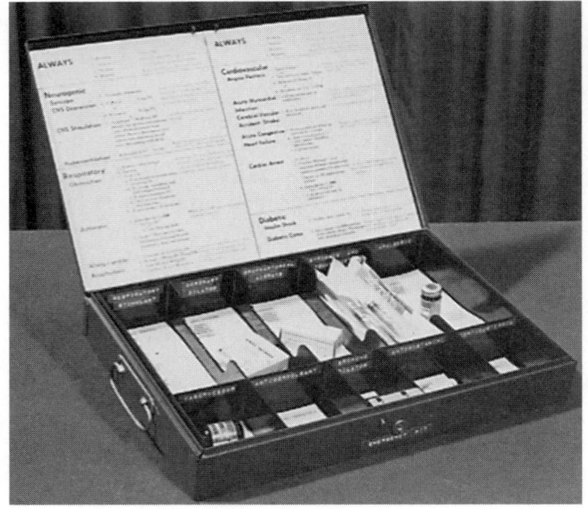

Figure 33-1 Emergency kit.

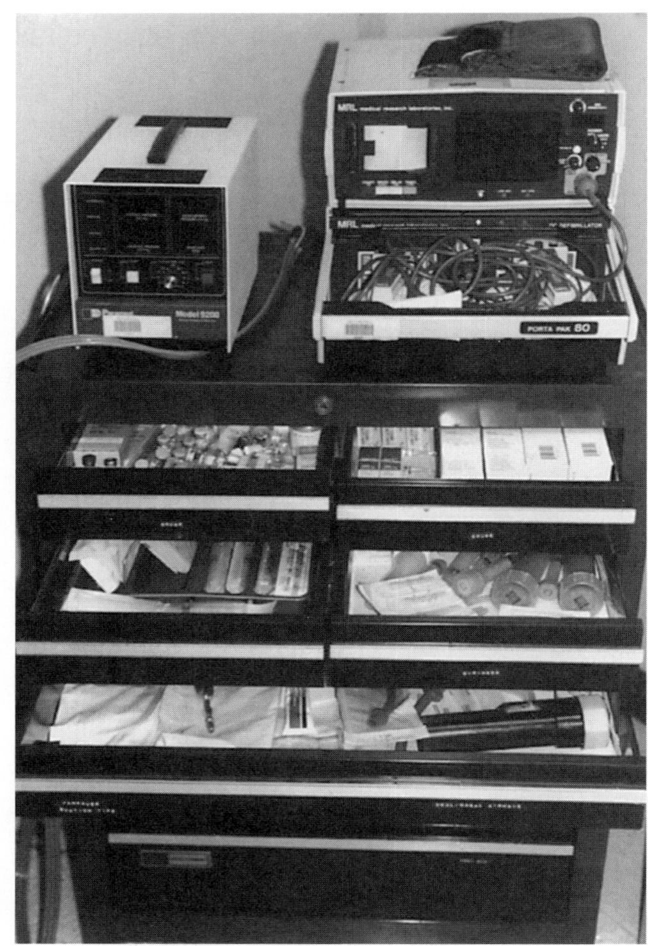

Figure 33-2 Fully equipped, mobile emergency kit. (Courtesy Department of Oral and Maxillofacial Surgery, University of Southern California, School of Dentistry.)

BOX 33-1

Emergency Drugs Required by California State Board of Dental Examiners for Conscious Sedation Permit and General Anesthesia

1. Vasopressor
2. Corticosteroid
3. Bronchodilator
4. Appropriate drug antagonists
5. Antihistaminic
6. Anticholinergic
7. Coronary artery vasodilator
8. Anticonvulsants
9. Oxygen
10. 50% dextrose or other antihypoglycemic
11. Muscle relaxant*
12. Intravenous medication for treatment of cardiopulmonary arrest*
13. Antidysrhythmic*
14. Antihypertensive*

*Use for general anesthesia only.

BOX 33-2 Suggested Emergency Equipment and Drugs

Suggested Equipment

A. Source of oxygen and equipment to deliver positive-pressure ventilation
B. Respiratory support equipment
   1. Oral airways/nasal airways
   2. Endotracheal tubes with stylets
   3. Laryngoscope and suitable blades (plus extra bulbs and batteries)
   4. Magill forceps or other suitable instruments
   5. Coniotomy set with connector
C. Stethoscope
D. Blood pressure cuff
E. Direct-current defibrillator
F. Electrocardiogram or electrocardioscope with leads and electropaste
G. Equipment to establish intravenous infusion
   1. Needles, syringes, intravenous sets, and connectors
   2. Intravenous cutdown set
   3. Tourniquets for venipuncture
   4. Adhesive tape
H. Pulse oximeter

Suggested Drugs

The following are examples of drugs that will be helpful in the treatment of anesthetic emergencies. The list should not be considered mandatory or all-inclusive.

A. Intravenous fluids
   1. Water for injection and/or mixing or dilution of drugs
   2. Intravenous fluids
B. Cardiotonic drugs
   1. Verapamil
   2. Digoxin
   3. Coronary dilators
      a. Amyl nitrite (ampules or pearls)
      b. Nitroglycerin (Nitrostat)
C. Vasopressors
   1. Dopamine hydrochloride (Intropin)
   2. Epinephrine 1:1000 or 1:10,000
   3. Dobutamine
   4. Isoproterenol (Isuprel)
   5. Phenylephrine (Neo-Synephrine)
D. Antidysrhythmic agents
   1. Atropine sulfate
   2. Lidocaine 2%
   3. Propranolol (Inderal)
   4. Procainamide
   5. Verapamil
   6. Verticillium or Bretylium
E. Antihypertensive agents (immediate)
   1. Diazoxide (Hyperstat)
   2. Chlorpromazine (Thorazine)
   3. Nitroprusside
   4. Nitroglycerin
F. Diuretics
   1. Furosemide (Lasix)
G. Antiemetics (Droperidol, Compazine)
H. Narcotic antagonist
   1. Naloxone (Narcan)
I. Anticholinergic antagonist
   1. Physostigmine salicylate (Antilirium)
J. Accessory drugs
   1. Dextrose 50%
   2. Hydrocortisone sodium succinate (Solu-Cortef)
   3. Dexamethasone (Decadron)
   4. Aminophylline
   5. Atropine sulfate
   6. Glycopyrrolate (Robinul)
   7. Diazepam (Valium)
   8. Methohexital 1% (Brevital)
   9. Sodium thiopental 2.5% (Pentothal)
   10. Diphenhydramine (Benadryl)
   11. Isuprel (Medihaler)
   12. Midazolam (Versed)
   13. Succinylcholine (Anectine)
   14. Morphine sulphate

Modified from American Association of Oral and Maxillofacial Surgeons, Committee on Anesthesia: *Office anesthesia evaluation manual*, ed 4, Rosemont, Ill, 1991, The Association.)

the emergency kit. Items of emergency equipment also have a very definite place in the management of life-threatening situations. As with drugs, however, it is important for the doctor to know his or her limitations when it comes to using this equipment. Improper use of emergency equipment may further complicate an already tenuous situation. There are two categories of emergency equipment: primary or basic equipment, which I believe should be available in every medical and dental office, and secondary or advanced equipment, for those persons who have received training and are experienced in its use.

Merely having items of emergency equipment available does not in and of itself make the office better equipped or the staff any more prepared to manage medical emergencies. Personnel expected to use emergency equipment must be trained in emergency management and in the proper use of these items.

Unfortunately, many emergency devices commonly found in dental and medical offices can prove to be useless or, more significantly, hazardous if used improperly or in the wrong situation. Training in the use of some items, such as the laryngoscope and oropharyngeal airway, may best be obtained only by caring for patients under general anesthesia, a situation usually not readily available. Many of the items of emergency equipment listed in this section are therefore recommended for use only by trained personnel. All of the secondary equipment falls into this category; unfortunately, several items listed as primary are also included (e.g., O_2 delivery system). Although all dentists and physicians should be trained in the use of O_2 delivery systems, courses in which these techniques are taught to clinical proficiency are particularly difficult to locate.

The types of drugs and equipment included in the emergency kit must be appropriate for the level of training of the office personnel who will be called on to use the kit. Table 33-1 lists drugs and equipment recommended for inclusion in a basic emergency kit.

LEVEL 1: BASIC EMERGENCY KIT

Injectable Drugs

The following two categories are considered to be primary critical drugs and should be included in *all* emergency kits:

1. Epinephrine (for management of acute allergic reactions)
2. Histamine blocker (antihistamine)

Epinephrine (Adrenalin) is the drug of choice in management of acute allergic reactions involving the respiratory or cardiovascular system. In addition, epinephrine administration is indicated in bronchospasm (asthma) and cardiac arrest. The minimum suggested for the emergency kit are one preloaded syringe (1:1000) (Figure 33-3) and three to four ampules of 1:1000 epinephrine. Preloaded epinephrine syringes are available in a 1:2000 concentration for administration to patients younger than 9 years of age. For doctors comfortable with venipuncture and intravenous (IV) drug administration, epinephrine is available as a 1:10,000 dilution (1 mg in 10 ml).

Several *histamine blockers* are available for parenteral administration. Most frequently used in emergency situations are diphenhydramine (Benadryl) and chlorpheniramine (Chlor-Trimeton). Indications for the administration of histamine blockers include management of delayed allergic response, definitive management of acute allergy, and as a local anesthetic when a history of allergy is present. Suggested for the emergency kit are several 1-ml ampules of either 10 mg/ml of chlorpheniramine or 50 mg/ml of diphenhydramine.

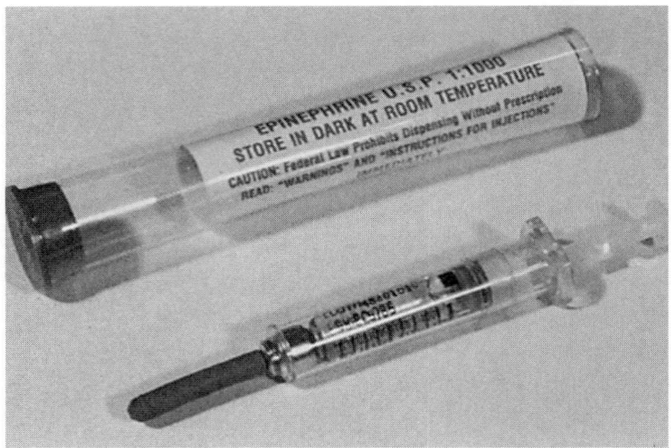

Figure 33-3 Preloaded epinephrine syringe.

Noninjectable Drugs

Five noninjectable drugs are recommended for all emergency kits. *Oxygen* is, arguably, the most important drug in the emergency kit. Although it is available in a variety of cylinder sizes (see Chapter 14), the "E" cylinder is most recommended for emergency availability. Therapeutic indications for the administration of O_2 include any situation in which respiratory distress is evident. The minimal suggested amount for the emergency kit is one "E" cylinder (an apparatus for O_2 delivery must also be available and is discussed later).

Vasodilators are administered in the immediate management of chest pain. The drug of choice is nitroglycerin as a translingual spray. Suggested for the emergency kit is one bottle of Nitrolingual Spray (0.4 mg/spray).

Bronchodilators are required for the definitive management of bronchospasm. Epinephrine, probably the most highly recommended bronchodilator, has been included in the emergency kit as an injectable drug. Other drugs, equally effective as bronchodilators (β_2 actions) but with fewer cardiovascular (β_1) side effects than epinephrine, are available and can be administered by aerosol inhalation directly into the bronchi (as can epinephrine). Recommended for use in the medical or dental office is albuterol, a drug with excellent β_2 effects but minimal β_1 actions. Therapeutic indications for administration of bronchodilators include respiratory distress as seen in asthma and allergic reactions with a significant respiratory component. Suggested for the emergency kit is one albuterol inhaler.

Hypoglycemia is not an uncommon occurrence. Most hypoglycemic patients, whether diabetic or not, remain conscious but exhibit bizarre behavior. Management involves the administration of an *antihy-*

TABLE 33-1 Module 1: Critical (Essential) Emergency Drugs and Equipment

	Primary Drug			*Recommended for Kit*	
Category	Generic	Proprietary	Alternative	Quantity	Availability
Injectables					
Antiallergy	Epinephrine	Adrenalin	None	One preloaded syringe and three to four 1-ml ampules	1:1000 (1 mg/ml)
Histamine blocker	Chlorpheniramine	Chlor-Trimeton	Diphenhydramine	Three to four 1-ml ampules	10 mg/ml
Noninjectables					
Oxygen	Oxygen		None	Minimum of 1 E cylinder	
Vasodilator	Nitroglycerin	Nitrolingual spray	Nitrostat SL tablets	One metered spray bottle	0.4 mg/dose
Bronchodilator	Albuterol	Proventil, Ventolin	Metaproterenol	One metered dose inhaler	
Antihypoglycemic	Sugar			Orange juice, nondiet soft drink	
Antiplatelet	Aspirin	Many	None	3 or 4 chewable (162 mg) tablets	162, 325 mg

Equipment	Description	Quantity
Emergency Equipment		
Oxygen delivery system	Positive-pressure and demand valve, or bag-valve-mask device and clear full-face masks of various sizes	Minimum of one oxygen delivery system with positive-pressure mask One portable bag-valve-mask device Minimum of one child, one small-adult, and one large-adult full-face masks
	Pocket mask	One pocket mask per employee
Syringes for drug administration	Disposable syringes	Two to four 2-ml syringes with attached needles for parenteral drug administration
Suction and suction tips	High-volume suction system	Office suction system
	Large-diameter, round-ended suction tips or tonsillar suction	Minimum of two
Tourniquets	Rubber or Velcro tourniquet, rubber tubing, or sphygmomanometer	Three tourniquets and one sphygmomanometer
Magill intubation forceps	Blunt-ended scissors with right-angle bend	One pediatric-size forceps

From Malamed SF: *Medical emergencies in the dental office*, ed 5, St Louis, 2000, Mosby.

poglycemic either intravenously, intramuscularly, or orally. Several commercial oral antihypoglycemic products are available, such as Glucola, Gluco-Stat, and Insta-Glucose. In addition, nondiet soft drinks, fruit juices, and simple sugar are available. Suggested for the emergency kit for management of the conscious hypoglycemic is some form of oral glucose.

Aspirin, an antithrombotic, is recommended for use in the prehospital phase of suspected acute myocardial infarction (AMI). Evidence indicates that aspirin reduces mortality in patients with AMI by 23% when used alone and by 42% when used in combination with thrombolytic therapy.[7] Suggested for the emergency kit is three or four "baby" or chewable aspirin (162 mg).

Primary (Basic) Emergency Equipment

The basic level of emergency equipment includes the following items:

1. O_2 delivery system
2. Suction and suction tips
3. Syringes for drug administration
4. Tourniquets
5. Magill intubation forceps

An *O_2 delivery system* adaptable to an E cylinder of oxygen must permit the delivery of positive-pressure O_2. Examples of this type of device include the positive-pressure/demand valve and the reservoir bag on all inhalation sedation units. The Robertshaw Valve and the Elder Valve (Figure 33-4) are examples of such devices. When properly placed, these devices provide O_2 on demand whenever the patient breathes spontaneously. The negative pressure created under the mask triggers the device to provide O_2 under positive pressure. In this regard the positive-pressure/demand valve operates similarly to a SCUBA (self-contained underwater breathing apparatus) mask and is readily usable by almost all rescuers. It is in the use of this device for controlled ventilation (positive-pressure ventilation) that potential difficulties arise. To properly ventilate an apneic patient using the positive-pressure mask, the rescuer *must* be able to maintain both a patent airway and an airtight seal with the mask on the patient's face using but one hand. The other hand is used to activate the valve that supplies O_2 to the patient. The positive-pressure/demand valve is one means of providing 100% O_2. For this device to be used, a source of 100% O_2 must be available. The positive-pressure/demand valve ceases to function once the O_2 cylinder is depleted.

A self-inflating bag-valve-mask device is a self-contained unit that is portable, easily transported to any site within the dental or medical office (Figure 33-5). It

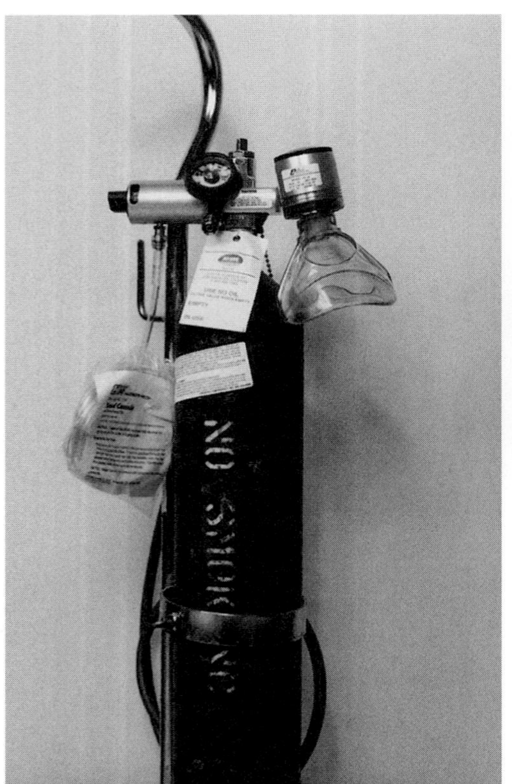

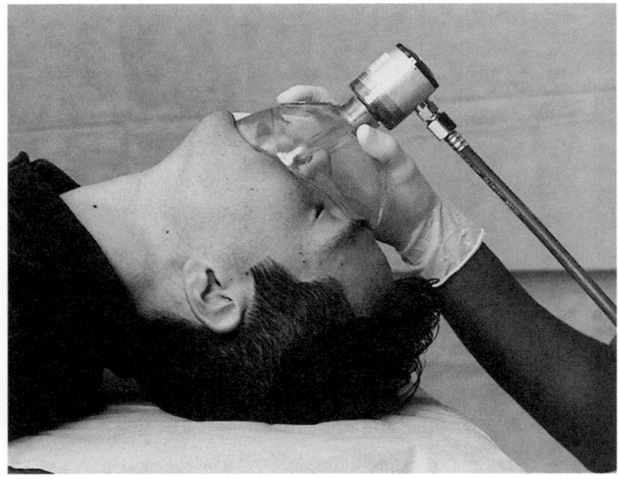

Figure 33-4 Positive-pressure O_2 system.

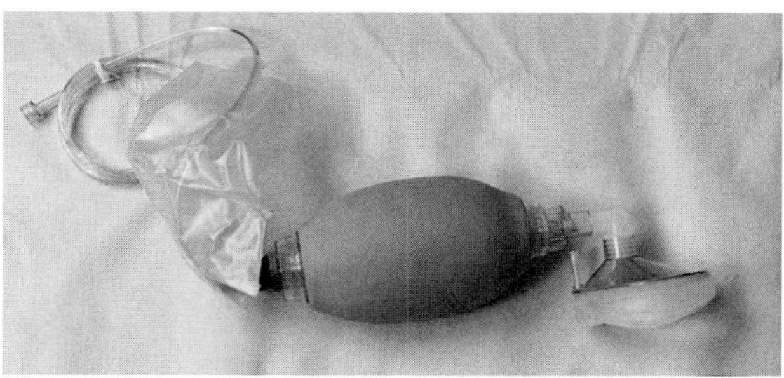

Figure 33-5 Self-inflating bag-valve-mask. Permits delivery of atmospheric air (21% oxygen) or oxygen-enriched air. Clear face mask is preferred to opaque.

does not require a compressed gas cylinder of O_2 to function and therefore has a wider area of potential use than the positive-pressure device. As with the positive-pressure device, the rescuer must be able to maintain both a patent airway and an airtight seal of the mask on the patient's face with but one hand, the other being used to squeeze the bellows bag and inflate the victim's lungs (Figure 33-6). This device has several proprietary names, including the Ambu bag and the Pulmonary Manual Resuscitator (PMR).

The self-inflating bag-valve-mask device may be used to deliver 21% O_2 (ambient or atmospheric air), or by attaching an O_2 delivery tube to the end of the bellows bag, enriched O_2 (greater than 21% but less than 100% O_2) may be supplied to the patient.

The self-inflating bag-valve-mask device is recommended for use in pediatric and smaller adult patients (because of their smaller lung capacity); however, the same device is not recommended for use in the larger-sized adult. Tests have demonstrated that even in the hands of well-trained ventilators these devices do not deliver an adequate volume of air to a large adult victim's lungs.[8] Addition of a reservoir bag that provides additional volume can make this device adequate for use in the large adult.

Face masks must be available if either the positive-pressure mask or bag-valve mask is to be used. A face mask should be constructed of a clear plastic or of rubber, which permits the efficient delivery of O_2 or air to the patient while permitting the rescuer to visually inspect the mouth for the presence of foreign matter (e.g., vomitus, blood) (Figure 33-7). Several sizes of face mask should be available. Suggested for the emergency kit is one portable O_2 cylinder (E cylinder) with a positive-pressure/demand valve and/or one portable self-inflating bag-valve-mask device.

Comment: Training is required for the safe and effective use of these devices.

It is essential that effective *suction* and *suction tips* be available in the office. The disposable saliva ejector is entirely inadequate in situations in which anything other than tiny objects must be evacuated from the mouth of a patient. Suction tips should be of large diameter and rounded so that there is little hazard of inducing bleeding should it become necessary to suction the hypopharynx. Plastic evacuators and tonsil suction tips are quite adequate for this purpose (Figure 33-8). The minimal suggested number for the emergency kit is two plastic evacuators or tonsil suction tips.

Plastic disposable syringes with an 18- to 21-gauge needle are required for drug administration. Many syringe sizes are available, but a 2-ml syringe is quite

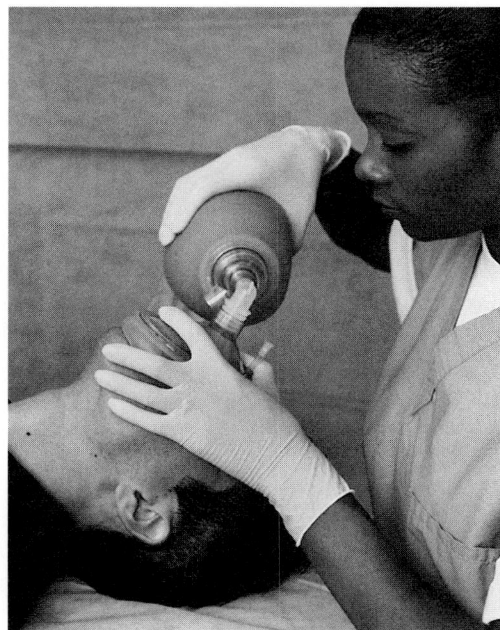

Figure 33-6 Hand positions with bag-valve-mask device.

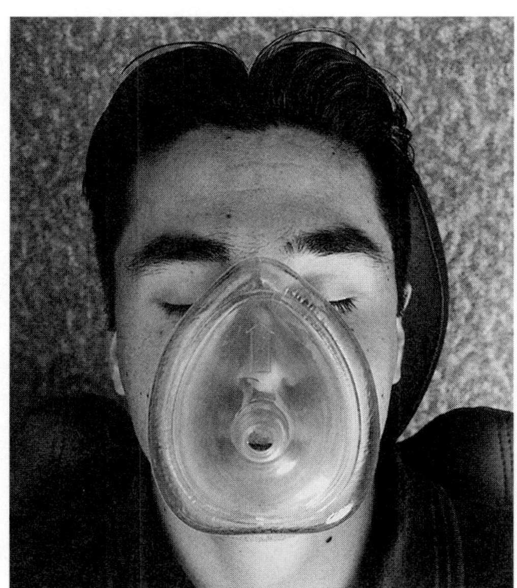

Figure 33-7 Pocket mask.

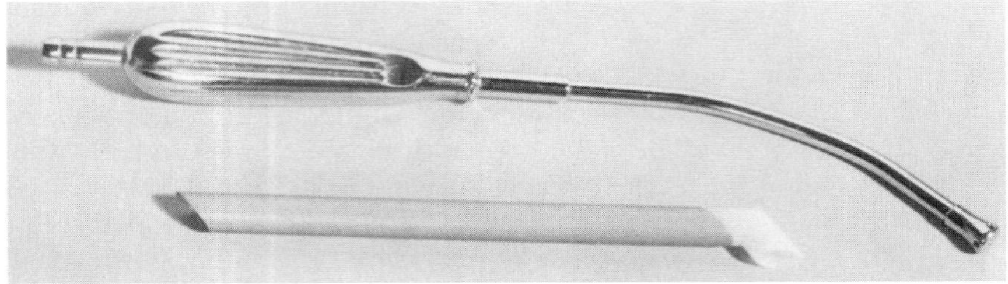

Figure 33-8 Primary emergency equipment: suction and suction tips.

adequate. Suggested for the emergency kit are two to three 2-ml disposable syringes with 18- to 21-gauge needles.

A *tourniquet* is required if IV drug administration is contemplated. In addition, three tourniquets will be required for management of acute pulmonary edema. A sphygmomanometer (blood pressure cuff) may be used as a tourniquet by inflating the cuff to a pressure that falls between the diastolic and systolic measurements. Suggested for the emergency kit are two to three tourniquets and a sphygmomanometer.

A *Magill intubation forceps* aids in the recovery of small objects that have fallen into the distal part of the oral cavity or pharynx (Figure 33-9). Table 33-1 summarizes the basic drugs and equipment recommended for the emergency kit.

LEVEL 2: SECONDARY (NONCRITICAL) DRUGS AND EQUIPMENT

Injectable Drugs

A number of injectable drugs—anticonvulsant, analgesic, vasopressor, corticosteroid, antihypoglycemic, antihypertensive, and anticholinergic drugs—are recommended for inclusion in the emergency kit of doctors who have advanced training in emergency medicine and/or anesthesia (Table 33-2). Such persons include oral and maxillofacial surgeons; dentist anesthesiologists; pedodontic, periodontic, endodontic, and other dental specialists who have completed a hospital training program; and general practitioners who have completed a general practice residency.

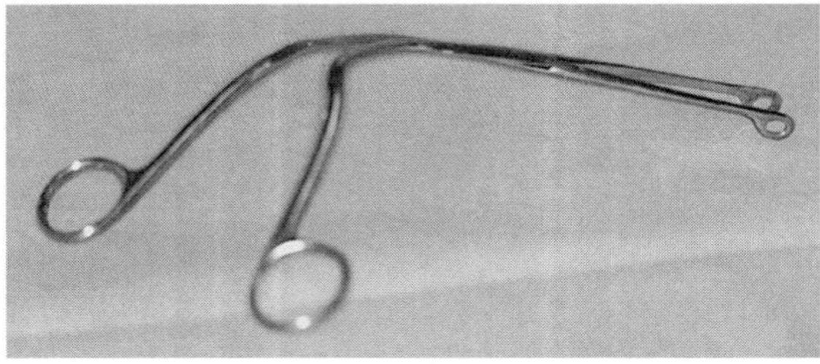

Figure 33-9 Magill intubation forceps.

The *anticonvulsant* of choice is a benzodiazepine, either diazepam or midazolam. Anticonvulsants are administered intravenously to terminate a tonic/clonic seizure, whether in a patient with a history of prior seizure disorders or in management of local anesthetic overdose. Other therapeutic indications for the emergency administration of a benzodiazepine include termination of febrile convulsions, hyperventilation (for sedation), and thyroid storm (for sedation). Suggested for the emergency kit is midazolam, 1 mg/ml in a 10-ml multidose vial.

An *analgesic* drug will be valuable during situations in which acute pain or anxiety is present. Management of pain during acute myocardial infarction represents an important indication for administration of analgesics. Other therapeutic indications include intense, prolonged pain or anxiety and as a sedative in the management of congestive heart failure (CHF). Opioid analgesics are the drugs of choice, with morphine sulfate most highly recommended. In recent years, however, the use of nitrous oxide–oxygen (N_2O-O_2) in management of pain during myocardial infarction has increased in popularity.[9] N_2O-O_2 is administered in a concentration of 35% N_2O and 65% O_2. If N_2O is not available, then morphine sulfate, 10 mg/ml (two to three 1-ml ampules), is recommended.

Vasopressors are administered to manage hypotension. One vasopressor, epinephrine, has already been included in the basic emergency kit; however, its administration in most cases of mild hypotension is not recommended. A vasopressor with less profound actions is usually desirable. Within this category many drugs are available; methoxamine is selected because of its ability to increase blood pressure with little secondary effect on the workload of the myocardium. Indications for vasopressor administration include management of hypotension as seen in syncopal reactions, drug-overdose reactions, postseizure states, acute adrenal insufficiency, and allergy. Recommended for the emergency kit is 10 mg/ml of methoxamine (two to three 1-ml ampules).

Parenteral *antihypoglycemics* are administered in definitive management of hypoglycemia and in the differential diagnosis of unexplained unconsciousness or seizures of unknown origin. A 50% dextrose solu-

TABLE 33-2 Module 2: Secondary (Noncritical) Drugs and Equipment

	Primary Drug			*Recommended for Kit*	
Category	Generic	Proprietary	Alternative	Quantity	Availability
Injectables					
Anticonvulsant	Midazolam	Versed	Diazepam	One 5-ml vial	5 mg/ml
Analgesic	Morphine sulfate	—	Meperidine	Two 2-ml ampules	10 mg/ml
Vasopressor	Methoxamine	Vasoxyl	Phenylephrine	Two or three 1-ml ampules	10 mg/ml
Antihypoglycemic	50% dextrose solution	—	Glucagon	One 50-ml vial (IV)	
Corticosteroid	Hydrocortisone sodium succinate	Solu-Cortef	—	One 2-ml vial	50 mg/ml
Antihypertensive	Esmolol	Brevibloc	Propranolol	Two 100-mg/ml vials	100 mg/ml
Anticholinergic	Atropine	—	—	Two or three 1-ml ampules or two 10-ml syringes	1.0 mg/10 ml
Noninjectables					
Respiratory stimulant	Aromatic ammonia	—	—	1-2 boxes	0.3 ml/Vaporole
Antihypertensive	Nifedipine	Procardia	—	1 bottle	10-mg capsules

Equipment	Description	Quantity
Emergency Equipment		
Cricothyrotomy equipment*	Scalpel or cricothyrotomy device	1 scalpel with disposable blade or cricothyrotomy device
Artificial airways*	Plastic or rubber oropharyngeal and nasopharyngeal airways	Assorted adult and pediatric airways
Equipment for endotracheal intubation*	Laryngoscope and blades (curved or straight)	Minimum of one and spare batteries
	Endotracheal tubes	Assorted adult and pediatric sizes

From Malamed SF: *Medical emergencies in the dental office*, ed 5, St Louis, 2000, Mosby.

*Use of these devices requires significant advanced training to ensure their safe and effective use.

tion is recommended; however, it must be administered intravenously. Recommended for the emergency kit is one vial (50 ml) of 50% dextrose. An alternative is glucagon, available as 1 mg/ml in a 2-ml ampule. Glucagon may be administered either intravenously or intramuscularly.

Corticosteroids are administered to manage the acute allergic reaction, but only after epinephrine and the histamine blockers have proved effective. Another indication for their administration is management of acute adrenal insufficiency. Recommended for the emergency kit is 50 mg/ml of hydrocortisone sodium succinate (one 2-ml vial).

The need to administer *antihypertensive* drugs to manage a hypertensive crisis (excessive elevations in blood pressure) is extremely uncommon. First, the incidence of extreme acute blood pressure elevations is quite rare, and second, other methods may be used to decrease blood pressure without the need for parenteral antihypertensive drugs. Oral drugs, such as nifedipine or nitroglycerin, may be administered in most situations to provide a minor depression of blood pressure. The inclusion of an antihypertensive drug is in response to state requirements for general anesthesia permits (and in a few states for parenteral sedation, too).

Esmolol (Brevibloc) is a β_1-selective adrenergic receptor-blocking agent with a very short duration of action and is the recommended parenteral drug for acute hypertensive episodes. It is available as a 10-mg/ml formulation, and two ampules of 100 mg/ml (with diluent) are recommended.

Atropine, a parasympathetic *anticholinergic* blocking agent, is recommended for the management of symptomatic bradycardia (adult heart rate of <60 beats per minute). Atropine is also considered an essential drug in ACLS, in which it is employed in the management of hemodynamically significant bradydysrhythmias (significant heart block and asystole). It is available as 0.5 mg/ml in 1-ml vials and 1 mg in a 10-ml syringe, and two or three ampules of 0.5 mg/ml (for intramuscular [IM] administration) and/or two 10-ml syringes of 1 mg per syringe (for IV administration) are recommended.

Noninjectable Drugs

Two noninjectable drugs, a respiratory stimulant and an antihypertensive, are recommended for doctors with some advanced training in emergency medicine. *Aromatic ammonia* is the recommended respiratory stimulant. Its use is not limited to persons with advanced training in emergency medicine. It is included as a secondary emergency drug because it does not represent a "critical" drug in emergency management. Available in a silver-gray Vaporole, it is crushed between the rescuer's fingers and held beneath the victim's nose. Indications for aromatic ammonia include respiratory depression not induced by opioid analgesics and vasodepressor syncope. Recommended for the emergency kit is one box of aromatic ammonia Vaporole.

COMMENT: Aromatic ammonia will be one of the most frequently used drugs in the emergency kit. It is suggested that one or two Vaporole be placed close to every treatment area so that required time will not be spent waiting for the emergency kit to arrive. Several Vaporole should remain in the emergency kit for use in other areas of the office (Figure 33-10).

Secondary (Advanced) Emergency Equipment

Several other items of equipment are available for use in emergency situations. Advanced training is required for the safe and effective use of these devices. It is therefore recommended that the following equipment *not* be included unless adequate training and experience have been obtained:

- Scalpel or cricothyrotomy needle
- Artificial airways
- Airway adjuncts

As a final step in attempting to manage an obstructed airway, cricothyrotomy may be necessary. Although this procedure is highly unlikely to ever be required, there are occasions in which the recommended procedures involving abdominal or chest thrusts may prove to be ineffective in opening an airway that has become obstructed by a foreign object.[10] One clinical situation in which the latter procedures will prove fruitless is laryngeal edema, a form of allergic response in which the soft tissues of the larynx swell, restricting the flow of air into and out of the trachea. The usual airway maneuvers (i.e., head-tilt/chin-lift) fail to provide a patent airway because a foreign object is not present. Cricothyrotomy is necessary to provide O_2 to the victim. It is recommended that in the office of a doctor who is trained in cricothyrotomy the emergency kit should contain a *scalpel* or a *cricothyrotomy needle* (Figure 33-11). The technique of cricothyrotomy is reviewed in Chapter 34. Suggested for the emergency kit is one scalpel with disposable blade and/or one 13-gauge–½-inch cricothyrotomy needle.

Plastic or rubber *oropharyngeal* and rubber *nasopharyngeal airways* assist in airway management. They are used routinely during and after general anesthesia to assist in airway maintenance in unconscious or semiconscious patients. The oropharyngeal airway is designed to lie between the base of the tongue and the posterior wall of the pharynx, lifting the tongue off of

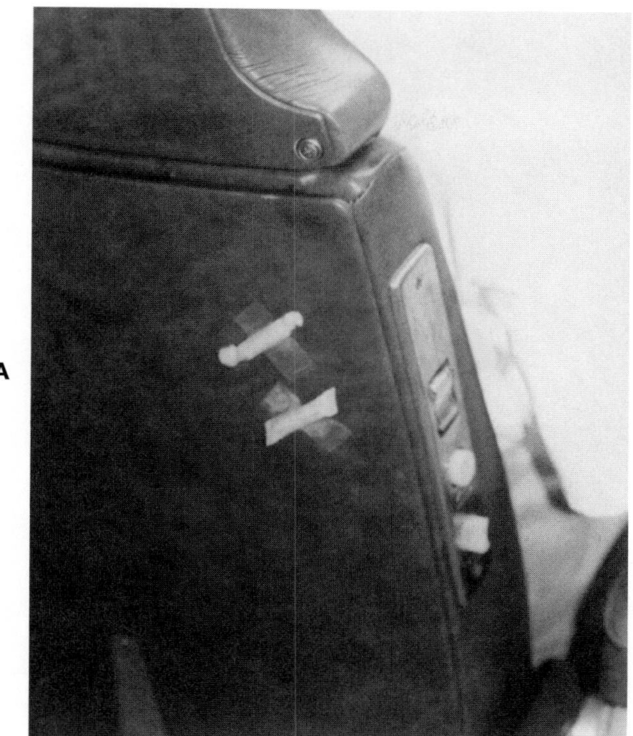

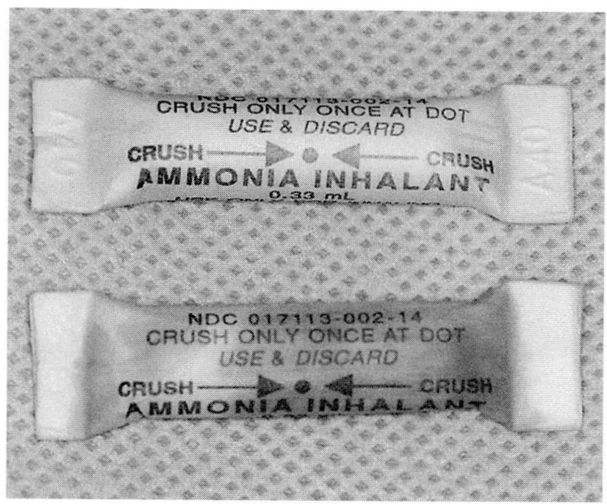

Figure 33-10 **A,** Aromatic ammonia Vaporole on back of dental chair. **B,** Aromatic ammonia Vaporole darkens (*bottom*) when used.

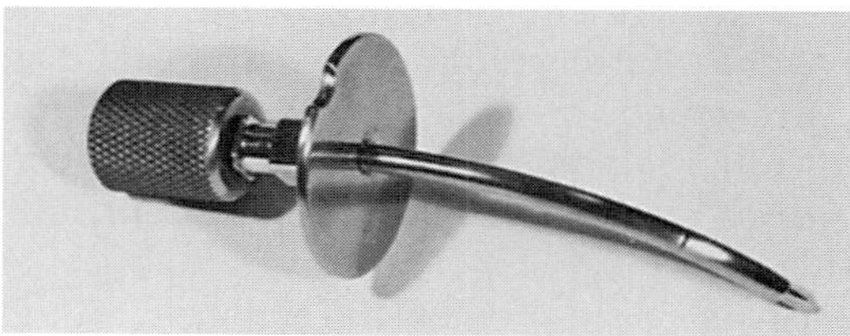

Figure 33-11 Cricothyrotomy needle.

the pharyngeal wall and thus aiding airway maintenance. Use of the oropharyngeal airway (Figure 33-12) must be restricted to persons trained in its insertion because improper placement will force the base of the tongue farther back into the pharynx, thereby adding to the degree of obstruction. If the oropharyngeal airway is placed into the pharynx of a patient who is not deeply unconscious, the patient will react to the presence of the airway by gagging (not too bad), vomiting or regurgitating (worse), or having a laryngospasm (worse yet). Placing an oropharyngeal airway in a still reactive patient is the equivalent of placing your finger deep down in your throat. In proper insertion of an oropharyngeal airway, the tip of the patient's tongue is held with a piece of gauze and pulled anteriorly while the airway is being inserted.

The nasopharyngeal airway is better tolerated by most patients. It is lubricated (K-Y Jelly or Xylocaine viscous) before insertion into one nostril (usually the right) and then gently advanced into position (Figure 33-13). Because it lies in the nasopharynx, not the oropharynx, gagging, vomiting, regurgitation, and laryngospasm rarely develop, even in a conscious patient.

Use of these airway adjuncts is recommended only when manual methods of airway maintenance have been ineffective. Training and experience in the use of oral and nasal airways is mandatory if they are to be used effectively and safely. Suggested for the emergency kit is a set of adult- and child-sized airways (either oropharyngeal or nasopharyngeal).

Endotracheal intubation using a *laryngoscope* and *endotracheal tube* provides the ultimate in airway maintenance. The use of endotracheal intubation must be strictly limited to persons who are well trained in this technique. Quite realistically this limits its usefulness to anesthesiologists, nurse anesthetists, trained paramedical personnel, and those few dentists and physicians who have received training in anesthesiology. The most common mistakes noted during intubation are accidental intubation of the esophagus and taking too long to intubate (it should take no longer than 15 seconds to intubate a patient). Table 33-2 summarizes the secondary emergency drugs and equipment.

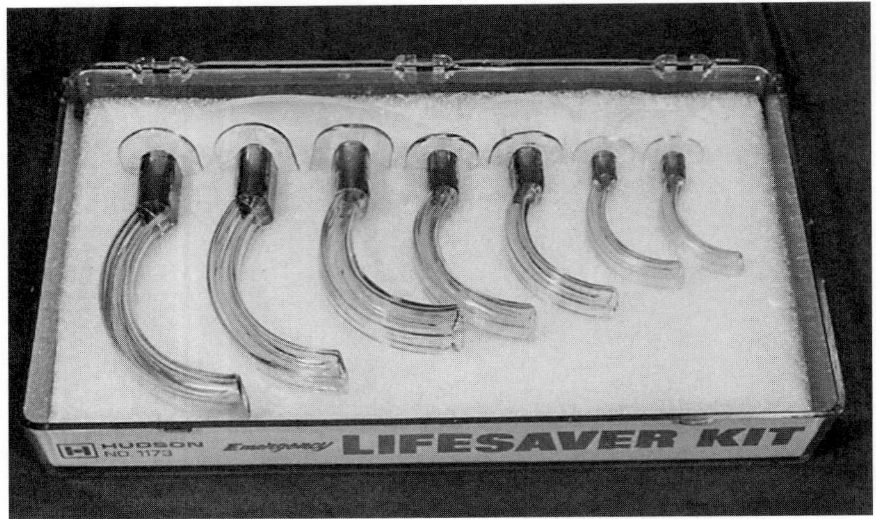

Figure 33-12 Oropharyngeal airways are available in a variety of sizes.

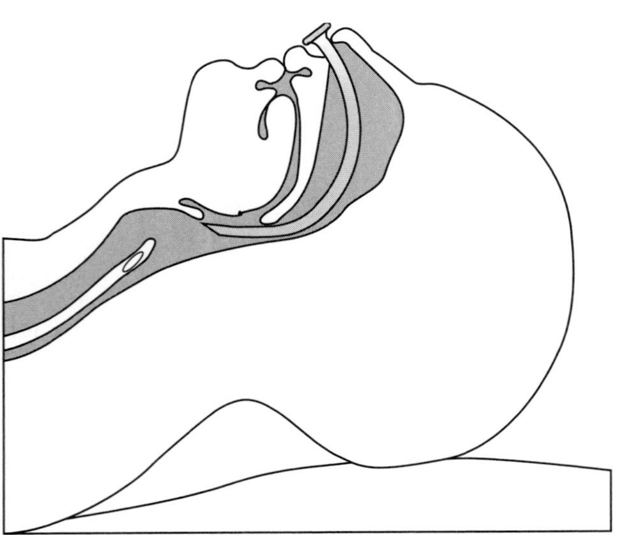

Figure 33-13 Nasopharyngeal airway.

LEVEL 3: ADVANCED CARDIAC LIFE SUPPORT

Drugs recommended by the International Consensus on Science for use in ACLS have recently undergone significant revision.[11] These drugs should be included in the emergency kit, or in a separate kit, in those offices in which the doctor has been trained in ACLS. The ACLS-trained doctor is referred directly to the most recent guidelines for more in-depth discussions of these drugs.[11]

LEVEL 4: ANTIDOTAL DRUGS

Antidotal drugs (Table 33-3) reverse some, or all, of the actions of other drugs that have been previously administered. Specific reversal agents should be available in the emergency drug kit where any technique of parenteral sedation is employed in patient management (IM, submucosal, IV, or general anesthesia). Only a brief description of each drug is given because the pharmacology of the antidotal drugs has been presented in Chapter 25. Antidotal drugs include opioid antagonists, a benzodiazepine antagonist, a drug for reversal of emergence delirium, and a vasodilator.

Opioid antagonists reverse the actions of opioid agonists (i.e., meperidine, morphine, and fentanyl). In clinical practice opioid antagonists are administered primarily to reverse unwanted respiratory depression produced by opioids. Naloxone (Narcan) is available as a 0.4 mg/ml dosage form (for adults). It is administered at a rate of 0.1 mg every 2 to 3 minutes to the adult up to 2.0 mg, with the patient's response being monitored constantly. In children an initial IV dose of 0.01 mg/kg is suggested.[12] One must never forget that in addition to reversing the respiratory depressant actions of opioid analgesics, naloxone also reverses its analgesic effects. Therefore patients who receive opioid analgesics for anesthesia and undergo their surgical procedure without the benefit of local anesthesia and then receive naloxone may experience severe postsurgical pain.[13] Nalbuphine, an opioid agonist/antagonist, has also been shown to be effective in reversing opioid-induced respiratory depression. A major advantage of nalbuphine over naloxone is that the analgesic properties of the opioid remain.[14]

TABLE 33-3 Module 4: Antidotal Drugs

Category	Primary Drug: Generic	Primary Drug: Proprietary	Alternative	Recommended for Kit: Quantity	Recommended for Kit: Availability
Injectables					
Opioid antagonist	Naloxone	Narcan	Nalbuphine	Two 1-ml ampules	0.4 mg/ml
Benzodiazepine antagonist	Flumazenil	Romazicon	—	One 10-ml multidose vial	0.1 mg/ml
Antiemergence delirium	Physostigmine	Antilirium	—	Two or three 2-ml ampules	1 mg/ml
Vasodilator	Procaine	Novocain	—	Two 2-ml ampules	10 mg/ml

From Malamed SF: *Medical emergencies in the office*, ed 5, St Louis, 2000, Mosby.

Recommended for the emergency kit is 0.4 mg/ml of naloxone (two to three 1-ml ampules) for use in adults. Naloxone is also available as a 0.02 mg/ml concentration for pediatric use.

The *benzodiazepine antagonist* flumazenil (Romazicon) reverses the clinical actions of diazepam and midazolam (as well as other benzodiazepines). Recovery from sedation is hastened, and the length of amnesia is decreased when flumazenil is administered.[15] It is recommended for IV use only; the initial dose of flumazenil is 0.2 mg administered intravenously over 15 seconds. Additional doses of 0.2 mg may be administered and repeated at 60-second intervals where necessary to a maximal dose of 1.0 mg. Most patients respond to 0.6 to 1.0 mg.[16] Suggested for the drug emergency kit is one 10-ml multidose vial of 0.1 mg/ml flumazenil.

Emergence delirium (central anticholinergic syndrome) is an uncommon ADR developing after administration of anticholinergics (primarily scopolamine) or benzodiazepines. Emergence delirium may be terminated through the administration of *physostigmine* (Antilirium). Dosage is 0.5 to 1.0 mg intramuscularly or intravenously. No more than 1 mg should be administered per minute. Additional doses may be administered every 10 to 30 minutes if the desired patient response is not obtained. Recommended for the emergency kit is 1.0 mg/ml of physostigmine (two to three 2-ml ampules).

A *vasodilator* is recommended for the emergency kit in the event that an extravascular injection of a tissue-irritating drug (e.g., diazepam, pentobarbital) occurs or in the extremely unlikely event of an intraarterial injection of a drug. Procaine (Novocain) remains the drug of choice because of its potent vasodilating and anesthetic actions. Recommended for the emergency kit are two to three 2-ml ampules of 1% procaine.

SUMMARY

The selection of emergency drugs and equipment for the dental or medical office must be based on the training and background of the doctor who is responsible for its use. Because of the diversity in emergency preparedness training among both dentists and physicians, no stereotyped emergency kit is appropriate for all practitioners. I have attempted to describe several levels of drugs and equipment that I believe would be appropriate with different degrees of expertise in emergency medicine. In addition, many states and provinces have credentialing bodies that regulate the use of conscious sedation and general anesthesia. Specific mandatory drug lists are included in many of these regulations. Regardless of the nature of drugs and equipment selected for the emergency kit, it is vital for the doctor to become familiar with the indications, contraindications, dosages, and method of administration of each of these drugs and to be able to correctly operate any available equipment.

REFERENCES

1. Malamed SF: *Medical emergencies in the dental office*, ed 5, St Louis, 2000, Mosby.
2. Pallasch TJ: This emergency kit belongs in your office, *Dent Management* 16:43, 1976.
3. Malamed SF: Drugs for medical emergencies in the dental office. In *ADA guide to dental therapeutics*, ed 2, Chicago, 2000, ADA Publishing.
4. American Dental Association Council on Dental Education: *Guidelines for teaching the comprehensive control of pain and anxiety in dentistry. Part II*, Chicago, 1992, The Association.

5. California State Board of Dental Examiners: *Conscious sedation and general anesthesia regulations.* Extract from California Code of Regulations. Title 16, Chapter 10, Article 5—General anesthesia and conscious sedation, 1993.
6. American Association of Oral and Maxillofacial Surgeons, Committee on Anesthesia: *Office anesthesia evaluation manual,* ed 4, Rosemont, Ill, 1991, The Association.
7. ISIS-2 (Second International Study of Infarct Survival Collaborative Group): Randomized trial of intravenous streptokinase, oral aspirin, both, or neither among 17,187 cases of suspected acute myocardial infarction. ISIS-2, *Lancet* 2:349, 1988.
8. Carden E, Hughes T: An evaluation of manually operated self-inflating resuscitation bags, *Anesth Analg* 54:133, 1975.
9. O'Leary U, Puglia C, Friehling TD et al: Nitrous oxide anesthesia in patients with ischemic chest discomfort: effect on beta-endorphins, *J Clin Pharmacol* 27:957, 1987.
10. Heimlich HJ: A life-saving maneuver to prevent food choking, *JAMA* 234:398, 1975.
11. International Consensus on Science: Guidelines 2000 for Cardiopulmonary Resuscitation and Emergency Cardiovascular Care, *Circulation* 102(suppl):112, 2000.
12. Naloxone, drug package insert, Du Pont Multi-Source Products, 1999.
13. Pallasch TJ, Gill CJ: Naloxone-associated morbidity and mortality, *Oral Surg* 52:602, 1981.
14. Hu C, Flecknell PA, Liles JH: Fentanyl and medetomidine anaesthesia in the rat and its reversal using atipamezole and either nalbuphine or butorphanol, *Lab Anim* 26:15, 1992.
15. Longmire AW, Seger DL: Topics in clinical pharmacology: flumazenil, a benzodiazepine antagonist, *Am J Med Sci* 306:49, 1993.
16. Romazicon, drug package insert, Roche Laboratories, April 1997.

CHAPTER 34

Management of Emergencies

CHAPTER OUTLINE

Despite efforts at prevention, complications and adverse drug reactions (ADRs) will arise during and after the administration of drugs for the management of pain or anxiety. In the office that has prepared for these situations before their occurrence, there is a greater likelihood of a successful outcome than in the unprepared or ill-prepared office. Many states, provinces, and specialty groups require that the dental office team be capable of correctly identifying and managing specific ADRs associated with parenteral sedation and general anesthesia.[1,2] These emergencies are reviewed in this chapter.

Pallasch[3] has proposed the following classification of ADRs:

- I. Toxicity related to direct extension of pharmacologic effects
  - A. Side effects
  - B. Abnormal dosage (overdosage)
  - C. Local toxic effects
- II. Toxicity related to altered recipient
  - A. Presence of pathology
  - B. Emotional disturbances
  - C. Genetic aberrations (idiosyncrasy)
  - D. Teratogenicity
  - E. Drug-drug interactions
- III. Toxicity related to drug allergy

According to Pallasch's system, there are three major methods by which drugs may produce adverse reactions:

1. A direct extension of the pharmacologic actions of the drug
2. A deleterious effect on a chemically, genetically, metabolically, or morphologically altered recipient
3. Initiation of an immune (allergic) response

Most ADRs are not life threatening. There are, however, potential responses that are life threatening, requiring immediate and effective management if the patient is to fully recover. These include the overdose reaction and the allergic response. A third, the idiosyncratic reaction, is also reviewed.

Overdose reaction refers to those signs and symptoms manifested as a result of an absolute or relative overadministration of a drug producing elevated blood or plasma levels of that drug in specific organs (termed *target organs*) of the body. For central nervous system (CNS)-depressant drugs an overdose occurs when the blood level of the drug becomes overly high in the cerebral circulation.[4] Clinical manifestations of an overdose are related directly to the normal pharmacologic actions of the agent. For example, in therapeutic doses, barbiturates produce a mild depression of the CNS that results in sedation or hypnosis (desirable effects). Barbiturate overdosage produces a more profound depression of the CNS, with respiratory or cardiovascular depression and a possible loss of consciousness.

Allergy is a hypersensitive state acquired through exposure to a particular allergen, reexposure to which brings about a heightened capacity to react.[5] Clinically, there are a variety of manifestations through which allergy expresses itself. These include drug fever, angioedema, urticaria, dermatitis, depression of blood-forming organs, photosensitivity, and anaphylaxis. Certain drugs are more likely than others to elicit allergic reactions, and allergic reaction is theoretically possible with any substance.

In contrast to overdose, in which clinical manifestations are related directly to the pharmacology of the causative agent, the clinical response observed in an allergic reaction is mediated by an exaggerated response of the immune system. The degree of this response determines the severity of the allergic reaction. Allergic responses to a barbiturate, a local anesthetic, an antibiotic, a bee sting, peanuts, and shellfish are produced by the same mechanism and may appear clinically similar. Management of all allergic reactions is basically the same, whereas overdose reactions to the first three agents listed are quite dissimilar clinically and require different management.

Idiosyncrasy or *idiosyncratic reactions* are those ADRs that cannot be explained by any known pharmacologic or biochemical mechanism. Another definition is that an idiosyncratic reaction is any ADR that is neither an overdose nor an allergic reaction. An example of an idiosyncratic reaction is CNS stimulation (excitation or agitation) produced after the administration of a known CNS depressant such as a barbiturate.

Idiosyncratic reactions span an extremely wide range of clinical expression. For example, depression after administration of a stimulant, stimulation after administration of a depressant, and hyperpyrexia after administration of a muscle relaxant are all idiosyncratic reactions. It is usually impossible to predict in whom such reactions will develop or, indeed, the nature of the resulting idiosyncratic reaction.

Because of the unpredictability of the nature and occurrence of idiosyncratic reactions, their management is of necessity symptomatic. Of primary importance in the management of idiosyncrasy is basic life support ($P \rightarrow A \rightarrow B \rightarrow C$): maintaining the airway and ensuring adequate ventilation and circulation. If seizures develop, management is based on airway maintenance and prevention of injury during the seizure.

It is thought today that virtually all instances of idiosyncrasy have an underlying genetic mechanism.[6] These genetic aberrations remain undetected until the individual receives a specific drug, such as succinylcholine, which then produces its bizarre (nonpharmacologic) clinical expression.

Two major forms of ADR, overdose and allergy, are reviewed in this chapter; in addition, other emergency situations are discussed. Successful demonstration of the management of these situations is frequently a requirement of the permitting process for parenteral sedation and general anesthesia. These complications are listed in Box 34-1.

OVERDOSE

Whenever CNS depressant drugs are administered, the possibility always exists that an exaggerated level of CNS depression might develop. This might be noted clinically as a slightly oversedated patient, or it could result in an unconscious, apneic patient.

BOX 34-1 Emergency Situations Identified for Parenteral Sedation and General Anesthesia

1. Airway obstruction, p. 508
2. Laryngospasm, p. 510
3. Bronchospasm, p. 496
4. Emesis and aspiration of foreign material under anesthesia, p. 512
5. Angina pectoris, p. 507
6. Myocardial infarction, p. 508
7. Cardiac dysrhythmias, p. 506
   a. Bradycardia
   b. Ventricular tachycardia
   c. Ventricular fibrillation
   d. Asystole
   e. Electromechanical dissociation (EMD)
8. Hypotension, p. 500
9. Hypertensive crisis, p. 504
10. Acute allergic reaction, p. 492
11. Seizures, p. 515
12. Hypoglycemia, p. 516
13. Syncope, p. 518
14. Hyperventilation, p. 513
15. Respiratory depression, p. 513

Data from California State Board of Dental Examiners: *Conscious sedation evaluation protocol*, Sacramento, 1993; and American Association of Oral & Maxillofacial Surgeons: *Office anesthesia evaluation manual*, ed 4, Rosemont, Ill, 1991, The Association.

The group of drugs most likely to produce an overdose is the barbiturates. Barbiturates represented the first major breakthrough in the pharmacologic management of anxiety, and because of this, adverse reactions, such as allergy, addiction, and overdose, were tolerated. In the 1960s, with the introduction of the benzodiazepines (drugs that do not possess the same potential for abuse and overdose), barbiturate use declined. However, barbiturates still remain a useful group in the dentist's and physician's armamentarium for the management of treatment-related anxiety.

Although the barbiturates present the greatest potential for adverse reaction, the opioid analgesics are involved with the greatest number of clinically significant episodes of overdose and respiratory depression. This is simply because opioids are more widely used than the barbiturates. As discussed elsewhere (see Chapters 7, 10, and 35), the use of opioids is popular in pediatric sedation. Opioids are often given intravenously, in conjunction with antianxiety drugs, to aid in sedation and pain control in the adult patient. Goodson and Moore[7] reported on 14 pediatric dentistry cases in which the administration of opioids (and other drugs) led to seven deaths and three instances of brain damage. Several opioids were implicated in these reactions: alphaprodine (7), meperidine (6), and pentazocine (1).

Predisposing Factors and Prevention

Because the barbiturates and opioids are commonly used for the management of pretreatment fear and anxiety, they are frequently administered orally or intramuscularly. The clinical efficacy of a drug depends, in large part, on its absorption into the cardiovascular system and on subsequent blood levels of the drug in various organs of the body. Only the inhalation and intravenous (IV) routes of drug administration permit titration. With oral and intramuscular (IM) drug administration, absorption is erratic, as demonstrated by the wide range of variability in clinical effectiveness. The normal distribution curve becomes important when drugs are administered via those nontitratable routes. "Average" drug doses are based on this curve; therefore secobarbital, 100 mg orally, provides a desired effect (mild sedation) in the majority of patients receiving it. For some patients (about 15% of the population), however, the 100-mg dose is ineffective; these patients require a larger dose to attain the same clinical level of sedation. These patients, termed *hyporesponders*, are not at risk for potential overdose when given an average dose because a lack of adequate sedation is the clinical result.

The potential danger in the use of drugs lies with patients for whom an average 100-mg dose of secobarbital is too great. These are persons who are quite sensitive (not allergic) to this drug and require smaller than usual doses to obtain clinically effective sedation, the so-called hyperresponders. It is normally not possible to predict the 15% of the population that will react in this manner. Only a history of an ADR may provide a clue to this occurrence. The medical history questionnaire should be examined carefully in relation to all prior drug reactions. When a history of drug sensitivity is obtained, great care should be exercised if barbiturates and opioid analgesics are to be used. Lower-than-average doses should be administered or different drug categories substituted. Nonbarbiturate sedative-hypnotic drugs, such as the benzodiazepines and the opioid agonist/antagonists, may be used in place of these drugs.

Although the clinical nature of the overdose cannot always be predicted, there is another way in which these drugs can produce this reaction—a way that is preventable. It relates entirely to the goal being sought by the doctor when these drugs are administered. Some clinicians administer barbiturates or opioids seeking deep levels of sedation in apprehensive patients. When these drugs are used in this manner via the oral or IM routes of drug administration, the potential for overdose increases. Most doctors who administer barbiturates in their practices have encountered patients who became uncooperative (less inhibited) after receiving these drugs. The planned procedure could not be completed because of the difficulty in managing a patient who was slightly overdosed on barbiturates. Larger doses of the barbiturate given to an anxious patient in an attempt to produce deeper levels of sedation may produce greater degrees of CNS depression, with possible loss of consciousness and significant respiratory depression.

Administering any CNS depressant to obtain deeper levels of sedation via routes of administration in which titration is not possible is foolhardy and an invitation to overdose. It cannot be condoned. Only those techniques allowing titration should be used when deeper levels of sedation are sought, and then only when the doctor and entire team are thoroughly familiar with both the technique and the drugs to be administered and are able to manage all possible complications associated with the procedure.

The inhalation and IV routes are the only routes that permit titration. A factor to be remembered regarding inhalation and IV sedation is that absorption of the drugs into the systemic circulation occurs rapidly, so drug responses (both therapeutic and adverse) develop quite suddenly. Titration remains the greatest safety feature these techniques possess and should always be used when possible. Table 34-1 summarizes the recommendations made throughout this book for the various routes of drug administration.

Clinical Manifestations

Barbiturate and Nonbarbiturate Sedative-Hypnotics. Barbiturates produce depression of a number of physiologic properties, including nerve tissue; respiration; and skeletal, smooth, and cardiac muscle. The mechanism of action (sedation and hypnosis) is depression at the level of the hypothalamus and the ascending reticular activating system (RAS), which produces a decrease in the transmission of impulses to the cerebral cortex. Further increases in barbiturate blood level produce depression at other levels of the CNS, such as profound cortical depression, depression of motor function, and finally depression of the medulla. This is represented diagrammatically as follows:

Sedation (calming) → Hypnosis (sleep) →
General anesthesia (unconsciousness with progressive respiratory and cardiovascular depression) →
Respiratory arrest

Conscious Sedation and Deep Sedation. At low (therapeutic) blood levels the patient appears calm and cooperative (conscious sedation). As the barbiturate level in the cerebral circulation increases, the patient falls into a rousable sleep (hypnosis). The doctor will notice the patient's inability to keep his or her mouth open despite reminders to do so. In addition, patients at this level of barbiturate-induced CNS depression tend to overreact to stimulation, especially that of a noxious nature. An unsedated adult patient may grimace in response to a painful stimulus; an adult deeply sedated with barbiturates demonstrates an exaggerated response, perhaps yelling or jumping. This reflects a loss of self-control over emotion that is associated with the CNS depressant action of the barbiturate.

TABLE 34-1 Summary of Routes of Drug Administration

	Control Over Technique		
Route of Administration	Titrate	Rapid Reversal	Recommended Safe Sedation Levels
Oral	No	No	Light
Rectal	No	No	Light
Intranasal	No	No	Light
Intramuscular	No	No	Adults: light to moderate Children: light, moderate, deep
Intravenous	Yes	Yes (opioids, benzodiazepines) No (other drugs)	Adults and children*: light, moderate, deep
Inhalation	Yes	Yes	Any sedation level

*There is usually little need for intravenous conscious sedation in normal, healthy children. Most children who will permit venipuncture will also permit intraoral local anesthetic administration. The intravenous route is of great benefit in managing children and adults with disabilities and those who are disruptive.

Hypnosis. With continued elevation of the barbiturate blood level, hypnosis (sleep) ensues, with a minor degree of respiratory depression (decreased depth and increased rate of ventilation). At this level of CNS depression there is usually no adverse action on the cardiovascular system, only a slight decrease in blood pressure and heart rate, similar to that occurring in normal sleep. Dental treatment cannot be continued at this level of CNS depression because the patient is unable to cooperate with the doctor by keeping his or her mouth open and may require assistance in maintaining airway patency (head-tilt). The patient still responds to noxious stimulation but in a sluggish manner.

General Anesthesia. With further elevation of the barbiturate blood level, the degree of CNS depression broadens so that the patient is now unconscious (incapable of response to sensory stimulation, loss of protective reflexes with attendant inability to maintain an airway). Spontaneous respiratory efforts are still present; however, with even further increase in barbiturate blood levels, medullary depression occurs, which is clinically evident as respiratory and cardiovascular depression. Respiratory depression is noted as shallow breathing movements at a slow or rapid rate. Ventilatory excursions of the chest are not an indication that air is entering or leaving the lungs but only that the patient is trying to bring air into the lungs. Cardiovascular depression is evident as a continued decrease in blood pressure (caused by medullary depression and direct depression of the myocardium and vascular smooth muscle) and an increased heart rate. The patient develops a shocklike appearance and has a weak and rapid pulse and cold, moist skin.

Respiratory Arrest. As the barbiturate blood level continues to increase, or if the patient is not managed adequately in the previous stage, respiratory arrest will occur. Respiratory arrest is readily managed with controlled ventilation. If ventilation is not adequately provided, cardiac arrest will ensue.

Other nonbarbiturate sedative-hypnotic drugs (i.e., benzodiazepines) also possess the potential to produce overdose, although this is not as likely to occur as with the barbiturates. The potential for overdose varies greatly from drug to drug, and to varying degrees all sedative-hypnotic drugs have this potential.

Opioid Agonists. Meperidine, morphine, fentanyl, alfentanil, and sufentanil are frequently used parenteral opioids. Meperidine and fentanyl are the most popular.

Meperidine, like most opioid agonists, exerts its chief pharmacologic actions on the CNS. Therapeutic doses of meperidine produce analgesia, sedation, euphoria, and a degree of respiratory depression. Of principal concern, of course, is the respiratory depressant action of the opioid agonists. They are direct depressants of the medullary respiratory center. In humans respiratory depression from opioid agonists is evident even at doses that do not disturb the level of consciousness. Respiratory depression produced by opioids is dose dependent: The larger the dose is, the greater is the level of respiratory depression. The opioid agonist/antagonists nalbuphine and butorphanol offer the combination of analgesia and sedation with minimal respiratory depression.

Death from opioid overdose almost always results from respiratory arrest. All phases of respiration are depressed: rate, minute volume, and tidal volume. The respiratory rate may fall below 10 breaths per minute. Rates of 5 to 6 breaths per minute are not uncommon. The cause of this decreased respiratory rate is a reduction in responsiveness of the medullary respiratory centers to increases in carbon dioxide tension (Pco_2) and also a depression of the pontine and medullary centers that are responsible for respiratory rhythm.

The cardiovascular effects of meperidine are not clinically significant when the drug is administered within its usual therapeutic dose range. Following IV administration of meperidine, however, there is normally an increase in the heart rate produced by the atropine-like vagolytic properties of meperidine. Even at overdose levels the blood pressure remains quite stable until late in the course of the reaction, when it falls, primarily as a result of hypoxia. The administration of O_2 at this time will produce an increase in blood pressure despite continued medullary depression. Overly high blood levels of opioid agonists can lead to loss of consciousness.

Overdose reactions to both the sedative-hypnotics and opioid agonists are produced by a progressive depression of the CNS that is manifested by alterations in the level of consciousness and as respiratory depression that ultimately results in respiratory arrest. The loss of consciousness produced by barbiturates or opioid agonists is not always the result of unintentional overdose—these drugs are commonly administered as the primary agents in general anesthesia (see Chapter 31). However, when conscious sedation is the goal, unintended loss of consciousness and respiratory depression/arrest must be considered as complications of drug administration.

The duration and the degree of this clinical reaction vary according to the route of administration, the dose administered, and the patient's individual sensitivity to the drug. In most situations oral and rectal administration result in reduced CNS depression but with a longer duration; IM, intranasal (IN), and submucosal administration result in a more profound level of depression of relatively long duration, whereas IV administration produces the most profound level of depression, but of shorter duration than that seen with the other techniques. The onset of respiratory depression after IV administration may be quite rapid, whereas that following oral or rectal administration is considerably slower. Onset is intermediate in IM and subcutaneous administration.

Management

Sedative-Hypnotic Drugs. Management of an overdose of a sedative-hypnotic drug is predicated on correcting the clinical manifestations of CNS depression. Of primary importance is the management of respiratory depression through the administration of basic life support (BLS). Unfortunately, there is no effective antagonist that can reverse the CNS depressant properties of the barbiturate sedative-hypnotics. Benzodiazepines, however, can be reversed through administration of flumazenil.

Diagnostic clues to the presence of an overdose of a sedative-hypnotic drug include the following[8]:

- Recent administration of sedative-hypnotic drug
- Decreased level of consciousness: sleepy → unconscious
- Respiratory depression (rapid rate, shallow depth)
- Loss of motor coordination (ataxia)
- Slurred speech

Step 1: Terminate Treatment. The rate at which clinical signs and symptoms of overdose develop will vary with routes of administration. Onset following IV administration will occur within minutes, within 10 to 30 minutes following IM administration, and within 45 minutes to an hour following oral administration.

Step 2: P—Position the Patient. The patient, who is either semiconscious or unconscious, is placed in the supine position with his or her legs elevated slightly (Figure 34-1). The goal in this situation, regardless of the level of consciousness, is to maintain adequate cerebral blood flow.

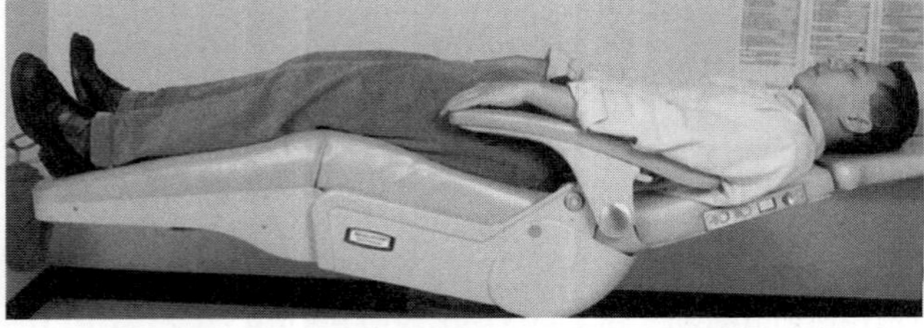

Figure 34-1 The unconscious patient should be placed in the supine position with the legs elevated slightly.

Step 3: A—Airway, B—Breathing, C—Circulation; Basic Life Support, as Indicated. A patent airway must be ensured and the adequacy of breathing assessed. Head-tilt or head-tilt/chin-lift may be required for airway patency at this time (Figure 34-2). The presence or adequacy of the patient's spontaneous ventilatory efforts is next assessed by the rescuer, who places his or her ear 1 inch from the patient's mouth and nose, listening and feeling for exhaled air while looking at the patient's chest to determine whether spontaneous respiratory efforts are being made. Maintaining a patent airway is the most important step in the management of this patient. Step 4b, providing adequate oxygenation, is contingent on successfully maintaining a patent airway.

Step 4: D—Definitive Care

Step 4a: Summon Medical Assistance, if Needed. In a situation in which the patient loses consciousness following barbiturate administration, it might be prudent to seek medical assistance immediately. The requirement for medical assistance varies depending on the doctor's training in airway management and anesthesiology. If the patient remains conscious but is overly sedated, seeking medical assistance is more of a judgment call by the doctor. When in doubt it is always wiser to seek assistance sooner rather than later.

Step 4b: Administer Oxygen. This patient may exhibit different types of breathing. He or she may be conscious but overly sedated, responding slowly to painful stimuli. In this situation the patient will probably be able to maintain his or her own airway and

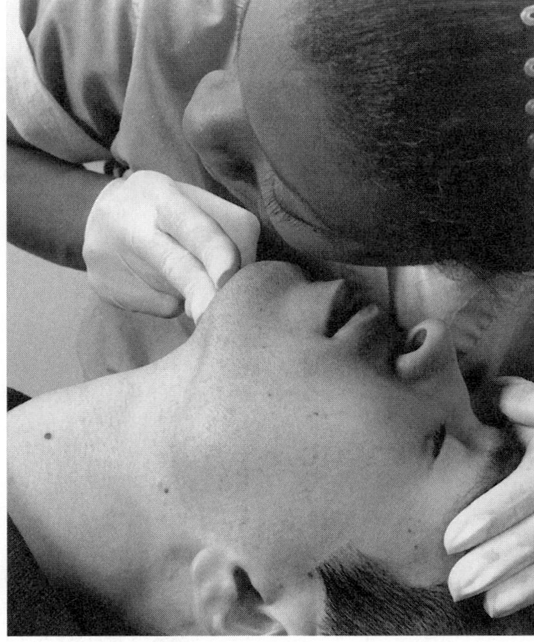

Figure 34-2 The head-tilt/chin-lift technique and "look-listen-feel."

will be breathing spontaneously and somewhat effectively. The rescuer need only monitor the patient, assist with airway maintenance (e.g., head-tilt/chin-lift) and, if desired, administer oxygen through a demand valve or nasal cannula.

The patient might be more deeply sedated and barely responsive to stimulation, with a partially or totally obstructed airway. In this situation assisted ventilation is essential in addition to airway maintenance. With patency of the airway ensured, the patient should receive oxygen via full-face mask. If spontaneous breathing is present but shallow, assisted positive-pressure ventilation is indicated. This is accomplished by activating the positive-pressure mask just as the patient begins each respiratory movement (just as the chest begins to expand). The positive-pressure mask is activated by depressing the button on top of the mask until the patient's chest rises and then releasing the button. With the self-inflating bag-valve-mask device, the bellows bag is squeezed at the start of each inhalation. With both devices, an airtight seal of the mask and head-tilt must be maintained at all times. If respiratory arrest is present, controlled artificial ventilation must be started immediately. The recommended rate for the adult is one breath every 5 seconds (12 per minute) and one breath every 3 seconds for the child aged 1 to 8 years (20 per minute) and the same rate for the infant younger than 1 year of age (20 per minute).[9] Expansion of the patient's chest is the only sure sign of successful ventilation. Overinflation is to be avoided because this leads to abdominal distention, which results in inadequate ventilation and increased risk of regurgitation.

Step 4c: Monitor Vital Signs. The patient's vital signs must be monitored throughout the episode. Blood pressure, heart rate and rhythm, and respiratory rate are monitored and recorded every 5 minutes. A member of the emergency team is assigned to this task. If the blood level of the sedative-hypnotic drug increases significantly, blood pressure will decrease while the heart rate increases. In the absence of blood pressure and pulse, chest compression must be initiated immediately.

In most cases of barbiturate or nonbarbiturate sedative-hypnotic drug overdose, the patient can be managed in this manner until the cerebral blood level of the drug decreases and consciousness returns or until emergency assistance arrives. Recovery occurs as a result of redistribution of the drug within compartments in the body, not biotransformation. The patient becomes more alert and responsive, breathing improves (becomes deeper), and if the blood pressure had been depressed, it returns to near baseline levels. The length of time for this process to occur depends on the drug administered (short-acting versus long-acting drug) and its route of administration.

Step 4d: Establish an Intravenous Line, if Possible. If an IV infusion has not previously been established, it is prudent to establish one at this time, if training and availability of equipment permit. Although there are no effective antidotal drugs for barbiturate overdose, hypotension may be treated effectively through intravenously administered solutions or drugs. As blood pressure decreases, however, veins become progressively more difficult to locate and to cannulate. Establishing venous access at the earliest possible time may prove invaluable later. Venipuncture should be attempted only if the doctor is trained in this technique, the necessary equipment is available, and the patient continues to receive adequate care (BLS) from other personnel. *A patent airway is more important than a patent vein.*

Step 4e: Definitive Management
Definitive management of sedative-hypnotic overdose produced by a *barbiturate* is based on maintenance of a patent airway and adequacy of ventilation until the patient recovers. Signs and symptoms of hypotension are evaluated by monitoring vital signs and determining the adequacy of tissue perfusion.*

Benzodiazepine overdosage may be reversed by the IV or IM administration of flumazenil, a specific benzodiazepine antagonist. Flumazenil is administered intravenously at a dosage of 0.2 mg in 15 seconds, waiting 45 seconds to evaluate recovery. If recovery is not adequate at 1 minute, an additional dose of 0.2 mg may be administered. This is repeated every 5 minutes until recovery occurs or a dose of 1.0 mg has been delivered.[10]

Step 5: Recovery and Discharge. In the event that the overdose is profound and requires the assistance of emergency personnel, the patient may require stabilization and transportation to a hospital for observation and full recovery. Should this be necessary, the doctor should always accompany the patient to the hospital. Box 34-2 outlines the steps to follow to manage sedative-hypnotic overdose.

In most cases sedative-hypnotic overdose is significantly less severe, with diminished responsiveness and slight respiratory depression. Management consists of positioning, airway maintenance, and assisted ventilation until recovery. Emergency medical assistance is not usually required. Before discharge in the custody of a responsible adult, the patient must be capable of standing and walking without assistance. Under no circumstances should the patient be discharged alone or if not adequately recovered.

*Adequacy of tissue perfusion may be determined by pressing on a nail bed or the skin and releasing pressure. Adequate perfusion is present when color returns in not more than 3 seconds. If 4 seconds or more is required for color to return, tissue perfusion is inadequate and consideration must be given to the immediate infusion of IV fluids.

BOX 34-2 Management of Sedative-Hypnotic Overdose

Terminate the dental procedure.
↓
P, Position the patient comfortably.
↓
ABC, Assess and perform basic life support, as needed.
↓
D, Initiate definitive care:
- Summon medical assistance, if required.
- Administer oxygen.
- Monitor vital signs.
- Establish an IV line, if possible.

Provide definitive management:
- Administer IV or IM flumazenil for benzodiazepine overdose
- Continue **P** → **A** → **B** → **C** for barbiturate overdose

↓
Permit recovery and discharge patient.

Drugs used in management include oxygen and, if benzodiazepines are the cause of the overdose, flumazenil. The need for medical assistance with altered consciousness varies with the training and experience of the doctor; with unconsciousness, medical assistance is needed.

Opioid Analgesics

Oversedation and respiratory depression are the primary clinical manifestations of opioid overdose. Cardiovascular depression normally does not develop until late in the opioid overdose reaction, especially with the patient in a supine position. Management of the patient who has received an absolute or relative overdose of an opioid is similar to that described for the sedative-hypnotic drugs with one major addition: A specific antagonist is available to reverse the clinical actions of opioid agonists.

Steps in the management of this patient follow. The clinical picture may vary from minor alterations in consciousness, with minimal respiratory depression, to the unconscious, apneic patient.

Diagnostic clues to the presence of an opioid overdose include the following[8]:

- Altered level of consciousness
- Respiratory depression (slow rate; normal to deep depth)
- Miosis (contraction of pupils of the eyes)

Step 1: Terminate the Treatment

Step 2: P—Position the Patient. The patient is placed in the supine position with the legs elevated slightly.

Step 3: A—Airway, B—Breathing, C—Circulation; Basic Life Support, as Indicated. A patent airway is ensured, and breathing is monitored. Opioids produce a decrease in the rate of breathing with little change in tidal volume. Therefore the depth of ventilation is increased.

In most cases of opioid overdose the patient remains conscious, although not fully alert and responsive. Assistance in airway maintenance may be desirable (e.g., head-tilt/chin-lift). With more profound depression, unconsciousness and respiratory arrest may occur, necessitating reassessment of airway and breathing. Because the cardiovascular system is relatively unaffected by opioid overdose, if oxygenation is maintained (airway patency and adequate ventilations are maintained), especially in the supine patient, the blood pressure and heart rate should remain close to baseline values.

Step 4: D—Definitive Care

Step 4a: Summon Medical Assistance, if Needed. Depending on the level of consciousness, the degree of respiratory depression, the training of the doctor in emergency care and anesthesiology, and the availability of equipment and drugs, it might be prudent to summon emergency medical assistance at this time. If unconsciousness and respiratory arrest are present, emergency medical assistance should be summoned immediately if the doctor is not well trained in anesthesiology. In the hands of a doctor well trained in emergency care and anesthesiology (e.g., general anesthesia), management of this patient may continue to include the administration of antidotal drugs (see following text).

Step 4b: Administer Oxygen. Oxygen and/or artificial ventilation is administered if necessary. The administration of oxygen is especially important in the early management of opioid overdose. Minimal cardiovascular depression is normally present and, when present, is a result of hypoxia secondary to respiratory depression. The administration of oxygen to a patient with a patent airway prevents or reverses opioid-induced cardiovascular depression, including dysrhythmias that may be evident.

Step 4c: Monitor and Record Vital Signs. Vital signs are monitored every 5 minutes and recorded. Should pulse and blood pressure be absent, cardiopulmonary resuscitation (P → A → B → C) is initiated immediately.

Step 4d: Establish an Intravenous Line, if Possible. With the cardiovascular system minimally effected by opioid overdose (with the patient in the supine position), it will be possible to establish an IV infusion in most patients. The availability of IV access will expedite definitive therapy.

Step 4e: Antidotal Drug Administration. Definitive management is available when an opioid is the likely cause of the overdose. Even when what could normally be considered a small dose of an opioid has been given (to a hyperresponding patient), an opioid antagonist should be administered to the patient if excessive respiratory depression (or apnea) has developed. No drug will be administered to this patient before the steps of BLS (P → A → B → C) have been assessed and performed, as needed. At this time an opioid antagonist is administered. *Naloxone* is the drug of choice and should, if possible, be administered intravenously to take advantage of the more rapid onset of action with this route. If the IV route is unavailable, IM administration is acceptable. The onset of action is slower after IM administration, but naloxone will prove to be effective if an opioid is responsible for the respiratory depression. Regardless of the route by which naloxone is administered, the emergency team must continue to provide the necessary steps of BLS from the time of naloxone administration until its onset of action (determined by increased patient responsiveness and more adequate and rapid ventilatory efforts).

Following IV administration, naloxone's actions are noted within 1 to 2 minutes (if not faster) and within 10 minutes following IM administration (in the presence of a near-baseline blood pressure). Naloxone is available in a 1-ml ampule containing 0.4 mg (adult dosage form) or 0.02 mg (pediatric dosage form). The drug is loaded into a plastic disposable syringe, and when the IV route is available, 3 ml of diluent (any IV fluid) is added to the syringe, producing a final concentration of 0.1 mg/ml of naloxone (adult) or 0.005 mg/ml (pediatric). The drug is then administered intravenously to the adult at a rate of 1 ml/min until the ventilatory rate and alertness increase. In children the IV dose is 0.01 mg/kg.[11] If naloxone is administered intramuscularly, a dose of 0.4 mg (adult) or 0.01 mg/kg (pediatric) is administered into a suitable muscle mass, such as the mid-deltoid (adult) or vastus lateralis (child or adult), or sublingually (if the patient is unconscious).

A potential problem with naloxone is the fact that its duration of clinical activity may be shorter than that of the opioid it is being used to reverse. This is especially true in cases in which longer-acting opioid agonists such as morphine are administered; it is less likely to occur with meperidine and still less likely with fentanyl and its analogs alfentanil, sufentanil, and remifentanil. When the opioid action is of greater duration than the intravenously administered naloxone, the doctor and staff will notice an initial improvement in the patient's clinical picture as the naloxone began to act and then see a recurrence of CNS depression approximately 10 minutes or more later (following IV administration of naloxone). Because the opioid producing the overdose continues to undergo redistribution and biotransformation during this time, in the event that such a rebound effect does occur, it would quite likely be much less intense than the initial response. In cases in which longer-acting opioids (e.g., morphine) have been administered intramuscularly or submucosally, it is recommended that the initial IV dose of naloxone be followed with an IM dose (0.4 mg [adult] or 0.01 mg/kg [pediatric]). In this way, as the clinical action of the IV naloxone dose is waning, the level of naloxone from the IM dose will be reaching a peak, minimizing the likelihood of a relapse of significant respiratory or CNS depression. The administration of naloxone in opioid overdose is important but not the most critical step in overall patient management (see following text).

Step 5: Permit Recovery. The patient is continuously observed and monitored after the administration of naloxone until clinical recovery becomes apparent. The patient may be transported to a recovery area within the dental office but should remain there under constant supervision for at least 1 hour. On the other hand, if the doctor considers it prudent, the planned dental treatment may continue. Once again, whether to continue treatment of this patient at this time is a judgment that can be made only by the doctor, and only after taking into consideration the status of the patient and the level of expertise of the doctor and staff in recognizing and managing this problem.

If any doubt exists, dental care should be discontinued. Vital signs are recorded every 5 minutes during the recovery period. Oxygen and suction must be available, and trained personnel must be present.

Step 6: Discharge. Patient discharge may require transport to a hospital facility for observation or follow-up care. In most cases hospitalization is unnecessary. Following an adequate period of recovery (minimum 1 hour of observation) in the dental or medical office, the patient can be discharged in the custody of a responsible adult companion, using the same recovery criteria established for parenteral sedation and general anesthesia.

Box 34-3 outlines the steps to follow in management of opioid overdose.

Drugs used in management include oxygen and naloxone.

The need for medical assistance in the presence of altered consciousness or unconsciousness depends on the doctor's training and experience.

Summary

The previous discussions dealt with overdose reactions of varying levels of severity that occur after the administration of a single drug. Although single-drug

BOX 34-3

Management of Opioid Overdose

Terminate the dental procedure.

↓

P, Position the patient supine with the legs elevated slightly.

↓

ABC, Assess and perform basic life support, as needed.

↓

D, Initiate definitive care:

- Summon medical assistance, if required.
- Administer oxygen.
- Monitor and record vital signs.
- Establish an IV line, if possible.
- Administer an antidotal drug (IV or IM naloxone).

↓

Permit recovery and discharge patient.

overdose can and does occur, especially after IM or submucosal administration (because of the inability to titrate to effect), many overdose reactions reported involve the administration of multiple drugs. In many of these cases, drugs such as an antianxiety drug are combined with an opioid to provide a level of sedation and some analgesia. A local anesthetic is then added to manage operative pain. Drugs in all three of these categories are CNS depressants. Added to this, in many cases, will be nitrous oxide (N_2O) and oxygen (O_2), adding yet another degree of CNS depression.

Whenever more than one CNS depressant drug is administered to a patient, the dosages of both drugs must be reduced from their usual dosage to prevent exaggerated, undesirable clinical responses. As demonstrated in Table 34-2, in most of the cases reported by Goodson and Moore, this step was not taken, with disastrous results often occurring.[7]

Another factor must be considered, one that most health professionals do not, as a rule, give much thought when using sedative techniques: Local anesthetics themselves are CNS depressants and can produce additive actions when administered in conjunction with drugs commonly used for sedation. The maximal dosage of local anesthetic to be administered to any patient, but especially to a child or lighter-weight adult, should be based on the patient's body weight in kilograms or pounds. When no other CNS depressants are being administered, this maximal dose could be reached without adverse effects if the patient is an American Society of Anesthesiologists (ASA) I and falls within the normal responding range on the bell-shaped curve. Table 34-3 presents the maximal recommended doses of the most commonly used local anesthetics. When a local anesthetic is administered with other CNS depressants, the local anesthetic dosage should be minimized.

A primary goal of conscious sedation is to produce a cooperative patient who still possesses protective reflexes (e.g., swallowing, coughing, maintenance of the airway). When possible, this goal should be achieved using the simplest technique available, as well as the fewest drugs possible. Polypharmacy, the combination of several drugs, is necessary in many patients to achieve the desired level of sedation and/or analgesia; however, if it is possible to reach this desired effect with but one drug, combinations ought not be used. The use of drug combinations increases the opportunity for ADRs and makes it less obvious which drug may be responsible for any problems that arise, thereby making management of the situation more difficult.

Within the individual techniques of sedation, it is suggested that single-drug regimens are preferable to combinations of drugs. Rational drug combinations are available for use in cases in which they are specifically indicated. With IV drug administration, the problem of severe ADRs should not occur if the technique of titration is strictly adhered to at all times. Titration is not possible with the IM, IN, and oral routes of administration. The doctor must modify individual drug dosages before their administration. Serious ADRs are more likely to occur when the technique used was one in which titration was not possible.

Consideration must also be given to the use of multiple techniques of sedation, as opposed to multiple drugs by one technique of administration. It is not uncommon for a patient who is a significant management problem to receive an oral antianxiety drug before arrival in the office, followed by either IM, submucosal, or IV sedation, as well as inhalation sedation and local anesthesia during the course of treatment. Whenever oral sedation with CNS depressants is used, the dosages of all subsequent CNS depressants should be evaluated carefully before their administration. This is critical when nontitratable routes of drug administration are used. With inhalation and IV sedation, careful titration of CNS depressant drugs to the patient who has previously received oral premedication will usually produce the desired level of clinical sedation with minimal risk of adverse response by the patient.

How, then, may overdose reactions best be prevented? Goodson and Moore made the following recommendations concerning the use of sedative techniques in which opioids are being administered[7]:

1. *Be prepared for emergencies.* The cardiovascular and respiratory systems should be monitored continuously. An emergency kit containing drugs such as epinephrine, oxygen, and naloxone should be readily available, in addition to equipment and

TABLE 34-2 Dose Administered Relative to Recommended Maximum Dose

Case	Narcotic Analgesics (%)*	Antiemetic Sedatives (%)*	Local Anesthetics (%)*	N_2O-O_2	Result
1	216	36	172	–	Fatality
2	173	145	237	–	Fatality
3	336	0	342	–	Fatality
4	127	27	267	+	Fatality
5	309	372	230	+	Brain damage
6	436	?	?	–	Fatality
7	100	136	107	–	Fatality
8	167	300	219	+	Brain damage
9	66	0	60	–	Recovery
10	66	92	?	+	Recovery
11	183	0	?	–	Recovery
12	200	558	0	–	Recovery
13	250	136	127	–	Brain damage
14	50	0	370	+	Fatality

From Goodson JM, Moore PA: *J Am Dent Assoc* 107:239, 1983. Copyright by the American Dental Association. Reprinted by permission.
*Expressed as a percentage of the maximal recommended dose for that patient.

trained personnel. In their paper, Goodson and Moore state that "because multiple sedative drug techniques can easily induce unconsciousness, respiratory arrest, and convulsions, practitioners should be prepared and trained to recognize and control these occurrences."

2. *Individualize the drug dosage.* When drugs are used in combination, the dosage of each drug must be selected carefully. The toxic effects of drug combinations appear to be additive. Drug selection must be based on the patient's general health history. The presence of significant systemic disease (ASA III or IV) usually indicates the need for a reduction of dosage. Because most sedative drugs are available in quite concentrated form and because children usually require very small dosages, extreme care must be taken when drugs are being prepared for administration.

   When possible, fixed-dose administration of drugs based on a range of ages (e.g., 4 to 6 years: 50 mg) should not be used. Dosages based on body weight or surface area of the patient, or titration, are preferred when possible.

   Should the selected drug dosage prove to be inadequate to produce the desired effect in the patient, it is prudent to consider a change in the sedation technique or in the drugs being used (at a subsequent appointment) rather than increasing the drug dosage to a higher and potentially more dangerous level at the same visit.

3. *Recognize and expect adverse drug effects.* When combinations of CNS depressants have been administered, the potential for excessive CNS and respiration depression is increased and should be expected.

TABLE 34-3 Maximum Recommended Doses of Local Anesthetics

	Dose		
Drug	mg/kg	mg/lb	Absolute Maximum Dose
Articaine	7.0	3.2	500
Lidocaine	4.4	2.0	300
Mepivacaine	4.4	2.0	300
Prilocaine	6.0	2.7	400
Bupivacaine	2.0	0.9	90
Etidocaine	8.0	3.6	400

The Dentists Insurance Company (TDIC), in a retrospective study of deaths and morbidity in dental practices over a 3-year period, concluded that in most of those incidents related to administration of drugs, there were three common factors.[12]

1. Improper preoperative evaluation of the patient
2. Lack of knowledge of drug pharmacology by the doctor
3. Lack of adequate monitoring during the procedure

These three factors greatly increased the risk of serious ADRs, with a negative outcome the usual result.

An overdose reaction to the administration of CNS depressant drugs may not always be a preventable complication; however, with care taken on the part of the doctor, the incidence of these events should be extremely low, with a successful outcome as the result virtually every time. With techniques such as IV and inhalation sedation, in which titration is possible, overdosage should be rare. With oral, IM, and IN drug administration, in which the doctor has little control over the drug's ultimate effect because of the inability to titrate, the doctor must expend greater care in the preoperative evaluation of the patient, in the determination of the appropriate drug dosage, and in monitoring during the procedure so that excessive CNS or respiratory depression may be identified and treated immediately. When the oral, IN, or IM routes are used, the onset of adverse reactions may be delayed. An adverse reaction may not develop until after the rubber dam is in place and the dental procedure has been started. Therefore monitoring of the patient throughout the procedure becomes extremely important to the patient's safety. My preferences, as of July 2002 in monitoring during parenteral sedation are as follows:

1. CNS
   a. Direct verbal contact with the patient
2. Respiratory system
   a. Pretracheal stethoscope
   b. Pulse oximetry
3. Cardiovascular system
   a. Continuous monitoring of vital signs
   b. Electrocardiogram (ECG)

ALLERGY

Allergy is a hypersensitive state acquired through exposure to a particular allergen, reexposure to which produces a heightened capacity to react. Allergic reactions cover a broad range of clinical manifestations, from mild, delayed-onset reactions occurring as long as 48 hours after exposure to immediate and life-threatening reactions developing within seconds of exposure. Although all allergic phenomena are important and require thorough evaluation by the doctor, only one form, the type I, or immediate, reaction is discussed here, for it may present the doctor with a life-threatening emergency situation. A classification of allergy types is presented in Table 34-4.

TABLE 34-4 Classification of Allergic Diseases (after Gell and Coombs)

Type	Mechanism	Principal Antibody or Cell	Time of Reactions	Clinical Examples
I	Anaphylactic (immediate, homocytotropic, antigen induced, antibody mediated)	IgE	Second to minutes	Anaphylaxis (drugs, insect venom, antisera) Atopic bronchial asthma Allergic rhinitis Urticaria Angioedema Hayfever
II	Cytotoxic (antimembrane)	IgG IgM (activated complement)	—	Transfusion reactions Goodpasture's syndrome Autoimmune hemolysis Hemolytic anemia Certain drug reactions Membranous glomerulonephrosis
III	Immune complex (serum sickness –like)	IgG (form complexes with complement)	6-8 hr	Serum sickness Lupus nephritis Occupational allergic alveolitis Acute viral hepatitis
IV	Cell-mediated (delayed) or tuberculin-type response	—	48 hr	Allergic contact dermatitis Infectious granulomas (tuberculosis, mycoses) Tissue graft rejection Chronic hepatitis

From Krupp MA, Chatton MJ: *Current medical diagnosis & treatment,* Stamford, Conn, 1984, Lange Medical Publications.

Allergic reactions are mediated through immunologic mechanisms that are similar regardless of the specific antigen responsible for precipitating the response. Therefore an allergic reaction to the venom of a stinging insect may be identical to that seen after aspirin or penicillin administration in a previously sensitized individual. Allergic reactions must be differentiated from the overdose, or toxic, reaction previously discussed, in which the observed signs and symptoms are a direct extension of the normal pharmacologic properties of the drug administered. Overdose reactions are much more commonly encountered than are allergic drug reactions. Of all ADRs, 85% result from the pharmacologic actions of drugs; 15% are immunologic reactions.[13] To the layperson, however, any adverse drug response is frequently labeled "allergic."

Allergy is a frightening word to those health professionals responsible for primary care of patients. Although none of the drugs commonly used for the management of pain and anxiety has a significantly high rate of allergenicity, allergic phenomena may still arise. The only drugs mentioned in this book that, to my knowledge, have never been shown to have produced allergy are N_2O and O_2. Although the concept of prevention has been stressed repeatedly throughout this book, in no other situation is this concept of greater importance than with allergy. Although allergy is not the most common ADR, it is frequently involved with the most serious of these reactions.

Of the many antianxiety drugs used, the barbiturates probably possess the greatest potential for sensitization of patients. Although not nearly as common as allergy to penicillin or aspirin, barbiturate allergy usually manifests itself in the form of skin lesions such as hives and urticaria or less frequently in the form of blood dyscrasias such as agranulocytosis or thrombocytopenia. Allergy to barbiturates occurs much more frequently in persons with a history of asthma, urticaria, and angioedema.[14] A documented history of allergy to any barbiturate represents an absolute contraindication to their administration.

Among the opioids, meperidine can release histamine locally. When meperidine is administered intravenously, this localized histamine release develops along the path of the vein through which the drug travels. This reaction is not allergy and requires no therapeutic management. The reaction resolves after the drug leaves the area of its administration. Use of meperidine is relatively contraindicated in asthmatic patients because of potential bronchospasm induced by histamine release when the drug enters the pulmonary circulation.

Following IV administration atropine, an anticholinergic, may produce flushing of a patient's face, neck, and upper chest. Known as *atropine flush*, this is not an allergic reaction and requires no therapeutic intervention because spontaneous resolution occurs within a brief time. Atropine flush is most often seen with overdose of atropine. However, in certain sensitive individuals (those who are hyperresponders on the bell-shaped curve), the usual therapeutic dose may provoke this response.

Prevention of Allergic Reactions

Whenever any drug or combination of drugs is being considered for administration, the doctor must question the patient about any prior exposure to that drug or members of the same drug family. In addition, the patient's medical history questionnaire must be evaluated. All questionnaires include questions concerning current drug use and prior ADRs. These two steps will, in most cases, enable the doctor to assess the possibility of an adverse drug response. Should a positive history be elicited, questioning is undertaken to determine the nature of the previous reactions. Although the questioning may vary, basic questions asked include the following:

1. What drug was used?
2. What happened? (The patient describes the sequence of events that ensued.)
3. What treatment was required? Was epinephrine or a histamine blocker administered? O_2 or aromatic ammonia?
4. Were the services of a physician or emergency paramedical personnel required? Were you hospitalized?
5. What is the name and address of the doctor (physician or dentist) who treated you at that time?

Knowledge of the signs and symptoms of the "reaction" and its management can go far in aiding the doctor in diagnosing the alleged "allergy."

The need for hospitalization or assistance of another health professional usually indicates a more serious ADR. If possible, it may be prudent to speak directly to the doctor involved with the patient at that time.

Following a thorough dialogue history and a review of the medical history questionnaire, it is usually possible to form a general opinion about the reaction. If the doctor is convinced that allergy did occur, other drugs that are structurally dissimilar to the offending drug should be selected for administration. In most cases, however, it will become obvious that the "allergy" was in fact a side effect of the drug (e.g., nausea from codeine) or that the response was psychogenic (i.e., induced by anxiety). If doubt remains as to the precise nature of the problem, the patient should be managed, at that time, with drugs unrelated to the one(s) in question, followed by consultation with an allergist (or other appropriate individual) so that more definitive testing may be undertaken.

Clinical Manifestations

Most allergic drug reactions are immediate, in particular the type I, or anaphylactic, reaction. The term *immediate*, relating to allergic phenomena, indicates the development of clinical signs and symptoms within 60 minutes of exposure to the allergen.

A number of organs and tissues are affected during immediate allergic reactions, particularly the skin, respiratory system, cardiovascular system, and gastrointestinal tract. Generalized, or systemic, anaphylaxis, by definition, affects all the systems mentioned. If hypotension is also a clinical component of the response, the term *anaphylactic shock* is correctly applied.

Immediate allergic reactions also manifest through any number of combinations involving these organs. Reactions involving one system are referred to as *localized anaphylaxis*, for example, asthmatic attack, in which the respiratory system is the sole target, or urticaria, in which the skin is the target organ.

Onset

The time elapsing between exposure of the patient to the antigen and the development of clinical signs and symptoms is of great importance. As a rule, *the more rapidly signs and symptoms evolve after exposure to an allergen, the more intense the ultimate response is.* Conversely, the greater the length of time is between exposure and onset, the less intense the reaction is. However, cases of anaphylaxis have been reported to arise many hours after exposure. Of importance, too, is the rate at which the signs and symptoms progress once they appear. If they appear and increase in severity rapidly, the reaction is more likely to become life threatening than one that progresses slowly or not at all.

Skin Reaction. Allergic skin reactions are the most common sensitization reaction to drug administration. Many types of allergic skin reaction may occur, the two most important types being localized anaphylaxis and drug eruption. Drug eruption constitutes the most common group of skin manifestations of drug allergy. Included in this category are urticaria, erythema (reddening), and angioedema (localized swelling).

Urticaria is associated with wheals (smooth, slightly elevated patches of skin) and often with intense itching (pruritus). Angioedema is a process in which localized swelling occurs in response to an allergen. Several forms of angioedema exist, but clinically they appear to be similar. The skin is usually of normal color (unless accompanied by urticaria or erythema) and temperature, and pain and itching are uncommon. The areas most commonly involved are the hands, face, feet, and genitalia. Of special concern is the potential involvement of the lips, tongue, pharynx, and larynx, leading to obstruction of the airway (laryngeal edema).

Allergic skin reactions, if the sole manifestation of allergy, are usually not considered life threatening. However, a skin reaction that develops rapidly after drug administration may be the first indication of the generalized reaction to follow.

Adhesive tape used during IV sedation is a fairly common cause of dermatologic reactions, the adhesive being the allergen. The usual response to this tape is erythema and urticaria developing around the site where the tape has been placed. In adhesive-allergic individuals, hypoallergenic tapes are recommended for use.

Respiratory Reactions. Clinical signs and symptoms of allergy may be related entirely to the respiratory tract, or signs and symptoms of respiratory tract involvement may develop along with other systemic responses. In a slowly developing generalized allergic reaction, respiratory tract involvement usually follows the skin response but precedes cardiovascular signs and symptoms. Bronchospasm is the classic respiratory manifestation of allergy. It represents the clinical result of constriction of bronchial smooth muscle. Signs and symptoms include respiratory distress, dyspnea, wheezing, flushing, possible cyanosis, perspiration, tachycardia, greatly increased anxiety, and the use of accessory muscles of respiration.

A second respiratory manifestation of acute allergy may be the extension of angioedema to the larynx, producing a swelling of the vocal apparatus with subsequent obstruction of the airway (laryngeal edema). Clinical manifestations include little or no air exchange from the lungs (chest is not moving, little or no air is felt); wheezing, indicative of partial airway obstruction; or no sound, indicating total obstruction. The occurrence of significant angioedema represents one of the most ominous of clinical signs. Acute airway obstruction leads rapidly to death of the patient unless immediately corrected.

Generalized Anaphylaxis. Generalized anaphylaxis is the most dramatic and acutely life-threatening form of allergy and may lead to clinical death within a few minutes. It may develop after the administration of an antigen via any route but is most likely to occur after parenteral administration. The time from antigenic challenge to the onset of reaction varies greatly, but typically the reaction develops rapidly, reaching a maximum within 5 to 30 minutes. Delayed responses of 1 hour or more have been reported. It is believed that this is the result of the rate at which the antigen enters into the circulatory system.

Signs and symptoms of generalized anaphylaxis are highly variable. Four major clinical syndromes are recognized: skin reactions, smooth muscle spasm (gastrointestinal and genitourinary tracts and respiratory smooth muscle), respiratory distress, and cardiovascular collapse. In typical generalized anaphylaxis, the symptoms progressively move through these four areas; however, in cases of fatal anaphylaxis, respiratory and cardiovascular disturbances predominate and are evident early in the reaction.

In the typical generalized anaphylactic reaction, the patient may begin to complain of feeling sick and intense itching, flushing, and giant hives may develop over the face and upper chest. Nausea, possibly followed by vomiting, may also occur. These early symptoms are primarily related to the skin. Other responses noted early in the reaction include conjunctivitis, vasomotor rhinitis (increased mucus secretion in the nose), and pilomotor erection (the feeling of hair standing on end).

Associated with the development of skin symptoms are various gastrointestinal and genitourinary disturbances related to spasm of smooth muscle. Severe abdominal cramps, nausea and vomiting, diarrhea, and fecal and urinary incontinence may occur.

Respiratory symptoms normally follow. However, in rapidly developing reactions, all symptoms may occur within a short time with considerable overlap. In particularly severe reactions respiratory and cardiovascular symptoms may be the only signs present.

Respiratory symptoms begin with a feeling of substernal tightness or pain in the chest. A cough may develop in addition to wheezing and dyspnea. If the respiratory disturbances are severe, cyanosis may develop, noted initially in mucous membranes and nail beds. Laryngeal edema may also develop, producing acute airway obstruction.

Signs and symptoms of cardiovascular disturbance follow and include pallor, lightheadedness, palpitation, tachycardia, hypotension, and cardiac dysrhythmias, followed by loss of consciousness and cardiac arrest. With loss of consciousness the anaphylactic reaction may more properly be called *anaphylactic shock.*

The duration of the anaphylactic reaction or any part of it may vary from minutes to a day or more. With prompt and appropriate therapy, the entire reaction may be terminated rapidly; however, the two most serious sequelae, hypotension and laryngeal edema, may persist for hours to days despite vigorous therapy. Death may occur at any time, the usual cause being upper airway obstruction produced by laryngeal edema.

Management

Skin Reactions. Allergic skin reactions may range from localized angioedema to diffuse erythema, urticaria, and pruritus. Management is based on the speed at which they appear after antigenic challenge (drug administration).

Delayed Skin Reactions. Skin reactions appearing more than 60 minutes after antigenic exposure that do not progress are considered non life threatening. These include a mild skin reaction after IM injection or localized reaction to adhesive tape.

When this occurs during parenteral sedation, the first step in management is the IM or IV administration of a histamine blocker such as diphenhydramine, 50 mg, or chlorpheniramine, 10 mg. The patient is then given a prescription for a histamine blocker to be taken orally for approximately 3 to 5 days. Medical consultation must follow with the patient's physician or an allergist to determine the nature of the allergy or allergies.

If the skin reaction is mild but the patient has left the office before it develops, the patient should be requested to return to the office, where the same therapy as described would be employed. Should the reaction be noted at a time when the patient is unable to return to the office for evaluation, the patient is advised to see a physician at a local hospital emergency room. The treating dentist should arrange to meet the patient at the hospital, if possible.

Histamine blockers inhibit the actions of histamine by occupying receptor sites on the effector cell (competitive antagonism), thereby preventing the agonist molecules (histamine) from occupying these same sites. The protective responses from histamine blockers include control of edema formation and itch. Other allergic responses, such as hypotension and bronchoconstriction, are influenced little, if at all, by histamine blockers. Histamine blockers are of value only in mild allergic responses in which only small quantities of histamine have been released or to prevent reactions in allergic individuals.

Immediate Skin Reactions. Allergic skin reactions developing in less than 60 minutes should be managed more vigorously. Other allergic symptoms of a relatively mild nature included in this section are conjunctivitis, rhinitis, urticaria, pruritus, and erythema.

Epinephrine is administered intravenously, intramuscularly, or subcutaneously in an adult dose of 0.3 mg. A histamine blocker (diphenhydramine or chlorpheniramine) is then administered. Medical consultation is requested.

When epinephrine administration was required, it is my belief that the patient should be fully evaluated before discharge from the office or hospital. In most cases the patient should be observed for at least 1 hour and, in the absence of a return of signs and symptoms, may be discharged home in the company of a responsible adult. If the reaction is more severe, medical consultation before discharge is indicated.

Respiratory Reactions

Bronchospasm. The most likely situations in dentistry in which an allergic reaction will manifest itself as a respiratory problem (bronchospasm) are (1) in the asthmatic patient who is allergic to bisulfites and comes into contact with them during dental care and (2) in the patient who is allergic to aspirin.

Diagnostic clues to the presence of an allergy involving bronchospasm include the following:

- Wheezing
- Use of accessory muscles of respiration

Bronchial smooth muscle constriction results in asthmalike reactions. Management of the acute asthmatic episode includes the following:

Step 1: Terminate the Treatment

Step 2: P—Position the Patient Comfortably. An upright or semierect position is usually preferred by the conscious patient who is exhibiting difficulty breathing.

Step 3: A—Airway, B—Breathing, C—Circulation; Basic Life Support, as Indicated. Assessment of airway and circulation will initially prove adequate. Breathing may demonstrate varying degrees of inadequacy, ranging from mild bronchospasm to almost complete obstruction and cyanosis.

Step 4: Remove Materials from the Patient's Mouth

Step 5: Calm the Patient. The conscious patient who experiences respiratory distress may become quite fearful. Try to allay any apprehensions.

Step 6: D—Definitive Care

Step 6a: Summon Medical Assistance. With clinically evident respiratory distress associated with wheezing and cyanosis, emergency medical care should be summoned immediately.

Step 6b: Administer a Bronchodilator. Albuterol may be administered by means of an aerosol inhaler (Ventolin or Proventil) or epinephrine by IM or subcutaneous injection (0.3 ml of a 1:1000 dilution for adults) or intravenously (0.1 ml of 1:10,000 every 15 to 30 minutes). The potent bronchodilating actions of epinephrine usually terminate bronchospasm within minutes of administration. Epinephrine is the drug of choice as an injected bronchodilator because it effectively reverses the actions of one of the major causes of bronchospasm—histamine; however, like the histamine blockers, epinephrine does not relieve bronchospasm produced by leukotrienes. Inhaled bronchodilators, such as albuterol, also act rapidly in the management of bronchospasm.

Step 6c: Monitor the Patient. The patient should remain in the dental office for observation because a recurrence of bronchospasm is possible as the epinephrine undergoes rapid biotransformation. Should bronchospasm reappear, epinephrine may be readministered intramuscularly or subcutaneously or albuterol administered by inhalation (aerosol).

Step 6d: Administer a Histamine Blocker. The IM administration of a histamine blocker minimizes the risk of a recurrence of bronchospasm as the histamine blocker occupies the histamine receptor site, preventing a relapse. Diphenhydramine, 50 mg intramuscularly (adults) or 2 mg/kg intramuscularly or intravenously (children), is suggested.

Step 6e: Recovery and Discharge. On arrival, emergency medical personnel will stabilize the victim and start any necessary definitive treatment. Additional treatment may involve the administration of one or more of the following: IV bronchodilators, atropine, or steroids (methylprednisolone); intubation and assisted ventilation may be necessary if bronchospasm is persistent and severe. In most cases a patient exhibiting an allergic reaction consisting primarily of respiratory signs and symptoms will require a variable period of hospitalization.

Box 34-4 outlines the steps to take in managing the respiratory allergic reaction.

Drugs used in the management of allergic reactions include oxygen, bronchodilators such as epinephrine (intravenously, intramuscularly, or subcutaneously),

BOX 34-4 Management of Respiratory Allergic Reaction

Terminate the dental procedure.

↓

P, Position the patient comfortably.

↓

ABC, Assess and perform basic life support, as needed.

↓

D, Initiate definitive care:

- Calm the patient.
- Summon medical assistance.
- Administer a bronchodilator, epinephrine (SC, IM, IV), albuterol (inhalation).
- Monitor vital signs.
- Administer a histamine blocker (IM).

↓

Hospitalize or discharge the patient.

albuterol (inhalation), and histamine blockers (intramuscularly).

Medical assistance is required if there is significant respiratory distress.

Laryngeal Edema. The second and usually more life-threatening respiratory allergic manifestation is the development of laryngeal edema. It may be diagnosed when little or no air movement can be heard or felt through the mouth and nose despite exaggerated spontaneous respiratory movements by the patient or when a patent airway cannot be obtained. A partially obstructed larynx in the presence of spontaneous respiratory movements produces the characteristically high-pitched crowing sound of stridor, in contrast to the wheezing of bronchospasm; total obstruction is accompanied by silence in the presence of spontaneous chest movement. The patient loses consciousness from lack of oxygen (e.g., hypoxia, anoxia). Fortunately, laryngeal edema is not common, but it may arise in any acute allergic reaction that involves the airway.

Diagnostic clues to the presence of laryngeal edema include the following:

- Respiratory distress
- Exaggerated chest movements
- High-pitched crowing sound—stridor (partial obstruction) or no sound (total obstruction)
- Cyanosis
- Loss of consciousness

Step 1: Terminate the Treatment

Step 2: P—Position the Patient. An upright or semi-erect position is usually preferred by the conscious patient exhibiting difficulty breathing. If the degree of edema is severe, the patient's level of consciousness will be significantly altered and the supine position with the feet elevated is most appropriate. If the patient is unwilling or unable to tolerate the supine position, he or she should be positioned based on comfort.

Step 3: A—Airway, B—Breathing, C— Circulation; Basic Life Support, as Indicated. Airway will be the most critical factor in managing laryngeal edema. Initial management should include extension of the neck (head-tilt/chin-lift or jaw-thrust/chin-lift), followed by insertion of either a nasopharyngeal tube or oropharyngeal airway. The conscious patient is usually able to tolerate a nasopharyngeal airway, but an oropharyngeal airway is likely to produce a gag reflex.

Step 4a: Summon Medical Assistance

Step 4b: Administer Epinephrine. The immediate administration of 0.3 ml of 1:1000 epinephrine intramuscularly (0.15 ml for child; 0.075 ml for infant) or 0.1 ml of 1:10,000 epinephrine intravenously over 5 minutes (adult), repeated every 3 to 5 minutes as necessary, is recommended. A maximum dose for 1:10,000 epinephrine of 5.0 ml every 15 to 30 minutes should not be exceeded.

Step 4c: Maintain Airway. In the presence of a partially obstructed airway, epinephrine administration may halt or even reverse the progress of laryngeal edema.

Step 4d: Administer Oxygen. Oxygen should be administered as soon as it becomes available.

Step 4e: Additional Drug Management. A histamine blocker (diphenhydramine, 50 mg for adults, 25 mg for children) and a corticosteroid (hydrocortisone, 100 mg) should be administered intramuscularly or intravenously following clinical recovery, which is noted by airway improvement: normal, or at least improved, breath sounds; absence of cyanosis; and fewer exaggerated chest excursions. Corticosteroids inhibit edema and capillary dilation by stabilizing basement membranes. They are of little immediate value because of their slow onset of action, even when administered intravenously. Corticosteroids have an onset of action approximately 6 hours after their administration. Corticosteroids are used to prevent a relapse, whereas epinephrine, a more rapidly acting drug, is used during the acute phase to halt or reverse the deleterious actions of histamine and other mediators of allergy.

These procedures (steps 1 through 4e) are normally adequate to maintain the patient. With the arrival of emergency medical assistance, the patient will be stabilized and transferred to a hospital for further observation and treatment.

Step 4f: Cricothyrotomy. A totally obstructed airway may not be reopened at all, or in adequate time, by the administration of epinephrine and other drugs. In this case an emergency airway must be created to maintain the patient's life. Time is of the essence, and it is not possible to delay action until medical assistance arrives. A cricothyrotomy is the procedure of choice for the establishment of an airway in this situation.[15] (The reader is referred to Chapter 11 of *Medical Emergencies in the Dental Office*[19] for a complete discussion of cricothyrotomy technique.) Once an airway is obtained, oxygen is administered, artificial ventilation initiated (if needed), and vital signs monitored.

Before the arrival of medical assistance, the drugs previously administered may halt the progress of the laryngeal edema and might even reverse it to a degree. The patient will require hospitalization following transfer from the dental office by the paramedics.

Box 34-5 outlines the steps in management of laryngeal edema.

Drugs used in management of laryngeal edema include oxygen, epinephrine (intravenously or intramuscularly),

BOX 34-5

Management of Laryngeal Edema

Terminate the dental procedure.
↓
P, Position the patient comfortably.
↓
ABC, Assess and perform basic life support, as needed.
↓
D, Initiate definitive care:
- Summon medical assistance.
- Maintain airway (head-tilt/chin-lift; jaw-thrust; use oropharyngeal or nasopharyngeal airways).
- Administer oxygen.
- Administer additional drugs: histamine blocker; corticosteroid.
- Perform cricothyrotomy as needed.

a histamine blocker (intramuscularly), and a corticosteroid (intravenously or intramuscularly).

Medical assistance is required.

Generalized Anaphylaxis. In generalized anaphylaxis a wide range of clinical manifestations may be noted; however, the cardiovascular system is involved in virtually all systemic allergic reactions. In rapidly progressing anaphylaxis, cardiovascular collapse may occur within minutes of the onset of symptoms. Immediate and aggressive management of this situation is imperative if the victim is to survive. In the dental office this reaction is most likely to occur during or immediately after administration of penicillin or aspirin to a previously sensitized patient. A more remote, although increasingly possible, cause might be latex sensitivity.

Two other life-threatening situations may develop during the injection of a local anesthetic that might on occasion mimic anaphylaxis: vasodepressor syncope and a local anesthetic overdose. In the immediate management of this situation, there must be an attempt to diagnose the actual cause of the problem.

Signs of Allergy Present

Should any clinical signs, such as urticaria, erythema, pruritus, or wheezing, be noted before or after the patient's collapse, the diagnosis is obvious: allergy. Management proceeds accordingly.

Step 1: P—Position the Patient. The unconscious, or conscious but hypotensive, patient is placed into a supine position with the legs elevated slightly.

Step 2: A—Airway, B—Breathing, C—Circulation; Basic Life Support, as Indicated. The airway is opened via head-tilt, and steps of BLS are carried out as needed.

Step 3: D—Definitive Care

Step 3a: Summon Medical Assistance. As soon as generalized anaphylaxis is considered a possibility, emergency medical services should be summoned.

Step 3b: Administer Epinephrine. The doctor should have previously called for the office emergency team. Epinephrine from the emergency drug kit (0.3 ml of 1:1000 for adults, 0.15 ml for children, and 0.075 ml for infants) is administered intramuscularly as quickly as possible. Because of the immediate need for epinephrine in this situation, a preloaded syringe of epinephrine should be available in the emergency kit. Epinephrine is the only injectable drug that need be maintained in a preloaded form (to minimize confusion when looking for it in this near-panic situation).

The site for IM injection should be based on muscle perfusion in the presence of what is likely to be profound hypotension. With decreased perfusion, the absorption of epinephrine from muscle will be delayed. It is recommended that consideration be given to the administration of epinephrine in this situation into the body of the tongue (intralingual) or the floor of the mouth (sublingual) (Figure 34-3). The needle may enter from either an extraoral or intraoral puncture site. The highly vascular oral cavity, even in the presence of hypotension, provides a more rapid onset of activity than seen in the more traditional IM sites (mid-deltoid, vastus lateralis).

Epinephrine, in one or more doses, usually produces clinical improvement in the patient. Respiratory and cardiovascular signs and symptoms should decrease in severity: Breath sounds improve as bronchospasm decreases and blood pressure increases.

Should the clinical picture fail to improve or continue to deteriorate (i.e., increasing severity of

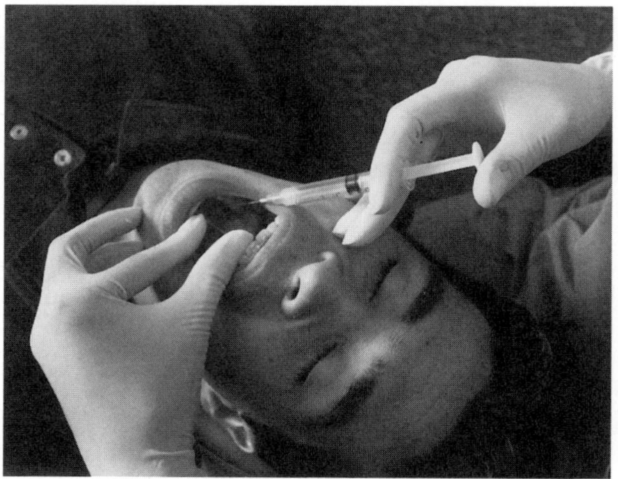

Figure 34-3 Sublingual epinephrine injection.

symptoms) within 5 minutes of the initial epinephrine dose, a second dose is administered. Subsequent doses may be administered as needed every 5 to 10 minutes if the potential risk of epinephrine administration (e.g., excessive cardiovascular stimulation) is kept in mind and the patient adequately monitored.

Step 3c: Administer Oxygen. Oxygen, at a flow of 5 to 6 L/min, can be delivered via nasal hood or full-face mask at any time during generalized anaphylaxis.

Step 3d: Monitor Vital Signs. The patient's cardiovascular and respiratory status must be monitored continuously. Blood pressure and heart rate (using the carotid artery) should be recorded at least every 5 minutes and chest compressions begun if cardiac arrest develops. During this acute, life-threatening phase of what is obviously an anaphylactic reaction, management consists of BLS, administration of oxygen and epinephrine, and continual monitoring of vital signs. Until improvement in the patient's status is noted, no additional drug therapy is indicated.

Step 3e: Additional Drug Therapy. Once clinical improvement is noted (e.g., increased blood pressure, decreased bronchospasm, return of consciousness), additional drug therapy is required. This includes the administration of a histamine blocker and a corticosteroid (both drugs intramuscularly or intravenously, if possible). These drugs function to prevent a recurrence of symptoms and to obviate the need for the continued administration of epinephrine. They are not administered during the acute phase of the reaction because they are too slow in onset and do not do enough immediate good to justify their use while the victim's life remains in danger. Epinephrine and oxygen are the only drugs to administer during the life-threatening phase of the anaphylactic reaction.

In the management of medical emergencies, it is stressed that definitive treatment of emergencies with drugs is of secondary importance to the PABCs of BLS. Drugs need not be administered in all emergency situations. Generalized anaphylaxis is the exception. Once a diagnosis of acute, generalized anaphylaxis is made, it is imperative that drug therapy (i.e., epinephrine) be initiated as soon as possible after the start of BLS. Review of clinical reports demonstrates the effectiveness of immediate drug therapy in anaphylaxis. Recovery from anaphylaxis is related to the rapidity with which effective treatment is instituted. Delay in treatment increases the mortality rate. Of those experiencing anaphylaxis provoked by bee stings, 87% survived if treated within the first hour, but only 67% of dying patients were treated in this first hour.[16]

On arrival in the office, emergency personnel will establish IV access, administer appropriate drugs (i.e., histamine blocker and corticosteroid), and stabilize and transport the victim to the hospital emergency room for definitive care.

BOX 34-6 Management of Generalized Anaphylaxis

(Signs and symptoms of allergy present)
Terminate the dental procedure.
↓
P, Position the patient (supine with the legs elevated).
↓
ABC, Assess and perform basic life support, as needed.
↓
D, Initiate definitive care:
- Summon medical assistance.
- Administer epinephrine (SC, IM, IV).
- Administer oxygen.
- Monitor vital signs.
- Administer additional drugs: histamine blocker; corticosteroid.

Box 34-6 outlines the steps to take to manage generalized anaphylaxis.

Drugs used in management of generalized anaphylaxis include oxygen, epinephrine (intravenously, intramuscularly, or sublingually), a histamine blocker (intramuscularly), and a corticosteroid (intravenously or intramuscularly).

Medical assistance is required for generalized anaphylaxis.

No Signs of Allergy Present

A second clinical picture of anaphylaxis might be one in which the patient receiving a potential allergen loses consciousness without any obvious signs of allergy being observed. This picture is disturbing because, in the absence of obvious clinical signs and symptoms of allergy, drug management for anaphylaxis is not indicated.

Step 1: Terminate Dental Treatment

Step 2: P—Position the Patient. Management of this situation, which might prove to result from any of a number of causes, requires immediate positioning of the patient in the supine position with the legs elevated slightly.

Step 3: A—Airway, B—Breathing, C—Circulation; Basic Life Support, as Indicated. Victims of vasodepressor syncope or postural hypotension rapidly recover consciousness once they are properly positioned and airway patency is ensured. BLS (breathing and circulation) should be continued in patients who do not recover at this point.

Step 4: D—Definitive Care

Step 4a: Summon Medical Assistance. If consciousness does not return rapidly after the steps of BLS have been initiated, emergency medical assistance should be sought immediately.

Step 4b: Administer Oxygen

Step 4c: Monitor Vital Signs. Blood pressure, heart rate and rhythm, and respiratory rate should be monitored at least every 5 minutes, and the elements of BLS should be started at any time they are required.

Step 4d: Definitive Management. On arrival, emergency medical personnel will seek to diagnose the cause of the loss of consciousness. If this is possible, appropriate drug therapy will be instituted, the patient stabilized, and the patient then transferred to a local hospital emergency room.

In the absence of definitive signs and symptoms of allergy (e.g., edema, urticaria, bronchospasm), epinephrine and other drug therapies are usually not indicated. Any of a number of other situations may be the cause of the unconsciousness, for example, drug overdose, hypoglycemia, cerebrovascular accident, acute adrenal insufficiency, myocardial infarction (MI), or cardiopulmonary arrest.

Continuing to apply the required steps of BLS until emergency medical assistance arrives is the most rational management of this situation.

Box 34-7 outlines the steps to take to manage generalized anaphylaxis without obvious signs of allergy being present.

The only drug used in management of this syndrome is oxygen. Medical assistance is always required.

Laryngeal edema is yet another possible development during the generalized anaphylactic reaction. Should ventilation become difficult despite adequate head-tilt and a clear pharynx (obtained by suctioning), it may become necessary to perform a cricothyrotomy to obtain an airway. Laryngeal edema is a manifestation of allergy. Once a patent airway has been assured (cricothyrotomy), epinephrine (0.3 mg) may be administered, followed by a histamine blocker and corticosteroid as outlined previously. Once stabilized, the patient must be transferred to a hospital for definitive management and observation.

BOX 34-7 Management of Generalized Anaphylaxis

(No signs and symptoms of allergy present)
Terminate the dental procedure.

↓

P, Position the patient (supine with the legs elevated).

↓

ABC, Assess and perform basic life support, as needed.

↓

D, Initiate definitive care:

- Summon medical assistance.
- Administer oxygen.
- Monitor vital signs.
- Provide definitive management.

Overdose and allergy represent the most serious complications associated with drug administration for anesthesia and sedation. Other complications may also produce life-threatening situations. These include hypotension, cardiac dysrhythmias, respiratory depression, and laryngospasm. The latter two have been reviewed previously in the discussion of complications of IV sedation (see Chapter 27).

HYPOTENSION

Slight decreases in a patient's blood pressure during general anesthesia or conscious sedation are not unusual. Such decreases in blood pressure are usually minimal, especially during conscious sedation. More significant reductions in arterial blood pressure are clinically important because of the necessity to maintain adequate tissue perfusion. A systolic blood pressure of 90 mm Hg in an ASA I adult might not require treatment, whereas the same blood pressure in an elderly hypertensive patient might constitute a life-threatening situation. The need to treat hypotension is based on the ability of the circulation to adequately perfuse the tissues. Clinical signs and symptoms associated with hypotension and inadequate tissue perfusion are found in Box 34-8 and include the presence of chest pain, dyspnea, or a systolic blood pressure (adult) below 90 mm Hg.[17]

BOX 34-8 Signs and Symptoms Associated with Significant Hypotension

Chest pain	Restlessness
Dyspnea	Anxiety
Hypotension (systolic blood pressure <90 mm Hg)	Disorientation
Congestive heart failure	Pallor
Ischemia	Cold, clammy skin
Infarction	Dilated pupils
	Prolonged capillary refill time

In the child, hypotension is characterized by the following[18]:

- Infants from 1 month to 12 months: systolic blood pressure (SBP) <70 mm Hg
- Children older than 1 year to 10 years: SBP <70 mm Hg + (2 × age in years)
- Beyond 10 years: a SBP <90 mm Hg

Always consider the difficulty in assessing blood pressure accurately in the smaller child. Use of a blood pressure cuff that is too small (narrow) for the arm produces artificially elevated readings, whereas use of too large a cuff (e.g., an adult cuff on a small child) produces artificially decreased readings. See Chapter 4 for a description of the proper technique of recording blood pressure.

In the conscious hypotensive patient, cerebral ischemia occurs secondarily and is associated with restlessness, anxiety, and disorientation. Circulatory inadequacy is suggested by pallor, cold and clammy skin, and dilated pupils. The rate of capillary refill can be used as a gauge of peripheral perfusion. In hypotensive states capillary refill time is prolonged.

During sedative procedures hypotension can be diagnosed in one or more of several ways:

1. Monitoring of blood pressure throughout procedure
2. Observation of and communication with the patient
3. Observation of the operative field during surgical procedures in which bleeding is normal. (The doctor and assistant will notice that the surgical field is considerably "cleaner" than usual. This should lead to an immediate evaluation of the blood pressure.)

If a blood pressure cuff is not immediately available, a quick estimate of SBP may be obtained through palpation of peripheral pulses at the radial, brachial, and/or carotid arteries. For example, if a carotid pulse is palpated but the brachial is absent, the SBP is greater than 60 mm Hg but lower than 70 mm Hg.

Pulse Palpated	*Systolic Blood Pressure Is at Least*
Radial artery	80 mm Hg
Brachial artery	70 mm Hg
Carotid artery	60 mm Hg

Causes of Hypotension

Possible causes of hypotension include the following:

- Excessive premedication
- The action of therapeutic drugs taken before the sedative/anesthetic procedure by the patient for preexisting disease
- Overdose of sedatives/anesthetics
- Reflex (light anesthesia, pain)
- Vascular absorption of local anesthetics
- Hemorrhage
- Positional changes of patient
- Hypoxia and hypercarbia
- Abnormalities of circulatory system
- Adrenocortical insufficiency
- Metabolic derangement (i.e., hypoglycemia or hyperglycemia)

Excessive premedication or the administration of a relative overdose to a "sensitive" patient may provoke hypotension. Following oral CNS depressant drug administration, this is unlikely to occur; however, hypotension has been documented after IM administration, especially of an opioid agonist. Opioids produce this effect through their depressant actions on the vasomotor center, reducing muscle tone, decreasing ventilation, and dilating peripheral blood vessels.

The influence of other *therapeutic drugs* being taken by the patient to manage preexisting disorders might result in hypotension. Drugs such as corticosteroids, antihypertensives, and tranquilizers such as chlorpromazine may produce hypotension.

Overdose of sedatives/anesthetics is unlikely to develop when these drugs are administered carefully via routes in which titration is available and is used. These include the inhalation and IV routes of administration. When these drugs are administered intramuscularly, intranasally, or submucosally, however, there is a greater likelihood of overdose and hypotension because of the lack of control over the drugs' ultimate effect. In addition, opioids are the drugs most often administered in these techniques, drugs that are more likely to produce hypotension if administered to excess. Conversely, *anesthesia that is too light or the presence of pain* is capable of reflexly inducing hypotension.

Vascular absorption of local anesthetics is another potential cause of hypotension. Many causes for local anesthetic overdose and hypotension exist, including overadministration (relative or absolute), intravascular administration, rapid absorption, slow elimination, or slow biotransformation. The primary means of preventing hypotension and overdose from local anesthetics are aspiration before every injection and slow administration of the smallest volume of solution that will provide adequate pain control. The reader is referred to other texts for a more in-depth description of local anesthetic overdose.[19]

Hemorrhage is unlikely to be severe enough during a dental procedure to produce a drop in blood pressure. However, this is not an uncommon cause of hypotension within the hospital during major surgical procedures.

Positional changes of the patient are more likely to produce postural or orthostatic hypotension, particularly in elderly patients, patients receiving certain drugs (Box 34-9), and those who have received CNS depressant drugs, particularly opioids.

Positional changes of the dental chair or the patient standing up from the chair should be accomplished gradually to permit the cardiovascular system to adapt to the increased effect of gravity as the patient becomes more upright. It has been mentioned throughout this book that the recommended position of the patient during procedures in which CNS depressants have been administered is supine with the legs elevated slightly or a semisupine position. The upright (erect) position should be avoided during treatment unless absolutely essential.

Hypoxia and *hypercarbia* are additional possible causes of hypotension. Adequate management of the patient's airway during deep sedation or general anesthesia is of critical importance.

Cardiovascular abnormalities are another possible cause of hypotension during sedative or anesthetic procedures. The occurrence of myocardial ischemia or infarction may result in a profound drop in blood pressure. In the conscious, albeit sedated, patient other clinical signs and symptoms would usually be available (e.g., pain radiating in a classic pattern, nausea, dusky appearance, cyanosis of mucous membranes) that would aid in diagnosis; however, in the unconscious patient such a diagnosis would be more difficult to establish. Other cardiovascular causes of hypotension, all of which are extremely unlikely to develop in the outpatient setting on ASA I or II patients, include embolism to the brain (cerebrovascular accident [CVA]) or lungs (pulmonary embolism), hypovolemia caused by the patient's poor physical condition before the start of the procedure (unlikely to be observed in the ambulatory outpatient setting), heart failure, and anaphylactic shock.

BOX 34-9 Drugs and Drug Categories Producing Postural Hypotension

Category
Adrenergic neuron blockers
α- and β-adrenergic blockers
Amiodarone
Angiotensin-converting enzyme inhibitors
Centrally acting antihypertensives
Calcium channel blockers
Diuretics
Ganglionic blockers
Levodopa
Vasodilators

Adrenocortical insufficiency may produce hypotension and shock. When a patient has received exogenous corticosteroid therapy in the recent past (the rule of twos, see Chapter 4), prophylactic corticosteroid administration before the start of any traumatic procedure is strongly recommended.

Metabolic derangements such as hyperglycemia (and ketoacidosis) or hypoglycemia are other possible causes of hypotension that should be considered. A history of diabetes mellitus in a hypotensive patient would provide an indication that this is a possible cause for the hypotension. Hypoglycemia is much more likely to be noted than hyperglycemia in the diabetic patient who is still conscious.

Management of Hypotension

Treatment of hypotension is directed to its cause. However, there are certain basic steps that must be carried out when hypotension occurs.

Step 1: P—Position the Patient. The procedure is terminated, and the patient is placed into the supine position with the feet elevated to increase blood flow to the brain and aid in return of venous blood from the legs.

Step 2: A—Airway, B—Breathing, C—Circulation; Basic Life Support, as Indicated. The patient will likely be attempting to breathe spontaneously, although the airway may or may not be patent. The pulse will be weak and probably rapid (tachycardia often accompanies hypotension). Blood pressure will be decreased from the patient's baseline values. O_2 may be administered to the patient at any time during management.

Step 3: D—Definitive Care

Step 3a. If an inhalation anesthetic such as N_2O (or any other gaseous agent) is being administered, its concentration is decreased. This step alone usually leads to an increase in blood pressure. Although the patient is receiving a concentration of N_2O that is within normal limits, a relative overdose of the drug may be administered if the patient is unusually sensitive to its actions.

If *barbiturates* have been administered intramuscularly or intravenously, general supportive measures (BLS) must be continued until the patient improves because no effective antagonistic drug for the barbiturates exists.

If *opioids* or a *benzodiazepine* has been administered, the appropriate antagonist (naloxone or flumazenil) may be administered intravenously or intramuscularly. Although the primary effect of naloxone is to improve respiratory depression induced by the opioids, a slight elevation in blood pressure may also be observed because the analgesic actions of the opioid also decrease and the patient begins to respond to painful stimuli if local anesthesia is absent.

Step 3b: Administer Fluids. When hypotension develops during an IV sedation procedure or if an IV infusion can be started, a relatively effective and safe means of managing hypotension is available, especially in the ASA I or II patient. The rapid IV infusion of solution (5% dextrose and water, physiologic saline, or lactated Ringer's solution) will provide extra fluid volume to the cardiovascular system and thereby increase the blood pressure. The 250-ml bag of solution should be opened and permitted to flow rapidly until it is observed that the blood pressure has increased. Mild decreases in systemic blood pressure may usually be reversed in this simple manner.

Step 3c: Administer Vasopressors. The administration of vasopressors is reserved for hypotension that is more severe and that persists after these preceding measures have been undertaken. A number of vasopressors are available. It was recommended in Chapter 33 that methoxamine or mephentermine be available in the emergency drug kit. Methoxamine exerts its effect by stimulating α-receptors, producing constriction in vascular smooth muscle in the skin, mucosa, kidney, and splanchnic region. *Methoxamine* has little or no direct effect on β-receptors that increase the workload of the heart. A reflex bradycardia may develop with methoxamine administration. Mephentermine increases blood pressure by enhancing cardiac contraction but does not increase peripheral resistance. Mephentermine is usually safe and effective for the management of unexplained hypotension during local or general anesthesia and sedation. In the absence of greater knowledge of the status of the patient's cardiovascular system and heart, the administration of other drugs (Table 34-5) with β actions or mixed α and β actions is not recommended.

Most vasopressors stimulate both α- and β-receptors, but the degree of stimulation by each drug varies. Table 34-5 summarizes clinical actions of the more commonly used vasopressors, and Box 34-10 lists the actions of the various receptors. Other vasopressors may be used in place of methoxamine, provided the doctor is knowledgeable of the pharmacology, indications, contraindications, precautions, adverse reactions, and recommended dosage of the drug. Methoxamine, in a dose of 5 to 10 mg intramuscularly or 2 to 5 mg intravenously, or mephentermine, 15 to 30 mg, is suggested. An IM dose is suggested; the IV route is reserved for emergency situations in which a more immediate response is required. The onset of activity is 15 minutes after IM administration and 2 to 3 minutes after IV administration. Duration of action is approximately 30 to 60 minutes (with the IV route). Box 34-11 outlines the steps to take to manage hypotension.

Hypotension in Patients Receiving Corticosteroid Therapy

Patients receiving corticosteroids or those having recently completed a prolonged course of steroid ther-

TABLE 34-5 Vasopressors: Summary of Actions on Receptors

				Usual Dose	
Agent	α	β_1	β_2	IV	IM
Epinephrine (most potent agent to α-receptor)	+	+	+	0.1 mg	0.2-0.3 mg
Norepinephrine bitartrate	+	+	+	Used as continuous IV drip	Not recommended IM
Isoproterenol	–	+	+	0.025 μg/kg/min IV drip	Not recommended IM
Phenylephrine	+	–	–	0.25-0.5 mg	2-3 mg
Mephentermine	+	+	+	5-15 mg	10-30 mg
Ephedrine	+	+	+	10-25 mg followed by IM dose	25-50 mg
Metaraminol	+	+	–	0.5-2 mg	2-5 mg
Methoxamine	+	–	–	2-5 mg	5-10 mg
Dopamine	–	+	–	Via continuous IV infusion (200 mg in 250 or 500 ml 5% dextrose and water)	
Propranolol		+	+	0.5-1 mg up to maximum of 2 mg IV	

BOX 34-10 Actions of α- and β-Receptors

α-Receptors
Peripheral vasoconstriction: skins, mucosa, intestine, kidney
Mydriasis
Myometrial contraction

β-Receptors
β-Receptors are subdivided into two groups: β_1- and β_2-receptors. Stimulation of these receptors produces the following reactions:
β_1-Receptors
Bronchodilation
Tachycardia
Palpitation
Hypertension
Insomnia
Tremor
Increased cardiac contractility
β_2-Receptors
Bronchodilation
Vasodilation

apy are more likely to develop hypotensive episodes during surgery and anesthesia. This is because of their inability to release adequate amounts of endogenous steroids into the circulation in response to the stress of surgery, leading to acute adrenal insufficiency. Preoperative administration of steroids (in consultation with the patient's physician) minimizes this risk. When hypotensive episodes develop during treatment, large IV doses of corticosteroids and vasopressors are required to prevent morbidity or death.

Hypotension in Patients Receiving β-Blockers

Patients receiving long-term β-blocker treatment are unable to respond to exercise with an elevation in their heart rate. When hypotension develops in these patients, management consists of the following[2]:

1. *Isoproterenol* (Isuprel), administered slowly intravenously at a rate of 0.2 mg at 1-minute intervals. The dose is determined by the patient's response. In the presence of total β-blockade, a large dose of isoproterenol may be required.
2. When the hypotensive episode persists despite isoproterenol administration, IV *glucagon* is administered.
3. *Atropine* (0.5 to 1.0 mg) is administered intravenously wherever severe bradycardia is present.

BOX 34-11 Management of Hypotension

Terminate the dental procedure,

P, Position the patient (supine with the legs elevated).

ABC, Assess and perform basic life support, as needed.
↓
D, Initiate definitive care.

Observe for possible cause of hypotension and manage as necessary:
- Decrease concentration of inhalation anesthetics.
- Reverse opioid actions with naloxone.
- Reverse benzodiazepine actions with flumazenil.
- If patient is diabetic, consider hypoglycemia and manage appropriately.
- Monitor and seek signs and symptoms of cardiovascular system involvement (e.g., angina, myocardial infarction).
- Determine history of recent corticosteroid therapy: IV administration of corticosteroids.

In absence of above, or continued hypotension:
- If IV route is available, administer IV infusate rapidly (up to 500 ml in ASA I, 250 ml in ASA II).
- If IV route is not available, or if hypotension is refractory to preceding steps, administer IM or IV vasopressor.

Summon medical assistance, as needed.

Administer oxygen.
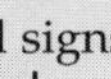
Monitor vital signs.
↓
Permit recovery and discharge the patient.

HYPERTENSIVE EPISODES

Elevations of blood pressure may be noted during surgical and dental procedures if the level of pain or anxiety control is inadequate. Transient elevations in blood pressure may be prevented through the administration (or readministration) of local anesthesia. Transient minor elevations in blood pressure (hypertensive urgencies) are usually well tolerated and of little danger to the patient. Sustained and/or significant elevations in blood pressure (hypertensive emergencies or crises) must be treated aggressively. Guidelines for the evaluation of blood pressure in both adult and pediatric patients were presented in Chapter 4.

Causes of episodes of high blood pressure during dental treatment, surgery, and anesthesia (sedation, general anesthesia) include the following[2]:

1. Light anesthesia or sedation
2. Pain
3. Hypercarbia
4. Hypoxia
5. Emergence delirium
6. Fluid overload (overhydration)
7. Hyperthermia

The most common causes of hypertension during dental procedures, surgery, and anesthesia are light anesthesia or sedation and the presence of pain. Management is directed at providing adequate sedation, anesthesia, and pain control. Blood pressure returns toward baseline levels as the quality of anesthesia improves.

Hypercarbia and hypoxia are the next most common causes of elevated blood pressure. Catecholamine release is increased with both hypercarbia and hypoxia. Airway management and ventilation reverse this cause of blood pressure elevation.

Postoperatively, pain, hypercarbia, and emergence delirium are common causes of elevated blood pressure. Strict management of the airway and O_2 administration preclude hypoxia and hypercarbia. Physostigmine administration terminates episodes of emergence delirium, and the use of local anesthesia or the administration of opioids or nonsteroidal antiinflammatory drugs (NSAIDs) helps manage posttreatment pain.

Fluid overload is an uncommon cause of high blood pressure in the dental outpatient, especially when the 250-ml bag of IV infusate is used. ASA III and IV patients with congestive heart failure (CHF) may be at risk for acute pulmonary edema when larger volumes of IV fluids are received.

Hyperthermia is associated with increased metabolic rates, increased heart rate, and increased blood pressure. Temperature should be recorded before conscious sedation when there is an indication that infection may be present or if the patient appears warm or flushed. Temperature should be recorded preoperatively and intraoperatively whenever general anesthesia is administered.

Management of a Hypertensive Crisis

A hypertensive crisis is said to exist when the SBP is 250 mm Hg or greater and/or the diastolic blood pressure (DBP) is 130 mm Hg or greater.[20] Hypertensive crises are most likely to occur in patients with chronic, stable hypertension. The goal in management is to avoid rapid changes in blood pressure without compromising cerebral perfusion.[21] To this end, antihypertensive therapy is not recommended in any patient unless there is severe hypertension (>200/130 mm Hg).[22] Hypertensive crisis must be distinguished from a modest and transient elevation in blood pressure from causes previously listed. Deepening of the anesthesia or eliminating pain through the readministration of local anesthetics will often bring with it a return of the elevated blood pressure toward baseline values. However, when elevated blood pressure does not return to acceptable levels within a few minutes of onset, or if it continues to increase, the possibility of a hypertensive crisis must be considered and steps initiated to manage it.

Among the possible acute causes of the hypertensive crisis are cardiovascular complications, such as MI and dissecting aortic aneurysm; recreational drug use (e.g., cocaine); monoamine oxidase inhibitor use; pheochromocytoma; and thyroid crisis.[21] It is important when evaluating the hypertensive crisis to distinguish whether the cause is cardiac or noncardiac.[2] When significant elevation is noted in the patient's blood pressure, proceed as follows.

Step 1: Terminate Dental Treatment and P—Position the Patient. Position the patient in an upright position (45 degrees or more upright).

Step 2: Assess A—Airway, B—Breathing, C—Circulation; Basic Life Support, as Indicated. Airway, breathing, and circulation are usually adequate.

Step 3: D—Definitive Care

Step 3a: Monitor Blood Pressure and Heart Rate and Rhythm Every 5 Minutes and Administer Oxygen.

Step 3b: Administer Fluids. Emergency medical personnel should be summoned.

Step 3c: Establish an IV infusion, if Not Already Present. Where the cause of the hypertensive crisis is cardiac, such as CHF, proceed as follows.

Step 3d: Titrate. Titrate nitroprusside (Nipride) at an infusion rate of 5 *mg*/kg/min until the blood pressure is lowered to a desired point. The average therapeutic range is between 0.5 and 10 μg/kg/min.

Where ischemic heart disease (MI) or CHF is present, proceed as follows:

Step 3d: IV Nitroglycerin, a Drug Similar to Nitroprusside, Is Administered as a 50-μg Bolus, Followed by an Infusion of 10 to 20 μg/min. The infusion may be increased 5 to 10 μg/min until the desired blood pressure response is noted.[2,21] When a noncardiac cause of the hypertensive crisis is present (e.g., anxiety, allergy, CVA), proceed as follows:

Step 3d: IV Diazoxide (Hyperstat) Should Be Administered in Doses of 1 to 3 mg/kg up to 150 mg. This dose may be repeated every 5 to 10 minutes up to 600 mg.

Step 4. When anxiety is a major component of the hypertensive crisis, midazolam or diazepam, titrated

TABLE 34-6 Parenteral Drugs Used in the Treatment of Hypertensive Crisis

Drug	Administration	Onset	Duration	Dosage	Side Effects
Sodium nitroprusside	IV fusion	Immediate	2-3 min	0.5-10 μg/kg/min	Hypotension, nausea, vomiting, apprehension
Diazoxide	IV bolus	q5-10min, up to 600 mg	1-5 min	6-12 hr 50-100 mg	Hypotension, tachycardia, nausea, vomiting, fluid retention; exacerbates myocardiac ischemia, heart failure, or aortic dissection
Nitroglycerin	IV infusion	1-2 min	3-5 min	5-100 μg/min	Headache, nausea, vomiting

IV, may be of some utility in managing the hypertension. Table 34-6 summarizes the drugs employed in management of the hypertensive crisis.

There may arise situations in which an IV infusion cannot be started and/or the appropriate parenteral antihypertensive drugs are not available for administration. In such instances the following regimen is suggested.

Step 1: Terminate Dental Treatment and P—Position the Patient. Position the patient in an upright position (45 degrees or more upright).

Step 2: Assess A—Airway, B—Breathing, C—Circulation; Basic Life Support, as Indicated. Airway, breathing, and circulation are usually adequate.

Step 3: D—Definitive Care

Step 3a. Monitor blood pressure and heart rate and rhythm every 5 minutes and administer oxygen.

Step 3b. Oxygen should be administered.

Step 3c. Emergency medical personnel should be summoned.

Step 3d. Sublingual nitroglycerin tablets (2 tablets of 0.4 mg) or two doses of Nitrolingual spray should be administered (spray medication onto the mucous membrane of the tongue). This dose may be repeated every 5 to 10 minutes if necessary.

Step 3e. On arrival of emergency medical assistance, an IV infusion will be established and appropriate antihypertensive drugs administered. The patient usually requires a period of hospitalization to ensure stabilization of the blood pressure.

CARDIAC DYSRHYTHMIAS

A dysrhythmia is any deviation from the normal sinus rhythm. It was reported as the most common intraoperative complication, occurring in 112,721 patients studied.[23] The incidence of perioperative dysrhythmias under general anesthesia has been reported by different sources to be from 4% to 60%.[24,25] Driscoll et al. have reported the incidence of dysrhythmias during extraction of erupted bicuspids in patients receiving local anesthesia and sedation to be 24.19%.[26]

Fortunately, the majority of dysrhythmias encountered during sedative and general anesthetic procedures rarely require drug intervention. Indeed, if bradycardia (<60 beats per minute) and tachycardia (>100 beats per minute) are discounted, the incidence of dysrhythmias requiring drug treatment is exceedingly low. However, the presence of a cardiac dysrhythmia can be a warning that some physiologic or pharmacologic problem exists that does require immediate management. DeRango[27] makes some generalizations about the incidence of cardiac dysrhythmias:

1. The majority of anesthetized patients who are continuously monitored (ECG) will demonstrate some dysrhythmia during the anesthetic period.
2. The incidence of dysrhythmias is higher in patients with a history of heart disease than in those without such a history.
3. The incidence of dysrhythmias is higher in patients whose tracheas are intubated.
4. The incidence of dysrhythmias is more frequent in patients undergoing surgery lasting more than 3 hours than in patients undergoing shorter procedures.
5. Patients receiving digitalis preoperatively have a higher incidence of dysrhythmias than patients not receiving digitalis.

From a review of the preceding information it appears that the incidence of cardiac dysrhythmias during outpatient procedures in ASA I or II patients should be considerably lower than that for in-hospital procedures. The very nature of the patient (healthier) and the type of procedure (shorter duration, trachea rarely intubated) are reasons for a decreased incidence of clinically significant dysrhythmias during outpatient procedures.

Precipitating Factors

Dysrhythmias may be produced in patients receiving anesthesia and sedation by the following means:

1. Anesthetic agents
2. Carbon dioxide (CO_2)
3. Stimulation under light planes of anesthesia
4. Vagal responses
5. Intubation
6. Anoxia
7. Duration of the procedure

Anesthetic agents may provoke dysrhythmias. Among commonly used inhalation anesthetics, halothane is associated with a greater incidence of dysrhythmias than enflurane, isoflurane, desflurane, and sevoflurane.

CO_2 retention (hypercarbia) is a common cause of dysrhythmias during anesthesia and sedation. The mechanism of dysrhythmia generation is the release of catecholamines by the increasing CO_2 tension in the blood. Many anesthetic drugs sensitize the myocardium to the effects of these catecholamines, and dysrhythmias are the result.

Stimulation of the patient during a procedure while the patient is under general anesthesia or sedation is a common cause of dysrhythmias. Stimulation (i.e., pain) leads to vagal and sympathetic responses that are ultimately responsible for most dysrhythmias. Management consists of either deepening the level of general anesthesia or sedation (to decrease patient response to stimulation) or providing more adequate pain control (local anesthesia).

Vagal responses produce a slowing of the sinus rate, which can lead to dysrhythmias such as sinus bradycardia, sinus arrest, junctional rhythms, and most frequently, premature ventricular contractions (PVCs). Vagal responses are much more likely to develop during general anesthesia than during sedative procedures. Most often, these responses occur in response to nondental surgical stimulation such as traction on intraabdominal structures, traction on extraocular muscles, pressure on the globe, and carotid sinus stimulation.

Tracheal intubation is probably responsible for the greatest incidence of dysrhythmias during general anesthesia, especially when the patient is in a light plane of anesthesia. Most often, the dysrhythmias seen are tachydysrhythmias associated with elevations in blood pressure. These tachydysrhythmias are normally transient and require no drug therapy. Management consists of adequate ventilation and a deepening of the level of anesthesia.

Anoxia or *severe hypoxia* during general anesthesia or sedation is another cause of dysrhythmias. Anoxia is associated with the development of hypercarbia (see previous discussion). Management consists of adequate ventilation.

The *duration of surgery* or of the procedure is related to the incidence of dysrhythmias. The incidence of dysrhythmias occurring during procedures that last less than 3 hours is considerably lower than that during procedures requiring more than 3 hours to complete. The body's ability to handle stress is compromised as the procedure lengthens. Increased levels of catecholamines appear in the blood, and dysrhythmias result.

Dysrhythmias are significant because they may indicate dysfunction of the myocardial conduction system, which, if the dysrhythmia is severe, may lead to cerebral, myocardial, or renal ischemia; CHF and pulmonary edema; MI; or ventricular fibrillation.

Again, the overwhelming majority of dysrhythmias occurring during general anesthesia and, especially during sedative procedures, are transient in nature and relatively benign, requiring no formal drug management. Management usually consists of ensuring adequate ventilation, increasing or decreasing (as appropriate) the level of anesthesia or sedation, and providing adequate pain control.

Continuous ECG monitoring of the patient receiving general anesthesia is required; however, the routine use of the ECG during sedative procedures is not necessary, although if available it should be employed in patients with a history of cardiovascular disease.

Dysrhythmias may be detected through the use of a pulse oximeter or other pulse-monitoring device, or more simply by keeping a finger on the patient's pulse. See Chapter 4 for a review of common dysrhythmias; advanced cardiac life support textbooks should be consulted for in-depth discussion of the significance and management of cardiac dysrhythmias.[2,28]

ANGINA PECTORIS

Stable angina pectoris is a characteristic thoracic pain, usually substernal, precipitated chiefly by exercise, emotion, or a heavy meal; relieved by vasodilator drugs and a few minutes of rest; and a result of a mild inadequacy of the coronary circulation.[5] Several anginal syndromes are identified, including stable angina (ASA III), vasospastic angina (coronary artery spasm, atypical angina, variant angina, Prinzmetal's angina: ASA III), and unstable angina (preinfarction or crescendo angina, intermediate coronary syndrome, and impending MI: ASA IV). Drugs used for the management of acute anginal episodes include nitroglycerin (sublingual tablets, translingual spray, or transdermal patch), which is used for the management of stable and vasospastic angina. Calcium channel blockers (nifedipine, diltiazem, and verapamil) are effective in managing the vasospastic component of angina.

Signs and Symptoms

The "pain" of angina is rarely described as such by the patient. More frequently, an acute anginal episode is described as a "tightness," "constricting feeling," or a "heavy weight" on the chest. The patient usually stops whatever he or she is doing and seeks relief by sitting upright and taking nitroglycerin. A typical anginal episode lasts but minutes with drug therapy but may persist for up to an hour. Chest pain of long duration, however, is more likely to lead to a presumptive diagnosis of MI than angina. Additional signs and symptoms associated with angina include palpitation, faintness, dizziness, dyspnea, and "indigestion."

It is important to note that *the pain of angina is quickly relieved by nitroglycerin administration and that it does not return.* Box 34-12 outlines the steps to take to manage chest pain with history of angina pectoris.

MYOCARDIAL INFARCTION

Prolonged ischemia of the myocardium produced by partial or complete occlusion of blood flow through one or more coronary arteries leads to necrosis of heart muscle. Severe chest pain and dysrhythmias commonly occur during MI. Cessation of effective cardiac function may occur, producing cardiac arrest and necessitating the immediate institution of BLS.

Signs and Symptoms

MI often mimics angina at its onset. One striking difference (in the nondental setting) is that 51% of patients are *at rest* when MI occurs, whereas angina is associated with an increase in myocardial activity.[29]

Patients experience a more severe and more prolonged pain that, although it may seem anginal at onset, progressively increases in severity. The patient is quite apprehensive and may exhibit weakness, diaphoresis, hypotension, and dysrhythmias. Dysrhythmias develop in 95% of MIs and increase the rate of morbidity and mortality associated with MI.[30] Hypotension is noted in 80% of patients with MI.[31]

Management

Management of MI progresses from that described for angina. Box 34-13 outlines the steps to take to manage chest pain.

AIRWAY OBSTRUCTION

The most common cause of airway obstruction during sedation or general anesthesia is posterior displacement of the tongue into the pharynx as muscle tonus is lost as a result of CNS depression produced by the administered drugs. The presence of a foreign object in the airway, such as a crown or tooth that becomes

BOX 34-12 Management of Chest Pain with History of Angina Pectoris

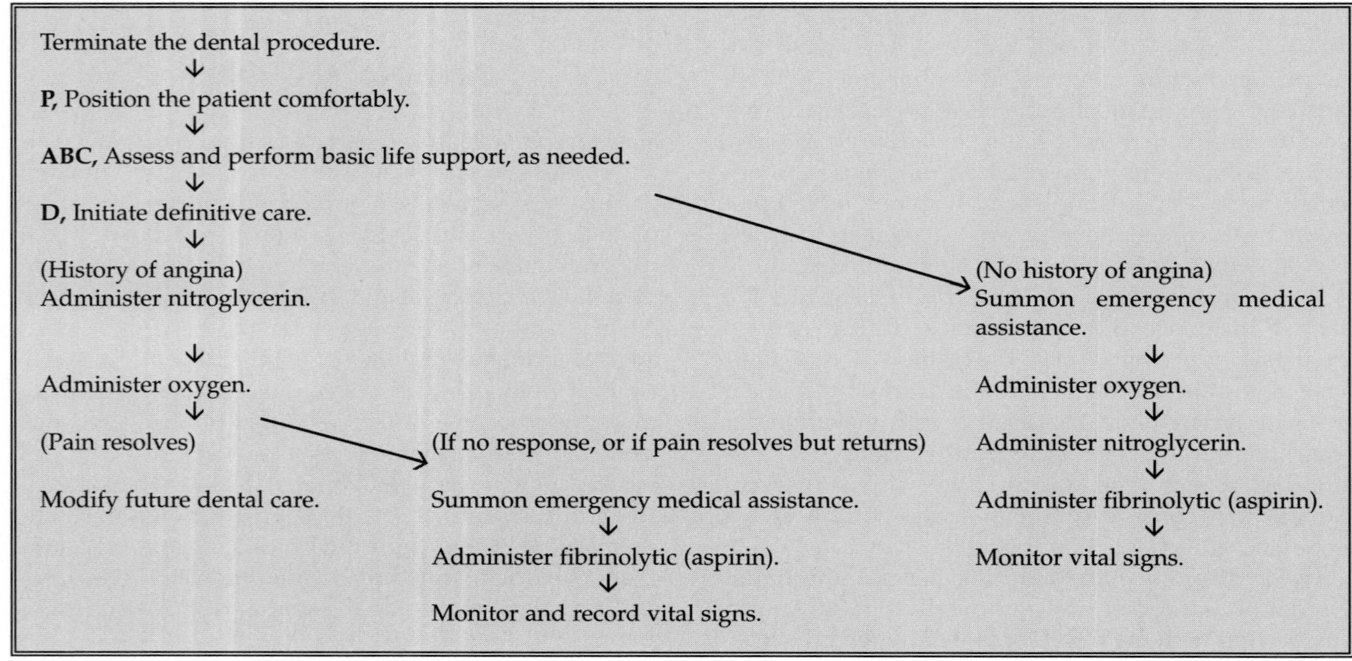

Terminate the dental procedure.
P, Position the patient comfortably.
ABC, Assess and perform basic life support, as needed.
D, Initiate definitive care.
(History of angina)
Administer nitroglycerin.
Administer oxygen.
(Pain resolves)
Modify future dental care.
(If no response, or if pain resolves but returns)
Summon emergency medical assistance.
Administer fibrinolytic (aspirin).
Monitor and record vital signs.
(No history of angina)
Summon emergency medical assistance.
Administer oxygen.
Administer nitroglycerin.
Administer fibrinolytic (aspirin).
Monitor vital signs.

BOX 34-13 Management of Chest Pain

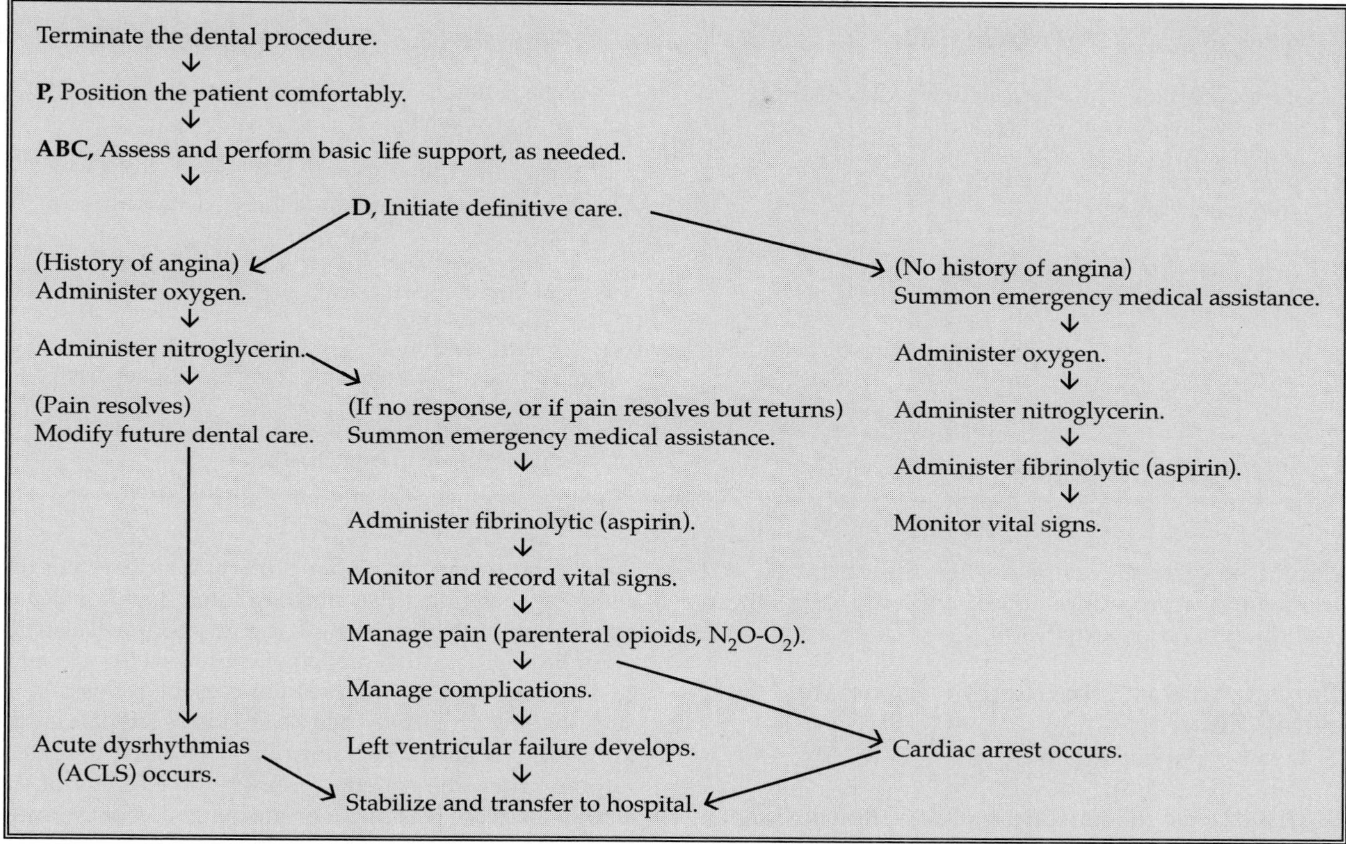
Terminate the dental procedure.
P, Position the patient comfortably.
ABC, Assess and perform basic life support, as needed.
D, Initiate definitive care.
(History of angina)
Administer oxygen.
Administer nitroglycerin.
(Pain resolves)
Modify future dental care.
(If no response, or if pain resolves but returns)
Summon emergency medical assistance.
Administer fibrinolytic (aspirin).
Monitor and record vital signs.
Manage pain (parenteral opioids, N_2O-O_2).
Manage complications.
Left ventricular failure develops.
Stabilize and transfer to hospital.
Acute dysrhythmias
(ACLS) occurs.
(No history of angina)
Summon emergency medical assistance.
Administer oxygen.
Administer nitroglycerin.
Administer fibrinolytic (aspirin).
Monitor vital signs.
Cardiac arrest occurs.

displaced, is a second possible cause of airway obstruction, although these often do not produce total obstruction but rather a partial airway obstruction. Fluids (blood, saliva, water, and vomitus) may also produce airway obstruction.

Partial or complete airway obstruction may occur. Distinctive sounds are associated with airway obstruction produced by various causes. These sounds must be detected, diagnosed, and managed as expeditiously as possible. Use of the pretracheal stethoscope during parenteral conscious or deep sedation and general anesthesia allows for instantaneous detection of airway problems.

Normal, unobstructed airflow through the mouth and nose has a very distinctive low whooshing sound. Movement of the chest during respiration is minimal and looks "smooth." Soft tissue retraction is not present. *Complete obstruction* of the airway is associated with the absence of sound. If the patient is attempting spontaneous ventilation, the observed respiratory movements appear exaggerated, with evident supraclavicular and intercostal soft tissue retraction. The use of abdominal muscles during respiration will also be evident. *Partial airway obstruction resulting from the tongue* being displaced posteriorly is associated with a snoring sound that often can be heard by all persons in the treatment room. The presence of *fluid in the airway* is detected by a gurgling or bubbling sound. One other sound that is heard is wheezing, which results from a partial obstruction of the lower airway caused by *bronchospasm.* Mild bronchospasm is associated with loud wheezing, whereas in more severe bronchospasm, in which little air is being exchanged, wheezing may be absent. Table 34-7 summarizes the sounds associated with breathing and their management.

Management

The doctor should proceed with each of the following steps until a patent airway is obtained, as will be noted by the return of sounds associated with spontaneous breathing. Box 34-14 lists the recommended sequences for removing airway obstruction.

Cricothyrotomy. When the preceding steps have failed to reestablish a patent airway, it may be necessary to perform a cricothyrotomy. Cricothyrotomy

TABLE 34-7 Breathing Sounds and Their Management

Sound	Probable Cause	Management
Quiet whooshing	Normal, unobstructed airway	None required
None/no respiratory efforts	Apnea	Controlled ventilation
None/exaggerated respiratory efforts	Complete obstruction	1. Head-tilt/chin-lift 2. Anterior displacement of tongue with hemostat or gauze 3. Pharyngeal suctioning 4. Abdominal thrusts 5. Cricothyrotomy
Snoring	Soft tissue (tongue) displaced in pharynx	1. Head-tilt/chin-lift 2. Anterior displacement of tongue with hemostat or gauze
Gurgling	Fluid in airway	Pharyngeal suction
Wheezing	Bronchospasm	Administration of bronchodilator

should be carried out only when the doctor is well trained in the procedure. Cricothyrotomy technique is described in other texts.[19]

Partial Airway Obstruction Associated with "Snoring"

1. Position patient supine.
2. Perform head-tilt/chin-lift.
3. Displace the tongue. Physically displace the tongue anteriorly by grabbing it with a hemostat or gauze sponge.

Partial Airway Obstruction Associated with "Gurgling"

1. Position the patient in the supine position.
2. Perform head-tilt/chin-lift.
3. Suction the airway. Using a tonsillar suction tip, suction the posterior pharynx until all fluids are removed.

Partial Airway Obstruction Associated with "Wheezing." The management of wheezing is discussed in the earlier section on respiratory allergic reactions. Administration of a bronchodilator is indicated.

LARYNGOSPASM

Laryngospasm is a protective reflex that functions to maintain the integrity of the airway by preventing foreign matter from entering into the larynx, trachea, and lungs. Laryngospasm is considered a complication associated with deep sedation and ultralight general anesthesia, not an emergency.[2]

Laryngospasm is extraordinarily uncommon during conscious sedation. By definition, in conscious sedation the patient retains his or her protective airway reflexes: coughing, gagging, or swallowing foreign matter to prevent its entry into the airway. Laryngospasm will also not occur during stage III (Guedel) of anesthesia (see Chapter 2). The degree of CNS depression present at this time is such that the protective reflexes are lost. Materials entering into the airway in stage III will not provoke a response from the patient. Ensuring the integrity of the airway therefore becomes a prime obligation of the anesthesiologist during general anesthesia.

Laryngospasm may be partial or complete. Partial laryngospasm is associated with a high-pitched crowing sound (stridor) and increased difficulty in ventilation, whereas a complete laryngospasm is associated with an (ominous) absence of sound in the presence of exaggerated respiratory efforts and soft tissue retraction in the supraclavicular and intercostal regions.

Management

On recognition of laryngospasm, the following steps should be taken.

Step 1: Position the Patient Supine

Step 2: Administer Oxygen. Administer 100% O_2 via a nasal hood. In most instances the patient will have already been receiving N_2O-O_2 during treatment. The doctor should simply terminate the flow of N_2O and increase the O_2 flow to about 5 to 8 L/min.

Step 3: Displace the Tongue. The doctor physically displaces the tongue anteriorly by grabbing it with a hemostat or gauze sponge.

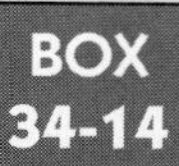

BOX 34-14 Recommended Sequences for Removing Airway Obstruction

For Adult Conscious Victim with Obstructed Airway
Identify complete airway obstruction: Ask, "Are you choking?"
↓
Identify yourself as someone who will help the victim: Say, "I can help you."
↓
Apply the Heimlich maneuver until foreign body is expelled or the victim becomes unconscious.
↓
Have medical or paramedical personnel evaluate the patient for complications before discharge.

For Adult Conscious Victim with Known Obstructed Airway Who Loses Consciousness
Place the victim in supine position with the head in a neutral position; call for help.
↓
Activate the EMS system (i.e., call 911) if a second person is available.
↓
Open the victim's mouth using tongue-jaw lift.
↓
Perform a finger sweep.
↓
Attempt to ventilate the patient; if ineffective:
↓
Perform 6 to 10 abdominal thrusts.
↓
Check for foreign body with finger sweep.
↓
Attempt to ventilate the patient; if ineffective:
↓
Repeat abdominal thrusts, finger sweeps, and attempted ventilations until effective.
↓
Have medical or paramedical personnel evaluate the patient for complications before dismissal.

For Adult Unconscious Victim, Cause Unknown
Rescuer manages unconscious victim in the usual manner.
Assess unresponsiveness.
↓
P, Position the victim in the supine position with the feet elevated.
↓
Call for help (office emergency team).
↓
A, Open the airway (head-tilt/chin-lift).
↓
B, Assess breathing (look, listen, feel)
↓
Attempt to ventilate. If unsuccessful:
↓
Activate EMS system (call 911).
↓
Perform Heimlich maneuver; 6 to 10 abdominal thrusts.
↓
Perform foreign body check: finger sweep.
↓
Attempt to ventilate; if ineffective:
↓
Repeat Heimlich maneuver, finger sweeps, and ventilation until successful.

EMS, Emergency medical services.

Step 4: Evaluate the Airway. All materials must be quickly removed from the patient's mouth. If bleeding is noted, the area should be packed with surgical gauze to prevent bleeding into the pharynx at this time. Using a tonsillar suction tip, the doctor completely and rapidly suction the oral cavity and posterior pharynx to remove any foreign matter.

Step 5: Reevaluate the Airway. Keeping an ear close to the patient's mouth and nose, the doctor pushes down on the patient's chest. If a rush of air is heard and felt, the spasm has been broken and the airway is patent. If no air is heard or felt, proceed to step 6. Oxygen saturation of the blood will decrease significantly, triggering the alarm on the pulse oximeter.

Step 6: Positive-Pressure Oxygen. Positive-pressure O_2 is administered in an effort to mechanically break the laryngospasm by physically forcing oxygen through the vocal cords. The absolute importance of effective suctioning before this step is evident as foreign material may be forced into the trachea by the positive-pressure oxygen flow.

Step 7: Administer a Muscle Relaxant. If the preceding steps are unsuccessful, succinylcholine administration is required. Succinylcholine should be administered only by doctors who have received prior training in its administration and who are able to manage the patient after its administration. An initial succinylcholine dose of 10 mg intravenously is recommended for the partial or incomplete laryngospasm, with a dose of 20 to 40 mg recommended for complete spasm or spasm that continues after the initial 10-mg dose is administered.

Step 8: Assess Ventilation and Control Ventilation, if Necessary. Following succinylcholine administration, apnea may be present for up to 4 minutes. Controlled ventilation is mandatory until spontaneous respiratory efforts return. Succinylcholine administration, especially in larger doses, produces hyperkalemia, which can provoke cardiac dysrhythmias (bradycardia and asystole). Monitoring of the blood pressure, heart rate, and heart rhythm should be continued throughout the recovery period.

EMESIS AND ASPIRATION OF FOREIGN MATERIAL UNDER ANESTHESIA

Emesis (vomiting) and possible aspiration of this material into the airway is one of the most frightening of potential emergencies arising during general anesthesia or deep sedation. Fortunately, it is also one of the least likely situations to develop when recommended patient management techniques are followed. When protective airway reflexes remain intact (conscious sedation), aspiration of vomitus is unlikely.

Vomiting itself is rarely a significant problem. The act of vomiting requires the forceful contraction of many muscle groups, including the diaphragm, resulting in a projectile expulsion of the vomitus from the patient's GI tract and mouth. Aspiration of vomitus, although possible, is unlikely. During deep sedation and general anesthesia, in which protective airway reflexes and muscle tonus are depressed or absent, vomiting does not occur. Regurgitation, a passive reflux of stomach contents into the esophagus and pharynx, can occur and presents a significant danger. Regurgitation is passive (no muscular contraction) and quiet. In nondental surgical situations, regurgitation may go unnoticed unless someone is actively monitoring the airway. A pretracheal stethoscope enables the gurgling sound associated with vomitus to be detected almost immediately. In dental situations vomitus will be observed in the posterior of the mouth or pharynx.

Stomach contents have an extremely low pH. Morbidity and death are more likely to occur the lower the pH of the aspirated materials.[32]

When vomitus is aspirated into the trachea, the potential for disaster exists. The makeup of the material aspirated has a profound effect on the resulting clinical situation. The aspiration of solid material may produce acute airway obstruction progressing to death unless it is managed immediately and aggressively.

When liquid is aspirated, the usual airway response is bronchospasm. Rales, dyspnea, tachycardia, partial airway obstruction, and cyanosis develop within seconds, followed shortly thereafter by hypotension.[2] Pulse oximeter values for oxygen saturation will be depressed (less than 90%) and are likely to remain depressed despite efforts to increase them.

Management

Step 1: Position the Patient. The patient should immediately be placed into the Trendelenburg position with a head-down tilt of at least 15 degrees. To assist gravity in directing the vomitus into the pharynx (not into the lungs), the patient should be turned onto his or her right side.

Step 2: Emergency Medical Services. The doctor should activate emergency medical services (EMS) as soon as possible after aspiration has been diagnosed.

Step 3: Suction. The pharynx should be suctioned, removing any vomitus that may be present.

Step 4: Secure the Airway. Intubation should be accomplished, if possible. The patient is turned onto his or her back for intubation.

Step 5: Oxygen. Oxygen, if not already administered, is administered at this time.

Step 6: Definitive Care

Step 6a: Tracheal Lavage. Tracheal lavage should be performed if the patient has been intubated. Following slight elevation of the patient's head, a bolus of 10 to 20 ml of either normal saline or sodium bicarbonate is administered into the endotracheal tube. Larger volumes of solution are contraindicated because this might propel the aspirated material further into the trachea and lungs. Immediately after lavage, suction and oxygenation are necessary. This procedure can be repeated several times.

Step 6b: Administer Intravenous Steroids. To minimize development of inflammation, edema, and aspiration pneumonitis, steroids should be administered. There is some controversy associated with steroid administration because of its ability to depress the immune response of these patients who may develop aspiration pneumonitis.

Step 7: Hospitalization. The patient who aspirated will usually be hospitalized for a variable time.

HYPERVENTILATION

In the dental environment hyperventilation usually represents an anxiety-induced response to a fear-provoking therapy. Losing control of breathing, the patient breathes more rapidly (tachypnea) and deeply (hyperpnea) than usual. Excessive CO_2 is eliminated, producing hypocapnia, which is associated with signs and symptoms such as a feeling of coldness and tingling that leads to paresthesias of the fingers, toes, and circumoral region. The patient may become lightheaded or experience a feeling of tightness in the chest (mimicking the discomfort of angina pectoris). This increases the patient's anxieties and intensifies his or her inability to control breathing. Continued hyperventilation may lead to a spasmodic contraction of the hands and feet, termed *carpopedal tetany*, and then to seizures and the loss of consciousness. Although hyperventilation may occur at any age, it appears that patients between their late teens and late thirties are more likely to hyperventilate.

Management

Management of hyperventilation is predicated on allaying the patient's anxieties and in elevating the CO_2 level of the blood to normal. The doctor elevates CO_2 levels by having the patient rebreathe his or her exhaled air. The preferred method of doing this is to have the patient cup his or her hands in front of the mouth and nose and simply rebreathe. This has two benefits. First, the warm, moist exhaled air will warm the patient's cold hands—a psychological boost to the frightened patient, and second, the CO_2 level of the patient's blood will increase, relieving the signs and symptoms noted. It is also possible to have a patient pinch one nostril closed and breathe through the remaining nostril with the mouth shut. The older technique of rebreathing exhaled air from a paper bag is no longer recommended.

In the unlikely event that hyperventilation continues, an IV infusion should be started with diazepam or midazolam titrated very slowly until the patient relaxes and his or her breathing becomes normal. Box 34-15 outlines the steps to take to manage hyperventilation.

BOX 34-15 Management of Hyperventilation

Terminate the dental procedure.

↓

P, Position patient comfortably (usually upright).

↓

ABC, Assess and perform basic life support, as needed.

↓

D, Initiate definitive care:

- Remove dental materials from the patient's mouth.
- Calm the patient.
- Correct respiratory alkalosis.
- Initiate drug management, if necessary.

↓

Perform subsequent dental treatment.

↓

Discharge the patient.

RESPIRATORY DEPRESSION

Respiratory depression may develop secondary to the administration of CNS depressant drugs. It is most likely to be observed during deep sedation and general anesthesia and when certain drug groups, such as the barbiturates and opioids, are used. Respiratory depression is less likely to occur during oral or inhalation conscious sedation and when benzodiazepines are used during parenteral sedation techniques.

Respiratory depression may be observed as a decreased rate of respiration (to apnea) and/or decreased ventilatory effort. Monitoring priorities during parenteral sedation and general anesthesia are based primarily on ensuring airway and ventilatory adequacy. The pretracheal stethoscope is the most significant monitor in this regard, permitting evaluation of each and every breath taken by the patient. Respiratory problems may be detected virtually instantaneously with the pretracheal stethoscope, which is suggested for parenteral conscious and deep sedation and general anesthesia cases. Pulse oximetry permits evaluation of the degree of oxygenation of the blood. Although it is effective, there is a 10- to 20-second time lag between respiratory changes and notification on the oximeter screen. In addition, CO_2 blood levels are not evaluated by the pulse oximeter. Use of the pulse oximeter is recommended for all parenteral conscious sedation, deep sedation, and general anesthesia cases. The capnograph permits virtually instantaneous (2- to 4-second delay) evaluation of the effectiveness of ventilation through monitoring of the end-tidal CO_2 of each breath. Airway obstruction and diminished ventilatory effort may be detected immediately, permitting corrective action to be instituted rapidly. Use of the capnograph is currently recommended for operating room general anesthesia but is gaining increasing acceptance in deep sedation and parenteral conscious sedation.

When respiratory depression results from drug administration, it may be possible to administer reversal agents. Naloxone effectively reverses opioid analgesics, and benzodiazepines may be reversed with flumazenil. No specific antagonists exist for either barbiturates or propofol. Propofol, a rapid-acting and short-acting drug, will rarely produce respiratory depression persisting longer than a few seconds.

Respiratory depression rarely represents a major problem when the doctor has received appropriate training in the administration of anesthetic drugs. Outside medical assistance is not usually required, for the period of respiratory depression is usually transitory, with no adverse effects to the patient occurring.

Management

Step 1: Terminate the Procedure

Step 2: Position. The patient should be placed in the supine position.

Step 3: Assess A—Airway, B—Breathing, C—Circulation; Basic Life Support, as Indicated. The doctor should provide airway maintenance and evaluate respiratory effectiveness (i.e., look, listen, and feel). In many instances assisted ventilation will be necessary to supplement the patient's inspired air volume. In a few instances in which apnea is present, controlled ventilation is necessary.

Step 4: D—Definitive Care

Step 4a. *Blood pressure and heart rate and rhythm should be monitored every 5 minutes and oxygen administered.*

Step 4b. *Start an IV infusion, if not already present.*

Step 4c. *Although their administration is not usually necessary, consider antidotal drug administration:*

- When *opioids* have been administered, slowly titrate *naloxone* at 0.1 mg/min until improved ventilation is noted. In children a dose of 0.005 mg/min is administered until improved ventilation is observed.[33]
- Following *benzodiazepine* administration, *flumazenil* should be considered at an IV dose of 0.2 mg/min until respiratory efforts improve. A usual adult dose of flumazenil is 0.5 mg.[34]
- When *barbiturates* have been administered, no effective antagonist exists. Continued assisted or controlled ventilation is necessary until spontaneous breathing returns.
- No effective antagonist exists for *propofol,* but prolonged respiratory depression is unlikely to be observed with this drug because of its extremely short duration of action.

Step 5: Recovery. Following return of ventilatory adequacy after a brief period of respiratory depression, it may be possible to continue with the dental treatment. If the period of respiratory depression was significant in depth or duration, the doctor may elect to terminate the dental procedure. At the end of the planned dental treatment or after termination of the treatment, the IM administration of an antidotal drug should be considered. In situations in which IM opioids or benzodiazepines have been administered, or in cases in which long-acting drugs such as morphine and lorazepam have been administered intravenously, the potential for a rebound depression exists (although this is highly unlikely to occur). IV antagonists have a rapid onset of clinical action, but their duration after IV administration may be shorter than that of the offending drug. An IM dose of either flumazenil or naloxone should be considered in these situations.

Step 6: Discharge. The patient will be discharged from the office in the custody of a responsible adult companion only when the treating doctor believes that the patient's recovery (from sedation or general anesthesia) is adequate to permit his or her safe dismissal from the office. Outside medical assistance is rarely required in respiratory depression.

Box 34-16 outlines the steps to take to manage sedative-hypnotic overdose. Box 34-17 outlines the steps to take to manage opioid overdose.

BOX 34-16 Management of Sedative-Hypnotic Overdose

Terminate the dental procedure.
↓
P, Position the patient comfortably.
↓
ABC, Assess and perform basic life support, as needed.
↓
D, Initiate definitive care:
- Summon medical assistance, if required.
- Administer oxygen.
- Monitor vital signs.
- Establish IV line, if possible.
- Provide definitive management:

Administer IV or IM flumazenil for benzodiazepine overdose.
Continue **P → A → B → C** for barbiturate overdose.
↓
Permit recovery and discharge the patient.

BOX 34-17 Management of Opioid Overdose

Terminate the dental procedure.
↓
P, Position the patient supine with the legs elevated slightly.
↓
ABC, Assess and perform basic life support, as needed.
↓
D, Initiate definitive care:
- Summon medical assistance, if required.
- Administer oxygen.
- Monitor and record vital signs.
- Establish IV line, if possible.
- Administer antidotal drug (intravenous or intramuscular naloxone).

↓
Permit recovery and discharge the patient.

SEIZURES

Seizures (or convulsions) are not uncommon during dental treatment. Patients with epilepsy are the most likely persons to have seizures in the dental environment because stressful situations may provoke seizures even in those with well-controlled epilepsy. More than 90% of patients with epilepsy have generalized tonic-clonic seizures, also known as *grand mal seizures.*[35] Local anesthetic overdose is another possible cause of seizures in the dental environment. The inadvertent intravascular (IV or intraarterial) administration of local anesthetics produces a seizure within seconds of injection. The administration of too large a total dose brings on a more gradual onset of seizure activity, the patient demonstrating increasingly severe signs and symptoms until frank tonic-clonic convulsions occur. Hyperventilation may be associated with seizures if the episode is permitted to continue for an extended period. Seizures are also associated with extreme hypoxia or anoxia and hypercarbia secondary to airway management problems or apnea, as well as with severe hypoglycemia.

Seizures are usually readily managed without resulting injury or mortality. The primary goals in seizure management are preventing injury to the patient during the seizure and ensuring the adequacy of ventilation. Ventilatory adequacy is of particular importance during the local anesthetic–induced seizure because pH changes alter the seizure threshold of the local anesthetic.[36] Acidosis, a result of hypoxia, hypercarbia, and lactic acid production during the seizure, lowers the threshold for local anesthetic–induced seizures, thereby prolonging the seizure and increasing the likelihood of serious postictal morbidity or death. Adequate ventilation will eliminate/prevent CO_2 retention and elevate the seizure threshold of the local anesthetic, thereby decreasing the duration of the seizure.

Anticonvulsants are rarely required to terminate seizures because most seizures are self-limiting, rarely lasting more than 2 to 5 minutes (grand mal epilepsy). However, EMS assistance will, on occasion, be recommended as a part of our management, for two reasons: first, to aid in the definitive management of the patient following the seizure, and second, to administer IV anticonvulsants if the seizure is still present on the patient's arrival.

Management

Step 1: Terminate the Procedure

Step 2: Position. The patient should be placed in the supine position.

Step 3: Assess A—Airway, B—Breathing, C—Circulation; Basic Life Support, as Indicated. During the clonic phase of a seizure, airway, breathing, and circulation need not be assisted.

Step 4: D—Definitive Care

Step 4a: Prevent Injury. The doctor must protect the patient during the clonic phase of the seizure (alternating generalized muscle contraction and relaxation). The doctor gently holds the patient's arms and legs. Movement of the limbs should be permitted, but within limits so as to prevent injury. Movement must not be restricted completely because this may cause injury to the patient. *DO NOT ATTEMPT TO PLACE ANY OBJECT INTO THE MOUTH OF A CONVULSING VICTIM* because this is the primary cause of injury to persons during seizures (fractured or avulsed teeth and injury to the soft tissues).

Step 4b: Activate EMS

Step 4c: Administer Oxygen. The doctor should ensure airway patency and administer oxygen to minimize hypoxia and hypercarbia.

Most *generalized tonic-clonic convulsions* cease spontaneously within 2 to 5 minutes. In some few cases a seizure may continue beyond 5 minutes, or a seizure may stop and recur before the patient recovers consciousness. These are the two definitions of status epilepticus, a situation representing an acutely life-threatening emergency.[37] Seizures secondary to *local anesthetic overdose* continue until the cerebral blood level of the local anesthetic falls below the seizure threshold for that drug. With adequate airway maintenance and oxygenation, local anesthetic–induced seizures do not persist for more than a few minutes. Although unlikely to occur, seizures occurring during *hyperventilation* continue until the CO_2 level of the blood is elevated to close to normal levels. Seizures secondary to *airway obstruction* or *anoxia* are associated with extreme morbidity or death. Airway patency and oxygenation must be ensured.

Step 4d: Intravenous Access. If the seizure persists, an IV infusion should be started, if possible. A catheter is recommended because its flexibility minimizes the risk of its being accidentally dislodged by the patient.

Step 4e: Anticonvulsant Administration. The administration of IV anticonvulsants should be considered if the seizure is prolonged. To be effective, anticonvulsants must be administered intravenously. Diazepam or midazolam should be titrated slowly (1 ml/min)—diazepam at a rate of 5 mg/min, midazolam at 1 mg/min—until seizure activity ceases. Anticonvulsant administration should be considered only if the doctor is well trained in management of the unconscious, apneic patient, for this is an entirely possible scenario in the postseizure state when anticonvulsants have been administered. IV barbiturates (e.g., thiopental, methohexital, pentobarbital) may also be administered, but the administration of these drugs increases the incidence of postseizure apnea.

Step 5: Postseizure Management. The epileptic patient who has not received anticonvulsants will normally be sleeping deeply and perhaps snoring in the immediate postseizure (postictal) state. Snoring is indicative of partial airway obstruction produced by the tongue. Management requires head-tilt/chin-lift and the administration of oxygen. The epileptic patient will also be mentally disoriented. The treating doctor should talk to the patient, explaining where the patient is, what has happened, and that everything is "all right." Complete recovery from a generalized tonic-clonic seizure requires several hours. EMS personnel will evaluate the patient to determine whether hospitalization is required or whether the patient may be discharged from the office in the custody of an adult companion.

Patients who have had a local anesthetic–induced seizure normally require hospitalization for an indefinite period so that their neurologic status can be better evaluated. Hospitalization may be suggested after hyperventilation-induced seizures, but the period of observation is usually minimal (several hours).

Seizures secondary to severe anoxia require hospitalization and intensive care for an undetermined period. Patients who have received anticonvulsant drugs to terminate their seizures are usually hospitalized.

Box 34-18 outlines the steps to take to manage generalized tonic-clonic seizure (GTCS). Box 34-19 outlines the steps to take to manage generalized convulsive status epilepticus.

HYPOGLYCEMIA

Hypoglycemia, or low blood sugar, is a not uncommon occurrence in patients with type 1, insulin-dependent diabetes mellitus (IDDM). Patients with type 2, non–insulin-dependent diabetes mellitus (NIDDM) are much less likely to become acutely hypoglycemic. Recent changes in the recommendations for management of type 1 diabetes suggest the more frequent administration of insulin (perhaps three to five times per day) as a means of preventing the onset of the chronic complications associated with diabetes. However, increased insulin administration brings with it an estimated threefold increase in the incidence of acute hypoglycemia.[38]

Inadequate cerebral blood levels of sugar lead to diminished CNS function. Clinical signs and symptoms associated with mild hypoglycemia include mental confusion, mild muscle tremor, diaphoresis, a feeling of being cold, and tachycardia. This is a likely scenario in a dental practice when the type 1 diabetic patient does not eat before a scheduled appointment. A telephone call the day before the scheduled dental appointment reminding the patient to eat should minimize this occurrence. If parenteral sedation or general anesthesia is scheduled, a period of fast is mandated. The patient's insulin needs will be decreased and should be so adjusted, either by the patient or after consultation with a physician. The

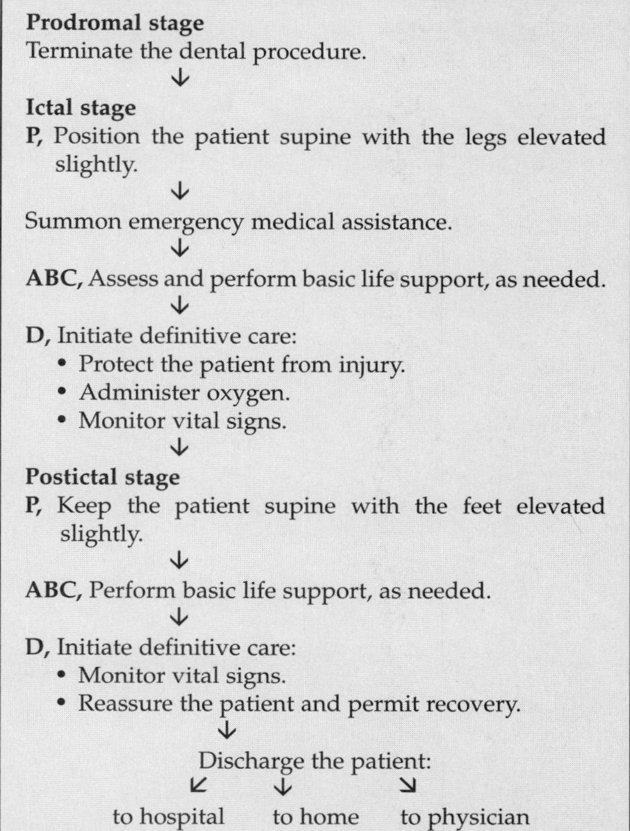

BOX 34-18 Management of Generalized Tonic-Clonic Seizure (Grand Mal)

Prodromal stage
Terminate the dental procedure.
↓
Ictal stage
P, Position the patient supine with the legs elevated slightly.
↓
Summon emergency medical assistance.
↓
ABC, Assess and perform basic life support, as needed.
↓
D, Initiate definitive care:
- Protect the patient from injury.
- Administer oxygen.
- Monitor vital signs.

↓
Postictal stage
P, Keep the patient supine with the feet elevated slightly.
↓
ABC, Perform basic life support, as needed.
↓
D, Initiate definitive care:
- Monitor vital signs.
- Reassure the patient and permit recovery.

↓
Discharge the patient:
↙ ↓ ↘
to hospital — to home — to physician

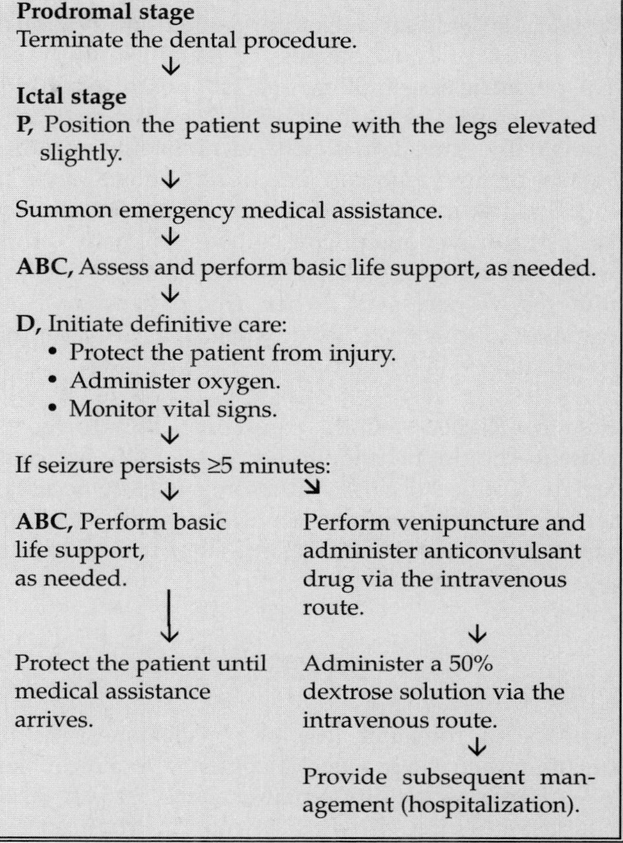

BOX 34-19 Management of Generalized Convulsive Status Epilepticus

Prodromal stage
Terminate the dental procedure.
↓
Ictal stage
P, Position the patient supine with the legs elevated slightly.
↓
Summon emergency medical assistance.
↓
ABC, Assess and perform basic life support, as needed.
↓
D, Initiate definitive care:
- Protect the patient from injury.
- Administer oxygen.
- Monitor vital signs.

↓
If seizure persists ≥5 minutes:
↓ ↘
ABC, Perform basic life support, as needed.
↓
Protect the patient until medical assistance arrives.

Perform venipuncture and administer anticonvulsant drug via the intravenous route.
↓
Administer a 50% dextrose solution via the intravenous route.
↓
Provide subsequent management (hospitalization).

use of 5% dextrose and water as the infusate is not contraindicated in the type 1 diabetic patient. The patient appears in the office slightly hypoglycemic after the fast, and 5% dextrose and water will provide a needed elevation in the blood sugar level.

When blood sugar levels fall too low, consciousness is lost and seizures are noted, although the latter should be unlikely in the dental situation. Mild hypoglycemia is easily managed with a rapid return to normal CNS functioning. The need for EMS and hospitalization is minimal. When hypoglycemia produces unconsciousness and/or seizures, EMS assistance is desirable and a period of hospitalization is the norm.

Management

Step 1: Terminate the Procedure

Step 2: Position. As soon as signs and symptoms of hypoglycemia are noted, the patient is placed into a comfortable position.

Step 3: Assess A—Airway, B—Breathing, C—Circulation; Basic Life Support, as Indicated

Step 4: D—Definitive Care. It should be determined whether the patient took an insulin dose and whether he has eaten food recently.

Step 4a: Administer "Sugar." If hypoglycemia is considered a possibility, the doctor should not hesitate to administer sugar to the patient orally. Most type 1 diabetic patients prefer orange juice, feeling that they recover faster than with other liquids (soft drinks). Permit the patient to drink 8 to 12 ounces of orange juice in 4-ounce increments over about 10 minutes. Return to normal CNS status is rapid. Some diabetic patients prefer candy bars. The planned dental care may continue if the doctor and patient agree.

Step 4b: Activate EMS. If the episode continues or if the patient loses consciousness, EMS should be summoned immediately.

Step 4c: Position. In the presence of unconsciousness, the patient must be placed into the supine position and BLS administered as needed. In most instances airway maintenance is all that is required.

Step 4d: Intravenous Access. An IV infusion, if not already present, should be established.

Step 4e: Administer an Antihypoglycemic. A dose of 30 ml of 50% dextrose is administered intravenously. The return of consciousness is usually quite rapid. The pediatric dose is 30 ml of a 25% dextrose solution. If an IV cannot be started or 50% (or 25%) dextrose is unavailable, glucagon may be administered intramuscularly or intravenously. The dose of glucagon is 0.5 to 1.0 mg administered subcutaneously, intramuscularly, or intravenously. Consciousness usually returns within 15 minutes, with the dose repeated every 15 minutes, if necessary. When the patient does not respond to glucagon, IV dextrose must be administered.[39]

Step 5: Recovery. Once consciousness returns, the patient should be monitored until EMS personnel arrive. A period of hospitalization is usually necessary when unconsciousness occurs secondary to hypoglycemia. Box 34-20 outlines the steps to take to manage hypoglycemia.

BOX 34-20 Management of Hypoglycemia

Conscious Patient

Recognize hypoglycemia.

↓

Terminate the dental procedure.

↓

P, Position the patient comfortably.

↓

ABC, Assess and perform basic life support, as needed.

↓

D, Initiate definitive care:

- Administer oral carbohydrates.

↓	↘
If successful:	If unsuccessful:
↓	↓
Permit the patient to recover.	Summon medical assistance.
↓	↓
Discharge the patient	Administer parenteral carbohydrates.
	↓
	Monitor the patient.
	↓
	Discharge the patient.

Unconscious Patient

Terminate the dental procedure.

↓

P, Position the patient supine with the legs elevated slightly.

↓

ABC, Assess and perform basic life support, as needed.

↓

D, Initiate definitive care:

- Summon emergency medical assistance.
- Administer carbohydrates:

IV 50% dextrose solution, 1 mg glucagon (via IM or IV route), transmucosal sugar, or rectal honey or syrup

↓

Allow the patient to recover and discharge per medical recommendations.

IM, Intramuscular; *IV,* intravenous.

SYNCOPE

Syncope, a transient loss of consciousness, is not uncommon in the practice of dentistry. In a recent survey of emergencies in dental practice, 53% of 30,000 emergencies were listed as syncope.[40] Produced by a sudden drop in heart rate leading to a drop in blood pressure, which decreases blood and oxygen delivery to the CNS, syncope is also referred to as *vasodepressor syncope, vasovagal syncope, common faint,* and *psychogenic syncope.*

During stressful situations, as might develop in the dental office, such as a sudden unexpected pain or the sight of blood or dental instruments (e.g., needles, the drill), blood is directed into the skeletal muscle of the legs and arms to prepare the body for the "fight or flight response." In the absence of movement, venous return of blood to the heart and blood flow to the brain decrease. Signs and symptoms of a slight decrease in cerebral blood flow include a feeling of warmth, the loss of color (pale or ashen gray skin tone), diaphoresis, complaints of feeling "bad" or "faint," and nausea, along with the development of a tachycardia. Tachycardia enables the body to compensate for the decrease in cardiac output and to maintain a minimally adequate blood flow to the brain, which maintains consciousness. In the absence of definitive treatment of this patient, decompensation occurs, consisting of a significant bradycardia (heart rate ± 20 beats per minute with periods of asystole frequently observed), which severely decreases cerebral blood flow and produces the loss of consciousness.[41] Placing the patient in the supine position with the legs elevated greatly increases venous return while airway maintenance ensures the delivery of oxygen to the blood. Recovery of consciousness is normally quite rapid, within 10 to 15 seconds following proper positioning and airway management. Rarely is either EMS or hospitalization necessary. Indeed, in a person who "felt faint" but never lost consciousness, the planned dental procedure may continue; however, when consciousness was lost for any period, the planned treatment should be rescheduled to a later date. Modifications in subsequent dental care should be considered so as to avoid recurrence of fainting.

Syncope is unlikely to occur in a sedated patient. More likely is the scenario of the fearful, nonmedicated patient collapsing in the reception area or in the dental chair on seeing the needle on the local anesthetic syringe. Pretreatment diagnosis of the patient's dental fears and modifications in dental care should prevent syncope from occurring. Most incidents of fainting occur with the patient seated in an upright position. With dental patients more often placed in a reclined position (or supine) in the dental chair, loss of consciousness from syncope is becoming less common.

Management

Step 1: Terminate the Procedure

Step 2: Position. The patient is placed into the supine position with the feet elevated.

Step 3: Assess A—Airway, B—Breathing, C—Circulation; Basic Life Support, as Indicated

Step 4: D—Definitive Care

Step 4a: All dental equipment should be removed from the patient's field of vision.

Step 4b: Administer Oxygen

Step 4c: Administer Ammonia. Ammonia inhalants should be available in every treatment room and in the emergency drug kit. Crushed between the rescuer's fingers, the inhalant is held under the patient's nose. Inhalation of ammonia, a noxious odor, provokes muscular movement of the arms and legs, thereby increasing the return of venous blood to the heart and increasing cardiac output and blood flow to the brain.

Step 5: Recovery. The episode will rapidly resolve, with the patient feeling considerably better once positioned and breathing oxygen. If both the doctor and the patient agree, the planned dental procedure may proceed. The doctor should consider modification of dental care to diminish any anxiety that may be present.

Step 6: Loss of Consciousness. Should unconsciousness occur, the patient is placed into the supine position with the feet elevated, and if not already done, head-tilt/chin-lift is performed and the airway assessed. The patient will usually be breathing spontaneously, and the heart rate will be slow (± 20 beats per minute).

Step 6a: Definitive Management. Consciousness should return within 10 to 15 seconds. The postsyncopal period is marked by the patient feeling poorly. The patient is nauseous (and will likely vomit), is achy all over, and will require approximately 24 hours to fully return to a normal state of function. Oxygen should be administered to the patient via nasal cannula or nasal hood during the recovery period. Vital signs should be monitored and recorded.

Step 6b: EMS. If consciousness does not return within 10 to 15 seconds, EMS should be activated. There are many other potential causes for unconsciousness that do not respond to the treatment described. Whenever unconsciousness persists for longer than 10 seconds, it is recommended that emergency assistance be sought immediately.

Step 7: Discharge. Discharge of the patient from the office should be considered only after a lengthy period of recovery (approximately 1 hour), during which time the patient remains under direct observation. Patients who have lost consciousness should not be permitted to leave the office alone or to drive a car or any other vehicle (e.g., bicycle, skate board). This patient should be discharged in the company of a responsible adult companion. There is rarely a need for EMS assistance

BOX 34-21 Management of Vasodepressor Syncope

Assess consciousness.

↓

Activate the office emergency system.

↓

P, Position the patient supine with the feet elevated slightly.

↓

ABC, Assess and open the airway; assess airway patency and breathing; assess circulation.

↓

D, Initiate definitive care:

- Administer oxygen.
- Monitor vital signs.
- Perform additional procedures:

Administer aromatic ammonia.
Administer atropine if bradycardia persists.
Maintain composure.

↓ ↘

(Postsyncopal recovery) Postpone further dental treatment. ↘

(Delayed recovery) Activate emergency medical services. ↙

Determine precipitating factors.

or for hospitalization in the common episode of faint. Box 34-21 outlines the steps to take to manage vasodepressor syncope.

SUMMARY

Emergency situations can and do arise in the dental and medical office. In this chapter several potential emergency situations associated with the administration of drugs for anesthesia, sedation, or pain control have been reviewed. The best treatment for these emergencies is their prevention. Adequate preoperative patient evaluation, adherence to recommended technique, intraoperative monitoring, and postoperative management will prevent virtually all of these complications.

Other medical emergencies that occur during medical and dental treatment were described. Patients who are at risk (ASA II, III, and IV) are unable to tolerate the stresses normally associated with operative or surgical procedures and are more likely to develop acute exacerbation of their underlying medical problems. The appropriate use of sedation and pain control in these patients will greatly decrease their risk during treatment.

REFERENCES

1. California State Board of Dental Examiners: *Conscious sedation evaluation protocol,* Sacramento, 1993.
2. American Association of Oral & Maxillofacial Surgeons: *Office anesthesia evaluation manual,* ed 4, Rosemont, Ill, 1991, The Association.
3. Pallasch TJ: *Pharmacology for dental students and practitioners,* Philadelphia, 1980, Lea & Febiger.
4. Dupont RL, Saylor KE: Depressant substances in adolescent medicine, *Pediatr Rev* 13:381, 1992.
5. *Mosby's medical, nursing, and allied health dictionary,* ed 6, St Louis, 2002, Mosby.
6. Boobis AR: Molecular basis for differences in susceptibility to toxicants: introduction, *Toxicol Lett* 64-65:109, 1992.
7. Goodson JM, Moore PA: Life-threatening reactions after pedodontic sedation: an assessment of narcotic, local anesthetic, and antiemetic drug interaction, *J Am Dent Assoc* 107:239, 1983.
8. Pollakoff J, Pollakoff K: *EMT's guide to signs and symptoms,* Los Angeles, 1991, Los Angeles Unified School District Vocational Education Program.
9. International Consensus on Science: Guidelines 2000 for Cardiopulmonary Resuscitation and Emergency Cardiovascular Care, *Circulation* 102(suppl):253, 2000.
10. Flumazenil, drug package insert, Roche Laboratories, 1993.
11. Naloxone, drug package insert, DuPont Multi-Source Products, 1993.
12. deJulien LF: Causes of severe morbidity/mortality cases, *J Calif Dent Assoc* 11:45, 1983.
13. Bates DW, Leape LLI, Petrycki S: Incidence and preventability of adverse drug events in hospitalized patients, *J Gen Intern Med* 8:289, 1993.
14. Dolovich J, Evans S, Rosenbloom D et al: Anaphylaxis due to thiopental sodium anesthesia, *Can Med Assoc J* 123:292, 1980.
15. Milner SM, Bennett JD: Emergency cricothyrotomy, *J Laryngol Otol* 105:883, 1991.
16. Peters GA, Karnes WE, Bastron JA: Near fatal and fatal reactions to insect sting, *Ann Allergy* 41:268, 1978.
17. American Heart Association: *Textbook of advanced cardiac life support,* Dallas, 1992, American Heart Association.
18. International Consensus on Science: Guidelines 2000 for cardiopulmonary resuscitation and emergency cardiovascular care, *Circulation* 102(suppl):295, 2000.
19. Malamed SF: *Medical emergencies in the dental office,* ed 5, St Louis, 2000, Mosby.
20. Hulyalkar AR, Miller ED Jr: Evaluation of the hypertensive patient. In Rogers MC, Tinker JH, Covino BC et al, eds: *Principles and practice of anesthesiology,* St Louis, 1993, Mosby.
21. Calhoun SC, Oparil S: Treatment of hypertensive crisis, *N Engl J Med* 323:1177, 1990.
22. Opie LH: Treatment of severe hypertension. In Kaplan NM, Brenner BM, Laragh JH, eds: *New therapeutic strategies in hypertension,* New York, 1989, Raven Press.
23. Cohen MM, Duncan PG, Pope WDB et al: A survey of 112,000 anaesthetics at one teaching hospital (1975-1983), *Can J Anaesth* 33:22, 1986.
24. Atlee JL: *Perioperative cardiac dysrhythmias: mechanisms, recognition, management,* ed 2, Chicago, 1989, Year Book Medical.
25. Wingard DW: What is a normal heart rate prior to surgery? *Anesthesiology* 63:130, 1985.
26. Driscoll EJ, Smilack ZH, Lightbody PM et al: Sedation with intravenous diazepam, *J Oral Surg* 30:332, 1972.
27. DeRango FJ: Management of common medical problems. In Lichtiger M, Moya F, eds: *Introduction to the practice of anesthesia,* ed 2, Hagerstown, Md, 1978, Harper & Row.
28. International Consensus on Science: Guidelines 2000 for cardiopulmonary resuscitation and emergency cardiovascular care, *Circulation* 102(suppl):86, 2000.
29. Phipps C: Contributory causes of coronary thrombosis, *JAMA* 106:761, 1936.
30. Ferraris VA, Ferraris SP, Gilliam HS et al: Predictors of postoperative ventricular dysrhythmias: a multivariate study, *J Cardiovasc Surg* 32:12, 1991.
31. Liau CS, Hahn LC, Tjung JJ et al: The clinical characteristics of acute myocardial infarction in aged patients, *J Formosan Med Assoc* 90:122, 1991.
32. Hollingsworth HM, Irwin RS: Acute respiratory failure in pregnancy, *Clin Chest Med* 13:723, 1992.
33. Barsan WG, Tomassoni AJ, Seger D et al: Safety assessment of high-dose narcotic analgesia for emergency department procedures, *Ann Emerg Med* 22:1444, 1993.

34. Kulka PJ, Lauven PM: Benzodiazepine antagonists: an update of their role in the emergency care of overdose patients, *Drug Safety* 7:381, 1992.
35. Earnest MP: Seizures, *Neurol Clin* 11:563, 1993.
36. Covino BG: Toxicity of local anesthetic agents, *Acta Anaesthesiol Belg* 39(suppl 2):159, 1988.
37. Treatment of convulsive status epilepticus: recommendations of the Epilepsy Foundation of America's working group on status epilepticus, *JAMA* 270:854, 1993.
38. The Diabetes Control and Complications Trial Research Group: The effect of intensive treatment of diabetes on the development and progression of long-term complications in insulin-dependent diabetes mellitus. *N Engl J Med* 329:977, 1993.
39. Glucagon, drug package insert, Eli Lilly, 1998.
40. Malamed SF: Managing medical emergencies, *JADA* 124:40, 1993.
41. van Lieshout JJ, Wieling W, Karemaker JM et al: The vasovagal response, *Clin Sci* 81:575, 1991.

SECTION VIII

SPECIAL CONSIDERATIONS

In this concluding section, several groups of patients for whom the management of pain and anxiety require greater attention are discussed. For these patients the overall risks of unwanted drug effects, acute medical problems, and unsuccessful results are greater than in other groups of patients. For these patients, too, the rewards for successful treatment (in terms of personal satisfaction and accomplishment) are infinitely greater.

The *pediatric patient* represents a group in which the various techniques of sedation and general anesthesia are frequently required. However, pediatric patients cannot be treated as though they were simply small adults. Drug dosages usually must be altered to meet the specific needs of the child patient. Unfortunately, a disproportionate number of the serious problems that have occurred in association with the use of sedative techniques in dental and medical outpatient practices over the past few years have occurred in the pediatric patient.[1] In Chapter 35 drugs and techniques that have proved successful in the pediatric patient are reviewed.

The *geriatric patient* also represents an increased risk of adverse drug response when central nervous system depressants (and other drugs) are administered.

Although the requirement for sedation is not usually as great in this rapidly growing segment of the population as in younger groups, there are some specific modifications in therapy that are appropriate in managing the geriatric patient.

In Chapters 37 through 39 *medically* and *physically compromised patients* are reviewed. Steadily increasing numbers of these patients are seeking treatment at dental and medical offices. The nature of the patient's underlying medical problem(s) may have a significant impact on the administration of drugs for the management of pain and anxiety. In some cases the patient may prove to be unable to communicate or to cooperate with the doctor, making monitoring during the procedure somewhat more difficult but ever more important. Most of the patients discussed in Chapters 38 and 39 can be successfully treated on an outpatient basis if specific treatment modifications are employed.

In prior chapters of this book specific contraindications to the administration of drugs were presented as the pharmacology of each drug was discussed. In this section the disease process is introduced, and the various techniques of sedation and specific drugs are reviewed as to their appropriateness for these patients.

REFERENCE

1. Goodson JM, Moore PA: Life-threatening reactions after pedodontic sedation: an assessment of opioid, local anesthetic, and antiemetic drug interaction, *J Am Dent Assoc* 107:239, 1983.

CHAPTER 35

The Pediatric Patient

CHAPTER OUTLINE

As important as patient management is in the realm of adult dentistry, it is in pediatric dentistry that proper patient management assumes the utmost importance. The young child, approaching a visit to the dentist for the first time, is influenced by a number of sources, some positive, some negative, that will affect his or her attitude and behavior during treatment. Some factors are controllable by the doctor and staff, but others are beyond their control. Proper patient management, especially in the younger, more impressionable patient, goes far toward producing a patient with positive attitudes about future dental and medical care; conversely, too many unfavorable influences will cause the patient to look on the prospect of future dental and medical care with increasing fear and trepidation.

In this chapter some of the basic concepts involved in the management of the pediatric patient are discussed briefly. For a more in-depth discussion of this subject, the reader is referred to the following textbooks:

McDonald RE, Avery DR: *Dentistry for the child and adolescent,* ed 7, St Louis, 1999, Mosby.

Pinkham JR: *Pediatric dentistry: infancy through adolescence,* ed 3, Philadelphia, 1999, WB Saunders.

Wei SH: *Pediatric dentistry: total child patient care,* Philadelphia, 1988, Lea & Febiger.

FACTORS INFLUENCING PATIENT RESPONSE

A number of factors interact to determine whether the pediatric patient will face a scheduled visit to the dentist or physician with eager anticipation or with fearful dread. These include the influences of the parent, of the child's peers, of the doctor, and of the office staff. The child's prior experience with health professionals is yet another factor.

Parental attitudes in general, and toward dentistry in particular, have a profound influence on a child's behavior. Factors thought to be of importance include the age of the parents and their level of maturity. Positive dental attitudes in parents create an environment for the child that is conducive to the acceptance of ideal dentistry. It is frequently heard that the greatest difficulty in patient management occurs when a child is accompanied to the dental office by the grandparent. The grandparents often represent the ultimate authority in the family and will do things as they see fit to do them, not as the doctor may desire. This may be a significant factor when decisions are made regarding the site and route of administration of sedative drugs.

The parents' prior experience with medical and dental health professionals will greatly influence their child's attitudes. Although few, if any, parents will intentionally tell their children of prior traumatic experiences they have had, such attitudes and feelings are transferred to the child nonverbally. Children may overhear their parents discussing their experiences or may see a parent suffering either before or after a dental appointment. Children are surprisingly astute observers and pick up the many clues that parents drop relating to their attitudes toward health care.

Parents may make statements to their children that influence the children's behavior or put the children on guard, expecting that something unpleasant might be in the offing. Simply telling a child, "If you behave yourself at the dentist I will buy you a treat later" may tell the child to anticipate the occurrence of something unpleasant.

The *influence of other children,* either siblings or acquaintances, must never be discounted. Such influence may be either positive or negative. In a family in which several children have undergone dental treatment without difficulty, younger children receive positive reinforcement before their visit. However, if prior appointments have been traumatic, such influence may be negative. The same is true for the friends of the child. I have found that young friends tend to accentuate the more negative aspects of dentistry and medicine.

Another factor influencing the child's behavior during treatment is *his or her own* prior experience with other health-care professionals. Traumatic experiences (e.g., a painful vaccination injection) provoke negative behavior in the patient, whereas positive experiences lead to a better-behaved child.

Some children are fearful at their very first visit to the dental office. The collective influence of the parents, siblings, and friends has produced this unwarranted apprehension. Although the goals of the doctor and staff will be somewhat more difficult to accomplish, the attitude of the office staff can dramatically change this child's feelings toward dentistry.

The factors that have been discussed thus far are truly out of the control of the doctor. Fortunately, the doctor is able to control several other factors. These include the attitudes of the doctor and staff and the environment (the office) in which the patient will be treated.

The *doctor* sets the behavior standard in the office. Kimmelman[1] has stated that firmness with kindness and a soft, clear voice is an asset in dealing with children. The dress of the doctor is important: White uniforms may provoke negative feelings in younger patients, whereas colorful uniforms or the absence of uniforms evokes a more positive response. With universal precautions (gloves, glasses, and masks being mandatory), explanations and role-playing with the child to make him or her comfortable with our safety garb are suggested.

The same guidelines are important for members of the *office staff.* In the management of the pediatric patient, the auxiliary may have significantly greater contact with the patient than does the doctor; therefore the attitude and attire of the staff are as important, if not more so, than the doctor's.

The time of day at which the appointment is scheduled may have bearing on a child's behavior, especially the younger child. Interference with a child's sleep or eating habits should be avoided, if possible. The young child accustomed to a midday nap may be irritable if he or she is in the dental chair instead of bed at that time. Younger patients are most easily managed early in the day. This is also true for the apprehensive adult patient (see Chapter 4). The basic concepts presented in the stress-reduction protocols are of great importance in managing the pediatric patient. The length of the appointment should not exceed the child's attention span. Younger patients are less able to tolerate longer appointments than are older, more mature children. Most children are able to tolerate 45-minute appointments with little difficulty.[2]

The *office environment* is another factor that influences the patient's behavior. An office in which many children are treated should offer an environment that appeals to children. Although most pediatric medical and dental offices are designed with this in mind, even in the office of the busy generalist a separate area of the reception area might be set aside for younger patients. The very fact that this area requires the patient to leave the parent will be more conducive to the separation from the parent that occurs at the time of dental treatment. The color of the office, soundproofing, and odors are important factors to consider in the design of the pediatric office and reception room. Many pediatricians and pediatric dentists offer their patients a gift as they leave the office. These gifts are used as a display of friendship, not as a reward for good behavior.

BEHAVIORAL EVALUATION OF THE PEDIATRIC PATIENT

Even though there are innumerable factors that interact to influence a child's behavior in the dental office, the doctor must still be able to evaluate the patient's ability to cope with the planned treatment. A number of systems have been developed to aid in classification of a child's behavior and the potential for successful dental treatment. Two of the most commonly used systems are the Frankl Behavioral Rating Scale[3] and the system devised by Wright.[4]

In the Frankl system the observer (doctor) places the child's behavior into one of four categories:

1. Definitely positive behavior
2. Positive behavior
3. Negative behavior
4. Definitely negative behavior

Johnson has stated that the Frankl scale appears to be closely related to the attitude of the parent toward dentistry.[5]

Wright's classification presents three major groups: (1) cooperative, (2) lacking cooperative ability, and (3) potentially uncooperative behavior, with multiple subgroups. Wright has stated that most doctors, either consciously or subconsciously, categorize the behavior of children into one of these groups. These classifications permit the doctor to more readily determine the appropriate means of overcoming the management problems presented by the patient[4]:

1. Cooperative: most children (can be treated by a tell-show-do approach)
2. Lacking cooperative ability
   a. Very young children with whom communication cannot be established nor comprehension expected
   b. Children with specific debilitating or handicapping conditions
3. Potentially uncooperative behavior
   a. Uncontrolled behavior: tantrums with flailing of arms and legs, suggestive of acute anxiety and fear (usually seen in young children 3 to 6 years old on the occasion of the first dental visit)
   b. Defiant behavior: may use passive resistance (most often seen in older children approaching adolescence)
   c. Timid behavior
      (1) May hide behind the parent, but usually little resistance to separation
      (2) Stalls or hesitates when given directions
      (3) Often withholds tears
      (4) Highly anxious
      (5) Does not always hear or comprehend instructions
   d. Tense cooperative behavior
      (1) Accepts treatment as it is provided
      (2) Voice may have a tremor when speaking
      (3) Body may tremble
      (4) Most often perspires noticeably on the palm of the hand or brow
      (5) Controls emotions
   e. Whining behavior
      (1) Allows dentist to proceed, but whines throughout
      (2) Frequently complains of pain
      (3) Emits sounds constantly

Successful treatment of the patient who lacks the ability to cooperate often requires the use of one of the techniques of sedation (conscious or deep). Should these fail to prove adequate, general anesthesia may be required.

The potentially uncooperative patient may or may not require sedation for successful treatment. The attitudes and technical abilities of the doctor and office staff will be the deciding factors with these patients.

DETERMINING THE NEED FOR SEDATION

The determination to use a technique of sedation should be made only following consideration of several factors:

1. Assessment of dental need
2. Patient cooperation
3. Parental cooperation and involvement
4. Economic considerations
5. Alternative treatment plans
6. Preoperative health evaluation
7. Preoperative behavioral assessment
8. Training and experience of doctor and staff

When only minimal treatment (e.g., one filling) is necessary, the need for sedation is negligible. This is especially true for the parenteral techniques (intramuscular [IM], subcutaneous [SC], intranasal [IN], and intravenous [IV]), which involve prolonged durations of drug effects. Inhalation sedation may be the most appropriate technique for this type of patient. If full-mouth treatment is necessary (e.g., nursing bottle syndrome), the use of IV deep sedation or general anesthesia might be considered.

Patient cooperation is obviously a factor in opting to use a sedation technique. It is the opinion of most pediatric dentists that at least one and preferably two attempts at treatment should be made before the use of sedation or general anesthesia is considered. With experience, it may become quite obvious to the doctor that a patient will require sedation or general anesthesia before the initiation of any treatment. Patients who are screaming as they walk through the parking lot to the dental office are more likely to be candidates for sedation. On the other hand, the patient who sits in the dental chair and cries throughout the treatment may be manageable without the use of adjunctive drug therapy. Crying, in the absence of overt disruptive behavior, may not be an indication for the administration of sedative drugs.

Parental attitudes must be taken into account when considering the use of sedation. Unfortunately, the use of sedation in dentistry has periodically received negative publicity, a factor that has conditioned some parents against the use of these techniques in their children. The desires of the parent should always be considered when formulating the patient's treatment plan; however, the doctor must always make the final decision. Several pediatric deaths have occurred in part because of the doctor's desires to accommodate the parent's wishes that all the dental treatment be completed at one visit. The parent's ability to follow directions must be determined if the doctor is considering the administration of oral drugs to the patient at home before the appointment. When doubt exists, the child should be scheduled early, with the drug administered by the doctor in the office.[6]

Economic considerations are also of importance in determining the nature of the sedative procedure to be used. One reason for the increased use of outpatient sedation in dentistry and medicine has been the high cost (in both financial and emotional terms) of hospitalization. Outpatient procedures are usually a fraction of the cost of the same procedure performed in a hospital. If the economic status of the family is such that they are unable to afford even the minimal fee for sedation, it might be prudent not to charge the patient for the service. The cooperation of the patient and family is readily obtained, and treatment becomes less traumatic for the entire staff and the patient.

Alternative modes of treatment should be considered. Which technique of sedation is most likely to be effective in this patient? Many doctors develop the disturbing practice of using the same technique (and in some cases the same drugs and dosages) on all patients. Consideration in selection of the technique and drugs involves multiple factors, including the degree of cooperation of the patient and the patient's medical history (i.e., allergies and illnesses). There is no one technique of sedation that will be effective in all patients. Indeed, in pediatric dentistry the failure rate for sedation is considerably greater than that seen in adults. Trapp has stated that a failure rate of 20% to 40% is not unusual unless the doctor is administering general anesthesia.[7] Recent experience with pediatric sedation has demonstrated a 20% to 40% failure rate with oral sedation but a 5% failure rate with IM/IV sedation. The greater the number of techniques available to the doctor, the greater the likelihood of a successful outcome.

The preoperative physical evaluation of the child will aid in determining the technique of choice for the patient. Among the items to be determined are the presence of allergies, medications being taken by the patient, and any prior hospitalizations. Behavioral evaluation also aids in a determination of the requirement for sedation or general anesthesia. In addition, training and experience of the doctor and staff are important in determining the appropriate sedative technique. Only those techniques with which the doctor and the staff are well acquainted should be considered for use. The requirements for adequate training in each of the commonly used techniques are discussed earlier in this text.

GOALS AND TECHNIQUES

All techniques of sedation discussed in this book may be used in the pediatric patient. In addition, drug administration by the submucosal (SM) route is occasionally used in pediatric dentistry. All of these techniques are reviewed with an eye toward their applicability in the pediatric patient.

Kopel[8] has stated that sedative premedication in the pediatric patient should be used to "train" or "retrain" the patient in an understanding of dental procedures and their importance. He continues by listing the following goals of pediatric premedication:

1. To make the child cooperative and comfortable
2. To decrease anxiety for the patient
3. To decrease strain, apprehension, and excessive fatigue for the doctor and staff
4. To minimize the need for hospitalization and its attendant problems

Listed are the techniques of patient management involving drug administration that are available in pediatric dentistry. These techniques are presented in the order of their desirability, from (in my opinion) most to least desirable:

1. Inhalation sedation with nitrous oxide–oxygen (N_2O-O_2)
2. Oral sedation
3. Oral and inhalation sedation
4. IV sedation with or without inhalation sedation
5. IM and IV sedation with or without inhalation sedation
6. IM, SM, or SC injection with or without inhalation sedation
7. Use of any of the aforementioned with body and oral restraints
8. General anesthesia in the hospital

The goal sought when using sedation in the pediatric patient is the same as with the adult: to use the most controllable and least profound technique that provides the desired goal.

Once a sedation technique is selected for the pediatric patient, the next task is to determine the appropriate dosage of the drug(s). Physiologic functions in children may vary considerably from those same functions in the older patient. The metabolic rate is increased in the younger patient. Conversely, enzyme systems responsible for the biotransformation of specific drugs may not yet be fully functional in certain younger patients. This factor and others lead to the increased possibility of higher blood levels developing when pediatric drug dosages are simply calculated from the adult dosage forms commonly supplied with drugs. Instances of morbidity and mortality have been reported in which drug doses within acceptable adult limits were administered to children.

There is no simple answer to the question of proper drug dosage. Many factors act to complicate drug selection and drug action in children. In addition, the desired level of drug action varies considerably from patient to patient and from doctor to doctor. The most reliable factor in predicting adequate drug effect is a patient's previous clinical experience with the drug in question. Once a drug has been administered to a patient, subsequent dosages can be modified according to this initial response. This is termed *titration by appointment.*[5] Although previous clinical experience can provide guidelines leading to safer and more effective drug administration, it is still necessary to determine a safe and effective drug dose for a first appointment.

Many drug package inserts provide prescribing information concerning pediatric dosages. However, many drugs introduced for the management of pain and anxiety in recent years have not undergone adequate clinical trials in children to permit recommendations concerning pediatric dosage. Conversely, many of these drugs provide only adult dosage forms or indicate that "information [in children] is inadequate to establish dosage." Wilson,[9] in a review of the 1963 *Physicians' Desk Reference,* found that 62% of listed drugs were not indicated for pediatric use, whereas an additional 16% were without recommendation for pediatric dosage. This number has steadily increased in recent years.

In those instances in which pediatric dosages were indicated, the dosages were those used in normal, nonstressful environments. Administration of this dosage form, although adequate to help a child to fall asleep at home, often proves to be entirely inadequate for sedation in a stressful environment such as the dental office. Most package inserts and pharmacology textbooks indicate the usual, nondental dosage of a drug. Pediatric dentistry texts should be consulted for appropriate dental treatment doses of these drugs.

Various factors govern the determination of drug dosages for children. These are generalizations, with exceptions to be anticipated:

1. *Age of the child:* In general, the older the child, the larger the dosage required to achieve the desired clinical action.
2. *Weight of the child:* This is very often used as the major factor in determining pediatric drug dosages, especially for parenterally administered drugs. In pediatric drug administration, more and more drugs are being prescribed in terms of body surface area, a factor thought to be a more reliable guide to drug dose than body weight.
3. *Mental attitude of the child:* The greater the degree of anxiety and fear, the larger the dose of drug(s) required.
4. *Level of sedation desired:* The individual doctor will seek to achieve ideal sedation in a given patient. However, the definition of ideal sedation varies considerably. To some doctors, ideal sedation exists only if a patient makes no movement or sound during treatment (i.e., deep sedation); others consider sedation ideal if the planned treatment can be completed in a more relaxed atmosphere (for the staff and patient), even with occasional movement and verbalization from the patient (i.e., conscious sedation). Light levels of conscious sedation may prove appropriate for the mildly apprehensive older child, whereas deep sedation may be required for the precooperative younger patient.
5. *Physical activity of the child:* The hyperactive, overly responsive child commonly requires increased drug dosages.
6. *Contents of the stomach:* Following oral administration, the presence of food in the stomach greatly influences the rate of drug absorption of some drugs into the cardiovascular system.
7. *Time of day:* Larger doses of drugs are required for sedation early in the day, when the patient is fresh and alert; lower doses are in order later in the day, when the patient is more fatigued.
8. *Ability to titrate:* When possible, drugs should be titrated. The ability to titrate eliminates guesswork from the calculation of the appropriate drug dosage for a patient. The two techniques of drug administration that permit titration, IV and inhalation, are increasingly popular in pediatric dentistry. Oral, IM, IN, and SM administration do not permit titration.

Formulas, such as Young's rule and Clark's rule, have been suggested as aids in determining pediatric drug dosages as a fraction of the adult dose. The success of such rules is haphazard at best and cannot be recommended.

Young's rule:

$$\frac{\text{Age of patient}}{\text{Age + 12}} = \text{Fraction of adult dose for children}$$

Clark's rule:

$$\frac{\text{Weight in pounds}}{150} \text{ or } \frac{\text{Weight in kilograms}}{70}$$

$$= \text{Fraction of adult dose for children}$$

Although age and weight are often used in determining pediatric drug dosage, they present certain problems. Because of significant variation in size among children of the same age, this factor (age) ought not be of primary consideration. Body weight is more commonly used in pediatric dose determination; however, the dose of many drugs is not always a simple linear function of body weight, and to calculate dosages as milligrams per pound or per kilogram leads to inaccuracies. Surface area, rather than body weight, has been shown to be a more accurate method of determining drug dosage for a patient. Unfortunately, manufacturers of virtually all drugs marketed today still present dosage recommendations in other units (e.g., mg/kg or mg/lb of body weight).

MONITORING

Monitoring of the sedated patient is discussed in Chapter 5. As important as monitoring is for all sedated patients, in the pediatric patient monitoring is possibly of even greater importance. Because of the relative lack of communication available between the doctor and the very young, precooperative or the handicapped patient, one of the most important means of communication—verbal—is often not present. In addition, because of the inability to titrate drugs administered orally, intramuscularly, or intranasally, the possibility of a relative overdose developing is somewhat enhanced. Constant monitoring of the patient is essential.

Baseline vital signs (blood pressure, heart rate and rhythm, and respiratory rate) should be recorded before treatment if the patient is cooperative. In the younger, precooperative patient, this often is not possible. Until the child has been sedated, it may be physically impossible to monitor the vital signs; however, while the child is screaming, yelling, and moving around, monitoring is actually being done by simply watching the child's reactions. As soon as the child becomes quiet (sedated), more objective monitoring must be initiated. Vital signs must be recorded and a pretracheal stethoscope placed in position and respirations monitored throughout the procedure.

The pretracheal stethoscope is probably the most valuable piece of monitoring equipment available (and the least expensive). With it the doctor is able to monitor continuously both breath sounds and, in many cases, heart sounds. The value of the pretracheal stethoscope cannot be overestimated.

Monitoring of breath sounds in the pediatric patient is of great value because the vast majority of complications seen in sedation of younger patients are associated with respiratory depression or airway management problems. Decreased or altered breath sounds or a slowed rate of breathing should alert the doctor to evaluate the patient's airway and respiratory status. Most cardiac problems in pediatric patients develop secondary to respiratory distress. Recommended monitoring for pediatric sedation includes the following:

1. Preoperative vital signs (if possible)
2. Vital signs periodically during treatment (recorded every 5 to 15 minutes)
   a. Heart rate and rhythm, monitored continuously
   b. Blood pressure, monitored every 5 minutes
3. Pretracheal stethoscope
4. Pulse oximetry

Optional monitoring for the pediatric patient includes the following:

1. End-tidal carbon dioxide ($ETCO_2$) monitoring
2. Electrocardiograph (ECG)

Supplemental O_2 or N_2O-O_2 administration via nasal hood or cannula is recommended for all pediatric sedation cases in which the patient tolerates it. Table 35-1 summarizes pediatric monitoring recommendations.

PHYSICAL RESTRAINT

It occasionally may become necessary to use physical restraints to treat the patient properly. Bed sheets may be tied around the patient and then secured with wide adhesive tape to provide restraint. Velcro strips and ties are also available. Parental informed consent *must* be obtained before any form of physical restraint is used in the pediatric patient. Use without prior consent has led to charges of assault and battery being filed against the doctor.[10]

Two devices are available and popular in pediatric dentistry. The Pedi-Wrap (Clark Associates, Inc., Worcester, Mass.) (Figure 35-1) is similar to the bed sheet but uses Velcro strips to secure the material. It is made of a netlike material that enables the patient to remain somewhat cooler while being restrained. Because the Pedi-Wrap is somewhat like a blanket, some children quiet down once secured in it. The Papoose Board (Olympic Medical Corporation, Seattle, Wash.) (Figure 35-2) is quite effective in restraining the head, torso, and upper limbs.

TABLE 35-1 Recommended Monitoring for Pediatric Patients

Monitor	Local Anesthesia			Technique: Oral			Technique: IM/SM			Technique: Inhalation			Technique: IV			General Anesthesia: Outpatient			General Anesthesia: Inpatient		
	Pr	*In*	*Po*	*Pr*	*In*	*Po*	*Pr*	*In*	*Po*	*Pr*	*In*	*Po*	*Pr*	*In*	*Po*	*Pr*	*In*	*Po*	*Pr*	*In*	*Po*
Heart rate[a]	**	0	*	**	**	**	**	**	**	**	**	**	**	**	**	**	**	**	**	**	**
					Cont.			Cont.			Cont.			Cont.			Cont.			Cont.	
Blood pressure[b]	**	*	*	**	**	**	**	**	**	**	**	**	**	**	**	**	**	**	**	**	**
					q15min			q15min			q15min			q5min			q5min			q5min	
Electrocardiograph (ECG)[c]	0	0	0	0	0	0	*	*	0	0	0	0	*	*	*	**	**	**	**	**	**
Respiration[d]	**	0	0	**	**	**	**	**	**	**	**	**	**	**	**	**	**	**	**	**	**
	V			V	PT		V	PT	V	V	V/PT	V	V	PT	V	V	PT	V	V	PT/E	V
Oximetry[e]	0	0	0	0	0	0	0	*	*	0	0	0	0	**	**	*	**	**	*	**	**
Temperature[f]	*	0	0	*	0	0	*	*	*	*	0	0	*	*	*	**	**	**	**	**	**

0, Not essential; ***, optional; ****, recommended; *Pr*, preoperative; *In*, intraoperative; *Po*, postoperative; *Cont.*, continuous; *V*, visual; *PT*, pretracheal stethoscope; *E*, esophageal stethoscope.

[a]Heart rate may be monitored by palpation in both the preoperative and postoperative periods; however, it is suggested that during intraoperative monitoring an electrical monitor providing a continuous reading be used. Devices such as the pulse meter, pulse oximeter, and ECG provide continuous heart rate monitoring.

[b]When blood pressure monitoring is recommended, I suggest that the blood pressure cuff be kept on the patient's arm throughout the entire procedure.

[c]By its very design the ECG provides continuous monitoring of the electrical activity of the heart as well as the heart rate.

[d]Visual implies a causal monitoring of the movements of the patient's chest for 30 to 60 seconds to obtain a respiratory rate. *PT* is the pretracheal stethoscope, providing continuous monitoring of respiratory sounds (and perhaps heart sounds as well). *E* is the esophageal stethoscope, a device inserted into the esophagus during general anesthesia that provides excellent sound quality for both heart and lung sounds.

[e]By its nature oximetry provides continuous monitoring of arterial oxygen saturation.

[f]Preoperative temperature monitoring may be done manually, but when intraoperative monitoring of body temperature is recommended, continuous monitoring is more readily accomplished with a rectal or esophageal probe.

These devices should not be wrapped too tightly, for the patient may become more agitated, but of greater importance, an overly tight wrap across the patient's chest may restrict respiratory movements that have already been somewhat compromised through the administration of central nervous system (CNS) depressants. The lower (abdominal and leg) restraints may be tightened if necessary.

The use of restraints also makes it more difficult for the doctor and assistant to monitor respiratory movements. The pretracheal stethoscope becomes even more important at these times.

MOUTH-STABILIZING DEVICES

Despite the fact that the patient has been restrained, it may still be difficult, if not impossible, for the doctor to examine and treat the patient safely and adequately. Several devices are used as aids to stabilize the mouth during treatment. Rubber bite blocks are available in a variety of sizes; when one is inserted between the teeth of the patient on the side opposite treatment, the patient may bite down onto the block but is unable to close the jaws. A long piece of dental floss should always be tied around the bite block and left outside the patient's mouth to aid in its retrieval, if necessary (Figure 35-3). A ratchet-type mouth prop (Molt prop) is also available. An advantage to the Molt prop is that the patient need open but a few millimeters for the device to be slipped between the teeth. Once in the mouth, the device can be opened to the desired level. When either device is used, the assistant should remain in contact with it to stabilize it and prevent its accidentally being dislodged.

DRUGS

Before discussing specific routes of drug administration and their use in pediatric dentistry, the drugs that are in most common use in pediatric sedation are

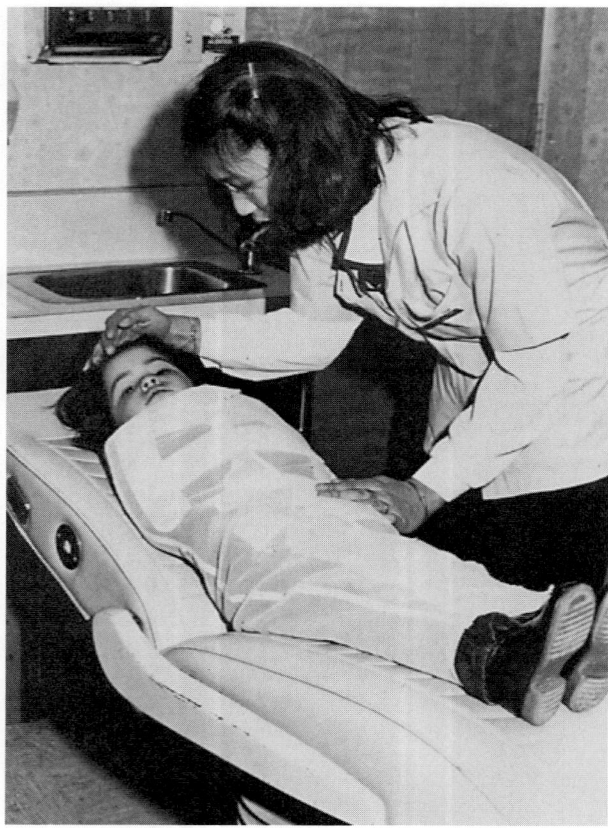

Figure 35-1 Pedi-Wrap restraint device.

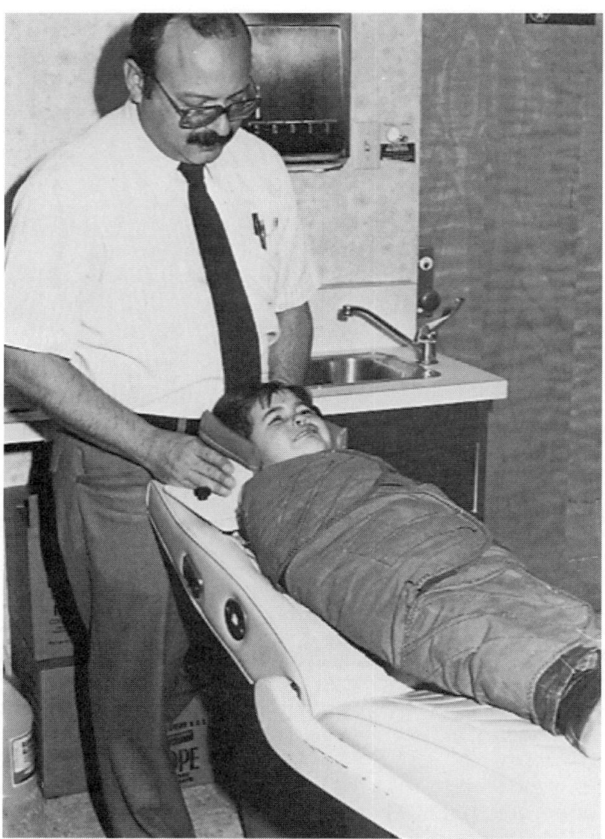

Figure 35-2 Papoose board restraint device.

listed (Table 35-2). These statistics are the results of a survey of 409 pedodontists.[11,12] Although this survey is more than 20 years old, the currently popular pediatric sedatives remain the same with only a few exceptions. Two routes of drug administration predominate, with more than 60% of the respondents indicating that they use the oral route and approximately 43% using inhalation sedation. It also becomes evident that although a variety of drugs are available for the management of anxiety, pediatric dentists and general practitioners who manage large numbers of children rely on a rather limited number of well-established drugs. Even more pronounced is the choice of drugs for combination therapy via the oral route, in which promethazine and meperidine stand virtually alone.

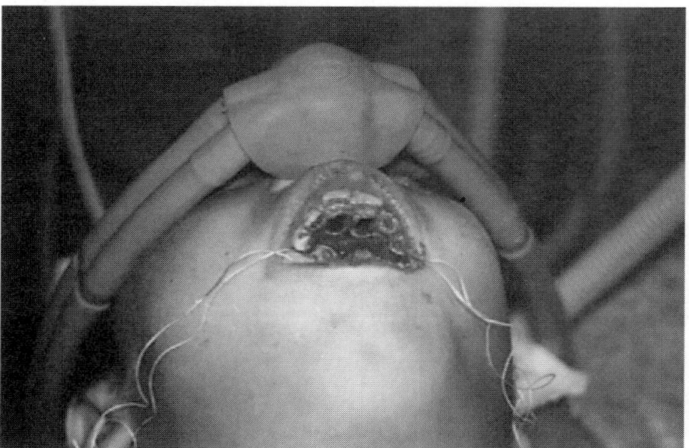

Figure 35-3 Strings of dental floss tied to two bite blocks placed into mouth of sedated patient permits their easy retrieval.

General Rules for Preoperative Medication

The usual preoperative and postoperative instructions given to the parent or guardian of children receiving drugs for the control of their dental fears are listed in Box 35-1. In addition to these instructions, Album also lists these general rules regarding the administration of sedatives to pediatric patients[13]:

1. There must be strict supervision of the patient while in the office.
2. Adequate time must be provided for the drug(s) to act.
3. A quiet environment is necessary.
4. Vital reflexes must not be impaired.
5. Drugs must not be administered during acute or chronic illness.

6. Parents must be informed of postoperative care.
7. The doctor must be familiar with side effects of medications.
8. Resuscitative equipment must be readily available.

Oral Sedation

Oral sedation is a valuable, although not entirely effective, technique in pediatric dentistry. Failure rates of up to 40% to 50% are to be expected if one is seeking conscious sedation via this route in younger children. One of its major advantages is the fact that there is no need for the use of a needle (in contrast to IM, SM, SC, and IV techniques) or of a nasal hood (as needed for inhalation sedation) to produce a clinical effect. In the past, it was common to have the parent or guardian of the patient administer the oral drug(s) at home before departing for the office. It is difficult to recommend this practice because of the numerous cases on record in which a parent has inadvertently oversedated the child, thinking perhaps that if 1 teaspoon of the drug is good, 2 or 3 teaspoons (or tablespoons) must be better.[6]

More highly recommended is the administration of the oral premedication in the dental office. The patient should be scheduled approximately 1 hour before the start of treatment and the oral drug administered by the doctor. Another consideration, when the drug has been administered in the office, is monitoring of the patient. If the office is busy, it must still be a staff member's responsibility to periodically check on the child (who is in the waiting room with his parent or guardian). In addition, a busy office environment is

TABLE 35-2 Drugs Commonly Used in Pediatric Dentistry

Proprietary Name	Approximate Percentage of Pediatric Dentists Prescribing
Agents Used Alone*	
Atarax	27
Chloral hydrate	24
Vistaril	23
Phenergan	16
Demerol	12
Valium	10
Seconal	8
Nisentil	7
Phenobarbital	5
Agents Used in Combination†	
Demerol	35
Phenergan	35
Atarax	19
Chloral hydrate	18
Vistaril	17
Nisentil	13
Thorazine	6
Seconal	5
Nembutal	5

Modified from Malamed SF. In Braham RL, Morris ME: *Textbook of pediatric dentistry.* © 1980, The Williams & Wilkins Co., Baltimore.
*Less than 5% prescribing Nembutal, Librium, Thorazine, Equanil, Miltown, pentothal, Sparine, and Trilafon.
†Less than 5% prescribing Equanil, Miltown, Valium, Sparine, pentothal, Trilafon, and Librium.

BOX 35-1 Pediatric Sedation

Preoperative Instructions

It is necessary to use sedative drugs to obtain dental care for your child. Please be aware of the following:

1. It is most important that you tell the doctor of any drug reactions, medical history, or illness and hospitalization your child has had.
2. The child must be accompanied by a parent or guardian for all appointments.
3. The first appointment will be necessary for adjustment of the proper drug dosage; therefore little dental work may be accomplished.
4. The child may remain sleepy for a time. Do not be alarmed; the drugs are "wearing off." Your child may be irritable as this occurs.
5. Do not allow the child to bit his or her lip, tongue, or cheek, if a local anesthetic has been used.
6. After dental care, your child should be under adult supervision and not be allowed to play near streets, stairways, and other areas where he or she may be injured by falling.
7. Cold drinks, such as ginger ale or colas, will help reduce any nausea and help stimulate your child become more alert.
8. Should any unusual situation arise, please call the doctor and notify him or her has soon as possible.

Modified from Kopel H: Lecture notes, AMED 750, August 1983.

not conducive to adequate sedation. A more quiet, relaxed environment is desirable during this waiting period. A quiet room, in which the patient and parent may stay, should be used for the administration of oral drugs and during the period of onset of drug action.

Younger children may not tolerate tablets and capsules well, with the parent having to fight with the child to administer the drug. Obviously, if the goal being sought is relaxation of the patient, this type of action is not recommended. Many of the drugs administered orally to children are available as an elixir or syrup, which may prove more palatable to the patient. If the child refuses to accept the liquid medication on a spoon, the drug may be administered through an irrigation syringe, the drug squirted into the buccal vestibule of the patient, not down the throat.

Drugs that have an unpleasant taste or odor may occasionally be mixed with other foods. Orange juice is commonly used; however, the addition of drugs may alter its taste. Acetaminophen (Tylenol) elixir is also commonly used to mask the taste of oral drugs. For smaller children, drugs may be mixed with applesauce, jellies, baby foods, or yogurt, although these may have an adverse effect on drug absorption from the gastrointestinal (GI) tract. Recently, midazolam elixir for oral administration has become available,[14] and fentanyl has been added to a lollipop.[15]

The drugs most frequently administered orally in pediatric dentistry are chloral hydrate, hydroxyzine, diazepam, midazolam,[16] the combination of chloral hydrate and promethazine, and meperidine in combination with chloral hydrate, hydroxyzine, diazepam, or promethazine. The pharmacology of these drugs was reviewed in Chapter 7. Pediatric use of these agents is discussed here.

Chloral Hydrate. Chloral hydrate is most effective for the very young patient and the patient with a mental or physical disability. Available orally as capsules, elixir, and rectal suppositories, it is most effective in the management of mild to moderate anxiety. The usual oral dosage form of the elixir is 500 mg/5 ml (1 teaspoon).

Initial Dosage. Chloral hydrate is administered 30 to 45 minutes before the planned appointment. The patient should have had nothing to eat or drink for 2 hours.

The dose of chloral hydrate may range from 500 to 2000 mg, with the usual range between 750 and 1500 mg (Table 35-3). The elixir forms of chloral hydrate usually contain syrups of orange or citric acid to mask its bitter taste. Because of its disagreeable taste and tendency to cause GI upset, chloral hydrate should be diluted still further with water, orange juice, or acetaminophen before being administered. Chloral hydrate must never be diluted in or added to alcohol. The duration of action of chloral hydrate is not more than 1 hour.

COMMENT: In the case of the very young child, it is suggested that a restraint such as a papoose board or a Pedi-Wrap be used during treatment.

Inhalation sedation with N_2O-O_2 may also be used as an alternative to increasing dosages of the oral drug if moderate to no success has been achieved with the original dosage. It is my belief, however, that when the first dose of a premedicating drug fails to provide the desired effect, additional doses should not be administered, nor should different drugs be given to the patient at that appointment. Rather, it is more prudent to discharge the patient and reschedule treatment for another day, reevaluating the choice of drugs and their dosage. The concept of "titration by appointment" suggests that a different dosage schedule be considered for subsequent appointments based on the response of the patient to the initial dose.

For maximum benefit to be obtained from the use of chloral hydrate, the scheduled appointment should not be longer than 1 hour. The parents of the patient should be advised of the possibility of a postoperative period of irritability or excitation as the effects of chloral hydrate wear off.

TABLE 35-3 Dose of Chloral Hydrate (to Nearest–Half-Teaspoonful)

Age (yr)	Weight (kg)	40 mg/kg	50 mg/kg	60 mg/kg	70 mg/kg
2-3	12-14	500	500-750	500-750	750-1000
3-4	14-16	500	750	750-1000	1000-1250
4-5	16-18	750	750-1000	1000-1250	1250-1500
5-6	18-21	750	1000-1250	1000-1250	1500
6-8	21-25	750-1000	1000-1250	1250-1500	1500-1750
8-10	25-30	1000-1250	1250-1500	1250-1500	1750-2000

Hydroxyzine. Hydroxyzine hydrochloride (Atarax) and hydroxyzine pamoate (Vistaril) are indicated for administration in patients who are older than 3 years, including adolescents. It is most effective in the management of very apprehensive, excited, agitated, and emotionally disturbed children. Additional indications for use of hydroxyzine include hyperactivity, autism, and severe behavioral problems.

Hydroxyzine hydrochloride is available as a syrup in 10 mg/5 ml (1 teaspoon). Hydroxyzine pamoate is available as an oral suspension as 25 mg/5 ml.

Dosage. For the nervous, apprehensive child, 50 mg should be administered 2 hours before the appointment, followed by the same dosage 1 hour before the appointment. In the hyperkinetic, agitated patient or patient with a behavioral problem, 25 mg is administered three times the day before treatment, and then 50 mg is administered 2 hours and then again 1 hour before treatment. In the less apprehensive patient, one dose of 50 to 75 mg hydroxyzine may be administered 1 hour before treatment. Another method of administering hydroxyzine is to give divided doses of the agent; for example, the patient receives 25 mg 1 hour before bed the evening preceding treatment, 25 mg on the morning of treatment, and another 25 mg 1 hour before the scheduled appointment (for an appointment between 11 AM and 1 PM). Hydroxyzine produces clinical actions within 30 to 60 minutes, with a maximal clinical duration of effective sedation between 1 and 2 hours.

Comment: Hydroxyzine is an excellent drug to give for the introduction of N_2O-O_2 to the apprehensive patient. The banana-flavored pamoate form of hydroxyzine, Vistaril, is more pleasant tasting to most patients than is the hydrochloride (vanilla flavored). Because of the relatively wide margin of safety observed with hydroxyzine, it may be used effectively with N_2O-O_2 and opioid analgesics, provided that reduced dosages of these drugs are used and that careful monitoring of the patient is maintained.

Promethazine. Promethazine (Phenergan) is most often used in combination with other drugs for preoperative sedation (e.g., chloral hydrate, hydroxyzine, meperidine). As a sole agent for sedation, promethazine is most often used to manage a child with mild anxiety. By itself it is not suitable for management of extreme apprehension or a disruptive, unmanageable child. Promethazine is available for oral administration as a tablet and syrup.

Initial Dosage. The oral dosage of promethazine is based on 1 mg/kg (Table 35-4).

TABLE 35-4 Dose of Promethazine

Age (yr)	Weight (kg)	Dose (mg)
2-3	12-14	12.5
3-4	14-16	12.5
4-5	16-18	25
5-6	18-20	25
6-8	20-25	25
8-10	25-30	37.5
10-12	30-36	37.5
12-14	36-45	50

Diazepam. Diazepam (Valium) is administered orally to the hyperactive, highly anxious, and excitable child older than 4 years. It is effective in patients with cerebral palsy, especially those with athetoid cerebral palsy, and in patients with mental retardation. Diazepam is available in tablet form and as a suspension in 5 mg/5 ml.

Initial Dosage. The initial dose of diazepam is 0.2 to 0.5 mg/kg. For the average child between the ages of 4 and 6 years, 2 to 5 mg is administered three times before treatment, with the last dose administered 1 hour before treatment. In children older than 6 years, 5 to 10 mg diazepam is administered three times before the appointment, with the last dose 1 hour before treatment. The actions of diazepam are noted within 1 hour and continue for approximately 2 hours longer.

Oral Combinations

Chloral Hydrate Plus Promethazine. Chloral hydrate is often combined with promethazine for administration to the patient younger than 3 years with rampant caries who is too young for the tell-show-do technique to be effective. Other indications for this combination are younger patients with mental or physical disabilities.

Initial Dosage. The dose for the 2- to 3-year-old patient is 1000 mg (2 teaspoons) chloral hydrate combined with 25 mg (1 teaspoon) promethazine. The dose for the 3- to 6-year-old patient is up to 1500 mg (3 teaspoons) chloral hydrate combined with 25 mg (1 teaspoon) promethazine. This combination is mixed together and then added to a fruit drink or soft drink and administered 30 to 45 minutes before the appointment. The patient should take nothing by mouth for 2 hours before its administration. Clinical effectiveness is noted within 45 minutes; maximal clinical benefit occurs at 1 hour.

COMMENT: The availability of a restraint, such as the Pedi-Wrap or Papoose Board, is recommended when managing the very young, apprehensive patient. For greatest benefit to be obtained from this combination of drugs, the maximal length of the appointment ought not to exceed 1 hour. The parents or guardian of the patient must be advised of the possibility of postoperative irritability or excitement as the drug effects wear off.

Promethazine Plus Meperidine. Meperidine (Demerol) and promethazine (Phenergan) are available as a premixed combination for both oral and parenteral administration. The combination is called Mepergan, and the oral form contains 25 mg promethazine and 50 mg meperidine. The combination is a rational one in that the opioid provides for a sedative and analgesic effect while promethazine potentiates the opioid effect and adds an antiemetic action (to counter any possible nausea produced by meperidine). Indications for the administration of this combination are (1) recalcitrant, defiant, and uncooperative behavior in children over 6 years of age who may require extensive treatment in a prolonged appointment and (2) severe mental retardation in children.

Initial Dosage. For the child weighing approximately 25 pounds (10 kg), the initial dose is 25 mg meperidine plus 12.5 mg promethazine. For the child weighing approximately 35 pounds (15 kg), the initial dose is 25 mg meperidine plus 25 mg promethazine. For the child weighing approximately 50 pounds (22 kg), the initial dose is 50 mg meperidine plus 25 mg promethazine. For ease of administration the contents of the capsule may be added to a flavored vehicle (liquid or food).

COMMENT: Opioid administration is associated with respiratory depression. The doctor should be experienced in the use of opioids, be able to recognize respiratory depression (monitoring the patient throughout the procedure), and have naloxone readily available whenever this combination is employed.

Because it is difficult to calculate the proper dosage in children when one uses a premixed combination (Mepergan), it is recommended that the doctor make the combination by simply mixing the two ingredients together in the appropriate dosages.

Parenteral Sedation

Parenteral sedation techniques in pediatric dentistry include the IM, IN, IV, and inhalation routes of drug administration. In this first section only IM and IN drug administration are discussed. Use of IM with IV and/or inhalation routes are discussed later in this chapter.

The IM and IN routes of drug administration are of greater importance in pediatric dentistry than for adult patients, primarily because of the decreased need for patient cooperation in these techniques. To administer a drug via these routes the patient merely need be restrained for a moment during the injection. As discussed in Chapters 3, 9, and 10, there are significant drawbacks to these techniques, the most significant of which is the lack of control over the ultimate drug action maintained by the doctor. Titration is not possible via these routes of drug administration; therefore the risk of oversedation is increased. Because the most commonly used drugs in these techniques have traditionally been the opioids, respiratory depression is an ever-present danger. The introduction of IM and IN midazolam has decreased this risk.

Both the IM and IN routes have equivalent onsets of action.[17] IM drug administration is popular because of its ease of administration, rapid onset of action, better absorption (than enteral routes), and greater predictability of the length of the latent period and duration of action. One disadvantage of the IM route is the patient's fear of receiving an injection. A disadvantage of IN drug administration is the potential for a burning sensation to occur in the nose with some drugs (e.g., midazolam) and a disagreeable taste if the drug should run into the patient's oropharynx. Use of an atomizer or a tuberculin syringe has been shown to minimize these problems.[18]

Monitoring of the patient receiving conscious or deep sedation via the IM or IN route is essential. The pretracheal stethoscope is an essential piece of equipment. Because these parenteral techniques are usually reserved for more difficult management problems, the use of physical restraint is required more often than not. The possibility of further respiratory embarrassment exists. Supplemental O_2 should always be administered throughout the procedure whenever IM or IN drugs are administered.

Meperidine Plus Promethazine. The combination of meperidine and promethazine, known as Mepergan, was discussed previously in the section on oral combinations. It is an effective combination for patients with severe management problems or severe mental retardation. This combination is especially recommended when procedures requiring 2 hours or more are planned.

Mepergan (Wyeth) is available in 10-ml vials and in 2-ml preloaded syringes. Each milliliter contains 25 mg meperidine and 25 mg promethazine.

Initial Dosage. The IM dose of this combination is based on 0.5 mg/lb or 1 mg/kg of body weight.

Lytic Cocktail. The combination of meperidine (Demerol), promethazine (Phenergan), and chlorpromazine (Thorazine) is termed the *lytic cocktail,* or DPT.[19] This combination has been used for many years in both pediatric dentistry and medicine. Its popularity is waning because of erratic patient responses; however, the lytic cocktail is still popular in pediatric medicine. *Clinical Practice Guideline: Acute pain management: operative or medical procedures and trauma* raises serious doubt as to the rationale for continued use of this technique.[20] The following is excepted from these guidelines:

> Exercise caution when using the mixture of meperidine (Demerol), promethazine (Phenergan), and chlorpromazine (Thorazine), also known as DPT. DPT—given intramuscularly—has been used for painful procedures. The efficacy of this mixture is poor when compared with alternative approaches, and it has been associated with a high frequency of adverse effects.[21] It is not recommended for general use and should be used only in exceptional circumstances.

The drugs are combined in one syringe and administered intramuscularly. The patient remains with his or her parent for a few minutes until becoming quiet and is then placed in the treatment environment, in a restraint. Monitoring devices are applied, supplemental O_2 and local anesthetic are administered, and the procedure is started.

Extrapyramidal reactions, especially tardive dyskinesia, are not uncommon side effects of the phenothiazines (promethazine and chlorpromazine). Should these develop, management requires the administration of diphenhydramine (see Chapter 7).

Midazolam. The water-soluble benzodiazepine midazolam has received considerable attention as an IM drug for pediatric sedation and has become the IM drug of choice in many institutions.[22] Midazolam has been used successfully intramuscularly as a sole agent for pediatric sedation, and it has been used in conjunction with IV midazolam. This technique is discussed in the section on pediatric IV sedation. The IM dose of midazolam that has been most successfully used is 0.15 to 0.2 mg/kg.[23,24] Midazolam produces a clinical effect within 10 minutes of its injection, so the patient may usually be placed in the dental chair with minimal difficulty. When it is used in conjunction with IV sedation, the duration of dental treatment is indefinite. As with all parenteral sedation techniques, monitoring is essential to patient safety.

The IN route of drug administration has received considerable interest in recent years as a technique that does not require an injection, yet provides a clinical effect equal to that achieved following IM drug administration.[17] Midazolam is one of two drugs (the other is sufentanil) that have received considerable attention via this route of administration. The IN administration of midazolam has proven to provide satisfactory sedation in a majority of cases, enabling child-parent separation to occur with minimal distress.[25] An IN dose of 0.2 mg./kg of midazolam is recommended. The drug should be administered slowly into each naris of the patient, preferably with a 1-ml tuberculin syringe (needleless) or an atomizer.[18] Once stimulation associated with dental treatment starts, IN-administered midazolam is not as effective as that by the IM route.[25]

Ketamine. Ketamine, a dissociative anesthetic most commonly used as a general anesthetic, has been administered with success in pediatric dentistry in subanesthetic doses.[26,27] When it is given intramuscularly, a dose of 3 to 7 mg/kg is administered, with an expected onset of dissociation within about 10 minutes. The patient can usually be discharged from the office within 90 minutes after the end of the procedure. It must be stated once again that ketamine should never be administered by anyone who has not been thoroughly trained in general anesthesia and in the management of the unconscious airway.

Inhalation Sedation

Inhalation sedation with N_2O-O_2 remains the most nearly ideal technique of sedation in pediatric dentistry. The advantages and indications for the administration of inhalation sedation in children are the same as for the adult patient. The major difficulties encountered with this technique in children are twofold: First, the lack of potency of N_2O-O_2 may render the technique ineffective in the management of the more apprehensive patient, and second, some children will object to the placement of the nasal hood. In most cases this second objection can be overcome by altering the usual technique of administration of N_2O-O_2 (see Chapter 15) to meet more realistically the requirements of the pediatric patient.

Dosage. The primary advantage of inhalation sedation is the ease with which it may be titrated. Concentrations of N_2O required to provide clinically adequate sedation in the child who readily accepts the nasal hood are virtually identical to those seen in adults. The overwhelming majority of children receiving N_2O-O_2 are adequately sedated at concentrations between 30% and 40% N_2O. Some patients may require less than 30%, and some few more than 40% N_2O.

Screaming and crying patients will breathe through their mouths to a much greater degree than is usual and therefore do not receive as great a volume of N_2O being delivered through the nasal hood. A means of overcoming this problem is demonstrated in Figure 35-4. The doctor removes the nasal hood from the patient's nose and holds it over the mouth so that as the child inhales he or she will receive greater volumes of N_2O. As illustrated in the figure, the patient is rather young (age 4) and has

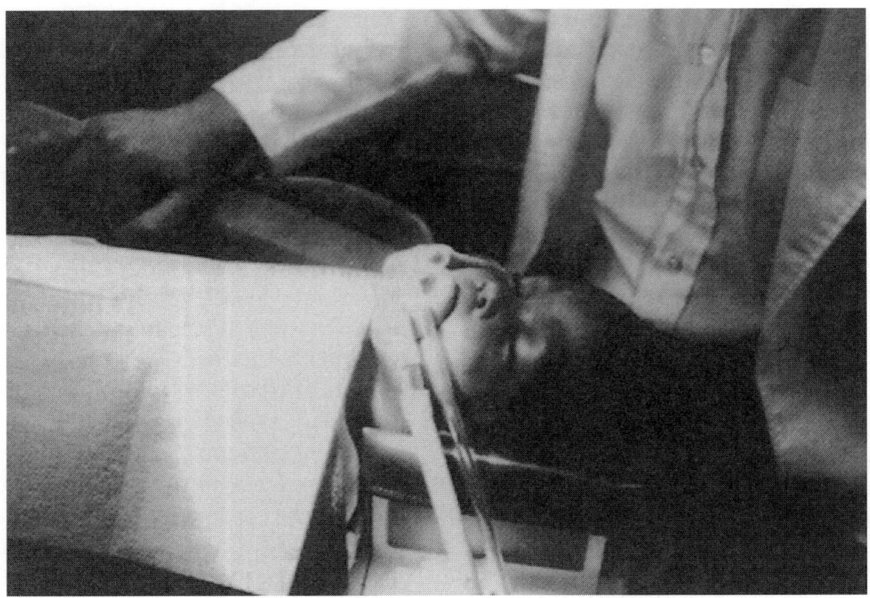

Figure 35-4 In a crying or screaming patient the nasal hood may be held over the patient's mouth, thereby increasing N_2O delivery.

been placed in a restraint. The nasal hood is held over the patient's mouth until he or she quiets down, at which time it is once again placed on the patient's nose and treatment continued. This process may need to be repeated throughout the dental treatment in some patients.

The patient who will not permit the nasal hood to be placed on the nose poses a greater problem. The following technique will, however, provide the doctor with an increased chance of success. With the child restrained, the nasal hood is placed as close to the child's face as is practical. The concentration of N_2O is maximal (70%), with a high-flow rate (10 to 15 L/min). The patient may be attempting to move his or her face away from the nasal hood and be crying or screaming; however, the patient will be receiving a high concentration of N_2O (not 70% because of air dilution) at this time. The nasal hood should be maintained close to, but not on, the face for a few moments until the child quiets. The nasal hood should then be placed onto the nose. At this time, the percentage of N_2O must be lowered to approximately 25% to 30% and then titrated to an appropriate level for the patient.

One of the more unpleasant problems when N_2O-O_2 is used in pediatric patients is vomiting. Although not common, the incidence of vomiting in pediatric patients is significantly greater than that seen in adults. Two reasons for this are (1) the lack of ability of the doctor to judge the level of the patient's sedation, which may lead to oversedation, and (2) the greater tendency of children to mouth breathe. Mouth breathing decreases the volume of N_2O being inhaled and lessens the level of sedation. When the patient returns to nose breathing, the sedation level deepens. Constant fluctuation in N_2O concentration is one cause of vomiting. Two techniques are available that decrease mouth breathing. First, simplest, and most effective is the use of the rubber dam. I strongly recommend its application whenever inhalation sedation (or for that matter any sedative technique) is used. It prevents mouth breathing almost entirely. Another method, used in the absence of a rubber dam, is to tell the mouth-breathing patient that some "special water" is being placed into the mouth and that he or she cannot swallow it. A small volume of water from the air-water syringe should be placed into the patient's mouth. To keep the water in the mouth, the patient will have to raise his or her tongue to the roof of the mouth, thereby eliminating mouth breathing.

Several methods of determining a younger patient's level of sedation are available. The first may be used with a patient who is somewhat cooperative and is able and willing to communicate with the doctor. The younger child may be unable to understand the terms usually used to describe the sensations associated with N_2O for the adult patient. The doctor will have to come to the level of the child's understanding. Playing a game with the child is an effective means of determining the level of sedation. The child pretends to be an astronaut, and the nasal hood is the space mask. As the child inhales through this space mask, the "astronaut" will begin to float in space. Questioning the child about his or her feelings can help determine the level of sedation (i.e., floating).

The second technique is used in situations in which the apprehensive child is less communicative. Titration of the N_2O-O_2 continues at the usual rate, the doctor observing the degree of tension in the patient's body. Watching and touching the patient's hands provides an excellent gauge of the level of sedation. It can be expected that the patient's hands will become more relaxed as sedation increases. The eyelids of the patient begin to close, and the patient may yawn occasionally. When the doctor believes that the patient is adequately sedated, treatment is attempted. Changes in N_2O-O_2 concentrations are based on the patient's response or lack of response to this treatment.

Nitrous Oxide–Oxygen with Other Techniques

N_2O-O_2 is often added to other techniques of sedation to increase their effectiveness. As discussed in Chapter 28, I believe that there is potential risk involved in this procedure if used by the inexperienced doctor who is not trained in recognizing unconsciousness and in airway management. When adequate operating room and outpatient conscious and deep sedation experience and training have been received (e.g., pediatric dentistry residency, general practice residency, anesthesiology residency), the combinations of oral plus inhalation sedation; IM or IN plus inhalation sedation; or IM and IV plus inhalation sedation may be used safely. Adequate monitoring of the patient, especially of the respiratory system, is essential. N_2O-O_2 must always be titrated; fixed concentrations should never be administered to all patients because not all patients react in the same manner.

Intravenous Sedation

Traditionally, the IV route has seldom been used in the management of pediatric dental or medical patients. Although this technique of drug administration is the most reliable and, when used as described, the safest, its use is seldom taught in pediatric dentistry training programs.

Because of the problems that have been associated with the administration of IM/SC/SM opioids in past years, alternative agents and techniques have been vigorously sought. With the introduction of midazolam into clinical use, a new group of drugs, the benzodiazepines, is now being used for IM/IN sedation in pediatrics.

When administered via these routes, these drugs have a fixed, somewhat short duration of clinical action (<1 hour). It was our thought to combine the administration of IM or IN midazolam (for initial patient management) with IV midazolam or other IV drugs (for continued patient management) in pediatric dental patients.

The technique for IV deep sedation is briefly described. Following a pretreatment visit at which the patient is thoroughly evaluated (medically, dentally, and psychologically) for suitability for sedation and after presedation instructions are given to the parent or guardian, the patient is brought to the dental office.

Pretreatment instructions include the necessity of taking nothing by mouth (being NPO) for a minimum of 4 to 6 hours before treatment, although smaller children require shorter NPO periods to prevent dehydration.

In a quiet room, with the lights turned down, the IM or IN dose of midazolam (usually 0.2 mg/kg) is administered to the patient (IM, lateral aspect of thigh) while he or she is being held in the parent's arms. A pulse oximeter probe is immediately placed on the patient's toe or finger, and the patient is left with the parent for approximately 10 minutes. The patient is monitored continuously (via pulse oximetry) during this induction period.

At 10 minutes the patient is placed into the dental chair, enveloped in a physical restraint, and inhalation sedation added (30% to 50% N_2O). The patient is usually somewhat cooperative but perhaps not relaxed enough to permit the dental treatment to commence. A venipuncture is performed in every patient, a continuous IV infusion (D_5W with pediatric infusion set) is established, and monitors are placed. These include the pretracheal stethoscope, ECG, and vital signs monitor in addition to the already placed pulse oximeter. Guidelines for parenteral sedation at the University of Southern California School of Dentistry (see Box 5-1) require the use of two continuous monitors at all times during pediatric parenteral sedation.

If possible, dental treatment is started at this time. However, in most situations the patient is not yet cooperative as the stimulation of treatment starts. Small incremental doses (0.5 to 1 mg) of midazolam or other IV drugs are added until the desired level of sedation is reached through titration. At this point, local anesthesia is administered and dental treatment can be started. If at a later time additional sedation is desired, additional doses of IV drugs are administered intravenously.

Meperidine is occasionally administered to these patients to aid in sedation and when a degree of analgesia is desirable at the conclusion of the dental procedure. Doses of 5 to 10 mg are administered intravenously as needed.

Propofol has been used during pediatric IV deep sedation when a rapid onset of short-duration sedation is required. In this manner propofol is being used as methohexital was during surgical procedures. Immediately (20 to 30 seconds) before the administration of a palatal local anesthetic, a dose of 5 to 10 mg of propofol is injected as a bolus. In addition, propofol is being administered toward the end of the procedure when the patient begins to get too light and movements interfere with the completion of the treatment. Increments of 10 mg of propofol enable the procedure to be completed successfully without prolonging the recovery period.

At the completion of treatment, the patient receives 100% O_2, the lights in the room are turned on, and the dental chair is positioned to make the patient somewhat uncomfortable. Our goal at this time is to arouse the patient and hasten his or her recovery and discharge. Monitoring is continued throughout the recovery period. When recovery is deemed adequate, the patient is dismissed in the custody of a parent or guardian. A telephone call to the family that evening to inquire as to the patient's status is mandated.

This technique should be used only by persons well versed in deep sedation, general anesthesia, and airway management. When deep sedation is used, a second individual should be solely responsible for the sedation while another does the required dentistry.

Using this technique of IM/IV and inhalation sedation, we have been able to manage the dental needs of patients ranging from 18 months to 10 years of age.

DISCHARGE FROM THE OFFICE

Pediatric patients who have received sedation may not be discharged from the office until the doctor is convinced that they have recovered adequately. The following are subjective discharge criteria for the pediatric patient:

1. The patient must be able to stand up and respond rationally to questioning and stimulation. If the child is unable to walk alone or must be carried, he or she should not be released from the office.
2. The patient's vital signs (blood pressure, heart rate and rhythm, respiratory rate, and O_2 saturation) must be stable.
3. In any situation in which the parent or guardian insists on taking the child before the doctor considers the patient adequately recovered, this must be immediately noted in the patient's chart, and it must be countersigned by a second person who is present. It is the doctor who must be the final judge of the patient's ability to be discharged safely from the office. Until such time, the patient should remain in the recovery area of the office. Figure 35-5 presents a list of objective criteria for discharge of the postsedation patient.

The following should be completed when considering the discharge of a patient following parenteral sedation. The patient postsedation score must be approximately equal to the baseline (presedation) score.

Patient's name: SSN: Date:

Physical Signs	(Pretreatment)	Baseline/Discharge Comments
A. MOVEMENT 2—able to walk (when appropriate) 1—able to move extremities 0—unable to move any extremity		
B. RESPIRATIONS 2—able to breathe deeply and cough 1—limited respiratory effort 0—no spontaneous respiratory effort		
C. CIRCULATION 2—systolic BP ±20% baseline level 1—systolic BP ±40% baseline level 0—systolic BP >±40% baseline level		
D. CONSCIOUSNESS 2—full alertness seen in ability to answer questions qppropriately 1—aroused when called by name 0—unresponsive to verbal stimulation		
E. COLOR 2—normal skin color and appearance 1—any alteration in skin color 0—frank cyanosis or extreme pale		
TOTAL SCORE: Dr's signature:		

Figure 35-5 Parenteral sedation discharge criteria. (Modified from *Guidelines for the use of parenteral sedation*, Los Angeles, 1991, The University of Southern California School of Dentistry.)

PEDIATRIC DENTISTRY OUTPATIENT SEDATION RECORD

Appendix 1

Date: ____ Sex: ____ Service Location: ____
Weight: ____ lb. Height: ____ ft. ____ in. Operating Dentist: ____
____ kg. Age: ____ yr. ____ mo. Assistant: ____
Hct: ____ % UA: ____ Anesthetist: ____
Preoperative Health Evaluation: ____
____ ASA 1 2 3 4 5 E
Preoperative Behavior Evaluation: ____
Frankl Scale: definitely + ☐, + ☐, − ☐, definitely − ☐
North Carolina Scale: Hands ☐, Legs ☐, Crying ☐, Physical resistance ☐
Reason for Sedation: ____
Preoperative Enternal Sedation Medication:
Drug: ____ Route: ____ dose (mg): ____ time: ____
Drug: ____ Route: ____ dose (mg): ____ time: ____
I.V.: arm ☐ hand ☐ foot ☐ foot ☐ R ☐ L ☐ B.P. Cuff ☐ P.C. Steth. ☐ Temp. Probe ☐
Other Monitoring Devices: ____

TIME																
Respiration rate/min.																
Pulse rate/min.																
Blood Pressure	S															
	D															
2% Xylo____ epi.	mg															
N_2O - O_2 (% Nitrous)	mg															
Alphaprodine (Nisentil)	mg															
Hydroxyzine (Vistaril)	mg															
Promethazine (Phenergan)	mg															
Diazapam (Valium)	mg															
Naloxone (Narcan)	mg															

Airway Support Needed ☐ Fluids: ____ Temp. preop.: ____ postop.: ____
Sedation Course: ____

Level of Sedation: ☐ Unconscious/unresponsive ☐ Heavily sedated/slightly passive
☐ Lightly sedated/moderately responsive ☐ Alert/very responsive
Behavior During Treatment: definitely + ☐, + ☐, − ☐, definitely − ☐
Treatment: Time started ____ Time completed ____ Elapsed time ____ hr. ____ min.
Services Provided: ____
Postoperative Course and Evaluation: ____
Disposition: ____
Time of Discharge: ____ Signature: ____

Patient Identification
#
Name
DOB

A

Figure 35-6 **A** and **B,** Pediatric sedation records. (**A,** Modified from Troutman KC: *Pediatr Dent* 4[special issue 1]:207, 1982.)

Continued

RECORDKEEPING

As with the adult patient, sedation records must be maintained for the pediatric patient. An example of one such form was presented in Chapter 26. Two other forms are shown in Figure 35-6.

GENERAL ANESTHESIA

Approximately 2% to 5% of pediatric patients will require general anesthesia for their dental care to be successfully completed. Dummett[28] lists the following indications for the administration of general anesthesia to the pediatric patient:

PEDIATRIC DENTISTRY OUTPATIENT SEDATION RECORD

Patient: ____________ Date: ________ Service Location: ____________

Student: ____________ # ___ Weight: ______ lb. ______ kg. Age: ______ yrs. ______ mo.

Faculty: ____________ Preoperative Health: ____________

Preoperative Behavior: Definitely pos. _____ Positive _____ Negative _____ Definitely neg. _____

(√) Reason for Medication: Immature _____ Apprehensive _____ Hysterical _____ Uncooperative _____
Fearful _____ Language _____ Retardation _____ Hyperactive _____ Other ____________

Medical Problem (specify) ____________

Preoperative Medication Drug ____________ Route ________ Dosage(mg) ________ Time ________
Drug ____________ Route ________ Dosage(mg) ________ Time ________

(√) Monitoring Devices: P.C. Steth. ________ B.P. Cuff ________ Temp. Probe ________
Other ____________

Vital Signs:

	Premed.	Before tx.	After tx.	Dismissal
Respiration rate/min.				
Pulse rate/min.				
Blood Pressure	S D	S D	S D	S D

Medication Administered:

	Dosage (mg)	Route (√): Oral	IM	SC	SM	Time Adminis.
2% Xylo _______ epi mg						
N_2O-O_2 (% Nitrous)						
Alphaprodine (Nisentil) mg						
Hydroxyzine (Vistaril) mg						
Promethazine (Phenergan) mg						
Diazapam (Valium) mg						
Chloral Hydrate (Noctec) mg						
Mereridine (Demerol) mg						
Naloxone (Narcan) mg						
Other ____________ mg						

Restraints: Yes _____ No _____ Papoose _____ Other ____________

(√) Level of Sedation: Unconscious/unresponsive _____ Heavily sedated/slightly passive _____
Lightly sedated/moderately responsive _____ Alert/very responsive _____

Airway support _____ Fluids _____ Temp. _____

(√) Side Effects: Nausea _____ Dizziness _____ Vomiting _____ Headache _____ Other ____________

(√) Behavior During tx.: Definitely pos. _____ Positive _____ Negative _____ Definitely neg. _____

Treatment time: Start ________ Completed ________ Elapsed time ________ hr. ________ min.

Services Provided: ____________ Efficiency of Med.: _____ good _____ fair _____ poor _____

(√) Next Visit: Same drug _____ Same dosage _____ Other drug ____________ No drug _____

(√) Discharge Evaluation: Unconscious _____ Drowsy _____ Alert _____ Time of discharge ____________ a.m./p.m.

Student Signature ____________

Faculty Signature ____________

B

Figure 35-6 cont'd For legend see p. 541.

1. Extensive dental needs in uncooperative children who resist all means of conventional management procedures, including premedication and restraints
2. Extensive dental needs in the young, immature, and precommunicative child whose behavior deters dental treatment
3. Multiple pulpally involved teeth in a child with cardiac disease where immediate treatment is indicated for the sake of the child's health
4. Extensive dental needs in patients with severely physical or sensorial disabilities (e.g., deafness and blindness), with whom communication cannot be achieved
5. Extensive dental needs in children with blood dyscrasias who may need transfusions
6. Extensive dental needs in children with mental retardation whose behavior deters dental treatment and impairs dentist-patient communication

As mentioned, before a decision is reached to use general anesthesia to complete treatment, at least two attempts should be made to treat the patient in the office using sedation techniques. Sedation combined with local anesthesia is a highly effective means of managing most patients. When attempts using these procedures have been unsuccessful and signs of progressive improvement in behavior and cooperation have not been demonstrated, general anesthesia should be considered.

Pediatric general anesthesia may be administered in one of three settings: in the dental office, in the hospital or outpatient surgical center as a day admission, or on an inpatient basis in the hospital. For the healthy American Society of Anesthesiologists (ASA) I pediatric patient, the potential trauma of separation from the parent in the strange environment of the hospital is a strong indication for the use of either in-office or outpatient day-admission procedures. If the child is ASA II, III, or IV, hospitalization and treatment as an inpatient are recommended.

REFERENCES

1. Kimmelman BB: Management of sensitive children in a general dental practice, *J Dent Child* 31:146, 1964.
2. Lenchner V: The effect of appointment length on the behavior of the pedodontic patient and his attitude toward dentistry, *J Dent Child* 33:61, 1966.
3. Frankl SN, Shiere FR, Fogelo HR: Should the parent remain with the child in the dental operatory? *J Dent Child* 29:150, 1962.
4. Wright GZ, ed: *Behavior management in dentistry for children,* Philadelphia, 1975, WB Saunders.
5. Johnson R: Lecture notes, AMED 750, August 1983.
6. Zendell E: Chloral hydrate overdose: a case report, *Anesth Prog* 19:6, 1972.
7. Trapp LD: Sedation of children for dental treatment, *Pediatr Dent* 4:164, 1982.
8. Kopel HM: Lecture notes, AMED 750, August 1983.
9. Wilson JT: Pediatric pharmacology: who will test the drugs? *J Pediatr* 80:855, 1972.
10. American Academy of Pediatrics Committee on Child Abuse and Neglect: Behavior management of pediatric dental patients, *Pediatrics* 90:651, 1992.
11. Wright GZ, McAuley DJ: Current premedicating trends in pedodontics, *J Dent Child* 40:185, 1973.
12. Malamed SF: Pharmacology and therapeutics of anxiety and pain control. In Braham RL, Morris ME, eds: *Textbook of pediatric dentistry,* Baltimore, 1980, Williams & Wilkins.
13. Album MM: Meperidine and promethazine hydrochloride for handicapped patients, *J Dent Res* 40:1036, 1961.
14. Midazolam elixir, drug information sheet, Roche Laboratories, Nutley, NJ, 2002.
15. Harrison P: Lollipop successful in providing analgesia to children before painful procedures, *Can Med Assoc J* 145:521, 1991.
16. Vetter TR: A comparison of midazolam, diazepam, and placebo as oral anesthetic premedicants in younger children, *J Clin Anesth* 5:58, 1993.
17. de Santos P, Chabas E, Valero R et al: Comparison of intramuscular and intranasal premedication with midazolam in children, *Rev Esp Anestesiol Reanim* 38:12, 1991.
18. Dabir PA, Dummett CO, Musselman RJ et al: Assessment of intranasal administration of midazolam for conscious sedation, using an atomizer, *J Am Acad Pediatr Dent* 23:168, 2001.
19. Benusis KP, Kapaun D, Furnam LJ: Respiratory depression in a child following meperidine, promethazine and chlorpromazine premedication: report of a case, *J Dent Child* 46:50, 1979.
20. Acute Pain Management Guideline Panel: *Acute pain management: operative or medical procedures and trauma, clinical practice guideline,* AHCPR Pub. No. 92-2, Rockville, Md, 1992, Agency for Health Care Policy and Research, Public Health Service, US Department of Health and Human Services.
21. Nahata M, Clotz M, Krogg E: Adverse effects of meperidine, promethazine, and chlorpromazine for sedation in pediatric patients, *Clin Pediatr* 24:558, 1985.
22. Silvasi DL, Rosen DA, Rosen KR: Continuous intravenous midazolam infusion for sedation in the pediatric intensive care unit, *Anesth Analg* 67:286, 1988.
23. Thiessen O, Boileau S, Wahl D et al: Sedation with intranasal midazolam for endoscopy of the upper digestive tract, *Ann Fr Anesth Reanim* 10:450, 1991.
24. Malamed SF, Quinn CL, Hatch HG: Pediatric sedation with intramuscular and intravenous midazolam, *Anesth Prog* 36:155, 1989.
25. Lam C: Midazolam premedication in children: a pilot study comparing intramuscular and intranasal administration, unpublished research thesis, University of Southern California School of Dentistry, Department of Pediatric Dentistry, 2001.
26. Rosen DA, Rosen KR, Elkins TE et al: Outpatient sedation: an essential addition to gynecologic care for persons with mental retardation, *Am J Obstet Gynecol* 164:825, 1991.
27. Ketamine IM, drug information sheet, Parke-Davis.
28. Dummett CO Jr: *Guidelines for hospital admission and discharge of pedodontic patients for restorative dentistry under general anesthesia,* New Orleans, 1976, Department of Pedodontics, Louisiana State University School of Dentistry.

CHAPTER 36

The Geriatric Patient

Christine L. Quinn

CHAPTER OUTLINE

When the United States was founded, life expectancy was about 35 years. By the mid–1800s it had increased to nearly 42 years. In 1950 life expectancy jumped to 68 years. As of the year 1991 the average life expectancy was 75.5 years. The Census Bureau has projected that by the middle of the twenty-first century, more than 40% of people aged 65 can be expected to live to the age of 90. Dentists can expect to be treating increased numbers of elderly patients as the life expectancy increases and individuals maintain their natural dentition.

Classically, age 65 is considered the beginning of the geriatric period. This is an arbitrary age cutoff that is thought to originate from two independent sources, the first of which was Imperial Germany. The Bismarck government decided that they had only enough money for those 65 years of age and older. The second source was a group of English physicians who decided to care exclusively for the elderly. They decided, based on population alone, that they would have time for only those older than 65 years.[1]

The geriatric population as a group is split into three parts: young-old, ages 65-74; old, ages 75-84; and oldest-old, age 85 and older. In 1998, 12.7% of the general population was 65 and older, and 1.5 % were 85 years and older. California has the largest population numbers of people older than 65, but Florida has the distinction of being the state with the largest percentage of residents older than 65 (18.3%).[2]

It is important to remember, though, that no matter what age is chosen as the beginning of the geriatric phase, everyone ages in two ways: chronologically and biologically.[1] This makes elderly individuals a physiologically diverse group because there is no correlation of biologic age with chronologic age because of the effects of concomitant diseases.

Almost 75% of young-old persons (in 1992) who were not institutionalized considered their health to be good, very good, or excellent, compared with almost two thirds of individuals older than age 75.[3] It has been found that an individual's perceived health is very important. Persons with chronic disease were more likely to die if they considered themselves to be in poor health compared with those who believed themselves to be in good health despite the presence of chronic disease.[3] At the time of the 1990 census, individuals reaching the age of 72 years or more made up the oldest 5% of our population. By the year 2000, that age had increased to 80 years.[4]

Although more people live to advanced age, they do so with increasing illness and disability. Many have diseases such as arthritis, diabetes, osteoporosis, and senile dementia. These chronic diseases are partially responsible for the functional limitations that some elderly individuals experience. Functional limitations may include difficulty with walking, getting outside, dressing, and other activities of daily living. Individuals with mild impairments usually are living within the community. As individuals acquire more impairments, the likelihood that they will be living in a care facility increases. In fact, the active life expectancy becomes an important concept in thinking about elderly individuals. The definition of *active life expectancy* is the expected years of physical, emotional, and functional well-being.[5]

The top five causes of death in elderly individuals are heart disease, malignant neoplasms, cerebrovascular disease, pneumonia and influenza, and chronic obstructive pulmonary disease. As individuals age, heart disease accounts for a larger percentage of the deaths (about 44% of deaths in individuals aged 85 years and older).[6,7]

The aging process involves both physiologic and pathologic changes that may alter patients' ability to respond to stress, as well as their response to drug administration (Table 36-1). Changes that occur with aging include a decrease in lean body mass, an increase in body fat (more so in women), and a decrease in total body water (more so in men).[4] As a result, the geriatric patient has a smaller central compartment (decreased body water), the rapidly equilibrating compartment is smaller (decreased lean body mass), and the slowly equilibrating compartment is larger (increased body fat).[4] The overall effect is that when a medication is given intravenously, there will be higher peak concentration because of the smaller central compartment. The volume of distribution should also be increased because of the body fat increases, and there may also be a longer duration of drug effect.[4] The question now is whether geriatric patients really have changes in their pharmacodynamics, or is it that there are changes in the early-phase pharmacokinetics that make the elderly patient seem more sensitive to medications?[8]

Adverse drug interactions are more common in elderly patients than in younger patients. The reason is that geriatric patients take medication to control the symptoms of age-related diseases. Approximately half of adults aged 75 years or older take at least two different prescription medications.[9]

Assessing the geriatric patient's physical status can be a challenge. Aging is a process rather than an age-related disease. Changes that are seen in all elderly patients, that are a function of altered tissue and organ system structure and function, represent aging, whereas changes occurring in tissue and organ system function that are not seen in all members of that population are probably age-related disease.[10] As mentioned, the aging process may alter patients' ability to respond to stress, as well as their response to drug

TABLE 36-1 Physiologic and Pathologic Changes in Geriatric Patients

Organ System	Anatomic Changes	Functional Changes
Body composition	Increased lipid fraction Loss of skeletal muscle and other components of lean body mass	Increased half-life for lipid-soluble drugs Decreased O_2 consumption, heat production, and cardiac output
Nervous system	Attrition of neurons Decreased neurotransmitter activity	Deafferentation, neurogenic atrophy, and decreased anesthetic requirement Impaired autonomic homeostasis
Cardiovascular system	Decreased arterial elasticity Ventricular hypertrophy Reduced adrenergic responsiveness	Increased impedance to ejection, widened pulse pressure Decreased maximal cardiac output
Pulmonary system	Loss of lung elastin Increased thoracic stiffness Reduced alveolar surface area	Increased residual volume Loss of vital capacity Impaired efficiency of gas exchange Increased work of breathing
Renal system	Reduced vascularity Tissue atrophy	Decreased plasma flow, glomerular filtration rate, drug clearance, and ability to handle salt and water loads
Hepatic system	Reduced tissue mass	Reduced hepatic blood flow and drug clearance

From Miller R: Effects of aging on body composition and major organ systems. In Miller R, ed: *Anesthesia*, ed 4, New York, 1994, Churchill Livingstone; and Muravchick S: Anesthesia for the elderly. In Miller R, ed: *Anesthesia*, ed 4, New York, 1994, Churchill Livingstone.

administration. It is for this reason that geriatric patients are potentially at increased risk during dental and medical procedures. An organ system approach to preoperative evaluation permits evaluation of the functional status of each major organ system, emphasizing the functional reserve of the systems most greatly affected by anesthetic medications (heart, lungs, central nervous system [CNS], and airway). Functional reserve is the difference between basal and maximum organ system function. Each individual organ system functional reserve should be evaluated by history review, laboratory data (when appropriate), and physical examination.[10]

Functional reserve is the margin that is needed to meet increased demands for cardiac output, carbon dioxide excretion, and other physiologic parameters. A patient's functional reserve declines with increasing age, no matter how fit an individual is.[10] Geriatric patients have a decreased functional reserve—their organs function at or near capacity during ordinary activities. However, when they are subjected to stress, this decrease in reserve contributes to an overall difficulty in handling a situation or illness. The organ systems most affected by anesthesia are the nervous system, the cardiovascular system, the respiratory system, the hepatic system, and the renal system.

Many physiologic and pathologic changes are encountered in the geriatric patient. A decrease in tissue elasticity is a major physiologic change that significantly affects organs throughout the body. For example, in patients 75 years of age, cerebral blood flow is 80% of what it was in patients at 30 years of age. Cardiac output has declined to 65%, renal blood flow has decreased to 45% of its volume, and hepatic blood flow has also decreased.[11] The decrease in renal perfusion has a potentially significant bearing on the actions of certain drugs, primarily those in which urinary excretion is a principal means of removing the drug and its metabolites from the body. This decrease is probably the most responsible for increased plasma drug concentrations. Drugs such as penicillin, tetracycline, and digoxin exhibit greatly increased β-half-lives.

The effect of aging on the nervous system includes cortical neuron loss and a reduction in neuron density. This does not affect daily function as much as it affects how the patient will respond to anesthetic agents and stress.[10] Brain atrophy occurs (about 30% of gross brain mass, mostly evident in the gray matter). There is also a generalized decrease in brain neurotransmitters, but there is no decrease in the affinity or density of CNS benzodiazepine receptors with age,[12] even though elderly patients seem to be more sensitive to the medication. There is some evidence that older adults may experience some cognitive dysfunction after anesthesia.[13] Autonomic functions change with age. Elevations in plasma epinephrine and norepinephrine are seen both at rest and in response to stress. This is to compensate for a reduction in responsiveness of autonomic end organs. In general the autonomic system is less self-regulated than in the younger adult. As a result, elderly patients are at greater risk for postural hypotension.

Age changes the mechanics of the heart but has little effect on the cardiac output.[4] Elderly patients develop some degree of hypertrophy but are able to maintain stroke volume by increasing preload and slightly decreasing the heart rate. The elderly heart, when compared with a young heart, is less tolerant of hypovolemia; it relies on ventricular filling to maintain the length-tension relationship to generate adequate cardiac effort.[14] This heart is more sensitive to the cardiac depressant effects of anesthetic medications. (Decrease in cardiac output associated with thiopental administration is correlated with a decreased dose requirement in elderly individuals.)[15,16]

In terms of the pulmonary system, elasticity in pulmonary tissues is lost and the intercostal muscles atrophy. The chest wall becomes less compliant as a result of fibrocalcification. In general, there is a decrease in vital capacity and an increase in residual volume.[10,17]

There is an overall decrease in clearance of anesthetic medications because of decreases in liver volume, blood flow, and intrinsic hepatic capacity. This reflects a loss of tissue mass. Anesthesia also decreases liver blood flow, so there is a reduced maintenance dose requirement with drugs that are cleared rapidly by the liver (i.e., propofol).[4]

Albumin concentration decreases with age, and β_1-acid glycoprotein increases with age. The influence of age depends on the site of plasma protein binding.[18] If a medication is highly protein bound, a decrease in albumin will result in a greater percentage of the drug being available to produce its actions. For example, diazepam is approximately 98.5% bound (1.5% free and available to exert its effect) in younger individuals. In elderly persons it is only 97% bound. This leaves twice as much diazepam available (3% versus 1.5%) to produce its clinical actions. Given the same drug dosage, the patient with diminished drug binding will exhibit more profound clinical actions. An example of this type of patient is an elderly patient who has poor nutrition.

As age increases, renal blood flow decreases because of tissue atrophy. The result is an increase in the elimination half-time of anesthetic medications that are cleared by the kidneys.[4,19]

COMMON HEALTH PROBLEMS

Some of the more commonly seen ailments and diseases of the geriatric population are discussed briefly in the following paragraphs, along with possible implications for dental treatment.

Arthritis

The arthritic patient may exhibit difficulty with positioning in the dental chair. Modification of positioning may be necessary for successful and comfortable treatment. The arthritic patient may also have decreased vital capacity because of a decrease in thoracic compliance. Drug management of arthritis commonly includes administration of salicylates, nonsteroidal antiinflammatory drugs (NSAIDs), and the newer COX-2 inhibitors.

Hypertension

Patients with hypertension are typically taking antihypertensive medications. A desirable level for blood pressure is below 140/90 mm Hg, without the patient experiencing unwanted symptoms. Side effects may be seen with all antihypertensive medications. Postural hypotension is the most commonly seen side effect, and the antihypertensive agents may accentuate this same effect produced by some of the CNS depressants used for sedation. Elderly patients are prone to hypotension even without the presence of antihypertensive medications because homeostasis is not as tightly regulated. Careful change of patient position and slow titration of sedative medications help minimize the significance of this side effect.

Heart Disease

Atherosclerotic heart disease (ASHD) is present in differing degrees in all patients older than 65 years. Heart disease is the number one cause of death in the elderly population. Possible signs and symptoms of ASHD include elevated blood pressure, irregularities in cardiac rhythm, undue fatigue, and "discomfort" in the chest on exertion. The administration of sedative medications may be indicated in these patients as a method of minimizing the development of potentially serious complications.

Angina is a common clinical manifestation of ASHD. Angina may also be seen in the post–myocardial infarction patient. This patient may be at greater risk of a medical emergency during treatment. Inhalation sedation with nitrous oxide–oxygen (N_2O-O_2) is an excellent sedative technique for this patient. Drug therapy for angina includes the administration of nitrates, which act as vasodilators. Postural hypotension may develop when these agents are administered in the management of an acute episode. Proper positioning minimizes the development of postural hypotension.

Emphysema

Emphysema is one form of chronic obstructive pulmonary disease (COPD) that may be seen in the geriatric population. Chronic exposure to pollutants (e.g., cigarette smoke, air pollution) is the most common cause of emphysema. Because the patient's respiratory reserves are quite diminished, stress reduction becomes important in patient management.

Glaucoma

Glaucoma is an abnormal accumulation of aqueous humor within the eye that leads to an increase in intraocular pressure. Patients with narrow-angle glaucoma may be treated with pilocarpine eyedrops. The medication constricts the pupils so that the aqueous humor may drain; however, when an anticholinergic medication such as atropine is administered, the iris folds back into the angle of the anterior chamber and blocks the outflow of the aqueous humor, increasing intraocular pressure. This effect usually requires larger-than-therapeutic doses of atropine (more than 1 mg). Atropine in the usual therapeutic dose (0.4 mg) is not absolutely contraindicated in these patients. Timolol, a β-adrenergic blocking agent, is used as an antiglaucoma agent. It is administered alone or in combination with other intraocular pressure–lowering agents.

MANAGEMENT OF PAIN AND ANXIETY

The need for adequate pain control during treatment is as compelling in the geriatric patient as in any other patient group. There are no specific contraindications in the geriatric patient to the administration of any local anesthetic or the use of any anesthetic technique in particular. It is, of course, incumbent on the operator to follow the American Dental Association (ADA) guidelines for the comprehensive control of anxiety and pain in dentistry, in terms of training and monitoring. These guidelines are discussed in Chapter 29. Local anesthesia drug dosages should be kept as low as possible in this age group because of the unknown degree of hepatic and renal dysfunction that may be present. The elimination half-life of the local anesthetic may be considerably prolonged, and plasma levels may remain elevated for extended periods. It is also important to be cognizant of all medications that the individual may be taking to prevent possible drug interactions. Block injections are preferred to infiltration because a smaller volume is used to achieve a wider area of anesthesia. The use of vasoconstrictors is not contraindicated in the normotensive patient or the patient with controlled hypertension. Caution should be exercised when using vasoconstrictors in the geriatric patient with untreated hypertension. The benefits should be weighed against the risk of increased heart rate, increased blood pressure, and possible dysrhythmias.[20]

The geriatric patient may also be dental phobic or noncooperative because of dementia. CNS depressant drugs may be indicated in these cases. Choice of anesthetic technique and medication depends on the severity of coexisting disease and age-related disease. The doctor must also keep in mind that the geriatric patient is more likely to develop adverse drug reactions than is the younger adult patient. The pharmacokinetics and pharmacodynamics of some medications may be profoundly influenced by age. For example, midazolam pharmacokinetics and pharmacodynamics are influenced by age. There is a 75% decrease in sedative dose from age 20 to age 90.[21,22]

Inhalation sedation with N_2O-O_2 is probably the most highly recommended technique of sedation for the geriatric patient. It offers the advantage of providing a light sedative technique with the benefits of supplemental oxygenation.

Oral sedation is indicated in geriatric patients. Age does not seem to affect absorption of oral medications. Because orally administered drugs cannot be precisely titrated, it is recommended that drugs be used in smaller dosages on the initial visit and then titrated by appointment, as necessary. Medications such as benzodiazepines and the newer nonbarbiturate sedative-hypnotics zolpidem and zaleplon are useful in managing mild anxiety. Benzodiazepines, such as oxazepam and triazolam, are indicated in the management of anxiety in the elderly patient because they are metabolized into inactive metabolites and do not have long half-lives. The newer nonbarbiturate sedative-hypnotics are chemically unrelated to benzodiazepines but work on a subset of the benzodiazepine receptor. They are both typically prescribed as sleep aids. Both of these medications have an onset of action in about 20 minutes and have relatively short half-lives. The listed half-lives for zolpidem and zaleplon are 2.5 hours and 1 hour, respectively. Barbiturates are not recommended for use because of their long duration of action and generalized CNS depressant effect. They may occasionally produce delirium in the geriatric patient. Antihistamines may also be used as antianxiety medications. See Chapter 7 for a complete discussion of the individual sedative medications.

Intramuscular (IM) sedation is generally not recommended because of the inability to titrate the medication. This technique is usually reserved for the induction of anesthesia in uncooperative patients. When required, midazolam is the medication of choice, keeping in mind the need to decrease the dose of drug in the elderly patient.

Intravenous (IV) sedation is recommended for patients with intense anxiety. Vascular access in the older patient may be more difficult because of the loss of elasticity and increase in fragility of the veins. Titration is the ultimate safeguard in IV sedation. Titration should occur even more slowly in the geriatric individual because of the pharmacokinetic changes that occur. The patient should be maintained at as light a sedative level as possible. Supplemental O_2 is recommended for all IV sedation procedures.

The use of *outpatient general anesthesia* depends on the overall health of the patient and the absence of significant systemic disease. The elderly patient with dementia is a typical patient requiring outpatient general anesthesia for dental care. This patient may be safely treated in an outpatient setting if he or she does not have significant systemic disease. It is also appropriate to consult the patient's primary care physician about the patient's overall health and presence of coexisting disease.

REFERENCES

1. Gambert SR: Aging: an overview, *Spec Care Dent* 3:147, 1983.
2. US Census Bureau: ST–98–40, *Population estimates for states by age, sex, race, and Hispanic origin*, July 1, 1998.
3. Rogers RC: Sociodemographic characteristics of long-lived and healthy individuals, *Population Dev Rev* 21:33, 1995.
4. Shafer SL: The pharmacology of anesthetic drugs in elderly patients, *Anesthesiol Clin North Am* 18:1, 2000.
5. Katz S, Branch LG, Branson MH et al: Active life expectancy, *N Engl J Med* 309:1218, 1983.
6. National Center for Health Statistics: *Health, United States, 1993*, Hyattsville, Md, 1994, Public Health Service.
7. National Center for Health Statistics: *Monthly vital statistics report*, vol 42, no. 2(S), Hyattsville, Md, 1993, Public Health Service.
8. Homer TD, Stanski DR: The effect of increasing age on thiopental disposition and anesthetic requirement, *Anesthesiology* 62:714, 1985.
9. Schecter BM, Erwin WG, Gerbino PP: The role of the pharmacist. In Abrams WB, Berkow R, eds: *The Merck manual of geriatrics*, Rahway, NJ, 1990, Merck Sharp & Dohme.
10. Muravchick S: Preoperative assessment of the elderly patient: geriatric anesthesia, *Anesthesiol Clin North Am* 18:71, 2000.
11. Stoelting RK, Dierdorf SF, McCammon RL, eds: Geriatric patients. In *Anesthesia and co-existing diseases*, ed 3, New York, 1993, Churchill Livingstone.
12. Barnhill JG, Greenblatt DJ, Miller LG et al: Kinetic and dynamic components of increased benzodiazepine sensitivity in aging animals, *J Pharmacol Exp Ther* 253:1153, 1990.
13. Moeller JT, the ISOPCD investigators: Long-term postoperative cognitive dysfunction in the elderly: ISPOCDI-1 study, *Lancet* 351:857, 1998.

14. Rooke GA: Autonomic and cardiovascular function in the geriatric patient, *Anesthesiol Clin North Am* 18:31, 2000.
15. Avram MJ, Sanghvi R, Henthorn TK et al: Determinants of thiopental induction dose requirements, *Anesth Analg* 76:10, 1993.
16. Christensen JH, Andreasen F, Jansen JA: Pharmacokinetics and pharmacodynamics of thiopentone: a comparison between young and elderly patients, *Anaesthesia* 37:398, 1982.
17. Zaugg M, Lucchinetti E: Respiratory function in the elderly, *Anesthesiol Clin North Am* 18:47, 2000.
18. Macklon AF, Barton M, James O et al: The effect of age on the pharmacokinetics of diazepam, *Clin Sci* 59:479, 1980.
19. Muravchick S: Anesthesia for the elderly. In Miller R, ed: *Anesthesiology*, ed 5, vol 2, New York, 2000, Churchill Livingstone.
20. Malamed SF: Anxiety and pain control in the older patient, *Spec Care Dent* 7:22, 1987.
21. Bell GD, Spickett GP, Reeve PA et al: Intravenous midazolam for upper gastrointestinal endoscopy: a study of 800 consecutive cases relating dose to age and sex of patient, *Br J Clin Pharmacol* 23:241, 1987.
22. Hughes MA, Glass PS, Jacobs JR: Context-sensitive half-time in multicompartment pharmacokinetic models for intravenous anesthetic drugs, *Anesthesiology* 76:334, 1992.

CHAPTER 37

The Medically Compromised Patient

CHAPTER OUTLINE

When we previously discussed the management of stress related to medical and dental treatment, it was mentioned that many patients are unable to tolerate the "usual" degree of stress related to dental therapy and, in some cases, with everyday existence. These persons usually have an underlying medical problem that limits their ability to handle stress in a normal manner. When such a patient is faced with a situation in which increased stress is present, there is an increased likelihood of this patient experiencing an acute exacerbation of the underlying disease process. Examples might include the patient with a history of coronary artery disease suffering from chest pain, the epileptic patient having a tonic-clonic seizure, or an asthmatic patient having an acute episode of bronchospasm during periods of increased stress, such as might occur during dental treatment.

Advances in medicine and pharmacotherapeutics have made it possible for more medically compromised patients to become increasingly functional to the degree that their existence is no longer limited to their home. Partially or fully ambulatory, they may now be gainfully employed and seek dental and medical care as would any other patient. These persons, however, do represent a greater degree of risk during stressful times. How then may the medically compromised patient be better managed? Reduction of stress associated with treatment is the primary goal in the successful dental management of these patients. Awareness and knowledge of the underlying disease process are essential. In this chapter disease entities that are more commonly seen in an ambulatory setting are reviewed. Following a brief description of each disease process, we list factors that tend to exacerbate it and review the methods available to successfully minimize perioperative stress in this patient.

CARDIOVASCULAR DISEASE

Cardiovascular disease ranks as the number one cause of death in the United States, United Kingdom, and other industrialized nations. It is estimated that the number of persons in the United States with signs and symptoms of cardiovascular disease exceeds 61.8 million. In 1999, 958,775 persons died from cardiovascular disease in the United States. Cancer, the second leading cause, was responsible for 549,838 deaths.[1]

Significant advances have occurred in both the surgical and pharmacologic management of many cardiovascular disorders. Patients who once suffered from extremely severe anginal pains caused by coronary artery disease are today asymptomatic as a result of coronary artery bypass and graft procedures. Newer drugs such as β-adrenergic blockers (e.g., propranolol), calcium channel blockers (e.g., verapamil, nifedipine), and angiotensin-converting enzyme (ACE) inhibitors (e.g., captopril) have enabled patients to lead more normal lives despite the continued presence of a serious cardiovascular disorder.

In view of the fact that more than 10% of the American population has signs and symptoms of clinically significant cardiovascular disease, it stands to reason that the dentist will be called on to manage the oral health needs of many cardiovascular-risk patients. Although there are many causes for the various cardiovascular diseases, there is one factor that, when present, is responsible for dramatically increasing the risk of an acute exacerbation. This is a myocardial oxygen (O_2) requirement that exceeds the supply capability of the coronary arteries. When myocardial O_2 requirements are not satisfactorily met, the patient responds with an acute exacerbation of the underlying disorder. For example, chest pain and/or dysrhythmias may develop in the patient with angina, and dyspnea will occur in the patient with congestive heart failure (CHF).

Patients at cardiovascular risk are usually able to tolerate elective and emergency dental care. Modifications in the planned dental treatment are based on the severity (American Society of Anesthesiologists [ASA] II, III, or IV) of the disease process as determined through physical evaluation of the patient (see Chapter 4). Sedation and pain control are of much greater importance in these patients than in ASA I patients. Specific details relating to the management of cardiovascular-risk patients are discussed in the following section.

Angina Pectoris

Angina pectoris is usually a result of arteriosclerotic heart disease but may occasionally occur in the absence of significant disease through coronary artery spasm, severe aortic stenosis, or aortic insufficiency. The basic mechanism involved in angina pectoris is a discrepancy between myocardial O_2 demand and O_2 delivery through the coronary arteries. Anginal pain is described as a squeezing or pressurelike pain, retrosternal or slightly to the left of the sternum, that appears suddenly during exertion and may radiate in a set pattern (Figure 37-1); it typically resolves with rest or the administration of nitrates. Patients with angina may be taking long-acting nitrates such as isosorbide dinitrate (Isordil, Sorbitrate) to prevent the occurrence of acute episodes.

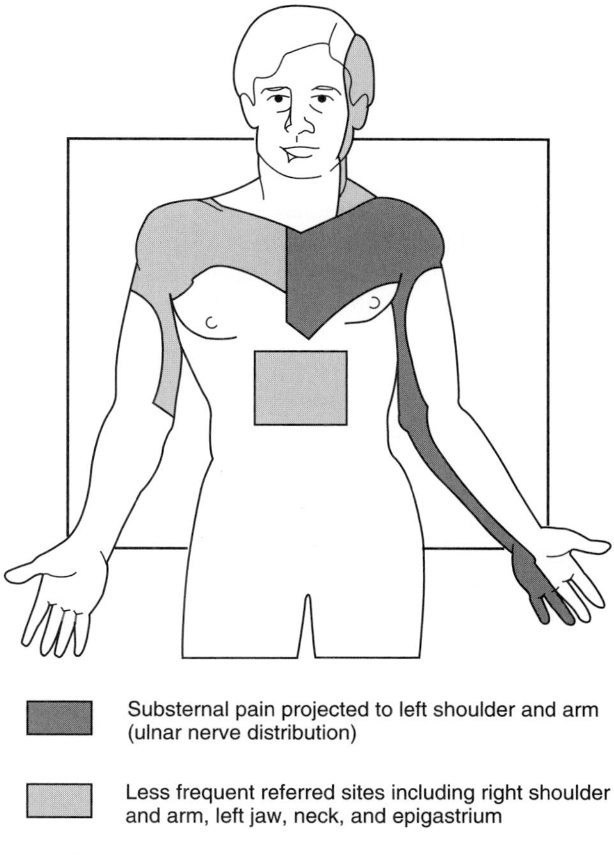

Figure 37-1 Radiation patterns of chest pain. (Redrawn from Jastak JT, Cowan FF Jr: *Dent Clin North Am* 17:363, 1973.)

Nitroglycerin is available for administration in several forms, including an intravenous (IV) form, translingual spray (Nitrolingual), transmucosal tablet, oral sustained-release form, topical ointment, transdermal patch, and the traditional sublingual tablet.[2]

The patient with stable angina represents an ASA III risk. Persons with easily managed and less frequent episodes might be classified as ASA II, and persons with daily (or more frequent) episodes or episodes that are increasing in frequency or severity (unstable angina) are categorized as ASA IV.

Factors increasing the likelihood of an acute exacerbation of anginal pain include the following:

- Physical activity
- Hot, humid environment
- Cold weather
- Large meals
- Emotional stress (e.g., argument, anxiety, sexual excitement)
- Caffeine ingestion
- Fever, anemia, thyrotoxicosis
- Cigarette smoking
- Secondhand smoke (smoke from other persons' cigarettes)
- Smog
- High altitudes

As with all patients, patients with a history of anginal pain may exhibit heightened anxiety before dental or surgical treatment. Sedation is especially indicated in these patients because of the effects of anxiety on the cardiovascular system. Increased blood levels of the catecholamines epinephrine and norepinephrine lead to an increase in the heart rate and an increase in the strength of each contraction. The net result is an increase in the O_2 requirement of the myocardium. In the presence of coronary artery disease this increased demand may not be met, resulting in an acute anginal episode. Dysrhythmias may also occur at this time. Minimizing stress and maximizing oxygenation of the patient are desired goals in preventing anginal episodes.

Oral conscious sedation is indicated. Light levels of sedation minimize possible clinically significant respiratory depression, which could induce myocardial ischemia. Although not essential, the continuous delivery of O_2 through a nasal cannula or nasal hood during treatment is recommended, especially in the ASA III or IV patient with a history of angina.

Intramuscular (IM) sedation is not usually indicated. The use of IM sedation in adult patients is rarely indicated, the IM route being used primarily in pediatric patients or adults with disabilities. Should an occasion necessitate the administration of IM sedation to a patient with angina, the level of sedation should be kept light to moderate. O_2 should be delivered via nasal cannula or nasal hood throughout the procedure and recovery period.

Inhalation sedation is highly recommended. Nitrous oxide–oxygen (N_2O-O_2) inhalation sedation is the preferred technique of sedation for patients with angina. Because anginal episodes are provoked by an unmet myocardial O_2 requirement, the administration of N_2O-O_2 serves the following beneficial purposes: (1) relaxes the patient; (2) increases the pain reaction threshold; and (3) increases oxygenation of the patient, including the myocardium. Not only does N_2O-O_2 minimize any increase in myocardial activity as a result of its sedative and analgesic properties, but also the typical patient will receive more than 50%, or at the least approximately 25%, O_2. This represents a 25% to 50% increase in O_2 delivery to the cells of the patient's body. N_2O-O_2 is the most nearly ideal sedative technique for the management of patients with angina.

IV conscious sedation is recommended for the more fearful patient with a history of angina. Levels of sedation should be kept as light as possible (e.g., diazepam or midazolam) to minimize potential respiratory depression, hypoxia, and myocardial ischemia. In addition, the patient should receive O_2 via nasal cannula or nasal hood throughout the procedure.

Elective general anesthesia is not recommended for all patients with angina. Outpatient general anesthesia in these patients is generally not indicated because of the increased risk of hypoxia during anesthesia and the inherent increased stress of general anesthesia and of the surgical procedure. Patients with angina who require general anesthesia are usually hospitalized, undergoing treatment as described earlier for inpatient procedures.

Unstable Angina

Unstable angina is also known as *intermediate coronary syndrome, preinfarction angina, premature* or *impending myocardial infarction* (MI), or *coronary insufficiency.* It is a syndrome intermediate in severity between angina pectoris and acute MI.

Because mortality from acute MI is greatest within the first hour, recognition of a syndrome that has an increased likelihood of impending MI mandates immediate hospitalization and monitoring of the patient in an intensive care unit to prevent sudden dysrhythmias and death. Many, if not most, unstable anginal patients are candidates for reperfusion therapy with either thrombolytics or primary balloon angioplasty and cardiac stent.

Unstable angina is recognized by the appearance of pain that is different in character, duration, radiation, and severity from the typical stable anginal episode or pain that, over a period of hours or days, demonstrates progressive ease of induction (decreased exercise tolerance) or that develops at rest or during sleep.

Patients with unstable angina who do not develop signs and symptoms of acute MI are considered to be in precarious balance between coronary artery supply and myocardial demand and should be managed as though they had suffered an MI.

Patients with unstable angina are considered ASA IV patients and therefore are not candidates for elective dental or surgical care. Immediate medical consultation is recommended. In the event that emergency care is required, hospitalization of the patient should be seriously considered. O_2 delivery via nasal cannula or nasal hood is recommended throughout the procedure, and N_2O-O_2 inhalation sedation is the only sedative technique recommended for this patient. Medical consultation is definitely indicated before any treatment is carried out on this very-high-risk patient.

Oral conscious sedation is indicated if absolutely necessary. Only light levels of central nervous system (CNS) depression should be sought. The administration of O_2 to this patient throughout the procedure is recommended.

IM sedation is not recommended in patients with unstable angina because of the possibility of hypotension, which further compromises coronary blood flow, and respiratory depression. Inhalation sedation is recommended because of the increased O_2 delivery to the patient throughout the procedure. IV conscious sedation is not recommended unless the occasion absolutely demands it. The possibility of hypotension and respiratory depression, although minimal, could further aggravate the precarious balance between coronary O_2 supply and demand. Lighter levels of conscious sedation, such as that seen with benzodiazepines, plus supplemental O_2 would best serve this patient.

Myocardial Infarction

MI is a clinical syndrome resulting from a deficient coronary arterial blood supply to a region of the myocardium, resulting in cellular death and necrosis. Synonyms for MI include *coronary occlusion, coronary thrombosis,* and *heart attack.*

More than 1.5 million Americans suffer acute MI annually. In 1985 ischemic heart disease and acute MI were responsible for 801,700 deaths in the United States.[3] It is the leading cause of death in the United States, responsible for 35% of deaths occurring in men between the ages of 35 and 50 years.

Patients who are status post-MI (have suffered an acute MI and survived) represent a definite risk during dental and surgical treatment. Immediately after an MI the incidence of reinfarction is high (36% reinfarction rate on surgical patients within 3 months of first MI).[4,5] With time and the formation of a myocardial scar, the incidence of reinfarction declines. Reinfarction rates fall to 16% at 5 months for post-MI patients undergoing surgical procedures and to 5% at 6 months after infarction. Reinfarction rates then level off at 5% and remain at that level indefinitely. By comparison, the risk of infarction during surgical procedures for a patient who has not had an MI is less than 0.1%.

Status post-MI patients may be receiving a number of drugs to manage post-MI complications such as CHF, angina, and dysrhythmias. Drug categories include anticoagulants, antidysrhythmics, digitalis, vasodilators (e.g., nitroglycerin), and various drugs to manage high blood pressure.

The status post-MI patient is considered an ASA III patient if more than 6 months have passed since the initial MI and no further cardiovascular complications have developed. In the event that cardiovascular complications have developed after the MI, medical consultation should be obtained. This patient is classified as either an ASA III or IV patient depending on the severity of the prior MI and the degree of cardiovascular dysfunction still present. For the 6 months immediately following the MI, the patient is considered an ASA IV patient, with all elective care deferred until a full 6 months after the infarction. In the event that emergency care is required, hospitalization should be given serious consideration.

An acute MI may be precipitated when the patient undergoes unusual stress, whether physical (pain) or emotional (anxiety). Unfortunately, the patient need not be undergoing any physical activity at the time of onset of the MI. Alpert and Braunwald[6] reported that 51% of patients were at rest and 8% were asleep when the signs and symptoms of MI initially developed. Of the patients, 18% were performing moderate or usual exertion, whereas only 13% were physically exerting themselves. It therefore appears to be more a matter of (bad) timing than a result of dental treatment when an acute MI develops in the dental office. Stress, however, does increase the risk to the status post-MI patient and must be considered.

Sedation in the status post-MI patient is extremely valuable because these patients are usually stress intolerant. Any unmet increase in myocardial O_2 demand can lead to serious complications, including anginal pain, increased severity of CHF, serious dysrhythmias, and reinfarction.

Oral conscious sedation is recommended for light levels of sedation (see Chapter 7). More profound (deep) sedation increases the risk of hypotension and respiratory depression with hypoxia. In the event that this does occur, airway management with supplemental O_2 administration is essential. IM sedation is not recommended unless other techniques are unavailable or ineffective, and then, only light to moderate sedation is indicated, with the administration of O_2 via nasal cannula or nasal hood encouraged.

Inhalation sedation is highly recommended. N_2O-O_2 inhalation sedation provides the myocardium with additional O_2 throughout the procedure. N_2O-O_2 has been used by paramedical and medical personnel for pain management during acute MI and has proved valuable in decreasing or eliminating the pain of MI.[7]

IV sedation is recommended in the post-MI patient when inhalation sedation has proved ineffective. Only lighter levels of sedation are recommended in the ASA III patient, with supplemental O_2 administered. Hospitalization is highly recommended for the ASA IV patient with angina for whom only emergency care is recommended, and then only in a controlled environment.

Both outpatient and inpatient general anesthesia for elective dental or medical procedures are relatively contraindicated in the status post-MI patient. The risk of reinfarction in this patient during general anesthesia is such that other (conscious) techniques should be attempted before considering the use of general anesthesia.

High Blood Pressure

Elevated blood pressure is not uncommon within the dental office because the stress associated with treatment leads to increased catecholamine release and subsequent elevations in heart rate and blood pressure. In Chapter 4, ASA classifications for blood pressure were presented. The two categories that must be reviewed are ASA III and IV. ASA III patients have a blood pressure of 160 to 199 mm Hg (ASA IIIa, 160 to 179 mm Hg; IIIb, 180 to 199 mm Hg) systolic and/or 95 to 115 mm Hg (IIIa, 95 to 104 mm Hg; IIIb, 105 to 115 mm Hg) diastolic. ASA III patients may receive elective dental care; however, steps should be taken to prevent any further elevation of blood pressure. Two of the most important steps are the management of pain through the effective use of local anesthesia (vasopressors are not contraindicated in the ASA III patient) and the management of fear and anxiety. ASA IV patients have a systolic blood pressure above 200 mm Hg and/or a diastolic blood pressure in excess of 115 mm Hg. Elective dental care is postponed until the blood pressure is better controlled. Emergency procedures may be performed; however, sedation and effective pain control are absolutely mandatory to prevent any further elevation in blood pressure. Hospitalization of the ASA IV patient who requires emergency dental care should be seriously considered.

Further elevation of the hypertensive patient's blood pressure may lead to a number of acute cardiovascular crises, including cerebrovascular accident (CVA; stroke), acute MI, acute renal failure, and acute heart failure (pulmonary edema). Most patients with high blood pressure are taking antihypertensive drug therapy to lower their blood pressure. Many drugs, each of which has its own side effects, are used to manage high blood pressure. The doctor must be aware of these side effects and any possible drug-drug interactions and take steps to minimize their occurrence or at least be able to manage them successfully. Table 37-1 lists the major categories of antihypertensive drugs and their more common side effects.

The primary side effects of antihypertensive drugs of concern during ambulatory patient care are orthostatic (postural) hypotension, CNS depression, and sedation. Prevention of clinically significant orthostatic hypotension requires that alterations in dental chair position occur gradually, allowing the patient to adapt to the increasing effect of gravity as the chair becomes increasingly elevated. Many CNS depressant drugs, especially opioids, enhance this effect of antihypertensive drugs. The use of CNS depressant drugs in patients who may be somewhat CNS depressed from their antihypertensive drugs must be managed with extreme care to prevent excessive sedation from occurring. Titratable techniques are, as always, preferred.

Elevations in a patient's blood pressure can be expected during dental procedures, especially those that are potentially traumatic. The stress-reduction protocols are especially valuable in these patients. Adequate pain control through the use of local anesthetics with vasopressors (if indicated) and anxiety reduction enable these patients to receive dental care with minimal risk.

In the hypertensive patient, increases in stress further elevate blood pressure. Increased blood pressure can precipitate acute medical crises. The use of sedation should minimize or eliminate blood pressure elevations and thereby decrease patient risk during treatment.

Oral conscious sedation is recommended. IM sedation is recommended. Opioid analgesics may enhance orthostatic hypotension associated with some antihypertensive drugs.

Inhalation sedation is recommended. Inhalation sedation may be used in patients in whom blood pressure readings are slightly above the ASA IV level (i.e., 206/112 mm Hg). N_2O-O_2 is titrated to the point at which the patient is comfortably relaxed. The patient's blood pressure is rechecked at this time. If it has fallen below the ASA IV level, the planned treatment may proceed; however, where the blood pressure remains in the ASA IV range (above 200/115 mm Hg), treatment should be canceled and the patient unsedated and dismissed.

IV conscious sedation is recommended. Opioid analgesics may enhance orthostatic hypotension produced by some antihypertensive drugs.

General anesthesia is indicated in ASA II or IIIa hypertensive patients for traumatic procedures in

TABLE 37-1 Side Effects and Drug Interactions of Antihypertensive Medications

Drug	Major Side Effects	Drug Interactions
ACE inhibitors	Hypotension Reversible renal insufficiency Reversible hyperkalemia	
Clonidine	Drowsiness Orthostatic hypotension Xerostomia	
Guanethidine	Orthostatic hypotension	Alcohol increases orthostatic hypotension
Hydralazine	Tachycardia Palpitation Increased angina Increased CHF	
Loop diuretics	Hypokalemia	
α-Methyldopa	Orthostatic hypotension Drowsiness Depression Xerostomia	
Potassium-sparing diuretics	Hyperkalemia Nausea (triamterene)	
Prazosin	Orthostatic hypotension with syncope Dizziness Weakness Blurred vision Nausea Headache Palpitation	
Propranolol	Bradycardia CHF Increased asthma Weakness Depression	Epinephrine may induce bradycardia
Reserpine	Drowsiness Sedation Weakness Depression Bradycardia	Hypotension with general anesthesia
Thiazide diuretics	GI upset Weakness Hypokalemia Hyperglycemia	

ACE, Angiotensin-converting enzyme; *CHF,* congestive heart failure; *GI,* gastrointestinal.

which sedative techniques are not indicated or have proved ineffective. The ASA II patient may be managed as an outpatient, whereas the ASA III and IV patient might be better managed as an inpatient.

Dysrhythmias

Myocardial rhythm disturbances are not uncommon. Fortunately, most dysrhythmias are of relatively benign nature in that the myocardium still functions effectively as a pump. However, some dysrhythmias are potentially more dangerous, requiring immediate treatment or referral to a physician.

Patients with clinically significant dysrhythmias will be receiving antidysrhythmic drugs. These drugs include quinidine, procainamide, disopyramide, flecainide, propafenone, and sotalol.[8]

In the absence of an electrocardiogram (ECG) and of training in its interpretation, the dentist is frequently unable to determine the precise nature of any dysrhythmia that might develop. Termination of dental treatment, administration of O_2, and consideration for immediate medical consultation are indicated in such cases.

Dysrhythmias may develop in patients with organic heart disease, for example, in the status post-MI patient, as well as in those with a "normal, healthy" heart. Stress, the ingestion (by the patient) of certain drugs and chemicals, or the administration (by the doctor) of certain drugs can precipitate or exacerbate cardiac dysrhythmias. Caffeine and nicotine are examples of two substances that may precipitate dysrhythmias, and several inhalation anesthetics, including halothane, sensitize the myocardium to catecholamines. Stress causes the release of significant amounts of the catecholamines epinephrine and norepinephrine into the blood, increasing myocardial work and inducing dysrhythmias.

Sedation is indicated in most patients with rhythm disturbances. Although any technique may be used, it is important that hypoxia and hypotension be avoided because of their dysrhythmogenic characteristics.

Oral sedation is recommended. IM sedation is recommended when other sedative techniques have proved ineffective. The use of supplemental O_2 delivered via nasal cannula or nasal hood is recommended when the IM route is used.

Inhalation sedation is recommended. N_2O-O_2 increases oxygenation, thereby eliminating a very common cause of dysrhythmias.

IV conscious sedation is recommended. O_2 supplementation is suggested to minimize the risk of hypoxia.

In patients in whom dysrhythmias are well controlled through the use of drugs and no other cardiovascular disease is evident, IV outpatient general anesthesia (e.g., propofol, methohexital) is a consideration, although this patient should be considered a candidate for hospitalization. ECG monitoring throughout the procedure is strongly recommended, as is administration of supplemental O_2. The administration of inhalation anesthetics such as halothane, which sensitize the myocardium to catecholamines, should be avoided, if possible. A commonly used general anesthesia technique for patients with dysrhythmias is N_2O-O_2 and IV opioids.

Local anesthesia is recommended for intraoperative and postoperative pain management. The use of vasopressor-containing local anesthetics is not contraindicated in most ASA II and III patients. Epinephrine-impregnated gingival retraction cord should be avoided in these patients. Box 37-1 lists contraindications (absolute and relative) to the inclusion of vasopressors in local anesthetic solutions.

BOX 37-1 Contraindications to Use of Vasoconstrictors

Absolute Contraindications

- Unstable angina pectoris (preinfarction angina, crescendo angina)
- Recent myocardial infarction (<6 mo)
- Recent coronary artery bypass surgery (<6 mo)
- Refractory dysrhythmias
- Untreated or uncontrolled severe hypertension (>200 and/or >115 mm Hg)
- Untreated or uncontrolled severe congenital heart failure
- Uncontrolled hyperthyroidism
- Uncontrolled diabetes
- Sulfite sensitivity
- Pheochromocytoma

Relative Contraindications

- Patients taking tricyclic antidepressants
- Patients taking phenothiazine compounds
- Patients taking monoamine oxidase inhibitors (MAOIs)
- Patients taking nonselective β-blockers
- Cocaine abuser

Modified from Perusse R, Goulet JP, Turcotte JY: *Oral Surg* 74:679, 1992.

Congestive Heart Failure

Heart failure is a pathophysiologic state in which an abnormality in cardiac function is responsible for the failure of the heart to pump blood in a volume adequate to meet the requirements of the metabolizing tissues of the body. Left-sided heart failure is associated with signs and symptoms associated with pulmonary vascular congestion; right-sided heart failure commonly exhibits signs and symptoms of systemic venous and capillary engorgement. Left- and right-sided heart failure can develop independently, or they may coexist. The term *CHF* refers to the combination of left- *and* right-sided heart failure in which there is evidence of both pulmonary and systemic congestion.

Pulmonary edema is usually an acute condition marked by excess serous fluid in the alveolar spaces or interstitial tissues of the lungs accompanied by extreme difficulty in breathing.

Heart failure may be produced by a number of etiologies, including coronary artery disease; myocarditis; hypertension; aortic or pulmonary valve stenosis; hypertrophic cardiomyopathy; aortic, mitral, or tricuspid valve insufficiency; thyrotoxicosis; anemia; pregnancy; and congenital left-to-right shunts. Heart failure is a common sequela of MI.

The annual rate of development of heart failure is 2.3 per 1000 men and 1.4 per 1000 women (Framingham study).[9] The incidence rises considerably after the age of 50 years. High blood pressure is a common precursor, with more than 75% of patients with CHF having a history of preexisting high blood pressure.

Patients with heart failure commonly take drugs to control their high blood pressure, as well as preparations of digitalis. Digitalis increases cardiac output, decreases right atrial pressure, decreases venous pressure, and increases the excretion of sodium and water.

There is considerable variation in the severity of heart failure. A commonly used method of classification of CHF is called the *functional reserve category.* Four classes are recognized, based on a patient's ability to climb a normal flight of stairs (Figure 37-2). The functional reserve classification is defined as follows:

1. Patient is able to climb a normal flight of stairs without pausing and can continue walking without resting.
2. Patient is able to climb a normal flight of stairs without pausing but must stop at the top of the stairs to catch his or her breath.
3. Patient is able to climb a normal flight of stairs but must pause before reaching the top of the stairs to catch his or her breath.
4. Patient is unable to climb a normal flight of stairs.

These numbers can be considered the ASA physical status classification for CHF.

Hypoxia or stress may increase the degree of heart failure by increasing the work of the myocardium and by increasing its oxygen requirement. The stress-reduction protocol is of considerable importance in the management of patients with CHF. Scheduling appointments early in the morning, when the patient is well rested; limiting the length of the appointment so as not to exceed the limit of the patient's tolerance; and monitoring vital signs preoperatively are recommended. If the weather becomes extremely warm or humid or if the patient appears somewhat fatigued before the start of treatment, it may be prudent to postpone the planned treatment to another day. Intraoperatively, the need for effective pain and anxiety control is quite important because increased stress produces an increased myocardial workload and an increase in the degree of heart failure.

Chair positioning of patients with CHF may require modification from that recommended for the sedated patient. Although the supine or semisupine position is strongly recommended for patients during sedative procedures, the patient with CHF may exhibit orthopnea, which precludes the use of this position. Should this occur, the patient should be placed in the most recumbent position in which he or she can still breathe comfortably.

Local anesthetics containing vasopressors *are* indicated for pain control in the patient with CHF. The recommended concentration of epinephrine is 1:100,000 or 1:200,000.

There are no contraindications to using any of the techniques of sedation in the patient with CHF. It is important to remember that the primary problem in this patient is the failure of the heart to deliver an adequate volume of blood (and O_2) to the tissues of the body. Because all sedative drugs are CNS, respiratory, and potentially cardiovascular depressants, it is essential that any additional hypoxia be prevented during the procedure. The ASA II patient with coronary heart disease is an excellent candidate for sedation with any technique, whereas the ASA III patient with CHF should be restricted to lighter levels of sedation by the oral or inhalation route.

Oral sedation is quite appropriate for the patient with CHF (ASA II or III) for preoperative anxiety control. Only light levels of sedation should be sought, such as that obtained with the benzodiazepines.

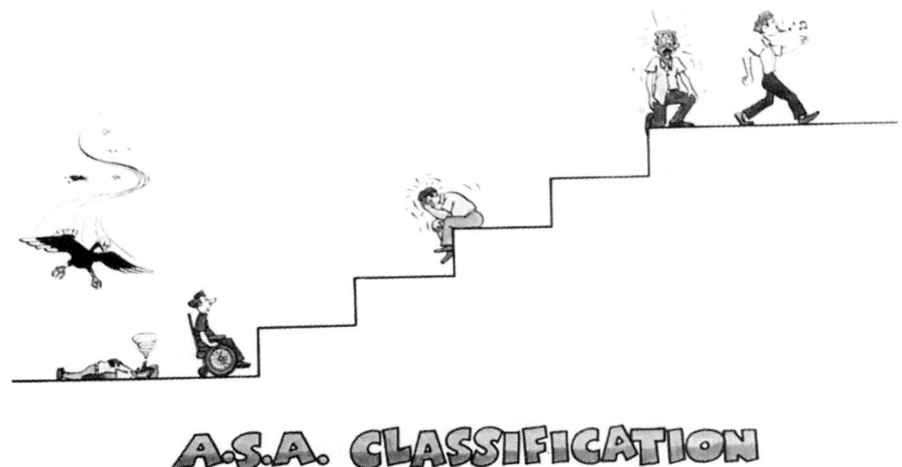

Figure 37-2 ASA classification for congestive heart failure. (Courtesy Dr. Lawrence Day.)

IM sedation should be reserved for the patient in whom other more controllable techniques have proved ineffective. Light to moderate levels of sedation may be sought, with O_2 supplementation provided throughout the procedure for the ASA II patient only. Potent respiratory depressants drugs such as opioids and barbiturates should be used with considerable care, if at all.

N_2O-O_2 inhalation sedation is an appropriate technique for the ASA II or III patient with CHF because it provides sedation and analgesia, as well as additional O_2 for the patient.

Light to moderate levels of IV sedation are recommended for the ASA II patient with CHF. Supplemental O_2 is recommended for all IV sedative procedures. The use of IV sedation is not recommended for use in the ASA III patient with CHF unless it is considered essential by the doctor, in which case only lighter levels of conscious sedation are recommended (with O_2 supplementation).

Outpatient general anesthesia is not usually recommended for the ASA II, III, or IV patient with CHF. In-hospital general anesthesia should be considered when other sedative techniques have proved inadequate in patient management.

BOX 37-2 Congenital Heart Lesions

Acyanotic Heart Lesions with Left-to-Right Shunts
Ostium secundum atrial septal defects
Anomalous pulmonary venous return
Endocardial cushion defects
Ostium primum atrial septal defect
Atrioventricular canal
Ventricular septal defects
Patent ductus arteriosus
Aorticopulmonary window and truncus arteriosus

Acyanotic Heart Disease with Obstructive Lesions
Coarctation of the aorta
Aortic stenosis
Pulmonary stenosis

Cyanotic Heart Lesions
Tricuspid atresia
Pulmonary atresia
Tetralogy of Fallot
Ebstein's anomaly of the tricuspid valve
Transposition of the great arteries

Congenital Heart Disease

The incidence of congenital heart disease is 9 per 1000 live births. Some defects develop as a result of genetic abnormalities; however, most congenital heart lesions occur in the absence of any detectable chromosomal abnormality. Although there are a large number of congenital lesions, those listed in Box 37-2 account for more than 80% of those seen in children with congenital heart disease. *Ventricular septal defects* account for approximately one third of all lesions, and *atrial septal defects* and *patent ductus arteriosus* account for 10% each; other relatively common defects include pulmonary stenosis and coarctation of the aorta. Less common are tetralogy of Fallot, aortic stenosis, and transposition of the great arteries.

Because great variation in clinical signs and symptoms and relevance toward dental care exists with congenital heart lesions, a thorough medical history, dialogue history, and clinical evaluation are absolutely essential. When a history of congenital heart disease is obtained, medical consultation with the patient's (child or adult) physician is recommended.

Primary concerns associated with dental management of this patient include the exacerbation of heart failure and cardiac dysrhythmias secondary to the stresses associated with dental treatment and the possibility of infection producing bacterial endocarditis. Consulting the most recent American Heart Association (AHA), American Medical Association (AMA), and American Dental Association (ADA) guidelines for prophylaxis, as well as possible medical consultation with the patient's primary care physician, will aid in determining the need for prophylactic antibiotics.[10] In many patients with surgically repaired defects, the need for antibiotic coverage during dental care exists for life.

As specifically relates to the management of pain and anxiety in patients with congenital heart disease, pain control through the use of local anesthetics is vitally important as a means of minimizing stress. The administration of vasopressor-containing local anesthetics is not contraindicated in these patients.

Sedative techniques are indicated as a means of minimizing intraoperative stress in this patient. The primary goal during the procedure is to provide adequate sedation without inducing hypoxia. The myocardium of the patient with congenital heart disease may be less able to tolerate hypoxic episodes than healthy heart muscle.

The oral route is indicated for light levels of sedation. Deep sedation via the oral route cannot be recommended.

IM sedation should be relegated to a last-choice technique for patients in whom other sedative procedures are unavailable or have proved ineffective. Only light to moderate sedation levels are recommended by the IM route, along with administration of supplemental O_2 throughout the procedure.

Inhalation sedation is an excellent sedation technique for these patients, primarily because of the additional levels of O_2 supplied throughout the procedure.

IV sedation is also recommended, provided the level of sedation remains light to moderate. Deep sedation is not recommended because of the increased likelihood of hypoxia and depression of respiratory and cardiovascular function. Supplemental O_2 should be administered when IV sedation is used.

Outpatient general anesthesia is not recommended in patients with congenital heart lesions, repaired or not. General anesthesia should be reserved for patients in whom sedative procedures have been ineffective. Because of the nature of the underlying disease, the patient is admitted to the hospital before the procedure to receive a more in-depth medical evaluation.

Valvular Heart Disease

Valvular heart disease is a common sequela of rheumatic fever. The incidence of valvular heart disease secondary to rheumatic fever has diminished in the past three decades; however, congenital valvular lesions are being diagnosed with increasing regularity. It is estimated that more than 18,000 cardiac valvular replacements are performed annually in the United States.[11]

Life expectancy is prolonged for most patients receiving valvular replacements. Along with this benefit, however, is the ever-present prospect of bacterial endocarditis. The reader is referred to the guidelines for prophylaxis, which present detailed antibiotic regimens for these patients.[10] The patient's primary care physician should be consulted before dental treatment.

The primary concern during the dental management of the patient with valvular heart disease is the prevention of bacterial endocarditis. In addition, stress should be minimized through the effective use of local anesthesia and sedation, as indicated. Hypoxia should be avoided.

The administration of local anesthetics with vasopressors is indicated in patients with valvular replacement.

Oral sedation is indicated in the management of lesser degrees of preoperative anxiety. Light levels of sedation only are recommended.

IM sedation is recommended when other sedative techniques are unavailable or have proved ineffective. Intraoperative O_2 administration is recommended for the light to moderate sedation recommended by the IM route.

Inhalation sedation with N_2O-O_2 is highly recommended for anxiety control in patients with valvular prostheses.

IV sedation is also recommended, with light to moderate levels only suggested. Intraoperative O_2 administration is suggested.

Outpatient general anesthesia is not recommended for the patient with a valvular prosthesis. Hospitalization and thorough workup are strongly suggested.

RENAL DISEASE

Glomerulonephritis, pyelonephritis, nephrotic syndrome, chronic renal insufficiency, and chronic renal failure are the most common disorders of renal function. Renal dialysis and transplantation are used in the management of chronic renal failure. In 2002 it was estimated that more than 200,000 persons were undergoing dialysis for end-stage renal disease.[12] Approximately 11,000 patients receive renal transplants annually in the United States.

Most renal failure patients may be safely managed in an outpatient setting, representing ASA II, III, or IV risks. Specific questioning and examination can determine the degree of risk.

All patients with altered renal function, especially those undergoing dialysis in the days just preceding their dialysis appointments, must be managed carefully because their blood chemistries may be in disarray. It is recommended that dental appointments be scheduled on the day following dialysis so that the patient's metabolic status is more optimal and the effects of systemic anticoagulation are minimal.

Prophylactic antibiotics may be required before dental care in the patient with renal disease, especially the renal transplant patient. Consultation with the patient's physician is strongly recommended to determine an appropriate antibiotic regimen.

Many patients with chronic renal disease, especially patients having undergone renal transplantation, receive long-term corticosteroid therapy. Such therapy diminishes the patient's capacity to respond appropriately to increased stress. The administration of supplemental corticosteroid may be recommended before particularly traumatic (emotionally or physically) procedures. Medical consultation is recommended.

Patients undergoing renal dialysis and renal transplant patients are considered at high risks for contracting hepatitis B and should be evaluated before the start of dental care. Patients who are surface-antigen negative and surface-antibody positive may be treated in the usual manner, whereas those who are surface-antigen positive should be treated using current recommendations to minimize transmission of hepatitis B. There is also an increased risk of human immunodeficiency virus (HIV) and acquired immunodeficiency syndrome (AIDS) infection. This increased risk should be considered before the use of parenteral techniques of sedation.

Most drugs are excreted through the kidneys, a percentage of the drug unchanged along with its major metabolites. Drugs such as cocaine and gallamine, which are excreted entirely unchanged in the urine, should not be administered to patients undergoing renal dialysis. Blood levels of these drugs would become overly high, increasing the risk of overdose (toxic reaction). Approximately 10% to 15% of most amide local anesthetics are excreted unchanged in the urine, whereas virtually no ester local anesthetic is found unchanged in the urine, having undergone biotransformation in the blood. Among drugs used for sedation, there is little problem in that only very small amounts of unchanged drug are found in the urine. Benzodiazepines and the opioids may be administered in the usual manner in both the patient with renal insufficiency and the functionally anephric patient. Aspirin must have its dosage regimen changed from the usual every 3 to 5 hours to every 4 to 6 hours in renal insufficiency and to every 8 to 12 hours in the anephric patient.

Amide local anesthetics may be administered normally. There are no contraindications to the inclusion of vasopressors.

Oral sedation is indicated for light to moderate levels of sedation.

IM sedation is indicated for light to moderate levels of sedation. The increased risk of hepatitis B or HIV in the dialysis patient must be considered before IM sedation.

Inhalation sedation is indicated.

IV sedation is indicated. The increased risk of hepatitis B or HIV in the dialysis patient must be considered before IV sedation.

General anesthesia on an outpatient basis is not recommended in the patient with chronic renal disease. Because of the potential presence of metabolic disorders, the patient should be hospitalized and thoroughly evaluated before general anesthesia.

RESPIRATORY DISEASE

The patient with respiratory disease must be evaluated carefully before dental treatment and especially before the administration of any CNS depressant drug that may further inhibit the patient's respiratory efforts. Many patients with chronic respiratory disorders have respiratory centers that are less sensitive to the normal stimulus for breathing: increased arterial carbon dioxide (CO_2) tension. Instead, these patients develop decreased arterial O_2 tension as their respiratory stimulus. Such patients may be described as hypercarbic (increased CO_2 tension) and hypoxic (decreased O_2 tension).

It is likely that many of these patients will be able to tolerate the stresses associated with their dental care with few, if any, modifications necessary in their treatment. However, the addition of stress can greatly increase the risk of an acute exacerbation of their disease process. Sedative drugs, which possess varying degrees of potential for respiratory depression, must be used with great care to minimize any further reduction in the respiratory drive of these patients.

Evaluation of patients with chronic respiratory disease revolves primarily around the patient's ability to exchange O_2 and CO_2 effectively. Inability to do so is demonstrated by the presence of clinical signs and symptoms. The most commonly observed respiratory disorders include asthma, chronic obstructive pulmonary disease (COPD), bronchiectasis, and pneumonia.

Asthma

Asthma is a clinical state of hyperreactivity of the tracheobronchial tree and is characterized by recurrent paroxysms of dyspnea and wheezing, which are the result of bronchospasm, bronchial wall edema, and hypersecretion by mucous glands. Several forms of asthma—extrinsic asthma (allergic asthma), intrinsic asthma (nonallergic asthma), drug-induced asthma, exercise-induced asthma, and occupational asthma—are recognized.

It is estimated that asthma affects 6 million to 8 million persons in the United States.[13] The typical asthmatic patient is asymptomatic between acute episodes but demonstrates varying degrees of respiratory distress during the acute asthmatic episode. Although the degree of respiratory distress is usually moderate, many persons die each year in the United States from asthma-related disorders.[14] The goal in the dental management of the asthmatic patient is to prevent the acute exacerbation.

The acute asthmatic episode may be triggered by any of the following items, probably the most significant of which in the dental management of this patient is increased stress:

- Psychological stress
- Antigen-antibody reaction (allergy)
- Bronchial infection
- Dust, fumes
- Climate (e.g., smog, cold)
- Drugs

Of primary importance to the doctor is to determine the type of asthma present and its degree of severity before the start of treatment. The typical asthmatic patient is classified as ASA II, with the ASA III asthmatic patient defined as a patient with a frequency of more than one acute episode per week or with episodes at any frequency that are difficult to manage without seeking medical attention.

Because the asthmatic patient appears asymptomatic between episodes, the doctor must be thorough in the dialogue history and physical examination. The doctor should determine which drugs the patient uses for management of acute episodes and request that the drugs be brought to all dental appointments. The acute asthmatic attack is in great part an episode of bronchial smooth muscle spasm (bronchospasm). To this are added bronchial wall edema and the secretion of copious volumes of mucus. The drugs used to manage the asthmatic episode are termed *bronchodilators;* the most common are listed in Table 37-2.

The use of sedative techniques in the asthmatic patient may be important in the prevention of acute episodes in clinical situations in which stress or anxiety levels are increased. However, some commonly used sedative drugs have the potential to provoke an acute episode of bronchospasm. Two examples are the barbiturates and opioids (especially meperidine), which are histamine-releasing drugs. These drugs should be avoided in the asthmatic patient.

Oral sedation is recommended for light to moderate levels of sedation. If possible, barbiturates and opioids should be avoided because of the potential for acute exacerbation. Chloral hydrate and hydroxyzine are frequently administered in the management of the asthmatic child, with good results.

IM sedation is recommended in the pediatric patient for whom other techniques are ineffective. Opioids and barbiturates, two commonly used drug groups, are relatively contraindicated in the asthmatic patient and should be avoided, if possible. Nasal O_2 throughout the procedure is recommended.

TABLE 37-2 Common Medications Used in Long-Term Management of Asthma

Drug Group	Examples (Generic Names)
Sympathomimetic amines	Epinephrine Isoproterenol Metaproterenol Ephedrine Pseudoephedrine Terbutaline
Xanthine derivatives	Aminophylline Theophylline Oxtriphylline Dyphylline
Corticosteroids	Hydrocortisone Prednisone Beclomethasone
Sodium cromoglycate	Cromolyn sodium
Steroids	Azmacort

Inhalation sedation with N_2O-O_2 is the most recommended sedative technique for both pediatric and adult asthmatic patients. Although N_2O does not possess bronchodilating properties similar to halothane, its sedative properties and the additional O_2 administered along with it effectively prevent the occurrence of acute asthmatic episodes. The occasional misguided medical consultant recommends against use of N_2O-O_2 because some individuals (mistakenly) believe that N_2O may provoke bronchospasm. Inhalation agents that irritate the respiratory mucosa are, in fact, capable of provoking bronchospasm; however, N_2O is not an irritating vapor and may be administered without increased risk (in fact, with decreased risk).

IV conscious sedation is recommended, with the addition of O_2 by nasal administration. Opioids and barbiturates are contraindicated (e.g., the Jorgensen technique) in the asthmatic patient.

Outpatient general anesthesia should be avoided in the asthmatic patient because of the increased risk of bronchospasm during general anesthesia. Dental and medical care for the patient with asthma who requires general anesthesia should be completed in the more controlled setting of the operating room of a hospital or day-surgery center.

Chronic Obstructive Pulmonary Disease

Chronic obstructive pulmonary (or lung) disease (COPD, COLD) is the most common cause of death and disability resulting from lung disease in the United States. Two primary disease entities comprise COPD: emphysema and chronic bronchitis. Unlike the asthmatic patient who is essentially asymptomatic in periods between acute episodes, the patient with COPD appears more debilitated and chronically ill, representing a greater risk during treatment. The typical patient with COPD is classified as an ASA III patient.

Emphysema

Emphysema represents a disease entity in which interalveolar septa (including blood vessels) are destroyed, producing a coalescence of air spaces to form abnormally large cystic or bullous areas in the lungs that do not function in gas exchange. The primary symptom presented in emphysema is a variable degree of dyspnea on exertion. The chest is often enlarged in a hyperinflated (barrel-chest) position. A chronic cough with sputum production may be present, although this is not characteristic of the disease.

There is no effective treatment for emphysema. Medical management is symptomatic, attempting to improve the patient's quality and length of life. Patients are cautioned to avoid all toxic inhalants such as cigarette smoke and toxic fumes. Minor pulmonary infection may readily lead to respiratory failure in these patients; therefore extraordinary care is maintained and vigorous treatment instituted at the first signs of infectious respiratory processes. Supplemental O_2 administered via a low-flow nasal cannula (2 to 3 L/min) at home using portable O_2 devices is frequently required for these patients.

Chronic Bronchitis

Chronic bronchitis is among the most common debilitating diseases in the United States. A strong relationship exists between chronic bronchitis and inhalation of irritating substances, most commonly cigarette smoke and various pollutants. Pathologic findings in chronic bronchitis include hyperplasia and hypertrophy of the submucosal bronchial mucous glands, hyperplasia of bronchiolar goblet cells, squamous metaplasia of bronchial mucosal cells, chronic and acute inflammatory infiltrates in the bronchial submucosa, profuse inflammatory exudates in the lumina of bronchi and bronchioles, and denudation of bronchial mucosa. Primary clinical symptoms include chronic cough and sputum production. Chronic bronchitis is most often seen in smokers older than 35 years. For a diagnosis of chronic bronchitis to be established, a productive cough must have been present for a minimum of 3 months a year in at least 2 consecutive years. As the disease progresses, it is marked by recurrent episodes of acute respiratory failure resulting from infectious exacerbations in the bronchi. These episodes are marked by increased cough, change in sputum from clear to purulent, fever, dyspnea, and varying degrees of respiratory distress; management consists of antibiotics, bronchodilators, and respiratory therapy.

Medical management of chronic bronchitis also includes cessation of cigarette smoking and exposure to toxic inhalants and the prevention or vigorous management of any respiratory infections. Other measures included in the management in some of these patients are home O_2 administration via nasal cannula and treatment of right-sided heart failure (with diuretics), which occasionally develops in chronic bronchitis.

The progression and prognosis of chronic bronchitis are quite variable; however, in general there is a progressive deterioration of pulmonary function, with increasing frequency of episodes of respiratory failure until death. The life expectancy in the typical patient, once severe symptoms develop, is rarely more than 5 to 10 years.

Typically, the patient with chronic bronchitis represents an ASA III risk; those with more mild symptoms are ASA II, but those who require supplemental O_2 at all times, have severe orthopnea, and a severe, productive cough are classified ASA IV. ASA IV patients should have elective dental care postponed until a time when their health improves. If dental care is urgent, hospitalization is recommended.

Dental management of patients with COPD usually requires alteration in patient positioning from the recommended supine position because of the presence of orthopnea. These patients should be positioned in the most recumbent position in which they are still able to breathe comfortably. Supplemental O_2 at low flows (2 to 3 L/min) may be administered via a nasal cannula or nasal hood throughout the dental appointment, whether or not a sedative procedure is used.

Local anesthesia is indicated for patients with COPD. Vasopressors are not contraindicated.

Oral sedation may be indicated, but only light levels of sedation. Opioids and barbiturates specifically are not recommended because of their greater propensity to depress respiration. Anticholinergics (atropine, scopolamine, and glycopyrrolate) and histamine blockers (hydroxyzine) are contraindicated because they increase the viscosity of secretions in the respiratory tract.

IM sedation is rarely considered in patients with COPD, primarily because these disease processes are almost always seen in older adults. Because of the ability of many IM-administered CNS depressant drugs to produce respiratory depression, this technique of sedation is not recommended. If IM sedation is used, opioids and barbiturates are contraindicated, anticholinergics and histamine blockers should be avoided, and O_2 must be administered in a 2- to 3-L/min flow throughout the procedure. Midazolam, a benzodiazepine, is the preferred IM sedative agent.

Inhalation sedation may be the only sedative technique that can be used in patients with COPD, with an expectation of clinical success that does not also increase the risk of acute respiratory failure. Theoretically, it is possible for the higher levels of O_2 administered with N_2O-O_2 to remove the stimulus for breathing in these patients (decreased arterial O_2 tension). In clinical practice, however, this situation is unlikely to develop, and N_2O-O_2 remains the sedative technique of choice in patients with COPD.

IV sedation is not recommended as a primary technique in patients with COPD because of the increased sensitivity of these patients to hypoxia and respiratory depression. Opioids, barbiturates, histamine blockers, and anticholinergics are contraindicated. Should IV sedation be necessary, light levels of sedation only, with drugs that do not produce significant respiratory depression (benzodiazepines), and the administration of 2- to 3-L/min nasal O_2 throughout the procedure are recommended.

Outpatient general anesthesia is contraindicated in patients with COPD. General anesthesia should be relegated to inpatient procedures within the operating room, where thorough preoperative evaluation is obtainable and patients can be observed both during and after the procedure before discharge.

NEUROLOGIC DISORDERS

Neurologic disorders, especially seizures, CVA, and myasthenia gravis, are of concern to the practicing dentist and physician. The patient who has a CNS disorder must be evaluated carefully, especially when the use of the CNS depressant drugs is contemplated.

Seizure Disorders

Seizure disorders are characterized by abrupt transient symptoms of a motor, sensory, psychic, or autonomic nature, often associated with changes in consciousness. These changes are secondary to sudden transient changes in brain function associated with excessive rapid electrical discharges in the gray matter.

The outline in Box 37-3 lists various types of seizure activity. The incidence of epilepsy (recurrent seizure activity) among the general population in North America is 0.5% to 1.0%.[15] It is estimated that more than 10 million persons have had at least one convulsion, and more than 2 million have had two or more episodes. It is also estimated that more than 200,000 Americans have seizures more than once a month despite medical treatment.

Seizures encountered most frequently and those possessing the greatest potential for morbidity and mortality are those in group II: generalized seizures or seizures without local onset. Within this group are the tonic-clonic convulsive episode, represented clinically as grand mal or major epilepsy, and petit mal or minor epilepsy (also termed an *absence attack*).

Among epileptic patients, 70% have only one type of seizure, the remainder having two or more types. Generalized tonic-clonic seizures are present in 90% of all epileptic patients (60% grand mal only; 30% grand mal plus others). Petit mal seizures are seen in 25% of patients with epilepsy (4% alone; 21% with other types). Petit mal is seen most often in children younger than 16 years. Psychomotor seizures are seen in approximately 18% of epileptic patients (6% alone; 12% mixed) and are minor seizures in which the victim loses contact with the environment for 1 or 2 minutes.

Anticonvulsant drugs are used to manage epilepsy, the goal being to prevent the occurrence of seizure activity by depressing the neuronal focus in the brain. Table 37-3 lists commonly prescribed anticonvulsants. Major dental treatment concerns with these patients are the prevention of seizure activity and patient management if a seizure does occur. Factors exacerbating seizures include psychological stress and fatigue. In the presence of apprehension over the planned procedure, sedative techniques should be considered. Alcohol is absolutely contraindicated in epileptic patients because it may precipitate seizure activity. No patient with a history of epilepsy should receive dental treatment if it is obvious that alcohol has recently been ingested. Alcohol should not be used as a sedative in epileptic patients. Most patients with well-controlled epilepsy (seizures developing rarely, less than one a month) are considered ASA II risks, with those having seizures more frequently considered ASA III risks. The degree of control over seizure activity is a primary factor in determining the risk involved in management of these patients.

Local anesthesia is indicated in the epileptic patient. Although the IV administration or the administration

BOX 37-3 International Classification of Epileptic Seizures

- Partial seizures (seizures beginning locally)
- Partial seizures with elementary symptoms (generally without impairment of consciousness)
- With motor symptoms (includes jacksonian seizures)
- With special sensory or somatosensory symptoms
- With autonomic symptoms
- Compound forms
- Partial seizures with complex symptoms (generally with impairment of consciousness), temporal lobe, or psychomotor seizures
- With impairment of consciousness only
- With cognitive symptoms
- With affective symptoms
- With "psychosensory" symptoms
- With "psychomotor" symptoms
- Compound forms
- Partial seizures secondarily generalized
- Generalized seizures (bilaterally symmetric and without local onset)
- Absences (petit mal)
- Bilateral massive epileptic myoclonus
- Infantile spasms
- Clonic seizures
- Tonic seizures
- Tonic-clonic seizures (grand mal)
- Atonic seizures
- Akinetic seizures
- Unilateral seizures (or predominantly)
- Unclassified seizures (due to incomplete data)

From Stefan H, Halasz P, Gil-Nagel A et al: *Eur J Neurol* 8:519, 2001.

TABLE 37-3 Drugs Used in Long-Term Management of Epilepsy

Generic Name	Proprietary Name	Type of Seizure	Side Effects
Acetazolamide	Diamox	Grand mal, petit mal	Drowsiness, paresthesia
Carbamazepine	Tegretol	Psychomotor, grand mal	Diplopia, transient blurred vision, drowsiness, ataxia, bone marrow depression
Clonazepam	Klonopin	Petit mal, atypical petit mal, myoclonic, akinetic	Drowsiness, ataxia, agitation
Ethosuximide	Zarontin	Petit mal	Drowsiness, nausea, vomiting
Methsuximide	Celontin	Petit mal, psychomotor	Ataxia, drowsiness
Mephenytoin	Mesantoin	Grand mal, some cases of psychomotor; effective when petit mal and grand mal coexist	Nervousness, ataxia, nystagmus, pancytopenia, exfoliative dermatitis
Phenacemide	Phenurone	Psychomotor	Hepatitis, benign proteinuria, dermatitis, headache, personality change
Phenobarbital	—	One of the safest drugs for all seizures; may aggravate psychomotor seizures	Drowsiness, dermatitis
Phenytoin sodium	Dilantin	Safest drug for grand mal and some cases of psychomotor epilepsy; may accentuate petit mal seizures	Gingival hypertrophy, rash, nervousness, ataxia, drowsiness, nystagmus
Primidone	Mysoline	Grand mal, especially in conjunction with other drugs	Drowsiness, ataxia
Valproic acid	Depakene	Petit mal, atypical petit mal, myoclonic, akinetic	Nausea and vomiting, drowsiness; interferes with platelets (similar to aspirin) and therefore may increase bleeding

of overly large doses of local anesthetics may provoke seizure activity (generalized tonic-clonic), it is unlikely that careful administration, following aspiration and slow injection of minimal volumes of the local anesthetic, will produce a problem. Vasopressors may be included in the local anesthetic.

The use of sedation in the epileptic patient is indicated, for it decreases the patient's fears of dentistry. It is important, however, that cerebral hypoxia be avoided because in the presence of cerebral hypoxia seizures may occur. Adequate oxygenation is therefore quite important for the epileptic patient.

Oral sedation is indicated for the preoperative management of anxiety. When it is used to produce light levels of CNS depression only, supplemental O_2 is not required.

IM sedation is indicated in patients in whom other techniques of sedation have proved ineffective. Supplemental O_2 is strongly recommended throughout the sedative treatment.

Inhalation sedation is an excellent technique for use in the epileptic patient. Occasional reports indicate that N_2O is capable of inducing seizure activity (it is allegedly epileptogenic) in seizure-prone patients.[16] Clinical experience with N_2O-O_2 over more than 100 years has conclusively proved its safety in the seizure-prone patient.[16,17]

IV conscious sedation is also recommended in the fearful epileptic patient. Techniques that include the administration of benzodiazepines or barbiturates are favored because these drugs are excellent anticonvulsants. The administration of supplemental O_2

throughout the procedure, to minimize the possibility of hypoxia, is strongly recommended. IV drugs such as ketamine, which provokes high-frequency electroencephalographic (EEG) activity, are not recommended in epileptic patients.

General anesthesia in the epileptic patient should be limited to in-hospital procedures.

Cerebrovascular Accident

CVA is a focal neurologic disorder caused by destruction of brain substance as a result of intracerebral hemorrhage, thrombosis, embolism, or vascular insufficiency. Synonyms for CVA include *stroke, brain attack,* and *cerebral apoplexy.*

CVAs are not uncommon in the adult population, although their occurrence in persons younger than age 40 is quite rare. In the United States approximately 400,000 new cases of acute CVAs are reported annually.[3] Although mortality rates from various types of CVA differ markedly, the overall rate is relatively high. More than 200,000 deaths are reported annually from CVA, making it the third leading cause of death in the United States (behind cardiovascular disease and cancer). The frequency with which CVA develops is emphasized by the fact that approximately 25% of routine autopsies (death from all causes) demonstrate evidence of prior CVA. CVAs are the most common form of brain disease. The average age of persons at the time of their first CVA is approximately 64 years. Fortunately, recent evidence demonstrates a declining incidence of CVA. For every 100 first episodes of CVA that occurred in a unit of adult population between 1945 and 1949, only 55 first episodes of CVA occurred between 1970 and 1974.[18] This decline occurs in both sexes and all age groups but is most notable in the elderly population.

A number of factors that increase the risk of CVA have been identified. These factors include high blood pressure, diabetes mellitus, cardiac enlargement, hypercholesterolemia, the use of oral contraceptives, and cigarette smoking. Consistently elevated blood pressure has been demonstrated to be a major risk factor in development of both hemorrhagic and atherosclerotic forms of CVA. Evidence from the Framingham study has led to the belief that high (systolic) blood pressure may be the major risk factor in the development of acute hemorrhagic CVA.[19] It is estimated that the risk of developing an acute CVA increases by 30% for every 10-mm Hg elevation in systolic blood pressure above 160 mm Hg.

The status post-CVA patient represents a significant risk within the dental or medical office during treatment. Survivors of CVAs have a good chance of recovering some degree of function. Gresham showed that 84% of CVA survivors live at home, 80% were capable of independent mobility, and 69% had total independence in the normal activities of daily living, yet only 10% exhibited no functional deficit.[20] With independent mobility the status post-CVA patient expects to receive dental and surgical care; however, it must be kept in mind that the recurrence rate of CVAs is high and that pain and anxiety only add to the risk presented by these patients.

Status post-CVA patients receive some or all of the following drugs: anticoagulants, antihypertensives, and aspirin. Anticoagulants are used in the status post-CVA patient primarily to minimize the risk of recurrent strokes. Antihypertensives are important in status post-CVA patients in whom high blood pressure is present. This includes approximately two thirds of all patients who have had a CVA. The treating doctor must be aware of the many side effects of the antihypertensive drugs (see Table 37-1). Low-dose aspirin therapy has been demonstrated to decrease the risk of CVA in men with transient cerebral ischemia (TCI).[20]

The typical status post-CVA patient represents an ASA II or III patient—ASA II if the patient has had a CVA more than 6 months previously and has no evidence of residual neurologic deficit, ASA III if the patient has had a CVA more than 6 months earlier but has some degree of neurologic deficit. The status post-CVA patient is classified as ASA IV if the CVA occurred less than 6 months earlier or if significant residual deficit remains.

Stress reduction is a top priority in the status post-CVA patient. The stress-reduction protocol, especially shorter appointments, effective pain control, and the management of apprehension, is of great importance in these patients.

All CNS depressants are relatively contraindicated in the status post-CVA patient. Any of these drugs may produce hypoxia, which may provoke increased confusion, aphasia, and other potentially serious complications, such as seizures. It has been my experience that lighter levels of sedation, as seen with inhalation sedation, are quite safe and highly effective in reducing stress in the status post-CVA patient. However, sedative techniques should be reserved for the status post-CVA patient in whom their use is truly justified.

Local anesthetics with vasopressors are not contraindicated in the status post-CVA patient provided that negative aspiration precedes the slow administration of the drug and that blood pressure is not overly elevated.

Oral sedation is quite valuable in the status post-CVA patient who demonstrates a greater degree of preoperative anxiety. Only light levels of sedation are recommended, using drugs such as the benzodiazepines. Medical consultation with the patient's physician is recommended before administration of these drugs.

IM sedation is contraindicated in the status post-CVA patient because of the lack of control maintained over the actions of the drugs and the increased potential for hypoxia.

Inhalation sedation is the most highly recommended sedation technique for the status post-CVA patient. Medical consultation before its administration is suggested because some physicians may object to the use of this technique because higher concentrations of O_2 may produce constriction of cerebral arteries, leading to decreased cerebral blood flow and possible hypoxia. However, when sedation is needed in the status post-CVA patient, inhalation sedation with N_2O-O_2 remains the preferred technique.

IV sedation should be reserved for only the most apprehensive status post-CVA patients, and then only following medical consultation. Once again an increased possibility of hypoxia after IV drug administration mitigates against use of this technique. When considered essential to the success of therapy, lighter levels of IV sedation, as obtained with benzodiazepines, are recommended. Supplemental O_2 is strongly recommended.

General anesthesia in the status post-CVA patient should be reserved for the hospital operating room environment, with the patient being admitted for a complete workup before the procedure and permitted to remain in the hospital until recovery is complete.

Myasthenia Gravis

Myasthenia gravis is a neuromuscular disorder characterized by a marked weakness and easy fatigability of muscles. Although almost any muscle within the body may be affected, muscles innervated by the bulbar nuclei (facial, oculomotor, laryngeal, pharyngeal, and respiratory muscles) are most often involved. The cause of myasthenia gravis is unknown, although investigators believe that it is an autoimmune response.[21] Muscle fatigability is worsened with exertion and improved with rest.

Myasthenia gravis occurs in 1 per 20,000 persons. It is more common in women (3:2 ratio) and appears most often between the ages of 20 and 30 years.

Clinical signs and symptoms include pronounced fatigability of muscles with subsequent weakness and paralysis. Weakness of extraocular muscles results in diplopia and strabismus. Ptosis of the eyelids becomes more pronounced later in the day. Difficulty with speech and swallowing may develop after prolonged use of these functions. The patient may have difficulty using the tongue and may have a high-pitched nasal voice. The so-called myasthenic smile, a snarling, nasal smile, may be evident. Fluctuations in the severity of the disease (exacerbations and remissions) are common and unpredictable. Muscle weakness is intensified by infection and certain drugs, such as increased dosages of anticholinesterases (e.g., physostigmine, neostigmine, edrophonium), aminoglycoside antibiotics (e.g., neomycin), and membrane stabilizers (e.g., procainamide, phenytoin).

BOX 37-4 Drugs Used in Myasthenia Gravis

Pyridostigmine bromide (Mestinon), especially effective in the treatment of bulbar muscle weakness
Neostigmine bromide
Ambenonium chloride (Mytelase), longer acting than neostigmine, with fewer side effects
Edrophonium bromide (Tensilon)
Ephedrine sulfate, administered with each dose of neostigmine; appears to enhance effectiveness of neostigmine

Patients with myasthenia gravis are managed with anticholinesterases (Box 37-4). In cases in which anticholinesterase drug management is ineffective, surgical removal of the thymus (thymectomy) or corticosteroid therapy is recommended. Side effects of anticholinesterase therapy include abdominal cramps, nausea, and vomiting. The addition of atropine or atropine-like drugs to the treatment regimen may alleviate or prevent side effects. In recent years plasmapheresis has been demonstrated to have a beneficial effect in the control of acute exacerbations of myasthenia gravis.[22]

The prognosis for myasthenia gravis is that approximately 75% of these patients improve after thymectomy, and many go into remission. Myasthenic crisis may occur, with sudden death from respiratory failure. Overtreatment with neostigmine or other anticholinesterases may produce extreme muscular weakness that may simulate myasthenic crisis. Physostigmine (Antilirium) is an anticholinesterase administered in the management of emergence delirium occurring following the administration of scopolamine or the benzodiazepines.

Exacerbation of myasthenia gravis occurs with infection and stress. A myasthenic crisis may be induced by a dental abscess or heightened anxiety about dental or surgical care. The myasthenic patient with a history of repeat crises should receive dental care within the confines of a hospital or other facility where acute airway management, including intubation, is readily available.

The administration of drugs with muscle-relaxant properties should be reserved for only essential situations. Few such occasions will arise in the typical outpatient dental or surgical setting.

Local anesthetics are the preferred drugs for the management of pain in myasthenic patients. Indeed, even in the hospitalized myasthenic patient, the use of regional nerve block anesthesia is preferred to general anesthesia. Vasopressors are not contraindicated.

Sedative techniques may be used, but care must be taken to avoid the administration of skeletal muscle relaxants such as diazepam and midazolam. Medical consultation is definitely indicated before the start of treatment in the myasthenic patient.

Oral, IM, inhalation, and IV techniques may be used on an outpatient basis if it is determined that they are absolutely necessary, and only following medical consultation. Drugs that produce muscle relaxation, especially nondepolarizing muscle relaxants, are contraindicated in the myasthenic patient.

LIVER DISEASE

Liver disease is of great importance because the liver is responsible, in large part, for the biotransformation of most drugs. Hepatic dysfunction may be responsible for prolonged and exaggerated effects of many drugs used for pain and anxiety control. A thorough history must be elicited when liver disease is suspected.

Probably the most recognizable sign of liver dysfunction is jaundice, a yellowish appearance of the skin and sclera. Jaundice is evidence of the accumulation of bilirubin in body tissues. Another, less common and less obvious sign of liver dysfunction is fetor hepaticus, a sweet, musty odor on the breath of the patient. Liver diseases of significance include viral hepatitis (type A, type B, and non-A, non-B), chronic hepatitis, alcoholic hepatitis, fatty liver, nodular cirrhosis, and biliary cirrhosis.

It is extremely unlikely that the dentist will be called on to treat the patient with active acute hepatitis. In the event that such an occasion arises, the primary concern on the part of the doctor and staff is to prevent cross-contamination. Precautions include masking and gloving, as well as sterilization of all equipment. Vaccination of the doctor and staff with hepatitis B vaccine is recommended. The degree of liver dysfunction present during the acute phase of hepatitis should be determined before treatment. Most local anesthetics (especially the commonly used amides) and CNS depressants undergo biotransformation in the liver. These drugs should be administered only if absolutely essential, and then only in the smallest effective dose. Medical consultation before treatment is suggested. During the acute phase of hepatitis, the patient may be quite debilitated and unable to tolerate additional stress. Treatment of an emergency nature only is recommended at this time.

Chronic hepatitis is a chronic inflammatory reaction of the liver that persists for more than 6 months. Although different forms of chronic hepatitis exist, the doctor must make a determination of the state of liver dysfunction in the patient before administering drugs. Chronic active hepatitis is characterized by progression to cirrhosis, although milder cases may resolve spontaneously. When deterioration of the patient's condition is evident, approximately 66% of patients die within 5 years of the onset of symptoms.

Alcoholic hepatitis is the most common form of chronic hepatitis. A history of heavy drinking over many years is always found. Parenchymal necrosis of the liver occurs as a result of alcohol abuse. Alcoholic hepatitis is the precursor of alcoholic cirrhosis. Alcoholic hepatitis may be reversible, depending on the degree of liver damage. In patients in whom the prothrombin time has been prolonged (to the degree at which liver biopsy cannot be performed), the mortality rate is 42%.

Drug-induced liver disease may result from toxic responses to the administration of various therapeutic agents. Drug-induced liver disease may mimic viral hepatitis or biliary tract obstruction. Examples of drug-induced liver disease follow:

- I. Viral hepatitis-like reactions
  - A. Halothane
  - B. Methoxyflurane
- II. Cholestatic reactions: inflammation of portal areas with features of allergy (eosinophilia)
  - A. Chlorpromazine
  - B. Prochlorperazine
  - C. Promazine
- III. Chronic active hepatitis
  - A. Chlorpromazine

The most common cause of nodular cirrhosis is the chronic abuse of alcohol. This disease involves hepatocellular injury, which leads to both fibrosis and nodular degeneration throughout the liver. Cirrhosis is a serious and irreversible disease that, when advanced, has a very poor prognosis. Response of the patient to most CNS depressant drugs may be exaggerated and prolonged.

Primary biliary cirrhosis is a chronic liver disease manifested by cholestasis. Insidious in onset, it is seen most frequently in women between the ages of 40 and 60 years. Its primary symptom is pruritus, with jaundice developing within 2 years of its onset. Secondary biliary cirrhosis follows chronic obstruction to bile flow, which is usually produced by a calculus, neoplasm, stricture, or biliary atresia.

The major concerns facing the doctor asked to manage a patient with liver disease include the possibly debilitated condition of the patient, the degree of hepatic dysfunction, and the possibility of cross-contamination of the office staff. ASA classifications for patients with liver disease range from ASA class II to

ASA class IV, based on signs and symptoms and the results of medical consultation.

In cases in which debilitation is obvious, elective dental care should be deferred until such time as the patient is better able to withstand the stresses involved in treatment. Emergency care should be considered only after consultation with the patient's physician and should be managed in the least traumatic manner. Definitive treatment may be instituted after the patient has returned to a better state of health.

The administration of drugs to the patient with serious liver damage increases the likelihood of adverse drug reactions because it is likely that the drug will undergo biotransformation into inactive metabolites at a considerably slower rate than usual. For example, the β-half-life of lidocaine in the healthy patient is 90 minutes, whereas with cirrhosis, lidocaine's half-life may approach 450 minutes.[23] Elevated blood levels of the drug develop, resulting in a prolonged duration of clinical action of CNS depressant drugs and a greater risk of side effects and overdose reactions. A significant percentage of the biotransformation of most drugs used in the management of pain and anxiety occurs in the liver. Dosages of these drugs must be determined after careful consideration of the effects of diminished liver function. In general, drug dosages should be decreased to approximately 50% of the usual dose in the patient with liver dysfunction. It is prudent to avoid the administration of such drugs when possible. The problem of cross-contamination has been previously discussed.

Local anesthesia is recommended in these patients. Vasopressors are not contraindicated. Because the half-life of amide local anesthetics may be considerably prolonged when significant liver disease is present, minimal volumes of amide local anesthetics should be administered. Nerve block is preferable to infiltration over large areas, except in patients in whom prothrombin times have increased because of their liver damage. In these patients infiltration or nerve blocks that have a minimal risk of hemorrhage are recommended.

Oral sedation is recommended as an excellent means of providing light levels of sedation. Drugs such as the benzodiazepines can be used with little increase in risk in the patient with hepatic dysfunction.

IM sedation should be avoided when possible in patients with hepatic dysfunction because the actions of the drugs may be prolonged and exaggerated. Opioids, drugs commonly used in IM sedation, demonstrate an exaggerated clinical action in the presence of liver dysfunction and should be avoided when possible.

Inhalation sedation with N_2O-O_2 is, without doubt, the safest and most effective sedative technique in patients with hepatic dysfunction. Neither gas undergoes biotransformation in the liver, and neither demonstrates exaggerated clinical actions in the presence of even significant liver dysfunction.

IV sedation is also relatively contraindicated in the presence of severe liver disease. Barbiturates and opioids may result in exaggerated and prolonged responses in these patients. The use of benzodiazepines is preferred in cases in which IV sedation is considered necessary.

Outpatient general anesthesia is also contraindicated in the presence of severe liver dysfunction. The patient for whom general anesthesia is contemplated should be hospitalized for a thorough preoperative evaluation, the condition stabilized, and the procedure completed in the operating room under careful monitoring.

ENDOCRINE DISORDERS

Several potentially important disease entities are related to dysfunction of the endocrine glands, including the thyroid, adrenal, pituitary, and parathyroid glands. Especially important to the practicing dentist and physician are disorders of the thyroid and adrenal glands, specifically hyperthyroidism, hypothyroidism, hyperadrenocorticism (Cushing's syndrome), and hypoadrenocorticism (Addison's disease).

Thyroid Gland Dysfunction

Located in the neck on either side of the trachea, the thyroid gland produces and secretes hormones that perform an important function in regulating the level of biochemical activity in most tissues of the body. Proper functioning of the thyroid gland is essential for normal growth and development.

Thyroid gland dysfunction is a relatively common medical disorder. If diabetes mellitus is excluded, thyroid dysfunction accounts for 80% of all endocrine disorders. Dysfunction of the thyroid gland may occur through overproduction (hyperthyroidism) or underproduction (hypothyroidism) of thyroid hormone. In both instances clinical manifestations cover a broad spectrum ranging from subclinical dysfunction to acute life-threatening situations. Fortunately, however, most patients with thyroid dysfunction have milder forms of the disease.

Hyperthyroidism

Hyperthyroidism is also known by several other names, including *thyrotoxicosis, toxic goiter* (diffuse or nodular), *Basedow's disease, Graves' disease, Parry's disease,* and *Plummer's disease.* It may be defined as a state of heightened thyroid gland activity associated with the production of excessive quantities of the thyroid hormones thyroxine (T_4) and triiodothyronine (T_3). Because thyroid hormones affect the cellular metabolism of virtually all organ systems, the signs and symptoms of hyperthyroidism may be noted in any part of the body. Untreated hyperthyroidism may lead to thyroid storm or crisis, which manifests itself, in part, as severe hypermetabolism.

The incidence of thyroid gland hyperfunction is 3 per 10,000 adults per year and has a female/male ratio of 5:1. Its peak incidence occurs between the ages of 20 and 40 years. Although its cause is unknown, hyperthyroidism is more common in areas of iodine deficiency and has been demonstrated to have familial (genetic) tendencies. It may manifest itself initially during periods of emotional and physical stress.

Patients with thyroid gland hyperfunction undergo treatment aimed at halting the excessive secretion of thyroid hormone. Management may involve surgical removal of all or part of the thyroid gland (total or subtotal thyroidectomy), long-term drug therapy with antithyroid drugs to achieve remission of the disease, or radioactive iodine therapy, rather than surgical excision. Frequently prescribed antithyroid drugs include thiouracil, propylthiouracil, methimazole (Tapazole), iothiouracil, and iodine.

Common signs and symptoms of hyperthyroidism are presented in Box 37-5. Mild degrees of thyroid hyperfunction may be mistaken for acute anxiety, with little increase in clinical risk to the patient. It must be noted that several cardiovascular disorders, primarily angina pectoris, are exaggerated in hyperthyroidism. Severe hyperfunction is an indication for immediate medical consultation. Dental care should not begin until the underlying metabolic disturbance has been corrected.

Additional considerations in hyperthyroid patients include contraindications to the administration of several drugs:

1. *Atropine and other anticholinergics,* because of their vagolytic properties, which produce an increase in heart rate: This may be a factor in precipitating thyroid crisis.
2. *Vasopressors,* drugs such as epinephrine, which act as cardiovascular stimulants: In the presence of a cardiovascular system already stimulated by the hyperthyroid state, cardiac dysrhythmias or thyroid storm may be precipitated. Local anesthetics with vasopressors may be used because they possess minimal epinephrine concentrations (1:100,000 and 1:200,000). Of greater risk, however, is racemic epinephrine cord used in gingival retraction. This more concentrated epinephrine formulation is more likely to precipitate undesirable side effects.

Mildly hyperthyroid patients might easily be mistaken for apprehensive patients. The use of conscious sedation is not contraindicated. Because the cause of this patient's apparent nervousness is not truly dental in origin, but hormonal, the efficacy of sedative drugs may be less than ideal.

BOX 37-5 Clinical Manifestations of Hyperthyroidism

Symptoms	*Signs*
Nervousness	Tachycardia
Increased sweating	Goiter
Hypersensitivity to heat	Skin changes
Palpitation	Tremor
Fatigue	Bruit over thyroid
Weight loss	Eye signs
Tachycardia	Atrial fibrillation
Dyspnea	
Weakness	
Increased appetite	
Eye complaints	

From Williams RH: *Textbook of endocrinology*, ed 6, Philadelphia, 1981, WB Saunders.

Hypothyroidism

Hypothyroidism is a clinical state in which the tissues of the body receive inadequate supplies of thyroid hormone. The clinical picture of hypothyroidism relates to the patient's age at the time of onset and to the degree and duration of hormonal deficiency. Cretinism is a clinical syndrome encountered in infants and children, resulting from deficiency of thyroid hormone during fetal and early life. Severe hypothyroidism developing in an adult is termed *myxedema.* Myxedema is the appearance of mucinous infiltrates beneath the skin. Severe, unmanaged hypothyroidism may ultimately lead to the loss of consciousness, a state termed *myxedema coma.*

Hypothyroidism in the adult usually develops as a result of idiopathic atrophy of the thyroid gland, a process currently thought to occur through an autoimmune mechanism. Other causes of hypothyroidism include total thyroidectomy, ablation following radioactive iodine therapy (both procedures are frequently used in the management of hyperthyroidism), and chronic thyroiditis. Hypofunction of the thyroid gland is much more common in women, with its incidence peaking about the time of menopause.

Patients with thyroid hypofunction receive thyroid extract or a synthetic preparation. The most frequently used drug and the one considered the drug of choice is levothyroxine sodium (Synthroid). Other drugs used in the management of hypothyroidism include liotrix (Euthyroid, Thyrolar) and dextrothyroxine (Choloxin).

Signs and symptoms of hypothyroidism are listed in Box 37-6. Clinically, hypothyroid patients may represent an increased risk during medical and dental treatment involving administration of CNS depressants. The hypothyroid patient is unusually sensitive to all CNS depressants, including sedatives, opioids, and local anesthetics. Normal therapeutic doses of these drugs may result in overdose reactions in the hypothyroid patient.

Before the start of treatment on the hypothyroid patient, the following are recommended:

1. Medical consultation with the patient's physician
2. Use of CNS depressants with extreme caution
3. Examination for the presence of cardiovascular disease

Note that hypothyroid patients have an increased incidence of cardiovascular disease, especially in cases that have persisted for many years.

The patient who is hypothyroid or hyperthyroid, is receiving medical treatment, and is presently asymptomatic represents an ASA II risk, whereas the patient with clinical signs and symptoms is considered ASA III. The following are recommendations for the use of pain- and anxiety-control techniques for both hypothyroid and hyperthyroid individuals.

Local anesthesia is recommended in both conditions. The use of vasopressors is not contraindicated in the hyperthyroid individual; however, minimal volumes of the least concentrated solution should be employed. In the clinically hypothyroid patient the volume of local anesthetic should be minimized to prevent local anesthetic blood levels from becoming elevated. Overdose thresholds for local anesthetics in the hypothyroid patient may be decreased.

BOX 37-6 Clinical Manifestations of Hypothyroidism: Symptoms

Weakness	Thick tongue
Dry skin	Edema of face
Coarse skin	Coarseness of hair
Lethargy	Pallor of skin
Slow speech	Memory impairment
Edema of eyelids	Constipation
Sensation of cold	Gain in weight
Decreased sweating	Loss of hair
Cold skin	Pallor of lips

From Williams RH: *Textbook of endocrinology*, ed 6, Philadelphia, 1981, WB Saunders.

Oral sedation is recommended in both patients. The use of CNS depressants is relatively contraindicated in the clinically hypothyroid patient. When oral sedation is necessary, the barbiturates and opioids should be avoided; instead, the benzodiazepines and other nonbarbiturate sedative-hypnotics are preferred.

IM sedation is recommended for use only when other techniques have proved inadequate. The use of opioids and barbiturates is not recommended in the hypothyroid individual.

Inhalation sedation is highly recommended because of the degree of control maintained over the drug's action. In the hypothyroid patient, lower-than-usual concentrations of N_2O often prove adequate, whereas the hyperthyroid individual may require greater than usual concentrations or the technique may prove to be unsuccessful. Careful titration of N_2O prevents accidental overdose in this technique.

IV conscious sedation should be administered with extreme care in the hypothyroid patient because the actions of most commonly used drugs will be exaggerated. This is especially so for the opioids and barbiturates but is also true, to a lesser degree, with benzodiazepines. Careful, slow titration minimizes the risk of adverse response. The hyperthyroid patient may prove difficult to sedate adequately within the dosage limits presented earlier (see Chapter 26). Failure of the IV technique to provide adequate sedation is preferable to administration of drug dosages in excess of those recommended.

Outpatient general anesthesia is contraindicated in the clinically hyperthyroid or hypothyroid patient. Hospitalization before the procedure, complete medical evaluation, and stabilization of the disease process should be considered before the administration of any general anesthetic in these patients.

Patients with thyroid gland dysfunction, whether hyperfunction or hypofunction, who are receiving or have received treatment, have normal levels of circulating thyroid hormones, and are asymptomatic are considered to be *euthyroid* (ASA II). Euthyroid patients may receive dental and medical treatment in the usual manner.

Adrenal Disorders

The adrenal gland is a combination of two glands, the cortex and the medulla, which, although fused together, remain distinct and identifiable. The adrenal cortex produces and secretes more than 30 steroid hormones. Cortisol, a glucocorticoid, is considered the most important product of the adrenal cortex. It permits the body to adapt to stress and is therefore extremely vital to continued survival.

Adrenal hypersecretion of cortisol leads to increased fat deposition in certain areas—the face (Figure 37-3, *A*)

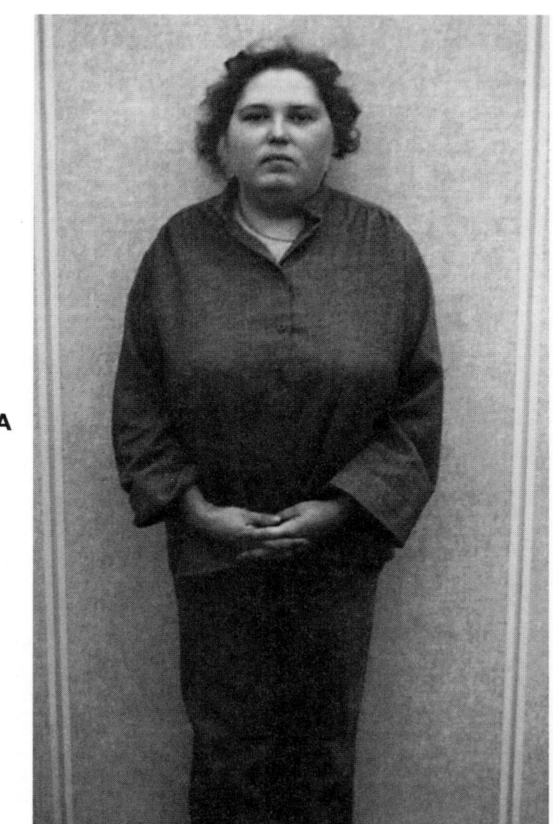

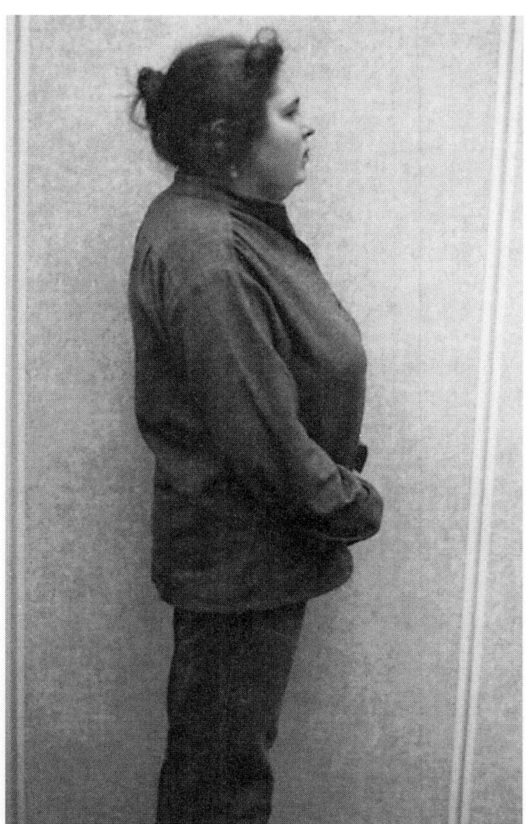

Figure 37-3 Hypersecretion of the adrenal cortex or chronic administration of corticosteroids leads to increased fat deposition in the face (**A**) and back (**B**).

and a "buffalo hump" (Figure 37-3, *B*) on the back, increases in blood pressure, and alterations in blood cell distribution (eosinopenia and lymphopenia). Clinically, cortisol hypersecretion, referred to as *Cushing's syndrome,* is usually readily corrected through surgical removal of part or all of the adrenal gland. Renal and adrenal surgery are important factors in the development of primary adrenal cortical insufficiency.

The patient with Cushing's syndrome is an ASA class II risk. The doctor should evaluate the patient carefully for the presence of high blood pressure, signs and symptoms of heart failure, diabetes mellitus, and possible emotional disorders (depression). The use of local anesthetics and other CNS depressants for sedation is not contraindicated in the patient with Cushing's syndrome. Medical consultation is recommended before therapy is started.

Inadequate production and secretion of cortisol, on the other hand, may lead to the relatively rapid development of signs and symptoms. Primary adrenocortical insufficiency is termed *Addison's disease,* an insidious and usually progressive disease. The incidence of Addison's disease is estimated at 0.3 to 1.0 per 100,000 persons, occurring equally in both sexes and throughout all age groups. Although all corticosteroids may be deficient in this disease state, it is important to note that the administration of physiologic doses of cortisol corrects most of the pathophysiologic effects. Clinical manifestations of adrenal insufficiency do not develop until at least 90% of the adrenal cortex has been destroyed.

Another form of adrenocortical hypofunction (secondary hypofunction) may occur through the administration of exogenous glucocorticosteroids to a patient with normal adrenal cortices. In the development of acute adrenal crisis, secondary adrenal insufficiency is a much greater potential threat than Addison's disease. Glucocorticosteroid drugs are widely prescribed in pharmacologic doses for the symptomatic relief of a variety of disorders. When used in this manner, glucocorticosteroid administration produces a disuse atrophy of the adrenal cortex, decreasing the ability of the adrenal cortex to produce the levels of corticosteroid necessary to cope with stressful situations, in turn leading to the development of signs and symptoms of acute adrenal insufficiency.

Patients with Addison's disease require corticosteroid administration in replacement (physiologic) doses for the remainder of their lives. However, patients receiving glucocorticosteroids for symptomatic treatment of their disorders commonly receive larger (pharmacologic or therapeutic) doses. These large doses may produce suppression of the normal adrenal cortex if continued for any length of time.

The "rule of two's" is valuable in determining risk in patients who are currently taking or have recently taken glucocorticosteroids.[24] It states that adrenocortical suppression should be suspected if a patient has received glucocorticosteroid therapy:

1. In a dose of 20 mg or more of cortisone or its equivalent daily
2. By the oral or parenteral route for a continuous period of 2 weeks or longer
3. Within 2 years of dental therapy

Following long-term exogenous corticosteroid therapy the adrenal cortex may require up to 9 months for a full recovery to normal function. Others have estimated that normal function may not return for as long as 2 years following long-term corticosteroid use.[25]

Because patients in these two categories are unable to adapt to stress in the usual manner, dental treatment must be modified to meet their needs. The stress-reduction protocol is extremely important in the overall management of these patients. In addition, both groups of patients require increased doses of their glucocorticosteroid drugs during and after the treatment period. Figure 37-4 is an example of a corticosteroid coverage protocol. Because stress represents a significant factor in increasing the risk involved in treatment of these patients, the requirement for adequate pain and anxiety control is critical.

Local anesthetics, with and without vasopressors, are indicated for use in these patients. All techniques of sedation are indicated. There are no contraindications to any technique or to specific drugs discussed previously.

Outpatient general anesthesia is contraindicated because of the increased stress associated with its administration, even in the best of situations. The patient with adrenal insufficiency, either primary or secondary, should be hospitalized for any general anesthetic procedure.

Card for Patient Receiving Corticosteroid Therapy

Mr.
Mrs.
Miss. ________ is being treated for (disorder)

with (corticosteroid) in a dose of (dose). In the event of "stress" the steroid dosage should be increased thus:

1. Mild "Stress" (e.g., common cold, single dental extraction, mild trauma): Use double doses daily.
2. Moderate "Stress" (e.g., flu, surgery under local anesthesia, several dental extractions): Use hydrocortisone, 100 mg, or prednisolone, 20 mg, or dexamethasone, 4 mg daily.
3. Severe "Stress" (e.g., general surgery, pneumonia or other systemic infections, high fever, severe trauma): use hydrocortisone, 200 mg, or prednisolone, 40 mg, or dexamethasone 8 mg daily.

When vomiting or diarrhea precludes absorption of oral doses, give dexamethasone 1 to 4 mg intramuscularly every 6 hours.

(Signed) ________ M.D.

(Address) ________

Figure 37-4 Sample corticosteroid coverage protocol for patient receiving corticosteroid therapy. (Redrawn from Streeten DHP: *JAMA* 232:944, 1975. Copyright 1975, American Medical Association.)

METABOLIC AND GENETIC DISORDERS

A number of disorders of metabolism and genetics are of potential importance in the management of pain and anxiety. The following disorders—diabetes mellitus, porphyria, malignant hyperthermia, and atypical plasma cholinesterase—are discussed here.

Diabetes Mellitus

Diabetes mellitus is a chronic systemic disease characterized by disorders in the production or utilization of insulin; in the metabolism of carbohydrate, fats, and protein; and in the structure and function of blood vessels. Diabetes is characterized by an inappropriately elevated level of glucose in the blood, termed *hyperglycemia.*

Diabetes mellitus is present in 1% to 2% of the population of the United States. This represents approximately 2 million to 4 million persons and includes only diagnosed diabetic persons. Another 1% to 2% of the population is believed to have undiagnosed or subclinical diabetes. Although diabetes is considered a disease of the elderly population (its incidence peaks in the fifth and sixth decades), it also occurs in young adults and children.

Two acute complications may develop in the diabetic patient: hyperglycemia (leading to diabetic coma) and, more important and much more common, hypoglycemia (leading to insulin shock). Whereas these complications must be looked for and managed if they develop, it is other, more chronic

TABLE 37-4 Chronic Complications of Diabetes Mellitus

Affected Part or Condition	Complication
Vascular system	Atherosclerosis
	Large blood vessel disease
	Microangiopathy
Kidneys	Diabetic glomerulonephritis
	Arteriolar nephrosclerosis
	Pyelonephritis
Nervous system	Motor, sensory, and autonomic neuropathy
Eyes	Retinopathy
	Cataract formation
	Glaucoma
	Extraocular muscle palsies
Skin	Xanthoma diabeticorum
	Necrobiosis lipoidica diabeticorum
	Pruritus
	Furunculosis
	Mycosis
Mouth	Gingivitis
	Greater incidence of dental caries and periodontal disease
	Alveolar bone loss
Pregnancy	Greater incidence of large babies, stillbirths, miscarriages, neonatal deaths, and congenital defects

complications that are responsible for the majority of deaths occurring in diabetic persons. Table 37-4 lists the chronic complications associated with diabetes mellitus. Three major categories of chronic complications are large blood vessel disease, small blood vessel disease (termed *microangiopathy*), and increased susceptibility to infection. The doctor treating the diabetic patient should carefully evaluate the patient for clinical signs and symptoms of cardiovascular disease, which is the most common cause of death in the diabetic patient.[26]

Knowledge on the part of the doctor of the type of diabetes—type 1, or insulin-dependent diabetes mellitus (IDDM), or type 2, non–insulin-dependent diabetes mellitus (NIDDM)—and the degree of control the patient maintains over his or her disease will enable the doctor to establish a risk factor for this patient. In general, the patient with well-controlled type 2 diabetes who demonstrates no associated disease is classified as an ASA II risk; patients with type 1 diabetes (patients with no β-cell activity) are ASA III or IV risks depending on the severity of the disease and their level of control.

It is important for the doctor to speak with the diabetic patient before treatment to discuss the possible effect of the dental care on the patient's eating habits. The diabetic patient must attempt to maintain a normal eating pattern so that he or she does not become hypoglycemic after insulin administration. With recent changes in recommendations for management of type 1 diabetes (increased frequency of insulin administration), it is expected that the incidence of hypoglycemic episodes will triple.[27] Alterations in insulin dosages may be required in some situations in which alterations in the patient's eating habits are unavoidable. Medical consultation may be indicated before adjustment of insulin dosage.

In the management of pain and anxiety, the diabetic patient does not present any unusual problems. Most techniques of pain and anxiety control are recommended for use in the diabetic patient. Treatment modification is required in the ASA III and IV diabetic patient according to the severity of the associated medical complications. The following relates to the diabetic patient who is classified as an ASA II risk.

Local anesthesia is recommended for use in the diabetic patient, with no restrictions regarding either the choice of local anesthetic or the vasopressor.

Oral sedation is recommended for use in the diabetic patient with no restrictions.

IM sedation is recommended for the diabetic patient when other techniques of sedation have proved ineffective. There are no specific contraindications to the administration of IM drugs.

Inhalation sedation is recommended for use in the diabetic patient, with no restrictions.

IV sedation is recommended in the diabetic patient, with no restrictions. The use of a 5% dextrose in water infusion will not produce any significant alteration in the patient's blood sugar level, especially when one considers that the patient receiving IV sedation will be NPO (nothing by mouth) for at least 4 to 5 hours before the procedure and will be slightly hypoglycemic.

Outpatient general anesthesia is usually contraindicated in the patient with type 1 diabetes. The patient with type 2 diabetes (NIDDM) is a good risk for outpatient general anesthesia. Most insulin-dependent diabetic patients who require general anesthesia should be hospitalized so that their diabetic condition can be stabilized and monitored closely both during and after the procedure.

Porphyria

Porphyrins are cyclic compounds that are the precursors of heme and other important enzymes and pigments. Heme is the complex of iron and porphyrin that unites with the protein globin to form hemoglobin. The porphyrias are disorders of porphyrin metabolism in which a marked increase in the production and excretion of porphyrins and their precursors is noted. Porphyria may be either hereditary or acquired. Porphyrias are classified in two main categories, hepatic porphyrias and erythropoietic porphyrias, depending on whether the excessive porphyrin production occurs within the liver or in the bone marrow.

It is important to be aware of the presence of latent or manifest porphyria because of the potential for some drugs to provoke episodes of acute intermittent porphyria. This rare disorder is exacerbated by the administration of barbiturates, sulfonamides, and griseofulvin, which cause a marked increase in porphyrin synthesis. Clinically, this is associated with acute episodes of abdominal pain, paresthesia, neuritic pain, convulsions, muscle paralysis, psychiatric disturbances, and the passage of a reddish urine. Death results from respiratory paralysis in up to 25% of patients with acute episodes. Such paralysis may not develop for several days after drug administration.

Patients who have porphyria are classified as either ASA II or ASA III patients, depending on the severity of the disorder and the incidence of acute exacerbations.

Local anesthetics with and without vasopressors are recommended in the patient with porphyria. Oral sedation is recommended; however, *barbiturates are absolutely contraindicated.* IM sedation is recommended, but administration of any barbiturate is absolutely contraindicated. Inhalation sedation is recommended in the patient with porphyria. IV sedation is recommended, but the administration of barbiturates is absolutely contraindicated.

Outpatient general anesthesia is contraindicated in the patient with porphyria. The patient with porphyria who requires a general anesthetic should be hospitalized before administration of the general anesthetic. Barbiturates are absolutely contraindicated in the patient with porphyria.

Malignant Hyperthermia

Malignant hyperthermia (MH; malignant hyperpyrexia) is a pharmacogenetic disorder in which a genetic variant in the patient alters their response to certain drugs. The problem is that before exposure to specific drugs it may be impossible to recognize an MH-susceptible patient. The genetic defect manifests itself as a flaw in the control of calcium levels in skeletal muscle when the normal intracellular environment is altered by certain drugs.[28] The concentration of calcium in the sarcoplasm is abnormally high. The list of drugs implicated as triggering malignant hyperthermia is large and includes many of the most commonly used general anesthetics:

- Halothane
- Enflurane
- Methoxyflurane
- Succinylcholine
- *d*-Tubocurarine
- Gallamine
- Ether
- Cyclopropane

Acute clinical manifestations of MH include the following: *Muscle rigidity,* which occurs in 80% of cases, may appear immediately after the administration of succinylcholine, a muscle relaxant. Masseteric rigidity is a common first sign. Rigidity may develop up to 2 hours after the beginning of a procedure when inhalation anesthetics are used. *Tachycardia* is almost universally present in MH. *Tachypnea* develops simultaneously with the tachycardia; however, in cases in which muscle relaxants have been administered, this symptom may be masked. *Fever* is the primary feature of MH. It is the rate of rise, not the absolute temperature, that is of importance in MH. In general anesthetic procedures, the use of a temperature probe is universally recommended. An elevation of temperature of more than 0.5° C should be suspect. Fever is usually a late sign, often noted after tachypnea and tachycardia. Other clinical signs include *dysrhythmias, cyanosis, dark venous blood* in the surgical field, *red urine,* and *hot skin.*

The mortality rate of patients with MH was 63% to 73% before the introduction of dantrolene sodium, an IV agent used to terminate episodes.[29] Dantrolene sodium inhibits the release of calcium from intracellular organelles such as mitochondria and the sarcoplasmic reticulum. Since its introduction the mortality rate from MH has decreased. Dantrolene sodium is also available in an oral form that has enabled susceptible patients to receive prophylaxis before their exposure to drugs that might induce MH.

The incidence of MH is approximately 1 per 15,000 children and 1 per 50,000 adults.[30] The majority of cases occur in children, adolescents, and young adults. Males develop MH more frequently than do females. MH is encountered with much greater frequency in certain areas of North America where families with the genetic trait have settled. Three areas of concentration include Toronto, Canada, and Wisconsin and Nebraska in the United States.

Patients with documented MH or those who are possibly susceptible are classified as ASA III risks. Definite treatment modification is in order to minimize risk for these patients during therapy. Medical consultation is recommended, discussing the proposed treatment, including drugs. The Malignant Hyperthermia Association of the United States (MHAUS) has an excellent web site (www.mhaus.org), which may be accessed for up-to-the-minute information regarding MH.

Local anesthetics of the amide group—articaine, lidocaine, mepivacaine, prilocaine, etidocaine, and bupivacaine—were considered absolutely contraindicated in MH patients. It was believed that these drugs were capable of triggering the MH response. Research has demonstrated conclusively that the *amide local anesthetics are not contraindicated* in the MH-susceptible patient,[31-33] nor is there any contraindication to the administration of the ester local anesthetics. The inclusion of vasopressors in the anesthetic solution is not contraindicated.

Oral sedation is recommended. Barbiturates, opioids, and benzodiazepines may be administered with no increased risk in patients with MH.

IM sedation may be administered, although I would probably have serious second thoughts about the administration of any parenteral sedation technique on an outpatient basis to a child with a history of malignant hyperpyrexia. Hospitalization would appear to be a more prudent approach to this patient's management.

Inhalation sedation with N_2O-O_2 is recommended in the patient with MH. Following consultation the use of inhalation sedation on an outpatient basis might prove to be most favored.

IV sedation is recommended; however, as with IM sedation, I personally believe that it is more prudent to consider hospitalization of the MH-susceptible patient who requires parenteral sedation, unless the patient's condition is well controlled with the administration of dantrolene sodium.

Outpatient general anesthesia is contraindicated in the patient with MH. Hospital-based care is recommended for the patient with MH who requires general anesthesia. Because of the risk involved in general anesthesia for this patient, the benefits to be gained by using general anesthesia should be carefully weighed against its risk before it is used.

Atypical Plasma Cholinesterase

Atypical plasma cholinesterase is another pharmacogenetic disorder. Two commonly used drugs—succinylcholine, a short-acting, depolarizing muscle relaxant used during intubation in general anesthesia, and the ester local anesthetics such as procaine, chloroprocaine, and propoxycaine—are metabolized by the enzyme plasma cholinesterase. A form of this enzyme, called atypical plasma cholinesterase, is found in 1 in 2820 persons.[34] Patients with atypical plasma cholinesterase are unable to metabolize these drugs at a normal rate and are therefore more likely to exhibit clinical signs and symptoms of (1) prolonged clinical activity and/or (2) drug overdose. When succinylcholine is administered, the clinical duration of muscular relaxation in these patients is considerably prolonged beyond the usual 5 minutes. In cases in which an ester local anesthetic has been administered, elevated blood levels, which increase the risk of drug overdose developing, are noted. Clinical duration of action (pain control) is not prolonged when local anesthetics are administered to these patients. Patients with atypical plasma cholinesterase are considered ASA II risks.

Amide local anesthetics are recommended in these patients. Vasopressors are not contraindicated. Ester local anesthetics should be avoided in patients with atypical plasma cholinesterase; however, if they must be administered, the smallest effective volume is recommended.

Oral, IM, and inhalation sedation are recommended without specific contraindications. IV sedation is recommended with the warning that succinylcholine not be administered to these patients.

Outpatient general anesthesia may be administered if succinylcholine is not administered to these patients. It is prudent, however, to consider hospitalization of these patients if general anesthesia is required.

HEMATOLOGIC DISORDERS

Several disorders of potential significance to the administration of drugs—anemia, sickle cell anemia, polycythemia vera, and hemophilia—are included in this category.

Anemia

Anemia is a condition in which an insufficient number of red blood cells (RBCs) produces a decrease in the total O_2-carrying capacity of the blood. Causes of anemia include hemorrhage (either external or internal), diminished manufacture of erythrocytes in the body, and a shortened life span of RBCs. McCarthy has listed the following three categories of anemia[35]:

1. Reduction below the normal number of erythrocytes: megaloblastic anemia, pernicious anemia, folic acid deficiency, aplastic anemia
2. Reduction in the quantity of hemoglobin: iron deficiency anemia, sickle cell anemia
3. Reduction in the volume of packed red cells: bleeding or destruction (hemolytic anemia)

Signs and symptoms of anemia include ease of fatigability, dyspnea, pallor, palpitation, angina pectoris, and tachycardia. With a normal adult hemoglobin level of 12 to 18 g/100 ml of blood, levels below 9 g/100 ml are considered indicative of anemia. The ASA risk categories for anemic individuals vary according to the severity of clinical signs and symptoms; however, in general, the anemic patient with a hemoglobin level above 9 g/100 ml is classified as ASA II, whereas the patient with a hemoglobin level below 9 g/100 ml is classified as ASA III.

Stress reduction is required for the anemic patient. The primary modification is the recommendation that the patient receive O_2 via nasal cannula throughout the treatment.

Local anesthetics are indicated with or without vasopressors. Prilocaine is relatively contraindicated in anemic individuals, especially those with methemoglobinemia.[36] Large volumes of prilocaine may produce cyanosis (managed with the administration of IV methylene blue).[37] Other amide and ester local anesthetics do not produce elevations in methemoglobin.

Oral sedation is recommended with no specific contraindications.

IM sedation is recommended. Supplemental O_2 administered via nasal cannula throughout the procedure is suggested.

Inhalation sedation is recommended. The supplemental O_2 administered along with the N_2O is quite beneficial to the patient.

IV sedation is indicated. Supplemental O_2 administered via nasal cannula is suggested.

Outpatient general anesthesia is relatively contraindicated in anemic patients because of the decreased O_2-carrying capacity of the blood. In patients with mild anemia and asymptomatic patients, outpatient general anesthesia may be contemplated. In most cases, however, patients with anemia should be hospitalized for the general anesthetic procedure.

Sickle Cell Anemia

Sickle cell anemia is a hereditary disorder seen almost exclusively in blacks. Abnormal hemoglobin is transmitted as a dominant trait. Heterozygous carriers have mixtures of normal and sickle hemoglobin in all of their RBCs. Sickling of erythrocytes occurs at a low O_2 tension, especially when the pH of blood is also low (acidosis). The S (sickle) hemoglobin (HbS), which is present in this disease, is less soluble in its deoxygenated (reduced) form, leading to an increase in the viscosity of whole blood. Increased viscosity results in stasis and obstruction of blood flow through capillaries, venules, and terminal arterioles, which results in pain and swelling in the involved organs.[38]

It is estimated that 50,000 Americans, primarily blacks, have sickle cell disease, in which HbSS is present in all RBCs. This is approximately 1 per 600 blacks. Sickle cell trait, which another 2 million black Americans may carry, rarely causes signs and symptoms because the RBCs contain both sickle and normal hemoglobin, HbAS.

The patient with sickle cell disease represents an increased risk during treatment, particularly treatment that involves the administration of drugs with the potential to produce respiratory depression. A sickle cell crisis might be precipitated by CNS depressant drugs, as well as by infection and extreme cold. When a sickle cell crisis occurs, the organs most often involved are the brain, kidneys, spleen, liver, and bones. The patient with sickle cell trait, although unlikely to develop crisis, may, in circumstances of extreme stress, such as physical exertion and general anesthesia, suffer a sickle cell crisis.

Most patients with sickle cell disease represent an ASA III risk during therapy. Those with sickle cell trait may be categorized as ASA II patients. Treatment modifications involve the provision for adequate oxygenation at all times in these patients, the prevention of acidosis, and the management of stress.

Local anesthetics are recommended either with or without vasopressors. No specific contraindications exist to any drug.

Oral sedation is recommended for light levels of preoperative anxiety control. Should moderate levels of sedation be sought by this route, the administration of supplemental O_2 via nasal cannula is recommended.

IM sedation is recommended when other techniques of sedation have been ineffective. O_2 administered via nasal cannula throughout the procedure is recommended.

Inhalation sedation with N_2O-O_2 is ideally suited for the patient with a history of sickle cell disease. Increased levels of O_2 are provided to the patient throughout the procedure.

IV sedation is recommended with no specific contraindications to any drugs. Supplemental O_2 administered via nasal cannula is recommended.

Outpatient general anesthesia is not recommended because the potential risk of hypoxia may be increased. Hospitalization of the patient is strongly recommended for the administration of general anesthesia.

Polycythemia Vera

Polycythemia vera is an overproduction of one or more types of blood cells, such as RBCs, white blood cells, or platelets. Symptoms are produced by an increased viscosity of blood and hypermetabolism. Although polycythemia vera may develop at any age, it is commonly observed after the age of 50 years. It is more common in men and is seen more often in Jews from Eastern Europe. Polycythemia vera is rarely encountered in blacks and Latin Americans.[39] Clinical signs and symptoms include headache, inability to concentrate, hearing loss, itching, pain in fingers and toes, a decreased feeling of well-being, and a loss of energy.

Complications of polycythemia vera include hemorrhage (gastrointestinal bleeding) and thrombosis, especially in uncontrolled polycythemia vera. Excessive bleeding is common during surgery. Management of polycythemia vera consists of administration of radiophosphorus and phlebotomy. Survival averages 13 years in properly treated patients. Acute leukemia causes the death of 5% of patients.

The typical patient with polycythemia vera represents an ASA II risk during treatment. Excessive bleeding is likely to occur during dental and surgical treatment. The use of supplemental O_2 is recommended during all treatment in these patients.

Local anesthesia is recommended, with no specific contraindications to any local anesthetic drug or vasopressor. Nerve block anesthesia, especially those techniques in which a high percentage of positive aspiration is likely to occur, such as inferior alveolar nerve block, should be avoided because of the potential risk of excessive bleeding. Alternative techniques such as the Gow-Gates mandibular block, periodontal ligament injection, or infiltration are preferred in these patients.

Oral sedation is recommended without specific contraindications.

Parenteral sedation techniques are relatively contraindicated because of the increased risk of excessive bleeding and venous thrombosis. IM sedation should be reserved for those patients in whom it is absolutely necessary and in whom the benefits of its use outweigh the potential risks. Supplemental O_2 is recommended.

Inhalation sedation is highly recommended.

IV sedation is relatively contraindicated because of the potential for increased bleeding and venous thrombosis. Risks should be carefully weighed against benefits when IV sedation is being considered. Supplemental O_2 is recommended.

Outpatient general anesthesia is relatively contraindicated in the patient with polycythemia vera. Hospitalization and treatment as an inpatient should be given careful consideration.

Hemophilia

Hemophilia is an inherited disorder of coagulation characterized by a lifelong history of abnormal bleeding. Hemophilia A and hemophilia B are the most common of the inherited bleeding disorders. Hemophilia A is classic hemophilia resulting from a deficiency of antihemophilic factor (AHF) activity. Because of its absence from plasma, thromboplastin formation is affected. Christmas disease, hemophilia B, is a deficiency in plasma thromboplastin component (factor IX).

Patients with hemophilia rarely have massive hemorrhages. Bleeding is usually a prolonged oozing that develops after minor surgery or trauma. Of special concern during dental care is the administration of local anesthesia for pain control (see following discussion). Management of patients with hemophilia consists primarily of the prevention of bleeding and the administration of the appropriate factor (VII or IX) to the patient either prophylactically before surgical procedures or when bleeding does occur, as after dental extractions.

Aspirin-containing analgesics should be avoided in persons with hemophilia because it prolongs bleeding for 24 to 48 hours. Acetaminophen, nonsteroidal anti-inflammatory drugs (NSAIDs), or other non–aspirin-containing analgesics may be used.

Local anesthesia is recommended, with no specific contraindications to the administration of any local anesthetic drug with or without a vasopressor. The administration of regional nerve block anesthesia, especially techniques with a greater incidence of positive aspiration (inferior alveolar nerve block, posterior superior alveolar nerve block, and mental [incisive] nerve block), should be avoided in the hemophiliac patient. Alternative techniques such as the Gow-Gates mandibular block, infiltration, periodontal ligament injection (PDL), and intraosseous are recommended.

Oral sedation is recommended with no specific contraindications.

IM sedation is contraindicated because of the increased potential for prolonged bleeding.

Inhalation sedation is recommended, with no specific contraindications.

IV sedation is recommended if the patient has received replacement therapy. Outpatient general anesthesia is contraindicated because of the increased risk of prolonged bleeding. Inpatient general anesthesia is preferred, with the patient well controlled before the procedure. Oral intubation is preferred to nasal intubation because of the reduced chance of bleeding.

REFERENCES

1. 2002 Heart and stroke statistical update. www.americanheart.org.
2. *Drug facts and comparisons (pocket edition),* ed 4, Philadelphia, 2000, Lippincott Williams & Wilkins.
3. American Heart Association: *1993 Heart Facts,* Dallas, 1993, The Association.
4. Tarhan S, Giuliani ER: General anesthesia and myocardial infarction, *Am Heart J* 87:137, 1974.
5. Weinblatt E, Shapiro S, Frank CW et al: Prognosis of men after first myocardial infarction: mortality and first recurrence in relation to selected parameters, *Am J Public Health* 58:1329, 1968.
6. Alpert JS, Braunwald E: Pathological and clinical manifestations of acute myocardial infarctions. In Braunwald E, ed: *Heart disease: a textbook of cardiovascular medicine,* ed 5, Philadelphia, 1997, WB Saunders.
7. Stern MS, Shine KI: Nitrous oxide and oxygen in coronary artery disease, *JAMA* 245:129, 1981.
8. Carey C, Lee H, Woeltje K: *The Washington Manual of Therapeutics,* ed 29, Philadelphia, 1998, Lippincott Williams & Wilkins.
9. Katz AM: Congestive heart failure, *N Engl J Med* 293:1184, 1975.
10. Dajani AS, Taubert KA, Wilson W et al: Prevention of bacterial endocarditis. Recommendations by the American Heart Association, *JAMA* 277:1794, 1997.
11. Atkins CW: Mechanical cardiac valvular prosthesis, *Ann Thorac Surg* 52:161, 1991.
12. National Kidney Foundation: 2002 Facts. www.kidney.org.
13. Burr ML: Epidemiology of asthma, *Monogr Allergy* 31:80, 1993.
14. Weiss KB, Gergen PJ, Wagener DK: Breathing better or wheezing worse? The changing epidemiology of asthma morbidity and mortality, *Annu Rev Public Health* 14:491, 1993.
15. Hauser WA: Seizure disorders: the changes with age, *Epilepsia* 33(suppl 4):S6, 1992.
16. Melon E, Homs JB: Nitrous oxide in neurosurgery: its safety in the seizure-prone patient, *Agressologie* 32:429, 1991.
17. Ito BM, Sato S, Kufta CV et al: Effect of isoflurane and enflurane on the electrocorticogram of epileptic patients, *Neurology* 38:924, 1988.
18. Manton KG, Corder LS, Stallard E: Estimates of change in chronic disability and institutional incidence and prevalence rates in the U.S. elderly population from the 1982, 1984, and 1989 national long term care survey, *J Gerontol* 48:S153, 1993.
19. Gresham GE, Fitzpatrick TE, Wolf PA: Residual durability in survivors of stroke: the Framingham study, *N Engl J Med* 293:954, 1975.
20. Sila CA: Prophylaxis and treatment of stroke: the state of the art in 1993, *Drugs* 45:329, 1993.
21. Oosterhuis HJ, Kuks JB: Myasthenia gravis and myasthenic syndromes, *Curr Opin Neurol Neurosurg* 5:638, 1992.
22. Genkins G, Sivak M, Tartter PI: Treatment strategies in myasthenia gravis, *Ann NY Acad Sci* 681:603, 1993.
23. Sawyer DR, Ludden TM, Crawford MH: Continuous infusion of lidocaine in patients with cardiac arrhythmias: unpredictability of plasma concentrations, *Arch Intern Med* 141:34, 1981.
24. McCarthy FM: Adrenal insufficiency. In McCarthy FM, ed: *Essentials of safe dentistry for the medically compromised patient,* Philadelphia, 1989, WB Saunders.
25. Streeten DHP: Corticosteroid therapy. II. Complications and therapeutic indications, *JAMA* 232:1046, 1975.
26. Fuller JH: Mortality trends and causes of death in diabetic patients, *Diabetes Metab* 19:96, 1993.
27. The Diabetes Control and Complications Trial Research Group: The effect of intensive treatment of diabetes on the development and progression of long-term complications in insulin-dependent diabetes mellitus, *N Engl J Med* 329:977, 1993.
28. Strazis KP, Fox AW: Malignant hyperthermia: a review of published cases, *Anesth Analg* 77:297, 1993.
29. Moore JL, Rice EL: Malignant hyperthermia, *Am Fam Physician* 45:2245, 1992.
30. Saleh KL: Practical points in the management of malignant hyperthermia, *J Post Anesthes Nurs* 7:327, 1992.
31. Dershwitz M, Ryan JF, Guralnick W: Safety of amide local anesthetics in patients susceptible to malignant hyperthermia, *J Am Dent Assoc* 118:276, 1989.
32. Jelic JS, Moore PA: Malignant hyperthermia and amide local anesthetics, *Penn Dent J* 55:35, 1988.
33. Minasian A, Yagiela JA: The use of amide local anesthetics in patients susceptible to malignant hyperthermia, *Oral Surg* 66:405, 1988.
34. Metrowitz MR, Mauro JV, Aston R et al: Prolonged succinylcholine-induced apnea caused by atypical cholinesterase: report of a case, *J Oral Surg* 38:387, 1980.
35. McCarthy FM: Physical evaluation and treatment modification. In McCarthy FM, ed: *Emergencies in dental practice,* ed 3, Philadelphia, 1979, WB Saunders.
36. Bellamy MC, Hopkins PM, Halsall PJ et al: A study into the incidence of methaemoglobinaemia after "three-in-one" block with prilocaine, *Anaesthesia* 47:1084, 1992.
37. Bhutani A, Bhutani MS, Patel R: Methemoglobinemia in a patient undergoing gastrointestinal endoscopy, *Ann Pharmacother* 26:1239, 1992.
38. Sansevere JJ, Milles M: Management of the oral and maxillofacial surgery patient with sickle cell disease and related hemoglobinopathies, *J Oral Maxillofac Surg* 51:912, 1993.
39. Murphy S: Polycythemia vera, *Dis Month* 38:153, 1992.

CHAPTER 38

The Physically Compromised Patient

Kenneth L. Reed

CHAPTER OUTLINE

Treatment of the physically compromised patient is not significantly different from treatment of any other dental patient. Although the level of knowledge of an internist is not necessary for proper dental treatment of this type of patient, the more information the dental professional has about these conditions, the more prepared and comfortable he or she will feel. As with all areas of dentistry, this area is rapidly changing. Understanding this, references in this chapter are Internet sites* because they generally have the most up-to-date information available concerning these conditions.

MULTIPLE SCLEROSIS

Multiple sclerosis (MS) is a chronic disease of the central nervous system (CNS). Symptoms may be relatively mild, such as paresthesia of the extremities, or they may be severe, such as blindness or paralysis.[1]

MS is an illness diagnosed in more than 350,000 people in the United States today.[2] MS is a demyelinating disease typically diagnosed between the ages of 20 and 40. There is such wide diversity in those afflicted that the final severity for any one individual cannot be determined at the initial onset of symptoms. A number of factors in combination are probably involved in MS.[3] The major theories of causes of MS are environmental, genetic, immunologic, and viral.[1]

Environmental

Those who are born in an area with a high incidence of MS and then move to an area with a lower risk appear to acquire the new risk, but only if the move occurs before the approximate age of puberty. It is possible that exposure to some environmental agent encountered before puberty may predispose a person to develop MS later in life.

Genetic

Although MS is known not to be hereditary per se, having a close relative with MS does increase one's risk of developing the disease. Some experts think that MS may develop as a result of a genetic predisposition, but only on reacting to an environmental antigen (actually an autoimmune response).

*Note: The web sites cited in this chapter are typically from professional organizations specializing in these areas or from educational institutions.

Immunologic

Most professionals agree that MS is primarily an autoimmune-modulated disease directed toward the myelin in the CNS; the exact antigen is unknown, but more is continually being learned. As the myelin sheath is damaged or destroyed, the nerve impulses are slowed or interrupted, leading to the symptoms of MS.

Viral

Some viruses of typical childhood exposure are known causes of demyelination and inflammation, so it is possible that a virus is the triggering factor in some cases of MS. Many viruses, including measles and herpes, have been evaluated to determine whether they might be associated with the development of MS, but at present, none have been proven causative. More recent studies, including one in Edinburgh, found no link between MS and measles or herpes.[4,5]

We know that worldwide, MS occurs with much greater frequency in latitudes above 40 degrees. In the United States specifically, MS occurs more frequently in states that are above the 37th parallel than in states below it. For informational purposes, the 37th parallel extends from approximately the southern border of Virginia to just south of San Francisco, California. It follows the northern border of North Carolina to the northern border of Arizona. The prevalence rate for those above the 37th parallel is approximately 125 cases per 100,000 people, whereas below the 37th parallel it is only around 70 cases per 100,000. MS is two to three times as common in women as in men.[1]

There are no particular concerns with local anesthetics in patients with MS, nor is inhalation sedation, oral sedation, or intravenous (IV) conscious sedation contraindicated. General anesthesia as performed in the dental office is normally acceptable as long as the stress of the procedure is minimized. Stress may influence the disease, so all efforts to minimize or eliminate stress are encouraged.

MUSCULAR DYSTROPHY

Muscular dystrophy is not one disease but a family of genetically transmitted diseases, each of which encompasses degeneration of musculature but with no definable nerve disturbances. The most common form is Duchenne muscular dystrophy (DMD) (also known as *pseudohypertrophic*).[6] It was first described by the French neurologist Guillaume Benjamin Amand Duchenne in the 1860s. Until the 1980s, little was known about the cause of any of the muscular dystrophies.

DMD occurs when a specific gene on the X chromosome does not manufacture a protein called *dystrophin;* therefore the disease affects only male subjects, but women may be carriers of the disease. The course of DMD is fairly predictable. Signs of muscle weakness may be seen as early as age 3.[7] Within the next 10 years, the heart and muscles of respiration can also be affected. Nearly all children with DMD lose the ability to walk sometime between ages 7 and 12.

Myotonic muscular dystrophy (DM, MMD, or Steinert's disease) is the most common adult form of muscular dystrophy, affecting more than 30,000 Americans.[8] This form of muscular dystrophy is quite unusual in that it also may trigger many other unrelated symptoms, such as hormonal problems, cataracts, heart disease, and myotonia (delayed relaxation of a muscle). Recently, researchers identified a new genetic form of myotonic muscular dystrophy (a mutation of a gene called *ZNF9*) that may shed light on the nature of mutations causing this and perhaps other diseases.

Muscular Dystrophy

Duchenne Muscular Dystrophy (DMD) (also known as *pseudohypertrophic*)
Onset: 2 to 6 years of age
Symptoms: generalized weakness and muscle wasting affecting limb and trunk muscles first; calves often enlarged

Becker Muscular Dystrophy (BMD)
Onset: adolescence or adulthood
Symptoms: almost identical to DMD but often much less severe; can be significant heart involvements

Emery-Dreifuss Muscular Dystrophy (EDMD)
Onset: childhood to early teens
Symptoms: weakness and wasting of shoulder, upper arm, and shin muscles; joint deformities common

Limb-Girdle Muscular Dystrophy (LGMD)
Onset: childhood to middle age
Symptoms: weakness and wasting affecting shoulder and pelvic girdles first

Facioscapulohumeral Muscular Dystrophy (FSH or FSHD) (also known as *Landouzy-Dejerine*)
Onset: childhood to early adulthood
Symptoms: facial muscle weakness, with weakness and wasting of the shoulders and upper arms

Myotonic dystrophy (MMD) (also known as *Steinert's disease*)
Onset: childhood to middle age
Symptoms: generalized weakness and muscle wasting affecting face, feet, hands, and neck first; delayed relaxation of muscles after contraction

Oculopharyngeal Muscular Dystrophy (OPMD)
Onset: early adulthood to middle age
Symptoms: first affects muscles of eyelid and throat

Continued

Muscular Dystrophy—cont'd

Distal Muscular Dystrophy (DD)
Onset: 40 to 60 years of age
Symptoms: weakness and wasting of muscles of the hands, forearms, and lower legs
Congenital Muscular Dystrophy (CMD)
Onset: at birth
Symptoms: generalized muscle weakness with possible joint deformities

Motor Neuron Diseases

Amyotrophic Lateral Sclerosis (ALS) (also known as *Lou Gehrig's disease*)
Onset: adulthood
Symptoms: generalized weakness and muscle wasting with cramps and muscle twitches common
Adult Spinal Muscular Atrophy (SMA)
Onset: 18 to 50 years of age
Symptoms: generalized weakness and muscle wasting with muscle twitches common; X-linked form affects men only and involves muscles of mouth and throat, as well as other muscles

Inflammatory Myopathies

Dermatomyositis (PM/DM)
Onset: childhood to late adulthood
Symptoms: weakness of neck and limb muscles; muscle pain and swelling common; skin rash typically affecting cheeks, eyelids, neck, chest, and limbs
Polymyositis (PM/DM)
Onset: childhood to late adulthood
Symptoms: weakness of neck and limb muscles; muscle pain and swelling common; sometimes associated with malignancy
Inclusion Body Myositis (IBM)
Onset: after age 50
Symptoms: weakness of arms, legs, and hands, especially thighs, wrists, and fingers; sometimes involves swallowing muscles

Diseases of the Neuromuscular Junction

Myasthenia Gravis (MG)
Onset: childhood to adulthood
Symptoms: weakness and fatigability of muscles of eyes, face, neck, throat, limbs, and/or trunk

Metabolic Diseases of Muscle

Phosphorylase Deficiency (MPD or PYGM) (also known as *McArdle's disease*)
Onset: childhood to adolescence
Symptoms: muscle cramps usually occurring after exercise; intense exercise can cause muscle destruction and possible kidney damage
Lactate Dehydrogenase Deficiency (LDHA)
Onset: childhood to adolescence
Symptoms: exercise intolerance with muscle damage and urine discoloration possible following strenuous physical activity

There are no particular concerns with local anesthetics in patients with muscular dystrophy, nor is inhalation, oral, or IV conscious sedation contraindicated. There may be some issues with patient positioning, but these are normally minor and of no disruption to the dental office. General anesthesia as normally performed in the dental office (without neuromuscular blocking agents) is acceptable in select circumstances after appropriate medical consultation, as needed.

PARKINSON'S DISEASE

Parkinson's disease (PD) is a degenerative neurologic disease that primarily affects the specific part of the brain (substantia nigra) that produces the neurotransmitter dopamine (Box 38-1). Symptoms include trembling (tremor), stooped posture, muscular stiffness (rigidity), and slowness of body movements (bradykinesia). The cause of PD is unknown, but some experts believe it may result from toxins, head traumas, or strokes.[9] Others believe PD results from the combination of a genetic predisposition and an as-yet unidentified environmental trigger.[10]

PD may appear at any age but is uncommon in those younger than 30; the risk of developing PD increases with increasing age. Men are affected slightly more often than women. Most patients do not experience the full range of symptoms just outlined.

Rigidity is always present unless it is temporarily ablated by anti-PD medications. This rigidity may lead to sensations of pain. The bradykinesia seen is caused by the brain's slowness in transmitting the instructions (chemically) to the appropriate parts of the body. Even when the instructions have been received, the body responds slowly in performing them.

Persons with PD may also have a long list of secondary symptoms. These may include depression, sleep disturbances, dizziness, constipation, and

BOX 38-1 Hoehn and Yahr Staging of Parkinson's Disease

Stage I
1. Signs and symptoms on one side only
2. Symptoms mild
3. Symptoms inconvenient but not disabling
4. Usually presents with tremor of one limb
5. Friends have noticed changes in posture, locomotion, and facial expression

Stage II
1. Symptoms are bilateral
2. Minimal disability
3. Posture and gait affected

Stage III
1. Significant slowing of body movements
2. Early impairment of equilibrium on walking or standing
3. Generalized dysfunction that is moderately severe

Stage IV
1. Severe symptoms
2. Can still walk to a limited extent
3. Rigidity and bradykinesia
4. No longer able to live alone
5. Tremor may be less than earlier stages

Stage V
1. Cachectic stage
2. Invalidism complete
3. Cannot stand or walk
4. Requires constant nursing care

Data from http://neurosurgery.mgh.harvard.edu/pdstages.htm.

dementia. They may also have trouble with speech, breathing, swallowing, and sexual function.

Levodopa is commonly prescribed for the treatment of PD. Structurally, it is a dopamine precursor. Some patients experience unacceptable side effects, including severe nausea and vomiting.[11] Levodopa/-carbidopa (Sinemet) represented a significant improvement. The addition of carbidopa delays levodopa biotransformation and allows more of the levodopa to reach the brain. A smaller dose of levodopa is then needed, and side effects are diminished.

Symmetrel (amantadine hydrochloride) is an indirect-acting dopamine agonist and is widely used as an early single-drug therapy. Sinemet is sometimes added to the Symmetrel regimen later in treatment. Anticholinergics act to decrease the activity of the balancing neurotransmitter acetylcholine. Because PD mainly involves a decreased activity of dopamine, one method of treatment has been to decrease the cholinergic system so that it no longer overpowers the dopaminergic system.[10] Selegiline (Eldepryl) has been shown to delay the need for Sinemet when prescribed very early in PD and is occasionally used in later stages to augment the effects of Sinemet.

COMT (catechol-*O*-methyltransferase) inhibitors represent a new class of medications used in the treatment of PD. These drugs require levodopa for efficacy. They simply prolong the duration of action of levodopa, requiring lower dosages and therefore diminishing its side effects.

There are no particular concerns with local anesthetics in patients with PD, nor is inhalation, oral, or IV conscious sedation contraindicated. Neuroleptics, phenothiazines, and butyrophenones are contraindicated during IV conscious sedation and general anesthesia, but the benzodiazepines, opioids, and alkylphenols are good choices.

BOX 38-2 Warning Signs of Stroke*

Sudden onset of the following:
- Numbness or weakness of the face, arm, or leg, especially on one side of the body
- Confusion, trouble speaking or understanding
- Trouble walking, dizziness, loss of balance or coordination
- Trouble seeing in one or both eyes
- Severe headache with no known cause

Data from http://www.strokeassociation.org.

*Every 53 seconds, someone in America has a stroke. Each year, about 600,000 Americans have a stroke, and 160,000 of them will die. Stroke is the number three cause of death and one of the leading causes of disability in the United States.[14]

STROKE

Stroke is a sudden loss of brain function caused by a blockage or rupture of a blood vessel to the brain, characterized by loss of muscular control, diminution or loss of sensation or consciousness, dizziness, slurred speech, or other symptoms that vary with the extent and severity of the damage to the brain (Boxes 38-2 and 38-3). It is also called *cerebral accident, cerebrovascular accident*, and *brain attack*.[12]

High blood pressure is the single most important risk factor for stroke.[13] *Stroke is a medical emergency; call 911!*

A stroke is a very specific type of brain injury and is typically caused by one of two mechanisms: (1) blockage of an artery (ischemic stroke) or (2) rupture of an artery (hemorrhagic stroke).

BOX 38-3 Permanent Neurologic Deficits That Are Commonly Produced by a Stroke

Weakness or paralysis, usually limited to one side of the body
Loss of sensation, usually limited to one side of the body
Problems with vision
Difficulty in talking or in understanding what is being said
Difficulty with organization
Clumsiness or lack of balance

Data from http://www.umassmed.edu/strokestop/.

Ischemic strokes are the result of arterial blockage. The primary problem is the diminution or elimination of blood flow (ischemia), which deprives the brain of necessary nutrients (oxygen and glucose). Secondarily, stroke slows the removal of waste products. The affected areas fail to thrive and may in fact die. The term *infarct* is commonly used (an area of tissue that undergoes necrosis as a result of obstruction of local blood supply, as by a thrombus or embolus).[12] About 80% of all strokes are the ischemic type.

A *transient ischemic attack* (TIA) can be an important predictor of stroke. A TIA is a temporary blockage of the blood supply to the brain caused by a blood clot; it usually lasts 10 minutes or less, during which dizziness, blurring of vision, numbness on one side of the body, and other symptoms of a stroke may occur.[11] In many ways TIAs resemble strokes, but the major difference is that in a TIA, no neurologic deficits remain once the attack has terminated because no brain tissue is permanently damaged.

In hemorrhagic strokes, bleeding can occur within the brain or around the brain. The bleeding produces injury through increased intracranial pressure, resulting in distortion, compression, and tearing of the surrounding brain tissue. About 20% of all strokes are the hemorrhagic type.[13]

Disorders of blood cells (e.g., sickle cell disease) or blood proteins can increase the chance of thrombus (a fibrinous clot formed in a blood vessel)[12] formation and therefore contribute to the risk of ischemic stroke.

An embolus (a mass, such as a detached blood clot that travels through the bloodstream and lodges so as to obstruct or occlude a blood vessel)[10] is most often a piece of a thrombus. Bits of plaque, fat, air bubbles, and other materials are also emboli. Often, an embolus travels with the blood until it encounters a constriction through which it cannot pass. When the embolus becomes lodged, it blocks the artery and reduces or eliminates blood flow and renders tissues ischemic.[13]

Local anesthetics themselves are not a problem in patients with a history of stroke, but the vasoconstrictors packaged with them can be a concern. Because hypertension is the single most important risk factor for stroke, most patients with a history of stroke also have a history of hypertension. It is very important to obtain baseline vital signs in this patient population before administration of local anesthetics. A stress-reduction protocol should be implemented.

Epinephrine should be limited to the least amount necessary to adequately perform the dental procedure; total elimination of epinephrine is not necessary. In general, up to 40 μg may safely be administered if done slowly and over an adequate time period. Forty micrograms is roughly the amount of epinephrine in two cartridges of 2% lidocaine with 1:100,000 epinephrine (U.S. volume of 1.8 ml of solution per cartridge) or four cartridges of local anesthetics containing 1:200,000 epinephrine (Marcaine, Duranest, Citanest Forte).[11] Periodic measurement of vital signs after administration of local anesthetics with or without vasoconstrictor is recommended for this group of patients.

Inhalation, oral, and IV conscious sedation are generally well tolerated and recommended in many instances because of their anxiolytic effects. The relaxation and slight reduction in blood pressure seen with these techniques are a benefit. Intramuscular sedation is not recommended because most patients with a history of stroke are taking anticoagulant medications of various types and efficacies. If there is no alternative to general anesthesia, recommended techniques would be those in which benzodiazepines and opioids are predominant, with alkylphenols administered as indicated.[15,16]

REFERENCES

1. National Multiple Sclerosis Society: www.nmss.org.
2. The Multiple Sclerosis Foundation: www.msfacts.org.
3. The International Multiple Sclerosis Support Foundation: www.msnews.org
4. The University of Edinburgh: Edinburgh study shows no link between MS and herpes virus: www.cpa.ed.ac.uk/news/research/15/3.html
5. The International Multiple Sclerosis Support Foundation: About the IMMS: www.imssf.org/weinrebherp.shtml
6. Muscular Dystrophy Association: www.mdausa.org
7. #310200 Muscular dystrophy, Duchenne type; DMD: www.ncbi.nlm.nih.gov/htbin-post/Omim/dispmim?310200
8. Parent Project Muscular Dystrophy: www.parentdmd.org
9. Parkinson's Information: www.parkinsonsinfo.com

10. Functional and Stereotactic Neurosurgery Staging of Parkinson's Disease: http://neurosurgery.mgh.harvard.edu/pdstages.htm
11. Physician's Desk Reference: www.pdr.net
12. Dictionary.com: www.dictionary.com
13. Strokestop: www.umassmed.edu/strokestop/
14. American Stroke Association: www.strokeassociation. org
15. Diprivan propofol: injectable emulsion: http://diprivan.com
16. Baxter Healthcare Corporation: http://baxftp.baxter.com/pub/product_info/propofol_pi.html

CHAPTER 39

Neurologic Illnesses and Other Conditions

Kenneth L. Reed

CHAPTER OUTLINE

Treatment of patients with various neurologic illnesses is many times more enjoyable than treatment of any other dental patient because patients with these special needs are genuinely a joy to be around. On the other hand, this patient population may present more challenges for the practitioner. As in Chapter 38, references in this chapter are Internet sites* because they generally have the most up-to-date information available about these conditions.

Persons with mental disabilities often suffer more dental disease than other dental patients. Financial considerations may make it difficult to obtain dental treatment, so sometimes it is delayed or avoided altogether. Those with neurologic illnesses may be unable to understand the consequences of poor dental hygiene and irregular care, or they may be uncooperative during dental treatment. Also, many of these disabilities interfere with the ability of the person to perform the fine motor skills needed to properly care for their dentition.[1]

ALZHEIMER'S DISEASE

> *The Oregonian*
> Saturday August 18, 2001
> HILLSBORO—*The Oregon Department of Justice reached a settlement Friday with a Hillsboro car dealership it said sold seven vehicles worth $244,708 in one month to an elderly Alzheimer's patient.*[2]

In dentistry the typical long-term relationships we have with patients allow us many times to see the patient's degradation of mental function over time in Alzheimer's. The informed consent we obtain before performing dentistry may sometimes come from a person other than the patient. Determining who the patient's guardian is and obtaining truly "informed consent" from that person is an absolute necessity.

The term *Alzheimer's disease* (AD) dates back to a 51-year-old woman admitted to the Frankfurt hospital in 1901 with signs of dementia. At a meeting held in 1906, Dr. Alois Alzheimer reported on this patient. The title of his lecture was "Über eiene eigenartige Erkrankung der Hirnrinde" (on a peculiar disorder of

*Note: The web sites cited in this chapter are typically from professional organizations specializing in these areas or from educational institutions.

the cerebral cortex). A few years later, presenile dementia was designated *Alzheimer's disease*.[3]

AD is the most common cause of dementia in older people. AD affects the parts of the brain that control thought, memory, and language. The cause of the disease still is unknown, and there is no cure.[4] About 10% of patients older than 65 years have AD, and almost 50% of those 85 and older have some signs of this disease. AD, however, is *not* a normal part of aging. Today, 4 million Americans have AD.[5]

People with AD may have trouble remembering recent events, activities, or the names of familiar people or things. As the disease progresses, symptoms are more obvious and become serious enough to cause those with AD, or more commonly their family members, to seek help. Later, people with AD may become anxious or aggressive, and they may wander away from home. Eventually, some patients will need complete, 24-hour nursing care.[4]

AD is a slowly progressing disease, starting with mild memory problems and ending with severe mental damage. Currently, there are no curative therapies for AD, but the drug tacrine (also called THA or Cognex) may alleviate some symptoms. There are other medications that may help with sleeplessness, agitation, wandering, anxiety, and depression. This symptomatic therapy can make a very positive difference for some of those with AD.

Scientists believe that genetic factors may be involved in more than half of the cases of AD. For example, the protein apolipoprotein E (ApoE) appears to be involved, but the exact mechanism of action is not completely understood.[6] AD probably is not caused by any one factor, however. It is likely that several factors in combination are involved.

The National Institute on Aging, the U.S. federal government's lead agency for AD research, funds Alzheimer's disease centers located throughout the United States. The centers carry out a wide range of research, including studies on the causes, diagnosis, treatment, and management of AD.[7]

Local anesthesia can be used in this patient population without specific concerns. Patients not severely affected with AD may benefit from some sort of sedation for dental therapy. Inhalation sedation is an excellent choice for patients mildly affected with AD and others who retain the ability to cooperate for the sedation and dental procedure. Oral sedation is generally not the first choice in this patient population because of its inherent lack of safety related to the inability to slowly and properly titrate the drug. Intravenous (IV) sedation is a good choice exactly because of the ability to slowly and precisely titrate the drugs to a clinical endpoint. Office-based general anesthesia would be a problem only because of another concomitant systemic disease, not because of AD itself.

To allow practitioners to keep current with these issues, the *Journal of Alzheimer's Disease* is available online.[8]

AUTISM

Pervasive developmental disorder (PDD) is a general category of disorders that are characterized by severe and pervasive impairment in several areas of development.[9] Among others, autism falls under this general category of disorders. Understanding of autism has grown tremendously since Dr. Leo Kanner first described it in 1943.[10] However, there is still no cure for the alterations in the brain that result in what we call autism. The more common other PDDs are listed in Box 39-1.[11]

Autism is a developmental disability that is typically diagnosed early in life. Autism and autistic-like behaviors may occur in as many as 1 in 500 individuals.[12] It is four times more prevalent in males than in females and is not related to racial, ethnic, or social groups. Family income, lifestyle, and educational levels do not affect the chance of autism's occurrence. Those with autism typically have difficulties with communication, social interactions, and leisure or play activities. Occasionally, aggressive and self-injurious behavior is seen.[11]

Autism is a disorder with a continuum of presentations, some mildly affected and others severely affected. Two children, both with the same diagnosis, can act very differently from one another and have varying skills. Therefore there is no standard "type" or "typical" person with autism.

BOX 39-1 Common Pervasive Developmental Disorders (PDDs)

Pervasive developmental disorder–not otherwise specified (commonly referred to as *atypical autism*): A diagnosis of PDD-NOS may be made when a child does not meet the criteria for a specific diagnosis but there is a severe and pervasive impairment in specified behaviors.

Rett's disorder: This is a progressive disorder that, to date, has occurred only in girls. There is a period of normal development and then a loss of previously acquired skills and loss of purposeful use of the hands replaced with repetitive hand movements beginning at the age of 1 to 4 years.

Childhood disintegrative disorder: This is characterized by normal development for at least the first 2 years, then significant loss of previously acquired skills.

Data from www.autism-society.org.

Current research links autism to organic alterations in the brain. There might be a genetic basis to the disorder, but to this point a specific gene has not been directly linked to autism. If there is a genetic basis to autism, it probably involves interactions among several genes. Some patients with autism may appear to have mental retardation, a behavior disorder, problems with hearing, or even odd and eccentric behavior (Box 39-2).[11]

Autism may coexist with other disorders that have neurologic effects, such as epilepsy, mental retardation, and Down syndrome. It may also coexist with genetic disorders such as fragile X syndrome, Landau-Kleffner syndrome, William's syndrome, or Tourette's syndrome.[13-16] It is not unusual for those with autism to test low in IQ. About 1 in 4 will develop seizures at some point.[11]

The more severely affected the individual is, the more difficulty he or she will have in cooperating with dental treatment. Autism itself infers no specific contraindications for using normal sedative and analgesic/anesthetic drugs. Local anesthesia, inhalation, oral and IV conscious sedation, and general anesthesia are all acceptable. As specific disease states are encountered secondary to autism (i.e., seizures), appropriate alteration to the anesthetic/sedative plan should be made.

BOX 39-2 Areas That May Be Affected by Autism

Communication: Language develops slowly or not at all; uses words without attaching the usual meaning to them; communicates with gestures instead of words; short attention span.

Social interaction: The child spends time alone rather than with others, shows little interest in making friends, and is less responsive to social cues such as eye contact or smiles.

Sensory impairment: Sensitivities in the areas of sight, hearing, touch, smell, and taste may be noted to a greater or lesser degree.

Play: The child does not participate in spontaneous or imaginative play, does not imitate others' actions, and does not initiate pretend games.

Behaviors: The child may be overactive or very passive; he or she throws tantrums for no apparent reason, perseverates (shows an obsessive interest in a single item, idea, activity, or person), apparently lacks common sense, may show aggression to others or self, and often has difficulty with changes in routine.

Data from www.autism-society.org.

CEREBRAL PALSY

Cerebral palsy (CP) is most often a developmental disability that manifests as an inability to fully control motor function, particularly muscle control and coordination (Box 39-3). CP is not communicable and is not a disease.[17]

There are several different types of cerebral palsy (Box 39-4).[18]

About 500,000 people in the United States have some form of CP; 8000 infants and 1500 preschool-age children are diagnosed with CP annually.[19] Adequate prenatal care may reduce the risk of some rare causes

BOX 39-3 Effects of Cerebral Palsy

Depending on which areas of the brain have been damaged, one or more of the following may occur:

- Muscle tightness or spasticity
- Involuntary movement
- Disturbance in gait or mobility
- Difficulty in swallowing
- Abnormal sensation and perception
- Impairment of sight, hearing, or speech
- Seizures
- Mental retardation
- Difficulties in feeding
- Bladder and bowel control
- Problems with breathing because of postural difficulties
- Skin disorders because of pressure sores
- Learning disabilities

Data from www.ucp.org.

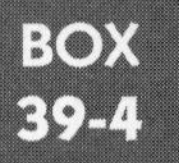

BOX 39-4 Types of Cerebral Palsy

Spastic Cerebral Palsy

This is the most common type of cerebral palsy.

Athetoid Cerebral Palsy

Athetosis is the word used for the uncontrolled movements that occur in this type of cerebral palsy.

Ataxic Cerebral Palsy

This is the least common type of cerebral palsy. *Ataxia* is the word used for unsteady shaky movements or tremor.

Mixed Types

Many children do not have just one type but rather a mixture of several of these movement patterns.

of CP; however, dramatic improvements over the last 15 years in obstetric care at delivery have not reduced the incidence of cerebral palsy. In most cases the injury causing the disorder may not be preventable.[20]

Early signs of CP usually appear before 3 years of age. Infants with CP are often developmentally delayed, such as in learning to roll over, sit, crawl, smile, or walk. Some affected children have hypotonia or hypertonia. The baby may seem flaccid and relaxed, even floppy, or may seem stiff or rigid. In some cases the baby has an early period of hypotonia that progresses to hypertonia after the first 2 to 3 months of life. Affected children may also have unusual posture or favor one side of their body.[21]

When one is discussing long-term goals in CP, *management* is a better word than *treatment.* Management of CP consists of facilitating the maximum in both growth and development. This requires involvement in the child's movement, learning, speech, hearing, and social and emotional development. Medications, surgical approaches, and braces may be used to improve nerve and muscle coordination and minimize dysfunction.

As children age, they may continue to require more assistance than others, including continuing physical therapy, special education, customized transportation devices, and modified employment opportunities. Those affected with CP may attend school, be productive in various jobs, raise families, and live independently.[22]

Local anesthesia and inhalation and/or oral conscious sedation can be used in this patient population as in any other dental patient. In fact, sedation is often beneficial in reducing spastic patient movement during dental procedures. In less cooperative patients, intramuscular (IM) or IV conscious sedation may be ideal, allowing patients to cooperate when they really want to but are just physically unable to sit still. If these measures fail, office-based general anesthesia may be safely and effectively performed in the majority of these patients using typical drugs and dosages.

DOWN SYNDROME

Sweatshirt noticed at a Down syndrome convention: *"The problem is not the way I look but the way you see me."*[1]

In 1866 John Langdon Down, an English physician, published an accurate description of a person with what came to be known as *Down's syndrome* and eventually *Down syndrome.* Down was superintendent of an asylum for children with mental retardation in Surrey, England, when he made the first distinction between children who were cretins (later to be found to have hypothyroidism) and what he referred to as "mongoloids."[23] In 1959 the French physician Jerome Lejeune identified Down syndrome as an abnormality of chromosomes. He found 47 chromosomes in each cell instead of the usual 46.[24]

Approximately 1 in every 1000 births results in an extra chromosome of the twenty-first group called *trisomy 21,* or *Down syndrome* (DS). DS affects more than a quarter of a million people in the United States.[23] There are three genetic mechanisms for trisomy 21. The first and most common is called *nondisjunction,* in which there is an entire extra chromosome 21 in all cells. This is the case for more than 90% of all patients with trisomy 21. The second is mosaic DS, in which trisomy 21 cells are mixed with a second cell line, usually "normal." The third is a translocation DS, about 3% to 5% of the total, in which part or all of chromosome 21 is translocated to another chromosome, usually 14.[25]

Box 39-5 lists genes that may *(no gene has yet been fully linked to any feature associated with Down syndrome)* have input into DS.[23]

About half of babies with DS have heart defects or visual or hearing impairment. These children are at increased risk of thyroid problems and leukemia. They also tend to have many colds, as well as bronchitis and pneumonia.[26] Whereas fewer than 10% of the general population will develop AD, about 25% of people with DS will suffer from this affliction. Patients with DS

BOX 39-5 Genes That May Have Input into Down Syndrome

Superoxide dismutase (SOD1): Overexpression of this gene may cause premature aging and decreased function of the immune system; its role in senile dementia of the Alzheimer's type or decreased cognition is still speculative.

COL6A1: Overexpression of this gene may be the cause of heart defects.

ETS2: Overexpression of this gene may be the cause of skeletal abnormalities and/or leukemia.

CAF1A: Overexpression of this gene may be detri mental to DNA synthesis.

Cystathionine β-synthase (CBS): Overexpression of this gene may disrupt metabolism and DNA repair.

DYRK: Overexpression of this gene may be the cause of mental retardation.

CRYA1: Overexpression of this gene may be the cause of cataracts.

GART: Overexpression of this gene may disrupt DNA synthesis and repair.

IFNAR: This is the gene for expression of interferon. Overexpression may interfere with the immune system, as well as other organ systems.

Data from www.ds-health.com.

have a life expectancy of approximately 55 years.[24] The most common traits of DS are listed in Box 39-6.[24]

Mouth breathing is common as a result of a small nasal airway. True macroglossia is rare; rather, a relative macroglossia is found in which the tongue is of normal size but the oral cavity is decreased in size as a result of the underdevelopment of the midface.[26]

Sleep apnea occurs more often in the DS population than in the general population. One in three children with DS may have an upper airway obstruction. The decreased airway size and lowered muscle tone predispose these patients to obstructive sleep apnea and airway compromise during anesthesia and sedation for dentistry.[23]

Sedative management of the dental patient with DS must consider both the primary disease and other medical problems as a result of or in conjunction with this disease. These patients can usually tolerate dental treatment as any other dental patient, with few if any modifications. All routes of conscious sedation (inhalation, oral, IM, IV) are perfectly acceptable for the patient with DS. Other coexisting medical problems may be cause for caution (e.g., sleep apnea, bronchitis, pneumonia). Patients with mitral valve prolapse (MVP) will probably require antibiotic prophylaxis before dental treatment. The thyroid condition of these patients should be considered. Office-based general anesthesia is an acceptable option, but one must keep in mind the special needs of this patient population related to various airway issues (e.g., relative macroglossia, small nasal airway) discussed earlier.

BOX 39-6 Most Common Traits of Down Syndrome

Muscle hypotonia (low muscle tone)
Flat facial profile (depressed nasal bridge and a small nose)
Oblique palpebral fissures (upward slant to the eyes)
Dysplastic ears (abnormal shape of the ears)
Simian crease (a single deep crease across the center of the palm)
Hyperflexibility (an excessive ability to extend the joints)
Dysplastic middle phalanx of the fifth finger ("pinky" finger has one flexion furrow instead of two)
Epicanthal folds (small skin folds on the inner corner of the eyes)
Relative macroglossia (enlargement of tongue in relation to size of mouth)
Excessive space between large and second toes

Data from www.ndss.org.

MENTAL RETARDATION

Mental retardation (MR) is not a physical limitation, as in an amputee or persons with CP or MS. It is not a physical condition such as being athletic or sedentary. MR is not like other problems; it is a cognitive level of functioning that begins early in life and is characterized by limitation in both intelligence and adaptive skills.[27] Three percent of the population of the United States suffers from MR. Those with MR can be expected to behave rationally at their functional level.[28]

The legal definition of MR is *an individual who exhibits significantly subaverage general intellectual functioning existing concurrently with deficits in adaptive behavior and manifested during the developmental period, which adversely affects a child's educational performance.*[29]

The definition of MR has three components: (1) intellectual functioning is subaverage (IQ of 70 to 75 range or below); (2) the deficit results from an injury, disease, or abnormality that existed before age 18; (3) the individual is impaired in his or her ability to adapt to the environment.[30] In addition to the legal definition presented earlier, MR is characterized by having related limitations in two or more of the following applicable adaptive skill areas[27]:

- Communication
- Self-care
- Home living
- Social skills
- Community use
- Self-direction
- Health and safety
- Functional academics
- Leisure
- Work

Chromosomal abnormalities are a more common cause of MR than are genetic, metabolic, and neurologic abnormalities, although the latter are also causes of MR. Trisomies involve an additional chromosome (47 chromosomes instead of the normal 46 chromosomes). DS, previously discussed and the most frequently occurring trisomy, results most often from a form of trisomy 21.

MR may result from many other chromosomal abnormalities, including the following:

- Partial deletion of a chromosome, e.g., of chromosome 5 in the *cri du chat* syndrome.
- Abnormalities in sex chromosomes, e.g., Klinefelter's syndrome (three sex chromosomes, two X and one Y sex chromosome [XXY], where normal is two sex chromosomes [either XX or XY]).
- Turner's syndrome (a single X sex chromosome only versus the normal XX or XY).[31]

Those with mild familial MR may have the fragile X syndrome; estimated to affect 1 in 2000 males and 1 in 4000 females. Physical features such as enlarged ears, long face with prominent chin, and macroorchidism are common.[13]

Congenital infections are a major cause of MR and may be secondary to rubella virus, cytomegalovirus (1 in about 750 live births), *Toxoplasma gondii,* and *Treponema pallidum.* Other viruses have been causally implicated, but at present, there are no scientific data to support such a position.[31]

Caution should be exercised when contemplating the use of long-acting local anesthetics because of possible lip and cheek biting. Other local anesthetics do not present any particular concern. Various techniques of conscious sedation (inhalation, oral, or parenteral) as used for other dental patients may be used in the patient with MR. IV sedation is particularly recommended because of its inherent safety afforded by slow titration. Office-based general anesthesia is typically not necessary for this patient population, but when it is indicated based on degree of difficulty of procedure or for patient management, it may be used safely.

SCHIZOPHRENIA

> "People do not cause schizophrenia; they merely blame each other for doing so."—E. Fuller Torrey[32]

Schizophrenia is the most common type of psychosis seen, characterized by thought disorder, delusions, and hallucinations. Thought disorder (an inability to think clearly and logically) is often manifested by disjointed and nonsensical language that renders those with schizophrenia incapable of participating in normal conversation. This contributes to alienation from family, friends, and society. Schizophrenia is now considered a group of mental disorders rather than a single entity.

Schizophrenia is a very disabling and emotionally devastating illness. Brain-imaging technology has demonstrated that schizophrenia is as much an organic brain disorder as is MS, PD, or AD. About 1% of the U.S. population has been diagnosed with schizophrenia. Although there is no known cure for schizophrenia, it is a very treatable disease. Most of those afflicted by schizophrenia respond to drug therapy, and many are able to lead productive and fulfilling lives.[32]

More than 2 million Americans have schizophrenia at any time. People with schizophrenia often suffer terrifying symptoms such as hearing voices or believing that others are reading their minds, controlling their thoughts, or intending to hurt them. Eighty percent of sufferers of this disease do not recover completely from this illness.[33]

Those with schizophrenia may suffer from "paranoid delusion" (a strongly held false belief exhibiting or characterized by extreme and irrational fear or distrust of others).[26] "Broadcasting" is a form of delusion in which the affected individual believes his or her thoughts can be heard by others. Hallucinations can be auditory, visual, or tactile; most often they take the form of voices heard only by the person.[32]

Who Gets Schizophrenia?

Genetic Associations

Genetic Link	*Probability of Developing Schizophrenia*
Neither parent has schizophrenia	1%
One parent has schizophrenia	13%
Both parents have schizophrenia	35%
Identical twin with schizophrenia	45%

Onset by Age

Age	*Probability of Developing Schizophrenia*
<16 yr	Rare
16-25 yr	75%
25-40 yr	20%
40+ yr	Rare

Onset by Sex

More men than women affected
More women than men affected

Data from: http://www.schizophrenia.com and http://www.nimh.nih.gov/publicat/schizoph.cfm.

Most people with schizophrenia are treated with and respond well to antipsychotic drugs. Some older antipsychotics (neuroleptics) such as haloperidol (Haldol) or chlorpromazine (Thorazine) may produce side effects that resemble some of the clinical symptoms of schizophrenia. Other commonly used medications include fluphenazine (Prolixin), thiothixene (Navane), trifluoperazine (Stelazine), perphenazine (Trilafon), and thioridazine (Mellaril). There is another drug class used to treat schizophrenia called atypical antipsychotics. The first drug in this line, clozapine (Clozaril), has been shown to be more effective than older medications, but because agranulocytosis (loss of the white blood cells that fight infection) is a side effect, the use of this drug requires that patients have blood tests every week or two.[26] Newer drugs such as olanzapine (Zyprexa), quetiapine (Seroquel), and risperidone (Risperdal), appear less likely to have this problem, but they do not appear to be as efficacious as clozapine.[32-34]

Tardive dyskinesia is the most unpleasant and serious side effect of the antipsychotic drugs. It may cause involuntary facial movements and jerking or twisting movements of other parts of the body. This usually develops in older patients, affecting 1 of 5 of those who have taken older antipsychotic drugs for many years. In most, but not all cases, the tardive dyskinesia slowly goes away when the medication is stopped.[32]

Antipsychotic drugs are often very effective in treating certain symptoms of schizophrenia, particularly hallucinations and delusions. Unfortunately, the drugs may not be as helpful with other symptoms, such as reduced motivation and emotional expressiveness.[33]

As with all medications patients are taking, reading and understanding the package inserts of these drugs is an absolute requirement. As an example, patients taking trifluoperazine (Stelazine) or haloperidol (Haldol) should have local anesthetics with epinephrine used cautiously because of the possibility of causing paradoxical hypotension.

Sedation for the dental patient with schizophrenia can be very tricky indeed. When possible, the avoidance of mind-altering drugs (essentially all sedatives used in dentistry) is highly recommended. If only a very light level of sedation is needed, inhalation sedation with nitrous oxide–oxygen is most appropriate, but it must be used with caution. Other routes of conscious sedation (oral, IM, and IV) are generally not indicated. Only after a thorough consultation with the physician managing the patient's antipsychotic medication regimen should these sedative regimens be considered. Office-based general anesthesia with ultrashort-acting medications (e.g., propofol, remifentanil) is generally preferable to conscious sedation because, during general anesthesia, the patient's consciousness is removed. This contrasts with only an altered conscious state seen in conscious sedation (attained through any of the various routes of administration). The fast offset of ultrashort-acting medications is beneficial in the dental patient with schizophrenia in rapidly returning to normal consciousness.

REFERENCES

1. The Resource Foundation for Children with Challenges: www.specialchild.com.
2. The Oregonian: www.oregonian.com/.
3. Eli Lilly and Company: Official prospect of Alzheimer's birthplace: www.kvkitzingen.brk.de/bereitschaften/marktbreit/m_alzhe.htm.
4. Alzheimer's Disease Education and Referral Center: www.alzheimers.org.
5. Alzheimer's Association: www.alz.org/.
6. American College of Medical Genetics, Bethesda, Md: www.faseb.org/genetics/acmg/pol–21.htm.
7. National Institute on Aging: www.nih.gov/nia/.
8. Journal of Alzheimer's Disease: www.j-alz.com/.
9. Pervasive developmental disorders: www.udel.edu/bkirby/asperger/pdd.html.
10. Johns Hopkins Hospital: Department of Psychiatry and Behavioral Sciences: www.med.jhu.edu/jhhpsychiatry/childresearch.htm.
11. Autism Society of America: www.autism-society.org.
12. National Center on Birth Defects and Developmental Disabilities: www.cdc.gov/ncbddd/dd/ddautism.htm.
13. The National Fragile X Foundation: www.nfxf.org/.
14. National Institute on Deafness and Other Communication Disorders: www.nidcd.nih.gov/health/pubs_vsl/landklfs.htm.
15. Tourette Syndrome Association, Inc.: www.tsa-usa.org.
16. Tourettes.com: www.tourettes.com.
17. United Cerebral Palsy: www.ucp.org.
18. UCP National: www.ucpa.org.
19. National Information Center for Children and Youth with Disabilities: www.nichcy.org/pubs/factshe/fs2txt.htm.
20. U.S. National Library of Medicine: www.nlm.nih.gov/medlineplus/ency/article/000716.htm.
21. National Institute of Neurological Disorders and Stroke: www.ninds.nih.gov/health_and_medical/pubs/cerebral_palsyhtr.htm.
22. Cerebral Palsy Facts & Figures: www.nettally.com/ucp/cerebral.htm.
23. Down syndrome: health issues: www.ds-health.com/.
24. National Down Syndrome Society: www.ndss.org/.
25. Risk and recurrence risk of down syndrome: nas.com/downsyn/benke.html.
26. Dictionary.com: www.dictionary.com.
27. American Association of Mental Retardation: www.aamr.org/index.shtml.
28. Public Images Network: www.publicimagesnetwork.org/diff.html.
29. The 'Lectric Law Library's Lexicon on Mentally Retarded: 192.41.4.29/def2/m027.htm.
30. Mental retardation: www.adoptions.dhr.state.ga.us/disable2.htm.
31. Merck & Co., Inc: www.merck.com/pubs/mmanual/section19/chapter262/262e.htm.
32. Schizophrenia.com: www.schizophrenia.com.
33. National Institute of Mental Health: www.nimh.nih.gov/publicat/schizoph.cfm.
34. Physician's Desk Reference.net: http://physician.pdr.net/physician/.

APPENDIX

Guidelines for the Use of Parenteral Sedation: University of Southern California School of Dentistry

This protocol was developed to provide guidelines for the safe and effective use of parenteral (intramuscular [IM] and intravenous [IV]) sedation procedures in the clinical environment. They are meant to be guidelines, flexible and dictated by the requirements of the specific clinical situation. In addition, these guidelines will require periodic revision as newer developments arise in the area of parenteral sedation.

PRELIMINARY EVALUATION

Candidates for parenteral sedation must be fully evaluated before the procedure to determine their physical status and need for sedation.

1. An approved medical history must be completed, must be dated, and must contain all indicated signatures.
2. Parenteral sedation is *not* contraindicated for use in the American Society of Anesthesiologists (ASA) I and II patient.
3. Parenteral sedation may be used in *selected* ASA III patients following evaluation and consent from the supervising faculty.

Appropriate written informed consent (or special behavior management consent form) must be obtained from the patient, parent, or guardian of the patient before the procedure. The medical history and planned sedation must be reviewed by the responsible faculty person and students.

Pretreatment instructions will be explained and a written form given to the patient, parent, or guardian of the patient. A sample of these instructions is provided later in this appendix (see Addendum A).

Before each treatment appointment, the medical history database is updated as necessary. Minimum questioning includes "Has there been any change in your medical history, health, or medicines since your last appointment?" All responses, positive and negative, are noted in a dated, signed treatment note. Minimum preoperative vital signs consisting of blood pressure and heart rate/rhythm must be measured at each treatment appointment and noted in the records.

It is understood that with some patients being discussed in this protocol, it may prove to be impossible to obtain preoperative vital signs. In such cases vital signs are monitored immediately upon induction of sedation.

MONITORING

All patients receiving parenteral sedation are monitored by direct observation (e.g., skin, mucous membrane color, respiratory movements). In addition, the following continuous monitoring must be employed:

- Pulse oximetry *and/or* capnography
  and
- Pretracheal stethoscope
  and
- Automatic vital signs monitor (every 5 minutes)
  - Blood pressure
  - Heart rate
  - Also the following when indicated:
    Electrocardioscope
    Capnograph

If an automatic vital signs monitor is not available, manual monitoring is performed every 5 minutes.

The information obtained must be recorded onto a suitable anesthesia/sedation record at appropriate intervals (every 5 to 15 minutes).

EMERGENCY DRUGS AND EQUIPMENT

In all parenteral sedation procedures, emergency equipment and drugs must be available. The following is included (as a minimum):

Emergency Drugs	Equipment
Epinephrine	Positive-pressure O_2
Antihistamine (e.g., diphenhydramine)	Face masks (p + a)*
Ephedrine	Laryngoscope
Anticonvulsant (e.g., midazolam)	Endotracheal tubes (p + a)*
Corticosteroid (e.g., hydrocortisone)	Lubricant jelly
	Suction tips
Vasodilator (e.g., nitroglycerin)	Oropharyngeal airways (p + a)*
Drug for emergence delirium (physostigmine)	Defibrillator
Narcotic antagonist (e.g., naloxone)	Blood pressure cuff (p + a + t)*
Hydralazine (Diazoxide)	Stethoscope
Bronchodilator (albuterol—as an inhaler)	Nasopharyngeal airways (p + a)*
(Epinephrine, aminophylline, Isuprel—IV drugs)	Magill forceps

Emergency equipment must be located either in the operatory or adjacent to the treatment area. Emergency procedure protocols should be available and monitored periodically.

TECHNIQUE

Preliminary Appointment

Evaluation of the following:

1. Need for parenteral sedation
2. Medical history obtained and reviewed
3. Dental treatment plan, if possible
4. Selection of IV/IM procedure
5. Check for presence of superficial veins (if IV procedure to be used)
6. Obtain baseline vital signs, if possible
7. Preoperative instructions to patient, parent/guardian (see Addendum A)
8. Patient education, as possible
9. Informed consent signed
10. Medical consultation, medically compromised patients at least annually; biannually for all other candidates for parenteral sedation or at discretion of supervising faculty

*a, Adult; p, pediatric; t, thigh.

Day of Treatment

The treatment team will consist of the following (minimal) personnel:

IV Sedation	Special Patient	Pediatric Patient
AMED IV student	AMED IV student	AMED IV student
AMED faculty	AMED faculty	AMED faculty
Dental assistant	Dental student	Pediatric dentistry student
Dental student	DMPH faculty Second dental student or dental assistant	Pediatric dentistry faculty Dental assistant

Oral & Maxillofacial Surgery (OMS)

OMS—resident*,†
SCSOMS program certified oral surgery assistant
OMS faculty

Suggested Protocol

1. Review informed consent, physical examination, medical history, and NPO status
2. Prepare drugs and equipment
3. Patient to restroom
4. Patient seated in dental chair (if possible)
   a. IM medications may be necessary in certain patients
5. Monitoring devices applied (see monitoring section)
6. Preoperative vital signs obtained
7. IV infusion started (if appropriate)
8. Supplemental oxygen or nitrous oxide–oxygen administered
9. Drugs are administered IM/IV

*Where OMS resident *has completed* an anesthesiology rotation, OMS faculty will be physically present in the operating room at the induction of sedation to baseline (acceptable sedation) levels, and again at discharge of the patient from the clinic.

†Where OMS resident has *not* completed an anesthesiology rotation, either the OMS faculty must be physically present in the operating room for the duration (induction to discharge) of the sedation or a second OMS resident, who has completed anesthesiology training, will be present throughout the procedure as the third member of the team, and is responsible solely for the sedation of the patient. In addition to the faculty supervisor trained in basic life support (BLS), there must be present at least one other member of the team.

10. Administer local anesthesia and commence dental treatment when adequate level of sedation is obtained.
11. Vital signs are monitored every 5 minutes throughout treatment and into the recovery period.
12. Vital signs are monitored and recorded at the termination of the dental treatment and the patient evaluated for recovery and discharge from the clinic (see discharge section).
13. Postoperative dentistry and sedation instructions are explained and a written form given to the patient and the patient's parent or guardian. A sample of these instructions is attached as Addendum C.
14. Patients will be dismissed from the clinic via wheelchair (when possible), in the custody of their parent or guardian, accompanied by an IV sedation student doctor and the treating dental student, and secured in their vehicle.
15. A posttreatment telephone call will be made by the treating dental or IV student that evening to ascertain the patient's posttreatment status and documented in the patient's chart.

MAXIMUM SEDATION/ANESTHESIA DRUG DOSAGES

The following are maximum intravenous dosages of the medications discussed in this protocol:

Drug	Maximum mg (IV. pedo. SP)	Maximum mg (OMS)
Diazepam	25	25
Midazolam	12.5 IV	12.5 IV
Midazolam	7.5 IM	7.5 IM
Meperidine	50	200*
Pentobarbital	200	200
Propofol	300	300
Nalbuphine	10	10
Butorphanol	2	2
Fentanyl	100 ug	150 ug*

Recovery

Following completion of the dental care, the patient must be permitted to recover from the sedation until such time as he or she is considered able to be safely dismissed from the clinic (see section on discharge). During the recovery period the patient will either remain in the treatment chair or be removed to a separate recovery area. In both cases there must be at least one person trained in anesthesia and sedation. Positive-pressure oxygen and a suction apparatus must be available in the recovery area.

*Administration of fentanyl or meperidine in excess of usual recommended doses requires authorization of, and direct presence in treatment room of, OMS faculty.

Discharge

Patients may be dismissed from the USCSD clinic following parenteral sedation when their postsedation discharge criteria are acceptable to the individuals responsible for recovery. These five categories are movement, respirations, circulation, consciousness, and color. Addendum B describes these criteria more fully. Postoperative dentistry and postoperative parenteral sedation instructions are explained and a written form given to the patient and to the patient's parent, guardian, or adult escort. A sample of the postoperative parenteral sedation instructions is attached as Addendum C.

Patients will be dismissed from the clinic via wheelchair (when possible), in the custody of their parent, guardian, or adult escort, and accompanied by an IV sedation doctor and the treating dental student. The latter two will remain with the patient until he or she is safely in the vehicle.

Posttreatment Follow-Up

A posttreatment telephone call will be made that evening to determine the patient's status. A note of this will be recorded into the patient's progress notes.

This contact is to be made by the dental student or resident of record. An AMED faculty will be available via telephone for consultation in the event of problems.

The student/resident should maintain a copy of the sedation record for evening review. The student resident should have the AMED or OMS faculty telephone number or air page alert. Faculty should be on air page alert for at least 24 hours after the sedation has been terminated.

ADDENDUM A

PRESEDATION INSTRUCTIONS

1. Arrangements must be made for a responsible adult to drive the patient home after IV/IM sedation. The patient will be unable to leave the clinic if unescorted.
2. The *adult* patient should have nothing to eat or drink for 8 hours prior to the procedure. *Pediatric* patients should not have anything to eat for 8 hours prior to the procedure and no liquids 4 hours prior for 0 to 3 years of age, 6 hours prior for 3 to 6 years

Patient's name: *SSN:* *Date:*

Physical Signs	(Pretreatment)	Baseline/Discharge Comments
A. MOVEMENT		
2—able to walk (where appropriate)		
1—able to move extremities		
0—unable to move any extremity		
B. RESPIRATIONS		
2—able to breathe deeply & cough		
1—limited respiratory effort		
0—no spontaneous respiratory effort		
C. CIRCULATION		
2—systolic BP ±20% baseline level		
1—systolic BP ±40% baseline level		
0—systolic BP >±40% baseline level		
D. CONSCIOUSNESS		
2—full alertness seen in ability to answer questions appropriately		
1—aroused when called by name		
0—unresponsive to verbal stimulation		
E. COLOR		
2—normal skin color and appearance		
1—any alteration in skin color		
0—frank cyanosis or extreme pale		
TOTAL SCORE:		
Dr's signature:		

of age, and 8 hours prior for 7 years and older (or unless specifically advised otherwise by the attending faculty).

3. The patient is advised to wear loose-fitting garments and a shirt/blouse with short sleeves.
4. The patient should plan to arrive in the office approximately 15 minutes before the scheduled appointment.
5. Should the patient develop a cold, flu, sore throat, or any other illness, the appointment should be rescheduled to a time when the patient is more physically fit. The patient, parent, or guardian should call the office if any of these symptoms develop.
6. If there are medications to be taken as part of the sedation treatment, they will be prescribed and the name of the drug, dosage, and instructions will be given to the patient.
7. The patient should continue to take his or her usual medications as prescribed for other conditions only after consultation with the supervising faculty. Such medications should be taken with minimal water if there is a morning or presedation dose.
8. The date, time, and place of appointment are given to the patient.

ADDENDUM B

PARENTERAL SEDATION DISCHARGE CRITERIA

The following should be completed when considering the discharge of a patient following parenteral sedation. The patient postsedation score must approximately equal his or her baseline (presedation) score.

ADDENDUM C

POSTSEDATION INSTRUCTIONS

1. Go home and rest for the remainder of the day.
2. Do NOT perform any strenuous activity. You should remain in the company of a responsible adult until you are fully alert.
3. Do not attempt to eat a heavy meal immediately. If you are hungry, a light diet (liquids or soft foods) will be more than adequate.

4. A feeling of nausea may occasionally develop after IV or IM sedation. The following may help you to feel better:
   a. Lying down for a while
   b. A glass of a cola beverage (or 7-Up)

   If nausea persists for more than 4 hours for adults or 1 hour for children, call the dentist who provided the sedation.
5. Do not drive a car or perform any hazardous tasks for the remainder of the day.
6. Do not take any alcoholic beverages or any medications for the remainder of the day unless you have contacted me first.
7. The following medications have been ordered for you by the doctor. Take them only as directed.
8. If you have any unusual problems or any questions you may call:
   a. The dentist who provided your sedation.
   b. If you are unable to contact the dentist who provided the sedation, please call one of the following appropriate emergency room numbers:

Adults:
Los Angeles County/U.S.C. Medical Center, (213) 226-2622 or (213) 226-7322

Children:
Children's Hospital of Los Angeles: (213) 669-2120
or
Long Beach Miller Memorial Medical Center: (213) 595-2133

Index

Page numbers followed by f indicate figure; t, tables; b, boxes

R

S